# Textbook of
# PERIODONTICS

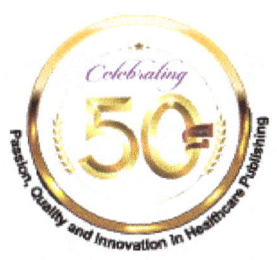

# Textbook of PERIODONTICS

**2 Edition**

**Shalu Bathla** MDS
Oral Implantologist, LASER Specialist
Professor
Department of Periodontology and Oral Implantology
MM College of Dental Sciences and Research
Mullana, Ambala, Haryana, India

*Assisted by*

**Manish Bathla** MD
Professor and Head
Department of Psychiatry
MM Institute of Medical Sciences and Research
Mullana, Ambala, Haryana, India

*Foreword*
**Rajeev Chitguppi** MDS (Periodontics)
Founder, Perioindia
Executive Editor, Dental Tribune South Asia
Research and Marketing Head, ICPA Health Products Ltd.

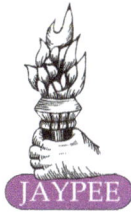

**JAYPEE BROTHERS MEDICAL PUBLISHERS**
The Health Sciences Publisher
New Delhi | London

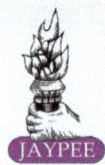 **Jaypee Brothers Medical Publishers (P) Ltd**

### Headquarters
Jaypee Brothers Medical Publishers (P) Ltd
EMCA House, 23/23-B
Ansari Road, Daryaganj
New Delhi 110 002, India
Landline: +91-11-23272143, +91-11-23272703
+91-11-23282021, +91-11-23245672
Email: jaypee@jaypeebrothers.com

### Corporate Office
Jaypee Brothers Medical Publishers (P) Ltd
4838/24, Ansari Road, Daryaganj
New Delhi 110 002, India
Phone: +91-11-43574357
Fax: +91-11-43574314
Email: jaypee@jaypeebrothers.com

### Overseas Office
J.P. Medical Ltd
83 Victoria Street, London
SW1H 0HW (UK)
Phone: +44 20 3170 8910
Fax: +44 (0)20 3008 6180
Email: info@jpmedpub.com

Website: www.jaypeebrothers.com
Website: www.jaypeedigital.com

© 2021, Jaypee Brothers Medical Publishers

The views and opinions expressed in this book are solely those of the original contributor(s)/author(s) and do not necessarily represent those of editor(s) of the book.

All rights reserved. No part of this publication may be reproduced, stored or transmitted in any form or by any means, electronic, mechanical, photocopying, recording or otherwise, without the prior permission in writing of the publishers.

All brand names and product names used in this book are trade names, service marks, trademarks or registered trademarks of their respective owners. The publisher is not associated with any product or vendor mentioned in this book.

Medical knowledge and practice change constantly. This book is designed to provide accurate, authoritative information about the subject matter in question. However, readers are advised to check the most current information available on procedures included and check information from the manufacturer of each product to be administered, to verify the recommended dose, formula, method and duration of administration, adverse effects and contraindications. It is the responsibility of the practitioner to take all appropriate safety precautions. Neither the publisher nor the author(s)/editor(s) assume any liability for any injury and/or damage to persons or property arising from or related to use of material in this book.

This book is sold on the understanding that the publisher is not engaged in providing professional medical services. If such advice or services are required, the services of a competent medical professional should be sought.

Every effort has been made where necessary to contact holders of copyright to obtain permission to reproduce copyright material. If any have been inadvertently overlooked, the publisher will be pleased to make the necessary arrangements at the first opportunity. The **CD/DVD-ROM** (if any) provided in the sealed envelope with this book is complimentary and free of cost. **Not meant for sale**.

**Inquiries for bulk sales may be solicited at:** jaypee@jaypeebrothers.com

*Textbook of Periodontics*

*First Edition :* 2017

*Second Edition :* **2021**

ISBN 978-93-90595-36-5

# Contributors

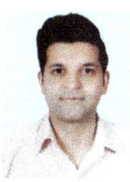

**Ajay Mahajan**
Professor
Department of Periodontology
HP Government Dental College and Hospital
Shimla, Himachal Pradesh, India

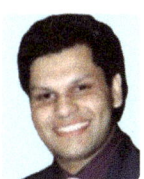

**Amit Aggarwal**
Professor and Head
Department of Oral Medicine and Radiology
MM College of Dental Sciences and Research
Mullana, Ambala, Haryana, India

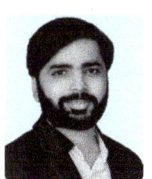

**Anuj Gandhi**
Consultant Implantologist
Smyle Dental Square
Borivali, Mumbai, India

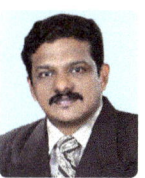

**Anil Melath**
Principal, Professor and Head
Department of Periodontology
MAHE Institute of Dental Sciences and Hospital
Puducherry, India

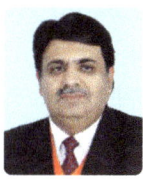

**Ashutosh Nirola**
Principal, Professor and Head
Department of Periodontics
Luxmibai Institute of Dental Sciences
Patiala, Punjab, India

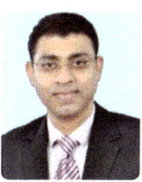

**Balaji Manohar**
Principal, Professor and Head
Department of Periodontology
Implantology
Kalinga Institute of Dental Sciences
Bhubneshwar, Odisha, India

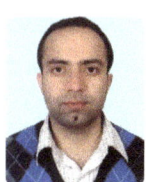

**Deepak Sharma**
Assistant Professor
Department of Periodontology
HP Government Dental College and Hospital
Shimla, Himachal Pradesh, India

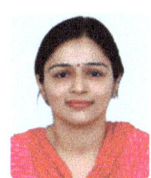

**Deepika Bali**
Associate Professor
DAV Dental College
Yamunanagar, Haryana, India

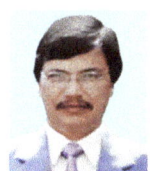

**Dhoom Singh Mehta**
Professor and Head
Department of Periodontics
Bapuji Dental College and Hospital
Davangere, Karnataka, India

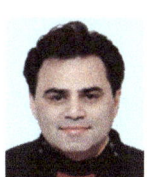

**Farhan Durrani**
Professor
Department of Periodontics
Faculty of Dental Sciences
IMS, Banaras Hindu University
Varanasi, Uttar Pradesh, India

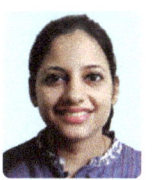

**Geetanjali Gandhi**
Reader
Department of Orthodontics
MM College of Dental Sciences and Research
Mullana, Ambala, Haryana, India

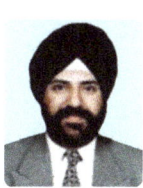

**Harpreet Singh Grover**
Consultant Periodontist
Dr Grover's Dental Clinic
New Delhi, India

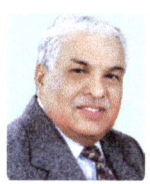

**Jagdish Chander Bathla**
Consultant Psychiatrist
Bathla Psychiatric Hospital
Karnal, Haryana, India

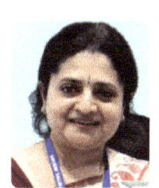

**Kanteshwari I Kumathalli**
Principal, Professor and Head
Department of Periodontics
Sri Aurobindo Dental College
Indore, Madhya Pradesh, India

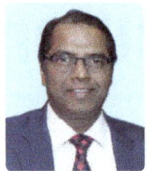
**Krishna K Gupta**
Professor and Head
Department of Periodontology Implantology
Vyas Dental College and Hospital
Jodhpur, Rajasthan, India

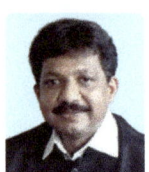
**MM Dayakar**
Professor and Head
Department of Periodontics
KVG Dental College
Sulia, Karnataka, India

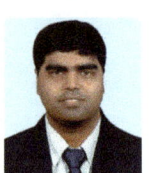
**Manikandan GR**
Consultant Periodontist
BR Hospital
Kollam, Kerala, India

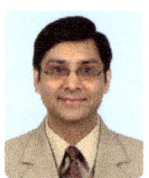
**Manish Bathla**
Professor and Head
Department of Psychiatry
MM Institute of Medical Sciences and Research
Mullana, Ambala, Haryana, India

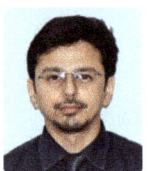
**Mayur Kaushik**
Professor and Head
Department of Periodontics
Subharti Dental College and Hospital
Meerut, Uttar Pradesh, India

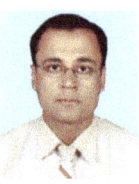
**Md. Jalaluddin**
Professor
Department of Periodontology
Kalinga Institute of Dental Sciences
Bhubaneshwar, Odisha, India

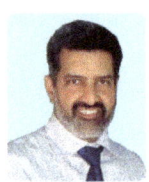
**Nageshwar Iyer**
Consultant Oral Surgeon
Smile Clinic
Yamunanagar, Haryana, India

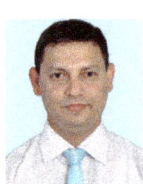
**Neeraj Deshpande**
Professor
Department of Periodontology
KM Shah Dental College and Hospital
Vadodara, Gujarat, India

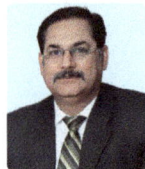
**Nikhil Srivastava**
Principal, Professor and Head
Department of Pediatric and Preventive Dentistry
Subharti Dental College and Hospital
Meerut, Uttar Pradesh, India

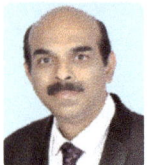
**Praveen Kudva**
Director Dental Studies
Principal and Dean
Sree Siddhartha Dental College
Agalkote, Tumakuru, Karnataka, India

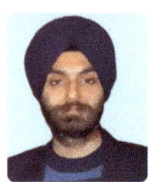
**Preetinder Singh**
Professor
Department of Periodontology and Oral Implantology
Swami Devi Dayal Hospital and Dental College
Barwala, Haryana, India

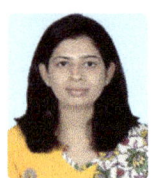
**Rachna V Prabhu**
Additional Professor
Department of Oral Medicine and Radiology
Yenepoya Dental College
Mangaluru, Karnataka, India

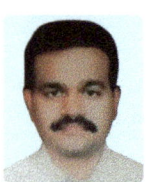
**Rajan Gupta**
Principal, Professor and Head
Department of Periodontics
Himachal Institute of Dental Sciences
Ponta Sahib, Himachal Pradesh, India

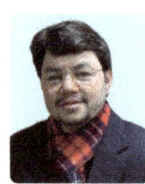
**Ramesh Fry**
Professor and Head
Department of Oral Surgery
MM College of Dental Sciences and Research
Mullana, Ambala, Haryana, India

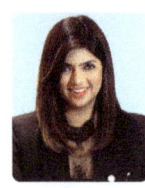
**Sana Farista**
Consultant Periodontist
Laser Specialist
Bandra (W), Mumbai, Maharashtra, India

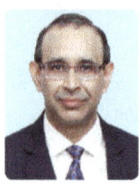
**Sanjay Kalra**
Consultant Endocrinologist
Bharti Hospital
Karnal, Haryana, India

# Contributors

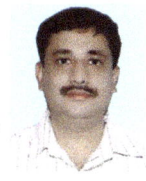
**Sanjeev Jain**
Principal, Professor and Head
Department of Periodontics
Guru Nanak Dev Dental College and Research Institute
Sunam, Punjab, India

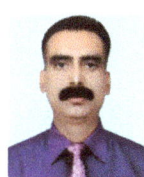
**Sanjeev K Salaria**
Principal, Professor and Head
Department of Periodontology
Kalka Dental College
Meerut, Uttar Pradesh, India

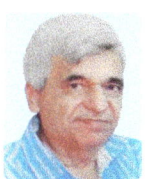
**Satish C Narula**
Professor and Head
Department of Periodontics
PGIMS, Government Dental College
Rohtak, Haryana, India

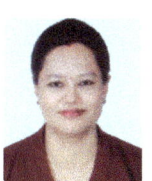
**Shaili Pradhan**
Professor
Department of Dental Surgery
National Academy of Medical Sciences
Kathmandu, Nepal

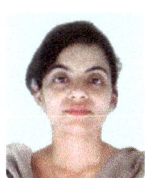
**Shailja Chatterjee**
Professor and Head
Department of Oral and Maxillofacial Pathology
Yamuna Institute of Dental Sciences and Research
Yamunanagar, Haryana, India

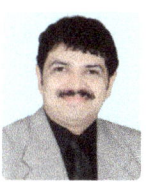
**Shashikant Hegde**
Professor and Head
Department of Periodontology and Oral Implantology
Yenepoya Dental College
Mangaluru, Karnataka, India

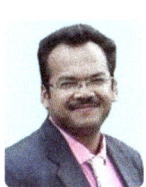
**Subash Chandra Raj**
Professor and Head
Department of Periodontics
SCB Government Dental College
Cuttack, Odisha, India

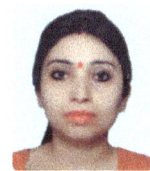
**Sumidha Rohatgi Bansal**
Professor
Department of Periodontics
Sudha Rustagi College of Dental Science and Research
Faridabad, Haryana, India

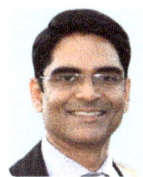
**Sushruth Nayak**
Professor and Head
Department of Oral Pathology
MM College of Dental Sciences and Research
Mullana, Ambala, Haryana, India

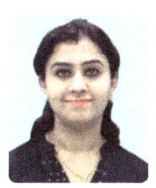
**Swantika Chaudhary**
Reader
Baba Jaswant Singh Dental College
Ludhiana, Punjab, India

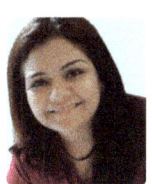
**Veenu Madaan Hans**
Associate Professor
ESIC Medical College and Hospital
Faridabad, Haryana, India

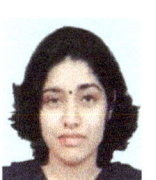
**Vishakha Grover**
Associate Professor
Department of Dentistry
HS Judge Institute of Dental Sciences
Punjab University
Chandigarh, India

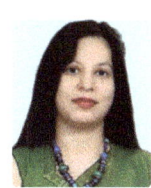
**Vineeta Nikhil Srivastava**
Dean
Professor and Head
Department of Conservative and Endodontics
Subharti Dental College
Meerut, Uttar Pradesh, India

# Foreword

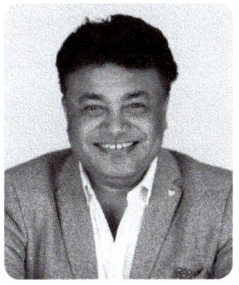

I am writing my first foreword for any book, and I am happy that I am doing it for a book that belongs to periodontology, my speciality. It also feels great to write it for my good friend and colleague, Dr Shalu Bathla, Oral Implantologist, LASER Specialist and Professor in Department of Periodontology and Oral Implantology, Maharishi Markandeshwar College of Dental Sciences and Research (MMCDSR), Mullana.

I know Dr Shalu since 2009 when I got the privilege of releasing her first book, *Tips and Tricks in Periodontology* in Agra, during the 12th Biennial International Academy of Periodontology Conference and 8th Postgraduate Workshop of Indian Society of Periodontology. I went through several sections of the book during the conference and was immensely impressed by it. I keep reading it even now as it has helped in many of my lectures. The book reflects the amount of hard work gone into its writing—to simplify the complex scientific concepts of periodontics and present them in an easy-to-remember format.

Over the last 12 years, I have witnessed Dr Shalu grow as a committed academician while remaining a keen student of the subject herself. She has also grown as an author and published two more books *Periodontics Revisited* in 2011 and *Textbook of Periodontics* (1st edition, 2017). Now, the second edition of *Textbook of Periodontics* is her fourth book.

Being an author myself, I know how difficult it is to write and publish a book. If a book goes into a second edition, it means that the readers have well received it. I know that whatever project Dr Shalu takes up, she executes it with total dedication. Her latest edition has 12 sections and 69 chapters. I am very confident that she has done complete justice to the book's content and presentation.

This textbook will immensely help the students, educators, and even practitioners. I sincerely hope that maximum students will read this book and improve their conceptual understanding of science. I wish this edition a great success, and I am sure we will see many more editions of this book in the coming years.

**Rajeev Chitguppi** MDS (Periodontics)
Founder, Perioindia
Executive Editor, Dental Tribune South Asia
Research and Marketing Head, ICPA Health Products Ltd.

# Preface to the Second Edition

The support provided to the first edition of the *Textbook of Periodontics* has motivated me to edit the book for the students in the field of periodontics.

This book is written keeping in mind the students particular needs for both postgraduates and undergraduates. The content is written as per the syllabus of the Dental Council of India (DCI). This edition too is a referenced textbook and is organized into 12 sections, with 69 chapters. The effort has been made to teach the subject efficiently using tables, easy-to-understand line diagrams, original colored photographs, flow diagrams, and points to ponder. Every chapter is supported by viva voce questions, and recent university questions.

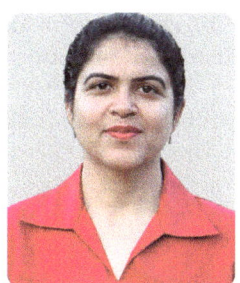

I hope that this edition will also stimulate insight and new trains of thought into the subject of periodontics, which will be immensely educative and helpful for the students and society at large.

Any suggestions and criticisms are most welcome at **HYPERLINK "mailto:periodonticsrevisited@gmail.com" periodonticsrevisited@gmail.com**

**Shalu Bathla**

# Preface to the First Edition

The support provided to "Periodontics Revisited" has motivated me to pen down another book for the students in the field of periodontics.

This book is written keeping in mind the special needs of the students such as the references, suggested readings and related landmark studies, that would be equally helpful for both postgraduates and undergraduates. The content is written as per the syllabus of the Dental Council of India.

The textbook is organized into 12 sections; and each section is further subdivided into several chapters. With the matter subdivided into smaller chapters, students will find easier to achieve their learning goals. Starting with the basics in section one, the text flows gradually from epidemiology; etiology; pathology; diagnosis; treatment including nonsurgical, surgical and implantology with the inclusion of interdisciplinary approaches onto the recent advances in the field of periodontology. The effort has been made to learn the subject in a simpler and easier way by the use of tables, easy-to-understand line diagrams, original colored photographs, flow diagrams and points to ponder in each chapter. Key information boxes are color coded to use as navigational aid for readers. This textbook is a referenced book with related landmark studies. Every chapter is supported by viva voce questions, university questions and suggested readings. This is the only book of periodontics that covers interdisciplinary relation between periodontics and seven other specialties.

Hoping that the content will be enough to stimulate insight and new trains of thoughts into the subject of periodontics which will be immensely educative and helpful for the students and for the society in large.

Any suggestions and criticisms are most welcome at periodonticsrevisited@gmail.com

**Shalu Bathla**

# Acknowledgments

*Dear Parents and GOD, I lay this book at your feet.*

I am extremely thankful to my teachers and mentors who have shaped my life and influenced me tremendously; Mrs Sangeeta Bhatia, Dr Sanjay Tewari, Dr SC Narula, Dr RK Sharma, and Dr Shikha Tewari.

I am grateful to par excellence researcher, Dr Rajeev Chitguppi, Founder, Perioindia; Executive Editor, Dental Tribune South Asia; Research and Marketing Head, ICPA Health Products Ltd., for writing the foreword of this book.

I would like to thank each of the contributors for devoting their time and effort towards this book. Thanks to the students, your questions and insights have challenged and strengthened me to present this work in a more friendly way to your desk.

I would like to thank my senior and colleagues; Dr Baljeet Singh, Dr Manish Khatri, Dr Ashish Kumar, Dr Ranjan Malhotra, Dr Pooja Palwankar, Dr Anoop Kapoor, Dr Vikram Blaggana, Dr Nikhil Sharma, Dr Dhirendra Singh, Dr Deepak Kochar, and Dr Priya V Gupta. I would also like to acknowledge Dr Mayur Davda, Dental Photography School, Mumbai, for giving me insight for the photography.

I would like to acknowledge Sh Tarsem Garg, Chancellor, MM Deemed to be University, Mullana, and the management who have given me a platform where I am today and full access to the library for my manuscript.

I thank Shri Jitendar P Vij (Group Chairman), Mr Ankit Vij (Managing Director), Mr MS Mani (Group President), Dr Madhu Choudhary (Publishing Head–Education), Ms Pooja Bhandari (Production Head), Ms Sunita Katla (Executive Assistant to Group Chairman and Publishing Manager), Dr Astha Sawhney (Development Editor), Ms Samina Khan (Executive Assistant to Publishing Head–Education), Mr Rajesh Sharma (Production Coordinator), Ms Seema Dogra (Cover Visualizer), Ms Geeta Barik (Proofreader), Mr Kulwant Singh (Typesetter), and Mr Nitesh Jain (Graphic Designer) of M/s Jaypee Brothers Medical Publishers (P) Ltd, New Delhi, India, who have done a great job "to put an icing on the cake" by way of their professional expertise to make my work reader-friendly and reach it to your desk.

I gratefully acknowledge my debt to my father-in-law Dr JC Bathla for nurturing the seeds of this endeavor at its infancy. I wish to express my gratitude to my parents, Smt Santosh Chandna and Sh GR Chandna; mother-in-law Smt Pushpa Bathla for their benevolent blessings. My brother Mr Pankaj Chandna, sister-in-law Mrs Neelu Chandna and nephew dear Raghav, has been there for me selflessly and lovingly. I also thank my sister-in-law Dr Reenu Khurana for encouraging me at every step.

I wish to express my deepest thanks to my husband Dr Manish Bathla, for outstanding assistance in compiling the manuscript and for his unconditional love and support. I am so thankful that I have you beside me, always pushing when I was ready to give up. Thanks for not just believing but knowing that I could do this!

The acknowledgment will not be complete if I do not express my thanks and love to my dear son Milind. He has grown up enough to give artistic inputs and suggestions regarding photographs and diagrams.

I dedicate this book to my dear son **MILIND** and my Husband **MANISH**!

# Contents

## Section 1: Normal Periodontium

**Chapter 1: Gingiva** — 3
*Shalu Bathla*
- Definition  *3*
- Macroscopic Features  *3*
- Microscopic Features  *6*
- Microcirculation  *12*
- Nerve Supply  *12*
- Clinical Criteria  *12*

**Chapter 2: Periodontal Ligament** — 16
*Shalu Bathla*
- Width and Structure  *16*
- Development  *16*
- Constituents  *16*
- Functions  *20*
- Blood Supply  *21*
- Nerve Supply  *21*
- Maintenance of Periodontal Ligament Space  *21*

**Chapter 3: Cementum** — 23
*Sushruth Nayak, Shalu Bathla*
- Development  *23*
- Functions  *23*
- Composition  *23*
- Classifications  *24*
- Various Junctions of Cementum  *25*
- Clinical Considerations  *26*

**Chapter 4: Alveolar Bone** — 28
*Shalu Bathla*
- Development  *28*
- Functions  *28*
- Structure  *29*
- Osseous Topography  *29*
- Composition  *31*
- Histology  *32*
- Coupling  *33*
- Bone Modeling and Remodeling  *33*
- Vascular Supply  *34*

**Chapter 5: Aging and Periodontium** — 36
*Shalu Bathla*
- Age Changes  *36*
- Effect of Aging on Tooth  *37*

## Section 2: Classification and Epidemiology

**Chapter 6: Classification of Periodontal Diseases** — 41
*Shalu Bathla*
- Rationale  *41*
- AAP 1986 Classification  *41*
- AAP 1989 Classification  *41*
- Ranney 1993 Classification  *42*
- AAP 1999 Classification  *42*
- 2017 Classification  *44*

**Chapter 7: Epidemiology** — 48
*Mayur Kaushik, Shalu Bathla*
- Aims  *48*
- Uses  *48*
- Epidemiological Studies  *48*
- Measurements  *49*
- Indices  *50*

## Section 3: Etiology

**Chapter 8: Periodontal Microbiology** — 61
*Shalu Bathla*
- Criteria for Defining Periodontal Pathogens  *61*
- Microbial Complexes in Subgingival Plaque  *62*
- Periodontal Pathogens  *62*
- Microorganisms Associated  *64*

**Chapter 9: Dental Plaque** — 68
*Shashikant Hegde, Shalu Bathla*
- Biofilm  *68*
- Definition  *69*
- Classification  *69*
- Clinical Assessment  *70*
- Composition  *71*
- Plaque Formation  *72*
- Microscopic Structure  *73*
- Metabolic Interactions  *73*
- Various Plaque Hypotheses  *73*
- Clinical Significance  *74*
- Other Tooth Deposits  *75*

**Chapter 10: Dental Calculus** — 78
*Ashutosh Nirola, Shalu Bathla*
- Definition  *78*
- Classification  *78*
- Composition  *79*
- Formation  *80*
- Clinical Assessment  *81*
- Attachment of Calculus to the Tooth  *82*
- Role of Calculus in Disease  *82*
- Local Contributing Factors  *82*

**Chapter 11: Immunity and Inflammation** — 87
*Deepak Sharma, Shalu Bathla*
- Cells of Immunity and Inflammation  *88*
- Leukocyte Functions  *91*
- Chemical Mediators of Inflammation  *93*
- Nonspecific and Specific Immunity  *94*
- Immune Mechanisms  *94*

- Antigen Processing and Presentation *96*
- Pathogen Associated Molecular Patterns *96*
- Pattern Recognition Receptors *97*

### Chapter 12: Pathogenesis and Host Response — 99
*Shalu Bathla*
- Microbiology and Immunology *99*
- Stages of Pathogenesis *99*
- Immunologic Aspects of the Microbial Interaction with the Host *102*
- Concepts of Pathogenesis *103*

### Chapter 13: Genetic Basis of Periodontal Diseases — 106
*Veenu M Hans, Shalu Bathla*
- Genetic Variance *106*
- Genetic Basis of Disease *106*
- Methods of Genetic Analysis *107*
- Disease and Polymorphism *107*
- Associated Problems *109*
- Clinical Implications *109*
- Nutrigenomics *110*

### Chapter 14: Systemic Factors and Periodontium — 112
*Balaji Manohar, Shalu Bathla*
- Hormonal Factors *112*
- Hematological Disorders *114*
- Immunodeficiency Disorders *116*
- Effect of Nutrition *117*
- Psychosomatic Disorders *120*
- Other Systemic Conditions *121*
- Drugs Induced Manifestations *121*

### Chapter 15: Periodontal Medicine — 124
*Praveen Kudva, Sanjay Kalra*
- Focal Infection Theory *124*
- Bacterial Reservoir *124*
- Effect on Cardiovascular System *125*
- Effect on Endocrine System *126*
- Effect on Reproductive System *126*
- Effect on Respiratory System *127*

### Chapter 16: Smoking and Periodontium — 129
*Shalu Bathla*
- Classifications *129*
- Constituents of Tobacco Smoke *129*
- Effects of Smoking *130*
- Smoking Cessation *132*

## Section 4: Pathology of Gingival and Periodontal Diseases

### Chapter 17: Defense Mechanisms of Gingiva — 137
*Shalu Bathla*
- Junctional Epithelium *137*
- Polymorphonuclear Leukocytes *138*
- Saliva *138*
- Gingival Crevicular Fluid *139*

### Chapter 18: Gingival Inflammation — 143
*Sanjeev K Salaria*
- Classifications *143*
- Stages of Gingivitis *144*
- Clinical Features *146*

### Chapter 19: Gingival Enlargement — 151
*Md. Jalaluddin, Shalu Bathla*
- Classifications *151*
- Scoring *151*
- Inflammatory Enlargement *151*
- Drug-induced Enlargement *152*
- Enlargement Associated with Systemic Diseases *155*
- Neoplastic Enlargement *157*
- False Enlargement *159*

### Chapter 20: Acute Gingival Conditions — 162
*Subash C Raj, Shalu Bathla*
- Necrotizing Ulcerative Gingivitis *162*
- Primary Herpetic Gingivostomatitis *166*
- Pericoronitis *167*

### Chapter 21: Soft and Hard Tissue Lesions — 171
*Shailja Chatterjee, Shalu Bathla*
- Desquamative Gingivitis *171*
- Metastatic Tumors of the Jaws *174*
- Malignant Lesions of Gingiva *175*
- Reactive Lesions of Gingiva *176*
- Peripheral Odontogenic Lesions *177*
- Granulomatous Gingivitis *178*
- Benign Neoplasms *179*
- Malignant Neoplasms *179*

### Chapter 22: Periodontal Pocket — 182
*Sanjeev Jain*
- Definition *182*
- Classifications *182*
- Clinical Features *183*
- Pathogenesis *184*
- Histopathology *184*
- Clinical Assessment *186*

### Chapter 23: Periodontal Abscess — 189
*Harpreet S Grover, Shalu Bathla*
- Definition *189*
- Classifications *189*
- Clinical Features *189*
- Microbiology *190*
- Pathogenesis and Histopathology *190*
- Diagnosis *190*
- Differential Diagnosis *191*
- Treatment *191*
- Complications *193*

### Chapter 24: Bone Defects — 194
*Sanjeev K Salaria*
- Factors Determining Bone Morphology *194*
- Etiology *194*
- Bone Defects *197*
- Diagnosis *201*

### Chapter 25: Periodontitis — 204
*Shalu Bathla*
- Status of Periodontitis in 1999 Classification *204*
- Chronic Periodontitis *204*
- Aggressive Periodontitis *208*
- Status of Periodontitis in 2017 Classification *213*

**Chapter 26: AIDS and Periodontium** 215
*Shalu Bathla*
- Structure of HIV  *215*
- Pathogenesis  *216*
- Periodontal Diseases in AIDS  *217*
- Periodontal Pathologies  *217*
- Diagnosis  *218*
- Treatment  *218*

**Chapter 27: Trauma from Occlusion** 221
*Sumidha R Bansal, Shaili Pradhan*
- Definitions  *221*
- Types  *221*
- Concepts  *222*
- Tissue Response  *223*
- Clinical Features  *223*
- Radiographic Features  *224*
- Role of Occlusal Trauma  *224*
- Treatment  *224*
- Effect of Trauma on Implants  *225*
- Pathologic Tooth Migration  *225*

**Chapter 28: Sex Hormones and Periodontium** 228
*Shalu Bathla*
- Effects on Periodontium  *228*
- Puberty  *229*
- Menstrual Cycle  *229*
- Pregnancy  *230*
- Oral Contraceptives  *232*
- Menopause  *232*
- Effects on Wound Healing  *232*

## Section 5: Diagnosis

**Chapter 29: Clinical Diagnosis** 237
*Shalu Bathla*
- Definition  *237*
- Types  *237*
- Key Stages  *237*
- History Taking  *237*
- Clinical Examination  *238*
- Investigations  *250*
- Diagnosis  *251*
- Treatment Plan  *251*

**Chapter 30: Radiographic Diagnostic Aids** 253
*Amit Aggarwal, Rachna V Prabhu*
- Ideal Requisites  *254*
- Radiographic Techniques  *254*
- Normal Radiographic Features  *255*
- Pathologic Radiographic Changes  *256*
- Limitations  *259*
- Advanced Radiographic Aids  *259*

**Chapter 31: Microbiological Diagnostic Aids** 262
*Vishakha Grover, Shalu Bathla*
- Indications  *262*
- Biomarkers  *262*
- Candidates for Biomarkers  *263*
- Limitations  *268*

**Chapter 32: Clinical Risk Assessment** 270
*Deepika Bali, Shalu Bathla*
- Definitions  *270*
- Risk Factors  *271*
- Risk Determinants  *271*
- Risk Indicators  *272*
- Risk Markers  *272*
- Risk Assessment  *272*

**Chapter 33: Prognosis** 276
*Rajan Gupta*
- Definition  *276*
- Prognostication Systems  *276*
- Prognostic Factors  *277*
- Diagnosis and Prognosis Interrelationship  *279*
- Prognosis of Patients  *279*

## Section 6: Treatment: Nonsurgical Therapy

**Chapter 34: Treatment Plan** 283
*Shalu Bathla*
- Phases of Periodontal Therapy  *283*
- Sequence  *284*
- Palliative Treatment  *285*
- Explaining the Treatment Plan to the Patient  *285*
- Referral  *285*

**Chapter 35: Halitosis** 287
*Shalu Bathla*
- Classification  *287*
- Etiology  *287*
- Pathogenesis  *288*
- Diagnosis  *289*
- Treatment  *291*

**Chapter 36: Dentin Hypersensitivity** 293
*Shalu Bathla*
- Definition  *293*
- Etiology  *293*
- Theories  *294*
- Diagnosis  *294*
- Hypersensitivity Measurement  *295*
- Management  *296*
- Prevention  *297*

**Chapter 37: Mechanical Plaque Control** 299
*Satish C Narula*
- Traditional Oral Hygiene Methods  *299*
- Toothbrushes  *299*
- Dentifrices  *305*
- Interdental Cleaning Aids  *306*
- Other Aids  *309*
- Oral Hygiene Methods Causing Trauma  *310*
- Assessment of Home Care  *310*
- Hawthorne Effect  *311*

**Chapter 38: Chemotherapeutic Agents** 314
*MM Dayakar, Shalu Bathla*
- Terminologies  *314*
- Chemotherapeutic Agents  *314*
- Chemical Antiplaque Agents  *314*

- Anticalculus Agents *318*
- Antimicrobials *319*
- Local Drug Delivery System *322*

### Chapter 39: Host Modulation — 327
*Shashikant Hegde, Manikandan GR*
- Host Modulatory Agents *328*

### Chapter 40: Periodontal Instruments — 333
*Shalu Bathla*
- General Characteristics *333*
- Parts of Instruments *333*
- Classification *335*

### Chapter 41: General Principles of Instrumentation — 352
*Shalu Bathla*
- Accessibility *352*
- Visibility, Illumination, and Retraction *353*
- Condition of the Instruments *353*
- Maintaining a Clean Field *356*
- Instrument Stabilization *356*
- Instrument Activation *358*
- Instrumentation Strokes *359*
- Principles of Scaling and Root Planing *360*

### Chapter 42: Manual Scaling and Root Planing — 362
*Shalu Bathla*
- Definition *362*
- Objectives *362*
- Scaling and Root Planing *362*
- Instrumentation Approaches *363*
- Full-Mouth Disinfection *368*
- Evaluation of Scaling and Root Planing *369*

### Chapter 43: Sonic and Ultrasonic Scaling — 371
*Shalu Bathla*
- Sonic Scalers *372*
- Ultrasonic Scalers *372*
- Tip Designs *372*
- Mechanism of Action *373*
- Ultrasonic Scaling Technique *373*
- Potential Hazards *374*
- Contraindications *375*

### Chapter 44: Splinting — 377
*Harpreet S Grover*
- Historical Perspective *377*
- Definition *377*
- Objectives *377*
- Indications *378*
- Contraindications *378*
- Advantages *378*
- Disadvantages *378*
- Classifications *378*

## Section 7: Treatment: Surgical Therapy

### Chapter 45: Surgical Anatomy — 385
*Nageshwar Iyer, Shalu Bathla*
- Anatomic Structures *385*
- Vital Structures *391*

### Chapter 46: General Principles of Periodontal Surgery — 394
*Shalu Bathla*
- Objectives *394*
- Preoperative Considerations *394*
- Intraoperative Considerations *395*
- Postoperative Instructions and Care *408*
- Postsurgical Complications *410*
- Wound Healing *411*

### Chapter 47: Gingival Curettage — 413
*Shalu Bathla*
- Terminology *413*
- Indications *413*
- Contraindications *413*
- Procedure *413*
- Present Concept *415*
- Healing after Curettage *415*

### Chapter 48: Gingivectomy — 417
*Dhoom S Mehta, Shalu Bathla*
- Historical Perspective *417*
- Definition *417*
- Objectives *417*
- Indications *417*
- Contraindications *417*
- Limiting Circumstances *418*
- Drawbacks *418*
- Gingivoplasty *418*
- Types *418*
- Postoperative Healing *422*

### Chapter 49: Periodontal Flap — 425
*Shalu Bathla*
- Definition *425*
- Objectives *425*
- Principles *425*
- Classifications *425*
- Incisions *426*
- Flap Procedures *429*

### Chapter 50: Resective Osseous Surgery — 438
*Shaili Pradhan, Shalu Bathla*
- Definitions *438*
- Objectives *438*
- Rationale *438*
- Osteoplasty Indications *438*
- Ostectomy Indications *439*
- Examination *439*
- Instruments *440*
- Procedure *440*
- Disadvantages *442*
- Postoperative Healing *442*

### Chapter 51: Regenerative Osseous Surgery — 444
*Shalu Bathla*
- Terminologies *444*
- Regenerative Surgical Management *444*
- Recent Advancements *452*
- Postoperative Tissue Changes *455*
- Factors Influencing Regenerative Procedures *456*
- Postoperative Healing *457*

**Chapter 52: Furcation** 460
*Shalu Bathla*
- Terminologies  460
- Classifications  460
- Etiology  462
- Factors Influencing Furcation Management  463
- Diagnosis  464
- Prognosis  465
- Management  465

**Chapter 53: Periodontal Plastic Surgery** 469
*Ajay Mahajan, Neeraj Deshpande*
- Objectives  469
- Selection Criteria  469
- Techniques for Increasing Attached Gingiva  470
- Root Coverage Gingival Recession  473
- Techniques for Frenectomy  480
- Techniques to Vestibular Extension  481
- Techniques for Papilla Reconstruction  482
- Techniques for Alveolar Ridge Augmentation  483

**Chapter 54: Periodontal Microsurgery** 486
*Shalu Bathla, Swantika Chaudhary*
- Historical Perspective  486
- Principles  486
- Magnification Systems  486
- Microsurgical Instruments  488
- Requirements of the Surgeon  489
- Role of Microsurgery in Periodontal Procedures  490

**Chapter 55: Periodontal Treatment of Medically Compromised Patients** 492
*Preetinder Singh*
- Cardiovascular Diseases  492
- Endocrine Disorders  496
- Renal Diseases  497
- Liver Diseases  498
- Pulmonary Diseases  498
- Immunosuppression and Chemotherapy  499
- Radiation Therapy  499
- Prosthetic Joint Replacement  500
- Pregnancy  500
- Hemorrhagic Disorders  501
- Blood Dyscrasias  503
- Infectious Diseases  503
- Patients on Bisphosphonate Therapy  505
- Epileptic Patients  506

## Section 8: Implantology

**Chapter 56: Implant Basics** 511
*Farhan Durrani, Shalu Bathla*
- Terminologies  511
- Indications  512
- Contraindications  512
- Classifications  512
- Biomaterials  514
- Soft Tissue—Implant Interface  514
- Implant—Bone Interface  515
- Evaluation of Osseointegrated Implants  516
- Diagnosis and Treatment Planning  517
- Osseous Considerations  518

**Chapter 57: Implant Surgical Procedures** 521
*Anuj Gandhi, Shalu Bathla*
- Armamentarium  521
- Surgical Protocol  524
- Two-stage Implant Surgery  524
- One-stage Implant Surgery  527
- Immediate Implant Placement  528
- Platform Switching  528

**Chapter 58: Advanced Implant Surgical Procedures** 532
*Ramesh Fry, Krishna K Gupta*
- Guided Bone Regeneration  532
- Socket Preservation  533
- Ridge Augmentation  534
- Socket Shield  535
- Sinus Elevation and Sinus Bone Grafting  536
- Nerve Repositioning  540

**Chapter 59: Peri-implantitis and Other Implant Related Complications** 543
*Anil Melath, Veenu M Hans*
- Definitions of Peri-implantitis  543
- Etiology of Peri-implantitis  543
- Classification of Peri-implantitis  544
- Diagnosis of Peri-implantitis  544
- Management of Peri-implantitis  545
- Supportive and Maintenance Therapy of Peri-implantitis  546
- Other Implant Related Complications  547
- Implant Failure  549

## Section 9: Interdisciplinary Approach

**Chapter 60: Periodontics-Prosthodontics** 555
*Shalu Bathla*
- Sequence of Treatment  555
- Application of Periodontics in Prosthodontics  555
- Periodontal Considerations in Complete Dentures and RPD  558
- Periodontal Considerations in FPD  558
- Periodontal Maintenance in the Prosthetic Patient  560

**Chapter 61: Periodontics-Endodontics** 563
*Vineeta N Srivastava, Shalu Bathla*
- Pathways of Communication  563
- Etiopathogenesis  564
- Classifications  565
- Diagnosis  567
- Treatment and Prognosis  568

**Chapter 62: Periodontics-Restorative Dentistry** 570
*Shalu Bathla*
- Inter-relationship  570
- Periodontal Considerations  571
- Maintenance  573

**Chapter 63: Periodontics-Orthodontics** 575
*Geetanjali Gandhi, Shalu Bathla*
- Indications  575
- Contraindications  575
- Benefits of Orthodontic Treatment  576

- Response to Tooth Movements  576
- Application of Orthodontics in Periodontics  577
- Application of Periodontics in Orthodontics  578
- Effects of Orthodontic Tooth Movement  579
- Systematics of Combined Treatment  580
- Maintenance  581

**Chapter 64: Periodontics-Pediatric Dentistry**  583
*Nikhil Srivastava, Shalu Bathla*
- Periodontium of Deciduous Dentition  583
- Gingivitis and Gingival Enlargement  583
- Periodontitis  588
- Periodontitis as a Manifestation of Systemic Diseases  588
- Anatomical Periodontal Problems  590
- Childhood Diseases Affecting Gingiva  590
- Maintenance  590

**Chapter 65: Periodontics-Oral Surgery**  593
*Ramesh Fry, Shalu Bathla*
- Inter-relationship  593
- Periodontal Considerations  594
- Maintenance  594

**Chapter 66: Periodontics-Psychiatry**  596
*Jagdish C Bathla, Manish Bathla, Shalu Bathla*
- Parafunctional Habits  596
- Psychosomatic Disorders  599
- Necrotizing Ulcerative Gingivitis and Stress  601
- Periodontal Aspects of Psychiatric Patients  601
- Implications of Psychiatric Medications  602
- Doctor–Patient Relationship  603

## Section 10: Recent Advances

**Chapter 67: Recent Advancements in Periodontics**  609
*Sana Farista, Veenu M Hans*
- Lasers  609
- Photodynamic Therapy  617
- Tissue Engineering  620
- Gene Therapy  622
- Nanotechnology  624
- Periodontal Vaccine  626
- Minimally Invasive Surgery  627
- Piezosurgery  628

## Section 11: Maintenance Phase

**Chapter 68: Supportive Periodontal Therapy**  635
*Kanteshwari I Kumathalli*
- Aims  635
- Maintenance Interval  635
- Maintenance Compliance  636
- Maintenance Program  636
- Retreatment of Selected Areas  637
- Maintenance for Implant Patient  638

## Section 12: Miscellaneous

**Chapter 69: Miscellaneous**  641
*Shalu Bathla*
- Sterilization  641
- Discoveries in Periodontics  645
- Prefix "Perlo" Used in Periodontics  647

**University Questions**  651
*Index*  659

# Section 1: Normal Periodontium

- Gingiva
- Periodontal Ligament
- Cementum
- Alveolar Bone
- Aging and Periodontium

# Chapter 1: Gingiva

Shalu Bathla

## Chapter Outline

- Definition
- Macroscopic Features
- Microscopic Features
- Microcirculation
- Nerve Supply
- Clinical Criteria

## INTRODUCTION

Oral mucosa consists of the masticatory mucosa, which includes the gingiva and the covering of the hard palate; the specialized mucosa, which covers the dorsum of the tongue; and the lining mucosa which covers the remaining part of the oral cavity. The gingiva is that part of the masticatory mucosa which covers the alveolar process and protects the underlying tissues. The attachment apparatus of periodontium consists of the periodontal ligament, cementum, and alveolar bone.

## DEFINITION

Gingiva is the part of oral mucosa that covers the alveolar processes of the jaws and surrounds the necks of the teeth.[1] Gingiva acts as a seal to teeth by firmly encircling them. This oral soft tissue is tightly bound to the underlying bone, both maxilla, and mandible.

## MACROSCOPIC FEATURES

Gingiva is divided anatomically into the following three domains **(Flowchart 1.1 and Fig. 1.1)**.

### Marginal Gingiva/Free Gingiva

Marginal gingiva is the terminal edge of the gingiva that covers the teeth in a collar-like fashion.[2] It is also termed as the free or unattached gingiva, as it is not fixed to the basal periosteum of alveolar bone. It is usually 1 mm wide and forms the soft tissue wall of the gingival sulcus.

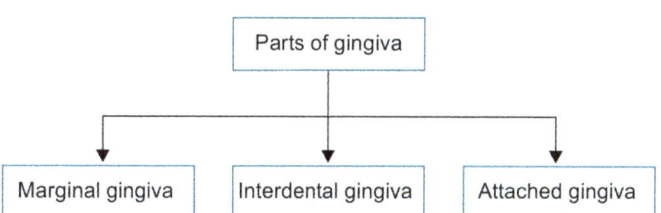

Flowchart 1.1: Division of gingiva.

### Gingival Sulcus

The gingival sulcus is a narrow space between the tooth and the free gingival margin. This V-shaped groove extends from the junctional epithelium (JE) at the base up to the free marginal gingiva. So functionally, one of its soft-tissue walls is formed by the free marginal gingiva. These are specialized tissues that separate the tooth from the normal gingival tissues. Gingival sulcus barely permits the entry of a periodontal probe, and its probing depth is 2–3 mm **(Fig. 1.2)**.

### Free Gingival Groove

Marginal gingiva is separated from attached gingiva by a shallow line called a free gingival groove. This indentation is located at a level corresponding to the level of cementoenamel junction (CEJ) **(Figs. 1.1A and B)**. Free gingival groove is present in only about 30–40% of adults.[3]

The presence or absence and the location of the gingival groove depends on the distinctness of the fan-shaped arrangement of the supra-alveolar collagenous fibers running from the cementum into the gingiva.

**Section 1:** Normal Periodontium

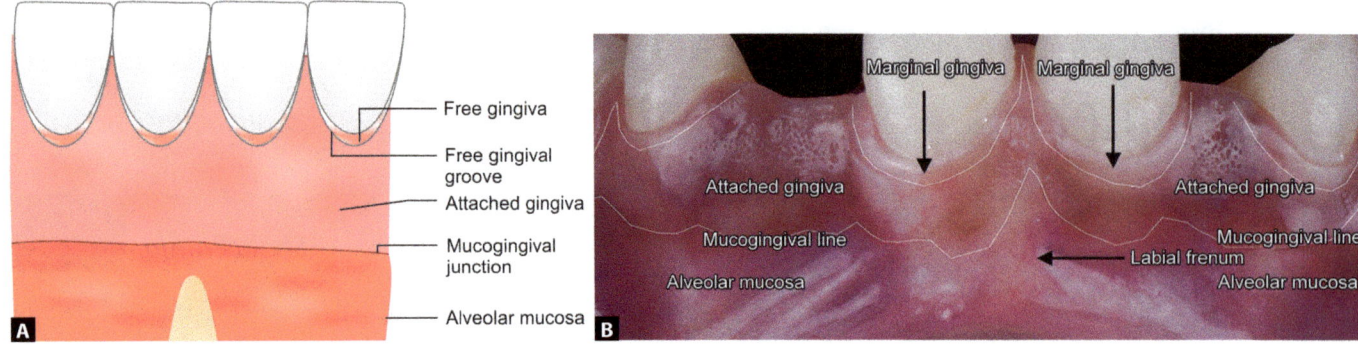

**Figs. 1.1A and B:** Schematic representation showing macroscopic features of the gingiva.
(CEJ: cementoenamel junction)
(*Courtesy:* Dr Anuj Gandhi)

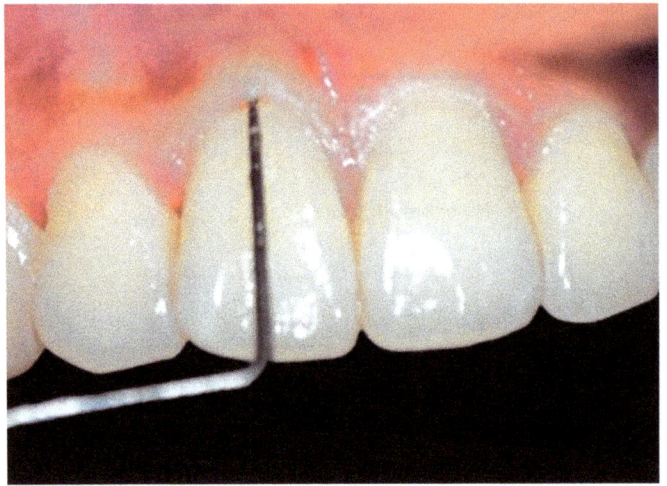

**Fig. 1.2:** Clinical picture showing normal clinical gingival sulcus depth.

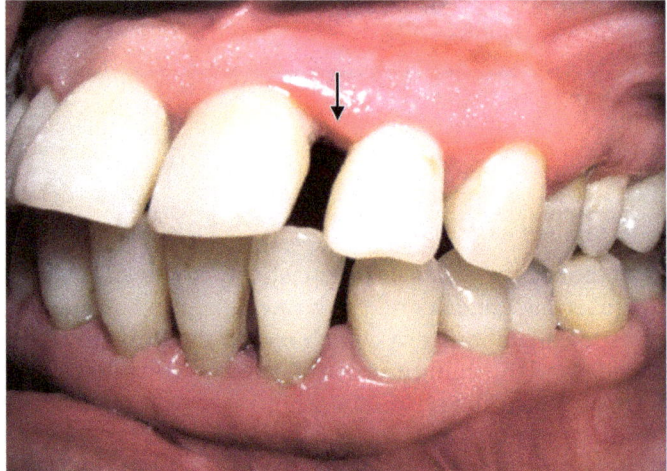

**Fig. 1.3:** Clinical picture showing an absence of interdental papilla in the diastema.

## Interdental Gingiva

Interdental gingiva, also known as the interdental papilla, is a portion of the gingiva which is located in the space between two adjacent teeth. However, interdental gingiva is not seen in cases of diastema **(Fig. 1.3)**.

## Col

It is a valley-like depression of the interproximal contact areas connecting lingual and buccal interdental papilla **(Fig. 1.4)**.[4] It is lined by nonkeratinized epithelium, which is gradually replaced by continuing cell division. Epithelium lining of the col is similar to junctional epithelium as both have the same origin, i.e., from the dental epithelium.

### *Significance*

As col has nonkeratinized epithelium, it is anatomically predisposed to the growth of oral microorganisms and susceptible to inflammation and disease progression.

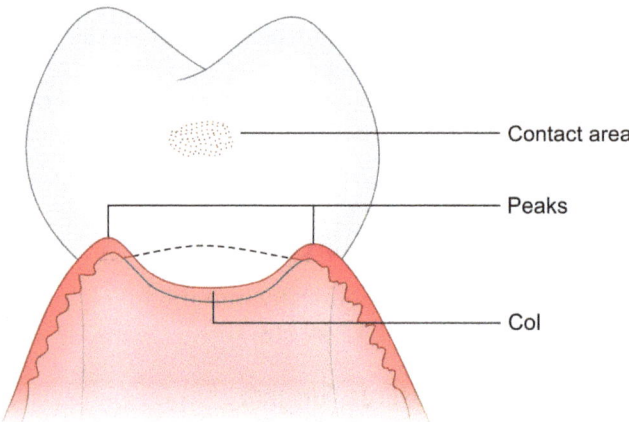

**Fig. 1.4:** Schematic representation showing col and peaks.

## Attached Gingiva

Attached gingiva is the part of the gingiva which is tightly attached to the underlying periosteum of alveolar bone and cementum by connective tissue fibers. It is a firm, resilient, and hence immovable portion of the gingiva. The attached gingiva is thus, firmly entrenched between two movable structures: the marginal gingiva coronally and the alveolar mucosa apically **(Table 1.1)**. The attached gingiva is different from keratinized gingiva and should not be confused with it. Keratinized part of the gingiva usually includes all, i.e., attached gingiva, marginal gingiva, and central portion of the interdental gingiva **(Fig. 1.5)**.

The width of the attached gingiva is measured as the distance between the mucogingival junction (MGJ) and the projection on the external surface of the bottom of the gingival sulcus/periodontal pocket. The dimensions of the attached gingiva vary from the anterior to the posterior teeth. The width of the attached gingiva is generally wider in the maxilla than in the mandible. The gingiva's narrowest zone is found in the region of the maxillary and mandibular first premolars and usually in connection with frenum and muscle attachments **(Table 1.2)**. The pattern of variation is approximately the same in deciduous and permanent teeth.

The width of the attached gingiva is wider in the supra erupted teeth.[5] It also increases with age.[6] This increase in dimension occurs as a result of an increase in the height of the alveolar process, which, in turn, is the result of the passive eruption.

**TABLE 1.1:** Differences between alveolar mucosa and attached gingiva.

|  | Alveolar mucosa | Attached gingiva |
|---|---|---|
| Color | Red | Pink |
| Surface texture | Smooth and shiny | Stippled |
| Epithelium | ♦ Thinner<br>♦ Nonkeratinized<br>♦ Rete pegs absent | ♦ Thicker<br>♦ Parakeratinized<br>♦ Rete pegs present |
| Connective tissue | ♦ More loosely arranged<br>♦ More blood vessels | ♦ Not so loosely arranged<br>♦ Moderate blood vessels |

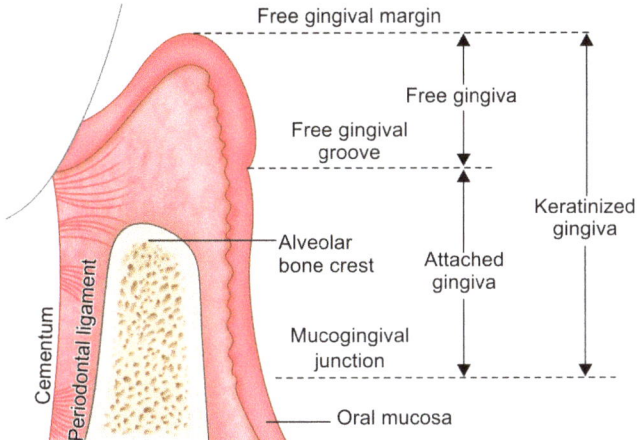

**Fig. 1.5:** Schematic representation showing keratinized gingiva.

**TABLE 1.2:** Dimensions of attached gingiva (on facial aspects).[2]

| Region | Dimensions (mm) |
|---|---|
| Maxillary incisor region | 3.5–4.5 |
| Mandibular incisor region | 3.3–3.9 |
| Maxillary 1st premolar | 1.9 |
| Mandibular 1st premolar | approx. 1.8 |

### Significance of Attached Gingiva

- It gives support to the marginal gingiva.
- It provides attachment or a solid base for the movable alveolar mucosa for the action of lips, cheeks, and tongue.
- It can withstand frictional and functional stresses of mastication and toothbrushing. When the marginal tissue is the alveolar mucosa, it does not resist the functional stresses of toothbrush trauma imposed on it. Frequently, the result is the apical shifting of the marginal tissue and additional recession. Attached gingiva is tightly attached to underlying periosteum and the alveolar bone with the densely organized connective tissue. Consequently, it is more resistant to the functional stresses placed upon it. Alveolar mucosa is a thin, delicate tissue, poorly attached to bone and cementum, and is not capable of withstanding these same functional stresses.
- It acts as a barrier to the passage of inflammation. In the presence of microbial flora, tooth having alveolar mucosa at its margin shows more clinical signs of inflammation than the corresponding tooth that has a sufficient band of the attached gingiva. Such marginal tissue appears to be more susceptible to the products of inflammation that may result in the pocket formation or apical migration of both attachment apparatus and marginal tissues.
- It provides resistance to tensional stresses. Attached gingiva serves as a buffer between the mobile free gingival margin and mobile alveolar mucosa. There are skeletal muscle fibers within the alveolar mucosa that exert a force in an apical direction on the attached gingiva. This force is dissipated by bound down keratinized tissue.

### Measurement of Width of Attached Gingiva

- *Anatomically*: Lip or cheek is stretched to delineate the mucogingival line and, at the same time, place the probe into the pocket to measure the depth. To determine the attached gingiva's width, measure the total width of the gingiva (gingival margin to the mucogingival line) and subtract pocket depth from it.
- *Functionally*:
    - Tension test: Stretch the lip or cheek outward and forward to mark the mucogingival line. Now to calculate the width of the attached gingiva, first

measure the total width of the gingiva from gingival margin to mucogingival line. Subtracting the sulcus or pocket depth from the gingiva's total width gives the width of the attached gingiva.

- Roll test: To conduct the roll test, mark the mucogingival line by pushing the adjacent mucosa coronally with a dull instrument. Measure the total width of the gingiva, i.e., distance from the gingival margin to the mucogingival line. Now subtract the sulcus or pocket depth from this total width of the gingiva to get the width of the attached gingiva.[7] A more reliable method of identifying the MGJ would be to take the side of a periodontal probe or similar blunt instrument and jiggle the alveolar mucosa in an apicoronal direction. Since the alveolar mucosa is mobile, it will roll up ahead of the blunt instrument.

- *Histochemically*: The iodine staining test is one of the histochemical tests that are useful for calculating the attached gingiva's width. In this test, you initially have to paint the gingiva and oral mucosa with Schiller's or Lugol's solution (iodine and potassium iodide solution). The presence of glycogen content in the alveolar mucosa imparts its brown color. However, the attached gingiva stays unstained as it is glycogen free. Measuring the total width of this unstained gingiva and subtracting the sulcus or pocket depth from the calculated total width gives us the width of the attached gingiva.

### Mucogingival Junction

The mucogingival junction is the vital landmark between the coronally positioned attached gingiva and the apically placed alveolar mucosa. It remains stationary throughout life. This anatomical feature is located on the three gingival surfaces, namely (1) facial gingiva of the maxilla and (2) facial and (3) lingual gingiva of the mandible. However, MGJ is absent on the maxilla's palatal gingiva due to an absence of a freely movable alveolar mucosa on the palate. Palatal gingiva of the maxilla extends with palatal tissue and bound to underlying palatal bones.

### Gingival Biotype

Gingival thickness is an essential determinant of periodontal health. Eger and Muller have classified gingival phenotype or biotype into thick and thin.[8] Thick gingival phenotype seems to be more conducive to periodontal health. A thin gingival phenotype predisposes to gingival recession and an increased tendency to gingival inflammation **(Fig. 1.6)**.

## MICROSCOPIC FEATURES

Histological examination of gingiva exhibited the following structures:
- Gingival epithelium
- Epithelium-connective tissue interface
- Gingival connective tissue or lamina propria

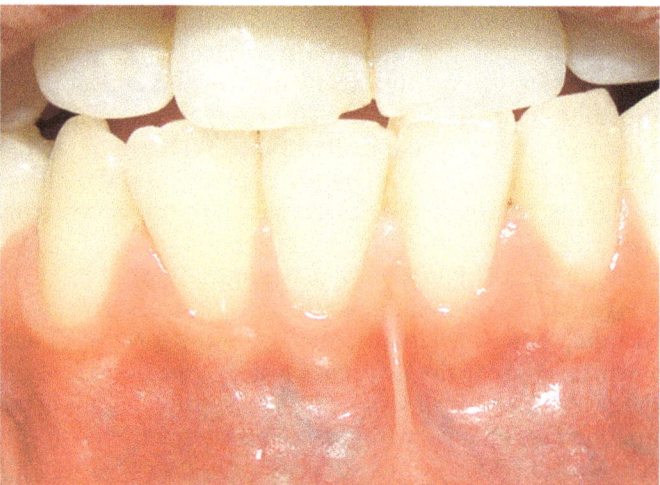

**Fig. 1.6:** Clinical picture showing the thin gingival phenotype.

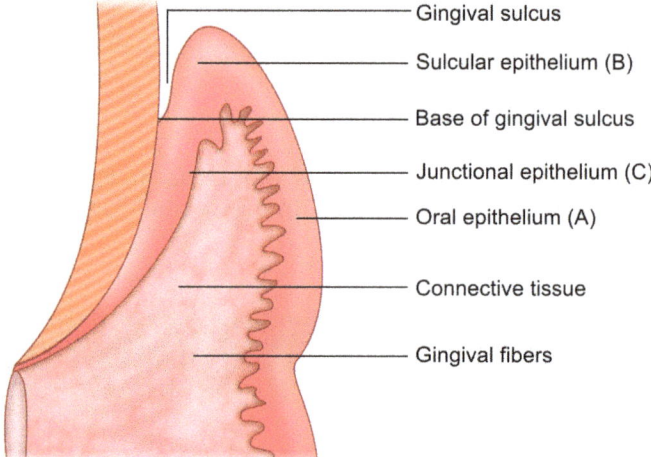

**Fig. 1.7:** Schematic representation showing gingival epithelium: (A) Oral epithelium, (B) Sulcular epithelium and (C) Junctional epithelium (JE).

### Gingival Epithelium

Typically, the gingival epithelium is divided into three types **(Fig. 1.7 and Table 1.3)**:
1. Oral epithelium
2. Sulcular epithelium
3. Junctional epithelium

### Oral Epithelium

The oral epithelium, also called an outer epithelium, is a keratinized stratified squamous type of epithelium. It covers the crest and outer surface of the marginal gingiva and surface of the attached gingiva.

The oral epithelium consists of following types of cellular layers **(Figs. 1.8 and 1.9)**:[3]
- *Stratum basale:* The cells of stratum basale are either cylindrical or cuboid. The basal cells are found immediately next to the connective tissue and are separated from connective tissue by a basement

| TABLE 1.3: Differences between oral, sulcular and junctional epithelium (JE). | | | |
|---|---|---|---|
| | Oral | Sulcular | Junctional epithelium (JE) |
| Keratinization | Keratinized | Nonkeratinized | Nonkeratinized |
| Rete pegs | Present | Absent | Absent |
| Strata granuloma and corneum | Present | Lacking | Lacking |
| Merkel cells | Present | Absent | Absent |
| Langerhans cells (LCs) | Present | Few | Absent |
| Type IV collagen in the basal lamina | Present | Absent | Absent |
| Tight junctions | More | Few | Few |
| Acid phosphatase activity | Present | Lacking | Lacking |
| Glycolytic enzyme activity | High | Lower | Lower |
| Intercellular space | Narrower | Narrower | Wider |

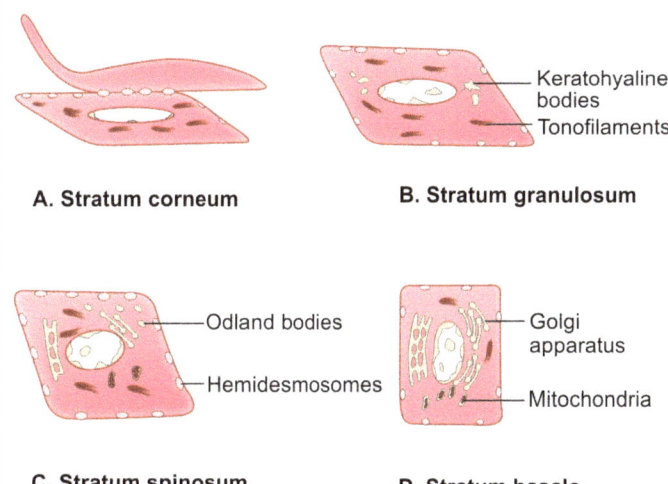

**Figs. 1.9A to D:** Schematic representation showing the cell of various layers of stratified squamous epithelium: (A) Stratum corneum; (B) Stratum granulosum; (C) Stratum spinosum; and (D) Stratum basale.

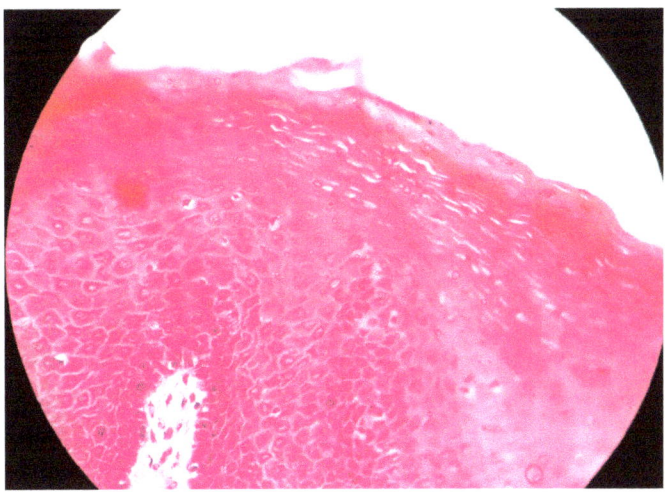

**Fig. 1.8:** Histological picture of stratified squamous epithelium showing stratum corneum, stratum granulosum, stratum spinosum and stratum basale.
(*Courtesy:* Dr Sushruth Nayak)

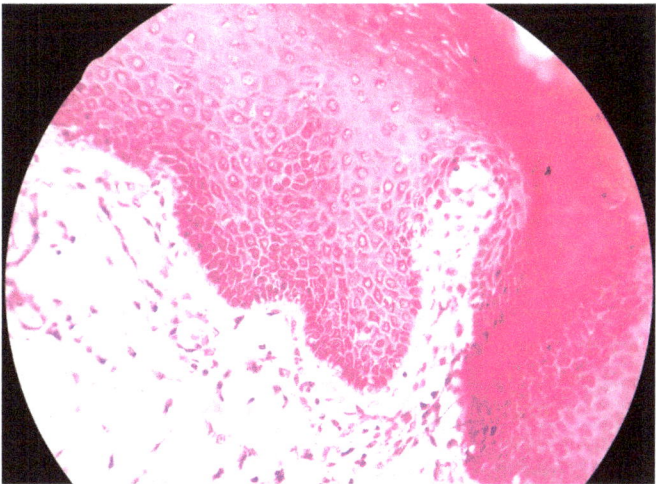

**Fig. 1.10:** Histological picture of stratified squamous epithelium showing stratum spinosum and stratum basale.
(*Courtesy:* Dr Sushruth Nayak)

membrane. It is the germinative layer and hence can divide. When two daughter cells have been formed by cell division, an adjacent older basal cell is pushed into the spinous cell layer and starts as a keratinocyte to traverse the epithelium. It takes approximately one month for a keratinocyte to reach the outer epithelial surface, where it is shed from the stratum corneum **(Fig. 1.10)**.

- *Stratum spinosum*: It is a prickle cell layer in which large polyhedral cells with short cytoplasmic processes are present. The uppermost cells from this layer contain granules called keratinosomes or Odland bodies. These are modified lysosomes, which contain a large amount of enzymes acid phosphatase that is involved in the destruction of organelle membranes **(Fig 1.10)**.

- *Stratum granulosum*: Cells of this layer are flattened in a plane parallel to the gingival surface. Keratohyalin granules, which are associated with keratin formation, are (1 μm in diameter) round in shape and appear within the cell's cytoplasm.

- *Stratum corneum*: It consists of closely packed, flattened cells that have lost nuclei and the most other organelles as they become keratinized. The cells are densely packed with tonofilaments. Clear, rounded bodies probably representing lipid droplets appear within the cytoplasm of the cell.

## Sulcular Epithelium

Sulcular epithelium is a nonkeratinized, stratified squamous epithelium that usually lines the gingival sulcus. It covers the area from the crest of the gingival margin up to the coronal end of the junctional epithelium.

### Junctional Epithelium

Junctional epithelium (JE) is composed of a collar-like band of the stratified squamous, nonkeratinized epithelium. It usually consists of two strata, namely stratum basale, and stratum suprabasale. The average length of JE is 0.25–1.35 mm. JE is composed of 15–30 cell layers coronally while only 1–3 cell layers apically and hence taper in apical direction.[1]

#### Development of Junctional Epithelium

Before the eruptive movements of the tooth begin, the crown of the tooth is lined with a double layer of epithelial cells. The inner layer of cells is called ameloblasts. It completes its formative function and develops hemidesmosomes and gets tightly bound to the enamel surface. The outer layer consists of more flattened cells, the remnants of all the remaining layers of the dental organ. These two layers, in combination, are termed as "reduced enamel epithelium." Once the process of tooth eruption starts in the oral cavity, the connective tissue present between reduced enamel epithelium and the overlying oral epithelium begins to breakdown and degenerates.[9] The basal cells from the oral epithelium as well as the cells of the outer layer of the reduced enamel epithelium start to proliferate and migrate into the degenerative connective tissue. In the end, they blend to form a mass of epithelial cells over the erupting tooth. Cell death in the middle of this epithelial plug leads to the formation of an epithelium-lined canal through which the tooth erupts without hemorrhage. From this mass of an epithelium along with the remaining reduced dental epithelium, the epithelial component of dentogingival junction is established. The reduced ameloblasts which have lost and do not regain the ability to divide change their morphology and are transformed into squamous epithelial cells that retain their attachment to the enamel surface. The cells of the outer layer of the reduced enamel epithelium retain their ability to divide and become basal cells of forming JE.

Initially, it was first named as an epithelial attachment (Epithelansatz) by Gottlieb. However, later it was examined electron microscopically and renamed as junctional or attachment epithelium by Stern. This epithelium synthesizes the material that attaches it to the tooth. Now this material, its morphology and mode, and mechanism of function are called the epithelial attachment. Thus, the cellular structure is referred to as junctional or attachment epithelium and its extracellular tooth attaching substance is called as the epithelial attachment.[10]

The junctional epithelium has three zones, namely (1) coronal, (2) middle, and (3) apical zones. The coronal zone is the most permeable zone of JE. The middle zone has the maximum adhesiveness among all the three zones.

The junctional epithelium has three surfaces: (1) internal surface facing the tooth surface; (2) external surface facing the gingival connective tissue and (3) coronal surface

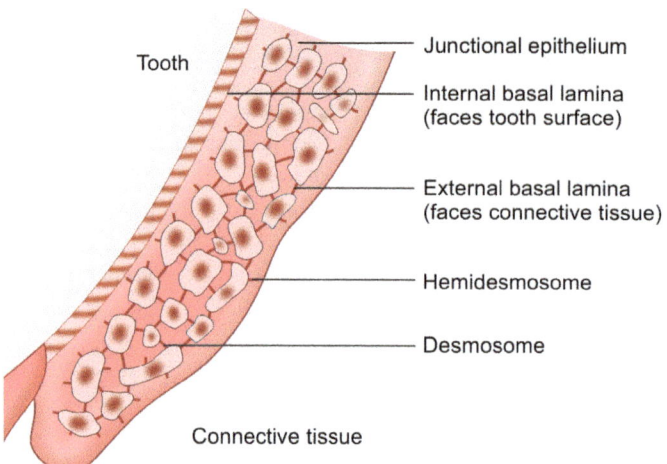

**Fig. 1.11:** Schematic representation showing junctional epithelium (JE).

forming the base of the sulcus. JE is bound to the tooth surface with internal basal lamina and to gingival connective tissue with external basal lamina **(Fig. 1.11)**.[11] The JE is attached to the tooth through the epithelial attachment apparatus. Ultramicroscopic examination of this apparatus reveals the presence of hemidesmosomes at the plasma membrane of the cells that directly attached to the tooth (DAT cells), and a basal lamina like an extracellular matrix called as the internal basal lamina on the tooth surface.[12]

The junctional epithelium is easily penetrated because of the following factors:
- Along with the JE, subepithelial vessels run parallel to the surface and consist mostly venules rather than capillaries. These venules have a greater disposition towards increased permeability as compared to capillaries and arterioles, and they are more susceptible to hemorrhage and thrombosis.
- Few tight intercellular junctions
- Minimal cytoplasmic filaments
- The higher number of intercellular spaces
- The lower number of desmosomes

#### Functions

Junctional epithelium serves many roles in regulating tissue health:
- It provides attachment to the tooth.
- It acts as an epithelial barrier against plaque bacteria. The external basement membrane laterally forms an effective barrier against invading microbes.
- Rapid cell division and funneling of junctional epithelial cells towards the sulcus hinder bacterial colonization, and repair of damaged tissue occurs rapidly.
- Junctional epithelium allows two-way movement of a variety of substances:
  - From connective tissue into crevice: Gingival fluid exudates, polymorphonuclear leukocytes (PMN), immunoglobulin (Ig), complement, and various cells of the immune system.

- From crevice to connective tissue: Foreign materials, such as carbon particles and trypan blue.
- Active antimicrobial substances are produced by junctional epithelial cells. These are defensins, lysosomal enzymes, calprotectin, and cathelicidin.
- Junctional epithelial cells which get activated by microbial substances secrete chemokines, such as interleukins (IL-1, IL-6, IL-8) and tumor necrosis factor-alpha (TNF-α) that attract and activate professional defense cells, such as lymphocytes and PMNs.[13]

### Cells Present in the Gingival Epithelium

Cells present in the gingival epithelium are namely keratinocytes and nonkeratinocytes.

*Keratinocytes:* These make up 90% of the total gingival cell population. They originate from the ectodermal germ layer. Structurally, they are like any other cells having cell organelles, such as the nucleus, cytosol, ribosomes, and golgi apparatus. They have melanosomes, which are the pigment-bearing granules present within these cells only and not in the other cells of the periodontium. The primary function of the gingival epithelium, i.e., protection and barrier against the oral environment is achieved by the proliferation and differentiation of the keratinocytes.[14]

Keratinization: It is defined as the transformation of living cells into horny material. Keratinocytes have to move from basal to superficial layers of the epithelium as the process of differentiation occurs in a basocoronal direction culminating in the formation of a keratin barrier. The microfilaments present in the keratinocytes help in cell motility and maintenance of the polarity.[15] Keratinocyte motility requires the following steps:
- Development of lamellipodia, i.e., extensions on the leading edge of the cell towards the direction of movement.
- Attachment of this portion of the cell to the substratum.
- Movement of the cytosolic material towards the leading edge of the cell.
- The detachment of the rear end.

*Nonkeratinocytes:* The various nonkeratinocytes or clear cells are Langerhans cells (LCs), Merkel cells, and melanocytes.
- *Langerhans cells*: They are modified monocytes belonging to reticuloendothelial systems, which reside chiefly in suprabasal layers. Paul Langerhans used the gold impregnation technique 100 years ago to visualize LCs. Langerhans cells can move in and out of the epithelium, unlike melanocytes. They are responsible for communication with the immune system by acting as antigen-presenting cells for lymphocytes and expressing receptors for C3 and Fc portion of immunoglobulin G (IgG). These cells contain specific elongated granules called as Birbeck's granules and have marked adenosine triphosphatase activity.[16]
- Merkel cells: They are usually found in the basal cell layer of the gingival epithelium. These cells either appear individually or in clusters. These are not dendritic cells as melanocytes and LCs.[17] These cells possess keratin tonofilaments and occasional desmosomes, which link them to adjacent cells. These cells are sensory in nature and respond to touch.[18]
- Melanocytes: They have their origin from neural crest cells located in the stratum basale of the oral gingival epithelium. Oral mucosal melanocytes were identified in the gingiva by Laidlaw and Cahn in 1932. Long dendritic processes from these cells are interposed between the keratinocytes of the epithelium. They lack tonofilaments and desmosomal connections to adjacent keratinocytes. Melanocytes are responsible for the barrier to ultraviolet (UV) damage and synthesize melanin, which is accountable for providing color to the gingiva. Melanin is synthesized in an organelle called premelanosomes or melanosomes in melanocytes from an amino acid called phenylalanine.[19] Melanosomes are transported along microtubules and actin filaments to the cell periphery. Melanocytes bind to the plasma membrane and transfer the melanosomes to adjacent keratinocytes **(Fig. 1.12)**. The precise mechanism is unknown but has been described as cytocrine secretion. Sometimes in the connective tissue, macrophages take up the melanosomes produced by melanocytes in the epithelium and are called melanophages or melanophores. Melanocytes may be classified as active or inactive, depending on the presence or absence of mature melanosomes. The ratio of melanocytes-to-keratinocytes producing epithelial cells is approximately 1: 36 cells.

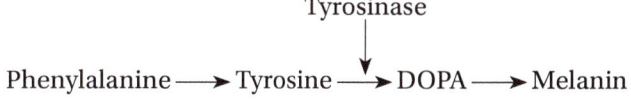

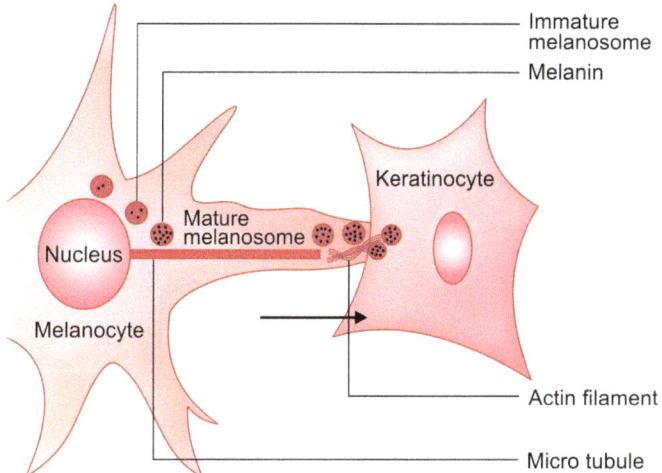

**Fig. 1.12:** Schematic representation showing the mechanism of melanosome transport.

## Section 1: Normal Periodontium

### Epithelium-Connective Tissue Interface

It is the boundary where epithelial tissue meets with connective tissue. Deep extensions of an epithelium that reach down into the connective tissue are called epithelial ridges or rete pegs. Finger-like extensions of connective tissue that extend up into the epithelium are called as connective tissue papillae **(Fig. 1.13)**.

Ultrastructurally, the epithelial-connective tissue interface is composed of *lamina lucida* and *lamina densa*. *Lamina lucida* is an electrolucent zone of 25–45 nm width and composed of glycoprotein laminin. *Lamina densa* is an electrodense zone of 40–60 nm where type IV collagen is present.[20]

From the lamina densa so-called anchoring fibrils project in a fan-shaped fashion into the connective tissue **(Fig. 1.14)**. These anchoring fibrils are of approximately 750 nm in length and form loops around collagen fibers.

### *Junctional Complexes*

The various junctional complexes present in the gingiva are:[21]
- Tight/occluding junctions are formed by the fusion of external leaflets of adjacent cell membranes at a series of points.
- *Adhesive junctions*:
  - Cell to cell:
    - Zonula adherens
    - Desmosomes: It is the most common type of junction, which consists of two adjacent attachment plaques, one from each cell that is separated by an interval of approximately 30 nm.
  - Cell to the matrix:
    - Focal adhesions
    - Hemidesmosomes
- *Communicating (gap) junctions*: They have intercellular pipes/channels that bridge both the adjacent membranes and intercellular space. The intercellular space in gap junction is approximately 3 nm and is the major pathway for direct intercellular communication.

### Gingival Connective Tissue or Lamina Propria

The gingival connective tissue, also called lamina propria, is composed of gingival fibers, various cells, and ground substances.

### *Gingival Fibers*

Human gingival fibers consist of collagen, reticulin, and elastin. Collagen fibers constitute more than 50% of the the volume of the human gingiva. Collagen fiber types I, III, IV, V, VI are commonly found in the gingiva.[22] Type I collagen predominates. The structural formula for type I collagen is [α1(I)]2' α2(I). Type III collagen is fetal collagen, which is important in the early phases of wound healing and remains in an unmineralized form. Type III collagen in the gingiva is partly responsible for the maintenance of space in the healing matrix. Lamina densa layer of the basement membrane of the epithelium consisted of type IV collagen. Type VI collagen is distributed with the elastin fibers along the blood vessels. Type VI collagen fibers impart rigidity required to maintain the elastic blood vessel wall from undergoing permanent deformation. Type VII collagen acts as anchoring fibrils and helps to reinforce epithelial attachment to the underlying connective tissue.[23]

Functions of Gingival Fibers
- To stabilize the attached gingiva to the alveolar process.
- To stabilize the attached gingiva to the tooth.
- It helps to maintain the epithelial seal to the tooth.
- To provide stability to the tooth.
- To brace marginal (free) gingiva firmly against the tooth and adjacent attached gingiva.
- To provide rigidity to withstand forces of mastication without being deflected away from the tooth surface.

Types of Gingival Fibers

Gingival fibers are arranged into the following groups **(Fig. 1.15)**:[24]
- *Dentogingival group*: These fibers extend from the cementum apical to JE and course laterally and coronally into lamina propria of the gingiva. These fibers provide gingival support.

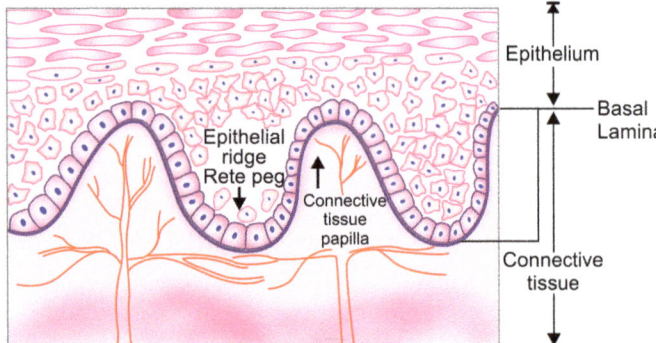

**Fig. 1.13:** Schematic representation showing epithelium-connective tissue interface.

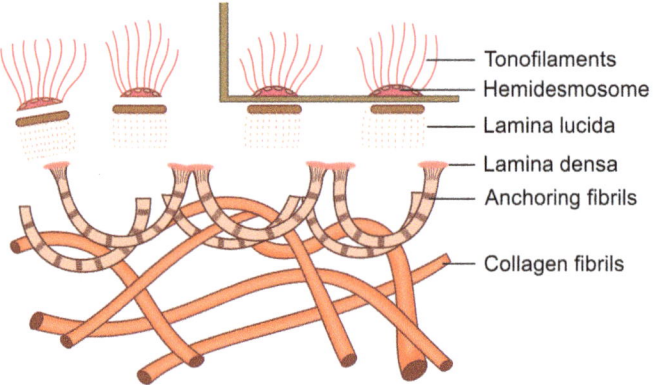

**Fig. 1.14:** Schematic representation showing basal lamina.

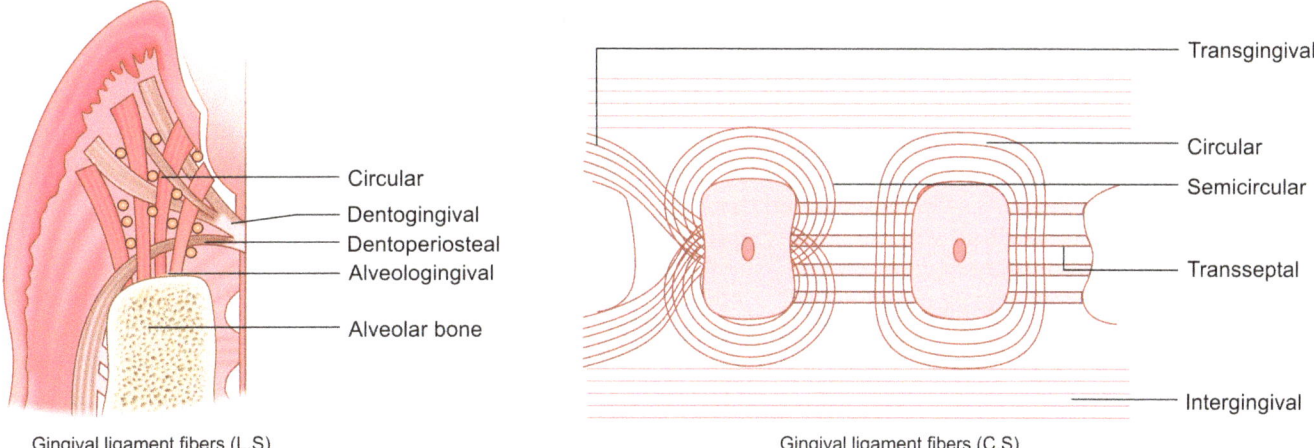

**Fig. 1.15:** Schematic representation showing gingival fibers.

- *Alveologingival group*: These fibers arise from the alveolar crest and insert coronally into the gingiva's lamina propria. These fibers connect the attached gingiva to the alveolar bone.
- *Circular group*: This group of fibers surrounds the teeth in a ring-like fashion. Such encircling of fibers helps to maintain the position and contour of the marginal gingiva.
- *Transseptal fibers*: These are the groups of prominent horizontal fibers. These are placed interproximally and extend from the cementum of one tooth to the cementum of the adjacent tooth. This helps to maintain a relationship of adjacent teeth and protects the interproximal bone. The transseptal fibers collectively form an interdental ligament connecting all the teeth of the arch. Though this ligament belongs to the supra-alveolar fiber apparatus, but appears to be uniquely important in maintaining the integrity of the dental arch. It is rapidly reformed after excision. Residual portions of transseptal fibers are seen even in advanced stages of resting periodontal disease.
- *Dentoperiosteal group*: On the oral and vestibular surfaces of jaws, the dentoperiosteal group of fibers extends from the tooth and passes over the alveolar crest to blend with fibers of the periosteum of the alveolar bone. These fibers anchor tooth to bone and protect periodontal ligament.
- *Semicircular group*: These are a group of fibers, which are attached at the proximal surface of a tooth immediately below the CEJ and go around the facial or lingual marginal gingiva of the tooth and get attached to the other proximal surface of the same tooth.
- *Transgingival group*: These fibers are usually attached to the proximal surface of one tooth, transverse the interdental space diagonally, go around the facial or lingual surface of the adjacent tooth, again traverse the interdental space diagonally and attach to the proximal surface of the next tooth. They secure the alignment of teeth in the arch.
- *Intergingival group*: These fibers run parallel to dentition on vestibular and oral surfaces. They provide contour and support for the attached gingiva.
- *Interpapillary group*: They are seen in the interdental gingiva extending in a faciolingual direction. They provide support for interdental gingiva.

Dentogingival, dentoperiosteal, and alveologingival fibers group provide the attachment of the gingiva to the tooth and the bony structure. Fibers of circular, semicircular, transgingival, intergingival, and transseptal bundles connect teeth.

## Cells Present in Gingival Connective Tissue

- *Fibroblasts*: These are derived from the undifferentiated progenitor mesenchymal cells that are present in the follicle.[25] These are elongated or spindle-shaped cells having prominent golgi apparatus, rough endoplasmic reticulum, mitochondria, vacuoles, and vesicles. Fibroblasts synthesize and secrete various cytokines, growth factors, and metabolic products. All these play a vital role in the development, maintenance and repair of the gingival connective tissue.[26]
- *Mast cells*: These are positioned perivascularly. They are identified by their unique cytoplasmic granules, which produce heparin and histamine.
- *Other cells*: They are eosinophils, macrophages, adipose, and inflammatory cells (neutrophils, plasma cells, and lymphocytes).

*Ground substance:* The cells, fibers, nerves, and vessels of the gingiva are embedded in a gel-like, viscous ground substance. The ground substance is composed of proteoglycans and glycoproteins, which facilitate cell movement and diffusion of various biologically active substances.

- Proteoglycans present in the gingival connective tissues are decorin, versican, biglycan, and syndecan.

- Glycoproteins present in gingival connective tissue are fibronectin, osteonectin, tenascin and laminin.[27]

## MICROCIRCULATION

Microcirculation to the gingiva, i.e., blood and lymph flow through the smallest blood vessels, is mediated through microcirculatory tracts, blood vessels, and lymphatic vessels. Microcirculation plays a vital role in tissue fluid drainage and the spread of inflammation. The methods commonly employed to detect microcirculation are immunohistochemical reactions, histoenzymatic reactions, perfusion of dyes, scanning electron microscopy, and laser Doppler flowmetry.

### Arterial Supply

There are three sources of blood supply to the gingiva, namely supraperiosteal arterioles, vessels of the periodontal ligament, and arterioles emerging from the crest of the interdental septa **(Fig. 1.16)**. Supraperiosteal arterioles mainly supply free gingiva and gingival sulcus. These arterioles are the terminal branches of the sublingual artery, mental artery, buccal artery, facial artery, greater palatine artery, infraorbital artery, and posterior superior dental artery. Vessels of periodontal ligament mainly supply col area. Arterioles emerging from the crest of the interdental septa mainly supply attached gingiva.

Dentogingival plexus is plexus of blood vessels beneath JE. The blood vessels in this plexus have a thickness of approximately 40 μm, which means that these are mainly venules. No capillary loops occur in healthy gingiva. Subepithelial plexus is plexus of blood vessels beneath the oral epithelium of free and attached gingiva and yield thin capillary loops of 7 μm to each connective tissue papilla.[3]

The venous and lymphatic vessels follow a course closely parallel to that of arterial supply. Lymphatic drainage starts in the connective tissue papillae and drains into regional lymph nodes. Buccal gingiva of maxilla, buccal and lingual gingiva of mandibular premolar and molar region drains into submandibular lymph nodes. Mandibular incisor region drains into submental lymph nodes, whereas third molars' region drains into jugulodigastric lymph nodes.[3] Their main function is to return fluids and filterable plasma components to the blood via the thoracic duct.

## NERVE SUPPLY

End branches of the trigeminal nerve innervate the various regions of the gingiva. The gingiva on the labial aspects of maxillary incisors, canines, and premolars are innervated by the superior labial branches from the infraorbital nerve. Buccal gingiva in the maxillary molar region is innervated by branches from the posterior superior dental nerve. Palatal gingiva is innervated by greater palatal nerve except for the incisors' area, which is innervated by the sphenopalatine nerve. Lingual gingiva in the mandible is innervated by sublingual nerve, a branch of lingual nerve. The mental nerve innervates gingiva on the labial aspects of mandibular incisors and canines. The buccal nerve innervates the buccal aspect of molars. Innervation of mandibular premolars is by both mental and buccal nerves. Krause type end bulbs, Meissner type tactile corpuscles, and encapsulated spindles are the types of neural terminals, which are present, mainly within the connective tissue but only a few endings occur between epithelial cells.[28]

## CLINICAL CRITERIA

Following are the clinical criteria of normal gingiva[1] **(Table 1.4)**.

### Color

The color of the gingiva is described as coral pink, which depends upon vascular supply, the thickness of the epithelium, degree of keratinization of the epithelium, and presence of pigment-containing cells **(Fig. 1.17)**.

A variation in gingival pigmentation is not produced by variation in the number of pigment forming melanocytes

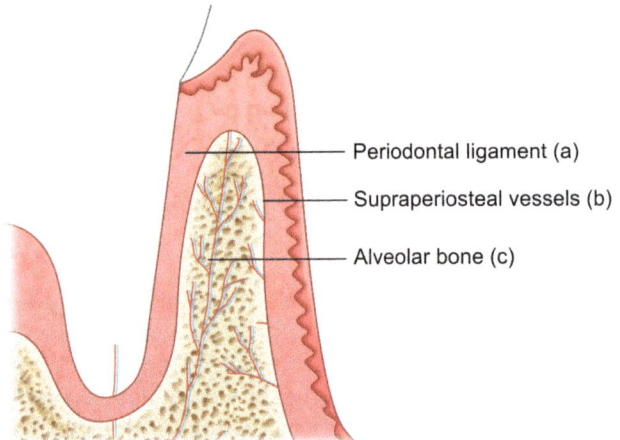

**Fig. 1.16:** Schematic representation showing gingival blood supply which derives from (a) Periodontal ligament, (b) Supraperiosteal vessels and (c) Alveolar bone.

**TABLE 1.4:** Clinical criteria.

| Clinical feature | Appearance in health |
|---|---|
| Color | Coral or pale pink |
| Surface texture | ◆ Free gingiva: Smooth<br>◆ Attached gingiva: Stippled |
| Contour | ◆ Marginal gingiva: Knife-edged<br>◆ Attached gingiva: Festooned |
| Shape | Interdental papilla: Pointed, pyramidal |
| Size | Fits snugly around the tooth |
| Consistency | Attached gingiva: Firm, resilient |
| Position | Fully erupted tooth: Margin is 1–2 mm above cementoenamel junction (CEJ) |

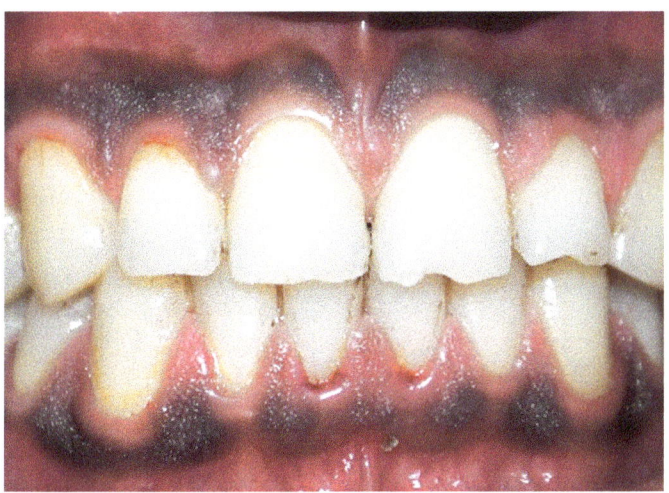

**Fig. 1.17:** Schematic representation showing generalized melanin pigmentation.

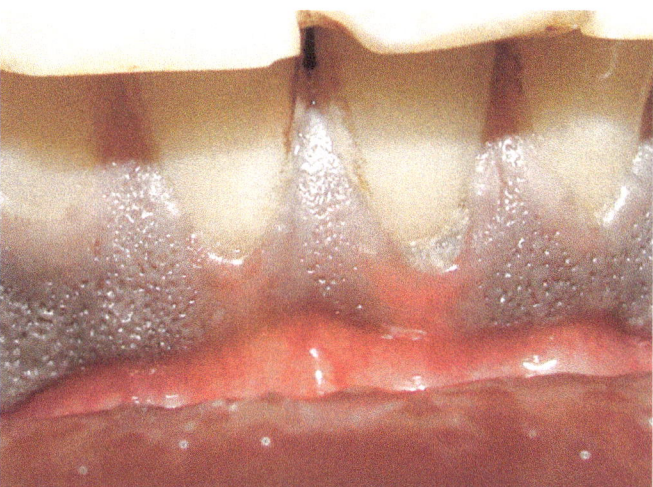

**Fig. 1.18:** Clinical picture showing stippling on attached gingiva and center of interdental papilla.

but by genetically determined variation in their pigment-producing capacity. Thus, variations in gingival pigmentation are related to complexion and race. It is lighter in blond individuals with a fair complexion as compared to dark complexion individuals. In the Caucasian individuals, pigmentation is minimal, in African or Asian individuals brown or blue-black areas of pigmentation are seen, while in Mediterranean people occasional patches of pigmentation are found.

*Melanin index for gingival pigmentation:*[19]
- *Category 0*: No pigmentation
- *Category 1*: Solitary unit(s) of pigmentation in the papillary gingiva without the formation of continuous ribbon between solitary units.
- *Category 2*: At least 1 unit of formation of continuous ribbon extending from two neighboring solitary units.

## Surface Texture

The free gingival surface is smooth while the attached gingival surface is stippled. Pitted surface texture giving orange-peel appearance is called stippling, which is more prominent on the labial than the lingual gingival surfaces. Stippling usually is present on the attached gingiva and center of the interdental papilla (**Fig. 1.18**). The intensity of stippling on an average is approximately 2.6 depressions/mm$^2$. It is best viewed by drying the gingiva and switching off the chair light. Stippling is more prominent in the maxillary labial area, and its intensity differs within different areas of the dentition. It varies with age also. It usually appears in children of about five years and increases with age but absent in old age. Stippling reflects the contours of the epithelial, connective tissue boundary in the healthy gingiva. In erythematous tissue, stippling may disappear, although it may be present in thick fibrotic tissue, which is diseased. It is not an absolute sign of health, and its absence is not necessarily a sign of disease.

*Histologically*: The bottom of the pits corresponds to deep ridges or projections of the epithelium into lamina propria of the connective tissue. The protruding parts correspond to a thinner epithelium over ridges or projections of the connective tissue. The ridge and the peg arrangements between the epithelium and connective tissue provide excellent mechanical stability between the two tissue components as well as large contact interphase for metabolic interchange.

## Contour

The marginal gingiva follows a scalloped outline typically and straight-line along with teeth with relatively flat surfaces. Attached gingiva has a festooned appearance with intermittent prominence corresponding to the contour of roots. When the teeth are placed more labially, the normal arcuate contour is accentuated, and gingiva is located further apically. When teeth are lingually placed, the gingiva is horizontal and thickened. Thus, the contour of the gingiva depends upon the shape and alignment of the teeth in the arch. Gingival contour also varies with the position and size of the area of proximal contacts along with dimensions of the embrasures.

## Shape

The contour of the proximal tooth surface, shape, and position of the proximal contact and dimensions of the gingival embrasures are an important determinant of the shape of the interdental gingiva. In normal contact areas and anterior regions, the interdental papilla is usually pointed and pyramidal. However, it is flat- or saddle-shaped in spaced teeth and molar regions.

## Size

The total of the bulk of cellular and intercellular elements and their vascular supply gives the size of the gingiva.

### Section 1: Normal Periodontium

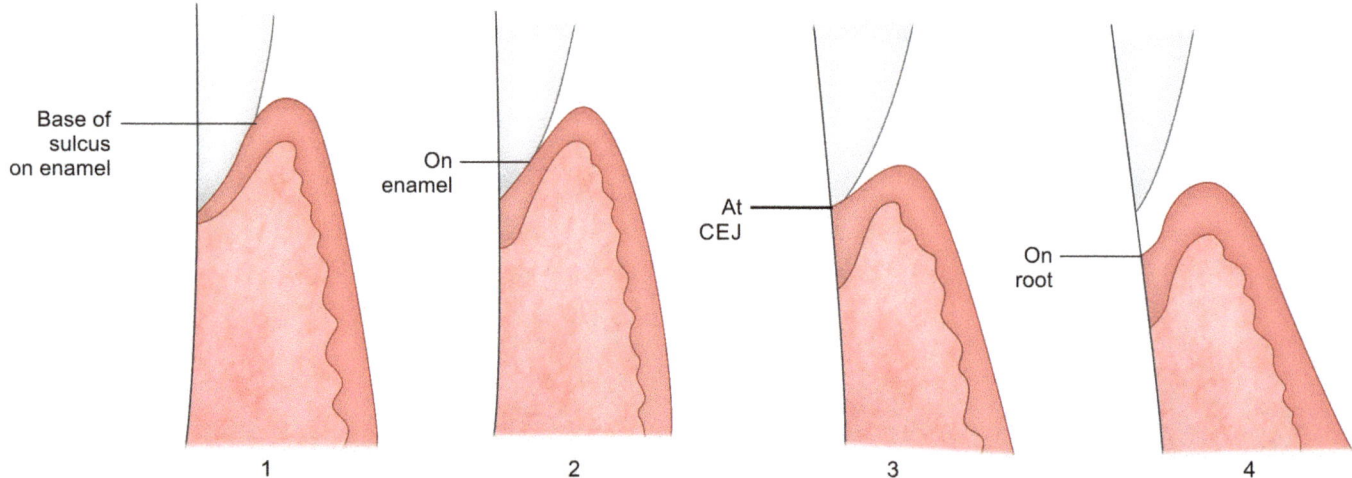

**Fig. 1.19:** Schematic representation showing four stages of passive tooth eruption.
(CEJ: cementoenamel junction)

## Consistency

On palpation with a blunt instrument, healthy attached gingiva should be firm, resilient, and tightly attached to the underlying bone. The presence of abundant collagen fibers and the noncollagenous protein in combination impart firm consistency to the gingiva.

## Position

The gingival position usually corresponds with the level of attachment of the gingival margin to the tooth. When the tooth erupts into the oral cavity, the margin and sulcus are at the crown's tip. As the eruption progresses, they are seen closer to the root.

## Continuous Tooth Eruption

The concept of continuous tooth eruption states that the eruption process remains continuous throughout life and does not stop even when teeth meet their functional antagonists. The process of continuous eruption involves two phases, such as active and a passive phase.

*Active eruption:* This phase involves the development of the teeth in the direction of the occlusal plane.

*Passive eruption:* It takes place due to the apical migration of the gingiva. This phase is divided into four stages (**Fig. 1.19**):[10]

1. *Stage 1*: The teeth reach the line of occlusion with JE and the base of the gingival sulcus, both are on the enamel.
2. *Stage 2*: The JE proliferates with its part both on the cementum and enamel. The base of the sulcus is still on the enamel.
3. *Stage 3*: The entire JE is on the cementum, while the base of the sulcus is at the cementoenamel junction. As the JE starts to proliferate from the crown onto the root, it does not remain at the cementoenamel junction any longer than at any other area of the tooth.
4. *Stage 4*: The JE has proliferated further on the cementum. The base of the sulcus is on the cementum, a portion of which is exposed. The JE's proliferation onto the root is accompanied by degeneration of gingival and periodontal ligament fibers and their detachment from the tooth.

### Points to Ponder

- The pH of the gingiva ranges from 6.5 to 8.5.
- Junctional epithelium and gingival fibers together form a functional unit called a dentogingival unit.
- The junctional epithelium is the only attachment in the body between soft tissue and calcified tissue, which is exposed to the external environment.
- Gingival fiber groups enable the gingiva to form a rigid cuff around the tooth that adds stability, especially when a significant portion of the periodontal ligament and alveolar support is lost. This explains the increased mobility in periodontally involved teeth immediately after surgical procedures (as these procedures disrupt or remove the gingival fiber groups).

## REFERENCES

1. Fiorellini JP, Kim DM, Ishikawa SO. The gingiva. In: Newman MG, Takei HH, Klokkevold PR, Carranza FA (Eds). Carranza's Clinical Periodontology, 10th edition. Philadelphia, PA, USA: WB Saunders; 2006. pp. 46-67.
2. Ainamo J, Löe H. Anatomical characteristics of the gingiva. A clinical and microscopic study of the free and attached gingiva. J Periodontol. 1966;37(1):5-13.
3. Lindhe J, Karring T, Araujo M. Anatomy of the periodontium. In: Lindhe J, Karring T, Lang NP (Eds). Clinical Periodontology and Implant Dentistry, 4th edition. Oxford, UK: Blackwell Munksgaard; 2003. pp. 3-49.
4. Cohen B. Morphological factors in the pathogenesis of the periodontal disease. Br Dent J. 1959;107:31-9.
5. Ainamo A, Ainamo J. The width of attached gingiva on supraerupted teeth. J Periodontal Res. 1978;13(3):194-8.
6. Ainamo J, Talari A. The increase with age of the width of the attached gingiva. J Periodontal Res. 1976;11(4):182-8.

7. Källestål C, Uhlin S. Buccal attachment loss in Swedish adolescents. J Clin Periodontol. 1992;19(7):485-91.
8. Seibert JS, Lindhe J. Esthetics and periodontal therapy. In: Lindhe J (Ed). Textbook of Clinical Periodontology, 2nd edition. Copenhagen, Denmark: Munksgaard; 1989. pp. 477-514.
9. Bosshardt DD, Lang NP. The junctional epithelium: from health to disease. J Dent Res. 2005;84(1):9-20.
10. Stern IB. Oral mucous membrane. In: Bhaskar SN (Ed). Orban's Oral Histology and Embryology, 11th edition. St. Louis: Mosby; 1991. pp. 260-336.
11. Eley BM, Manson JD. The periodontal tissues. In: Periodontics, 5th edition. Edinburgh, Scotland: Wright Publishing; 2004. pp. 1-20.
12. Pollanen MT, Salonen JI, Uitto VJ. Structure and function of the tooth epithelial interface in health and disease. Periodontol 2000. 2003;31:12-31.
13. Hassell TM. Tissues and cells of the periodontium. Periodontol 2000. 1993;3:9-38.
14. Hefti AF. Aspects of cell biology of the normal periodontium. Periodontol 2000. 1993;3:64-75.
15. Galvin S, Loomis C, Manabe M, Dhouailly D, Sun TT. The major pathways of keratinocyte differentiation as defined by keratin expression: an overview. Adv Dermatol. 1989;4:277-99.
16. DiFranco CF, Toto PD, Rowden G, Gargiulo AW, Keene JJ, Connelly E. Identification of Langerhans cells in human gingival epithelium. J Periodontol. 1985;56(1):48-54.
17. Winkelmann RK, Breathnach AS. The Merkel cell. J Invest Dermatol. 1973;60(1):2-15.
18. Ness KH, Morton TH, Dale BA. Identification of Merkel cells in oral epithelium using antikeratin and antineuroendocrine monoclonal antibodies. J Dent Res. 1987;66(6):1154-8.
19. Hanioka T, Tanaka K, Ojima M, Yuuki K. Association of melanin pigmentation in the gingiva of children with parents who smoke. Pediatrics. 2005;116(2):e186-90.
20. Squier CA, Finkelstein MW. Oral mucosa. In: Ten Cate AR, Richard A, Nanci A (Eds). Ten Cate's Oral Histology: Development, Structure and Function, 8th edition. St. Louis: Elsevier-Mosby; 2013. pp. 278-310.
21. Farquhar MG, Palade GE. Junctional complexes in various epithelia. J Cell Biol. 1963;17:375-412.
22. Bartold MS, Narayanan AS. Biology of the Periodontal Connective Tissues. Chicago, USA: Quintessence Publishing; 1998.
23. Bartold PM. Connective tissues of the periodontium. Research and clinical implications. Aust Dent J. 1991;36(4):255-68.
24. Grant DA, Stern IB, Listgarten MA. Gingiva and dentogingival junction. In: Periodontics, 6th edition. St. Louis: CV Mosby; 1988. pp. 25-55.
25. Giannopoulou C, Cimasoni G. Functional characteristics of gingival and periodontal ligament fibroblasts. J Dent Res. 1996;75(3):895-902.
26. Bartold PM, Walsh LJ, Narayanan AS. Molecular and cell biology of the gingiva. Periodontol 2000. 2000;24:28-55.
27. Mariotti A. The extracellular matrix of the periodontium: dynamic and interactive tissues. Periodontol 2000. 1993;3:39-63.
28. Avery JK, Rapp R. Pain conduction in human dental tissues. Dent Clin North Am. 1959;489.

## VIVA VOCE

**Q1. What is internal basement lamina and external basement lamina?**
Ans. Internal basement lamina is a junctional epithelium- tooth interface. External basement lamina is a junctional epithelium-connective tissue interface.

**Q2. What is the ratio of melanocytes to keratinocytes producing epithelial cells?**
Ans. The ratio of melanocytes-to-keratinocytes producing epithelial cells is 1: 36 cells.

**Q3. What is the oxygen consumption of healthy gingiva?**
Ans. The oxygen consumption of healthy gingiva is $QO_2$ (oxygen) = 1.6 ± 0.37. The respiratory activity of epithelium is approximately three times greater than that of connective tissue, and the respiratory activity of the sulcular epithelium is approximately twice that of the whole gingiva.

**Q4. Where is the mucogingival junction (MGJ) usually absent?**
Ans. The palatal gingiva of the maxilla is continuous with the palate's tissue, which is bound down to the palatal bones. Because the palate is devoid of freely movable alveolar mucosa, there is no mucogingival junction.

**Q5. Where melanin is formed and stored?**
Ans. Melanin is synthesized in an organelle called premelanosomes/melanosomes in melanocytes cells. It is stored in melanophages/melanophores.

**Q6. What are desmosomes and hemidesmosomes?**
Ans. The cell membrane of the epithelial cells facing the lamina lucida harbors several electron-dense, thicker zones appearing at various intervals along the cell membrane. These structures are called as hemidesmosomes. A desmosome is made up of two hemidesmosomes facing one another. Separated by a zone containing electron-dense granulated material.

**Q7. Which keratins are found in the outer epithelium?**
Ans. K1, K2, and K10 in the orthokeratinized area and less in the parakeratinized area. K19 is found in the parakeratinized area and less in orthokeratinized areas.

**Q8. What is the significance of col?**
Ans. Col has nonkeratinized epithelium; thus, it is anatomically predisposed to the growth of oral microorganism and susceptible to inflammation and disease prcogression.

**Q9. In which cells Birbeck's granules found?**
Ans. Langerhans cells.

**Q10. Classify the gingival phenotype or biotype.**
Ans. Eger and Muller classified the gingival phenotype into thick and thin.

# Chapter 2

# Periodontal Ligament

*Shalu Bathla*

## Chapter Outline

- Width and Structure
- Development
- Constituents
- Functions
- Blood Supply
- Nerve Supply
- Maintenance of Periodontal Ligament Space

## INTRODUCTION

The attachment apparatus of the tooth includes the periodontal ligament, cementum, and alveolar bone. The periodontal ligament is the soft, specialized connective tissue situated between the cementum covering the root of the tooth and bone forming the socket wall.[1] The synonyms of periodontal ligament are periodontal membrane, alveolodental ligament, desmodont, pericementum, dental periosteum, and gomphosis.[2]

## WIDTH AND STRUCTURE

Width of periodontal ligament ranges from 0.15 mm to 0.38 mm.[3] Its shape is like an hour-glass apicocoronally, corresponding to the rotation point of the tooth.[4] It is thinnest in the middle, at the axis of rotation, and widens coronally and apically. The thickness of the periodontal ligament seems to be maintained by the functional movements of the tooth. In functionless and embedded teeth, it is thinner and wider in teeth under excessive occlusal stresses.[2]

## DEVELOPMENT

During the process of normal tooth eruption, when the crown commences the oral mucosa, the fibroblasts of the dental follicle become active and start producing collagen fibrils.[5] Initially, these fibers lack orientation but soon acquire an orientation oblique to the tooth. The first collagen bundles appear in the region immediately apical to the cementoenamel junction and give rise to the gingivodental fiber groups. As tooth eruption progresses, additional oblique fibers appear and get attached to the newly formed bone and cementum. The alveolar crest and transseptal fibers develop when the tooth emerges into the oral cavity. Alveolar bone deposition coincides with the periodontal ligament organization (**Figs. 2.1A to D**). During the eruption, cemental Sharpey's fibers appear first, followed by Sharpey's fibers emerging from the bone. Sharpey's fibers of bone are fewer in number and more widely spaced than those emerging from the cementum.[4] At a later stage, alveolar fibers extend into the middle zone to join the lengthening cemental fibers and attain their classic orientation, thickness, and strength when the occlusal function is established.[3]

## CONSTITUENTS

Following are the constituents of the periodontal ligament (**Flowchart 2.1**):

### Cellular Elements

- *Connective tissue cells*:
  - Synthetic cells:
    - Fibroblasts: These are the most predominant connective tissue cells. They are spindle-shaped or stellate cells with an oval-shaped nucleus containing one or more nucleoli.[6] They originate from mesenchymal cells. They have the ability to synthesize and secrete a wide range of extracellular molecules, such as collagen fibers,

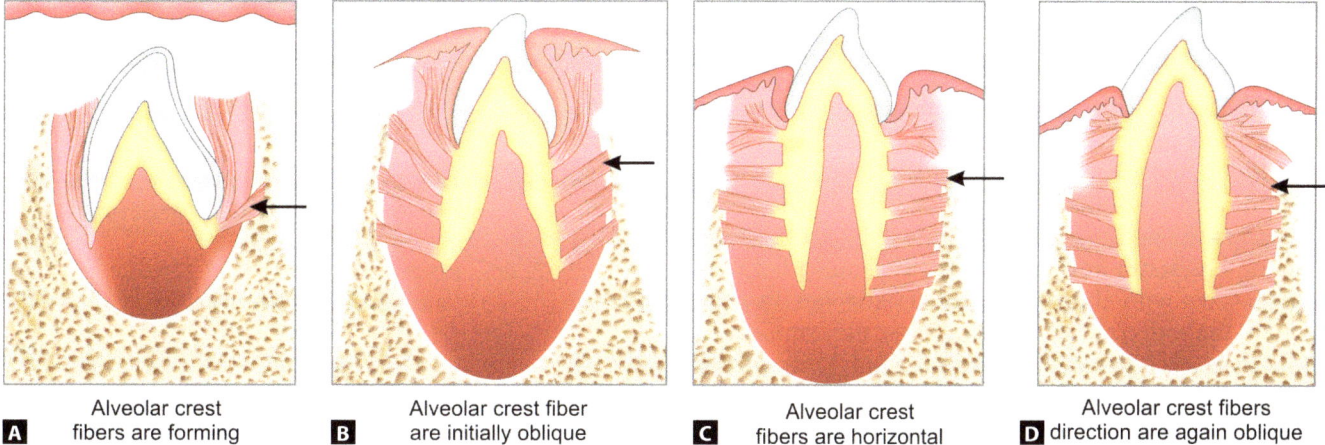

**Figs. 2.1A to D:** Schematic representation showing the development of principal periodontal ligament fibers; (A) Alveolar crest fibers are forming; (B) Alveolar crest fibers are initially oblique in direction; (C) Alveolar crest fibers are horizontal in direction; and (D) Alveolar crest fibers direction are again oblique (but in opposite directions).

**Flowchart 2.1:** Constituents of the periodontal ligament.

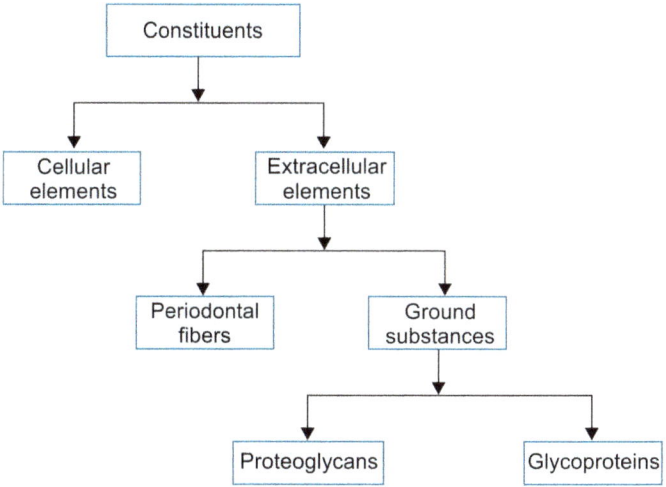

elastic fibers, proteoglycans, glycoproteins, growth factors, and enzymes (collagenase). They also have the capacity to synthesize and degrade collagen.[7]

- Cementoblasts: These cells actively secrete the organic matrix of cementum within the periodontal ligament.
- Osteoblasts: These are the cells that are found on the surface of the alveolar bone. Their ultrastructure and gross appearance are similar to other osteoblasts that are found elsewhere in the body.[8]
- *Resorptive cells*:[9]
  - Osteoclasts: These are bone-resorbing cells, which are formed by the fusion of mononuclear cells arising from bone marrow.
  - Fibroblasts: These cells are also responsible for degrading collagen fibers.
  - Cementoclasts: These are mononuclear cells resembling osteoclast located in Howships lacunae.

- *Epithelial cells*: These are cuboidal in shape and arranged in clusters called rests. They are considered as remnants of Hertwig's root sheath. These cells are located all over the periodontal ligament and close to the cementum. They are more in cervical and apical areas of the periodontal ligament. On stimulation, cells proliferate and contribute to the formation of periapical cysts and lateral root cysts. It has been reported that epithelial cell rests of Malassez (ERM) has a significant role in the maintenance of periodontal ligament space.[10] In physiologic conditions, it is thought that ERM may contribute to maintaining a nonmineralized area as they are devoid of any mineralization propensity. These cells are involved in the pathogenesis of several disorders, including pocket formation. The presence of c-Met receptors in the ERM suggests that these cells can respond to the inflammatory cytokine and hepatocyte growth factor. This scatter factor is thought to be capable of aiding migration of these cells and hence aid in the pathogenesis of pocket. These cells are also thought to be responsible for cementum repair as they are found in areas of resorption when a mechanical injury was created in experimental animals. It has been suggested that cells retain the capacity to differentiate into cementoblasts and lay down the matrix. Thus, ERM is thought to have a potential role in the physiological maintenance of periodontal ligament space.[11] It may also contribute to the pathogenesis of pocket formation and probably may mediate the process involved in regeneration.
- *Immune system cells*: Various defense cells present in periodontal ligament are neutrophils, lymphocytes, macrophages, mast cells, and eosinophils.
- *Cells associated with neurovascular elements*
- *Progenitor cells*

## Extracellular Elements

### Periodontal Ligament Fibers

In human tooth, the periodontal ligament is made up of two types of fibers namely, collagen and oxytalan.[12]

1. *Oxytalan*: These are immature elastic fibers. The orientation of these fibers is different from collagen fibers. Oxytalan fibers run in axial direction instead of collagen fibers, which run from bone to tooth. One end of these fibers is embedded in cementum or bone and the other end in the wall of a blood vessel. Thus, they support the blood vessels of the periodontal ligament. These are numerous and dense in the cervical region of the ligament.
2. *Collagen*: It is a triple helix protein composed of different types of amino acids, such as glycine, proline, hydroxylysine, and hydroxyproline. It always contains hydroxylysine and hydroxyproline.[13] There are at least 19 recognized collagen types encoded by 30 separate genes dispersed among at the minimum 12 chromosomes.[14]

Types I, III, V, VI, XII (FACIT) of collagen are present in the periodontal ligament.

*Collagen synthesis and assembly* **(Flowchart 2.2)**: Fibroblasts, chondroblasts, osteoblasts, odontoblasts, and other cells play a vital role in the synthesis of collagen.[3] The formation and secretion of collagen molecule take approximately 35–60 minutes.

It is secreted in an inactive form called procollagen, which is then converted into tropocollagen.[3] In the extracellular space, tropocollagen is polymerized into collagen fibrils, which are then aggregated into collagen bundles by the formation of cross-linkages **(Fig. 2.2)**. There is a rapid turnover rate of periodontal ligament collagen, with a half-life of only 10–15 days, which is about five times faster than gingival collagen.

## Principal Fibers of Periodontal Ligament

The principal fibers of periodontal ligament are arranged in six groups **(Fig. 2.3)** and are named according to their location and direction of attachment **(Table 2.1)**:[3]

1. *Transseptal group*: These fibers run into the interproximal space over the crest of alveolar bone and get inserted in the cementum of a neighboring tooth. These constitute the bulk of the interdental gingiva. As they are without osseous attachment, they are assumed to be a part of the gingiva. They have the innate capacity to reconstruct themselves in periodontal disease even there is the destruction of the alveolar bone. This unique property of fibers is responsible for returning teeth to their original state after orthodontic therapy.
2. *Alveolar crest group (apico-oblique)*: These fibers run obliquely just below junctional epithelium and extend from the crest of an alveolar process up to the cervical part of cementum. This fiber groups help to avoid extrusion and lateral tooth movements.

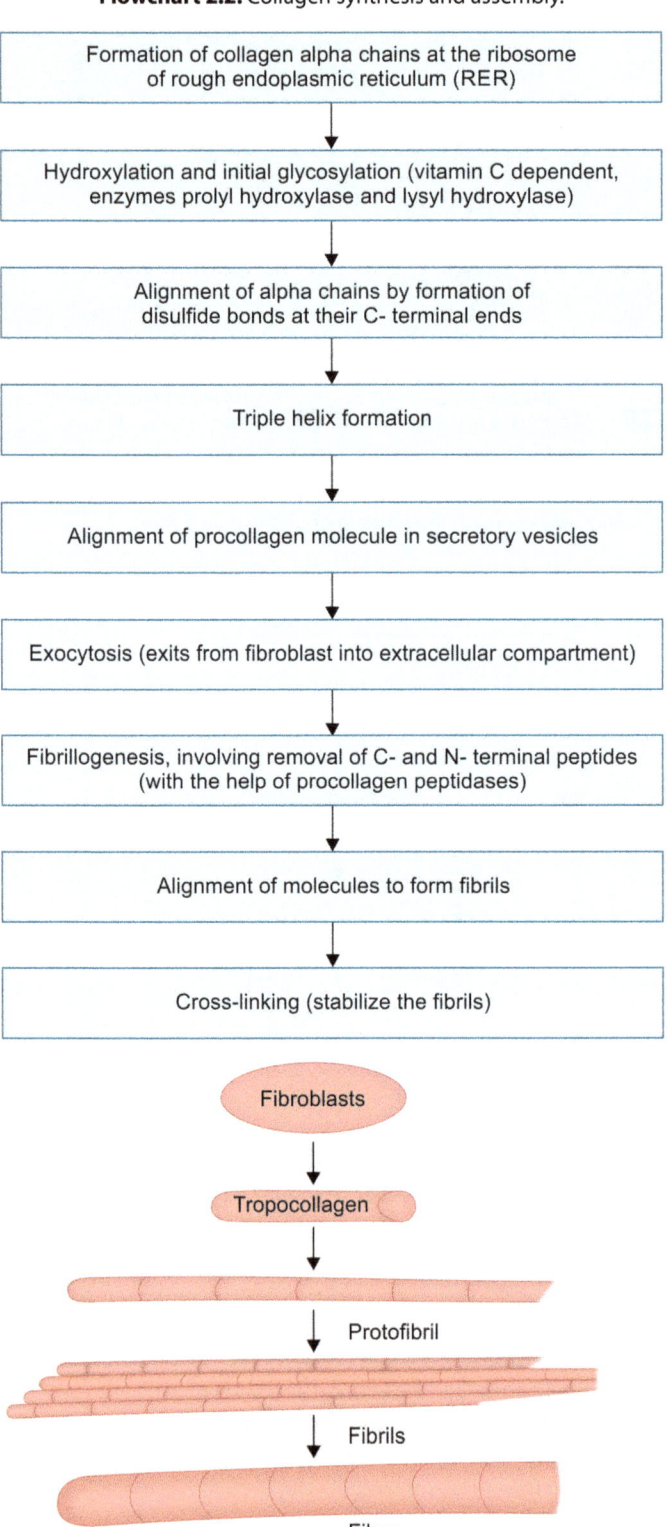

**Flowchart 2.2:** Collagen synthesis and assembly.

**Fig. 2.2:** Schematic representation showing the formation of collagen fiber.

3. *Horizontal group*: This group of fiber radiate at right angles to the long axis of the tooth and runs from cementum to the alveolar bone. This fiber resists horizontal pressure against the crown of the tooth.

## Chapter 2: Periodontal Ligament

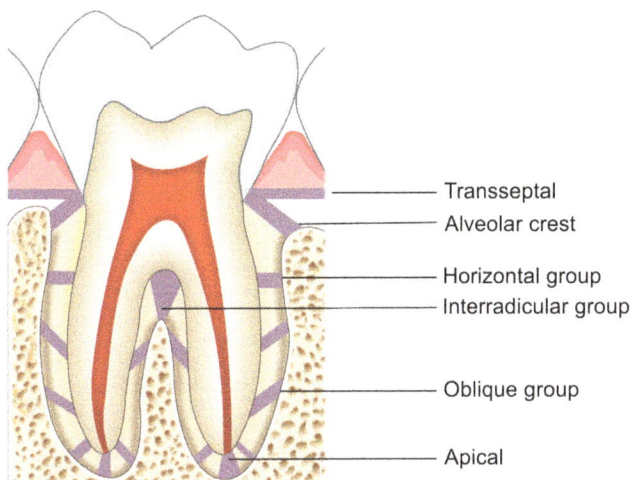

**Fig. 2.3:** Schematic representation showing principal periodontal ligament fiber groups.

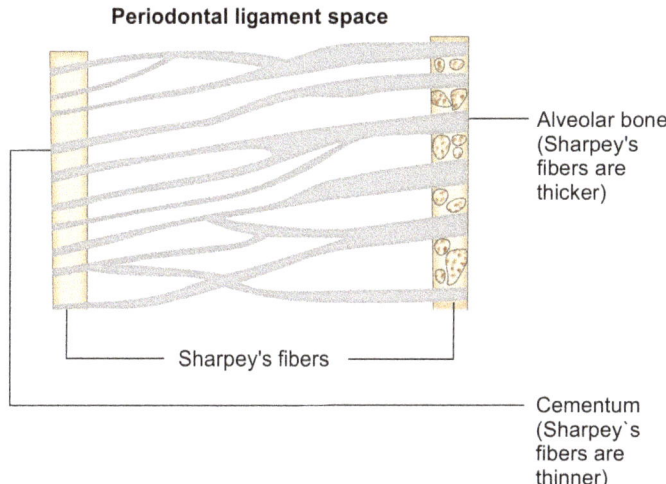

**Fig. 2.4:** Schematic representation showing Sharpey fibers.

**TABLE 2.1:** Principal fibers of the periodontal ligament.

| Principal fibers | Location | Functions |
|---|---|---|
| Alveolar crest | Cervical root to the alveolar crest of alveolar bone proper | Prevent extrusion and lateral tooth movements |
| Horizontal | Mid root to adjacent bone proper | Resists horizontal forces |
| Oblique | Apical one-third of root to adjacent bone proper | Resists vertical masticatory stresses and convert them into tension on alveolar bone |
| Apical | Apex of root to fundic proper | Prevent tooth tipping, resist luxation and protect neurovascular supply to the tooth |
| Interradicular | Between roots to alveolar bone proper | Prevent luxation, torquing and tooth tipping |

4. *Oblique group (coronal-oblique)*: These fibers radiate from the cementum in a coronal direction and placed obliquely to the bone. This fiber group is the largest, making up two-thirds of the fibers. They can withstand the vertical masticatory stress and transform them into tension on the alveolar bone.
5. *Apical group*: They run irregularly and get extended from the cementum to bone at the socket's apical region. They prevent tooth tipping, resist luxation, and protect neurovascular supply to the tooth.
6. *Interradicular group*: These are found only between roots of multirooted teeth running from cementum into bone, forming the crest of interradicular septum. They prevent luxation, tooth tipping, and torquing.

### Sharpey Fibers

In 1846, Scottish anatomist William Sharpey described Sharpey fibers. Sharpey's fibers are the ends of the periodontal fibers that are inserted in cementum and alveolar bone. It is also called as perforating fibers. On the cementum side, these Sharpey's fibers are much thinner in diameter and inserted at closer intervals than the alveolar bone side **(Fig. 2.4)**. These differences in the pattern of insertion have clinical importance in the distribution of forces that are generated within the periodontal ligament during occlusion, traumatic forces, and tooth movement. These forces are more evenly distributed along the cementum surface and are more concentrated along with the more widely spaced insertions on the alveolar bone side.[4] As a result, in response to mechanical forces, there is generally a remodeling of the periodontal housing on the alveolar bone side and not on the cementum side, preventing the possibility of significant cementum and root resorption.

### Ground Substance

Ground substance is an amorphous, nonfibrous, and noncellular matrix-forming major component of the periodontal ligament. It helps in the exchange of water, ions, and nutrients across the connective tissue cells. This function is essential for the maintenance of the normal function of connective tissue. Thus, it imposes a significant effect on the tooth's stability undergoing various degrees of stress.[15]

The main constituents are protein-carbohydrate macromolecules. These complexes are divided into proteoglycans and glycoproteins.

### *Proteoglycans*

They are the large group of extracellular macromolecules composed of a protein core with the attachment of glycosaminoglycan chains. The proteoglycans, namely decorin and biglycan involved in the organization and regulation of collagen fibers and are abundantly present in the periodontal ligament.[16] Decorin especially is presently bound to collagen and is vital to regulate fibrillogenesis.

Decorin is also bound to transforming growth factor-beta (TGF-β) and prevents excessive fibrosis. This property prevents undue cross-linking of the collagen fibers.[17]

### Glycoproteins

They are the macromolecules with carbohydrate core. They have adhesive properties, which bind cells to extracellular elements. These glycoproteins are grouped into two: fibronectin and tenascin. Fibronectin is a large protein that binds cells to collagen and proteoglycans. It promotes the adhesion of fibroblasts to the extracellular matrix and plays a role in the alignment of collagen fibers.[18]

## Cementicles

Cementicles are globular masses of cementum arranged in concentric lamellae that lie free in the periodontal ligament or adhere to the root surface. These cementicles may develop from calcified epithelial rests or calcified thrombosed vessels or calcified Sharpey's fiber within periodontal ligament.[13]

## FUNCTIONS

Periodontal ligament serves the following functions:[13]
- *Supportive functions*:
  - Establishing a strong attachment of teeth to the bone.
  - Maintaining the conventional relationship of gingival tissues to the teeth.
  - Protecting blood vessels and nerves from trauma induced by mechanical forces.
  - Transmitting occlusal forces to the underlying bone: The principal periodontal ligament fibers are arranged in a similar fashion to a suspension bridge or hammock.[19] On loading axial forces, the wavy principle oblique fibers of periodontal ligament spread out in their full length to resist the significant part of the forces and tooth gets depressed in the socket. Hence, the periodontal ligament can readily absorb axial forces induced on it. However, rotational and lateral forces are absorbed less easily. On the tension side, periodontal fibers extend and bone deposits, while on the pressure side, fibers get compressed and bone resorbs.
  - Resisting impact of occlusal forces and thus acts as a shock absorber. There are three different theories to explain the mechanism of tooth support:
    1. *Tensional theory*: This theory assumes that the principal fibers of periodontal ligament play a major role in tooth support and transmission of forces to the bone **(Flowchart 2.3)**.
    2. *Viscoelastic system theory*: According to this theory, the displacement of the tooth is largely controlled by fluid movement, and fibers play a secondary role **(Flowchart 2.4)**.

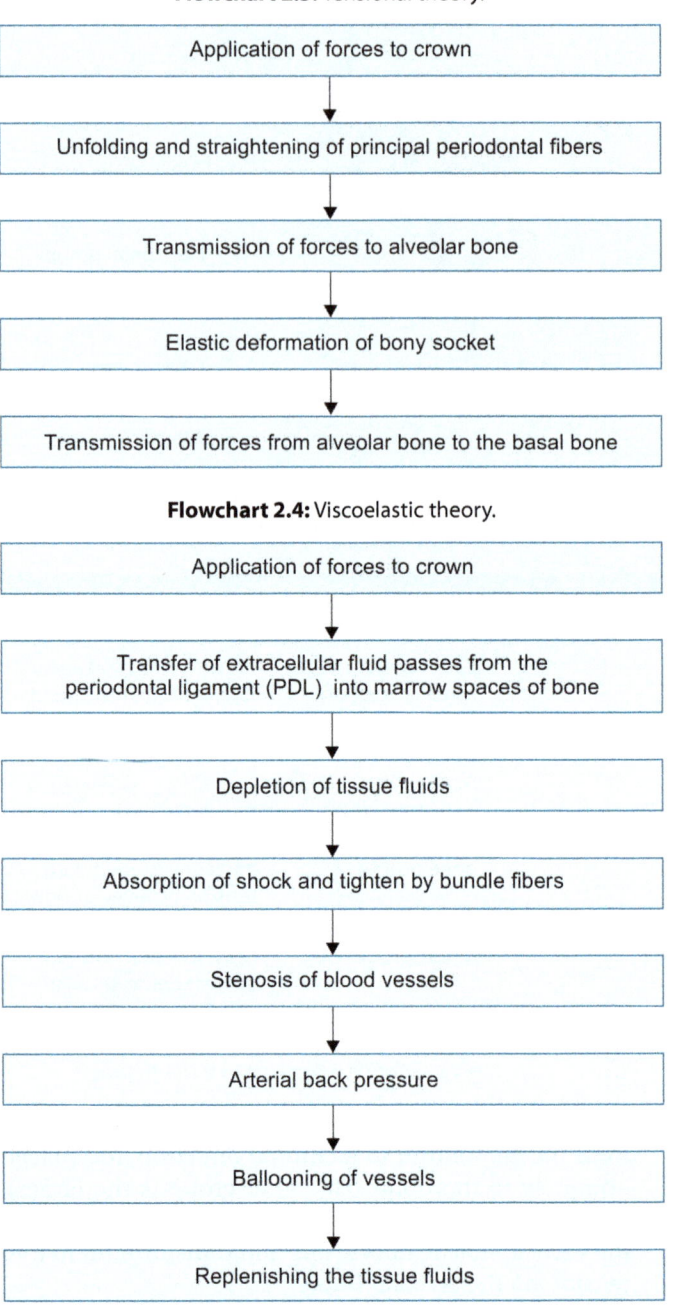

**Flowchart 2.3:** Tensional theory.

Application of forces to crown → Unfolding and straightening of principal periodontal fibers → Transmission of forces to alveolar bone → Elastic deformation of bony socket → Transmission of forces from alveolar bone to the basal bone

**Flowchart 2.4:** Viscoelastic theory.

Application of forces to crown → Transfer of extracellular fluid passes from the periodontal ligament (PDL) into marrow spaces of bone → Depletion of tissue fluids → Absorption of shock and tighten by bundle fibers → Stenosis of blood vessels → Arterial back pressure → Ballooning of vessels → Replenishing the tissue fluids

3. *Thixotropic theory*: According to this theory, the periodontal ligament has the rheological behavior of a thixotropic gel (i.e., the property of becoming fluid when shaken/stirred and then becoming semisolid again).
- *Sensory functions*: Periodontal ligament is capable of transmitting tactile, pressure, and pain sensations by trigeminal pathways.
- *Nutritive functions*: It supplies nutrients to cementum, bone, and gingiva through blood vessels and lymphatics.
- *Formative functions*: The tissues have the regenerative capacity in providing the cell lineage, namely osteoblast, cementoblast, and fibroblast. Thus, it helps in the

formation and resorption of cementum and bone during physiologic tooth movement and repair of injuries.
- *Homeostasis*: With the presence of both formative and resorptive activity, the periodontal ligament provides homeostasis in the tissue environment.

## BLOOD SUPPLY

The blood supply is derived from the inferior and superior alveolar arteries to mandible and maxilla, respectively. Blood supply reaches the periodontal ligament from three sources:
1. Apical vessels
2. Penetrating vessels from the alveolar bone
3. Anastomosing vessels from the gingiva

Blood vessels are present in the interstitial spaces of loose connective tissue between the principal fibers and are connected in the net-like plexus that runs longitudinally. These blood vessels are closer to the bone than to cementum. The blood supply increases from the incisors to the molars; is greatest in the gingival third of single-rooted teeth, less in the apical third, and least in the middle; is equal in the apical and middle thirds of multirooted teeth. Comparing the surfaces, it is slightly greater on the mesial and distal surfaces than on the facial and lingual; and is greater on the mesial surfaces of mandibular molars than on the distal.[13]

The capillaries of other connective tissues are continuous, while in the periodontal ligament, they are fenestrated. Due to fenestration, they have a greater ability of diffusion and filtration, which is related to high metabolic requirements of periodontal ligament and its high rate of turnover.

The venous drainage of the periodontal ligament accompanies the arterial supply. Venules receive the blood through the abundant capillary network; there are also, arteriovenous anastomoses that bypass the capillaries. These are more frequent in apical and interradicular regions.

## NERVE SUPPLY

Sensory nerves that supply the periodontium arise from maxillary and mandibular divisions of the trigeminal nerve. These fibers are capable of transmitting tactile, pressure, and pain sensations by the trigeminal pathways.[20] Nerve bundles pass into the periodontal ligament from the periapical area and through channels from the alveolar bone that follow the blood vessels' course. They divide into single myelinated fibers, which ultimately lose their myelin sheaths and end in one of four types of neural termination:[13]
1. Free endings are the first and most frequent that carries pain sensation. They spread out in a fashion of tree branches and are placed uniformly throughout the length of the root. They are derived from unmyelinated fibers. However, they carry with them a Schwann cell envelope with processes that project into the surrounding connective tissue. Such endings are thought to be nociceptors and mechanoreceptors.
2. Ruffini endings are slowly adapting, low-threshold mechanoreceptors located mainly in the apical areas. They appear dendritic and have ensheathing Schwann cells that are especially close to collagen fibers bundles.
3. Coiled Meissner's corpuscles are mechanoreceptors found mainly in the mid-root region. The function and ultrastructure have not been determined yet.
4. Spindle-like pressure and vibration endings with the lowest frequency are surrounded by a fibrous capsule and located mainly at the root apex.

Within the periodontal ligament, 75% of the mechanoreceptors have their cell bodies in the trigeminal ganglion, and 25% of the mechanoreceptors have their cell bodies in the mesencephalic nucleus.[3]

## MAINTENANCE OF PERIODONTAL LIGAMENT SPACE

Periodontal ligament plays a unique role in maintaining periodontal space though it is constantly exposed to mechanical forces or orthodontic tooth movement.[21] Following factors have been thought to contribute to this maintenance of periodontal ligament space **(Table 2.2)**:[15]

**TABLE 2.2:** Factors maintaining periodontal ligament space.

| Cellular factors | Molecular factors (biochemical) | Genetic factors |
|---|---|---|
| Fibroblasts | Osteocalcin | Runx2 |
| Epithelial cell rests of Malassez | Bone sialoprotein | Msx2 |
| | Osteonectin | PLAP1 |
| | Nitrous oxide (NO) | Twist gene |
| | Osteoprotegrin (OPG) | |
| | Periostin | |
| | Growth factors | |
| | S100 Protein | |

### Points to Ponder

- Intermediate plexus (Sicher 1966): Fibers arising from cementum and bone are joined in the mid-region of periodontal ligament space, giving rise to a zone of distinct appearance in the light microscope. It was believed that the intermediate plexus provides a site where rapid remodeling of fibers occurs, allowing adjustment in the ligament to be made to accommodate small movements of the tooth. However, evidence derived from an electron microscope provided no support for this and was believed to be an artifact.
- Fibroblasts are described as architects, builders, and caretakers of connective tissue and play a dual role incollagen synthesis and degradation.
- The shape of the periodontal ligament is hour-glass.
- The width of the periodontal ligament is 0.15–0.38 mm.
- Supportive, nutritive, regenerative, and sensory are the main functions of the periodontal ligament.

## REFERENCES

1. Grant DA, Stern IB, Listgarten MA. Periodontal ligament. In: Periodontics, 6th edition. St. Louis: CV Mosby; 1988. pp. 56-75.
2. Melcher AH, McCulloch CA. Periodontal ligament. In: Bhaskar SN (Ed). Orban's Oral Histology and Embryology, 11th edition. St. Louis: Mosby; 1992. pp. 203-38.
3. Freeman E. Periodontium. In: Ten Cate AR, Richard A, Nanci A (Eds). Ten Cate's Oral Histology: Development, Structure, and Function, 5th edition. St. Louis: Elsevier-Mosby; 1998. pp. 253-88.
4. Lindhe J, Karring T, Araujo M. Anatomy of the periodontium. In: Lindhe J, Karring T, Lang NP (Eds). Clinical Periodontology and Implant Dentistry, 4th edition. Copenhagen, Denmark: Blackwell Munksgaard; 2003. pp. 3-49.
5. Moxham BJ, Grant DA. Development of the periodontal ligament. In: Berkovitz BK, Moxham BJ, Newman HN (Eds). The Periodontal Ligament in Health and Disease, 2nd edition. St. Louis: Mosby-Wolfe; 1995. pp. 161-81.
6. Giannopoulou C, Cimasoni G. Functional characteristics of gingival and periodontal ligament fibroblasts. J Dent Res. 1996;75(3):895-902.
7. Berkovitz BK, Schore RC. Cells of the periodontal ligament. In: Berkovitz BK, Moxham BJ, Newman HN (Eds). The Periodontal Ligament in Health and Disease, 2nd edition. St. Louis: Mosby-Wolfe; 1995. pp. 9-33.
8. Hassell TM. Tissues and cells of the periodontium. Periodontol 2000. 1993;3:9-38.
9. Hefti AF. Aspects of cell biology of the normal periodontium. Periodontol 2000. 1993;3:64-75.
10. Xiong J, Gronthos S, Bartold PM. Role of the epithelial cell rests of Malassez in the development, maintenance and regeneration of periodontal ligament tissues. Periodontol 2000. 2013;63(1):217-33.
11. Rincon JC, Young WG, Bartold PM. The epithelial cell rests of Malassez—a role in periodontal regeneration? J Periodontol Res. 2006;41(4):245-52.
12. Beertsen W, McCulloch CA, Sodek J. The periodontal ligament: a unique, multifunctional connective tissue. Periodontol 2000. 1997;13:20-40.
13. Bernard GW, Carranza FA. The tooth supporting structures. In: Newman MG, Takei HH, Carranza FA (Eds). Carranza's Clinical Periodontology, 9th edition. Philadelphia, PA, USA: WB Saunders; 2003. pp. 36-57.
14. Rodwell VW, Kennelly PJ. Proteins: higher orders of structure. In: Murray RK, Granner DK, Rodwell VW. Harper's Illustrated Biochemistry, 27th edition. Philadelphia, PA, USA: McGraw-Hill Publishing; 2006. pp. 30-40.
15. Arun KV. Organization of the matrix. In: Molecular Biology of Periodontium, 1st edition. New Delhi, India: Jaypee Brothers Medical Publishers; 2010. pp. 35-69.
16. Bartold PM. Connective tissues of the periodontium. Research and clinical implications. Aust Dent J. 1991;36(4):255-68.
17. Bartold PM, Narayanan AS. Biology of the Periodontal Connective Tissues. Chicago, USA: Quintessence Publishing; 1998.
18. Holmstrup P. The microanatomy of the periodontium. In: Wilson TG, Kornman KS (Eds). Fundamentals of Periodontics. Chicago, USA: Quintessence Publishing; 1996. pp. 27-46.
19. Davies WR, Picton DC. Dimensional changes in the periodontal membrane of monkey's teeth with horizontal thrusts. J Dent Res. 1967;46: 114.
20. Linden RW, Billar BJ, Scott BJ. The innervations of the periodontal ligament. In: Berkovitz BK, Moxham BJ, Newman HN (Eds). The Periodontal Ligament in Health and Disease, 2nd edition. St. Louis: Mosby-Wolfe; 1995. pp. 133-59.
21. Bartold PM, Narayanan AS. The biochemistry and physiology of the periodontium. In: Wilson TG, Kornman KS (Eds). Fundamentals of Periodontics. Chicago, USA: Quintessence Publishing; 1996. pp. 61-108.

## VIVA VOCE

**Q1.** How is periodontal ligament unique among the various ligament and tendon systems of the body?
**Ans.** It is the only ligament to span two distinct hard tissues, namely, tooth cementum and alveolar bone.

**Q2.** What is the width of the periodontal ligament?
**Ans.** The width of the periodontal ligament is 0.15–0.38 mm.

**Q3.** What is the shape of periodontal ligament space?
**Ans.** Hour-glass shape: Periodontal ligament is thinnest at the axis of rotation in the middle and widens coronally and apically.

**Q4.** Which is the largest group of periodontal ligament fibers?
**Ans.** The oblique group is the largest group of periodontal ligament fibers.

**Q5.** Which is the group of periodontal ligament fibers found only between the roots of a multirooted tooth?
**Ans.** Interradicular group of periodontal ligament fibers is found only between roots of multirooted teeth.

**Q6.** Which periodontal fibers are consistent and reconstructed even after the destruction of the alveolar bone?
**Ans.** Transseptal fibers are consistent and reconstructed even after the destruction of the alveolar bone.

**Q7.** What are cementicles?
**Ans.** They are calcified masses found in the periodontal ligament. They are caused by calcification of epithelial rest, Sharpey's fibers, or thrombosed vessels.

**Q8.** Name amino acids present in collagen.
**Ans.** Glycine, proline, hydroxylysine, and hydroxyproline. It always contains hydroxylysine and hydroxyproline.

**Q9.** Which type of collagen is present in periodontal ligament?
**Ans.** Types I, III, V, VI, XII (FACIT).

**Q10.** In which structure type IV collagen is present?
**Ans.** Basement membrane.

# Cementum

*Sushruth Nayak, Shalu Bathla*

## Chapter Outline

- Development
- Functions
- Composition
- Classifications
- Various Junctions of Cementum
- Clinical Considerations

## INTRODUCTION

*Cementum is calcified avascular mesenchymal tissue that forms the outer covering of the anatomic root.*[1] Two pupils of Purkinje in 1835 first demonstrated cementum microscopically.[2] The hardness and calcification of cementum, when it is fully mineralized, is less than that of dentin. Cementum is light yellow, with a dull surface. It cannot remodel and is resistant to resorption.

## DEVELOPMENT

The enamel organ, including the epithelial root sheath as it develops, is surrounded by a layer of connective tissue known as the dental sac. The zone immediately in contact with the dental organ and continuous with the ectomesenchyme of the dental papilla is called the dental follicle, which consists of undifferentiated fibroblasts. The rupture of Hertwig's root sheath allows the mesenchymal cells of the dental follicle to contact the dentin, where they start forming a continuous layer of cementoblasts. Cementum formation begins by deposition of a meshwork of irregularly arranged collagen fibrils sparsely distributed in a ground substance or matrix called precementum or cementoid. This is followed by a phase of matrix maturation, which subsequently mineralizes to form cementum. Cementoblasts, which are initially separated from the cementum by uncalcified cementoid, sometimes become enclosed within the matrix and are trapped. Once they are enclosed, they are referred to as cementocytes and will remain viable in a fashion similar to that of osteocytes.[3]

## FUNCTIONS

- Cementum provides attachment to the collagen fibers of periodontal ligament to the root surface.
- It functions as a covering for the root surface, a seal for the open dentinal tubules thus, preventing dentinal sensitivity.
- It aids in maintaining the teeth in functional occlusion.
- It contributes to the process of repair after damage to the root surface.[2]

## COMPOSITION

- *Inorganic*: 45–50%
    - The inorganic portion consists mainly of calcium and phosphate in the form of hydroxyapatite.[4] Trace elements are also found in cementum. It has the highest fluoride content of all the mineralized tissue.[2]
- *Organic*: 50–55%
    - Collagen type I (90%), III, V, XII [FACIT (Fibril Associated Collagens with Interrupted Triple Helices)], XIV are present in cementum. The sources of collagen fibers are fibroblasts that produce extrinsic Sharpey's fibers and cementoblasts that produce intrinsic fibers of the cementum matrix.[5]
    - Noncollagenous: Fibronectin, bone sialoprotein, osteopontin, osteocalcin, osteonectin, and alkaline phosphatase.[6] Osteocalcin is a mineral regulatory protein related to bone matrix formation and mineralization which is expressed by cementoblasts

lining the roots of developing and fully formed teeth.[7]
- Formative cells: Cementoblast.
- Degradative cells: Cementoclast/odontoclast
- Adhesion molecule: Cementum attachment protein (CAP) is present on the outer surface of the cementum. CAP is known to play a role in chemotaxis and differentiation of cementoblasts before laying down the cementoid matrix. Also, CAP mediates the attachment of the periodontal ligament fibers to the root surface.[8]
- Growth factor: Insulin-like growth factor.

## CLASSIFICATIONS

Cementum can be classified as:
- *According to the location (Fig. 3.1)*:[9]
    - Radicular cementum: It is the cementum that covers the root and forms the bulk of the cementum.
    - Coronal cementum: It is the cementum that is found on the enamel, which is thin and poorly developed.
- *According to cells present (Table 3.1)*:[10]
    - Acellular cementum: It is the first cementum to be formed before the tooth reaches the occlusal plane. It does not contain cells and covers the cervical third or half of the root. **(Fig. 3.2)**
    - Cellular cementum: It forms after the tooth has reached the occlusal plane. It contains cementocytes in individual spaces (lacunae) that communicate with each other through a system of anastomosing canaliculi. **(Fig. 3.3)**
- *According to fibers present*: Schroeder through light and electron microscopy, has enabled cementum to be classified into five different subtypes based on the source of collagen fibers:[11]
    - Acellular afibrillar cementum (AAC): 1–15 µm. It consists of an only mineralized matrix, which is a

**TABLE 3.1:** Differences between acellular and cellular cementum.

| Parameters | Acellular cementum | Cellular cementum |
|---|---|---|
| Formation | Forms before tooth reach the occlusal plane | Forms after tooth reach the occlusal plane |
| Cells | Does not contain any cells | Contains cementocytes |
| Location | Coronal portion of the root | Apical portion of the root |
| Rate of formation | Slower | Faster |
| Incremental lines | More | Sparse |
| Function | Forms after regenerative periodontal surgical procedure | Contributes to the length of root during growth |
| Calcification | More calcified | Less calcified |
| Sharpey's fibers | More | Less |
| Regularity | Regular | Irregular |
| Thickness | 20–50 µm near the cervix, 150–200 µm near the apex | Thickness of 1 mm to several mm |

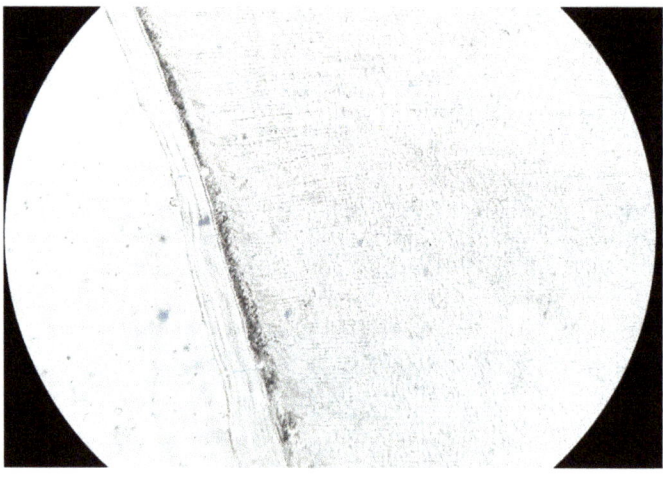

**Fig. 3.2:** Histological picture acellular cementum.
(*Courtesy*: Dr Sushruth Nayak)

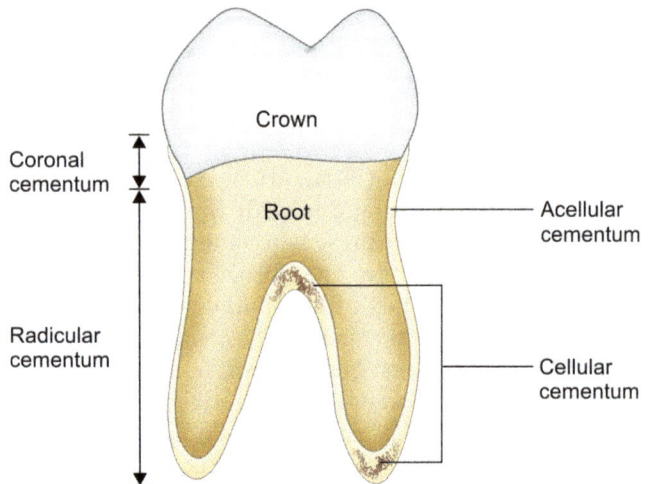

**Fig. 3.1:** Schematic representation showing the distribution of cementum on the tooth surface.

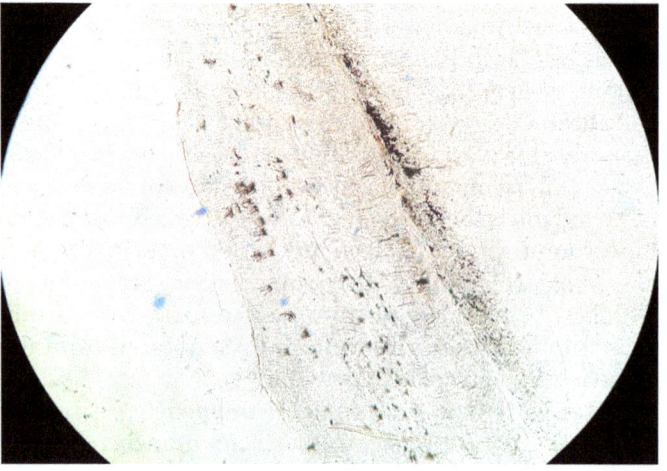

**Fig. 3.3:** Histological picture cellular cementum.
(*Courtesy*: Dr Sushruth Nayak)

product of cementoblasts. Both cells and collagen (extrinsic and intrinsic) fibers are absent. It forms coronal cementum. Loss of the cervical part of the reduced enamel epithelium at the time of tooth eruption may place portions of mature enamel in contact with the connective tissue, which then will deposit over it an acellular afibrillar type of cementum
- Acellular extrinsic fiber cementum (AEFC): 30–230 μm. It consists of only extrinsic, i.e., Sharpey's fibers, which is a product of fibroblasts. This type of cementum lacks cells and is found in the cervical third of the root. It is primarily responsible for the anchorage of the tooth in the alveolus.
- Cellular mixed stratified cementum (CMSC): 100–1,000 μm. It consists of both extrinsic and intrinsic collagen fibers, which are the product of fibroblasts and cementoblasts. It also contains viable cells, i.e., cementoblasts and cementocytes. It is found primarily in the apical third of the roots and furcation region.
- Cellular intrinsic fiber cementum (CIFC) or reparative cementum: It consists of cells and intrinsic fibers, lacking extrinsic collagen fibers, which is a product of cementoblasts. It repairs and fills resorption areas.
- Intermediate cementum or layer of Hopewell Smith: 10–20 μm. It was initially described in 1920 by Hopewell Smith,[12] but Bencze gave the definitive name in 1927.[13] Intermediate cementum is an ill-defined zone near the cementodentinal junction of certain teeth. The clinical significance of this layer is that it contains enamel-like protein, i.e., amelogenin, which is a product of the Hertwig's epithelial root sheath.

## Thickness of Cementum

The thickness of cementum varies from 16 μm to 60 μm (thickness of hair) near the cervix to 150–200 μm (thickest) near the apex. Cementum is thicker in distal surfaces than mesial surfaces due to functional stimulation during mesial drift/migration. It is a continuous process, and the rate varies throughout their life.[1]

## VARIOUS JUNCTIONS OF CEMENTUM

### Cementodentinal Junction

It is the interface between dentin and cementum. The collagen fibers of cementum and dentin intervene at their interface in a very complex manner. The dentin's collagen fibrils are arranged haphazardly, with each fibril running an independent course, whereas, in acellular cementum, the fibril runs in the same direction and more or less perpendicular to cementum surface. But still, it is not possible to determine which fibrils are cemental in origin and which are of dentinal origin.[2]

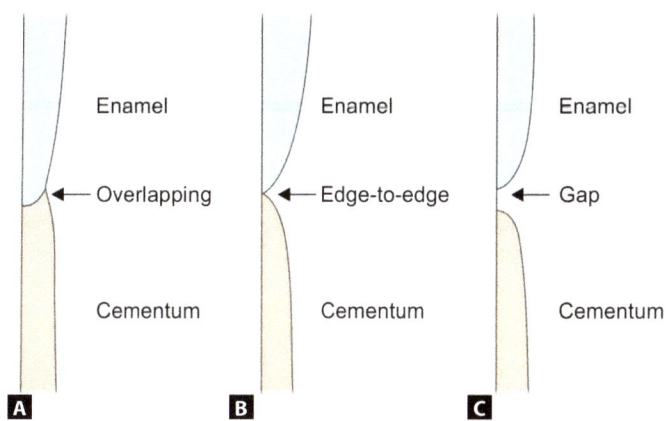

**Figs. 3.4A to C:** Schematic representation showing cementoenamel junctions (CEJ): (A) Cementum overlaps enamel (60–75%); (B) Edge-to-edge (30%); and (C) Enamel and cementum do not meet (5–10%).

### Cementoenamel Junction

The relation between cementum and enamel at the cervical region of teeth is variable **(Figs. 3.4A to C)**.[1] Although, one of these patterns may predominate in an individual tooth, all forms can also be present.
- In about 60–75%, cementum overlaps enamel, and this occurs when the enamel epithelium degenerates at its cervical termination permitting connective tissue to come in direct contact with the enamel surface.
- In about 30%, the edge-to-edge butt joint is there.
- In about 5–10%, space is present between cementum and enamel, and there is no cementoenamel junction (CEJ), the cervical portion of the root is delayed in its separation from dentin.[1]
- Recently another pattern seen in about 1.6% of teeth is the overlapping of the enamel on cementum.[14,15] This was observed under an optical microscope. From an embryological standpoint, odontogenesis does not explain the fourth possible type of CEJ, namely enamel over cementum, since cementogenesis is initiated only after completion of enamel formation. Muller and van Wyk demonstrated that an optical illusion causes it. Therefore, the existence of this pattern (i.e., enamel overlapping cementum) is controversial.

*Methods of Cementoenamel Junction Location*

Various methods for location of CEJ are represented through **Flowchart 3.1**.[16]

*Clinical Importance of Cementoenamel Junction*
- *Helps in determining the clinical attachment level (CAL)*: CEJ is a significant static landmark for measuring CAL, i.e., the level of the attachment of fibers to the tooth root, in the presence of periodontal disease.[16]
- *Assess alveolar bone destruction*: CEJ-bone crest distance is measured to assess alveolar bone destruction.

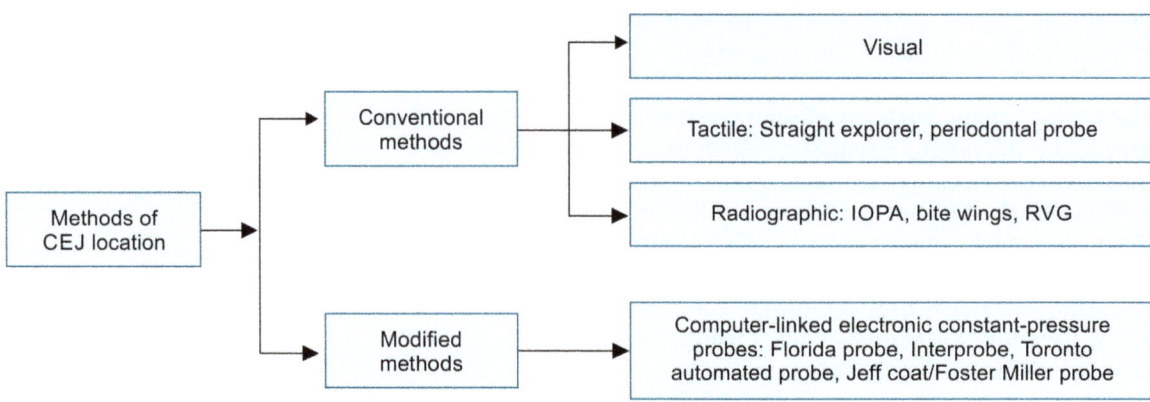

Flowchart 3.1: Methods for the location of cementoenamel junction (CEJ).

(IOPA: intraoral periapical; RVG: radiovisiography)

- *Role of CEJ in gingival recession management*: Identification and location of CEJ help to assess visible and hidden gingival recession. Measurement of the gingival recession is thus helpful in determining the dimensions of graft needed to cover it.
- CEJ is vital for the placement of various membranes during surgical procedures.
- *CEJ, a landmark to diagnose cervical enamel projections (CEPs)*: CEJ serves as an essential reference for the diagnosis of CEPs. Masters and Hoskins classified these unusual anatomical structures based on the degree of extension of enamel beyond the CEJ and depending on their location in relation to furcation topography. These are the extensions of enamel from the CEJ onto the root surface.
- *Role of CEJ in furcation areas*: Enamel spurs projecting from CEJ into the furcation act as etiological factors for furcation defects. The furcal surface closest to the CEJ of the tooth is the most susceptible area to bone denudation as a result of periodontal disease.
- *Determination of furcation*: CEJ distance, helps in treatment planning.[17]
- In the case of wasting diseases, tooth resorption often starts at CEJ.
- *Implications in restorative dentistry*: Special care should be taken with the CEJ area to avoid dentin hypersensitivity and cervical resorption.

## CLINICAL CONSIDERATIONS

- *Repair and resorption of cementum*: Generally, root cementum is protected from relatively extensive remodeling because it is avascular and not exposed to the osteoclast-like precursor cells in the circulation. But cementum on the root surface can undergo resorption and repair alternately according to the change in the environment faced by it. There may be local or systemic causes of cemental resorption.
  - Local causes: Trauma from occlusion, cysts, and tumors, periapical pathology, excessive orthodontic forces, embedded teeth, replanted and transplanted teeth, idiopathic, pressure from malaligned erupting teeth, and teeth without functional antagonists.
  - Systemic causes: Deficiency of calcium, deficiency of vitamin A and D, hypothyroidism and hereditary fibrous osteodystrophy.[1]
- *Cementum anomalies* (Table 3.2):
  - Hypercementosis refers to a prominent thickening of the cementum.[2] It may be localized to one tooth or affect the entire dentition. It occurs as a generalized thickening of the cementum, with nodular enlargement of the apical third of the root. Hypercementosis of the entire dentition may occur in patients with Paget's disease.
  - Cementoblastoma is the only neoplasm of cementum.
  - Cementoma is not a true neoplasm, but it is a fibro-osseous lesion.
  - Cementicles are the calcified round or ovoid bodies sometimes seen in the periodontal ligament. These are present singly or in multiple numbers near the cemental surface. There are two types of cementicles—free cementicles (lie free in the periodontal ligament) and attached cementicles (attached to the root surface).[2]
- *Ankylosis*: Fusion of the cementum and alveolar bone with obliteration of the periodontal ligament is termed as ankylosis. It occurs in teeth with cemental resorption, which suggests that it may represent a form of abnormal repair.

**Clinical Tip**

Cementum is painless to scale because of the absence of nerves, unlike bone, but like bone, it is a living tissue containing cells.

**TABLE 3.2:** Cementum formation altered in diseases.

| Diseases | Cementum anomalies |
| --- | --- |
| Paget's disease | Hypercementosis |
| Hypopituitarism | Decrease |
| Cleidocranial dysplasia | Defective |
| Hypophosphatasia | Total absence |

- *Exposure of cementum to the oral environment*: In cases of gingival recession and loss of attachment, cementum becomes exposed to the oral environment. The cementum is sufficiently permeable to be penetrated in these cases by inorganic ions, organic substances, and bacteria. Bacterial invasion of the cementum occurs commonly in periodontal disease.
- *Root sensitivity*: When there is a gap between cementum and enamel, the patient may experience root sensitivity during instrumentation/exposure to extreme temperature.
- *Enamel matrix protein*: These proteins stimulate the differentiation of surrounding mesenchymal cells into cementoblasts, forming acellular cementum. Once a new cementum layer is formed, collagen fibers form in the adjacent periodontal ligament, attaching into the new cementum.[18]

### Points to Ponder

- Acellular extrinsic fiber cementum type of cementum is desired following a regenerative periodontal surgical procedure.
- Both acellular cementum and cellular cementum are arranged in lamellae separated by incremental lines parallel to the root's long axis. These lines represent rest periods in cementum formation.
- Acellular extrinsic fiber cementum (AEFC) is more desirable than cellular intrinsic fiber cementum due to the presence of cementum attachment protein (CAP).

## REFERENCES

1. Bernard GW, Carranza FA. The tooth supporting structures. In: Newman MG, Takei HH, Carranza FA (Eds). Carranza's Clinical Periodontology, 9th edition. Philadelphia, PA, USA: WB Saunders; 2003. pp. 36-57.
2. Armitage GC. Cementum. In: Bhaskar SN (Ed). Orban's Oral Histology and Embryology, 11th edition. St. Louis: CV Mosby; 1991. pp. 180-202.
3. Freeman E. Periodontium. In: Ten Cate AR, Richard A, Nanci A (Eds). Ten Cate's Oral Histology: Development, Structure, and Function, 5th edition. St. Louis: Elsevier-Mosby; 1998. pp. 253-88.
4. Bartold PM, Narayanan AS. The biochemistry and physiology of the periodontium. In: Wilson TG, Kornman KS (Eds). Fundamentals of Periodontics, 2nd edition. Chicago, USA: Quintessence Publishing; 2003. pp. 61-108.
5. Lindhe J, Karring T, Araujo M. Anatomy of the periodontium. In: Lindhe J, Karring T, Lang NP (Eds). Clinical Periodontology and Implant Dentistry, 4th edition. Oxford, UK: Blackwell Munksgaard; 2003. pp. 3-49.
6. Bartold PM. Connective tissues of the periodontium. Research and clinical implications. Aust Dent J. 1991;36(4):255-68.
7. Bartold PM, Narayanan AS. Biology of the Periodontal Connective Tissues, 1st edition. Chicago, USA: Quintessence Publishing; 1998.
8. Arun KV. Organization of the matrix. In: Molecular Biology of Periodontium, 1st edition. New Delhi, India: Jaypee Brothers Medical Publishers; 2010. pp. 35-69.
9. Grant DA, Stern IB, Listgarten MA. Cementum. In: Periodontics, 6th edition. St. Louis: CV Mosby; 1988. pp. 76-93.
10. Bosshardt DD, Selvig KA. Dental cementum: the dynamic tissue covering of the root. Periodontol 2000. 1997;13:41-75.
11. Schroeder HE. The Periodontium, 1st edition. Berlin, Germany: Springer-Verlag; 1986.
12. Hopewell-Smith A. Concerning human cementum. J Dent Res. 1920;2:59-76.
13. Blackwood HJ. Intermediate cementum. Br Dent J. 1957;102:345-50.
14. Arambawatta K, Peiris R, Nanayakkara D. Morphology of the cemento- enamel junction in premolar teeth. J Oral Sci. 2009;51(4):623-7.
15. Ash MM, Nelson SJ. Development and eruption of the teeth. In: Wheeler's Dental Anatomy, Physiology and Occlusion, 9th edition. St. Louis: Saunders-Elsevier; 2010. pp. 21-44.
16. Vandana KL, Gupta I. The location of cementoenamel junction for CAL measurements: A clinical crisis. J Indian Soc Periodontol. 2009;13(1):12-5.
17. Vandana KL, Haneet RK. Cementoenamel junction: An insight. J Indian Soc Periodontol. 2014;18(5):549-54.
18. Hammerström L. Enamel matrix, cementum development and regeneration. J Clin Periodontol. 1997;24(9 Pt 2):658-68.

### VIVA VOCE

**Q1. Who first demonstrated cementum microscopically?**
**Ans.** Two pupils of Purkinje first demonstrated cementum microscopically in 1835.

**Q2. Which types of collagen are present in cementum?**
**Ans.** Collagen type I (90%), III, V, XII (FACIT), XIV are present in cementum.

**Q3. What are the sources of collagen fibers of cementum?**
**Ans.** The sources of collagen fibers of cementum are:
- Fibroblasts which produce extrinsic Sharpey's fibers.
- Cementoblasts which produce intrinsic fibers of the cementum matrix.

**Q4. Which type of cementum is desired following the regenerative periodontal surgical procedure?**
**Ans.** Acellular extrinsic fiber cementum (AEFC) is desired following the regenerative periodontal surgical procedure.

**Q5. Which is the mineral regulatory protein present in cementum?**
**Ans.** Osteocalcin is the mineral regulatory protein present in cementum.

**Q6. What kind of cementum is present in resorption areas?**
**Ans.** Cellular intrinsic fiber cementum (CIFC).

**Q7. Which disease shows hypercementosis of the entire dentition?**
**Ans.** Paget's disease.

**Q8. What is intermediate cementum?**
**Ans.** It is an ill-defined zone near the cementodentinal junction of individual teeth.

**Q9. Which cementum covers the cervical third of the root?**
**Ans.** Acellular cementum.

**Q10. What are the cervical enamel projections?**
**Ans.** These are the extensions of enamel from the CEJ onto the root surface.

# Chapter 4

# Alveolar Bone

Shalu Bathla

## Chapter Outline

- Development
- Functions
- Structure
- Osseous Topography
- Composition
- Histology
- Coupling
- Bone Modeling and Remodeling
- Vascular Supply

## INTRODUCTION

Alveolar bone is the part of maxilla and mandible that forms and supports the sockets of teeth (alveoli).[1] It is a specialized connective tissue, i.e., mainly composed of the mineralized organic matrix. Together with the root cementum and periodontal ligament, the alveolar bone constitutes the teeth' attachment apparatus. The main function is to distribute and reabsorb forces generated by mastication and other tooth contacts. In addition, the jaw bones consist of the basal bone, which is the portion of the jaw located apically but unrelated to the teeth (Fig. 4.1).

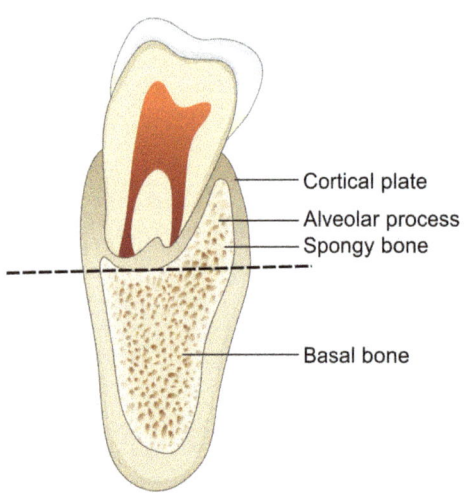

**Fig. 4.1:** Schematic representation showing the dotted line indicates the separation between the alveolar bone and basal bone.

## DEVELOPMENT

The alveolar bone begins to first form by an intramembranous ossification within the ectomesenchyme surrounding the developing tooth. This first bone formed called woven bone is less organized and is replaced with a more organized lamellar bone. When a deciduous tooth is shed, its alveolar bone is resorbed. The succedaneum permanent tooth moves into place, developing its alveolar bone from its dental follicle. As the tooth root forms and the surrounding tissues develop and mature, alveolar bone merges with the separately developing basal bone, and the two become one continuous structure. Although alveolar bone and basal bone have different intermediate origins, both are ultimately derived from neural crest ectomesenchyme. Mandibular basal bone begins mineralization at the exit of the mental nerve from the mental foramen, whereas the maxillary basal bone begins at the exit of the infraorbital nerve from the infraorbital foramen.[2]

## FUNCTIONS

- *Protection*: Alveolar bone forms the tooth socket and provides a good range of protection from various forces imposed on the tooth.
- *Attachment*: It provides good surface area for the insertion of principal fibers of the periodontal ligament.
- *Support*: Alveolar bone acts as good support for the tooth roots both on the facial and palatal (lingual) sides.
- *Shock absorber*: By transmitting the forces to underlying tissues, it acts as a shock absorber and protects the tooth from direct stress or tension.

**Flowchart 4.1:** Structural division of alveolar bone.

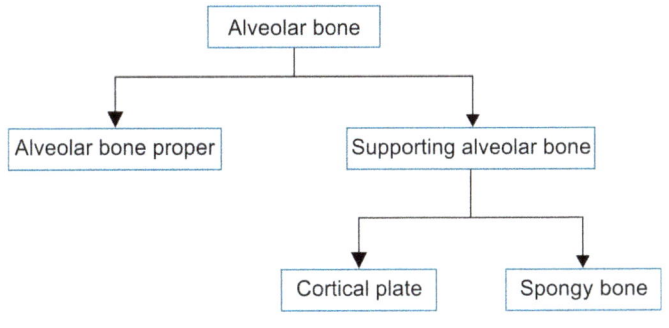

## STRUCTURE

Based on the anatomic feature, the alveolar process is divisible into separate areas **(Flowchart 4.1)**, but it functions as a unit with all parts interrelated in support of the teeth.

## Alveolar Bone Proper

It is the thin layer of compact or dense bone that forms an inner wall of the tooth socket. It is a continuation of the cortical plate that encircles the root of the tooth and provides attachment to principal fibers of the periodontal ligament[3] **(Box 4.1)**.

- *Cribriform plate*: The alveolar bone proper is also termed as a cribriform plate as many foramina perforate it. These minute openings transmit the branches of the interalveolar blood vessels and nerves into the periodontal ligament.[2]
- *Bundle bone*: This is the part of alveolar bone proper that provides attachment to the principal fibers of the periodontal ligament, also called Sharpey's fibers.[4] This bone contains few fibrils in the intercellular substances. This bone is not unique to the jaws. It occurs throughout the skeletal system wherever ligament and muscles are attached.
- *Lamina dura*: Radiographically, this bundle bone appears as a thin radiopaque line surrounding the roots of teeth and is called as lamina dura.[5] Lamina dura appears denser than the adjacent supporting bone. This radiographic density may be due to the mineral orientation around the fiber bundles and the apparent lack of nutrient canals. However, there is no difference in mineral content between lamina dura and the supporting bone. It is evaluated clinically for periodontal or periapical pathology. It disappears after the extraction of the tooth. In several systemic diseases that resulted in structural changes in the jaws, the lamina dura may also change.

**BOX 4.1:** Different terminology for alveolar bone proper.

- Cribriform plate (anatomic term)
- Bundle bone (histologic term)
- Lamina dura (radiographic term)

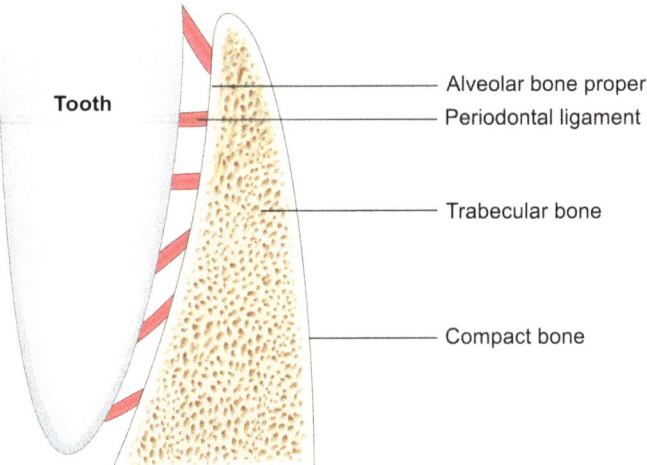

**Fig. 4.2:** Schematic representation showing the tooth-supporting alveolar process.

**BOX 4.2:** Different terminology for supporting alveolar bone.

- Spongy bone (anatomic term)
- Trabecular bone (radiographic term)
- Cancellous bone (histologic term)

## Supporting Alveolar Bone

It is a part of alveolar bone that encircles the alveolar bone proper and provides support to the tooth socket **(Fig. 4.2)**. It is composed of two parts:

- *Cortical plates*: These are the compact bones and constitute the alveolar bone's outer and inner plates.[2]
- *Spongy bone*: Also termed as cancellous bone, this is situated in the area between the alveolar bone proper and cortical plates. Cancellous bone has many irregular open spaces joined by flat bones known as trabeculae. Cancellous bone is more in the maxilla as compared to the mandible. Most of the facial and lingual portions of the sockets are formed by compact bone alone. Cancellous bone surrounds the lamina dura in apical, apicolingual, and inter radicular areas1 **(Box 4.2)**.

## OSSEOUS TOPOGRAPHY

Height and thickness of facial and lingual bony plates are affected by the alignment of the teeth, angulations of the root to the bone, and occlusal forces.[2]

- *Normally*: The bone contour conforms to the prominence of the roots, with intervening vertical depressions that taper towards the margin.
- *On teeth in labial version*: The margin of the labial bone is located farther apically than on teeth in proper alignment. The bone margin is thinned to a knife-edge and presents an accentuated arc in the direction of the apex.
- *On teeth in lingual version*: The facial bony plate is thicker than normal. The margin is blunt and rounded and horizontal rather than arcuate.

## Interdental Septum

The interdental septum consists of cancellous bone bordered by the socket wall cribriform plates (lamina dura or alveolar bone proper) of approximating teeth and the facial and lingual cortical plates.[1] If the interdental space is less than 0.5 mm, i.e., in kissing roots, cancellous bone is lacking **(Fig. 4.3)**. The septum may consist of only the cribriform plate leading to the diminished blood supply. If roots are too close together, and irregular "window" can appear in the bone between adjacent roots **(Fig. 4.4)**. The mesiodistal angulation of the interdental septum's crest is usually parallel to the line drawn between the cementoenamel junctions of the approximating teeth. The mesiodistal and faciolingual dimensions and shape of the interdental septum may vary with the alignment of the tooth and convexity of the crowns of the two approximating teeth **(Fig. 4.5)**. In young adults, the distance between the cementoenamel junction and the crest of the alveolar bone varies between 0.75 mm and 1.49 mm (average 1.08 mm).[6]

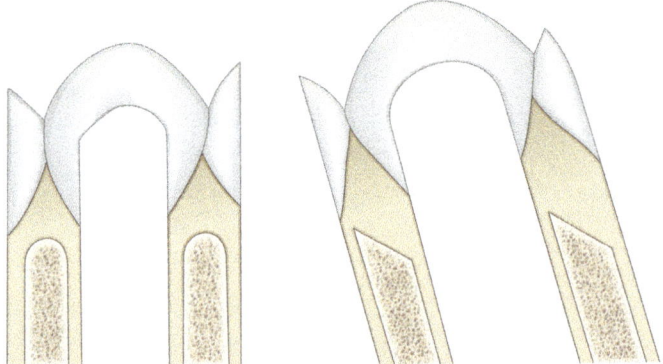

**Fig. 4.5:** Schematic representation showing variations in the shape of interdental alveolar crest according to the position of teeth.

## Fenestration and Dehiscence

The anatomy of the alveolar processes depends upon the alignment and position of the teeth. When the teeth are in extreme buccal or lingual versions, the alveolar processes are extremely thin or missing on that side of the teeth. Fenestrations are the isolated areas in which root ais denuded of bone, and marginal bone is intact. Dehiscences are the denuded areas that extend through the marginal bone **(Figs. 4.6 and 4.7)**. Dehiscence and fenestration are both associated with the extreme buccal or lingual version of teeth. It occurs in 20% of all teeth.[1]

These are more frequent over anterior than posterior teeth. The root in such defects is covered only by periosteum and the overlying gingiva. According to Elliot and Bowers, dehiscences were usually noticed in the mandible, and fenestrations are more common in the maxilla.[7]

### *Methods to Detect*

- *Tactile method*: Run a finger over the prominent root in apicocoronal and mesiodistal directions. The crest of the bone at the apical extent of the defect may be felt, as may the lateral border. As the finger is moved coronally, the bone's bridge may be felt at the coronal part of a fenestration but not in dehiscence.
- *Bone sounding/transgingival probing*: It is done by anesthetizing the tissue locally and inserting the probe horizontally and walking along with the tissue tooth interface so that the operator can feel the bony topography. It may be used to differentiate between two types of defects. The sensation transmitted through the probe on touching the tooth is solid and sharp, one whereas bone gives a softer and mushy feeling. If the sense is like touching tooth, the probe is moved halfway to the free margin and is pressed through the soft tissue. If the bone is touched, the defect is a fenestration, and if not, then it is dehiscence.
- *Radiographs*: Cone-beam computed tomography (CT) images can show bone dehiscences and fenestrations.

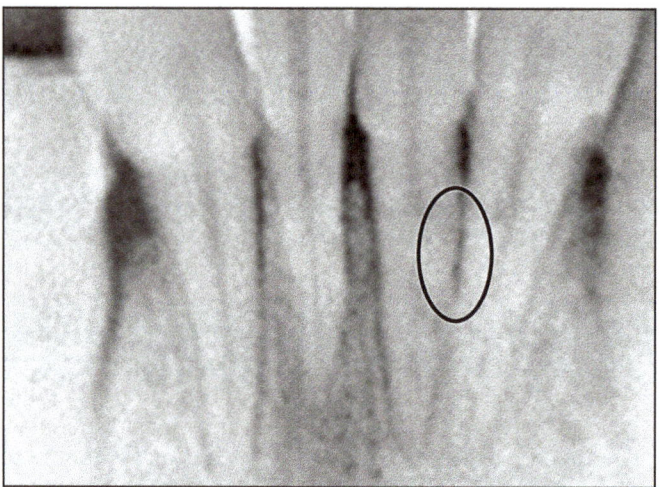

**Fig. 4.3:** Schematic representation showing kissing roots where the cancellous bone is lacking.

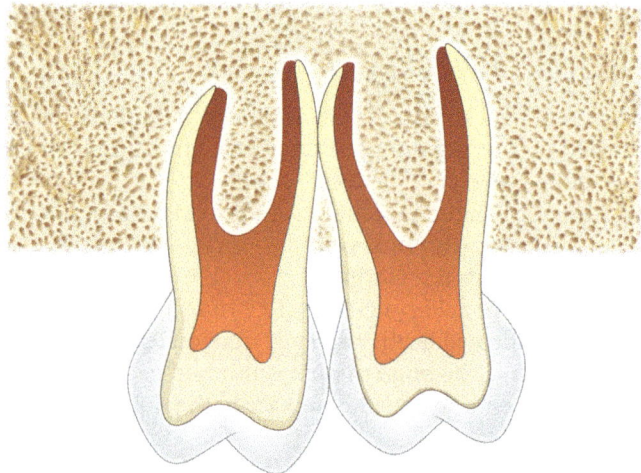

**Fig. 4.4:** Schematic representation showing boneless window between adjoining close roots of molars.

Chapter 4: Alveolar Bone

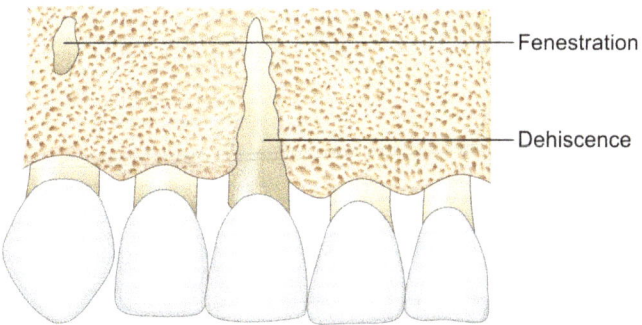

Fig. 4.6: Schematic representation showing dehiscence and fenestration.

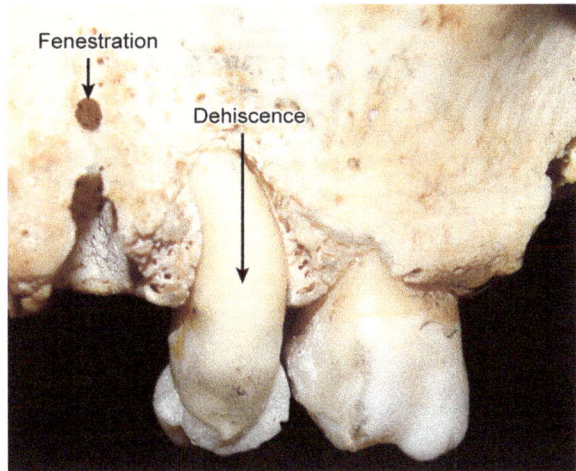

Fig. 4.7: Clinical picture showing dehiscence and fenestration.

## Clinical Importance

- The defects are significant clinically because where they occur, the root is covered only by the periosteum and overlying gingiva, which may atrophy under irritation and expose the root.
- Before any mucogingival surgical procedure, especially lateral pedicle existence of osseous dehiscence or fenestration should be ruled out.
- In the case of gingival grafting procedure, if the receptor site has fenestration defect, soft tissue is capable of reattaching to the exposed surface with higher predictability than dehiscence.
- If the abutment tooth has dehiscence or fenestration, the partial denture will damage the abutment and abutment loss will occur in a short period.

## COMPOSITION

Composition of alveolar bone is as follows (**Flowchart 4.2**):

## Extracellular Components

- *Inorganic (67%)*: The inorganic matter is composed principally of the minerals: calcium and phosphate,

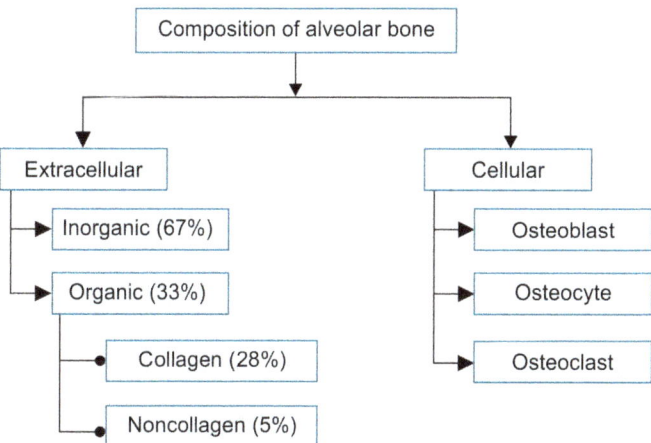

Flowchart 4.2: Composition of alveolar bone.

along with hydroxyl, carbonates, citrate, traces of sodium, magnesium, and fluorine. The mineral salts are mainly in the form of hydroxyapatite crystals.[2]
- *Organic (33%)*:
  - Collagen (28%): Type I (mainly), type III, V, XII, and XIV.
  - Noncollagenous protein (5%): The various noncollagenous proteins are osteonectin, osteopontin, bone sialoprotein, osteocalcin, bone proteoglycan, biglycan, bone proteoglycan II decorin, thrombospondin and bone morphogenetic proteins (BMPs).[8,9]

## Cellular Components

### Osteoblasts

These are mononucleated cells forming a large part of bone surfaces. They are usually cuboidal or slightly elongated in shape.[10] They synthesize both collagenous and noncollagenous bone proteins and are thought to be derived from multipotent mesenchymal cells. These cells exhibit a high level of alkaline phosphatase on the outer surface of their plasma membrane. This enzyme is used as a cytochemical marker to distinguish preosteoblasts from fibroblasts. Functions of osteoblast are bone formation by synthesizing organic matrix of bone, cell-to-cell communication and maintenance of bone matrix and bone resorption by producing proteases, which are involved in matrix degradation and maturation.[5]

Osteoblasts produce type I collagen and various noncollagenous proteins (osteopontin, osteocalcin, and osteonectin) and multiple proteoglycans. These also produce cytokines and growth factors like BMPs (BMP-2 and BMP-7),[11] transforming growth factor-beta (TGF-β), insulin-like growth factor (IGF), and platelet-derived growth factor (PDGF).

### Osteocytes

They are modified osteoblasts, which got entrapped in lacunae during the secretion of the bone matrix. The transformation of osteoblasts into osteocytes is mainly dependent on the speed of bone formation. As the speed of bone formation increases, the number of osteocytes per unit volume also increases. The osteocyte extends processes called canaliculi that radiate from the lacunae. These canaliculi bring oxygen and nutrients to the osteocytes through blood and remove metabolic waste products.[12] They are smaller cells than osteoblasts, having a decreased quantity of secretory and synthetic organelles in it.

*Bone lining cells* originate from inactive osteoblasts that line almost a significant part of the bone surface.[13] The cells are flattened, elongated, spindle-shaped with the presence of a round/oval nucleus. Bone-forming cells, their connecting cell processes, and osteocytes form an extensive homeostatic network of cells. This network plays an essential role in the regulation of plasma calcium concentration.[14]

## Osteoclasts

These are multinucleated giant cells of 50–100 µm size. These are irregular oval- or club-shaped, having branching processes. They are derived from hematopoietic tissue and formed by the fusion of circulating blood cell monocytes.[15] They are found in bay-like depressions in the bone called Howship's lacunae. The part of the cell in contact with bone shows the convoluted surface, the ruffled border, which is the site of great activity due to ion transport and protein secretion. The ruffled border is surrounded by a clear zone that has no organelles other than microfilaments **(Fig. 4.8)**. The peripheral region of the apical membrane is tightly juxtaposed to the matrix called a sealing zone. Both clear and sealing zones help in the attachment of osteoclast to the bone matrix. The basolateral membrane is the major site for the receipt and integration of regulatory signals. The enzymes released by osteoclast are acid phosphatase, arylsulfatase, β-glucuronidase, several cysteine proteinases, such as cathepsin B and L, tissue plasminogen activator (TPA), matrix metalloprotease (MMP-1) and lysozymes.

*Osteoprogenitor cells*: They are long, thin stem cell populations to generate osteoblast.

## HISTOLOGY

Bone whether compact or trabecular are deposited in layers or *lamellae*, each lamella being about 5 µm thick. Lamellae are made up of osteocytes found within empty spaces called lacunae. Three distinct types of lamellae are **(Fig. 4.9)**:[11]
1. *Circumferential lamellae* which surround the entire bone-forming its outer perimeter.
2. *Concentric lamellae* make up for the bulk of the bone and osteon.
3. *Interstitial lamellae* are found between the adjacent concentric lamellae.

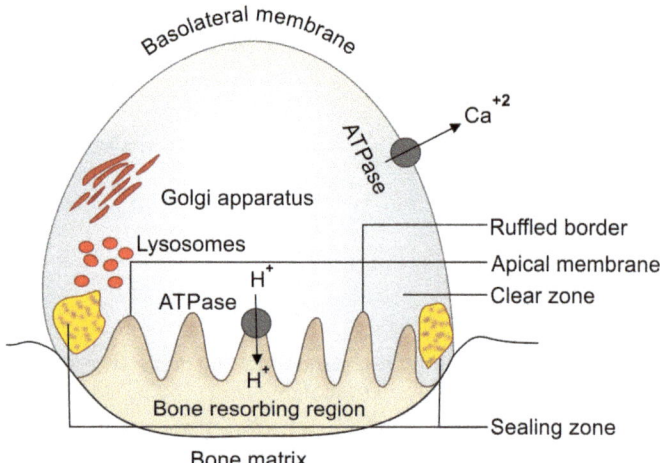

**Fig. 4.8:** Schematic representation showing activated osteoclast.

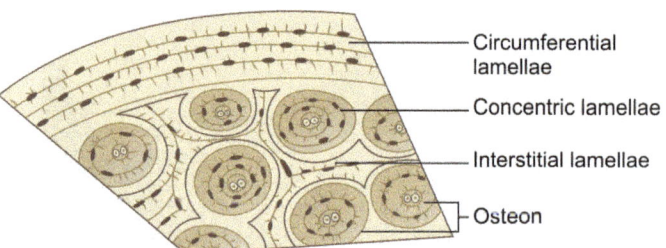

**Fig. 4.9:** Schematic representation showing different types of lamellae.

Osteocytes are usually detected in lacunae of bone and are joined with each other through canaliculi. It takes part in the formation of Haversian canals by encircling around the neurovascular bundles. This whole unit is called osteon, which is the remarkable feature of compact bone. It is cylindrical in structure and runs along the parallel axis of the bone. Volkmann's canals are small channels placed perpendicular to the Haversian canals. Volkmann's canals connect adjacent osteons and carry nerves and blood vessels **(Fig. 4.10)**.[12]

"Haversian canals can be considered as elevators of a tall building and the Volkmann's canals as hallways on specific floors."

*Periosteum*: The outer aspect of cortical bone is surrounded by a connective tissue membrane called the periosteum. It consists of an inner layer of osteoblasts surrounded by osteoprogenitor cells, which have the potential to differentiate into osteoblasts.[1] The outer layer of the periosteum consists of vascular and neural components. It also contains collagen fibers, which penetrate the bone and bind the periosteum to the bone. Periostin is a recently identified protein that is termed so because it was initially identified in the periosteum. It is a secreted cell adhesion protein that is 90 kDa in size. Structurally, it is a disulfide-linked protein that favors osteoblast attachment and spreading. Osteoblast adherence is mediated through the presence

Chapter 4: Alveolar Bone

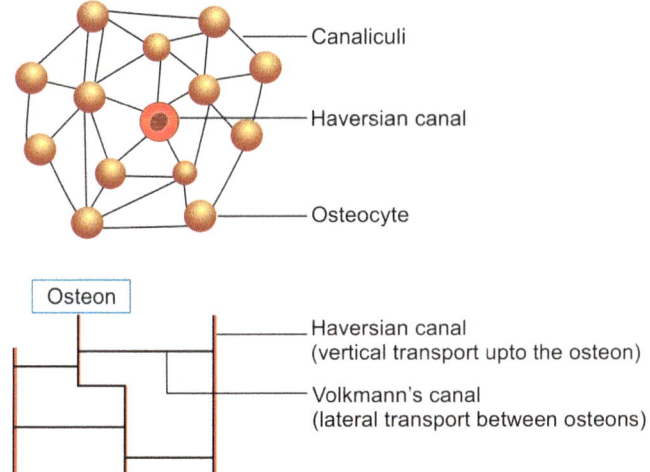

Fig. 4.10: Schematic representation showing osteocytes and osteon.

of αvβ3 and αvβ5 integrins that are upregulated in the presence of periostin.[16]

*Endosteum*: The tissue lining the internal bone cavities is called endosteum. It is composed of a single layer of osteoblasts and a small amount of connective tissue. The inner layer is the osteogenic layer, and the outer is the fibrous layer.[1]

## COUPLING

It is the interdependency of osteoblasts and osteoclasts in the remodeling of the bone **(Fig. 4.11)**.

### Osteoblast-Osteoclast Coupling

The development of osteoclasts is controlled by the stromal cells through the receptor activator of nuclear factor-kappa (RANK)/RANK ligand (RANKL)/osteoprotegerin (OPG) axis. RANK is activated through its ligand RANKL which is produced from the osteoblasts/stromal cells. Upon RANK/RANKL binding, activation of osteoclasts occurs, which subsequently leads to bone resorption. On the other hand, OPG is also produced by various mesenchymal cells and acts as a soluble decoy receptor of RANKL. OPG binds to RANKL and prevents downstream activation. As downstream signaling does not occur, there is no activation of transcription factors and therefore, no osteoclastogenesis.[17]

## BONE MODELING AND REMODELING

The process by which the overall size and shape of the bone are established is called bone modeling. It extends from embryonic bone development to the pre-adult period of human growth, which is continuous and covers a large surface. It is an adaptation in the initial bone architecture of mineralized bone without any change in tissue morphology.

Bone remodeling or a bone turnover occurs in order to allow the replacement of old bone by new bone. It does not stop when adulthood is reached, although its rate slows down, which is cyclic and usually covers a small area. It involves two processes: bone resorption and bone apposition. Thus, modeling and remodeling occur throughout life to allow the bone to adapt to the external and internal demands.[5]

As the osteoclasts move through the bone, the leading edge of resorption is termed as the cutting cone and is characterized in cross-section by a scalloped array of Howship's lacunae, each housing osteoclasts. When a portion of an earlier osteon is left unresorbed, it becomes an interstitial lamella. Behind the cutting, the cone is the migration of mononucleated cells onto the roughened cylinder. As these cells differentiate into osteoblasts, they

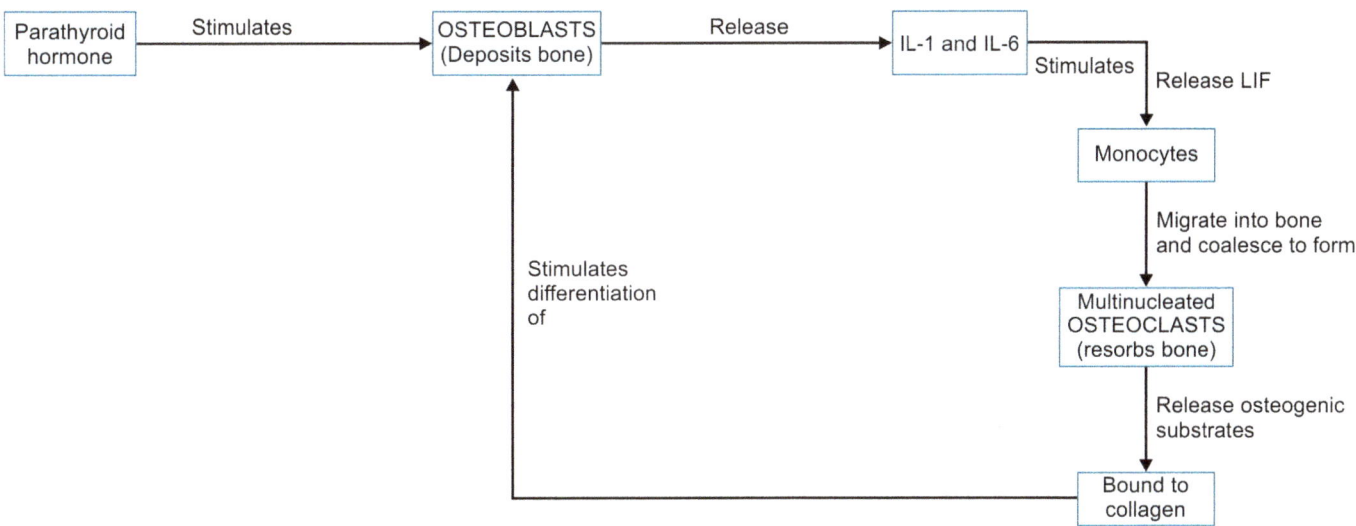

Fig. 4.11: Schematic representation showing the coupling mechanism.
(IL: interleukin; LIF: leukemia-inhibiting factor)

produce a coating termed as the cement or reversal line. It is a thin layer of glycoproteins comprising bone sialoprotein and osteopontin that acts as a cohesive, mineralized layer between the old bone and the new bone to be secreted.

Osteoblasts begin to lay down the new bone matrix on top of the cement line, mineralizing it from the outer to the inner side. The entire area of the osteon where active formation occurs is termed as the filling cone. As formation proceeds, some osteoblasts become osteocytes. Once the formation is complete, the Haversian canal contains a central blood vessel and a layer of inactive osteoblasts, the lining cells that communicate by means of cell processes with the embedded osteocytes.

The repeated deposition and removal of bone tissue accommodate the growth of a bone without losing function or its relationship to neighboring structures during the remodeling phase.[18]

The various bone-resorbing factors are:
- *Systemic factors*: Parathyroid hormone, vitamin $D_3$ and thyroid hormone.
- *Local factors*: Prostanoids, lipoxygenase metabolites, interleukin-1 (IL-1), IL-6, tumor necrosis factors alpha, and beta (TNF-α and β).
- *Growth factors*: Transforming growth factor-alpha (TGF-α), TGF-β, epidermal growth factor (EGF), Platelet-derived growth factor (PDGF).
- *Bacterial factors*: Lipopolysaccharides, lipoteichoic acids, peptidoglycans.[1]

Ten Cate described the sequence of events in the resorptive process as below:[5]
- Osteoclasts get attached to the mineralized surface of the bone.
- The proton pump's action creates a sealed acidic environment that helps in the demineralization of bone and exposure of the organic matrix.
- The organic matrix of bone breaks down into its constituent amino acids under the influence of released enzymes, such as cathepsin and acid phosphatase.
- Mineral ions and amino acids get sequestered within the osteoclast. Rest is explained in "Chapter 24: Bone Defects".

## VASCULAR SUPPLY

The vascular supply to the bone enters the interdental septa through nutrient canals together with veins, nerves, and lymphatics. Dental arterioles, which branch off the alveolar arteries, send tributaries through the periodontal ligament. Some small branches enter the bone marrow spaces through the perforations in the cribriform plate. Small vessels emanating from the facial and lingual compact bone also enter the marrow and spongy bone.[1]

### Points to Ponder
- Fenestration is a window-like circumscribed defect, whereas dehiscence is a cleft-like split defect.
- Osteoblasts are bone builders, whereas osteoclasts are bone consumers.
- Matrix Gla protein is a negative regulator of mineralization.

## REFERENCES

1. Bernard GW, Carranza FA. The tooth supporting structures. In: Newman MG, Takei HH, Carranza FA (Eds). Carranza's Clinical Periodontology, 9th edition. Philadelphia, PA, USA: WB Saunders; 2003. pp. 36-57.
2. Bhaskar SN. Maxilla and mandible (alveolar process). In: Orban's Oral Histology and Embryology, 11th edition. St. Louis: Mosby; 1991. pp. 239-59.
3. Grant DA, Stern IB, Listgarten MA. Alveolar process. In: Periodontics, 6th edition. St. Louis: CV Mosby; 1988. pp. 94-118.
4. Weinmann JP, Sicher H. Bone and bones. In: Fundamentals of Bone Biology, 2nd edition. St. Louis: Mosby; 1955.
5. Freeman E. Periodontium. In: Ten Cate AR, Richard A, Nanci A (Eds). Ten Cate's Oral Histology: Development, Structure, and Function, 5th edition. St. Louis: Elsevier-Mosby; 1998. pp. 253-88.
6. Gargiulo AW, Wentz FM, Orban B. Dimensions and relations of the dentogingival junction in humans. J Periodontol. 1961;32:261-7.
7. Elliot JR, Bowers GM. Alveolar dehiscence and fenestration. Periodontics. 1963;1:245-8.
8. Bartold PM, Narayanan AS. The biochemistry and physiology of the periodontium. In: Wilson TG, Kornman KS (Eds). Fundamentals of Periodontics. Chicago, USA: Quintessence Publishing; 1996. pp. 61-108.
9. Sodek J, Mckee MD. Molecular and cellular biology of alveolar bone. Periodontol 2000. 2000;24:99-126.
10. Hefti AF. Aspects of cell biology of the normal periodontium. Periodontol 2000. 1993;3:64-75.
11. Wozney JM. The bone morphogenic protein family and osteogenesis. Mol Reprod Dev. 1992;32:160-7.
12. Lindhe J, Karring T, Araujo M. Anatomy of the periodontium. In: Lindhe J, Karring T, Lang NP (Eds). Clinical Periodontology and Implant Dentistry, 4th edition. Oxford, UK: Blackwell Munksgaard; 2003. pp. 3-49.
13. Deldar A, Lewis H, Weiss L. Bone lining cells and hematopoiesis: an electron microscopic study of canine bone marrow. Anat Rec. 1985;213(2):187-201.
14. Matthews JL, Wiel CV, Talmage RV. Bone lining cells and the bone fluid compartment, an ultrastructural study. Adv Exp Med Biol. 1978;103:451-8.
15. Ko JS, Bernard GW. Osteoclast formation in vitro from bone marrow mononuclear cells in osteoclast-free bone. Am J Anat. 1981;161(4):415-25.
16. Romanos GE, Asnani KP, Hingorani D, Deshmukh VL. PERIOSTIN: role in formation and maintenance of dental tissues. J Cell Physiol. 2014;229(1):1-5.
17. Arun KV. Cells of the periodontium. In: Molecular Biology of Periodontium, 1st edition. New Delhi, India: Jaypee Brothers Medical Publishers; 2010. pp. 1-34.
18. Saffar JL, Lasfargues JJ, Cherruau M. Alveolar bone and the alveolar process: the socket that is never stable. Periodontol 2000. 1997;13:76-90.

## VIVA VOCE

**Q1. Which is the least stable periodontal tissue?**
**Ans.** Alveolar bone is the least stable periodontal tissue.

**Q2. What is the distance between the crest of the alveolar bone and the cementoenamel junction in young adults?**
**Ans.** It varies between 0.75 mm and 1.49 mm (average 1.08 mm).

**Q3. Which cell produces RANKL?**
**Ans.** RANKL is produced from the osteoblasts/stromal cells.

**Q4. What is coupling?**
**Ans.** It is the interdependency of osteoblasts and osteoclasts in the remodeling of the bone.

**Q5. Why is bone lining the socket called bundle bone?**
**Ans.** Bone lining the socket is called bundle bone as it provides attachment for periodontal ligament fiber bundles.

**Q6. What is endosteum?**
**Ans.** The tissue lining the internal bone cavities is called endosteum.

**Q7. What is periosteum?**
**Ans.** The outer aspect of cortical bone surrounded by a connective tissue membrane called the periosteum.

**Q8. What are fenestrations?**
**Ans.** Fenestrations are the isolated areas in which root is denuded of bone, and marginal bone is intact.

**Q9. What are dehiscences?**
**Ans.** These are the denuded areas that extend through the marginal bone.

**Q10. Which types of collagen are present in alveolar bone?**
**Ans.** Type I (mainly), type III, V, XII, and XIV.

# Chapter 5: Aging and Periodontium

*Shalu Bathla*

## Chapter Outline

- Age Changes
- Effect of Aging on Tooth

## INTRODUCTION

Aging is slowing of a natural function, a disintegration of the balanced control and organization that characterizes the young adult. General features of aging found in all tissues are tissue desiccation, reduced elasticity, altered cell permeability, and diminished reparative capacity. The vasculature, gingiva, periodontal ligament, cementum, and alveolar bone all demonstrate the age changes.

## AGE CHANGES

### Gingiva

Stippling usually disappears with age. The width of the attached gingiva increases with age **(Fig. 5.1)**.

- *Gingival epithelium*: Aging results in:[1]
  - Thinning and decreased keratinization
  - Flattening of rete pegs
  - Migration of junctional epithelium (JE) to more apical position
  - Reduced oxygen consumption
  - Decreased resistance to functional trauma
  - Increased epithelial permeability to various microbial antigens.
- *Gingival connective tissue*: Aging results in:[2]
  - Speeding up the conversion of soluble to insoluble collagen
  - Hastening the mechanical strength of collagen
  - Elevating the denaturing temperature of collagen
- Decreasing the rate of synthesis of collagen
- Greater collagen content.

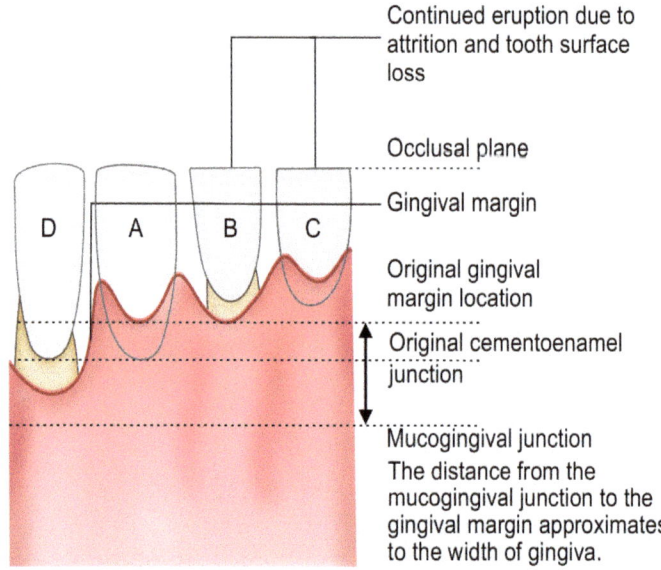

**Fig. 5.1:** Schematic representation showing the relationship between gingival margin and crown and root surface.
A. In normal human tooth, the gingival margin is located at 1–2 mm above the cementoenamel junction (CEJ)
B. In a clinical recession case with the beginning of the attrition of the incisal edge and continuous tooth eruption, the gingival margin stays at the same level as in position A. Hence the tooth surface gets exposed. However, there is no change in the width of the attached gingiva.
C. As the process of wearing off the incisal edge and tooth eruption continues, the gingival margin has shifted with the tooth, and the entire dentogingival complex has transferred coronally, increasing the width of the attached gingiva.
D. With no attrition of incisal edge, gingiva has shifted apically with a reduction in the attached gingiva's width, and clinical recession is evident.

## Periodontal Ligament

Aging results in:[1]
- Decreased number of fibroblasts
- More irregular structures
- Decreased organic matrix production
- Decreased epithelial cell rests of Malassez (ERM)
- Elevated bulk of elastic fibers.

## Cementum

Aging results in:[3]
- Increase in cemental width (5–10 times)
- Decrease in permeability.

## Alveolar Bone

Aging results in:[1]
- Bone undergoes osteoporosis with aging
- Reduction in bone metabolism
- *Decreased*:
    - Vascularity
    - Healing capacity
    - The ability of alveolar bone to withstand occlusal forces, after the age of 30 years.

## EFFECT OF AGING ON TOOTH

The most obvious change in the teeth with aging is a loss of tooth substance caused by the attrition.[4] Occlusal wear cause reduction in cusp height and inclination. Wear of teeth also occurs on the proximal surfaces, accompanied by mesial migration of the teeth. Attrition and proximal wear results in a reduced maxillary, mandibular overjet in the molar area and an edge-to-edge bite anteriorly **(Figs. 5.2 and 5.3)**.[5]

## Bacterial Plaque

Dentogingival plaque accumulation has been suggested to increase with age. Supragingival plaque does not show any qualitative differences in plaque composition between young and older individuals.[6] The subgingival plaque shows some qualitative differences in plaque composition. There is an increase in the number of enteric rods and pseudomonads in older adults.[7]

It has been speculated that an ecological shift occurs in certain periodontal pathogens with age, specifically including an increased role of *Porphyromonas gingivalis* and a decreased role of *Aggregatibacter actinomycetemcomitans*.[8]

## Progression of Periodontal Diseases

Several studies have been conducted to understand the influence of aging and the progression of periodontal diseases. According to one proposed theory, a tooth from advanced periodontal disease areas may get lost at an early age. This indicates that old age is not a true risk factor for periodontal disease. Furthermore, advanced age does not decrease plaque control. Thus, age has been assumed to be an associated factor, but not as a significant risk factor for periodontitis.[9] During periodontitis, the biological changes in periodontal tissue cells are affected by age. Still, they are not the result of the aging process.[10]

Maintenance of good oral hygiene is always a major issue in older people. Various illnesses, medication use, altered mental status, and decreased body mobility and dexterity worsens the problem of poor dental hygiene at old age. A habit of tooth brushing and oral cleaning gets hampered in the elderly due to physical and sensory limitations, such as visual disturbances, disabilities, and loss of memory. Moreover, frail people suffering from hemiplegia and arthritis with hand deformities always find it difficult to perform regular brushing.[11]

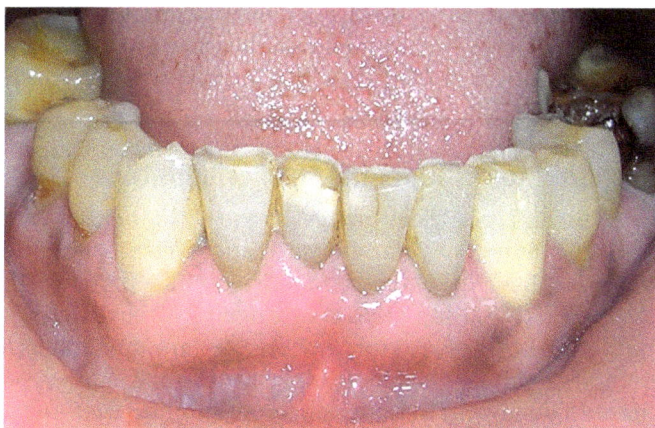

**Fig. 5.2:** Clinical picture showing attrition associated with aging.

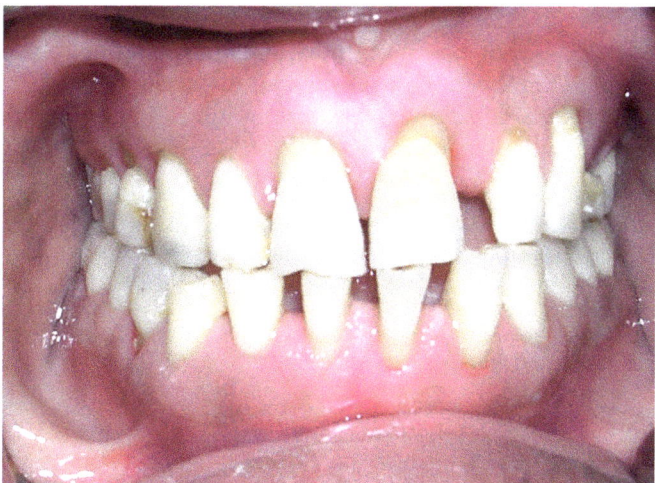

**Fig. 5.3:** Clinical picture showing periodontal changes associated with aging.

## Response to Treatment of the Periodontium

Despite the histological changes in the periodontium with aging, no differences in response to nonsurgical or surgical treatment have been shown for periodontitis patients.[13,14] Periodontal healing and recurrence of disease are not influenced by age. Factors to consider are medical and mental health status, medications, functional status, and lifestyle behaviors that influence periodontal treatment. For older adults, a nonsurgical approach is often the first treatment of choice. Depending on the nature and extent of periodontal disease, surgical therapy may be indicated. The surgical technique should minimize the amount of additional root exposure. Individuals responding best to surgical therapy are those who can maintain the surgical result. Thus, age alone is not a contraindication to surgery and implant placement.[11]

In such a scenario, the use of newer equipment, such as lightweight, electric-powered toothbrushes proves to be a better option for oral hygiene in older adults with physical impairments.[12]

### Points to Ponder

Common age changes in all periodontal tissues:
- Narrowing of the vessel lumen
- Thickening of vessel walls
- Loss of cellularity
- Increasing fibrosis

## REFERENCES

1. Van der Velden U. Effect of age on the periodontium. J Clin Periodontol. 1984;11(5):281-94.
2. Mackenzie IC, Holm-Pedersen P, Karring T. Age changes in the oral mucous membranes and periodontium. In: Holm-Pedersen P, Walls AW, Ship JA (Eds). Textbook of Geriatric Dentistry, 2nd edition. Copenhagen: Munksgaard; 1996.
3. Berglundh T, Lindhe J, Sterrett JD. Clinical and structural characteristics of periodontal tissues in young and old dogs. J Clin Periodontol. 1991;18(8):616-23.
4. Grant DA, Stern IB, Listgarten MA. Periodontal structure in aging humans. In: Periodontics, 6th edition. St. Louis: CV Mosby; 1988. pp. 119-34.
5. Eley BM, Manson JD. The periodontal tissues. In: Outline of Periodontics, 5th edition. Edinburgh: Wright; 2004. pp. 1-20.
6. Holm-Pedersen P, Agerbaek N, Theilade E. Experimental gingivitis in young and elderly individuals. J Clin Periodontol. 1975;2(1):14-24.
7. Newman MG, Grinenco V, Weiner M, Angel I, Karge H, Nisengard R. Predominant microbiota associated with periodontal health in the aged. J Periodontol. 1978;49(11):553-9.
8. Mombelli A. Aging and the periodontal and peri-implant microbiota. Periodontol 2000. 1998;16:44-52.
9. Page RC, Beck JD. Risk assessment for periodontal diseases. Int Dent J. 1997;47(2):61-87.
10. Needleman I. Aging and the periodontium. In: Newman MG, Takei HH, Carranza FA (Eds). Carranza's Clinical Periodontology, 9th edition. Philadelphia, PA, USA: WB Saunders; 2003. pp. 58-63.
11. Fedele DJ, Niessen LC. Periodontal treatment for older adults. In: Newman MG, Takei HH, Carranza FA (Eds). Carranza's Clinical Periodontology, 9th edition. Philadelphia, PA, USA: WB Saunders; 2003. pp. 551-7.
12. Johnson BD, Mulligan K, Kiyak HA, Marder M. Aging or disease? Periodontal changes and treatment considerations in the older dental patient. Gerontology. 1989;8:109-18.
13. Axelsson P, Lindhe J, Nyström B. On the prevention of caries and periodontal disease. Results of a 15-year longitudinal study in adults. J Clin Periodontol. 1991;18(3):182-9.
14. Lindhe J, Socransky S, Nyman S, Westfelt E, Haffajee A. Effect of age on healing following periodontal therapy. J Clin Periodontol. 1985;12(9):774-87.

### VIVA VOCE

**Q1.** What happens to the stippling with age?
**Ans.** Stippling usually disappears with age.

**Q2.** What is the effect of aging on the width of the attached gingiva?
**Ans.** The width of the attached gingiva increases with age.

**Q3.** What are the effects of aging on periodontal ligament?
**Ans.** The number of fibroblasts and epithelial cell rests of Malassez decreases with age.

**Q4.** What are the effects of aging on cementum?
**Ans.** Cemental width increases, whereas permeability decreases with age.

**Q5.** What is the most obvious change in the teeth with aging?
**Ans.** Loss of tooth substance caused by the attrition.

**Q6.** What are the effects of aging on junctional epithelium?
**Ans.** Junctional epithelium migrates to a more apical position.

**Q7.** What are the effects of aging on the alveolar bone?
**Ans.** Bone undergoes osteoporosis with aging.

**Q8.** Does supragingival plaque show any qualitative differences in plaque composition between young and older individuals?
**Ans.** No.

**Q9.** What happens to rete pegs with age?
**Ans.** Flattening of rete pegs occurs with age.

**Q10.** What are the effects of aging on periopathogens?
**Ans.** The ecological shift occurs in certain periodontal pathogens with age, an increased role of *Porphyromonas gingivalis* and a decreased role of *Aggregatibacter actinomycetemcomitans*.

# Section 2

# Classification and Epidemiology

- ❖ Classification of Periodontal Diseases
- ❖ Epidemiology

# Chapter 6: Classification of Periodontal Diseases

*Shalu Bathla*

## Chapter Outline
- Rationale
- AAP 1986 Classification
- AAP 1989 Classification
- Ranney 1993 Classification
- AAP 1999 Classification
- 2017 Classification

## INTRODUCTION

The classification should be a systematic arrangement of groups that possess common attributes. This arrangement should provide insight into the relationship between groups and members of the same group. Classification of disease is necessary to separate conditions into distinct categories to aid clinical and laboratory diagnosis and specific treatments. A system of classifying or grouping the pathologic processes affecting the periodontium serves to identify the etiology and to facilitate communication among clinicians, students, and epidemiologists. Over the years, several classification systems have been developed to organize and name various disease entities or conditions affecting the periodontium.

## RATIONALE

The purposes of classification systems include:[1]
- Communicating clinical findings accurately to other dental healthcare providers and dental insurance providers.
- Presenting information to the patient about his/her disease
- Formulating individualized treatment plan
- Predicting treatment outcomes

## AAP 1986 CLASSIFICATION

The American Academy of Periodontology (AAP) has classified periodontal diseases into four groups:[2]
1. *Juvenile periodontitis*:
    - Prepubertal
    - Localized juvenile periodontitis
    - Generalized juvenile periodontitis
2. Adult periodontitis
3. Necrotizing ulcerative gingivo-periodontitis
4. Refractory periodontitis

## AAP 1989 CLASSIFICATION

In 1989, the Third World Workshop of the AAP was held in Princeton (California, USA), and there periodontal diseases and conditions were classified.[3] This classification was a refinement of one that had been proposed by Page and Schroeder in 1982.

AAP World Workshop in clinical periodontics classified periodontal diseases into five categories:
1. Adult periodontitis
2. *Early-onset periodontitis*:
    - Prepubertal:
        - Localized
        - Generalized
    - Juvenile:
        - Localized
        - Generalized
    - Rapidly progressive
3. *Periodontitis associated with systemic diseases*:
    - Down syndrome
    - Papillon–Lefèvre syndrome
    - Diabetes type I
    - Acquired immunodeficiency syndrome (AIDS)
    - Other diseases
4. Necrotizing ulcerative periodontitis (NUP)
5. Refractory periodontitis

## Main Features

This classification was based on the infection/host response paradigm depended heavily on the age of the affected patients (prepubertal and juvenile periodontitis), rate of progression (adult and early periodontitis), host factors (periodontitis associated with systemic disease) and response to the conventional therapy (refractory periodontitis).

## Drawbacks

Drawbacks associated with 1989 AAP classifications are as follows:[4]
- No separate category of gingivitis/gingival disease.
- Periodontitis categories had non-validated age-dependent criteria.
- There was an extensive crossover in rates of progression of the different categories of periodontitis. Rapidly progressive periodontitis was a heterogeneous category.
- There was extensive overlap in the clinical characteristics of the different categories of periodontitis.
- Refractory periodontitis and prepubertal periodontitis were heterogeneous categories.
- Finally, different forms of periodontitis proposed in the classification shared many microbiologic and host response features, which suggested extensive overlap and heterogeneity among the categories.

# RANNEY 1993 CLASSIFICATION

This classification system included not only forms of gingivitis and periodontitis caused by plaque, but also modifying factors, such as aggravating factors and general disease status. Compared to the AAP 1989 classification, this system eliminated two categories, i.e., refractory periodontitis and periodontitis associated with systemic disease.[5]

- *Gingivitis*:
  - Gingivitis, plaque bacterial:
    - Nonaggravated
    - Systemically aggravated by sex hormones, drugs, and systemic diseases
  - Necrotizing ulcerative gingivitis (NUG):
    - Systemic determinants unknown
    - Related to human immunodeficiency virus (HIV)
  - Gingivitis, non-plaque:
    - Associated with skin diseases, infectious, allergic
- *Periodontitis*:
  - Adult periodontitis
    - Nonaggravated
    - Systemically aggravated (neutropenias, leukemias, lazy leukocyte syndrome, AIDS, diabetes mellitus, Crohn's disease, Addison's disease)
  - Early-onset periodontitis:
    - Localized early-onset periodontitis: Neutrophil abnormality
    - Generalized early-onset periodontitis: Neutrophil abnormality; immunodeficient
    - Early-onset periodontitis related to systemic diseases—leukocyte adhesion deficiency, hypophosphatasia, Papillon-Lefèvre syndrome, neutropenias, leukemias, Chediak-Higashi syndrome, AIDS, diabetes mellitus type I, trisomy 21, histiocytosis X, Ehlers-Danlos syndrome (type VIII).
    - Early-onset periodontitis, systemic determinants unknown
  - NUP:
    - Systemic determinants unknown
    - Related to nutrition
    - Related to HIV
    - Periodontal abscess

# AAP 1999 CLASSIFICATION

In November 1999, the First International Workshop for Classification of Periodontal Diseases and Conditions was held in Oak Brook (Illinois, USA). The following classification of periodontal diseases was proposed.[6]

1. *Gingival diseases*:
   - Dental plaque-induced gingival diseases
   - Non-plaque-induced gingival diseases
2. *Chronic periodontitis*:
   - Localized chronic periodontitis
   - Generalized chronic periodontitis
3. *Aggressive periodontitis*:
   - Localized aggressive periodontitis (LAP)
   - Generalized aggressive periodontitis (GAP)
4. Periodontitis as a manifestation of systemic diseases
5. *Necrotizing periodontal diseases*:
   - Necrotizing ulcerative gingivitis (NUG)
   - Necrotizing ulcerative periodontitis (NUP)
6. *Abscesses of the periodontium*:
   - Gingival abscess
   - Periodontal abscess
   - Pericoronal abscess
7. *Periodontitis associated with endodontic lesions*:
   - Periodontal-endodontic lesion
   - Endodontic-periodontal lesion
   - Combined lesion
8. *Developmental/acquired conditions and deformities*:
   - Occlusal trauma
   - Localized tooth-related factors that predispose to plaque-induced gingival diseases/periodontitis
   - Mucogingival conditions and deformities around teeth
   - Mucogingival conditions and deformities on edentulous ridges.

Chapter 6: Classification of Periodontal Diseases

## Gingival Diseases

*Dental plaque-induced gingival diseases*: These diseases may occur on a periodontium with no attachment loss or on one with attachment loss that is stable and not progressing.
- *Gingivitis associated with dental plaque only*:
  - Without local contributing factors
  - With local contributing factors
- *Gingival diseases modified by systemic factors*:
  - Associated with the endocrine system:
    - Puberty-associated gingivitis
    - Menstrual cycle-associated gingivitis
    - Pregnancy-associated:
      - Gingivitis
      - Pyogenic granuloma
    - Diabetes mellitus-associated gingivitis
  - Associated with blood dyscrasias:
    - Leukemia-associated gingivitis
    - Others
- *Gingival diseases modified by medications*:
  - Drug-influenced gingival diseases:
    - Drug-influenced gingival enlargements
    - Drug-influenced gingivitis:
      - Oral contraceptive-associated gingivitis
      - Others
- *Gingival diseases modified by malnutrition*:
  - Ascorbic acid deficiency gingivitis
  - Others

*Non-plaque-induced gingival diseases*:
- *Gingival diseases of specific bacterial origin*:
  - *Treponema pallidum*
  - *Neisseria gonorrhea*
  - Streptococcal species
  - Others
- *Gingival diseases of viral origin*:
  - Herpes virus infections:
    - Primary herpetic gingivostomatitis
    - Recurrent oral herpes
    - Varicella-zoster
  - Others
- *Gingival diseases of fungal origin*:
  - Candida-species infections: Generalized gingival candidiasis
  - Linear gingival erythema
  - Histoplasmosis
  - Others
- *Gingival diseases of genetic origin*:
  - Hereditary gingival fibromatosis
  - Others
- *Gingival manifestations of systemic conditions*:
  - Mucocutaneous lesions:
    - Lichen planus
    - Pemphigoid
    - Pemphigus vulgaris
    - Erythema multiforme
    - Lupus erythematosus
    - Drug-induced
    - Others
  - Allergic reactions:
    - Dental restorative materials:
      - Mercury
      - Nickel
      - Acrylic
      - Others
    - Reactions attributable to:
      - Toothpaste or dentifrices
      - Mouthrinses or mouthwashes
      - Chewing gum additives
      - Food and additives
      - Others
- *Traumatic lesions (factitious, iatrogenic/accidental)*:
  - Chemical injury
  - Physical injury
  - Thermal injury
- Foreign body reactions
- Not otherwise specified

## Chronic Periodontitis

[Slight: 1–2 mm CAL (clinical attachment loss); moderate: 3–4 mm CAL; severe: >5 mm CAL]
- Localized
- Generalized (>30% of sites are involved)[7]

## Aggressive Periodontitis

(Slight: 1–2 mm CAL; moderate: 3–4 mm CAL; severe: >5 mm CAL)
- Localized
- Generalized[8]

## Periodontitis as a Manifestation of Systemic Diseases

- *Hematologic disorders*:
  - Leukemias
  - Acquired neutropenia
  - Others
- *Genetic disorders*:
  - Down syndrome
  - Familial and cyclic neutropenia
  - Leukocyte adhesion deficiency syndromes
  - Chediak-Higashi syndrome
  - Papillon-Lefèvre syndrome
  - Glycogen storage disease
  - Histiocytosis syndromes
  - Ehlers-Danlos syndrome
  - Cohen syndrome
  - Hypophosphatasia
  - Infantile genetic agranulocytosis
  - Others
- Not otherwise specified

## Developmental/Acquired Deformities and Conditions

- *Localized tooth-related factors that modify or predispose to plaque-induced gingival diseases or periodontitis*:
  - Tooth anatomic factors
  - Dental restorations or appliances
  - Root fractures
  - Cervical root resorption and cemental tears
- *Mucogingival deformities and conditions around teeth*:
  - Gingival or soft-tissue recession:
    - Facial or lingual surfaces
    - Interproximal (papillary)
  - Lack of keratinized gingiva
  - Decreased vestibular depth
  - Aberrant frenum or muscle position
  - Gingival excess:
    - Pseudopocket
    - Inconsistent gingival margin
    - Excessive gingival display
    - Gingival enlargement
    - Abnormal color
- *Mucogingival deformities and conditions on edentulous edges*:
  - Vertical and/or horizontal ridge deficiency
  - Lack of gingiva or keratinized tissue
  - Gingival or soft-tissue enlargements
  - Aberrant frenum or muscle position
  - Decreased vestibular depth
  - Abnormal color
- *Occlusal trauma*:
  - Primary occlusal trauma
  - Secondary occlusal trauma

## Main Features

Main features of AAP 1999 classification system are as follows:[4,9]

- *Addition of gingival disease component*: Comprehensive section of gingival diseases is included in this classification.
- *Replacement of adult periodontitis with chronic periodontitis*: There is a replacement of the term "adult periodontitis" with chronic periodontitis since epidemiological evidence suggests that chronic periodontitis may also be seen in adolescents.
- *Discontinuation of term "refractory periodontitis"*: There is the elimination of separate categories of rapidly progressive periodontitis and refractory periodontitis because of the lack of evidence that they represent different conditions.
- *Replacement of early-onset periodontitis with aggressive periodontitis*: The term juvenile periodontitis was replaced by aggressive periodontitis. This replacement is because of the clinical difficulties in determining the age of onset in many of these cases. The term "aggressive" was added as tissue and bone destruction occurs rapidly as compared with other periodontitis.
- Replacement of NUP with necrotizing periodontal diseases.
- A new classification group of periodontitis as a manifestation of the systemic disease has been added, and this includes those cases of prepubertal periodontitis directly resulting from known systemic diseases.
- Addition of new group categories of abscesses of the periodontium and periodontic–endodontic lesions.
- Addition of a new category of developmental/acquired conditions/deformities.

## Drawbacks: Critical Analysis

Following are the disadvantages associated with the 1999 AAP classification:[1,2]

- Extensive: Although this classification is one of the most scientifically sound and widely accepted classification of periodontal diseases and conditions, but from the clinical aspect, it appears complex and too comprehensive having too many subclassifications that it is difficult to remember the details of the classification.
- As given by Lang for aggressive periodontitis, primary criteria need detailed systemic investigations, familial history, and rate of progression, which are difficult to access in clinical practices.
- Diabetes mellitus has not been given place for the systemic condition modifying the periodontal disease.
- There is no description of the environmental factors (smoking) affecting the periodontitis, despite many proven studies available.
- As chronic and aggressive periodontitis are polymicrobial and polygenic, multiple forms of periodontitis need to be subclassified into discrete microorganism/host genetic polymorphism groups, such as:
  - Group A: Set number 1 of microorganism + Set number 1 of genetic polymorphism.
  - Group B: Set number 2 of microorganism + Set number 2 of genetic polymorphism.
- The classification has not discussed implant-related problems/conditions.

## 2017 CLASSIFICATION

The 2017 World Workshop, a combined collaboration by the European Federation of Periodontology (EFP) and the American Academy of Periodontology (AAP), held in Chicago on November 9 to 11, 2017, has culminated in a new classification system for periodontal and peri-implant diseases and conditions.[10]

## Chapter 6: Classification of Periodontal Diseases

A. **Periodontal Health, Gingival Diseases, and Conditions**
A1. *Periodontal health and gingival health*
  1. Clinical gingival health on an intact periodontium
  2. Clinical gingival health on a reduced periodontium
     2a. Stable periodontitis patient
     2b. Non-periodontitis patient
A2. *Gingivitis*: Dental biofilm induced
  1. Associated with dental biofilm alone
  2. Mediated by systemic or local risk factors
     2.1. Systemic risk factors
        a. Smoking
        b. Hyperglycemia
        c. Nutritional factors
        d. Pharmacological factors
        e. Sex steroid hormones
           ○ Puberty
           ○ Menstrual cycle
           ○ Pregnancy
           ○ Oral contraceptives
        f. Hematological conditions
     2.2. Local risk factors predisposing factors
        a. Dental plaque biofilm retention factors (e.g., Prominent restoration margins)
        b. Oral dryness
  3. Drug-influenced gingival enlargement
A3. *Gingival diseases*: Non-dental biofilm-induced
  1. Genetic/developmental disorders
     1.1. Hereditary gingival fibromatosis (HGF)
  2. Specific infections
     2.1. Bacterial origin
        ♦ Necrotizing periodontal diseases (*Treponema* spp., *Selenomonas* spp., *Fusobacterium* spp., *Prevotella intermedia*, and others)
        ♦ *Neisseria gonorrhoeae* (gonorrhea)
        ♦ *Treponema pallidum* (syphilis)
        ♦ *Mycobacterium tuberculosis* (tuberculosis)
        ♦ Streptococcal gingivitis (strains of streptococcus)
     2.2. Viral origin
        ♦ Coxsackie virus (hand-foot-and-mouth disease)
        ♦ Herpes simplex 1/2 (primary or recurrent)
        ♦ Varicella-zoster virus (chickenpox or shingles affecting V nerve)
        ♦ Molluscum contagiosum virus
        ♦ Human papilloma virus (squamous cell papilloma, condyloma acuminatum, verruca vulgaris, and focal epithelial hyperplasia)
     2.3. Fungal
        ♦ Candidasis
        ♦ Other mycoses (e.g., histoplasmosis, aspergillosis)
  3. Inflammatory and immune conditions and lesions
     3.1. Hypersensitivity reactions
        ♦ Contact allergy
        ♦ Plasma cell gingivitis
        ♦ Erythema multiforme
     3.2. Autoimmune diseases of skin and mucous membranes
        ♦ Pemphigus vulgaris
        ♦ Pemphigoid
        ♦ Lichen planus
        ♦ Lupus erythematosus
     3.3. Granulomatous inflammatory conditions (orofacial granulomatosis)
        ♦ Crohn's disease
        ♦ Sarcoidosis
  4. Reactive processes
     4.1. Epulides
        ♦ Fibrous epulis
        ♦ Calcifying fibroblastic granuloma
        ♦ Pyogenic granuloma (vascular epulis)
        ♦ Peripheral giant cell granuloma (or central)
  5. Neoplasms
     5.1. Premalignant
        ♦ Leukoplakia
        ♦ Erythroplakia
     5.2. Malignant
        ♦ Squamous cell carcinoma
        ♦ Leukemia
        ♦ Lymphoma
  6. Endocrine, nutritional, and metabolic diseases
     6.1. Vitamin deficiencies
        ♦ Vitamin C deficiency (scurvy)
  7. Traumatic lesions
     7.1. Physical/mechanical insults
        ♦ Frictional keratosis
        ♦ Toothbrushing-induced gingival ulceration
        ♦ Factitious injury (self-harm)
     7.2. Chemical (toxic) insults
        ♦ Etching
        ♦ Chlorhexidine
        ♦ Acetylsalicylic acid
        ♦ Cocaine
        ♦ Hydrogen peroxide
        ♦ Dentifrice detergents
        ♦ Paraformaldehyde or calcium hydroxide
     7.3. Thermal insults
        ♦ Burns of mucosa
  8. Gingival pigmentation
        ♦ Gingival pigmentation/melanoplakia
        ♦ Smoker's melanosis
        ♦ Drug-induced pigmentation (antimalarials; minocycline)
        ♦ Amalgam tattoo

**B. Periodontitis**

B1. *Necrotizing periodontal diseases*
   1. Necrotizing gingivitis
   2. Necrotizing periodontitis
   3. Necrotizing stomatitis

B2. *Periodontitis*
   1. Stages: Based on severity and complexity of management
      Stage I: Initial periodontitis
      Stage II: Moderate periodontitis
      Stage III: Severe periodontitis with potential for additional tooth loss
      Stage IV: Severe periodontitis with potential for loss of the dentition
   2. Extent and distribution: Localized, generalized, molar-incisor distribution
   3. Evidence or risk of rapid progression, grades: anticipated treatment response
      a. Grade A: Slow rate of progression
      b. Grade B: Moderate rate of progression
      c. Grade C: Rapid rate of progression

There is no evidence of a specific pathophysiology that enables the differentiation of cases as "aggressive" or "chronic" periodontitis or provides guidance for different kinds of intervention. There is little consistent evidence that aggressive and chronic periodontitis are different diseases. The forms of the disease previously described as "chronic" and "aggressive" are now described under the single category of "periodontitis." Three forms of periodontitis have been identified: 1. Periodontitis; 2. Necrotizing periodontitis; 3. Periodontitis as a direct manifestation of systemic diseases.

However, there is evidence that multiple factors, and the interactions between them, influence clinically observable disease outcomes (phenotypes) at the individual level. On a population basis, the average (mean) rates of periodontitis progression are consistent across all observed populations in the world. However, there is evidence that specific segments of the population exhibit different levels of disease progression. A classification system based only on disease severity fails to capture important dimensions of an individual's disease, including complexity (which influences approaches to therapy) and risk factors (which influence disease outcomes). A multidimensional system of stages and grades has been devised further to describe the different manifestations of periodontitis in individual cases. Stages describe the severity and the extent of the disease; grades describe the likely rate of progression.

B3. *Periodontitis as manifestation of systemic diseases*
   Classification of these conditions should be based on the primary systemic disease according to the International Statistical Classification of Diseases and Related Health Problems (ICD) codes.

**C. Periodontitis as a manifestation of systemic diseases and developmental and acquired conditions.**

C1. Systemic diseases or conditions affecting the periodontal supporting tissues

C2. *Other periodontal conditions*
   1. Periodontal abscesses
   2. Endodontic-periodontal lesions

C3. *Mucogingival deformities and conditions around teeth*
   1. Gingival phenotype
   2. Gingival/soft tissue recession
   3. Lack of keratinized gingiva
   4. Decreased vestibular depth
   5. Aberrant frenum/muscle position
   6. Gingival excess
   7. Abnormal color
   8. Condition of the exposed root surface

The new case definitions related to treatment of gingival recession are based on interproximal loss of clinical attachment and also incorporate the assessment of the exposed root and cementoenamel junction. The consensus report presents a new classification of gingival recession that combines clinical parameters including the gingival phenotype as well as characteristics of the exposed root surface. In the consensus report the term periodontal biotype was replaced by periodontal phenotype.

C4. *Traumatic occlusal forces*
   1. Primary occlusal trauma
   2. Secondary occlusal trauma
   3. Orthodontic forces

*Traumatic occlusal force*, replacing the term *excessive occlusal force*, is the force that exceeds the adaptive capacity of the periodontium and/ or the teeth. Traumatic occlusal forces can result in occlusal trauma and excessive wear or fracture of the teeth.

C5. *Prosthesis and tooth-related factors that modify or predispose to plaque-induced diseases/ periodontitis*
   1. Localized tooth-related factors
      a. Tooth anatomic factors
      b. Root fractures
      c. Cervical root resorption, cemental tears
      d. Root proximity
      e. Altered passive eruption
   2. Localized dental prosthesis-related factors
      a. Restoration margins placed within the supracrestal attached tissues
      b. Clinical procedures related to the fabrication of indirect restorations
      c. Hypersensitivity/toxicity reactions to dental materials

The section on prostheses-related factors was expanded in the new classification. Supracrestal attached tissues replaced the term biologic width. Clinical procedures involved in the fabrication of indirect restorations were added because of new data indicating that these procedures may cause recession and loss of clinical attachment.

**D. Peri-implant diseases and conditions**
- D1. Peri-implant health
- D2. Peri-implant mucositis
- D3. Peri-implantitis
- D4. Peri-implant soft and hard tissue deficiencies

So, the salient features are:
1. Introduction of the term "gingival pigmentation".
2. Identifying smoking and diabetes as the major potential risk factors that can alter the staging of periodontal disease.
3. Recognition of "periodontitis as a manifestation of systemic disease", such as Papillon-Lefèvre syndrome.
4. Systemic conditions affecting the periodontium when not related to dental plaque will be considered as "Systemic Diseases or Conditions Affecting the Periodontal Supporting Tissues".
5. Management protocol of gingival recession based on the inter proximal attachment loss.
6. The term periodontal phenotype replaced the periodontal biotype and supracrestal attachment is the new term replacing the biological width.
7. Introduction of the term traumatic occlusal force.

## REFERENCES

1. van der Velden U. Purpose and problems of periodontal disease classification. Periodontol 2000. 2005;39:13-21.
2. American Academy of Periodontology. Glossary of periodontic terms. J Periodontol. 1986; Suppl:1-3.
3. American Academy of Periodontology (AAP). Consensus Report and Discussion: Section I. In: Nevins M, Becker W, Kornman K (Eds). Proceedings of the World Workshop in Clinical Periodontics. Chicago, IL, USA: American Academy of Periodontology; 1989. pp. I23-32.
4. Armitage GC. Classifying periodontal diseases—a long-standing dilemma. Periodontol 2000. 2002;30:9-23.
5. Ranney RR. Classification of periodontal diseases. Periodontol 2000. 1993;2: 13-25.
6. 1999 International Workshop for a Classification of Periodontal Diseases and Conditions. Papers. Oak Brook, Illinois, October 30- November 2, 1999. Ann Periodontol. 1999; 4:i, 1-112.
7. Consensus Report: Chronic Periodontitis. 1999 International Workshop for a Classification of Periodontal Diseases and Conditions. Ann Periodontol. 1999;4: 38.
8. Consensus Report: Aggressive Periodontitis. 1999 International Workshop for a Classification of Periodontal Diseases and Conditions. Ann Periodontol. 1999;4: 53.
9. Novak MJ. Classification of diseases and conditions affecting the periodontium. In: Newman MG, Takei HH, Carranza FA (Eds). Carranza's Clinical Periodontology, 9th edition. Philadelphia, PA, USA: WB Saunders; 2003. pp. 64-73.
10. Papapanou PN, Sanz M, et al. Periodontitis: Consensus report of Workgroup 2 of the 2017 World Workshop on the Classification of Periodontal and Peri-Implant Diseases and Conditions. J Clin Periodontol. 2018;45(Suppl 20):S162-S170.

## VIVA VOCE

**Q1.** In which classification system, gingival diseases were not included?
**Ans.** In 1989 AAP Classification, gingival diseases were not included.

**Q2.** What was the fundamental difference between AAP 1989 and Ranney 1993 classification system?
**Ans.** AAP 1989 classification system eliminated "Refractory periodontitis" and "Periodontitis associated with systemic disease" categories.

**Q3.** In which classification system were abscesses of the periodontium added?
**Ans.** Abscesses of the periodontium were added in 1999 AAP Classification.

**Q4.** What is the major drawback associated with the 1999 AAP Classification?
**Ans.** It is very extensive and comprehensive.

**Q5.** In which classification system, the term "Aggressive periodontitis" was introduced?
**Ans.** 1999 AAP Classification.

**Q6.** In which classification system, early-onset periodontitis was replaced with aggressive periodontitis?
**Ans.** 1999 AAP Classification.

**Q7.** Why was the term early-onset periodontitis replaced with aggressive periodontitis?
**Ans.** The term early-onset periodontitis was replaced by aggressive periodontitis because of the clinical difficulties in determining the age of onset in these cases.

**Q8.** What are the systemic diseases related to early-onset periodontitis?
**Ans.** Leukocyte adhesion deficiency, hypophosphatasia, Papillon–Lefèvre syndrome, neutropenias, leukemias, Chediak–Higashi syndrome, AIDS, diabetes mellitus type I, trisomy 21, histiocytosis X, Ehlers–Danlos syndrome (type VIII).

**Q9.** In which classification system, gingival pigmentation was added?
**Ans.** 2017 Classification.

**Q10.** Which term replaced biologic width in 2017 Classification?
**Ans.** Supra crestal attached tissues.

# Chapter 7: Epidemiology

*Mayur Kaushik, Shalu Bathla*

## Chapter Outline

- Aims
- Uses
- Epidemiological Studies
- Measurements
- Indices

## INTRODUCTION

John M Last (1988) defined epidemiology as "the study of the distribution and determinants of health-related states or events in specified populations and the application of this study to the control of health problems".[1]

## AIMS

Following are the three aims of epidemiology, which were put forward by Lowe and Kostrzewski in 1973:[2]
- To describe the disease and health-related problems and events in a specified population.
- To provide the data for planning, implementing, and evaluating health services for the prevention, control, and treatment of diseases.
- To understand the causation of disease.

## USES

Following are the seven uses of epidemiology identified by Morris:[3]
1. Studying the rise and fall of disease in the population
2. Diagnosis at the community level
3. Evaluation and planning
4. Evaluation of an individual's risks
5. Identifying syndrome
6. Completing the natural history of the disease
7. Searching for causes and risk factors

## EPIDEMIOLOGICAL STUDIES

Following are the two broad types of epidemiological studies (**Flowchart 7.1**):[4-6]
1. Observational epidemiological studies
2. Experimental epidemiological studies

**Flowchart 7.1:** Epidemiological studies.

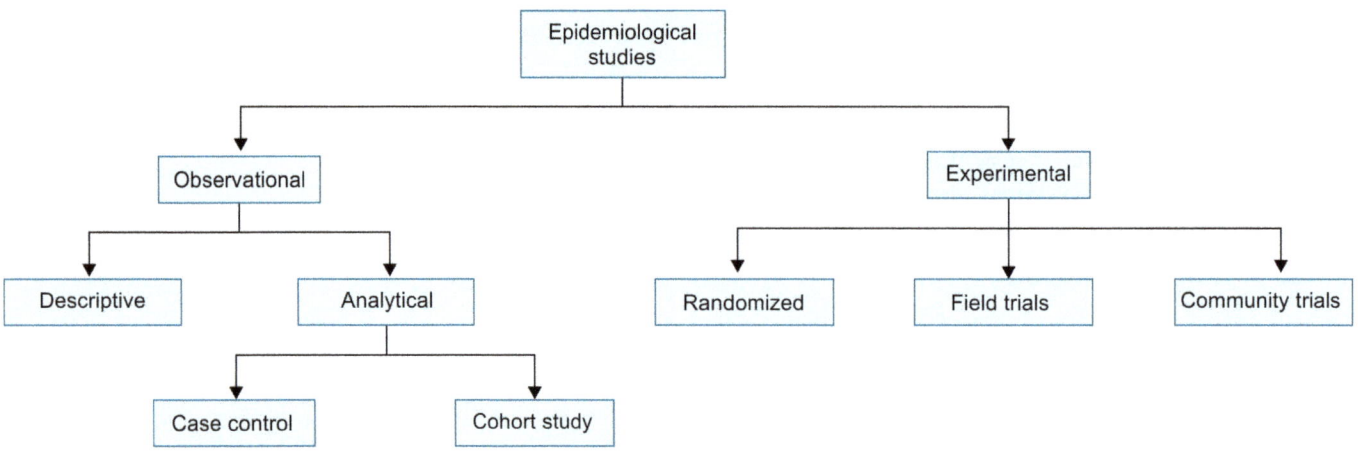

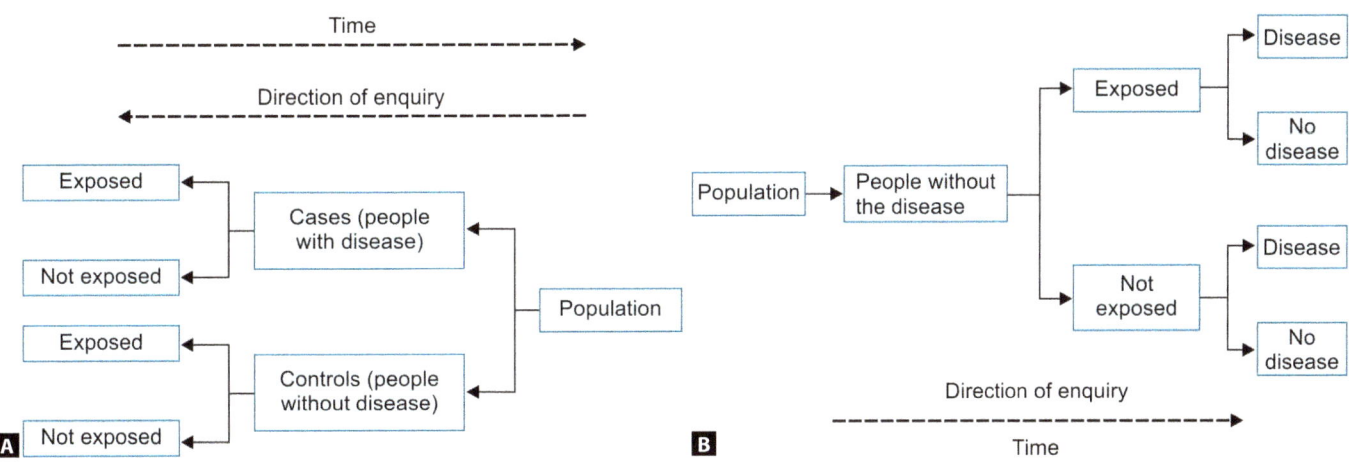

**Figs. 7.1A and B:** Schematic representation showing analytical epidemiology: Design of (A) case-control study; (B) cohort study.

## Observational Epidemiological Studies

These are of two kinds, namely descriptive and analytical epidemiological studies.

### Descriptive Epidemiological Studies

Descriptive studies are used to observe and document the occurrence, progression, and distribution of a disease or condition in population concerning host, agent, and environmental factors. The first phase of any epidemiological investigation includes these descriptive studies.

### Analytical Epidemiological Studies

Analytical studies are used to investigate hypotheses derived from descriptive epidemiologic studies or other data sources. Case-control and cohort studies are the two types of analytical observational studies.[5,7,8]

*Case-control study:* In a case-control study, the unit is the individual rather than the group. This study involves a group of individuals who already have the disease (patients), i.e., cases and groups of individuals who are free from a similar disease, i.e., controls. The focus is on the disease or some other health problem that has already developed. Thus, these are basically comparison studies. Case-control studies are useful for studying risk factors associated with relatively rare diseases. In case-control studies, it is possible to select a group of cases and an appropriate group of controls (matched or unmatched) and investigate exposure or risk factors thought to be associated with the occurrence of disease **(Fig. 7.1A)**. The usual measure of association is the odds ratio. A case-control study can provide important information about the association between exposure levels for rare diseases but cannot provide estimates of disease occurrence. The odds ratio is a measure of the strengths of the association between risk factors and outcomes. It can be derived from a case-control study. It is the ratio of exposure among the cases to exposure among the controls.

*Cohort study:* Repeated observations on the same subject over a period of time. It is also called a longitudinal, prospective, or follow-up study. The cohorts are identified before the disease's appearance under investigation, and the study proceeds from cause to effect **(Fig. 7.1B)**. The cohort study design is useful for comparing disease incidence for relatively common diseases among groups having different exposure levels or risk factors.

## Experimental Epidemiological Studies

Experimental epidemiology is used to test the hypothesis further by introducing a preventive or therapeutic agent and comparing the outcome in test subjects with concurrent observations in control groups.

Experimental epidemiology includes clinical trials, which may be categorized as follows:
- Randomized controlled trials
- Field trials
- Community trials

In 1986, Lindhe et al., stated that there are certain minimum requirements for the design of acceptable clinical trials:[9]
- The hypothesis should be testable.
- The number of subjects should be adequate.
- Two separate groups: Control and test groups
- Subjects should be randomly assigned to these groups
- To assess the effects of therapy, measurements should be reproducible and appropriate.
- Appropriate statistical methods should be employed to test the hypothesis.

## MEASUREMENTS

### Cross-sectional Study

A study carried out at one point in time. Cross-sectional study designs are often used to investigate the association between risk factors and disease prevalence in situations where less is known concerning the form or type of association. It is also known as a prevalence study. This is the most commonly used study design. The focus is on the prevalence of the disease, not the incidence.[10]

### Incidence

It is defined as the number of new cases of a specific disease occurring in a defined population during a specified period of time.

$$\text{Incidence} = \frac{\text{Number of new cases of a specific disease during a given time period}}{\text{The population at risk}} \times 1{,}000$$

### Prevalence

It refers to all the cases both old and new present currently in the population at a given time or during a given period of time in a given population.

Prevalence = Incidence × Mean duration

## INDICES

According to Russell, an index has been defined as a "numerical value describing the relative status of a population on a graduated scale with definite upper and lower limits, which are designed to permit and facilitate comparison with other populations classified by the same criteria and methods".[11]

Methods that express clinical observations in numerical values are known as indices. There are many indices for recording and quantifying periodontal and gingival conditions, which can be used with reproducible accuracy. Indices may allow a more straight forward approach to gather and interpret data.

Indices may be classified as:[12]
- *According to the reversibility of the index*:
  - Reversible index: Index that measures changeable conditions, e.g., papillary marginal attached (P-M-A) index, gingival index (GI).
  - Irreversible index: Index that measures unchangeable conditions, e.g., dental caries index.
- *According to the extent of the area measured*:
  - Simplified index: Index that measures only a demonstrative sample of the dental apparatus. Greene and Vermillion's oral hygiene index simplified (OHI-S).
  - Full-mouth index: Index that measures the patient's entire dentition or periodontium, e.g., Russell's periodontal index (PI).
- *According to the entity which they measure*:
  - Symptom Index: Sulcular or gingival bleeding index.
  - Disease index: The decay portion (D) of the DMF decayed, missing, filled (DMF) index.
  - Treatment index: The filled portion (F) of the DMF index.

## Gingival Indices

### Papillary Marginal Attached Index

In 1944, Massler and Schour developed the PMA index.[13] In this index, the number of gingival units affected was counted rather than the severity of the inflammation.

*Teeth examined*: All of the facial gingival tissues surrounding all the teeth were assessed except 3rd molars. Around a tooth, the facial surface of gingiva was divided into three parts:
1. Papillary gingiva (P)
2. Marginal gingiva (M)
3. Attached gingiva (A)

*Method*: The examination starts from the left maxillary 2nd molar around to the right maxillary 2nd molar and then from the right mandibular 2nd molar to the left mandibular 2nd molar.

For prevalence studies, each PMA unit is scored 0 or 1 for the absence or presence of inflammation, respectively. The P, M, and A numerical values for all teeth are totaled separately and then added together to calculate the PMA index score per person.

### Gingival Index

In 1963, Loe and Silness[14] developed the gingival index (GI). In this index, based on gingival consistency, color, and bleeding on probing, the severity of gingivitis is assessed.

*Teeth examined*: GI can be determined for selected teeth or the entire dentition. The selected teeth or index teeth are: 16, 11, 24, 36, 31, 44 [Federation Dentaire Internationale (FDI) system].

*Method*: Systematically for each tooth, four gingival areas, i.e., (i) distal, (ii) facial, (iii) mesial and (iv) lingual are examined. Bleeding is assessed by running a periodontal probe circumferentially along the tissue wall of the gingival sulcus.

*Calculation of index*: Add the scores of four gingival areas of the tooth and divide by four to get a tooth score. Then, total the tooth scores together and divide them by the number of teeth examined to obtain an individual's GI score **(Tables 7.1 and 7.2)**.

| TABLE 7.1: Criteria for gingival index (GI). | |
|---|---|
| Score | Criteria |
| 0 | Normal gingiva |
| 1 | Mild inflammation: Slight change in color and slight edema. No bleeding on probing |
| 2 | Moderate inflammation: Redness, edema, and glazing. Bleeding on probing |
| 3 | Severe inflammation: Marked redness, edema, and ulceration. The tendency towards spontaneous bleeding |

**TABLE 7.2:** Scoring criteria for gingival index (GI).

| Gingival scores | Condition |
|---|---|
| 0.1–1.0 | Mild gingivitis |
| 1.1–2.0 | Moderate gingivitis |
| 2.1–3.0 | Severe gingivitis |

**TABLE 7.3:** Scoring criteria of the modified gingival index (MGI).

| Score | Criteria |
|---|---|
| 0 | Absence of inflammation |
| 1 | Mild inflammation: Slight change in color, little change in the texture of any portion but not the entire marginal or papillary gingival unit |
| 2 | Mild inflammation: Criteria as above but involving the entire marginal or papillary gingival unit |
| 3 | Moderate inflammation: Glazing, redness, edema, and/or hypertrophy of the marginal/papillary gingival unit |
| 4 | Severe inflammation: Marked redness, edema, and/or hypertrophy of the marginal/papillary gingival unit; spontaneous bleeding, congestion, or ulceration |

## *Modified Gingival Index*

In 1986, Lobene et al. developed a modified gingival index (MGI).[15] Following are the modifications in this index:
- Elimination of gingival probing to assess the absence or presence of bleeding. Thus, the noninvasive index allows repeated evaluations and permits intra-calibration, and inter-calibration of examiners.
- Redefinition of the scoring system for mild and moderate inflammation.

The developers of the MGI decided to eliminate probing, which could disturb plaque and irritate the gingiva. The presence of periodontal pockets or attachment loss cannot be assessed by this index **(Table 7.3)**.

## Bleeding Indices

The bleeding indices are based on the objective diagnostic signs of inflammation. These detect early inflammatory changes, which occur before any changes in gingival color, form, and texture. They also detect inflammatory lesions at the base of the periodontal pocket, an area that is inaccessible to visual examination. They can be used to enhance the patient's motivation for plaque control because the patient can easily understand.

The disadvantages of the gingival bleeding index are as follows:
- Types of the probe, angulation depth, and probing force may vary and may bring discrepancy in the results.
- Bleeding from gingival sulcus may be associated with other forms of periodontal disease, not only gingivitis.

## *Sulcus Bleeding Index*

In 1971, Muhlemann and Son developed the sulcus bleeding index (SBI) for the assessment of gingival bleeding.[16]

**TABLE 7.4:** Scoring criteria of sulcus bleeding index (SBI).

| Score | Criteria |
|---|---|
| 0 | Healthy appearance of P and M; no bleeding upon sulcus probing |
| 1 | Apparently healthy P and M showing no color or contour change and no swelling, but bleeding from sulcus on probing |
| 2 | Bleeding on probing and color change caused by inflammation (reddening); no swelling or macroscopic edema |
| 3 | Bleeding on probing, change in color, slight edematous swelling |
| 4 | Bleeding on probing, color change, obvious swelling |
| 5 | Spontaneous bleeding on probing, color change, marked swelling with or without ulceration |

This index detects early inflammatory gingival disease by locating areas of gingival sulcus bleeding by gentle probing.

*Method*: This is based on the evaluation of gingival bleeding on probing, gingival color and gingival contour changes. Four gingival units are scored systematically for each tooth; the labial and lingual marginal gingiva (M units) and the mesial and distal papillary gingiva (P units). The probing of the four areas should be carried out under proper illumination. For M units, the probe should be held parallel to the tooth's long axis, but for P units, it should be directed towards the col area. After probing, wait for 30 seconds before scoring the apparently healthy gingival units. The gingiva should be dried gently to observe color changes.

*Scoring criteria*: Assessment of gingival bleeding is done according to **Table 7.4**.

*Calculation*: Each of the four gingival units (P and M units) is scored from 0 to 5 to obtain the SBI of the area. The four units' scores are totaled and then divided by 4 to obtain the SBI for the tooth. By totaling scores for individual teeth and the number of teeth, the SBI is determined.

## *Papillary Bleeding Index*

In 1977, Muhlemann developed papillary bleeding index (PBI).[17] Gentle probing of the interdental papilla is done to assess the bleeding.

*Method*: This is performed by sweeping the papillary sulcus on the mesial and distal aspects with a periodontal probe. Right maxillary and left mandibular quadrants probed lingually, and the left maxillary and right mandibular quadrants probed buccally. On the papilla's mesial and distal aspects, the blunt periodontal probe is inserted into the gingival sulcus at the base of the papilla and then moved coronally to the papilla tip. The intensity of bleeding was recorded on a scale of 0–4.

*Scoring criteria*: Assessment of gingival bleeding is done by PBI using **Table 7.5**.

*Calculation*: Each papilla is scored according to the criteria. The scores are added and then divided by the number of papilla examined.

**Section 2:** Classification and Epidemiology

**TABLE 7.5:** Scoring criteria for papillary bleeding index (PBI).

| Score | Criteria |
|---|---|
| 0 | No bleeding after probing |
| 1 | A single discrete bleeding point appears after probing |
| 2 | Several isolated bleeding points or a single fine line of blood appears |
| 3 | The interdental triangle fills with blood shortly after probing |
| 4 | Profuse bleeding occurs after probing; blood flows immediately into the marginal sulcus |

## Gingival Bleeding Index

In 1974, Carter and Barnes developed gingival bleeding index (GBI) to record the presence or absence of gingival inflammation as determined by bleeding from interproximal gingival sulci.[18]

*Method*: All interproximal areas having a mesial and distal sulcus component are considered to be susceptible to gingival inflammation, and these areas are recorded as total risk areas. Each interproximal area has two sulci, which either are scored as one interdental unit or maybe scored individually. Certain areas may be excluded from scoring because of accessibility, tooth position, a diastema, or other factors, and if exclusions are made, a consistent procedure should be followed for an individual and group, if a study is to be conducted. 3rd molars are usually excluded, and 26 interdental units are scored.

*Procedure*: Unwaxed dental floss is passed interproximally first on one side and then on the other side of the papilla. The floss is then curved around the adjacent tooth and brought below the gingival margin. The floss is moved up and down carefully without lacerating gingiva in one stroke. For each area, a new length of floss is used. Retract for visibility of bleeding from both facial and lingual aspects. A gap of 30 seconds should be allowed for reinspection of an area that does not show blood immediately either in the area or on the floss.

*Scoring criteria*: Bleeding indicates the presence of disease. No attempt is made in this index to quantify the severity of bleeding because no bleeding represents healthy tissues.

## Bleeding Time Index

In 1981, Nowicki et al.[19] developed the bleeding time index (BTI). For this index, the Michigan "0" probe is inserted in the sulcus till slight resistance is felt, and then the gingiva is stroked back and forth once over an area of approximately 2 mm. The scoring criteria are given in **Table 7.6**.

## Quantitative Gingival Bleeding Index

In 1985, Garg and Kapoor developed quantitative gingival bleeding index (QGBI) which has virtuous reliability and reproducibility.[20]

**TABLE 7.6:** Scoring criteria of bleeding time index (BTI).

| Score | Criteria |
|---|---|
| 0 | No bleeding within 15 seconds of second probing (i.e., 30 seconds total time) |
| 1 | Bleeding within 6–15 seconds of second probing |
| 2 | Bleeding within 11–15 seconds of first probing or 5 seconds after second probing |
| 3 | Bleeding within 10 seconds after initial probing |
| 4 | Spontaneous bleeding |

**TABLE 7.7:** Scoring criteria of the quantitative gingival bleeding index (QGBI).

| Score | Criteria |
|---|---|
| 0 | No bleeding on brushing; bristles free from bloodstains |
| 1 | Slight bleeding on brushing; bristle tips stained with blood |
| 2 | Moderate bleeding on brushing; about half of bristle length from the tip downwards stained with blood |
| 3 | Severe bleeding on brushing; entire bristle length of all bristles including brush head covered with blood |

*Method*: Index takes into consideration the magnitude of bloodstains covering toothbrush bristles on brushing and squeezing gingival tissue units in a segment, with one score for entire one segment (canine to canine, or left or right premolars and molars in maxillary or mandibular arches—six segments in all). Bleeding is generally immediately evident on the bristles of the brush; however, 30 seconds are allowed for reinspection of each segment **(Table 7.7)**.

## Plaque Indices

### Plaque Component of the Periodontal Disease Index

In this index, six Ramfjord teeth 16, 11, 24, 36, 31, 44 (FDI system) are stained with Bismarck brown solution.[21] The criteria are to measure the presence and extent of plaque on a scale of 0–3, looking specifically at all interproximal, facial and lingual surfaces of the index teeth **(Table 7.8)**.

$$\text{Plaque score of an individual} = \frac{\text{Total score}}{\text{Number of teeth examined}}$$

This index is used in longitudinal studies of periodontal diseases and clinical trials of preventive or therapeutic agents.

**TABLE 7.8:** Scoring criteria of plaque component of the periodontal disease index (PDI).

| Score | Criteria |
|---|---|
| 0 | No plaque present |
| 1 | Plaque present on some but not all interproximal, buccal and lingual surfaces of the tooth |
| 2 | Plaque present on all interproximal, buccal and lingual surfaces, but covering less than one-half of the surfaces |
| 3 | Plaque extending over all interproximal, buccal and lingual surfaces and covering more than one-half of these surfaces |

| TABLE 7.9: Scoring criteria of plaque index (PI). | |
|---|---|
| Score | Criteria |
| 0 | No plaque in the gingival area |
| 1 | A film of plaque adhering to the free gingival margin and adjacent area of the tooth. The plaque may be recognized only by running a probe across the tooth surface |
| 2 | Moderate accumulation of soft deposits within the gingival pocket and on the gingival margin and/or adjacent tooth surface that can be seen by the naked eye |
| 3 | The abundance of soft matter within the gingival pocket and/ or on the gingival margin and adjacent tooth surface |

## Plaque Index

Plaque index (PI) assesses only the thickness of plaque at the gingival area of the tooth.[14]

*Method*: The evaluation or scoring is done on the entire dentition or on selected teeth. The surfaces examined are the four gingival areas of the tooth, i.e., distofacial, facial, mesiofacial, and lingual surfaces. The light source, mouth mirror, dental explorer, and air drying of the teeth and gingiva are used in the scoring of this index **(Table 7.9)**.

$$\text{Score for area} = \frac{\text{Total of the four scores per tooth}}{4}$$

$$\text{Score for person} = \frac{\text{Plaque index scores per tooth}}{\text{No. of teeth examined}}$$

## Patient Hygiene Performance Index

In 1968, Podshadley and Haley[22] developed the patient hygiene performance (PHP) index to assess an individual's oral hygiene performance. It is a simplified index used as an educational and motivational tool for the patient **(Table 7.10)**.

*Method*: Apply a disclosing agent before scoring. Instruct the patient to swish and expectorate for 30 seconds and not to rinse. The examination is made using a mouth mirror. Each tooth surface to be evaluated is divided longitudinally into mesial, middle, and distal thirds. The middle third is then subdivided horizontally into occlusal or incisal, middle, and gingival thirds **(Fig. 7.2)**.

*Debris scores for each subdivision*: According to the presence of stained debris, each of the five subdivisions are scored as follows:
- 0: No debris (or questionable)
- 1: Debris definitely present

Patient hygiene performance (PHP) index
$$= \frac{\text{Total debris score}}{\text{Number of teeth scored}}$$

*Rating of PHP index*:
- 0: Excellent
- 0.1–1.7: Good
- 1.8–3.4: Fair
- 3.5–5.0: Poor

| TABLE 7.10: Teeth and surfaces to be examined: Six index teeth. | | |
|---|---|---|
| Index teeth | Tooth | Surface |
| 16 | Upper right 1st molar | Buccal |
| 11 | Upper right central incisor | Labial |
| 26 | Upper left 1st molar | Buccal |
| 36 | Lower left 1st molar | Lingual |
| 31 | Lower left central incisor | Labial |
| 46 | Lower right 1st molar | Lingual |

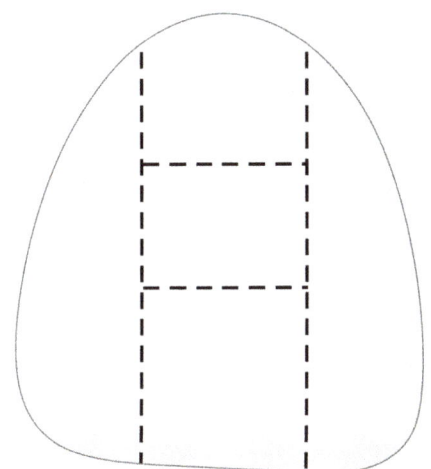

Fig. 7.2: Schematic representation showing patient hygiene performance (PHP) index tooth.

## Turesky Modification of the Quigley–Hein Plaque Index

In 1970, Turesky, Gilmore, and Glickman modified Quigley–Hein plaque index.[23] After using the basic fuchsin disclosing agent, plaque is assessed on the teeth' facial and lingual surfaces. The scoring criteria for this index are given in **Table 7.11**.

$$\text{Plaque score per person} = \frac{\text{Total of all plaque score}}{\text{Number of surface examined}}$$

| TABLE 7.11: Scoring criteria of Turesky modification of Quigley–Hein plaque index. | |
|---|---|
| Score | Criteria |
| 0 | No plaque |
| 1 | Separate flecks of plaque at the cervical margin of the tooth |
| 2 | A thin, continuous band of plaque (up to 1 mm) at the cervical margin of the tooth |
| 3 | A band of plaque wider than 1 mm, but covering less than one-third of the crown of the tooth |
| 4 | Plaque covering at least one-third, but less than two-thirds of the crown of the tooth |
| 5 | Plaque covering two-thirds or more of the crown of the tooth |

**TABLE 7.12:** Scoring criteria of calculus component of the periodontal disease index (PDI).

| Score | Criteria |
|---|---|
| 0 | Absence of calculus |
| 1 | Supragingival calculus extending only slightly below the free gingival margin (not >1 mm) |
| 2 | A moderate amount of supragingival and subgingival calculus or subgingival calculus alone |
| 3 | An abundance of supragingival and subgingival calculus |

## Calculus Indices

### Calculus Component of the Periodontal Disease Index

In 1959, Ramfjord[21] described the calculus index as one of the components of the periodontal disease index.

*Method*: In this index, to determine the presence and extent of calculus on the facial and lingual surfaces of the six index teeth are evaluated. Dental explorer and/or a periodontal probe and mouth mirror are the instruments used in this index **(Table 7.12)**.

*Calculation*: To obtain a calculus score per person, the calculus score per tooth are added and then divided by the number of teeth examined.

### Calculus Surface Index

In 1961, Ennever, Sturzenberger, and Radike developed a calculus surface index (CSI).[24] It is used to determine rapidly whether a specific agent has any effect on reducing or preventing supragingival or subgingival calculus.

Index teeth 32, 31, 41, 42 (mandibular incisors) are examined for the absence or presence of calculus by visual and tactile examination **(Table 7.13)**. This index shows good intraexaminer reproducibility, in a relatively short period of time.

### Simplified-Oral Hygiene Index

In 1964, Greene and Vermillion developed a simplified-oral hygiene index (OHI-S).[25] It is a composite index which deals with both calculus and oral debris together.

Following are the surfaces of six index teeth:
1. The buccal surface of 16 (right maxillary 1st molar)
2. The labial surface of 11 (right maxillary central incisor)
3. The buccal surface of 26 (left maxillary 1st molar)
4. Lingual surface of 36 (left mandibular 1st molar)
5. Labial surface of 31 (left mandibular central incisor)
6. Lingual surface of 46 (right mandibular 1st molar)

**TABLE 7.13:** Scoring criteria of calculus surface index (CSI).

| Score | Criteria |
|---|---|
| 0 | Indicates the absence of calculus |
| 1 | Indicates the presence of calculus |

**TABLE 7.14:** Scoring criteria of the simplified debris index (DI-S).

| Score | Criteria |
|---|---|
| 0 | No debris or stain present |
| 1 | Soft debris covering not more than one-third of the tooth surface or the presence of extrinsic stain without other debris regardless of surface area covered |
| 2 | Soft debris covering more than one-third, but not more than two-thirds of the exposed tooth surface |
| 3 | Soft debris covering more than two-thirds of the exposed tooth surface |

**TABLE 7.15:** Scoring criteria of the simplified calculus index (CI-S).

| Score | Criteria |
|---|---|
| 0 | No calculus present |
| 1 | Supragingival calculus covering not more than one-third of the exposed tooth surface |
| 2 | Supragingival calculus covering more than one-third, but not more than two-thirds of the exposed tooth surface or the presence of individual flecks of subgingival calculus around the cervical pattern of the tooth or both |
| 3 | Supragingival calculus covering more than two-thirds of the exposed tooth surface or a continuous heavy band of subgingival calculus around the cervical portion of the tooth or both |

*Method*: The OHI-S has two components, the simplified debris index (DI-S) and the simplified calculus index (CI-S).

*Oral debris index*: The surface area covered by debris is estimated by running the side of an explorer (Shepherd's hook) along the tooth surface being examined **(Table 7.14)**.

After debris scores are recorded, the teeth are then examined for calculus **(Table 7.15)**.

Calculation of the index: DI-S and CI-S scores are obtained by calculating the index as follows:
- 0.0–0.6: Good
- 0.7–1.8: Fair
- 1.9–3.0: Poor

For each individual, the DI-S and CI-S scores are totaled and divided by the number of tooth surfaces examined.

Simplified debris index (DI-S) score
$$= \frac{\text{Total score}}{\text{Number of surfaces examined}}$$

Simplified calculus index (CI-S) score
$$= \frac{\text{Total score}}{\text{Number of surfaces examined}}$$

Once the DI-S and CI-S scores are calculated separately, then they are added together to get the OHI-S score. OHI-S scores are as follows:
- 0.0–1.2: Good
- 1.3–3.0: Fair
- 3.1–6.0: Poor

## Volpe–Manhold Calculus Assessment

In 1965, Volpe and Manhold developed the Volpe–Manhold index (VMI) to assess the presence and severity of calculus formation, especially the newly formed supragingival calculus, following an oral prophylaxis.[26] It is used for longitudinal studies.

*Method*: A periodontal probe graduated in millimeter divisions is used to measure the deposits in calculus on the lingual surfaces of the six mandibular anterior teeth.

To obtain VMI scores, the three-tooth planes, the mesial, distal and gingival, on the lingual surface of the lower six anterior teeth are examined. The periodontal probe is used to measure the linear extent of the supragingival calculus by placing the flat calibrated end of the probe always at the most inferior visible border of the calculus formation. Volpe–Manhold index (VMI)

$$= \frac{\text{Total VMI score}}{\text{Number of lower anterior teeth examined}}$$

## Marginal Line Calculus Index

In 1967, Muhlemann and Villa developed a marginal line calculus index (MLC-I). This index is used in short-term clinical trials (i.e., <6 weeks) of anticalculus agents.[27]

This index is used to assess the supragingival calculus along the gingiva margins on the lingual aspects of the four mandibular incisors. The examination is done using a mouth mirror, after drying the tooth surfaces with air. The various calculus indices are summarized in **Table 7.16.**

## Periodontal Disease Indices

### Periodontal Index

In 1956, Russell developed this index.[28]

*Teeth examined*: All the teeth present are examined. This is a composite index because it measures reversible as well as irreversible aspects of periodontal disease **(Table 7.17)**. Scoring values (0, 1, 2, 6, and 8) is chosen to relate the stages of the disease in an epidemiological survey to the clinical conditions observed.

### Russell's Rule

The Russell's rule states that "When in doubt assign the lower score"; scores obtained as per Russell's rule are as follows:
- 0–0.2: Clinically normal supportive tissues
- 0.3–0.9: Simple gingivitis
- 1.0–1.9: Beginning destructive periodontal disease
- 2.0–4.9: Established destructive periodontal disease
- 5.0–8.0: Terminal disease

### Periodontal Disease Index

The PDI is a modification of Russell's PI for epidemiological surveys of periodontal diseases.[21] This index's characteristic feature is that it measures the periodontal attachment related to the cementoenamel junction (CEJ) of the teeth.

*Components of PDI*: The PDI comprises of three components, namely:
1. Plaque
2. Calculus and gingival component
3. Periodontal component

**TABLE 7.16:** Various calculus indices.

| Name | Year | Authors | Method |
|---|---|---|---|
| Calculus surface index (CSI) | 1961 | Ennever, Sturzenberger, Radike | Use air, mirror, and explorer to detect calculus |
| Calculus index simplified (CI-S), part of a simplified- oral hygiene index (OHI-S) | 1964 | Greene and Vermillion | With an explorer, detect calculus around the cervical portion of the tooth |
| Volpe–Manhold index (VMI) calculus assessment | 1965 | Volpe, Manhold, and Hazen | Measure with the probe in three planes |
| Marginal line calculus index (MLC-I) | 1967 | Muhlemann and Villa | Divide tooth in half (mesial and distal); with air, visualize minute areas of supramarginal calculus next to gingiva on the lingual surface of four mandibular incisors |

**TABLE 7.17:** Scoring criteria of periodontal index.

| Score | Stages of disease | Criteria |
|---|---|---|
| 0 | Negative | Neither overt inflammation in the investing tissues nor loss of function due to destruction of supporting tissues |
| 1 | Mild gingivitis | Overt area of inflammation in the free gingiva, but this area does not circumscribe the tooth |
| 2 | Gingivitis | Inflammation completely circumscribes the tooth, but there is no apparent break in the epithelial attachment |
| 6 | Gingivitis with pocket formation | The epithelial attachment has been broken, and there is a pocket. There is no interference with normal masticatory function, the tooth is firm in its socket, and has not drifted |
| 8 | Advanced destruction with loss of masticatory function | The tooth may be loose, drifted, may sound dull on percussion with a metallic instrument, or maybe depressible in its socket |

## Section 2: Classification and Epidemiology

**TABLE 7.18:** Scoring criteria of periodontal disease index (PDI).

| Score | Criteria |
|---|---|
| 0 | Absence of inflammation |
| 1 | Mild-to-moderate inflammatory gingival changes not extending all around the tooth |
| 2 | Mild-to-moderately-severe gingivitis extending all around the tooth |
| 3 | Severe gingivitis, characterized by marked redness, tendency to bleed and ulceration |
| 4 | The gingival crevice in any of the four measured areas (mesial, distal, buccal, lingual), extending apically to the cementoenamel junction (CEJ), but not >3 mm |
| 5 | The gingival crevice in any of the four measured areas extending apically, 3–6 mm from CEJ |
| 6 | The gingival crevice in any of the four measured areas extending apically, >6 mm from CEJ |

*Scoring methods*: The six-selected index teeth are called Ramfjord teeth which include:
1. The 16 maxillary right 1st molar
2. The 21 maxillary left central incisor
3. The 24 maxillary left 1st premolar
4. The 36 mandibular left 1st molar
5. The 41 mandibular right central incisor
6. The 44 mandibular right 1st premolar. Scoring criteria are given in **Table 7.18**.

Periodontal disease index (PDI)

$$= \frac{\text{Total number of individual tooth scores}}{\text{Number of teeth examined}}$$

*The score for an individual*: Add the individual PDI scores and then divide by the number of people examined to obtain the PDI score for a group.

## Community Periodontal Index of Treatment Needs

Joint Working Committee of the World Health Organization (WHO) and FDI by Ainamo et al.[29] developed community periodontal index of treatment needs (CPITN) in 1982. This index was developed primarily to survey and evaluate periodontal treatment needs rather than determining past and present periodontal status, i.e., the recession of the gingival margin and alveolar bone. This index records gingival inflammation, periodontal pocket, dental calculus, and other plaque retentive factors.

CPITN probe is designed for two purposes, namely measurement of pocket depth and detection of subgingival calculus. Color coding with a black mark starting at 3.5 mm and ending at 5.5 mm allows the measurement of pocket depth. 0.5 mm of ball tip present over the probe helps in the detection of subgingival calculus **(Fig. 7.3)**.

*Procedure*: For assessment of periodontal treatment needs, the whole dentition is divided into sextants, and then each sextant is given a score **(Table 7.19)**.

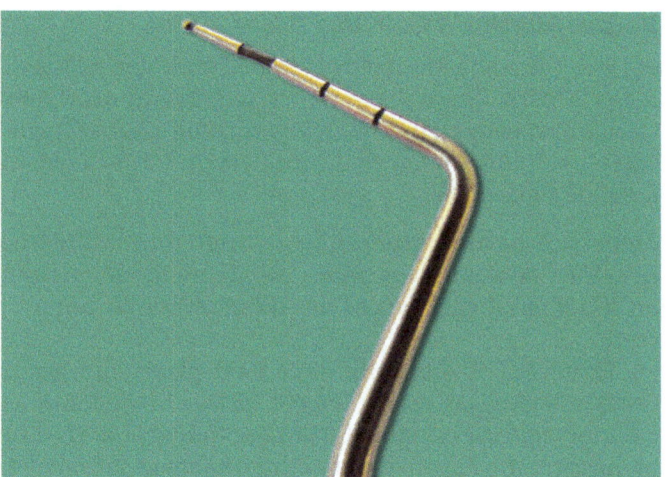

**Fig. 7.3:** Photograph showing community periodontal index of treatment needs (CPITN) probe.

**TABLE 7.19:** Criteria for the community periodontal index of treatment needs (CPITN).

| Periodontal status | | Treatment needs | |
|---|---|---|---|
| Score | Criteria | Score | Criteria |
| 0 | Healthy periodontium | 0 | No treatment needed |
| 1 | Bleeding observed, directly or by using mouth mirror after sensing | I | Oral hygiene needs improvement |
| 2 | Calculus felt during probing, but the entire black area of the probe is visible | II | I + Professional scaling |
| 3 | Pocket 4 mm or 5 mm (gingival margin is situated on the black area of the probe) | II | I + professional scaling |
| 4 | Pocket >6 mm (black area of probe not visible) | III | I + II + complex treatment |

*Index teeth*: For individuals of ages 20 years or more, only ten index teeth, namely 17, 16, 11, 26, 27, 31, 36, 37, 46, and 47 (FDI system), are examined. These teeth have been considered as the best estimators of the worst periodontal condition of the mouth. For individuals of age up to 19 years, six index teeth, i.e., 16, 11, 26, 31, 36, and 46, are examined.

*Probing procedure*: A tooth is probed to detect subgingival calculus and bleeding response and to measure pocket depth. The probing force can be divided into:
- Working component: It is used for determining and measuring pocket depth.
- Sensing component: It is used for detecting subgingival calculus.

The working force should not be more than 20 g. The probe is inserted in the gingival sulcus, and pocket depth is measured against measuring lines or color code. The ball

Chapter 7: Epidemiology

**TABLE 7.20:** Various periodontal disease indices.

| Name | Year | Authors | Method |
|---|---|---|---|
| Periodontal index (PI) | 1956 | Russell | Do not use probe; weigh scores and combine gingival and periodontal status |
| Periodontal disease index (PDI) | 1967 | Ramfjord | Select the "Ramfjord" teeth (16, 21, 24, 36, 41 and 44) and score for gingiva, attachment loss, calculus and plaque |
| Community periodontal index treatment needs (CPITN) | 1982 | Ainamo et al. | Epidemiological index: Use O'Leary's sextants with specified index teeth or worst tooth, WHO probe, 0–4 codes per sextant; evaluate bleeding, deposits and pocket depth |
| Extent and severity index[30] | 1986 | Carlos, Wolfe, and Kingman | Epidemiological index: Estimates the attachment level from probe depths—14 sites in each of 2 contralateral quadrants |

end of the probe should be kept in contact with the root surface. For sensing subgingival calculus, the lightest force is used. Recommended probing sites are distal, midline, and mesial of facial and lingual/palatal surfaces. Withdrawing the probe between each probing or with the probe tip remaining in the sulcus, the probe may be walked around the tooth.

### Points to Ponder

- Prospective or forward studies are cohort studies, while retrospective or backward studies are case-control studies.
- Cross-sectional studies are like photographs, and longitudinal studies are cine films.
- Case-control studies can be more prone to bias than cohort studies.
- Clinical trials avoid bias and confounding through the processes of randomization and blinding.
- *G index*: This periodontal index is a colorimetric test to measure gingival inflammation based on the saliva's hemoglobin content. Abbott and Caffesse in 1978 formed a correlation between the G index values, gingival index, and crevicular fluid flow.
- Various periodontal disease indices are periodontal index, periodontal disease index, community periodontal index treatment needs, and extent and severity index **(Table 7.20)**.

## REFERENCES

1. Last JM. What is "clinical epidemiology"? J Public Health Policy. 1988;9(2):159-63.
2. Lowe CR, Kostrzewski J. Epidemiology: a guide to teaching methods. Edited for the International Epidemiological Association, in collaboration with the World Health Organization. Edinburgh: Churchill Livingstone; 1973.
3. Morris JN. Uses of epidemiology. 1955. Int J Epidemiol. 2007;36(6):1165-72.
4. Park K. Textbook of Preventive and Social Medicine, 17th edition. Kolkata, India: Banarsidass Bhanot Publishers; 2002. pp. 44-107.
5. Peter S. Epidemiology, etiology, and prevention of periodontal diseases. In: Essentials of Preventive and Community Dentistry, 4th edition. New Delhi, India: Arya (Medi) Publishing House; 2004. pp. 110-3.
6. Greene JC. General principles of epidemiology and methods for measuring prevalence and severity of the periodontal disease. In: Genco RJ, Goldman HM, Cohen DW (Eds). Contemporary Periodontics. St. Louis: CV Mosby; 1990. pp. 97-105.
7. Kingman A, Albandar JM. Methodological aspects of epidemiological studies of periodontal diseases. Periodontol 2000. 2002;29:11-30.
8. Beck JD, Arbes SJ, Jr. Epidemiology of gingival and periodontal diseases. In: Newman MG, Takei HH, Carranza FA (Eds). Carranza's Clinical Periodontology, 9th edition. Philadelphia, PA, USA: WB Saunders; 2003. pp. 74-95.
9. Lindhe J, Socransky S, Wennström J. Design of clinical trials of traditional therapies of periodontitis. J Clin Periodontol. 1986;13(5):488-99.
10. Loe H, Morrison E. Epidemiology of periodontal disease. In: Genco RJ, Goldman HM, Cohen DW (Eds). Contemporary Periodontics. St. Louis: CV Mosby; 1990. pp. 106-16.
11. Russell AL. Epidemiology and the rational bases of dental public health and dental practice. In: Young WO, Striffler DF, Russell AL (Eds). The Dentist, His Practice, and His Community, 2nd edition. Philadelphia, PA, USA: WB Saunders; 1969. pp. 35-62.
12. Peter S. Indices in dental epidemiology. In: Essentials of Preventive and Community Dentistry, 4th edition. New Delhi, India: Arya (Medi) Publishing House; 2004. pp. 311-59.
13. Massler M. The P-M-A index for the assessment of gingivitis. J Periodontol. 1967;38(6):592-601.
14. Löe H. The gingival index, the plaque index, and the retention index systems. J Periodontol. 1967;38(Suppl):610-6.
15. Lobene RR, Weatherford T, Ross NM, Lamm RA, Menaker L. A modified gingival index for use in clinical trials. Clin Prevent Dent. 1986;8(1):3-6.
16. Mühlemann HR, Son S. Gingival sulcus bleeding--a leading symptom in initial gingivitis. Helv Odontol Acta. 1971;15(2):107-13.
17. Mühlemann HR. Psychological and chemical mediators of gingival health. J Prev Dent. 1977;4(4):6-17.
18. Carter HG, Barnes GP. The gingival bleeding index. J Periodontol. 1974;45(11):801-5.
19. Nowicki D, Vogel RI, Melcer S, Deasy MJ. The gingival bleeding time index. J Periodontol. 1981;52(5):260-2.
20. Garg S, Kapoor KK. The quantitative gingival bleeding index. J Indian Dent Assoc. 1985;57(3):112-3.
21. Ramfjord SP. The periodontal disease index (PDI). J Periodontol. 1967;38(6):602-10.
22. Podshadley AG, Haley JV. A method for evaluating oral hygiene performance. Public Health Rep. 1968;83(3): 259-64.
23. Turesky S, Gilmore ND, Glickman I. Reduced plaque formation by the chloromethyl analogue of vitamin C. J Periodontol. 1970;41(1):41-3.
24. Ennever J, Sturzenberger OP, Radike W. The calculus surface index method for scoring clinical calculus studies. J Periodontol. 1961;32:54-7.

**Section 2:** Classification and Epidemiology

25. Greene JC, Vermillion JR. The simplified oral hygiene index. J Am Dent Assoc. 1964;68:7-13.
26. Volpe AR, Manhold JH. A method of evaluating the effectiveness of potential calculus inhibiting agents. N Y State Dent. 1962;28:289-90.
27. Mühlemann HR, Villa PR. The marginal line calculus index. Helv Odontol Acta. 1967;11(2):175-9.
28. Russell AL. A system of classification and scoring for prevalence surveys of periodontal disease. J Dent Res. 1956;35(3):350-9.
29. Ainamo J, Barmes D, Beagrie G, Cutress T, Martin J, Sardo-Infirri J. Development of the World Health Organization (WHO) community periodontal index of treatment needs (CPITN). Int Dent J. 1982;32(3):281-91.
30. Carlos JP, Wolf MD, Kingman A. The extent and severity index: a simple method for use in epidemiologic studies of periodontal disease. J Clin Periodontol. 1986;13(5): 500-5.

## VIVA VOCE

**Q1.** What are the advantages of the modified gingival index (MGI) over the gingival index (GI)?
**Ans.** The advantages of MGI over GI are as follows:
1. MGI is a non-invasive index.
2. MGI is more sensitive than GI.

**Q2.** Which disclosing agent is used in the plaque component of the periodontal disease index (PDI) and Turesky–Gilmore–Glickman plaque index?
**Ans.** The disclosing agent used in:
1. Plaque component of PDI: Bismarck brown solution
2. Turesky–Gilmore–Glickman plaque index: Basic fuchsin.

**Q3.** Which epidemiologic index has a true biologic gradient?
**Ans.** The periodontal index by Russell has a true biologic gradient.

**Q4.** Why Russell's index is called a composite index?
**Ans.** Russell's index is called a composite index because it records both reversible changes due to gingivitis and irreversible changes brought by periodontal disease.

**Q5.** What are the drawbacks of the CPITN index?
**Ans.** CPITN index does not record irreversible changes, i.e., recession, tooth mobility, and attachment loss.

**Q6.** What are the types of observational epidemiological studies?
**Ans.** Descriptive and analytical epidemiological studies.

**Q7.** When are experimental, epidemiological studies carried out?
**Ans.** Experimental epidemiology is used to test the hypothesis by introducing a preventive or therapeutic agent and comparing the outcome in test subjects with concurrent observations in control groups.

**Q8.** What are the types of experimental, epidemiological studies?
**Ans.** Randomized controlled trials, field trials, and community trials.

**Q9.** What are the types of analytical observational studies?
**Ans.** Case-control and cohort studies.

**Q10.** What is the Odds ratio?
**Ans.** It is the ratio of exposure among the cases to exposure among the controls.

# Section 3

# Etiology

- ❖ Periodontal Microbiology
- ❖ Dental Plaque
- ❖ Dental Calculus
- ❖ Immunity and Inflammation
- ❖ Pathogenesis and Host Response
- ❖ Genetic Basis of Periodontal Diseases
- ❖ Systemic Factors and Periodontium
- ❖ Periodontal Medicine
- ❖ Smoking and Periodontium

# Chapter 8: Periodontal Microbiology

*Shalu Bathla*

## Chapter Outline
- Criteria for Defining Periodontal Pathogens
- Microbial Complexes in Subgingival Plaque
- Periodontal Pathogens
- Microorganisms Associated

## INTRODUCTION

Microbial etiology of gingival and periodontal diseases needs to be well understood because of two major reasons: First, the identification of etiological agents of periodontal diseases would help determine suitable treatment strategies. Second, it would provide a useful therapeutic approach to control and prevent periodontal diseases, e.g., the manufacturing of vaccines against various pathogens before the onset of diseases.[1] However, periodontal diseases' microbiology is difficult to understand and study due to difficulty in sample collection, cultivation, and identification of isolates. Periodontal infections are mixed infections, and microbiota is very complex, making it hard to distinguish between secondary invaders and true pathogens. Periodontal disease appears to be episodic, and thus, there is a difficulty in differentiating between active and inactive sites for sampling.[2]

## CRITERIA FOR DEFINING PERIODONTAL PATHOGENS

### Koch's Postulates

Koch formulated the following four criteria in order to accept microorganism as the causative agent of an infectious disease (**Fig. 8.1**):[3]

1. *Association*: The microorganisms must be constantly present in every lesion of the disease.
2. *Isolation*: The microorganism must be isolated in pure culture from the diseased lesions of the host.
3. *Inoculation and reproduction of the lesion*: This pure culture of microorganism should reproduce the lesions of the specific disease when inoculated into a suitable animal model.
4. *Reisolation*: The microbes must be reisolated in pure culture from the lesions produced in the experimental animals.

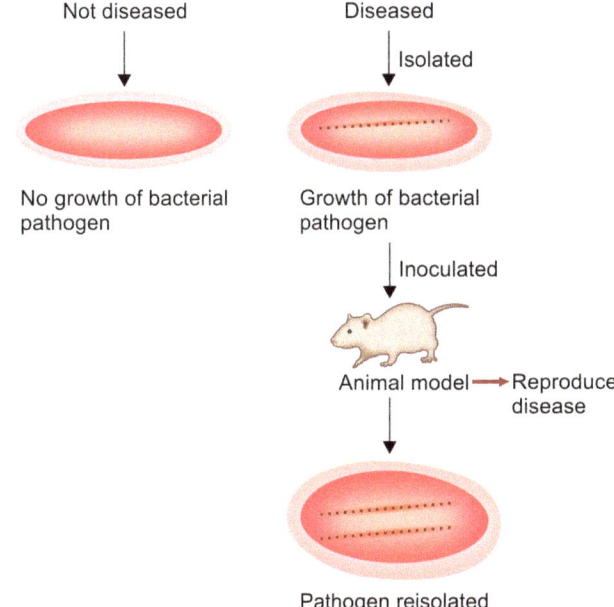

**Fig. 8.1:** Schematic representation showing Koch's postulates.

In the case of periodontal diseases, Koch's postulates have certain limitations:
- *Inability to culture all the organisms*: Practically it is difficult to grow large-sized spirochetes in pure culture in periodontitis cases.
- Applying postulates in periodontal disease is unable to determine the exact state of disease progression.

- *Lack of a good model system*: In many microbial cases, the host range is limited to animal species or to humans. In such cases, causative bacteria do not reproduce (*Porphyromonas gingivalis* are usually unable to colonize in animals).[4]

Thus, Koch's postulates only deal with microbes as a causative agent for disease and lack the role of the environment or the host's influence in disease development and progression.

## Socransky's Criterion

Sigmund Socransky, a researcher at the Forsyth Dental Center in Boston, proposed five criteria by which periodontal microorganisms may be judged to be potential pathogens:[5]

1. *Association of the suspected organism with the lesion*: Association is the first requirement for a microbe to cause a periodontal lesion. Pathogen should be associated with the disease, with an increased number of organisms at diseased sites.
2. *Elimination of the suspected organism*: Organism should be eliminated or decreased in sites where the clinical resolution of disease with treatment has occurred.
3. *Host response to organism*: Microbe should be able to demonstrate an altered host humoral or cellular immune response.
4. *Animal studies*: Pathogens should be capable of causing the same disease in experimental animal models.
5. *Virulence factors*: Potential pathogens should be capable of producing virulence factors, which destroy the periodontal tissues.

## MICROBIAL COMPLEXES IN SUBGINGIVAL PLAQUE

In 1998, Socransky SS et al., conducted a study to define various microbial complexes in subgingival plaque.

Five major microbial complexes identified in the respective study were (**Fig. 8.2**):
1. Yellow complex: *Streptococcus spp., S. sanguinis, S oralis, S. mitis, S. intermedius, S. gordonii*
2. Purple complex: *A. odontolyticus, V. parvula*
3. Green complex: *A. actinomycetemcomitans* serotype a, *Capnocytophaga spp., E. corrodens*
4. Orange complex: *F. nucleatum, Campylobacter gracilis, C. rectus, P. intermedia, P. micros*
5. Red complex: *P. gingivalis, T. denticola, T. forsythia*

## Significance

Microbes from yellow, purple, and green complexes colonize first in subgingival plaque. Microbes from the orange complex are assumed to fill early colonizers. Red complex members are associated with bleeding on probing and are active at advanced stages of plaque development. Green and orange complexes include species recognized as pathogens in both periodontal and nonperiodontal infections.[6]

## PERIODONTAL PATHOGENS

The World Workshop in Periodontology (Consensus Report 1996) identified three microbes as important periodontal pathogens, namely *Aggregatibacter actinomycetemcomitans, P. gingivalis,* and *Tannerella forsythia.*

### *Aggregatibacter Actinomycetemcomitans (Actinobacillus Actinomycetemcomitans)*

In 1912, *A. actinomycetemcomitans* was first isolated by German microbiologist Klinger from a lesion of cervicofacial actinomycosis. The microorganism was isolated together with *Actinomyces israeli*. Hence, the species name

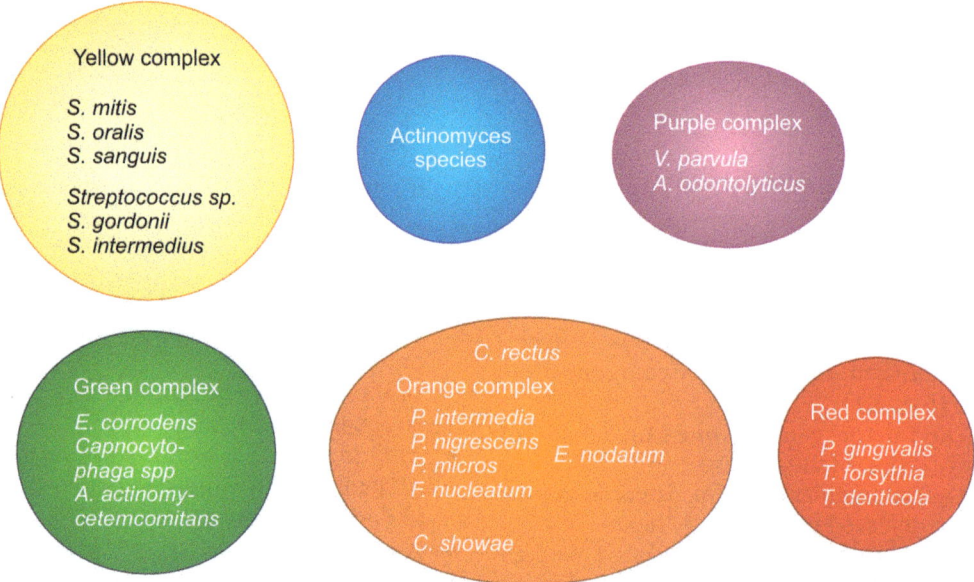

**Fig. 8.2:** Schematic representation showing microbial complexes in subgingival plaque.

actinomycetemcomitans means together with *Actinomyces*. Genus names Actinobacillus: *Actino* referring to star-shaped internal morphology of the colonies and *bacillus* referring to cell shape (rod-shaped).

*Morphological characteristics*: It is a member of the family *Pasteurellaceae*. Its size is approximately $0.4 \pm 0.1 \times 1.0 \pm 0.4$ μm. It is nonsporulating, nonmotile, gram-negative coccobacillus.

It is capnophilic, which requires an atmosphere of 5–10% carbon dioxide ($CO_2$) for its good growth. The solid media growth of small, smooth, convex, circular, and translucent colonies ranging in a diameter of 0.5–1.0 mm appears. They have a slightly irregular edge, and internal morphology has a star-shaped appearance.

*Biochemical characteristics*: A. actinomycetemcomitans is nonhemolytic, fermentative, oxidase, and catalase-positive. It does not produce indole.

*Ultrastructure*: Ultrastructurally, this microbe has outer- and inner-cytoplasmic membranes with periplasmic space in between them. The important features of *A. actinomycetemcomitans* that favor bacterial virulence are the presence of fimbriae, vesicles, and extracellular amorphous material. Fimbriae are the small cell surface filamentous appendages. They are arranged in the form of peritrichous arrays and help in bacterial colonization on host tissues. Vesicles are membrane blebs and lipopolysaccharide in nature. They originate from and become continuous with the outer membrane. The vesicles act as delivery vehicles for *A. actinomycetemcomitans* toxic materials due to its adhesive properties, bacteriocin, endotoxin, and bone resorption activity. Certain *A. actinomycetemcomitans* cells have amorphous material on their surface that frequently embeds adjacent cells in a matrix.

*Serological characteristics*: In 1983, Zambon et al., divided *A. actinomycetemcomitans* into three serotypes as a, b and c.[7,8] Serotype a and b are common in the human oral cavity, and serotype c constitutes approximately 10% of *A. actinomycetemcomitans* human oral isolates. Kaplan et al., in 2001, divided *A. actinomycetemcomitans* into six serotypes from a to f.

*Virulence factors*: It elaborates a myriad of virulence factors in order to maintain itself in the oral cavity.
- Factors interfering with host defense mechanisms are leukotoxin (Ltx), chemotaxis inhibitor, Fc binding protein, and immunosuppressive factors. Ltx has the ability to kill human polymorphonuclear cells (PMNs), lymphocytes, and monocytes. LtxA (116-kDa protein) belongs to the pore-forming toxin family.
- Factors facilitating microbial colonization and existence in the human oral cavity are bacteriocin, adhesins, invasins.
- Factors that destroy host tissues are endotoxin, collagenase, cytotoxin, cytolethal distending toxin, and epitheliotoxin.
- Factors inhibiting host tissues repair are inhibitors of bone formation and fibroblast inhibitory factor.[9]

### *Porphyromonas Gingivalis*

In the late 1970s, the black-pigmented *Bacteroides* was found to contain highly saccharolytic species, namely *Prevotella melaninogenica*, intermediate level of carbohydrate fermenter, i.e., *P. intermedia* or asaccharolyticus, i.e., *Porphyromonas gingivalis*. *P. gingivalis* is an anaerobic, gram-negative, asaccharolytic, nonmotile rod-shaped bacteria, which produce black-pigmented colonies.[1]

*Virulence factors*: *P. gingivalis* produces virulence factors, such as collagenase, endotoxin, fatty acids, ammonia ($NH_3$), hydrogen sulfide ($H_2S$), indole, hemolysin, fibrinolysin, phospholipase A and bone resorption inducing factor. Virulence of *P. gingivalis* is facilitated with its ability to get attached to other bacteria, epithelial cells and connective tissue components, fibronectin, and fibrinogen. The fimbriae have a significant role in the microbial colonization and activation of cytokine production. *P. gingivalis* causes chemokine paralysis by inhibiting the production of interleukin-8 (IL-8) by epithelial cells, which is chemotaxin for PMNs. Thus, it inhibits PMN migration.[10]

*Gingipains*: This is the important virulence factor of *P. gingivalis*. Travis and colleagues originally coined the term "gingipain." These extracellular cysteine proteinases are arginine-specific proteinase, i.e., RgpA and RgpB and other lysine-specific proteinases, i.e., Kgp. Three different genes encode these gingipains, i.e., RgpA, RgpB, and kgp.[11]

Functions of these enzymes are to:
- Activate kallikrein/kinin system
- Downregulate polymorphonuclear neutrophils
- Activate the blood clotting system
- Disturb host defense system: Gingipains degrade different components of the complement system.
- Stimulate and activate matrix metalloproteinases (MMPs): Gingipain directly activates latent MMPs. Rgp stimulates the expression of MMP-1.

### *Tannerella Forsythia (Bacteroides Forsythus)*

In the mid of 1970s, *T. forsythia* was first isolated at the Forsyth Institute from the patient with progressing advanced periodontitis and was described as Fusiform Bacteroides by Tanner et al. It is an anaerobic, gram-negative, spindle-shaped, highly pleomorphic rod. This species is difficult to grow alone, and for its growth, it requires N-acetylmuramic acid.[12] Its growth is enhanced by cocultivation with *Fusobacterium nucleatum*.[13]

*Virulence factors*: The various virulence factors produced by *T. forsythia* are fatty acid, endotoxin, and methylglyoxal.

## Others

Spirochetes are anaerobic, gram-negative, motile, helical-shaped rods of 5–15 μm long with a diameter of 0.5 μm organisms. They have 3–8 irregular spirals. Classified species of spirochetes include *Treponema pallidum* (associated with secondary syphilis); *T. denticola, T. vincentii, T. socranskii* (often associated with periodontitis). The virulence factors of *T. denticola* are proteolytic enzymes that destroy immunoglobulins, mainly immunoglobulin A (IgA), immunoglobulin M (IgM), immunoglobulin G (IgG) and complement factors. They penetrate epithelium and connective tissue, degrade collagen and dentin and destroy complement factors and immunoglobulins. Two major difficulties associated with spirochetes species are: (i) isolation and cultivation of spirochetes species, and (ii) difficulty in identifying and understanding different oral spirochetes species. Cultivable treponemes require growth medium enriched with infusions of animal organs, trypsin digests of casein, various fatty acids, and accessory growth factors. Along with this, some cultivable species need persistent anaerobic culture for proper growth.[14]

*Fusobacterium nucleatum* is an anaerobic, gram-negative, cigar-shaped bacillus with pointed ends. Because Fusobacterium coaggregate with most oral microorganisms, they are believed to be important bridging organisms between the primary (early) and secondary (late) colonizers during colonization. This organism can induce apoptotic cell death in mononuclear and PMNs and can trigger the release of elastase, cytokines and oxygen radicals from leukocytes.[15]

*Prevotella intermedia* is an anaerobic, gram-negative and short round-ended rod.

*Campylobacter rectus* is a gram-negative anaerobic vibrio. It is short but motile. When cultured on blood agar plates, it forms small convex, corroding, or pitting colonies. It produces leukotoxin and is capable of stimulating fibroblasts.

*Peptostreptococcus micros* are gram-positive and grow obligate anaerobically. It is one of the rare cocci in periodontitis.[16]

## Viruses

Viruses are much smaller than bacteria. The involvement of viruses in periodontitis is assumed for a long time. The presence of virion defines the significant role of the virus in disease causation. The virion is an extracellular infectious virus particle (30–150 nm), which forms an infective form of the virus. It is composed of nucleic acid, which is either deoxyribonucleic acid (DNA) or ribonucleic acid (RNA). A protein shell surrounds this nucleic acid called a capsid. The capsid, along with the enclosed nucleic acid, is called a nucleocapsid. The capsid is either icosahedral, i.e., cubical or helical.

There are mainly four viral families associated with oral viral diseases:

1. *Herpes viruses*: Herpes virus virion size is approximately 120–250 nm, and the capsid is icosahedral, composed of 162 capsomers and enclose linear double-stranded DNA genome.[3] There are eight human herpes virus species, namely: (1) herpes simplex virus-1 (HSV-1), (2) herpes simplex virus-2 (HSV-2), (3) varicella-zoster virus (VZV), (4) Epstein–Barr virus (EBV),(5) human cytomegalovirus (HCMV), (6) herpes simplex virus-6 (HSV-6), (7) herpes simplex virus-7 (HSV-7), and (8) herpes simplex virus-8 (HSV-8). Herpes simplex virus may cause primary acute herpetic gingivostomatitis (AHGS). EBV-1 and HCMV are present in Papillon–Lefevre syndrome periodontitis, localized aggressive periodontitis (LAP), and in severe chronic periodontitis patients.

   Herpes viruses can cause periodontal tissue destruction through two pathways: (i) a direct cytopathic effect was produced due to virus infection and replications on fibroblasts, endothelial cells, keratinocytes, and other inflammatory cells. HCMV specifically infects macrophages and T cells, and EBV infects B cells. HCMV modulate antigen-specific T lymphocyte leading to increase CD8 suppressor cells, and (ii) indirect result is produced due to virus-associated impairment of the immune-defense mechanism. This enhances the virulence of bacterial periopathogens. *A. actinomycetemcomitans* counts get elevated in cases of LAP lesions when associated with active human cytomegalovirus infection. In chronic periodontitis, due to the presence of HCMV or EBV-1, there is the elevated occurrence of various periopathogens, such as *P. gingivalis, P. intermedia, T. denticola, T. forsythia,* and *C. rectus* (Flowchart 8.1).[17]
2. *Human papillomaviruses*: They are small, non-enveloped, icosahedral, double-stranded DNA viruses.
3. *Retroviruses.*
4. *Picornaviruses*: These are small, nonenveloped, icosahedral RNA viruses like coxsackie.[3]

## MICROORGANISMS ASSOCIATED

### Periodontal Health

Beneficial species of the host affect the disease progression by preventing the colonization/proliferation of pathogenic microorganisms, e.g., hydrogen peroxide produced by *S. sanguinis* is lethal to *A. actinomycetemcomitans*. Sometimes, these species also degrade the virulence factors produced by the pathogens. Following are the beneficial microorganisms:[2]

- *S. sanguinis*
- *S. mitis*
- *Capnocytophaga* sp.
- *Veillonella*
- *Atopobium* sp.
- *Gemella* sp.

**Flowchart 8.1:** Herpes virus causing periodontal tissue destruction.

```
Bacteria plaque --Causes--> Gingivitis
                                |
                              Causes
                                ↓
          Influx of inflammatory cells containing latent herpes viruses
                                ↓
Immunosuppression, stress, infection ---> Herpes virus activation
                                          |
                    ┌─────────Causes──────┼──────────────────┐
                    ↓                     ↓                  ↓
            Direct cytotoxicity    Immunosuppression    Overgrowth of pathogenic bacteria
                    └─────────────────────┼──────────────────┘
                                          ↓
                            Periodontal tissue destruction
```

## Chronic Gingivitis/Dental Plaque-induced Gingivitis[15]

- Gram-positive organisms:
  - *S. sanguinis*
  - *S. oralis*
  - *S. mitis*
  - *S. intermedius*
  - *A. viscosus*
  - *A. naeslundii*
  - *Peptostreptococcus micros*
- Gram-negative organisms:
  - *P. intermedia*
  - *Veillonella parvula*
  - *F. nucleatum*
  - *Haemophilus*
  - *Campylobacter* sp.
  - *Capnocytophaga*

## Chronic Periodontitis[15]

- *P. gingivalis*
- *P. intermedia*
- *T. forsythia*
- *F. nucleatum*
- *Eikenella corrodens*
- *C. rectus*
- *A. actinomycetemcomitans*
- *Treponema*
- *P. micros*
- *Eubacterium* sp.
- Herpes virus group: EBV-1, HCMV[18]

## Localized Aggressive Periodontis[19, 20]

- *A. actinomycetemcomitans*
- *P. gingivalis*
- *C. rectus*
- *F. nucleatum*
- *E. corrodens*
- *Capnocytophaga* sp.

- *Eubacterium brachy*
- *B. capillus*
- Spirochetes
- Herpes viruses including EBV-1, HCMV[18]

## Necrotizing Periodontal Disease[21]

- Spirochetes
- *P. intermedia*

## Abscesses of Periodontium[22]

- *P. intermedia*
- *P. gingivalis*
- *F. nucleatum*
- *T. forsythia*
- *P. micros*

**TABLE 8.1:** New names of various periodontal bacteria.

| Previous name | Current name |
| --- | --- |
| *Wolinella recta* | *Campylobacter rectus* |
| *Bacteroides intermedius* | *Prevotella intermedia* |
| *Bacteroides gingivalis* | *Porphyromonas gingivalis* |
| *Bacteroides melaninogenicus* | *Prevotella melaninogenica* |
| *Bacteroides forsythus* | *Tannerella forsythia* |
| *Actinobacillus actinomycetemcomitans* | *Aggregatibacter actinomycetemcomitans* |
| *Streptococcus sanguis* | *Streptococcus sanguinis* |

### Points to Ponder

- Ecosystems/niches present in the oral cavity are:
  - Supragingival hard surfaces: (teeth, implants, restoration, and prostheses), periodontal/peri-implant pocket, buccal epithelium, palatal epithelium, epithelium of the floor of the mouth and dorsum of the tongue.
  - Subgingival ecologic niches present in the oral cavity are: Tooth/implant surface, gingival exudate fluid medium, the surface of epithelial cells, and a superficial portion of the pocket epithelium.
- New names of various periodontal bacteria are mentioned in **Table 8.1**.

## REFERENCES

1. Zambon JJ. Microbiology of periodontal disease. In: Genco RJ, Goldman HM, Cohen DW (Eds). Contemporary Periodontics. St. Louis: CV Mosby; 1990. pp. 147-60.
2. Haake SK, Newman MG, Nisengard RJ, Sanz M. Periodontal Microbiology. In: Newman MG, Takei HH, Carranza FA (Eds). Carranza's Clinical Periodontology, 9th edition. Philadelphia, PA, USA: WB Saunders; 2003. pp. 96-112.
3. Ananthanarayan P. Historical introduction. In: Ananthanarayan P. Textbook of Microbiology, 6th edition. New Delhi, India: Orient Longman; 2002. pp. 1-6.
4. Socransky SS, Haffajee AD. The bacterial etiology of destructive periodontal disease: current concepts. J Periodontol. 1992;63(4 Suppl):322-31.
5. Socransky SS, Haffajee AD. Microbiology of periodontal disease. In: Lindhe J, Karring T, Lang NP (Eds). Clinical Periodontology and Implant Dentistry, 4th edition. Blackwell Munksgaard; 2003. pp. 106-49.
6. Socransky SS, Haffajee AD, Cugini MA, Smith C, Kent RL. Microbial complexes in subgingival plaque. J Clin Periodontol. 1998;25(2):134-44.
7. Zambon JJ. Actinobacillus actinomycetemcomitans in human periodontal disease. J Clin Periodontol. 1985;12(1):1-20.
8. Slots J, Reynolds HS, Genco RJ. Actinobacillus actinomycetemcomitans in human periodontal disease: a cross-sectional microbiological investigation. Infect Immun. 1980;29:1013-20.
9. Fives-Taylor PM, Meyer DH, Mintz KP, Brissette C. Virulence factors of Actinobacillus actinomycetemcomitans. Periodontol 2000. 1999;20:136-67.
10. Darveau RP, Belton CM, Reife RA, Lemont RJ. Local chemokine paralysis, a novel pathogenic mechanism for Porphyromonas gingivalis. Infect Immun. 1998;66(4):1660-5.
11. Pandit N, Changela R, Bali D, Tikoo P, Gugnani S. Porphyromonas gingivalis: Its virulence and vaccine. J Int Clin Dent Res Organ. 2015;7(1):51-8.
12. Wyss C. Dependence of the proliferation of Bacteroides forsythus on exogenous N-acetylmuramic acid. Infect Immun. 1989;57(6):1757-9.
13. Socransky SS, Haffajee AD, Dzink JL. Relationship of subgingival microbial complexes to clinical features at the sampled sites. J Clin Periodontol. 1988;15(7):440-4.
14. Ellen RP, Galimanas VB. Spirochetes at the forefront of periodontal infections. Periodontol 2000. 2005;38:13-32.
15. Moore WE, Moore LV. The bacteria of periodontal diseases. Periodontol 2000. 1994;5:66-77.
16. Nishihara T, Koseki T. Microbial etiology of periodontitis. Periodontol 2000. 2004;36:14-26.
17. Slots J. Herpesviruses in periodontal diseases. Periodontol 2000. 2005;38:33-62.
18. Contreras A, Slots J. Herpesviruses in human periodontal disease. J Periodontal Res. 2000;35(1):3-16.
19. Kornman KS, Robertson PB. Clinical and microbiological evaluation of therapy for juvenile periodontitis. J Periodontol. 1985;56(8):443-6.
20. Moore WE. Microbiology of periodontal disease. J Periodontal Res. 1987;22(5):335-41.
21. Listgarten MA. Electron microscopic observations on the bacterial flora of acute necrotizing ulcerative gingivitis. J Periodontol. 1965;36:328-39.
22. Herrera D, Roldan S, Gonzalez I, Sanz M. The periodontal abscess (I). Clinical and microbiological findings. J Clin Periodontol. 2000;27(6):387-94.

## VIVA VOCE

**Q1.** Who discovered *Tannerella forsythia*?
**Ans.** *Tannerella forsythia* was first isolated at the Forsyth Institute from subjects with progressing advanced periodontitis in the mid-1970s and was described as Fusiform Bacteroides by Tanner et al.

**Q2.** Who discovered *Actinobacillus actinomycetemcomitans*?
**Ans.** *Actinobacillus actinomycetemcomitans* was first isolated by German microbiologist Klinger, in 1912 from a lesion of cervicofacial actinomycosis. The microorganism was isolated together with *A. israelli*. Hence, the species name actinomycetemcomitans means together with Actinomyces. Genus name *Actinobacillus*, "actino," referring to star-shaped internal morphology of the colonies and bacillus referring to cell shape (rod-shaped).

**Q3.** What are the various species of Bacteroides?
**Ans.** The various species of Bacteroides are as follows:
- Asaccharolytics: *P. gingivalis*
- Intermediate level of carbohydrate fermenter: *P. intermedia*
- Highly saccharolytic: *P. melaninogenica*.

**Q4.** Name the bacteria which invade epithelial cells.
**Ans.** Bacteria invading epithelial cells are as follows:
- *P. gingivalis*
- *A. actinomycetemcomitans*
- Spirochetes (*T. pallidum*)
- *F. nucleatum*

**Q5.** Name the motile bacteria.
**Ans.** Motile bacteria are:
- *Spirochetes*
- *C. rectus*
- *Selenomonas*

**Q6.** **Name the bacteria which produce leukotoxin (Ltx).**
**Ans.** Bacteria producing leukotoxin are:
- *A. actinomycetemcomitans*
- *C. rectus*

**Q7.** **Name various gingipains produced by *P. gingivalis*.**
**Ans.** Arginine-specific proteinase, i.e., RgpA and RgpB and lysine-specific proteinase, i.e., Kgp.

**Q 8.** **Name various virulence factors produced by *P. gingivalis*.**
**Ans.** Collagenase, endotoxin, fatty acids, ammonia, hydrogen sulfide, indole, hemolysin, fibrinolysin, phospholipase A and bone resorption are inducing factors.

**Q9.** **Name various virulence factors produced by *A. actinomycetemcomitans*.**
**Ans.** Leukotoxin, chemotaxis inhibitor, Fc binding protein, and immunosuppressive factors.

**Q10.** **What are the differences between transmission, contagious, and translocation?**
**Ans.** Following are the differences between transmission, contagious, and translocation:

| | |
|---|---|
| Transmission: | ◆ Passing of microorganisms directly from one person to another |
| | ◆ Periopathogens are transmissible within the members of the family |
| | ◆ Transmission of cariogenic species from mother to child |
| Contagious: | This refers to the likelihood of a microorganism causing disease after being transmitted from an infected to an uninfected host |
| Translocation: | Intraoral transmission of bacteria from one niche to another. Also called as cross-infection |

# Chapter 9

# Dental Plaque

Shashikant Hegde, Shalu Bathla

## Chapter Outline

- Biofilm
- Definition
- Classification
- Clinical Assessment
- Composition
- Plaque Formation
- Microscopic Structure
- Metabolic Interactions
- Various Plaque Hypotheses
- Clinical Significance
- Other Tooth Deposits

## INTRODUCTION

A biofilm is defined as a single cell and microcolonies enclosed in a highly hydrated, predominately anionic exopolymer matrix. These sessile cells behave in different ways from their free-floating planktonic ones.[1]

Biofilms are the microbial colonization of diverse microorganisms usually located on hard nonshedding material, including tooth surface areas. Biofilm formation occurs on both living and nonliving materials due to microbial adherence to wetted surfaces. Oral cavity, contact lenses, medical implant devices, water pipes and aquatic systems including boats and docks, are common places favoring biofilm formation.[2]

## BIOFILM

Each microbial colony from the biofilm cluster is an independent and well-organized community. Each microcolony is sessile and mushroom-shaped with its own customized living environment. In biofilms, microcolonies of bacterial cells are distributed in the glycocalyx matrix.[3] Presence of water channels in between the microcolonies permits the exchange of nutrients and bacterial products throughout the biofilm.[4]

Biofilm bacteria adapted certain properties due to its natural biofilm environment. These bacterial characteristics are different from their planktonic state. This helps to understand dental plaque as a biofilm and not as bacteria in the planktonic state.

## Properties Adapted by Biofilm

The properties adapted by biofilm bacteria are as follows:

### Quorum Sensing

Quorum sensing is a way of the cell to cell communication that regulates gene expression by sharing information on cell-population density. It is the chief method of sharing information by biofilm-associated bacteria. It involves bacteria-induced production and release of signaling compounds that mediate intercellular communication and elicit the regulation of specific gene expression. These signaling compounds are known as autoinducer and exist in two forms, namely 1 and 2. Autoinducer 2 is released by both Gram-positive and Gram-negative bacteria and encoded by the *luxS* gene. In *Streptococcus gordonii*, *luxS* facilitates the expression of *sspA* and *sspB* genes and encodes for a protein that provides a binding site for the attachment of major fimbriae *Porphyromonas gingivalis*. Thus, *S. gordonii* acts as an early colonizer and provide preferential attachment to *P. gingivalis* which function as a secondary colonizer.[5]

### Gene Transfer

The process of horizontal gene transfer has great potential to exchange genetic information in biofilm bacterial communities. In the case of *S. mutan* intercellular communications via quorum sensing is facilitated through competence stimulating peptide (CSP). Genes of the CSP signaling system such as *comC*, *comD*, *comE*, *comX* mediate various functions like biofilm formation and competence, i.e., ability to accept foreign deoxyribonucleic acid (DNA) and acid tolerance.[6]

### Antimicrobial Resistance

In comparison to planktonic counterpart, biofilm bacteria have stronger resistance (1,000–1,500 times) to biocides and antimicrobial agents. In this regard, the possible hypothesis explaining the increased resistance to antimicrobials is as follows:[7]

- *First*: The exopolysaccharide from the biofilm matrix impede the diffusion of antimicrobial agents.
- *Second*: Due to physiological differences among biofilm bacteria, only a part of biofilm bacteria is usually susceptible to growth-dependent antibiotics.
- *Third*: Due to genetic changes that happened in the transition from planktonic to biofilm bacteria, such bacteria become insensitive to various biocides and antimicrobial agents.
- *Fourth*: A slower rate of growth of biofilm organisms due to nutrient limitation may also lead to antimicrobial resistance.
- *Finally*: Extracellular enzymes, such as β-lactamase and formaldehyde dehydrogenase becomes concentrated in the extracellular matrix and inactivates some antibiotics.

### Regulation of Gene Expression

Biofilm living has found to possess great potential in controlling differential gene expression processes. In the oral cavity, exposure of *S. gordonii* to saliva induces *sspA/B* genes, which mediate host surface binding and coaggregation with *P. gingivalis* and *Actinomyces* spp. Likewise, in biofilm-associated *S. mutans* genes encoding glucan (*gtf*) and fructan (*ftf*) synthesis are differentially regulated.[8]

### Biofilm-associated Bacterial Antigens and Virulence Factors

- Heat shock proteins (HSPs): HSPs belong to the family of stress proteins which are usually synthesized by bacterial cells, when exposed to the environment. It is a bacterial-cellular way to respond to diverse environmental stresses, such as temperature, pH, infection, inflammation, and redox potential. Selected HSPs act as molecular chaperones and play a vital role in the assembly and folding of proteins. Hence, HSPs are better known for their cytoprotective role by protecting the cell from the damaging effects of environmental stress. HSPs are classified based on their molecular weight. HSP60, HSP70, and HSP80 refer to families of HSPs on the order of 60 kDa, 70 kDa, and 80 kDa in size, respectively. In *Aggregatibacter actinomycetemcomitans*, HSPs at lower doses stimulate osteoblast activation and epithelial proliferation while are cytotoxic at high doses. Microbial HSPs are usually related to an array of autoimmune diseases, such as rheumatoid arthritis and atherosclerosis. Accumulative pieces of evidence reported the link between prolonged exposures to HSPs and the occurrence of periodontitis and subsequent role in promoting autoimmune disease.[6]
- Lipopolysaccharides, fimbriae, and extracellular proteolytic enzymes.

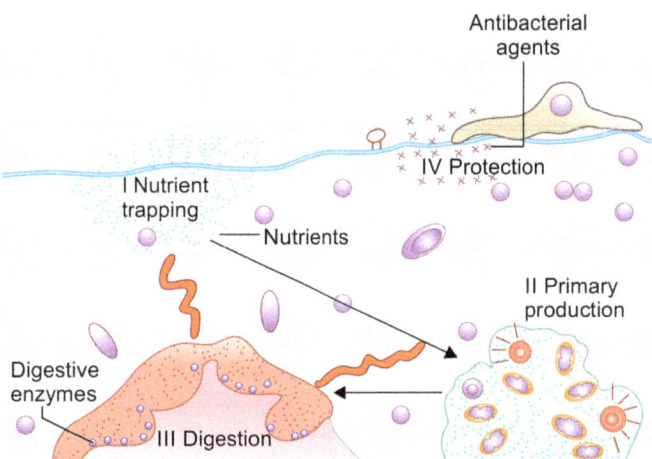

**Fig. 9.1:** Schematic representation showing characteristic features of plaque biofilm: I—Nutrients are trapped; II—Own nutrients are produced; III—Nutrients are digested and IV—Protected from antibacterial agents.

### Functions of Biofilm

Functions of biofilm are to **(Fig. 9.1)**:[3]

- Facilitate processing and uptake of nutrients
- Protect and cross-feed one species
- Provide nutrients for another species

## DEFINITION

According to World Health Organization (WHO) in 1978, "Dental plaque is defined as a specific but highly variable structural entity resulting from sequential colonization and growth of microorganisms on the surfaces of teeth and restoration consisting of microorganisms of various strains and species are embedded in the extracellular matrix, composed of bacterial metabolic products and substance from serum, saliva, and blood."

Dental plaque can be defined as the soft deposits that form the biofilm adhering to the tooth surface or other hard surfaces in the oral cavity, including removable and fixed restorations.[9]

Plaque can be described as the soft, tenacious material found on tooth surfaces which is not readily removed by rinsing with water.[10]

## CLASSIFICATION

Based on the position on the tooth and implant surface **(Flowchart 9.1, Fig. 9.2 and Table 9.1)**:

- *Supragingival plaque*: Plaque present above or at the level of marginal gingiva.[11]
    - Coronal: Plaque present above the level of the marginal gingiva

**Section 3:** Etiology

**Flowchart 9.1:** Classification of plaque based on the position of plaque on the tooth or implant surface.

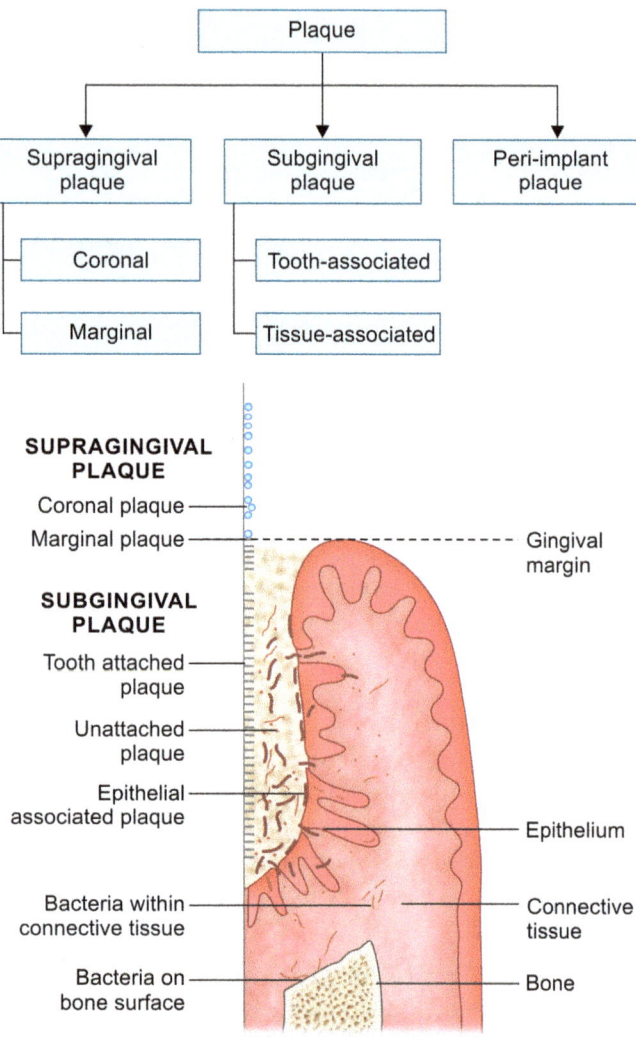

**Fig. 9.2:** Schematic representation showing supragingival and subgingival plaques.

- Marginal: Plaque present at the level of marginal gingiva.
- *Subgingival plaque*: Plaque located between the tooth and the gingival sulcular tissue just beneath the marginal gingiva **(Fig. 9.2 and Tables 9.2 and 9.3)**.[11]
    - Tooth-associated subgingival plaque
    - Tissue-associated subgingival plaque
- *Peri-implant plaque*: Plaque presents around the exposed threads or textured surfaces of the implant.

## CLINICAL ASSESSMENT

The following methods can assess plaque:
- *Direct vision*: Plaque becomes detectable with naked eyes after an uninterrupted formation for 1–2 days.
- *Using explorer/probe*: With the help of an explorer or probe, the tooth surface can be scraped to detect plaque.
- *Using disclosing agents*: Plaque can be easily detected by using a disclosing solution or tablet **(Fig. 9.3)**. Disclosing

**TABLE 9.2:** Differences between tooth and tissue associated subgingival plaque.

| Parameters | Subgingival plaque | |
| --- | --- | --- |
| | **Tooth-associated** | **Tissue-associated** |
| Extension | Does not extend to the junctional epithelium | Extends to the junctional epithelium |
| Penetration | May penetrate cementum | May penetrate epithelium and connective tissue |
| Microorganisms predominate | Gram-positive bacteria: S. mitis, S. sanguinis, A. naeslundii, Eubacterium | Gram-negative bacteria: S. oralis, P. micros, P. gingivalis, P. intermedia, T. forsythia, F. nucleatum |
| Clinical significance | Associated with calculus formation and root caries | Associated with gingivitis and periodontitis |

**TABLE 9.1:** Differences between supragingival and subgingival plaques.

| Parameters | Supragingival plaque | Subgingival plaque |
| --- | --- | --- |
| Location | Coronal to the margin of free gingiva | Apical to the margin of free gingiva |
| Origin | Salivary glycoprotein and salivary microorganisms | Downgrowth of bacteria from supragingival plaque |
| Distribution | Areas left uncleaned, cervical third and proximal surfaces | Attached plaque covers calculus, and unattached plaque extends to the periodontal attachment |
| Retention | The rough surface of teeth or restoration, malposition teeth, and carious lesion | Overhanging margins of filling and periodontal pockets |
| Structure | Adherent, densely packed microbial layer over pellicle on the tooth surface | Tooth surface-attached plaque; unattached plaque; epithelium-attached plaque |
| Predominate microorganisms | Primarily gram-positive, aerobic population, cocci | Primarily gram-negative, anaerobic population, motile, spirochetes, rods |
| Source of nutrients for bacterial proliferation[12] | Saliva and ingested food | Gingival crevicular fluid (GCF), exudate and leukocytes |
| Clinical significance | Causes gingivitis, supragingival calculus, and dental caries | Causes gingivitis, periodontal infection and subgingival calculus |

**TABLE 9.3:** Plaque microorganisms associated with tooth and tissue.

| Tooth associated plaque microorganisms: | • *Streptococcus sanguinis*<br>• *S. mitis*<br>• *Actinomyces viscosus*<br>• *A. naeslundii*<br>• *Eubacterium* sp. |
|---|---|
| Tissue associated plaque microorganisms: | • *Staphylococcus intermedius*<br>• *S. oralis*<br>• *P. micros*<br>• *P. gingivalis*<br>• *P. intermedia*<br>• *F. nucleatum*<br>• *T. forsythia* |

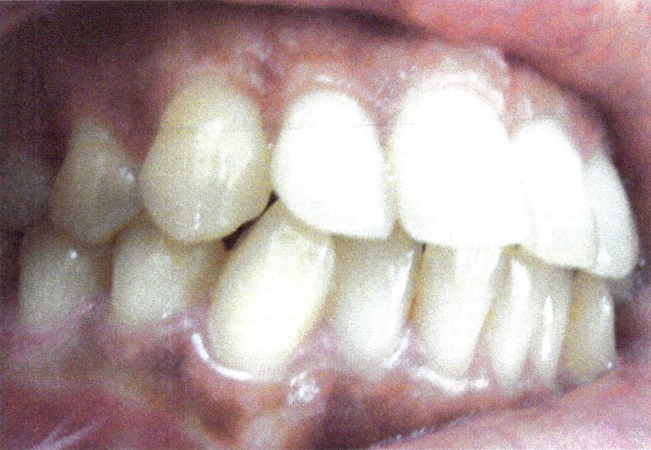

**Fig. 9.4:** Clinical picture showing plaque not visible through the naked eye.

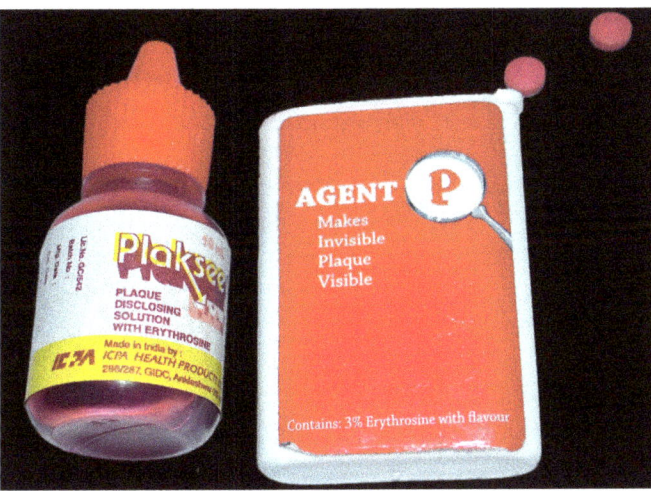

**Fig. 9.3:** Photograph showing disclosing agents: liquid and tablet form. (*Source*: ICPA Health Products Ltd.)

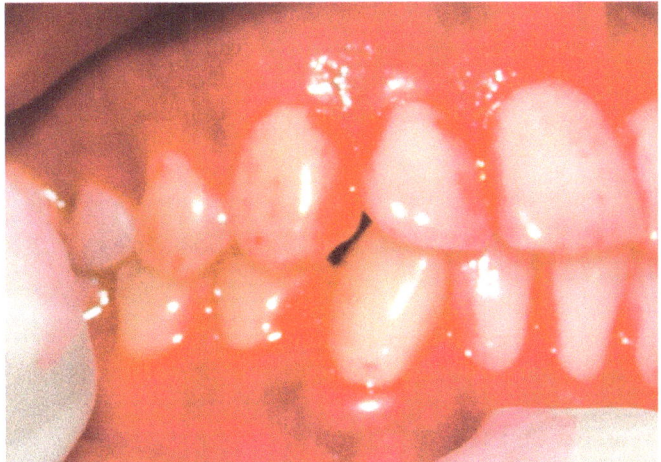

**Fig. 9.5:** Clinical picture showing plaque visible through the use of disclosing agent.

solution contains a dye or other coloring substance, which imparts its color to calculus, plaque, and films on the surface of teeth, tongue, and gingiva **(Figs. 9.4 and 9.5)**. Such characteristics are due to interaction resulting from differences between the polarity of the plaque components and the dyes. The particles are bound to the surface by electrostatic interaction (proteins) and hydrogen bonds (polysaccharides). The various disclosing agents are Skinner iodine solution, iodine disclosing solution, basic fuchsin, Bismarck brown, erythrosin [United States Federal Food, Drug, and Cosmetic Act (FDC) Red No. 3], two-tone dye (FDC Red No. 3 and FDC Green No. 3).[12]

- *Clinical records*: There are various indices for recording and scoring plaque, which is explained in "Chapter 7: Epidemiology".

## COMPOSITION

Dental plaque is mainly composed of microorganisms. The material present between the bacteria in the dental plaque is called an intermicrobial matrix, which is approximately 20–30% of the plaque volume.[11] Plaque microbes, saliva, and gingival exudates are the sources that contribute to the intermicrobial matrix **(Flowchart 9.2)**.

- *Microorganisms*:
  - Bacterial: There are approximately 700 distinct bacterial species and approximately $2 \times 10^8$ bacteria are present in 1 mg of dental plaque.[13]
  - Nonbacterial: Mycoplasma, yeasts, protozoa and viruses.[14]
- *Intercellular matrix*:
  - Host cells: Intermicrobial matrix constitutes a range of host cells, including epithelial cells, macrophages, and leukocytes.
  - Organic compounds: These are polysaccharides, proteins, glycoproteins, and lipid materials. Polysaccharides, mainly dextran, are produced by bacteria. Albumin originates from the crevicular fluid. Saliva contains glycoproteins, which form an essential component of the pellicle. It is also known to initially coat a clean tooth surface. The lipid material is composed of disrupted bacterial and host cell membrane debris.[11]

**Section 3:** Etiology

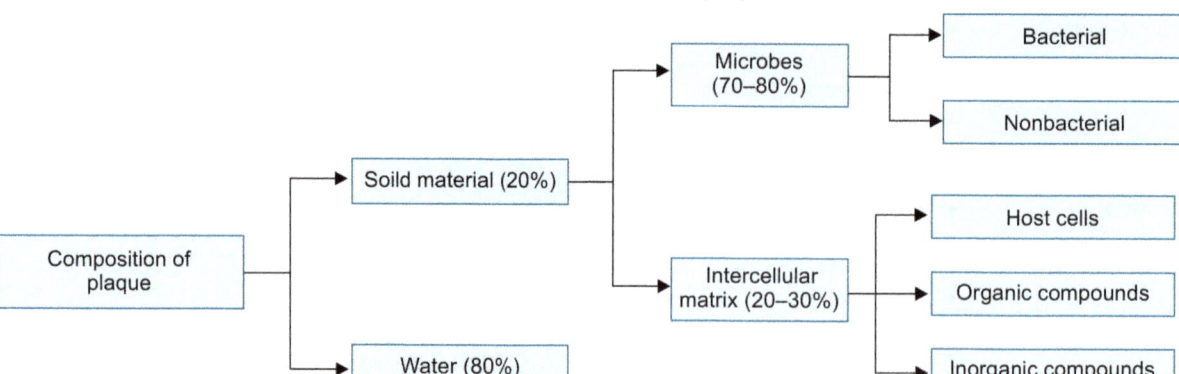

Flowchart 9.2: Composition of plaque.

- Inorganic compounds: These are calcium, phosphorus, fluoride, sodium, and potassium. Saliva is the prime source of inorganic constituents of supragingival plaque. Once the mineral content increases, the plaque mass becomes calcified to form calculus. The inorganic component of subgingival plaque is derived from crevicular fluid.[11]

## PLAQUE FORMATION

The plaque formation is divided into three phases (Fig. 9.6):[11]
1. Pellicle formation
2. Initial colonization of microorganisms
3. Secondary colonization and maturation of microbes

### Phase I: Pellicle Formation

Pellicle formation is the prerequisite for the development of plaque. The pellicle is composed of a variety of salivary glycoproteins (mucins) that are derived from saliva, crevicular fluid, bacterial, and host tissue cells. Van der Waal forces, electrostatic forces, and hydrophobic forces play a crucial role in pellicle formation. Hydrophobic macromolecules adsorb on the tooth surface to form this conditioning film called acquired pellicle. Three types of time-dependent adsorption of salivary proteins take place to progress the pellicle formation process. Salivary proteins, such as proline-rich protein-3 (PRP-3), PRP-4, and statherin, get adsorb very fast onto hydroxyapatite (HAP) while amylase, glycosylated PRP (PRG) and cystatins bind slowly. The third type of protein adsorption is noted in PRP-1, PRP-2, and histatins. It is a two-step process with rapid adsorption involving the direct binding of proteins to HAP, followed by slow adsorption with protein-protein interactions.[15] This pellicle then alters the charge and free energy of the tooth surface, which in turn increases the efficiency of bacterial adhesion.

### Phase II: Initial Colonization of Microorganisms

Early/initial colonizers are gram-positive facultative microbes, such as *Actinomyces viscosus* and *S. sanguis*.[16]

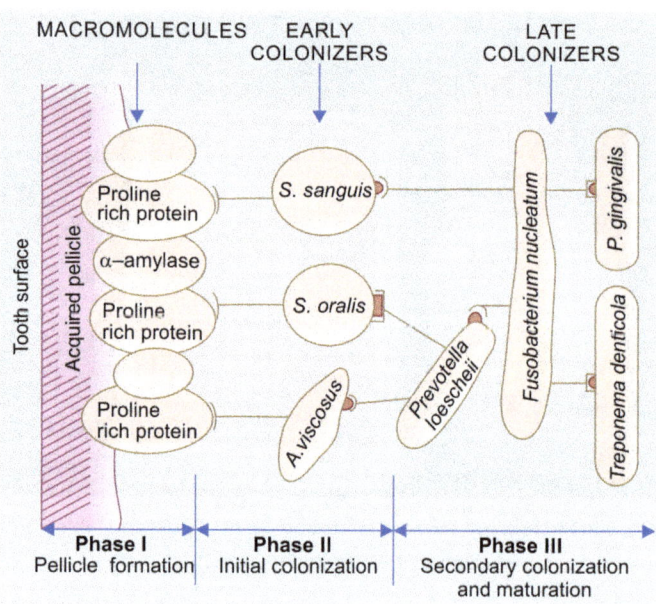

**Fig. 9.6:** Schematic representation showing phases of plaque formation.

Both get attached variably to the pellicle-coated tooth surfaces. Some possess specific attachment structures, such as extracellular polymeric substances and fimbriae, which enable them to attach rapidly upon contact. There is an interaction of receptors of the dental pellicle and adhesins of the bacterial surface. *A. viscosus* has fimbriae on which protein adhesins bind specifically to proline-rich proteins (PRPs) found in the dental pellicle.

### Phase III: Secondary Colonization and Maturation of Microbes

Late/secondary colonizers are gram-negative bacteria (*P. intermedia, P. gingivalis, Fusobacterium nucleatum*),[17] which do not initially colonize clean or pellicle-coated tooth surfaces but may get attach to early colonizers or among themselves by the process called coaggregation. Coaggregation is the characteristic of various species and genera of plaque microbes to adhere to each other. *F. nucleatum* is believed to be important in bridging between primary and secondary colonizers. Examples of the interaction of secondary colonizers with early colonizers are *F. nucleatum* with *S. sanguis*;[18] *Prevotella loescheii* with *A. viscosus*;[19] *Capnocytophaga ochraceus* with *A. viscosus*.[20] The examples of interaction among secondary colonizers are *F. nucleatum* with *P. gingivalis*; *F. nucleatum* with *Treponema denticola*.[21]

## MICROSCOPIC STRUCTURE

### Supragingival Plaque

Corncob structures are common at the surface of the supragingival deposits. These structures have an inner core of rod-shaped bacterial cells (*F. nucleatum*) and over the surface of which is attached to the coccal cells (*Streptococci* or *P. gingivalis*).[22] The term corncob was coined by Jones in 1971 because they resembled an ear of corn **(Fig. 9.7)**.[23]

### Subgingival Plaque

With increasing thickness of plaque, diffusion in and out becomes more and more difficult. An oxygen gradient develops as a result of rapid utilization by the superficial bacterial layers and poor diffusion of oxygen through the matrix. Completely anaerobic conditions eventually emerge in the deeper layers of the deposits. This leads to the transition from gram-positive to gram-negative microorganisms. In the subgingival plaque, test tube brush or bristle brush structures are common. These are composed of filamentous bacteria to which gram-negative rods adhere **(Fig. 9.8)**.[24] Tissue-associated subgingival plaque microorganisms are *S. intermedius*, *S. oralis*, *P. micros*, *P. intermedia*, *P. gingivalis*, *T. forsythia* and *F. nucleatum*.[11]

## METABOLIC INTERACTIONS

Metabolic interactions among different bacterial species found in plaque are **(Flowchart 9.3)**:
- Synergistic/agonistic interactions:[25]
  - *Streptococcus* and *Actinomyces* produce lactate and formate as metabolic byproducts, which are used in the metabolism of *Veillonella* and *Campylobacter*, respectively.
  - *Veillonella* produces menadione, which is used by *P. gingivalis* and *P. intermedia*.
  - *Campylobacter* produces protoheme, which is used by *P. gingivalis*.
  - *P. gingivalis* produces isobutyrate, which is utilized by *Treponema*.
  - *Treponema* and *Capnocytophaga* produce succinate, which is used by *P. gingivalis*.
- Antagonistic interactions:[26]
  - *S. sanguinis* produces hydrogen peroxide ($H_2O_2$), which kills *Aggregatibacter actinomycetemcomitans*.
  - *A. actinomycetemcomitans* produce bacteriocin, which kills *S. sanguinis*.

Metabolic interactions between the host and microorganisms are found in plaque. The host acts as an essential source of nutrients. The breakdown of host hemoglobin provides hemin iron, which is essential in the metabolism of *P. gingivalis*. Bacteria are using ammonia released by the degradation of host protein by bacterial enzymes as nitrogen source.[27]

## VARIOUS PLAQUE HYPOTHESES

### Nonspecific Plaque Hypothesis

In 1976, Walter J Loesche proposed a hypothesis regarding the formation of nonspecific plaque. According to this hypothesis, periodontal infection occurs due to release of noxious products by the entire plaque flora.[28] **(Table 9.4 and Flowchart 9.4)** The shortcomings of respective the hypothesis was as follows:
- Some individuals with a constant amount of plaque and calculus never developed destructive periodontitis.
- Some sites were not affected, whereas advanced disease was found in adjacent sites.

### Specific Plaque Hypothesis

According to this hypothesis, only specific plaque portions are pathogenic that result in periodontal infection. Moreover, this pathogenicity is affected by the presence of or increase in specific microorganisms, as in the case of well-known exogenous bacterial infections of man, such as tuberculosis, syphilis. The shortcoming was that there were occasions when either disease was diagnosed in the absence of the putative pathogens or when pathogens were present with no evidence of disease **(Table 9.4 and Flowchart 9.4)**.

### Modern Version of Specific Theory

Socransky described it in 1979. According to this theory, approximately 6–12 bacterial species have a potential role in the development of significant cases of destructive periodontitis, while additional species may be responsible for the small number of other cases.

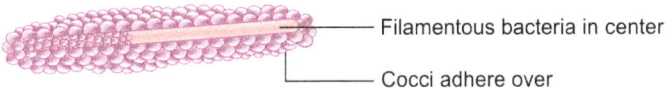

**Fig. 9.7:** Schematic representation showing corncob formation.

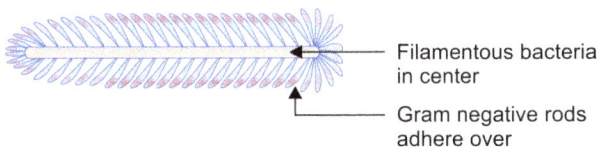

**Fig. 9.8:** Schematic representation showing test tube brush formation.

**Flowchart 9.3:** Metabolic interactions among different bacterial species in the plaque biofilm.

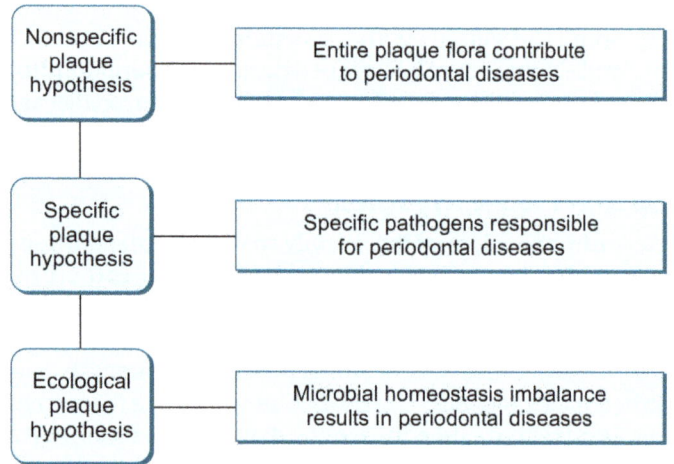

| TABLE 9.4: | Clinical implication of plaque hypotheses. |
|---|---|
| Nonspecific plaque hypothesis | This hypothesis implies that periodontal disease may be treated by reducing plaque to an acceptable level and maintaining healthy plaque or total plaque control. |
| Specific plaque hypothesis | This hypothesis implies that therapy should be directed at the elimination of specific pathogens, for instance, by appropriate antibiotics. |
| Ecological plaque hypothesis | According to this hypothesis, controlling the environmental factors that bring ecological shifts and eradicating the putative pathogen reduces diseases. |

**Flowchart 9.4:** Various plaque hypotheses.

- Nonspecific plaque hypothesis → Entire plaque flora contribute to periodontal diseases
- Specific plaque hypothesis → Specific pathogens responsible for periodontal diseases
- Ecological plaque hypothesis → Microbial homeostasis imbalance results in periodontal diseases

## Ecological Plaque Hypothesis

In 1991, PD Marsh proposed the ecological concept of plaque formation. According to this hypothesis, periodontitis is an opportunistic endogenous infection due to ecological shift in the plaque biofilm involving the predominant transition of gram-positive facultative anaerobic bacteria to gram-negative obligate anaerobic bacteria.[29] This ecological shift is mainly due to development of anaerobic environment from the result of host-microbial and microbe-microbe interactions, and it favors further bacterial growth. Ecological changes in the environment may determine the pathogenicity and virulence mechanisms of a particular organism, and hence any bacterial species may be pathogenic in that environment[30] **(Table 9.4 and Flowchart 9.4).**

## Unified Theory

Theilade described the unified theory in 1986. It is the modern version of nonspecific and specific plaque hypothesis. According to this theory, all bacterial plaque may contribute to the pathogenic potential of the subgingival flora to a greater or lesser extent. This is due to its ability to colonize and evade host defenses and provoke inflammation and tissue damage.[31]

## Keystone Pathogen Hypothesis

In 2012, George Hajishengallis et al., proposed the hypothesis of the keystone pathogen. According to it, certain low abundance microbial pathogen increases the quantity of normal microbiota and changes their composition that can lead to inflammatory disease.[32]

## CLINICAL SIGNIFICANCE

Marginal plaque plays a crucial role in the development of gingivitis. Along with this, supragingival plaque and tooth-associated subgingival plaque is associated with calculus formation and root caries.

Tissue-associated subgingival plaque is essential in the soft-tissue destruction that characterizes different forms of periodontitis. The pathogenic potential of tissue-associated subgingival plaque is due to the microorganism invasion into connective tissues and release of endotoxins and inflammatory substances.[11]

## Plaque Accumulation and Retention

The various plaque retentive areas are:
- *Natural areas/factors*:
  - Supragingival: Supragingival calculus, cavitated carious lesions, and exposed cementum.
  - Subgingival: Subgingival calculus, cavitated carious lesions, furcation involvement, root grooves, rough unplaned cementum, deep, narrow pockets, and enamel projections.
- *Iatrogenic factors*: Overhanging restoration margins, orthodontic bands, over contoured and inadequate crown margins, and portions of the removable prosthesis that impinge on the gingiva.

Plaque accumulates more rapidly on rough surfaces of teeth, restoration, and calculus. Plaque accumulation around crowded teeth is much greater than the teeth in proper alignment, especially in mandibular anterior teeth. Teeth that are not in use during mastication also show more plaque accumulation. Patients who are not motivated and cooperative show more plaque deposition.

## Control and Removal of Plaque

Dental plaque cannot be easily washed away by vigorous rinsing or water sprays. It also resists disruption by antimicrobial agents that cannot easily penetrate the protective polysaccharide matrix barrier characteristic of biofilms. Therefore, dental plaque is removed by scaling and root planing. It can also be removed by the individual mechanical intervention (tooth-brushing, flossing) and chemical intervention (antiplaque agents). Rest is explained in "Chapter 37: Mechanical Plaque Control" and "Chapter 38: Chemotherapeutic Agents".

## OTHER TOOTH DEPOSITS

Other than plaque, the tooth surface is also prone to certain deposits, such as pellicle, material alba, food debris **(Table 9.5)**, stains, and calculus.
- *Pellicle*: This is an organic film deposited on the tooth surface. It is mainly derived from the saliva. During the initial stages of deposition, it is with few or no bacteria. However, after a few hours, bacteria from the oral cavity start depositing on the pellicle and change its composition.
- *Materia alba*: This is a yellow or grayish-white and soft deposit on the tooth surface. It is a collection of microorganisms, desquamated epithelial cells, leukocytes, and a mixture of salivary proteins and lipids with few or no food particles. It is easily displaced with a water spray.[11]
- *Calculus*: This is a hard deposit on the tooth surface. Mineralization of dental plaque that is surrounded by a layer of unmineralized plaque results in calculus.[11] Rest is explained in "Chapter 10: Dental Calculus".

**TABLE 9.5:** Differences between plaque, materia alba, and food debris.

| Characteristic | Plaque | Materia alba | Food debris |
|---|---|---|---|
| Structures | Definite, regular | Amorphous | No structure |
| Effect of rinsing | Do not dislodge | Dislodged by forceful rinsing | Dislodged readily |
| Adherence | Close | Loose | None |

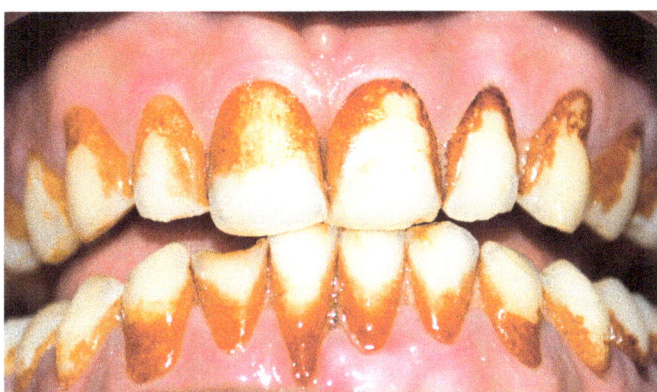

**Fig. 9.9:** Clinical picture showing extrinsic stains

- *Dental stains*: These are the pigmented deposits on the tooth surface. Such stains are not associated with gingivitis but can cause aesthetic problems. Frequent use of tobacco products, coffee, tea, certain mouth rinses, and pigments in foods leads to staining of the tooth surface **(Fig. 9.9)**.

*Green stains*: They may occur on the gingival third of the facial surface of anterior maxillary teeth. *Penicillium* and *Aspergillus* have been suggested as the responsible chromogenic organisms. These are common in children more often in boys than girls.[33]

*Brown stains*: Brown color is usually due to the presence of tannin. It is a thin and translucent acquired pigmented pellicle, which is free from bacteria. It occurs in individuals who do not brush sufficiently or those who use dentifrice with inadequate cleansing action. Such stains develop on the buccal surface of the maxillary molars and the lingual surface of the mandibular incisors.[34]

*Orange stains*: Occasionally, light and thin deposit of material of brick red or orange color are seen on facial and lingual surfaces of anterior teeth. *Serratia marcescens* and *Flavobacterium lutescens* have been suggested as the responsible chromogenic organisms for orange stains. As compared to green and brown stains, orange stains are usually rare.

*Black stains*: Chromogenic bacteria, i.e., *Actinomyces* species have been implicated as the causative agent for black stain. A person with good oral hygiene develops black stain as a thin black line on facial and lingual surfaces of the teeth near the gingival margin and as a diffuse patch on the proximal surfaces. These are common in women.

**Section 3:** Etiology

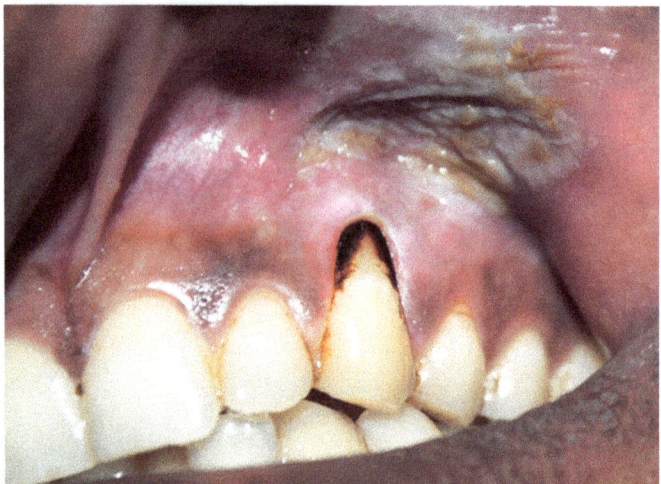

**Fig. 9.10:** Clinical picture showing tobacco stains.

*Tobacco stains*: They range in appearance from light brown to dark brown or black and cover approximately the cervical one-third to half of the most affected teeth. Stain usually occurs on the lingual and palatal surfaces and is commonly found in pits, fissures, and other enamel irregularities. Tobacco staining is directly proportional to the number of cigarettes smoked per day. These are found in individuals who smoke pipes or cigars and also those who use smokeless tobacco, i.e., snuffs **(Fig. 9.10)**.

*Metallic stains*: These are explained in "Chapter 18: Gingival Inflammation."

*Chlorhexidine stains*: Frequent use of chlorhexidine preparation leads to dark yellow or brownish stain formation on both artificial and natural teeth. Stains are more severe when chlorhexidine is used in higher concentrations.[33] Rest is explained in "Chapter 38: Chemotherapeutic Agents".

### Points to Ponder

- Dental plaque can be defined as the soft deposits that form the biofilm adhering to the tooth surface or other hard surfaces in the oral cavity, including removable and fixed restorations.
- Based on position on the tooth, plaque is of two types: (1) supragingival plaque—plaque present above or at the level of marginal gingiva; and (2) subgingival plaque—plaque located between the tooth and the gingival sulcular tissue just beneath the level of marginal gingiva.
- Materia alba differs from dental plaque as it lacks an organized internal structure due to which material alba can be easily displaced with water spray.

### REFERENCES

1. Busscher HJ, Evans LV (Eds). Oral Biofilms and Plaque Control. India: Harwood Academic Publishers; 1998.
2. Carlsson J. Bacterial metabolism in dental biofilms. Adv Dent Res. 1997;11(1):75-80.
3. Socransky SS, Haffajee AD. Dental biofilms: difficult therapeutic targets. Periodontol 2000. 2002;28:12-55.
4. Lang NP, Mombelli A, Attstrom R. Dental plaque and calculus. In: Lindhe J, Karring T, Lang NP (Eds). Clinical Periodontology and Implant Dentistry, 4th edition. Oxford, UK: Blackwell Munksgaard; 2003. pp. 81-105.
5. Frias J, Olle E, Alsina M. Periodontal pathogens produce quorum-sensing signal molecules. Infect Immun. 2001;69(5):3431-4.
6. Tatakis DN, Kumar PS. Etiology and pathogenesis of periodontal diseases in periodontology: present status and future concepts. Dent Clin North Am. 2005;49:493-7.
7. Xu KD, McFeters GA, Stewart PS. Biofilm resistance to antimicrobial agents. Microbiology. 2000;146(Pt 3):547-9.
8. Chandki R, Banthia P, Banthia R. Biofilms: a microbial home. J Indian Soc Periodontol. 2011;15(2):111-4.
9. Bowen WH. Nature of plaque. Oral Sci Rev. 1976;9:3-21.
10. Dawes C, Jenkins GN, Tonge CH. The nomenclature of the integuments of the enamel surface of teeth. Brit Dent J. 1963;115:65-8.
11. Haake SK, Newman MG, Nisengard RJ, Sanz M. Periodontal microbiology. In: Newman MG, Takei HH, Carranza FA (Eds). Carranza's Clinical Periodontology, 9th edition. Philadelphia, PA, USA: WB Saunders; 2003. pp. 96-112.
12. Wilkins EM. Bacterial plaque and other soft deposits. In: Clinical Practice of the Dental Hygienist, 8th edition. Philadelphia, PA, USA: Lippincott Williams & Wilkins; 1999. pp. 264-76.
13. Socransky SS, Gibbons RJ, Dale AC, Bortnick L, Rosenthal E, Macdonald JB. The microbiota of the gingival crevice area of man. Total microscopic and viable counts of specific microorganisms. Arch Oral Biol. 1963;8:275-80.
14. Contreras A, Slots J. Herpes viruses in human periodontal disease. J Periodontal Res. 2000;35(1):3-16.
15. Kleinberg I. Biochemistry of the dental plaque. Arch Oral Biol. 1970;4:43-90.
16. Fachon-Kalweit S, Elder BL, Fives-Taylor P. Antibodies that bind to fimbriae block adhesion of Streptococcus sanguis to saliva-coated hydroxyapatite. Infect Immun. 1985;48(3):617-24.
17. Kolenbrander PE, London J. Adhere today, here tomorrow: oral bacterial adherence. J Bacteriol. 1993;175(11):3247-52.
18. Kaufman J, DiRienzo JM. Isolation of a corncob (coaggregation) receptor polypeptide from *Fusobacterium nucleatum*. Infect Immun. 1989;57(2):331-7.
19. Weiss EI, London J, Kolenbrander PE, Andersen RN, Fischler C, Siraganian RP. Characterization of monoclonal antibodies to fimbria-associated adhesins of *Bacteroides loescheii* PK1295. Infect Immun. 1988;56(1):219-24.
20. Weiss EI, Eli L, Shenitzki B, Smorodinsky N. Identification of the rhamnose-sensitive adhesin of *Capnocytophaga ochracea* ATCC 33596. Arch Oral Biol. 1990;35(Suppl):127S-130S.
21. Kolenbrander PE, Parrish KD, Andersen RN, Greenberg EP. Intergeneric coaggregation of oral *Treponema spp.* with *Fusobacterium spp.* and intrageneric coaggregation among *Fusobacterium spp*. Infect Immun. 1995;63(12):4584-8.
22. Gibbons RJ, Nygaard M. Interbacterial aggregation of plaque bacteria. Archives of Oral Biology. 1970;15:1397-1400.
23. Grant DA, Stern IB, Listgarten MA. Microbiology (plaque). In: Periodontics, 6th edition. St. Louis: CV Mosby; 1988. pp. 147-97.
24. Listgarten MA. Structure of the microbial flora associated with periodontal health and disease in man. A light and electron microscopic study. J Periodontol. 1976;47:1-18.
25. Grenier D. Nutritional interactions between two suspected periodontopathogens, *Treponema denticola,* and

*Porphyromonas gingivalis.* Infect Immun. 1992;60(12): 5298-301.
26. Socransky SS, Haffajee AD. The bacterial etiology of destructive periodontal disease: current concepts. J Periodontol. 1992;63(4 Suppl):322-31.
27. Carlsson J. Microbiology of plaque-associated periodontal disease. In: Lindhe J (Ed). Textbook of Clinical Periodontology, 1st edition. Oxford, UK: Blackwell Munksgaard; 1983.
28. Heijl L, Lindhe J. Effect of selective antimicrobial therapy on plaque and gingivitis in the dog. J Clin Periodontol. 1980;7(6):463-78.
29. Marsh PD. Dental plaque: biological significance of a biofilm community lifestyle. J Clin Periodontol. 2005;32(Suppl 6):7-15.
30. Marsh PD. Dental plaque as a biofilm and a microbial community-implications for health and disease. BMC Oral Health. 2006;6(Suppl 1): S14.
31. Theilade E. The nonspecific theory in microbial etiology of inflammatory periodontal diseases. J Clin Periodontol. 1986;13(10):905-11.
32. Hajishengallis G, Darveau RP, Curtis MA. The keystone-pathogen hypothesis. Nat Rev Microbiol. 2012;10(10): 717-25.
33. Carranza FA, Newman MG, Klokkevold PR, Takei HH. Carranza's Clinical Periodontology, 12th edition. Philadelphia, PA, USA: WB Saunders; 2006. pp. 111-20.
34. Hamilton PH. A sialolith in the submaxillary duct: report of a case. Oral Surg Oral Med Oral Pathol. 1950;3(11):1388-9.

## VIVA VOCE

**Q1.** Who coined the term biofilm?
**Ans.** Bill Costerton, in 1978 coined the term biofilm.

**Q2.** Which organism is believed to be important in bridging between primary and secondary colonizers during plaque maturation?
**Ans.** *F. nucleatum* is believed to be important in bridging between primary and secondary colonizers during plaque maturation.

**Q3.** Give examples of coaggregation.
**Ans.** Examples of coaggregation are:
  A. Interaction of secondary colonizers with early colonizers: Corncob and test tube brush are the examples of coaggregation:
  - *F. nucleatum* with *S. sanguinis*
  - *P. loescheii* with *A. viscosus*
  - *C. ochraceus* with *A. viscosus*
  
  B. Interaction among secondary colonizers:
  - *F. nucleatum* with *P. gingivalis*
  - *F. nucleatum* with *T. denticola*

**Q4.** What are the corncob structures?
**Ans.** Corncob structure: Structures that have an inner core of rod-shaped bacterial cells, such as *F. nucleatum* and over the surface of which attach the coccal cells, such as *Streptococci* or *P. gingivalis*.

**Q5.** What is cryptitopes?
**Ans.** These are hidden receptors for bacterial attachment. Hidden segments of salivary acidic proline-rich proteins (PRPs) become exposed when the molecules undergo a conformational change as they adsorb to the apatitic mineral of the tooth (*cryptic*, meaning hidden, and *topo*, meaning place).
Certain bacteria keenly bind to salivary acidic PRPs adsorbed onto apatitic surfaces, and they do not interact with PRPs in solution. PRP molecules undergo a conformational change when they adsorb to hydroxyapatite, and these hidden segments become exposed, and these adhesins of bacteria recognize cryptic segments.

**Q6.** What is quorum sensing?
**Ans.** It is a way of a cell to cell communication that regulates gene expression by sharing information on cell-population density.

**Q7.** What are heat shock proteins (HSPs)?
**Ans.** HSPs belong to the family of stress proteins, which are usually synthesized by bacterial cells when exposed to the environment.

**Q8.** Who gave the ecological plaque hypothesis?
**Ans.** In 1991, PD Marsh gave the ecological plaque hypothesis.

**Q9.** What are the phases of plaque formation?
**Ans.**
- Pellicle formation
- Initial colonization of microorganisms
- Secondary colonization and maturation of microbes

**Q10.** Which phase is the prerequisite for the development of plaque?
**Ans.** Pellicle formation is the prerequisite for the development of plaque.

# Chapter 10

# Dental Calculus

Ashutosh Nirola, Shalu Bathla

## Chapter Outline

- Definition
- Classification
- Composition
- Formation
- Clinical Assessment
- Attachment of Calculus to the Tooth
- Role of Calculus in Disease
- Local Contributing Factors

## INTRODUCTION

Arabian physician and surgeon Albucasis (936–1013 AD) put forth the significant association between calculus and dental disease. He defined and explained this association and described the need and the way to remove calculus from teeth.[1] The theory "Doctrine of Calculus" was given by Paracelsus (1493–1541). He stated that pathologic calcification occurred in a variety of organs. These disease conditions occur due to metabolic disturbance when the body takes nourishment from food and rejects the refuse as "tartarus," a material that cannot be broken. The tartar consists of gravel and glue-like components derived from barley, peas, milk, meat, fish, and drinks, such as wine and fruit juice. He recognized the extensive formation of tartar on the teeth and related this to toothache. In the ensuing period of the 1960s, dental calculus was considered as one of the etiological agents for periodontitis. This was attributed to the roughness of calculus that irritates gingiva followed by secondary bacterial infection.[2] According to current knowledge, dental plaque is considered as the precursor of calculus, which exists in the form of mineralized plaque. The resulting calculus is always covered with a plaque on its surface.

## DEFINITION

Dental calculus is an adherent, calcified, or calcifying mass that forms on the surfaces of teeth and dental appliances.

## CLASSIFICATION

Based on the relationship to the gingival margin, dental calculus is classified as supragingival and subgingival calculus (**Table 10.1**).[3]

### Supragingival Calculus

It is a mineralized oral biofilm, usually white or whitish-yellow. It is formed coronal to the gingival margin and hence can be seen in the oral cavity. It can be separated easily from the underneath tooth surface (**Fig. 10.1**).

### Subgingival Calculus

It is a mineralized oral biofilm formed below the free gingival margin, often on the root surface (**Fig. 10.2**). Unlike supragingival calculus, subgingival calculus is more likely to have a dark-green, brown-black color owing to the absorption of blood pigments from the gingival sulcus or diseased periodontal pocket.

The various forms of subgingival calculus are shown in **Figure 10.3**.

- *Spicules*: These are small isolated pieces of calculus which are frequently located at line angles and interdental areas.
- *Ledge*: It is a larger deposit that forms on a section of the tooth and is approximately parallel to the cementoenamel junction (CEJ).

**TABLE 10.1:** Differences between supragingival and subgingival calculus.

| Parameters | Supragingival calculus | Subgingival calculus |
|---|---|---|
| Location | Coronal to the gingival margin **(Fig. 10.1)** | Below the crest of the marginal gingiva **(Fig. 10.2)** |
| Color | White or whitish-yellow | Brown or black |
| Shape | Amorphous bulky,[4] shapes of calculus is determined by the contour of the gingival margin, anatomy of teeth, and pressure of tongue, lips, and cheeks | May be thin, finger- and fern-like.[5] Flattened to conform to pressure from the pocket wall |
| Consistency | Moderately hard | Brittle, flint-like |
| Attachment | Easily detached from the tooth | Attached firmly to the tooth surface |
| Visibility | Visible on routine clinical examination | Not visible on routine clinical examination |
| Composition | Salivary proteins are present; lesser magnesium whitlockite; more brushite and octacalcium phosphate; sodium content is lesser | Salivary proteins are absent; more magnesium whitlockite; lesser brushite and octacalcium phosphate;[6] sodium content increases with the depth of the pocket |
| Source | Formed from salivary secretions | Formed from gingival exudate |
| Distribution | The symmetrical arrangement on teeth, more on the facial surface of maxillary molars and lingual surface of mandibular anterior due to openings of salivary glands ducts **(Fig. 10.4)** | Related to pocket depth, heaviest on proximal surfaces |

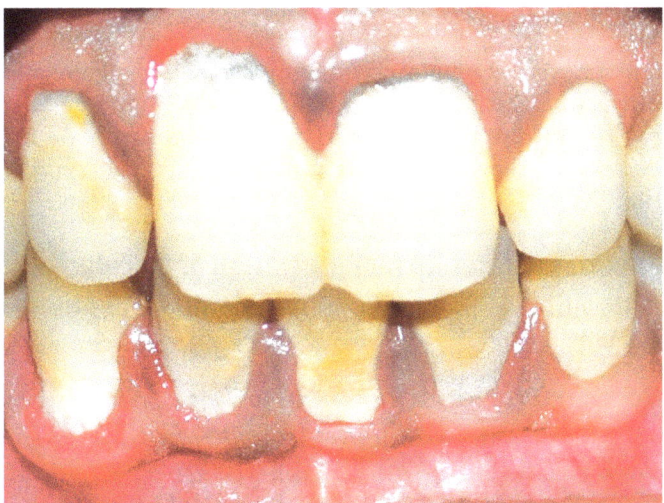

**Fig. 10.1:** Clinical picture showing supragingival calculus.

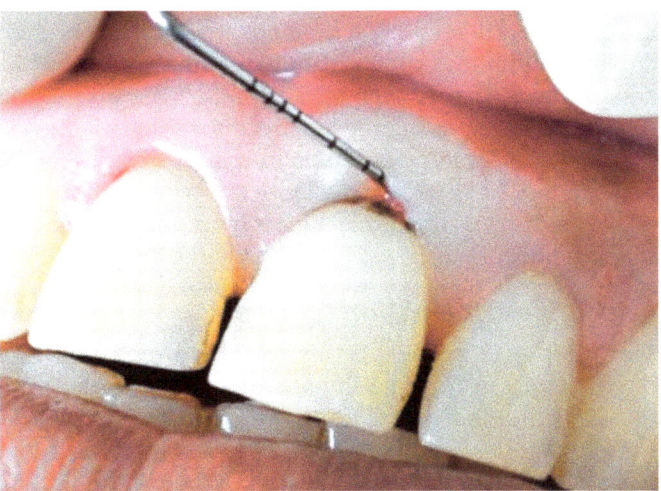

**Fig. 10.2:** Clinical picture showing subgingival calculus revealed by deflecting pocket wall.

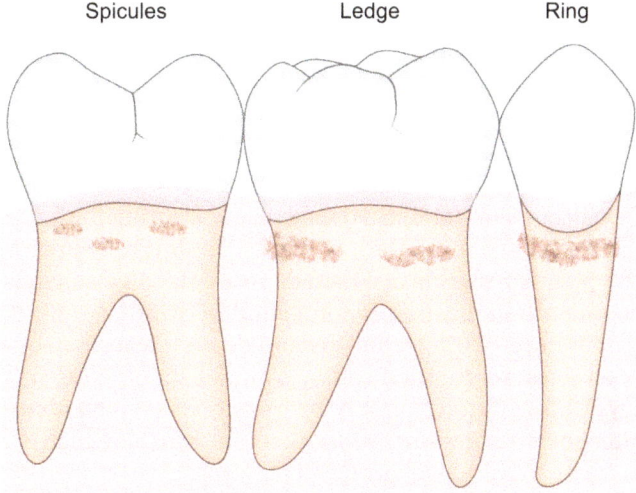

**Fig. 10.3:** Schematic representation showing forms of subgingival calculus.

- *Ring form*: It is a ledge-like deposit that encircles the tooth, forming a ring of calculus.

## COMPOSITION

- *Inorganic content*:
    - Elements:
        - Calcium (39%)
        - Phosphorus (19%)
        - Carbon dioxide (1.9%)
        - Magnesium (0.8%)
        - Traces of sodium, strontium, zinc, bromine, manganese, copper, gold, tungsten, aluminum, silicon, fluorine, iron.[7]
    - Compounds:
        - Calcium phosphate (75.9%)
        - Calcium carbonate (3.1%)

- Traces of magnesium phosphate and other metals[8]
- Crystals: Four main forms of crystals are as follows:[9]
  - Hydroxyapatite $[Ca_{10}(PO_4)_6(OH)_2]$ (58%)
  - Magnesium whitlockite $[Ca_9(FeH_2MgO_{32}P_8]$ (21%)
  - Octacalcium phosphate $[Ca_8H_2(PO_4)_6 \cdot 5H_2O]$ (12%)
  - Brushite $[CaHPO_4 \cdot 2H_2O]$ (9%)

Hydroxyapatite and octacalcium phosphate are found most frequently in supragingival calculus. In the mandible, brushite is more common in the anterior region and magnesium whitlockite in the posterior areas.[3]

- *Organic content:*[10]
  - Carbohydrates (1.9–9.1%): Glucose, galactose, rhamnose, galactosamine, glucuronic acid, mannose, arabinose, galacturonic acid, glucosamine
  - Proteins (5.9–8.2%)
  - Lipids (0.2%): Neutral fats, fatty acids, cholesterol, phospholipids, cholesterol esters
  - Protein polysaccharide complexes, desquamated epithelial cells, leukocytes, and microorganisms.

## FORMATION

Calculus is a mineralized dental plaque. During the first 14 days of plaque formation, mineral salts start to deposit on soft plaque resulting in a hard deposition.[11] 50% calcifying plaque mineralization is completed in two days, and the remaining 60–90% get finished in 12 days.[12] Not all plaques need to undergo calcification. Mineralization consists of crystal formation, namely hydroxyapatite, octacalcium phosphate, magnesium whitlockite, and brushite, each with a characteristic developmental pattern.

Supragingival calculus gets mineralized from saliva, while subgingival calculus mineralization takes place through the gingival crevicular fluid.[13] Calcium is the driving force for plaque mineralization. A dental plaque can concentrate calcium 2–20 times higher as compared to its level in saliva. The calcification process and the rate of calculus accumulation are usually person-specific and vary from person to person. Even in the same individual, this process can vary with respect to teeth and times. Based on individual differences for calculus formation, persons are classified as heavy, moderate, or slight calculus formers or as noncalculus formers. Heavy calculus formers are characterized by a high salivary concentration of calcium and phosphorus as compared to light calculus formers. Light calculus formers have higher levels of parotid pyrophosphate, which inhibit the calcification process. Early plaque of heavy calculus formers is characterized by precipitation of high calcium, three times more phosphorus, and less potassium than that of noncalculus formers.[14] This provides a reasonable explanation for phosphorus as a significant element than calcium in plaque mineralization.

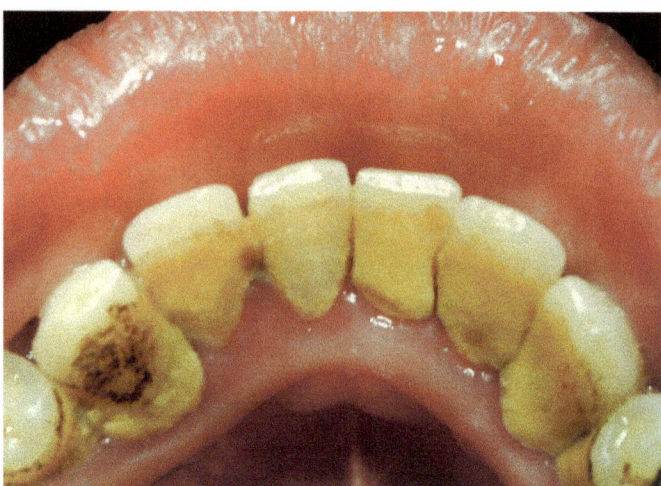

**Fig. 10.4:** Clinical picture showing heavy calculus at lingual surfaces of mandibular anterior teeth in relation to Wharton duct.

Calcification means deposition and binding of calcium ions to the carbohydrate-protein complexes of the organic matrix and the precipitation of crystalline calcium phosphate salts. The crystal formation takes place inside the intercellular matrix, on the bacterial surface, and finally inside the bacteria.[15] The mineralization process is considered the same for both supragingival and subgingival calculus.

## Theories Related to Mineralization of Calculus

Following are the theories related to mineralization of calculus:[16]

### Booster/Precipitation Theory

An increase in the pH due to the loss of carbon dioxide and the formation of ammonia (NH) leads to the precipitation of calcium phosphate salts **(Flowchart 10.1)**.

Urea is a metabolic byproduct of nitrogen-containing substances. The action of urease hydrolyzes bacterial urea. At a neutral pH, urease hydrolyzed urea into $NH^+$ and bicarbonate. In acidic pH, aqueous and gaseous carbon dioxide equilibrates with bicarbonate while in alkaline pH, aqueous and gaseous $NH_3$ coexists with $NH^+$. NH formed during the ureolysis of urea led to an increased plaque pH that facilitates natural calculus formation. The ureolytic pH response (an increase in plaque pH by the production of $NH_3$ from urea) favors calculus formation by enhancing calcium phosphate precipitation in plaque fluid.

### Epitactic or Nucleation Concept

This theory is based on the concept that small foci of calcification induced by seeding agents enlarge to form a "calcified mass." This theory is also known as "heterogeneous nucleation." The process starts with the removal of calcium from the saliva by carbohydrate-protein complexes and binding with it to form nuclei to facilitate subsequent mineral deposition **(Flowchart 10.2)**.

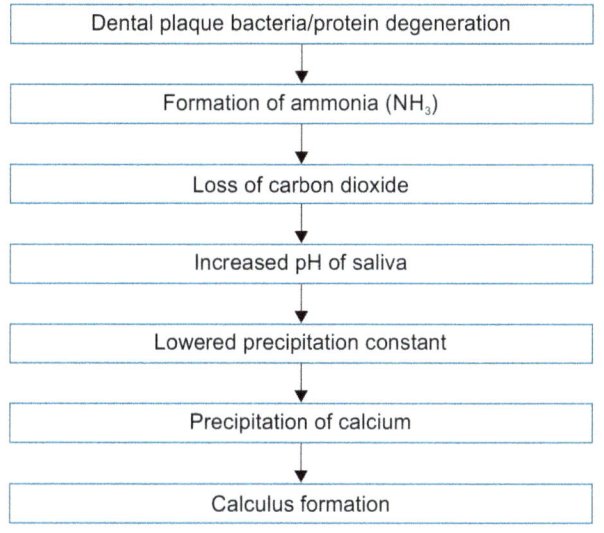

Flowchart 10.1: Booster theory of calculus formation.

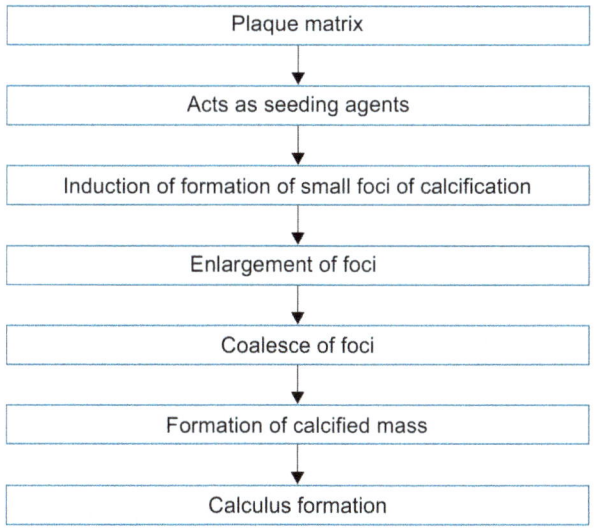

Flowchart 10.2: Seeding theory of calculus formation.

### Inhibition Theory

Calcification occurring only at a specific site is because of the existence of an inhibiting mechanism at noncalcifying sites. Where calcification occurs, the inhibitor is altered or removed. The inhibiting substance is thought to be pyrophosphate, and among the controlling mechanism is the enzyme alkaline pyrophosphatase, which can hydrolyze the pyrophosphate to phosphate. The pyrophosphate inhibits calcification by preventing the initial nucleus from growing, possibly by "poisoning" the growth centers of the crystal.

### Transformation Theory

Amorphous noncrystalline deposits and brushite can be transformed to octacalcium phosphate and then to hydroxyapatite.

## Role of Microorganisms in the Mineralization of Calculus

Bacterial plaque plays a significant role in calculus mineralization by forming phosphatases. Phosphatases are responsible for changes in the plaque pH and subsequent mineralization.[17] But other studies stated that these bacteria are only passively involved, as calculus may develop in germfree animals too.[18]

Previous studies reported the role of filamentous microorganisms in the formation of supragingival calculus, while microorganisms of diverse morphologies are associated with plaque adjacent to subgingival calculus. Filamentous organisms, diphtheroid, and *Bacterionema* and *Veillonella* species play a part in intracellular apatite crystals formation. The process of calculus formation continues until the matrix, and bacteria get calcified.

According to Little et al. (1966), calculus never contains deoxyribose and ribose, indicating the lack of nucleic acids in calculus. The absence of nucleic acids in calculus is suggestive of the concept that the oral microorganisms may undergo extensive degradation and leave only the cell walls for calculus formation **(Table 10.2)**.[10]

## CLINICAL ASSESSMENT

The clinical assessment can be done by:
- *Visual examination by use of compressed air:* Small amounts of unstained supragingival calculus are frequently invisible when they are wet with saliva. Blowing air down the gingival crevice helps to detect subgingival calculus deposits. The dark edge of calculus may be seen at or just beneath the gingival margin.
- *Exploring:* An explorer may be used when the visual examination is not definite. A fine subgingival explorer "TU-17" can detect the subgingival calculus.
- *Probing:* A fine calculus probe [World Health Organization (WHO) 621] or ball end of the CPITN (Community Periodontal Index of Treatment Needs) probe with a light touch is used to detect the subgingival calculus. While probing for sulcus or pocket, a rough subgingival tooth surface can be felt when calculus is present. Although there are other causes of roughness, subgingival calculus is the most common.
- *Radiographs:* Although the calculus deposit is visible on radiographs but is not always reliable for diagnosis. Radiographs may be useful in the diagnosis of subgingival calculus **(Fig. 10.5)**. The calculus location

**TABLE 10.2:** Calcification promoters and inhibitors.

| Calcification promoters | Calcification inhibitors |
|---|---|
| Urea | Pyrophosphate salts |
| Fluoride | Zinc salts |
| Silicon | Triclosan with a PVM/MA copolymer |

(PVM/MA: polyvinyl methyl ether/maleic acid)

**Section 3:** Etiology

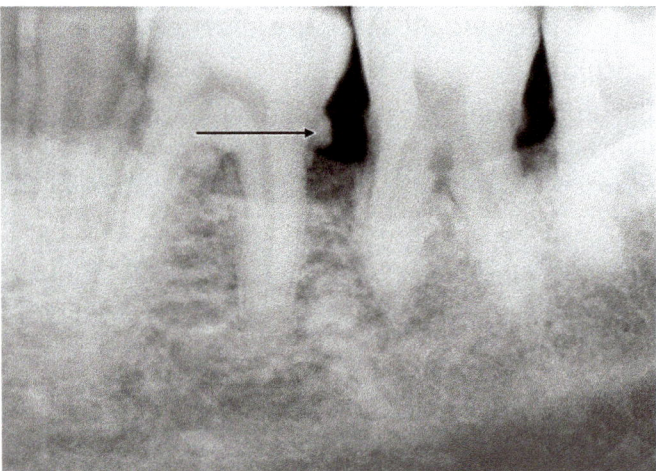

**Fig. 10.5:** Radiographic image showing interproximal subgingival calculus.

does not indicate the bottom of the periodontal pocket because the most apical plaque is not sufficiently calcified to be visible on radiographs.
- *Clinical records*: The various indices for recording and scoring calculus are explained in "Chapter 7: Epidemiology".

## ATTACHMENT OF CALCULUS TO THE TOOTH

Zander HA reported four types of calculus attachment[19] **(Figs. 10.6A to D)**. Later on, Shroff mentioned that the type of attachment of calculus probably depends on the time duration since the calculus formed on the tooth.

Four modes of calculus attachment to the tooth surface are:
1. Calculus attachment with an organic pellicle.
2. Attachment with the mechanical locking system into surface irregularities, such as resorption lacunae and caries. This type of attachment makes the removal of calculus difficult as calculus embedded beneath the cementum surface penetrates the dentin.
3. Penetration of calculus bacteria into cementum.
4. The close adaptation of calculus undersurface depressions to the gently sloping mounds of the unaltered cementum surface.

The attachment of calculus to pure titanium implant is less intimate than to root surface.

## ROLE OF CALCULUS IN DISEASE

Calculus may be harmful both physically and chemically to adjacent gingiva. It is permeable and, thus, may absorb and adsorb toxic products. It is rough and porous,[20] which facilitates the retention of dental plaque. It is always covered with unmineralized plaque providing subsequent retention and promotion for new plaque accumulation.[21] It causes periodontal destruction in the following manner:
- It brings bacterial overlay closer to the supporting tissues.
- It interferes with the local self-cleansing mechanism.
- It provides a nidus for continuous plaque accumulation.
- It makes plaque removal more difficult.

## LOCAL CONTRIBUTING FACTORS

### Anatomic Factors

#### Proximal Contact Relation

The position and coherence of the proximal contacts along with the contour of the marginal ridges and developmental grooves help to avoid interproximal food impaction. Food impaction is the forceful wedging of food into the periodontium by occlusal forces. Hirschfeld in 1930 classified vertical food impaction relative to etiological factors:[22]
- *Class I*: Occlusal wear
- *Class II*: Loss of proximal support
- *Class III*: Extrusion of a tooth beyond the occlusal plane

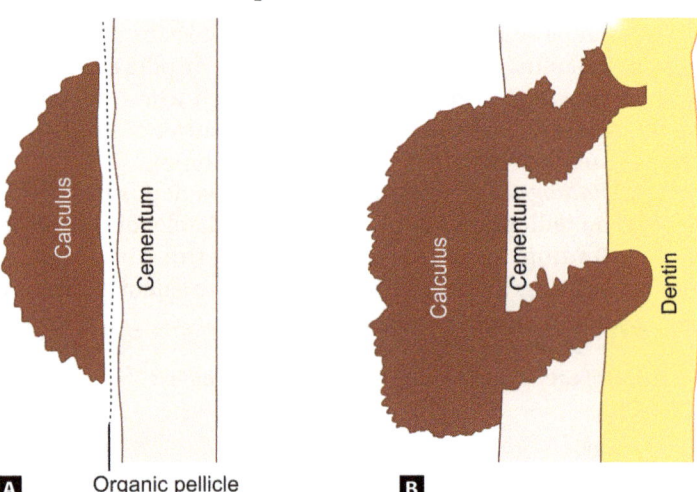
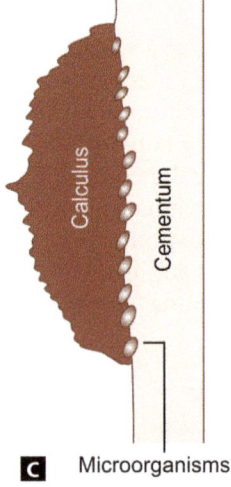
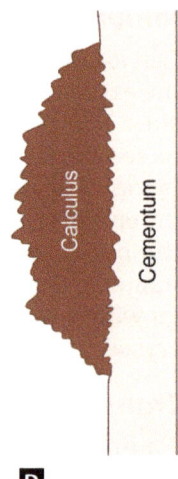

**Figs. 10.6A to D:** Schematic representation showing modes of attachment of calculus.

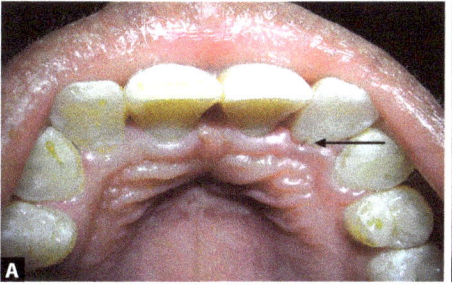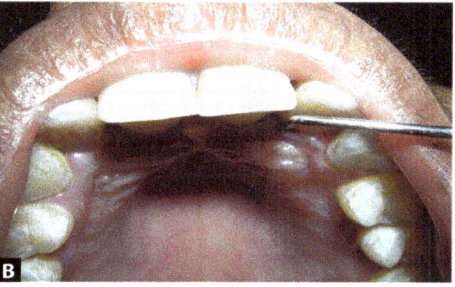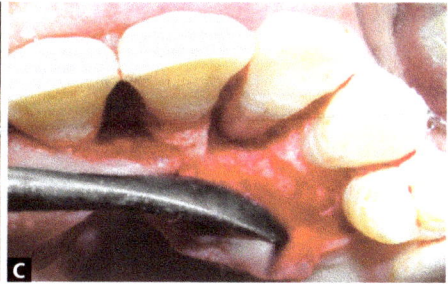

**Figs. 10.7A to C:** Clinical picture showing (A) Palatogingival groove at the cingulum of maxillary lateral incisor; (B) Pocket associated with palatogingival groove and (C) Bone loss associated with palatogingival groove.

- *Class IV*: Congenital morphologic abnormalities
- *Class V*: Improperly constructed restorations

Sequelae of food impaction:
- Feeling of pressure and the urge to dig the material from between the teeth
- Vague pain which radiates deep in the jaws
- Gingival inflammation with bleeding and a foul taste in the involved area
- Gingival recession
- Periodontal abscess formation
- Varying degree of inflammatory involvement of the periodontal ligament with an associated elevation of the tooth in its socket, prematurity in functional contact, and sensitivity to percussion
- Destruction of alveolar bone
- Caries of the tooth

Plunger cusps usually wedge food forcibly into interproximal embrasures of opposing teeth. Distolingual cusps of maxillary molars are the most common plunger cusp. Plunger cusp effect may occur with wear, or it may be the result of a shift in tooth positions following the failure to replace a missing tooth.

### Cervical Enamel Projection and Enamel Pearls

Cervical enamel projection (CEP) and enamel pearls are narrow wedge-shaped extensions of enamel projecting from the CEJ towards the furcation area. These are usually plaque retentive and can predispose to furcation involvement.

### Intermediate Bifurcation Ridge

It is a convex excrescence of cementum running longitudinally in between the mesial and distal roots of a mandibular molar. It is positioned at the midpoint between the buccal and lingual surfaces of the root division area or may present in a more lateral position. They are commonly found on 1st molars. These ridges cause difficulty in the removal of plaque and calculus. Their inadequate removal increases the possibility of failure of furcation treatment, especially regenerative therapy.

### Palatogingival Groove

The palatogingival groove, also termed as the palatoradicular groove, extends from the base of cingulum in apical direction for a variable distance (**Fig. 10.7A**). It is usually present in maxillary lateral incisors. Deep pocketing of maxillary incisors, especially isolated, helps in the examination of palatogingival grooves (**Fig. 10.7B**). When palatogingival grooves are presented with bone loss and attachment loss, removing the groove through odontoplasty or reducing its depth helps to minimize plaque retention (**Fig. 10.7C**).

### Root Proximity

The close proximity of tooth roots in an association with thin interproximal septum enhances the risk for periodontal destruction.

### Iatrogenic Factors

Inadequate dental procedures which lead to the destruction of periodontal tissues are referred to as iatrogenic factors.

### Restorative Dentistry

Laceration of gingiva due to improper use of rubber dam clamps, matrix bands, and burs causes a varying degree of mechanical trauma and inflammation. Improperly conducted restorations can harm the patient's oral health (**Fig. 10.8**). Overhanging margins of restorations and crowns facilitate further plaque development by limiting the patient's access.

### Prosthesis

Poorly designed clasps, prosthesis saddles, and pontics can directly traumatize periodontal tissues (**Fig. 10.9**). Thus, prosthesis acts as iatrogenic irritants for periodontal tissues.

### Orthodontic Procedures

Orthodontic therapy directly injures the gingiva due to the use of overextended bands, chemical irritation by exposed cement (**Fig. 10.10**) and by creating excessive, unfavorable forces, or both. This damages periodontium and favors plaque retention.

### Extraction of Impacted Third Molar

The extraction of impacted 3rd molars usually results in the formation of vertical bone defects distal to the 2nd molars. Careless use of elevators or forceps during extraction results in the crushing of alveolar bone.

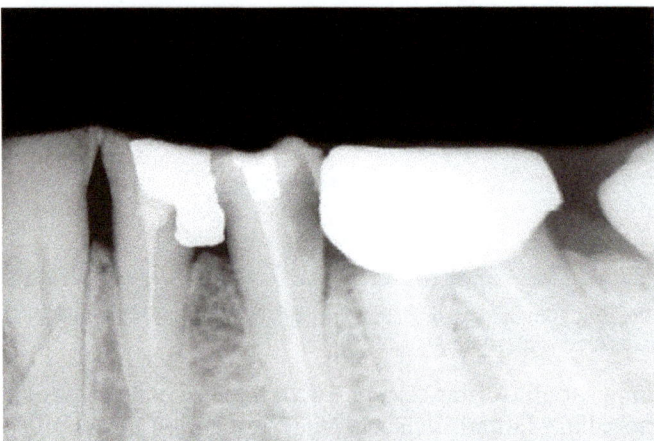

**Fig. 10.8:** Radiographic image showing interproximal bone loss associated with overhanging restoration.

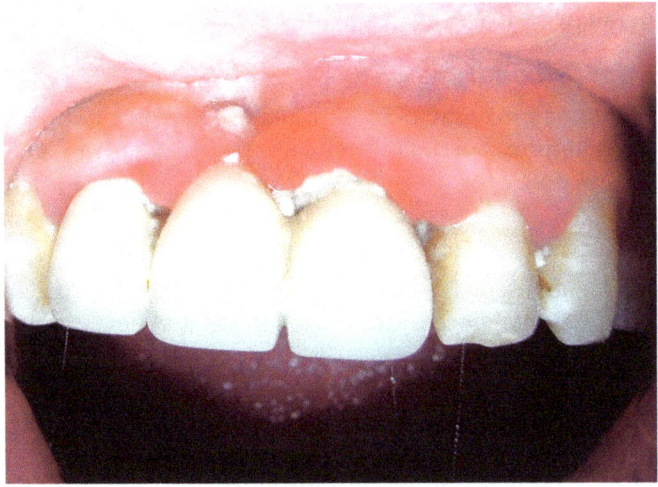

**Fig. 10.9:** Clinical picture showing inflammatory gingival changes around fixed partial prosthesis.

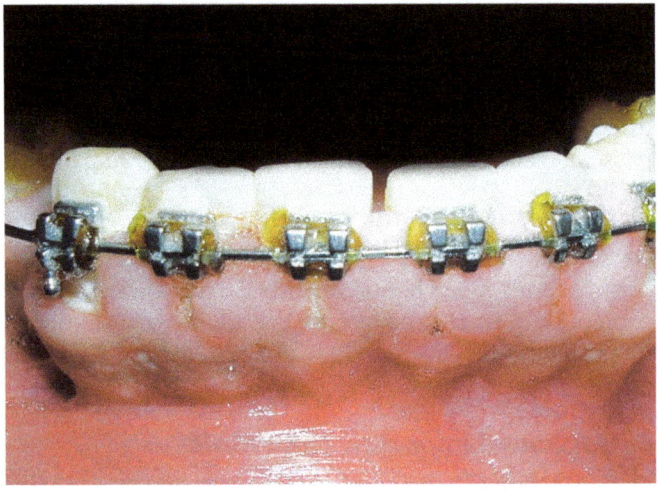

**Fig. 10.10:** Clinical picture showing gingival hyperplasia in lower anterior due to chemical irritation by excess resin cement.

## Malocclusion as Contributing Factors

Crowded or malaligned teeth are always difficult to clean as compared to the properly aligned counterpart. In deep bite, maxillary incisors impinge on the mandibular labial gingiva of mandibular incisors on the palatal gingiva causing gingival and periodontal inflammation **(Figs. 10.11A and B)**. The inability to replace missing posterior teeth imposes adverse effects on periodontal support for the remaining teeth. On extracting the mandibular 1st molar, the initial change occurs is a mesial drifting and tilting of the mandibular 2nd and 3rd molars along with extrusion of the maxillary 1st molar. Once the mandibular 2nd molar drifts mesially, its distal cusps extrude and act as plungers. The distal cusps of the mandibular 2nd molar get choked between 1st and 2nd maxillary molars and open the contact by deflecting the maxillary 2nd molar distally. This leads to food impaction along with gingival inflammation and eventual loss of the interproximal bone between the maxillary 1st and 2nd molars.

## Habits as Contributing Factors

### Toothbrush and Floss Trauma

The improper habit of toothbrushing usually damages dental soft and hard tissues. Typically, a new toothbrush, especially a hard one, can damage the mucosal epithelium resulting in painful ulcerations on the gingiva. If the thin marginal gingiva gets abraded, it can result in gingival recession and exposure of the root surface. The abrasives in toothpaste also play an essential role in gingival abrasion. The defect usually manifests as V-shaped notches at the level of the CEJ **(Fig. 10.12)**. Flossing can also cause damage to dental hard and soft tissues. When the floss is forcefully snapped through the contact point, it gives rise to flossing clefts as it cuts into the gingiva. Also, an aggressive up and down cleaning motion can produce an injury to the gingiva.

### Mouth Breathing and Tongue Thrusting

The habit of mouth breathing dehydrates the gingival tissues and enhances the possibility of inflammation. The development of dental plaque may or may not be seen in such cases, and some cases may present with gingival enlargement. Professional cleaning and plaque control measures help to control the gingival inflammation up to some extent only. Tongue thrusting, also called the reverse swallow or immature swallow, is commonly associated with an anterior open bite. It occurs due to an orofacial muscular imbalance. Here, the tongue gets thrust forwards against the teeth instead of facing against the palate during swallowing. If the pressure against the teeth is high, it can lead to tooth mobility and enlargement of the anterior teeth' spacing.

Chapter 10: Dental Calculus

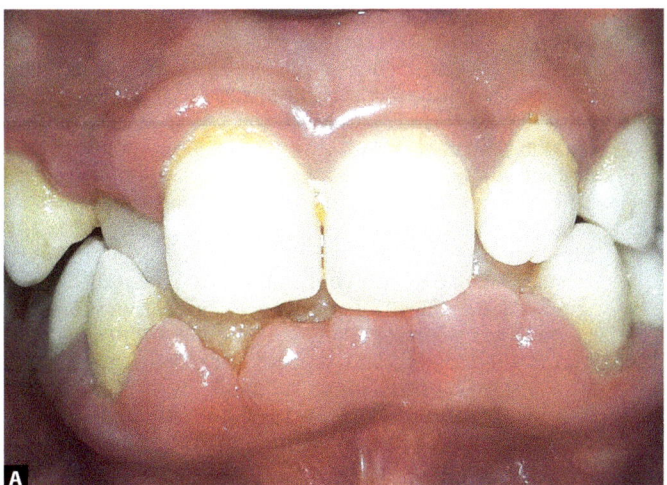
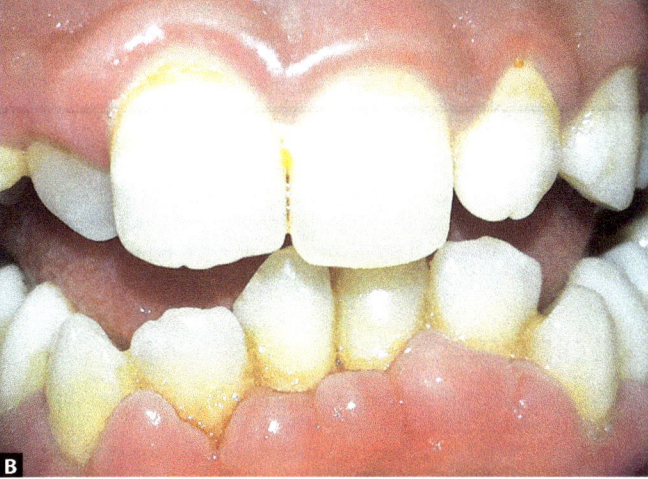

**Figs. 10.11A and B:** Clinical picture showing deep bite causing gingival and periodontal inflammation.

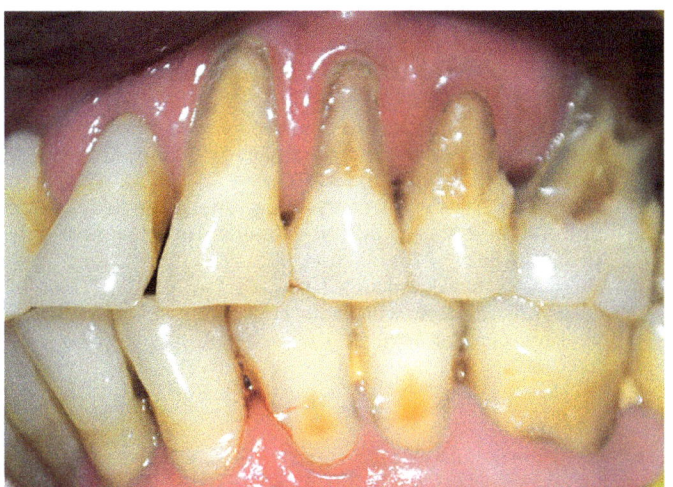

**Fig. 10.12:** Clinical picture showing toothbrushing abrasion.

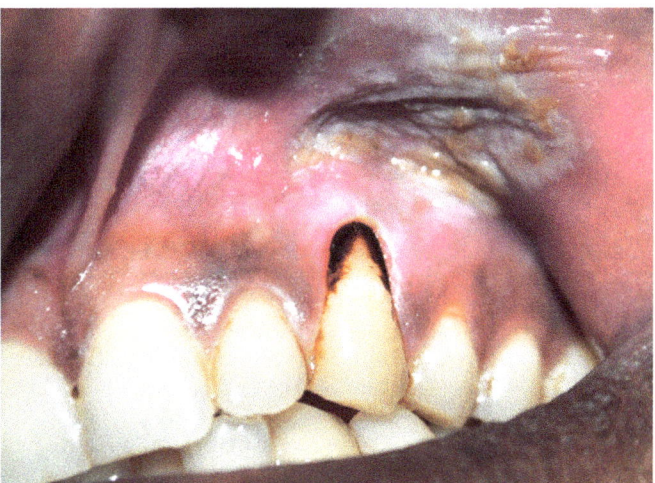

**Fig. 10.13:** Clinical photograph showing tobacco stains.

The problem should be identified during the diagnostic phase as it can lead to the potential destruction of periodontal tissues.

## Tobacco Use

Currently, smoking is reported as a significant risk factor for the development and progression of periodontitis **(Fig. 10.13)**. Rest is explained in "Chapter 16: Smoking and Periodontium".

## Factitious Injuries

Factitious injuries are self-inflicted injuries produced by patients themselves. Such injuries are challenging to diagnose because of their unusual presentation. Such injuries are commonly produced by pricking the gingiva with a fingernail **(Fig. 10.14)**, with knives and by using toothpicks or other oral hygiene devices.

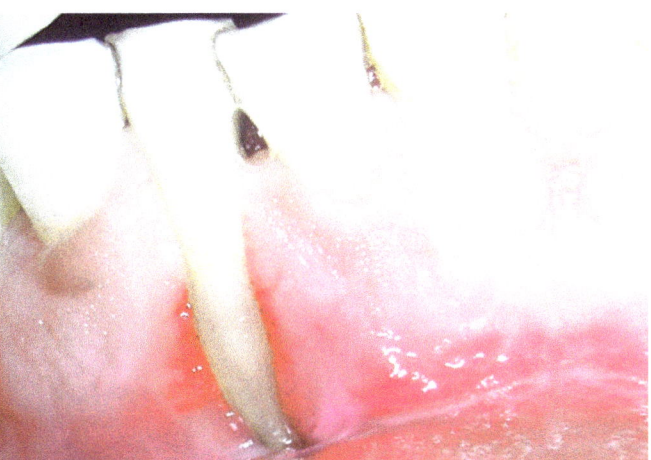

**Fig. 10.14:** Clinical picture showing localized gingival recession due to pricking of the gingiva with a fingernail.
(*Source:* Dr Ajay Mahajan)

## Section 3: Etiology

> **Points to Ponder**
> - Calculus is the most prominent plaque retentive factor and is a secondary etiologic factor for periodontitis.
> - It can also occur readily in germfree animals.
> - Calculocementum is the deeply embedded calculus in the cementum and looks morphologically similar to cementum.[23]
> - The reversal phenomenon is the decline from maximal calculus accumulation. It is attributed to the tendency of bulky calculus to mechanical wear from food, cheeks, lips, and tongue.

## REFERENCES

1. Fairbrother KJ, Heasman PA. Anticalculus agents. J Clin Periodontol. 2000;27(5):285-301.
2. Mandel ID, Gaffar A. Calculus revisited. A review. J Clin Periodontol. 1986;13(4):249-57.
3. Hinrichs JE. The role of calculus and other predisposing factors. In: Newman MG, Takei HH, Carranza FA (Eds). Carranza's Clinical Periodontology, 9th edition. Philadelphia, PA, USA: WB Saunders; 2003. pp. 182-203.
4. Wilkins EM. Dental calculus. In: Clinical Practice of the Dental Hygienist, 8th edition. Philadelphia, PA, USA: Lippincott Williams & Wilkins; 1999. pp. 277-84.
5. Grant DA, Stern IB, Listgarten MA. Calculus. In: Periodontics, 6th edition. St. Louis: CV Mosby; 1988. pp. 198-215.
6. Rowles S. The inorganic composition of dental calculus. In: Blackwood HJ (Ed). Bone and Tooth. Oxford, UK: Pergamon Press; 1964. pp. 175-83.
7. Mühler J, Ennever J. Occurrence of calculus through several successive periods in a selected group of subjects. J Periodontol. 1962; 33: 22.
8. White DJ. Dental calculus: recent insights into the occurrence, formation, prevention, removal, and oral health effects of supragingival and subgingival deposits. Eur J Oral Sci. 1997;105(5 Pt 2):508-22.
9. Jin Y, Yip HK. Supragingival calculus: formation and control. Crit Rev Oral Biol Med. 2002;13(5):426-41.
10. Little MF, Bowman L, Casciani CA, Rowley J. The composition of dental calculus. 3. Supragingival calculus—the amino acid and saccharide component. Arch Oral Biol. 1966;11(4):385-96.
11. Tibbetts L, Kashiwa H. A histochemical study of early plaque mineralization. Abstract No. 616. J Dent Res. 1970;19: 202.
12. Muhlemann HR, Schroeder HE. Dynamics of supragingival calculus formation. Adv Oral Biol. 1964;1:175-203.
13. Stewart R, Ratcliff P. The source of components of subgingival plaque and calculus. Periodont Abstr. 1966;14: 102.
14. Mandel I. Biochemical aspects of calculus formation. J Periodont Res. 1969;4(Suppl):7.
15. Zander HA, Hazen SP, Scott DB. Mineralization of dental calculus. Proc Soc Exp Biol Med. 1960;103:257-60.
16. Mandel ID. Dental calculus. In: Genco RJ, Goldman HM, Cohen DW (Eds). Contemporary Periodontics, 1st edition. St. Louis: CV Mosby; 1990. pp. 135-46.
17. Mandel I. Calculus formation. The role of bacteria and mucoprotein. Dent Clin North Am. 1960;4: 731.
18. Gustafsson BE, Krasse B. Dental calculus in germfree rats. Acta Odontol Scand. 1962;20:135-42.
19. Zander H. The attachment of calculus to root surfaces. J Periodontol. 1953;24: 16.
20. Friskopp J, Hammarström L. A comparative, scanning electron microscopic study of supragingival and subgingival calculus. J Periodontol. 1980;51(10):553-62.
21. Schroeder HE. Crystal morphology and gross structures of mineralizing plaque and of calculus. Helv Odontol Acta. 1965;9:73-86.
22. Hirschfeld. Food impaction. J Am Dent Assoc. 1930;17:1504-11.
23. Selvig KA. Attachment of plaque and calculus to tooth surfaces. J Periodontal Res. 1970; 5(1): 8-18.

## VIVA VOCE

**Q1. What is the reversal phenomenon of calculus?**
**Ans.** The reversal phenomenon is the decline from maximal calculus accumulation due to the vulnerability of bulky calculus to mechanical wear from food, cheeks, lips, and tongue.

**Q2. Why is subgingival calculus dark green or dark brown?**
**Ans.** Subgingival calculus is dark green or dark brown because of the presence of blood products (iron heme pigments) associated with subgingival hemorrhage.

**Q3. Why supragingival calculus forms most readily on the lingual surface of lower anterior teeth?**
**Ans.** Supragingival calculus forms most readily on the lingual surface of lower anterior teeth due to following reasons:
- The abundant supply of urea from the major salivary gland (submandibular gland) secretions tends to increase pH in plaque and promote calcium and phosphate ions precipitation.
- Due to the presence of submandibular gland Wharton's duct on the lingual surface of lower anterior teeth, higher salivary film velocity promotes clearance of acid and salivary sugar from plaque leading to higher pH of lingual area.

**Q4. Which is the essential plaque retentive factor?**
**Ans.** Calculus is the essential plaque retentive factor as it retains and harbors plaque on its rough surface.

**Q5. Which mineral is more critical in plaque mineralization?**
**Ans.** Phosphorus.

**Q6. Who gave the theory "Doctrine of Calculus"?**
**Ans.** Paracelsus.

**Q7. Which explorer is used to detect subgingival calculus?**
**Ans.** A fine subgingival explorer "TU-17" can detect the subgingival calculus.

**Q8. Name various calcification promoters.**
**Ans.** Urea, Fluoride, Silicon.

**Q9. Name various calcification inhibitors.**
**Ans.** Pyrophosphate salts, Zinc salts, and Triclosan with a PVM/ MA copolymer.

**Q10. Why does the location of calculus not indicate the bottom of the periodontal pocket?**
**Ans.** The most apical plaque is not sufficiently calcified to be visible on radiographs.

# Chapter 11: Immunity and Inflammation

*Deepak Sharma, Shalu Bathla*

## Chapter Outline

- Cells of Immunity and Inflammation
- Leukocyte Functions
- Chemical Mediators of Inflammation
- Nonspecific and Specific Immunity
- Immune Mechanisms
- Antigen Processing and Presentation
- Pathogen Associated Molecular Patterns
- Pattern Recognition Receptors

## INTRODUCTION

Inflammation refers to tissue injury or irritation, initiated by the entry of pathogens or other irritants.[1]

## Cardinal Signs

Four cardinal signs or hallmarks of inflammation are as follows:[1]
1. Rubor (redness)
2. Tumor (swelling)
3. Calor (heat)
4. Dolor (pain)
   The fifth clinical sign is *functio laesa* (loss of function).

## Types of Inflammation

Inflammation is grouped into two basic forms:
1. Acute inflammation
2. Chronic inflammation **(Table 11.1)**

**TABLE 11.1:** Features of acute and chronic inflammation.

| Feature | Acute inflammation | Chronic inflammation |
|---|---|---|
| Onset | Fast minutes or hours | Slow days |
| Cellular infiltrate | Mainly neutrophils | Monocytes/macrophages and lymphocytes |
| Tissue injury | Mild and self-limiting | Severe and progressive |
| Local and systemic signs | Prominent | Less |

## Immune System

The immune system is a network designed for the homeostasis of large molecules (oligomers) and cells based on specific recognition processes. Recognition of the structural features of an oligomer by receptors on immune cells is a crucial component of the specificity of the immune system.

Immunity is the resistance produced by the host against injury caused by microorganisms and their products.[2]

## Types of Immune Responses

Immune responses are categorized as follows.[3]

### Nonspecific/Innate Immune Responses

It is considered as the first line of defense without antigenic specificity. These do not adapt to repeated exposure to the same pathogen. It has two major components: cellular and humoral. The cellular component consists of neutrophils, macrophages, dendritic cells, and natural killer (NK) cells. The humoral component is comprised of the complement system.

### Specific/Adaptive Immune Responses

It is characterized by antigenic specificity, which will increase after exposure to a pathogen, and maintains higher levels for years. It has two major components: cellular and humoral. T-cells mediate the cellular component, and the humoral component consists of antibodies formed by B-cells.

## CELLS OF IMMUNITY AND INFLAMMATION

### Macrophages

These are modified monocytes, which exit from bone marrow after two days and increase in size to about 22 μm and thus, are called macrophages. They are essential because they secrete interleukin (IL: IL-1, IL-6, IL-8, IL- 10), tumor necrosis factor-alpha (TNF-α), interferon-alpha (INF-α) and interferon-gamma (INF-γ) and insulin-like growth factor.[1] They also produce prostaglandins, cyclic adenosine monophosphate (cAMP) and collagenase in response to stimulation by bacterial endotoxin, immune complexes, or lymphokines **(Fig. 11.1)**. Macrophages possess CR1, CR3, CR4, C5aR receptors and plays important role in antigen presentation (MHC Class II receptor, CD1).

### Mast Cells

These cells are among the most effective cells in alerting the endothelium of a local problem. They carry receptors for the Fc portion of immunoglobulin E (IgE) [Fc-epsilon receptors (FcεR)] and immunoglobulin G (IgG) [Fc- gamma receptors (FcγR)] and complement components (C3a and C5a). They contain cytoplasmic granules called lysosomes, which store histamine, heparin, slow-reacting substances of anaphylaxis (SRS-A), TNF-α, leukotriene $C_4$, neutrophilic chemotactic factor, and eosinophil chemotactic factor.[4] The mast cells release granule contents into the extracellular compartment without loss of cell viability. Endotoxins, injury and exposure to certain toxins, lipopolysaccharide (LPS) and immunologic reactions are various stimuli which may lead to mast cell degranulation.[1]

### Neutrophils

Neutrophils account for about 60% of the total circulating leukocytes. They are the initial leukocytes recruited into the gingiva. They exit the circulation and migrate into the junctional epithelium and GCF, where they provide the first cellular host defense mechanism to contact and control periodontal bacteria. They act as a double-edged sword. Neutrophils that differentiate almost entirely within the bone marrow in 14 days and retain their small size of 10 μm when they exit from bone marrow are called microphages. Neutrophils are the first leukocytes gather at the site of inflammation. They are always the dominant cell type within the junctional epithelium and the gingival crevice. Hence, they play a crucial role in controlling the periodontal microbiota.[1]

Neutrophils possess receptors CR1, CR3, CR4, C5aR and also receptors for IgG antibody (FcγR).

Each neutrophil contains two types of granules **(Fig. 11.2)**:[5]
1. Specific granules are lysozyme, lactoferrin, and $B_{12}$-binding protein (cobalophilin).
2. Azurophilic granules are defensins, serprocidin, elastase, proteinase 3, azurocidin, cathepsin G and lysozyme.

### Lymphocytes

Three main types of lymphocytes identified based on antigen receptors are: (1) T lymphocytes, (2) B lymphocytes, and (3) natural killer (NK) cells.

#### T Lymphocytes

T lymphocytes, also called T-cells, play an essential role in cell-mediated immunity. These cells get mature and differentiate in the thymus gland situated in the neck. The presence of a low-affinity transmembrane complex called T-cell antigen receptor (TCR) on the cell surface helps to recognize diverse antigens. Four main types of T lymphocytes are: (1) T helper cells (TH cell), (2) cytotoxic T-cells, (3) suppressor T-cells (regulatory cells) and (4) memory cells.[6]

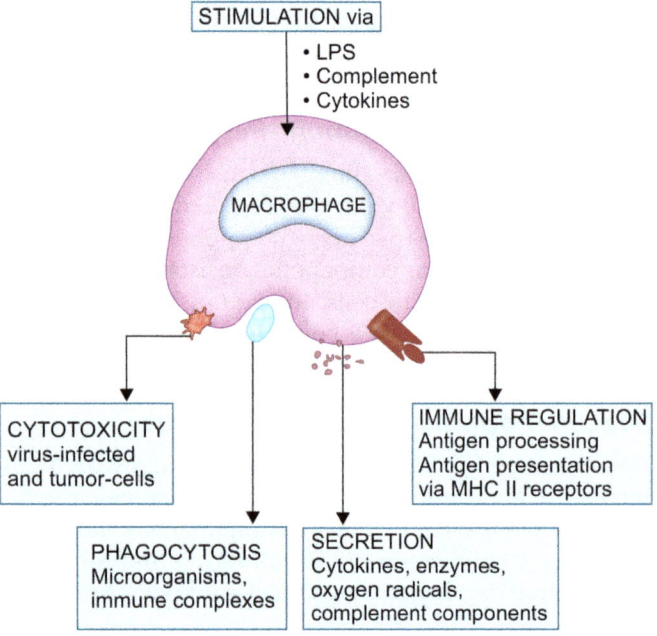

**Fig. 11.1:** Schematic representation showing functions of macrophage.
(LPS: lipopolysaccharide; MHC: major histocompatibility complex)

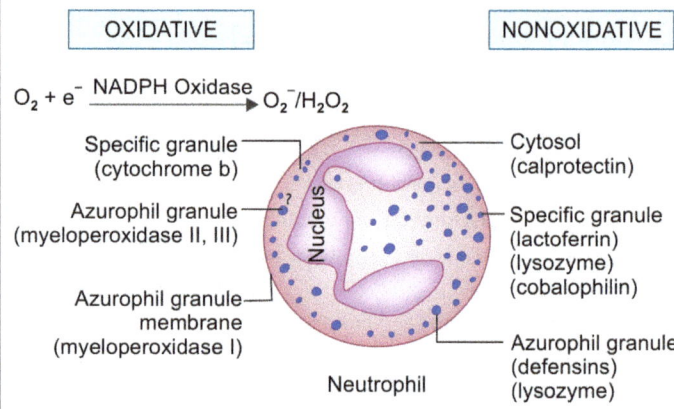

**Fig. 11.2:** Schematic representation showing the antimicrobial system of neutrophils.

## B Lymphocytes

B lymphocytes, which are derived from liver, spleen, and bone marrow, are the precursor for plasma cells, and play a role in humoral immunity. They recognize diverse antigens using a high-affinity transmembrane complex called B-cell antigen receptor (BCR). When coming in contact with antigens and get activated via TH cells, B lymphocytes differentiate into antibody-producing plasma cells.[6]

## Antigen-presenting Cells

Antigen-presenting cells (APCs) are immune cells that mediate the cellular immune response by processing and presenting antigens for recognition by certain lymphocytes, such as T-cells. Classical APCs are dendritic cells, macrophages, Langerhans cells, and B cells. Langerhans cells reside in the suprabasilar portions of the squamous epithelium of gingiva. They express high levels of MHC Class II molecules, CD1, adhesion molecules, and costimulatory factors.

## Natural Killer Cells

Natural killer cells, also called NK cells/K cells/killer cells, are the lymphocyte subset. They are an essential component of the innate immune response and have a role in host rejection. They are usually larger than small lymphocytes and consist of abundant azurophilic granules, and hence known as a large granular lymphocyte. They do not express TCR or Ig. They possess several classes of antigen receptors, including killer-inhibitory receptors and killer-activating receptors. These receptors will recognize antigen associated with major histocompatibility complex (MHC) class I molecules, and certain other surface glycoproteins. NK cells recognize and kill particular tumor and virus-infected cells and also secrete cytokines that activate macrophages to destroy ingested microbes with the help of a phenomenon known as antibody-dependent cell-mediated cytotoxicity (ADCC).

Antibody-dependent cell-mediated cytotoxicity is the nonphagocytic killing of an antibody-coated target cell by a cytotoxic effector cell. It is a process of cell-mediated immune defense and usually associated with the release of the content of cytotoxic granules or by the expression of cell death-inducing molecules. The classical NK cells-mediated ADCC involves the interaction of NK cells and target-bound antibodies. NK cell expresses Fc receptor commonly known as CD16 or FcγR-III receptor. It identifies and binds to the Fc portion of a target-bound antibody, such as IgG. Binding of Fc receptor of NK cells to the Fc region of IgG triggers the release of cytokines, such as TNF-α and IFN-γ from NK cells, resulting in the lysis of target cells **(Fig. 11.3)**.

A significant increase in the NK cell levels is noted in diseased periodontal tissues, suggesting their involvement in the immune response to plaque accumulation. Systemic conditions associated with periodontitis, such as Papillon–Lefèvre syndrome, Chédiak–Higashi syndrome, and smoking, are associated with functionally impaired NK cell. This favors the opinion of the protective function of NK cells in the periodontium.[7]

Plasma cells are the terminal cells in the progression from B-cells. They occur in germinal centers and tissues, where they produce immunoglobulins and antibodies, the effector cells for systemic and local immunity, respectively.

*Immunoglobulins*: Based on structural differences human immunoglobulins are divided into five classes as (1) IgG, (2) IgM, (3) IgA, (4) IgE, and (5) IgD. Immunoglobulin molecules are composed of either two κ or two λ light (small) chains and one of five types of heavy (large) polypeptide chains.

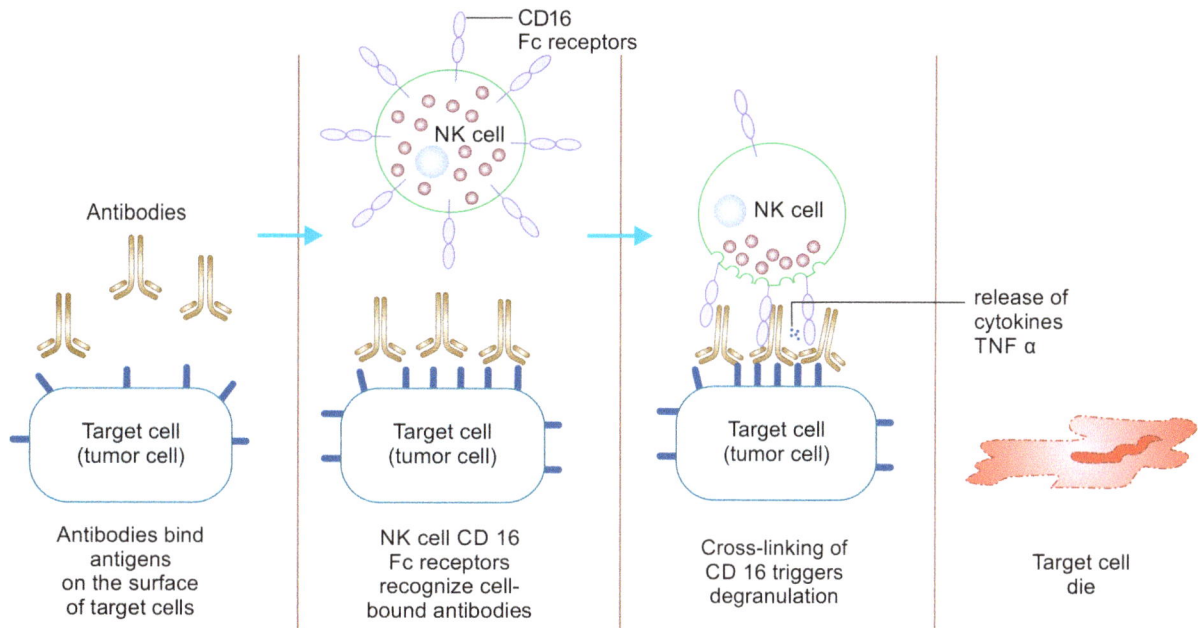

**Fig. 11.3:** Schematic representation showing antibody-dependent cell-mediated cytotoxicity (ADCC).

**Section 3:** Etiology

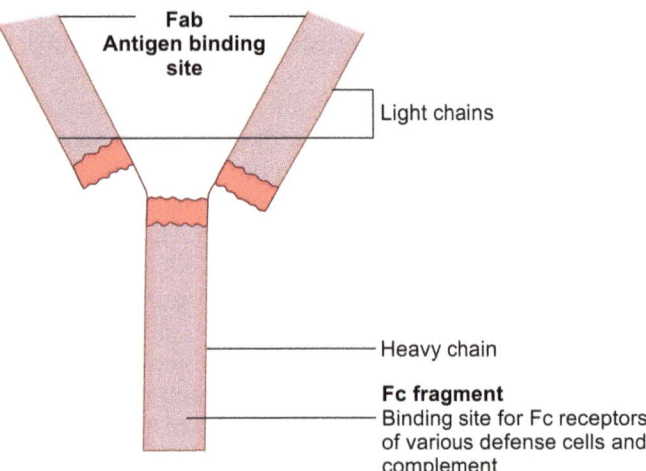

**Fig. 11.4:** Schematic representation showing immunoglobulin molecule: Y-shaped glycoprotein with heavy and light chains.

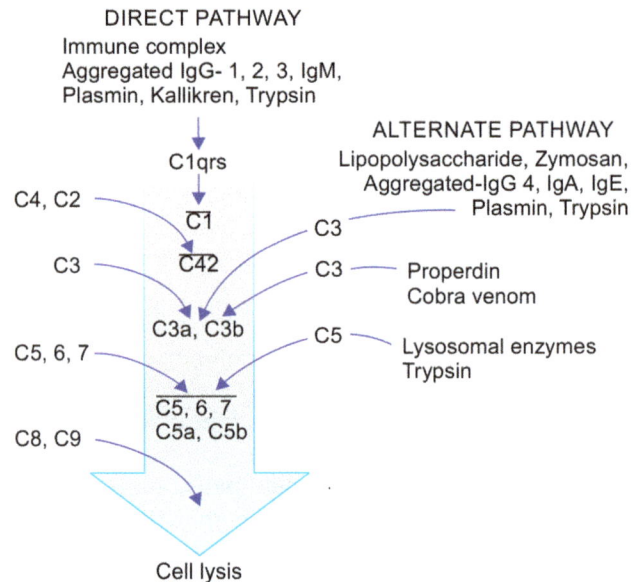

**Fig. 11.5:** Schematic representation showing complement cascade (direct and alternate pathways).

The type of heavy chain determines the class. The basic immunologic structure appears to be Y-shaped. The tail of Y contains the ends of two heavy chains and is referred to as Fc fragment. It is in this region where complement binding takes place. The remaining area of the Y-shaped molecule is composed of the light chains and the remainder of the heavy chains. This is the Fab or antigen-binding site **(Fig. 11.4)**.[3]

Properties of secretory IgA antibodies make them unique and influence their function on mucosal surfaces. Secretory IgA is more resistant to digestion by proteolytic enzymes than other immunoglobulins. It has been suggested that the secretory component of a polypeptide chain attached to the Fc portion of secretory IgA stabilizes this portion of the molecule, facilitating its transport across the glandular epithelium. It is also possible that the J chain, the fourth type of polypeptide chain associated with secretory IgA may function in making secretory IgA more resistant to proteolysis.[3]

Functions of immunoglobulins are:
- Opsonization of microorganisms
- Complement activation
- Antigen binding: Antigen-antibody complex
- Toxin neutralization
- Neutralization of viruses
- Hypersensitivity reactions (type I-III)

## Complement System

The complement system is the complex of series of heat-labile components present in normal serum. It consists of a large number of distinct plasma proteins (C1–C9), which get activated by antigen-antibody interaction. It is a part of the innate immune system and carries biologically significant consequences.[3]

The complement cascade is activated by two parallel, but independent mechanisms called as classical/direct and alterative or properdin pathway. The reaction sequence in the activation of the complement system has a cascading type pathway.[8] After one component of the complement system is bound with the Fc portion of the antibody in the antibody-antigen complex, the other components of the complement system react in an ordered sequence.

The classical pathway is initiated with antigen antibodies (IgG or IgM) reactions and by aggregated immunoglobulins. The classical sequence includes the involvement of C1, C4, C2, C3, C5, C6, C7, C8, and C9. The complex C42 cleave C3 into C3a and C3b. C3a exhibit biological activity while C3b binds to the cell membrane **(Fig. 11.5)**.[8]

An alternative pathway for complement activation also exists. Aggregated antibodies of the IgG, IgA and IgE classes, endotoxin, fungi, yeast cell walls, viruses, parasites, and other substances can initiate the complement sequence by direct activation of C3 which is the third component of complement without triggering the beginning of the cascade starting with C1. The alternative pathway initiated with C3 cleavage after the conversion of the C3 proactivator. Once the C3 gets activated, the remaining sequence is similar to the classical pathway: C5, C6, C7, C8, and C9.[8]

Bacterial endotoxins and dextran polysaccharides can also act as activators of the alternative pathway. Dental plaque and pure bacteria cultures can also initiate complement cascade by the alternative pathway, even in the absence of antibodies. On activation of complement by endotoxin, biologically-active fragmentation products are released.

Complement mediates immunological membrane damage and amplifies the inflammatory responses.

The biologic effects of the complement system are:
- *Chemotaxis*: C3a, C5a and C5b67
- *Kinin production*: C2a
- *Opsonization*: C3b
- *Cell lysis*: C6, C7, C8, and C9

# Chapter 11: Immunity and Inflammation

- *Activation of B lymphocytes*: C3b
- *Enhancement of blood clotting*: C6
- *Increased vascular permeability*: C3a, C5a
- *Promotion of clot lysis*: C3, C4

## LEUKOCYTE FUNCTIONS

For neutrophils to effectively control bacterial infections, their functions including transendothelial migration, chemotaxis, transepithelial migration, opsonization, phagocytosis and intraphagolysosomal killing must be intact **(Box 11.1 and Fig. 11.6)**.

Disorders of neutrophils are associated with invasive periodontal infection, and aggressive periodontitis, severe periodontal destruction involving both the primary dentition and permanent dentition is evident in individuals with disorders affecting neutrophil chemotaxis and phagocytosis. Also, otherwise, healthy individuals with severe periodontal problems may have subtle defects in neutrophil function.

### Transendothelial Migration

It is the selective interaction between leukocytes and endothelium that results in the leukocyte pushing its way between endothelial cells to exit the blood and enter the tissues.

Sequential phases of transendothelial migration of neutrophils are **(Fig. 11.7)**:[9]

- *Rolling*: Leukocytes L-selectin interacts with addressins on the lumenal surface of endothelial cells, pauses to inspect the endothelium.

> **BOX 11.1:** Functions of neutrophil.
> - Generation of acute-phase signals: Involves activation of serum complement components
> - Chemotaxis: Directed migration to the site of infection
> - Phagocytosis of microbial invaders
> - Antimicrobial system: Killing off bacteria

- *An insult to local tissue*: Local insult triggers the release of inflammatory mediators IL-1β, TNF-α from mast cell.
- *Signaling the endothelium*: TNF-α, C5a, LPS can stimulate endothelial cells to express P-selectin and E-selectin on their lumenal surface.
- *Increased rolling*: P-selectin and E-selectin on the endothelial cells interact with glycosaminoglycan [(GAG) carbohydrate molecules] of leukocytes. This increases the number of leukocytes attached to the lumenal surface of the endothelium.
- *Chemokine signaling*: The release of chemokine IL-8 by stimulated endothelium causes the leukocyte to shed L-selectin. Thus, chemokine functions as a signal for rolling arrest.
- *Rolling arrest*: Leukocyte function-associated antigen-1 (LFA - 1) binds to intercellular cell adhesion molecule 2 (ICAM-2), which results in arresting of rolling. Thus, this rolling arrest occurs because phagocyte becomes firmly associated with endothelium.
- *Zipper phase*: Clusters of differentiation 31 (CD31), an adhesion molecule, present on both endothelial cells and leukocytes. The binding of these two molecules helps leukocytes migrate on the boundaries between endothelial cells.

About 1–2% of all neutrophils migrate across the junctional epithelium daily. This transepithelial migration requires a chemotaxis gradient. The junctional epithelium expresses the chemotactic cytokine (chemokine) IL-8 and ICAM-1. A gradient of the membrane-bound ICAM-1 and the soluble IL-8 molecules are formed, with increased expression towards the tissue's outer surface. This distribution is ideal for the migration of neutrophils into the gingival sulcus. Neutrophils may use their adhesions LFA-1 (leukocyte function-associated antigen 1), Mac-1 (macrophage-1 antigen), or both to bind intercellular cell adhesion molecule-1 (ICAM-1) on the epithelial cell in the process of epithelial transmigration.

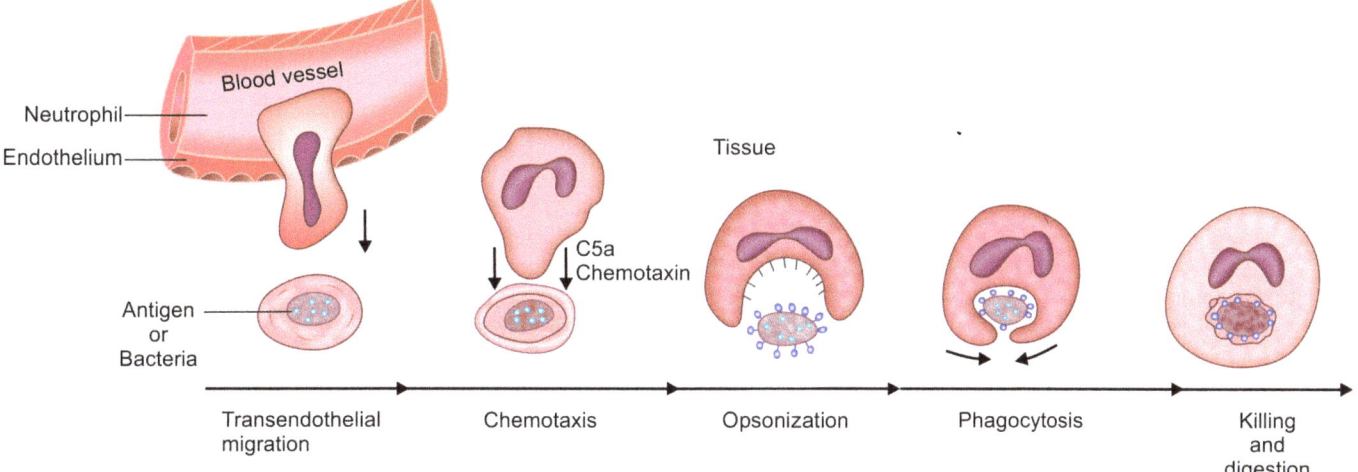

**Fig. 11.6:** Schematic representation showing functions of neutrophil.

**Section 3:** Etiology

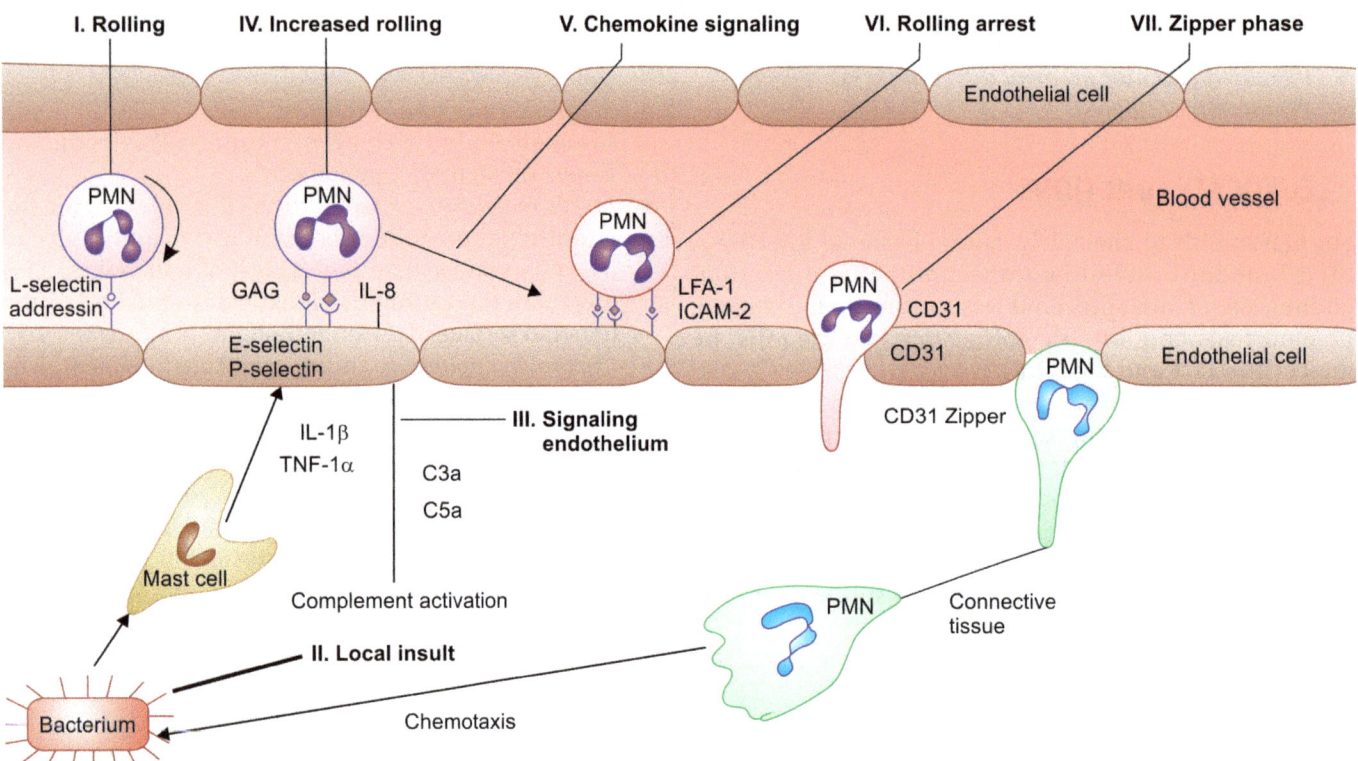

**Fig. 11.7:** Schematic representation showing transendothelial migration.
(PMN: polymorphonuclear leukocyte; CD31: clusters of differentiation 31; IL-1: interleukin-1; TNF: tumor necrosis factor-alpha; GAG: glycosaminoglycan; ICAM-2: intercellular cell adhesion molecule 2; LFA-1: leukocyte function-associated antigen 1)

## Chemotaxis

Inside the connective tissue location and migration of leukocyte is guided by a biological process known as chemotaxis. Chemotaxis is the characteristic movement of motile cells or organisms under the influence of a specific chemical signal. The process is receptor-mediated and initiated by chemotactic factors forming a concentration gradient to attract and accumulate phagocytic cells at the site of the reaction.[10]

The chemoattractants can be exogenous chemoattractants (bacterial products) or endogenous chemoattractants (C5a and IL-8). The chemotaxins for neutrophils are TNF-α, IL-8, platelet-activating factor, leukotriene B4, C5a, neutrophilic chemotactic factor, IL-1, IFN-α, and N- formyl-methionyl peptides.

## Opsonization

Opsonization refers to the process of coating a particle with recognizable molecules to enable phagocytic ingestion. The two types of opsonins are complement metabolite (C3b) and IgG.[3]

## Phagocytosis

Phagocytosis is the engulfment of particulate matters or microbial parasites by the external cell membrane of the phagocyte, resulting in an intracellular, membrane-delimited structure termed as a phagosome. Bacteria within the phagosome and phagolysosome may be killed by oxidative or nonoxidative mechanisms.[5]

## Killing and Digestion

There are two killing mechanisms: one is the oxidative mechanism, and other is nonoxidative mechanism.[9]

### Oxidative Mechanism

There is the formation of superoxide anion with the help of nicotinamide adenine dinucleotide phosphate (NADPH) oxidase enzyme of neutrophil, and this is superoxide which is capable of diffusing across the membrane. Hydrogen peroxide ($H_2O_2$) is reduced to hydroxyl radical, which is capable of causing DNA damage. Myeloperoxidase catalyzes $H_2O_2$ and chloride to hypochlorous acid (HOCl) **(Fig. 11.8)**. This HOCl molecule has antimicrobial properties.

### Nonoxidative Mechanism

Nonoxidative mechanism of killing involves phagosome-lysosome fusion, resulting in secretion of bactericidal substances, such as lysozyme, cathepsin G, and a- defensins **(Fig. 11.2)** into the phagolysosome containing the ingested bacterium.

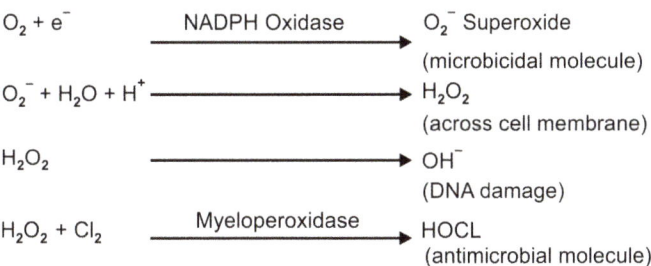

**Fig. 11.8:** Schematic representation showing the oxidative mechanism. (NADPH: nicotinamide adenine dinucleotide phosphate-oxidase; $H_2O_2$, hydrogen peroxide; HOCl: hypochlorous acid)

## CHEMICAL MEDIATORS OF INFLAMMATION

Chemical mediators of inflammation are the substances released from the cells, plasma, or damaged tissue itself. They are broadly classified into two groups **(Flowchart 11.1)**:[1]
1. Cell-derived mediators: Mediators released by cells
2. Plasma-derived mediators: Mediators originating from plasma

### Cell-derived Mediators

#### Histamine

Histamine is an amine released by mast cells as a part of the local immune response to a variety of stimuli such as trauma, heat or immune reactions, and certain cytokines. The main actions of histamine are vasodilation and increase vascular permeability.

#### Serotonin

Serotonin, also known as 5-hydroxytryptamine (5-HT), is a preformed mediator present in platelet granules. Its release is stimulated by platelet aggregation. It shows effects similar to histamine.

#### Prostaglandins

Prostaglandins are lipid autocoids synthesized from arachidonic acid by the action of cyclooxygenase (COX) isoenzymes. Prostaglandin $E_2$ ($PGE_2$), prostacyclin ($PGI_2$), prostaglandin $D_2$ ($PGD_2$), prostaglandin $F_2\alpha$ ($PGF_2\alpha$), and thromboxane $A_2$ ($TXA_2$) are principal prostaglandin mediating pathogenic mechanisms in inflammation.

### Cytokines

The word "cytokine" is derived from the Greek terminology "Kyttaro" meaning *cells* and "Kinisi" meaning *movement*. Cytokines are a broad category of low-molecular-weight polypeptides weighing 5–70 kDa. They are released by macrophages, B lymphocytes, T lymphocytes, and mast cells. Chemokines, interferons, ILs, lymphokines and TNF is an important cytokine involved in cell signaling and regulating the activity of other cells **(Table 11.2)**.[11]

- *Interleukin-1*: IL-1 is a group of 11 cytokines involved in regulation of inflammatory responses. It is found in two proinflammatory forms as IL-1α and IL-1β encoded by separate genes. Both are the significant elements of the "osteoclast activating factor." IL-1 is mainly released from activated macrophages or lymphocytes. It is also produced from mast cells, fibroblasts, keratinocytes, and endothelial cells. Bacterial LPS is a potent activator of macrophage IL-1 production, whereas TNF-α and IL-1 itself also can activate macrophage IL-1 production.

**TABLE 11.2:** Actions of various cytokines.

| Actions | Cytokines |
|---|---|
| Proinflammatory | IL-1, IL-6, IL-8, TNF-α, IFN-γ |
| Anti-inflammatory | IL-4, IL-10, IL-13, TGF-β |
| Scarring | IL-6, TGF-β |
| Antiscarring | IL-10 |
| Angiogenic | IL-8, angiogenins, VEGF |
| Antiangiogenic | IL-10 |

(IL: interleukin; TNF-α, tumor necrosis factor-alpha; IFN-γ: interferon-gamma; TGF-β: transforming growth factor-beta; VEGF: vascular endothelial growth factor)

**Flowchart 11.1:** Chemical mediators of inflammation.

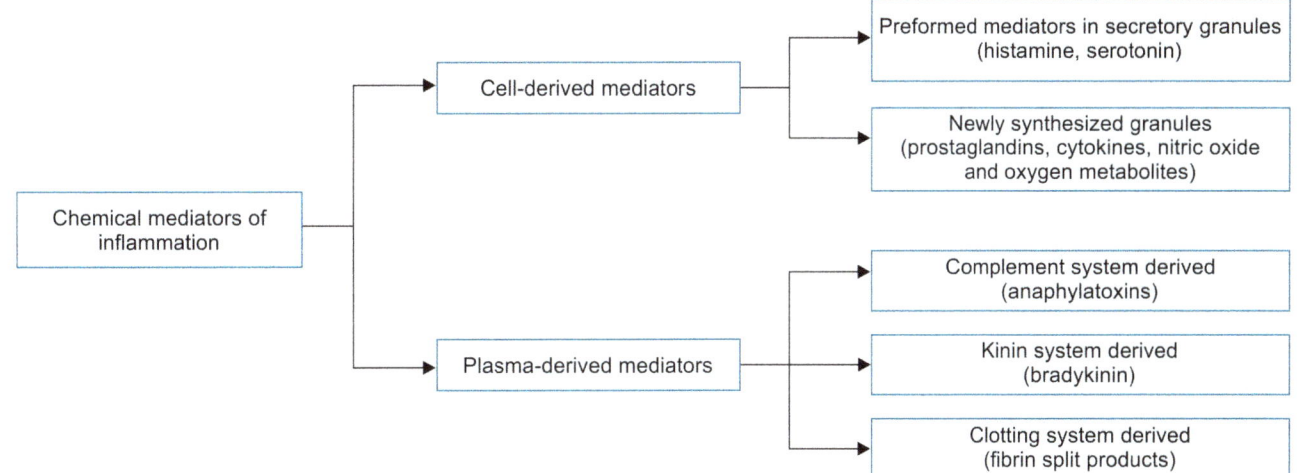

IL-1 stimulates the process of osteoclast proliferation, differentiation, and activation.[11]
- *Interleukin-6*: IL-6 is proinflammatory cytokine synthesized by macrophages, fibroblasts, lymphocytes, and endothelial cells. IL-1 and bacterial LPS induce the production of IL-6 while estrogen and progesterone inhibit production. IL-6 plays a significant role in bone resorption by causing the fusion of monocytes and forming multinuclear cells.
- *Interleukin-10*: IL-10 has a significant effect in suppressing immune and inflammatory responses. The activation of T-cells (human Th0, Th1, and Th2 cells), B cells, monocytes, and macrophages initiate the release of IL-10. It has shown to play a central role in inhibiting the antigen-presenting capacity of macrophages by downregulating class II MHC expression.[12]
- *Tumor necrosis factor-α*: This multipotential cytokine is released primarily by macrophages. Similar to IL-1, TNF-α produces a wide variety of biological effects. The proinflammatory effects of IL-1 and TNF-α include: stimulation of endothelial cells to express selectins that facilitate recruitment of leukocyte, (2) activation of macrophage IL-1 production, and (3) induction of $PGE_2$ by macrophages and gingival fibroblasts causing bone resorption. Both IL-1 and TNF-α gets accumulated in significant concentrations in gingival crevicular fluid (GCF) at periodontally diseased sites, thus suggesting their role in periodontal infection. Successful management of periodontitis case is found to be associated with reduced IL-1 concentration.

### Nitric Oxide

Nitric oxide (NO) is a short-acting, soluble-free radical gas produced by a variety of cells. It causes vascular smooth muscle relaxation (vasodilation), antagonism of all stages of platelet activation (antiplatelet activating agent), and microbicidal action. Its synthesis occurs de novo from L-arginine, molecular oxygen, and NADPH under the influence of enzyme nitric oxide synthase. Nitric oxide can affect only cells that are close to the source where it is generated.

### Oxygen-derived Free Radicals

They are synthesized via the NADPH oxidase pathway.

## Plasma-derived Mediators

### Anaphylatoxins

These are complement peptides C3a, C4a, C5a, which can cause smooth muscle contraction, increase vascular permeability, and histamine release from mast cells.

### Bradykinin

It is a short-lived, vasoactive peptide that is able to induce vasodilation, increase vascular permeability, cause smooth muscle contraction, and induce pain.

### Plasmin

It is a proteolytic enzyme that acts to break down fibrin clots, cleave complement protein C3, and activate factor XII.

### Thrombin

It is a serine protease that converts soluble fibrinogen into insoluble fibrin.

## NONSPECIFIC AND SPECIFIC IMMUNITY

Nonspecific immunity, also known as innate immunity, is the first line of defense response from the host. The cellular components of nonspecific immunity comprise phagocytic cells, namely neutrophils, monocytes, NK cells, complement system, mast cells, and additional inflammatory mediators.

Specific immunity, also known as acquired immunity, represents the host's second line of defense mechanism. The specific immune system is constituted by T lymphocytes, B lymphocytes, plasma cells, and immunoglobulin.

Interaction between nonspecific and specific immunity is well explained in **Figure 11.9**.

## IMMUNE MECHANISMS

Immune mechanisms are the defense mechanism exhibited by the host against the range of foreign substances, including bacteria and viruses. These protective responses consist of several types of overreaction or hypersensitivity that usually result in local tissue destruction. Sensitized the host may present with tissue damage (immune-pathologic changes) when exposed continuously to the sensitizing antigen.[13]

Hypersensitivity reactions occurring as a part of immune mechanisms have been divided into four types as type I, II, III, and IV. Type I, II, and III reactions are humoral and are termed as immediate reactions because they occur in minutes to hours. Type IV reactions are cellular or cell-mediated and are called as delayed reactions because they occur within days.[3]

### Anaphylactic Reaction (Type I)

Immunoglobulin E plays a direct role in its pathogenesis through its ability to sensitize the skin. This sensitizing capability is referred to as reaginic and the IgE antibody as reagin. IgG antibody combines with antigen in the circulation before it can bind to IgE in mast cells or basophils and prevents sensitization. These IgG antibodies are referred to as blocking antibodies.

Immunoglobulin E antibodies involved in anaphylactic reaction attach strongly at the Fc portion of the antibody to receptors found on mast cells and basophilic leukocytes primarily in gingival connective tissues (**Fig. 11.10**). This antibody-antigen reaction causes the release of pharmacologically active substances from the sensitized cells. These substances cause the response and have the potential to induce tissue damage in periodontal disease.

# Chapter 11: Immunity and Inflammation

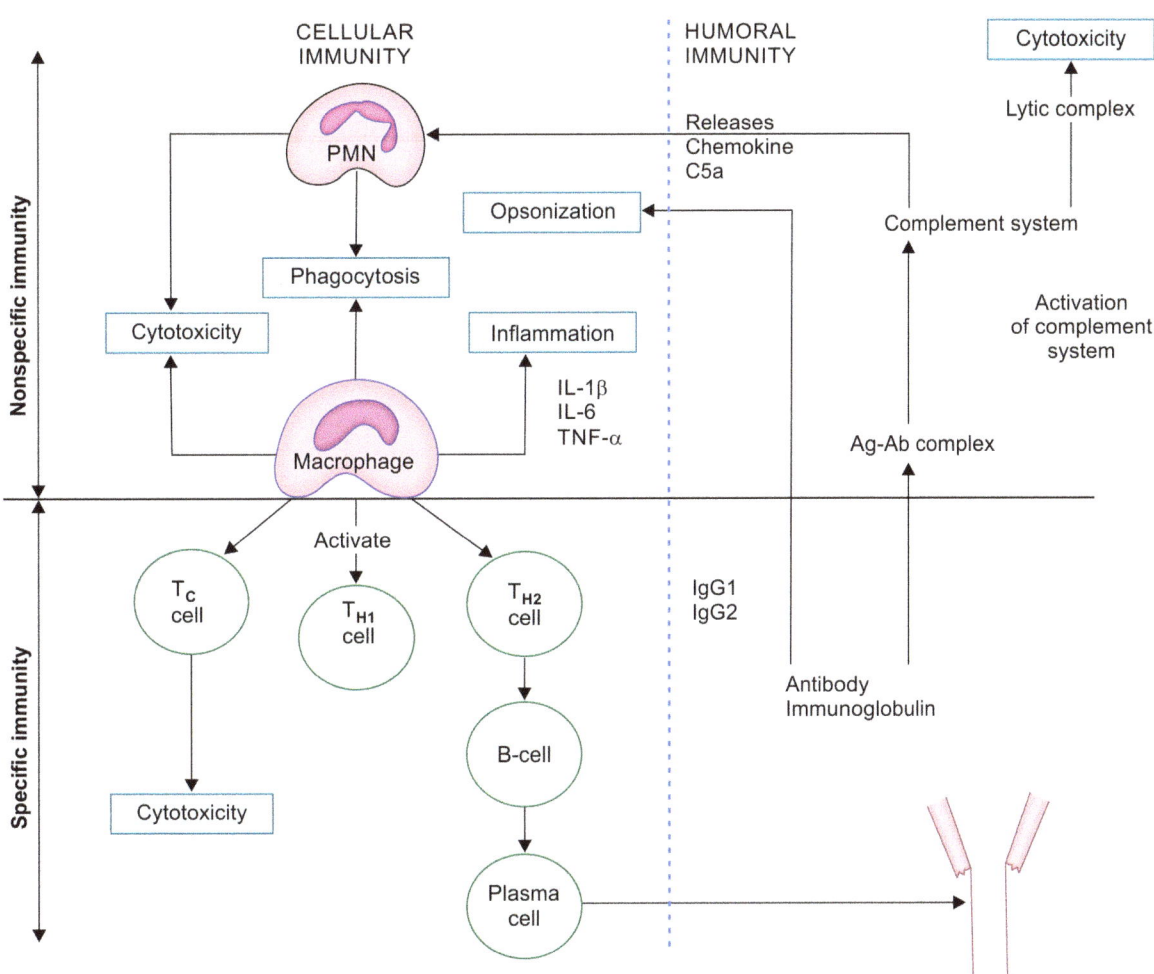

**Fig. 11.9:** Schematic representation showing the interaction between nonspecific and specific immunity.
(PMN: polymorphonuclear leukocyte; IL: interleukin; TNF-α: tumor necrosis factor-alpha)

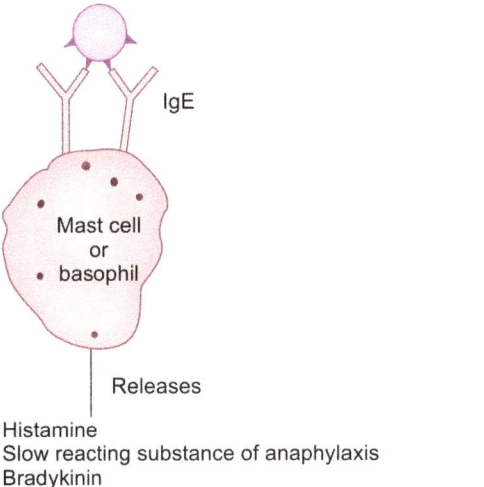

**Fig. 11.10:** Schematic illustration showing anaphylactic reaction type I.

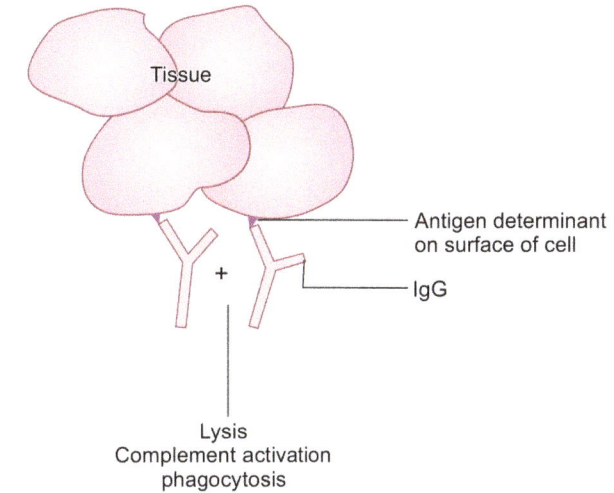

**Fig. 11.11:** Schematic illustration showing cytotoxic reaction type II.

## Cytotoxic Reaction (Type II)

The cytotoxic reaction is a combination of IgG (or rarely IgM) antibodies with the antigenic determinants on the cellular surface resulting in cytotoxic/cytolytic effects **(Fig. 11.11)**.

## Immune Complex (Arthus) Reaction (Type III)

When high levels of antigen to which the host has been sensitized are present and persist without being eliminated. Antigen-antibody (IgG and IgM) complexes precipitate in and around small blood vessels, and with subsequent complement activation causes tissue damage at the site of local reaction. This may result in inflammation, hemorrhage, and necrosis. The release of lysosomal enzymes from polymorphonuclear leukocytes (PMNs), mast cell activation, platelet agglutination, microthrombi formation, and neutrophil chemotaxis result in tissue destruction. This reaction is referred to as an immune complex or Arthus reaction and commonly mediated by IgM or IgG antibodies. The ability of these antibodies to fix complement, which is partially responsible for the chemotactic attraction of the PMNs, has been found to play a significant role in the Arthus reaction (**Fig. 11.12**).

## Cell-mediated Immunity or Delayed Hypersensitivity (Type IV)

The phenomenon of delayed hypersensitivity belongs to the class of immune responses known as cell-mediated immunity. These reactions are referred to as type IV reactions. Cellular immunity does not involve circulating antibodies but is based on antigens' interaction with the surface of T lymphocytes releasing lymphokines that cause biological effects on leukocytes, macrophages, and tissue cells. Lymphocytes that can develop into plasma cells that produce antibodies are designated as B-cells. T and B lymphocytes have been shown to produce biologically active lymphokines (**Fig. 11.13**).

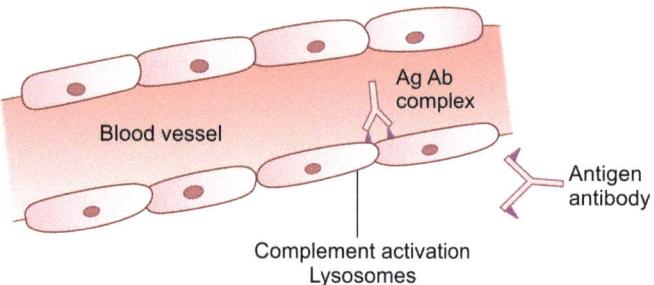

**Fig. 11.12:** Schematic representation showing immune complex reaction type III.

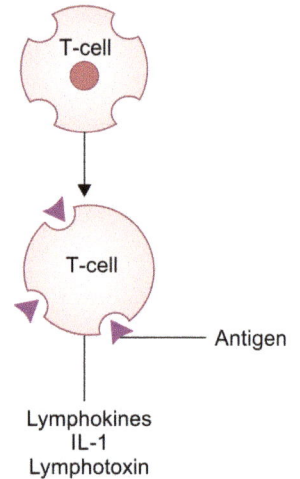

**Fig. 11.13:** Schematic representation showing delayed hypersensitivity reaction type IV.

## ANTIGEN PROCESSING AND PRESENTATION

Major histocompatibility complex is a locus on the short arm of chromosome 6 that encodes for two molecules, namely MHC I and MHC II. MHC I molecule is encoded by HLA A, B, and C genes, and the MHC II molecule is encoded by the HLD gene. MHC I molecules are present on nucleated cells consisting of two nonidentical chains which interact with cytotoxic T-cell having CD 8 receptors. MHC II molecules are present on antigen-presenting cells consisting of two identical chains that interact with helper T-cells having CD 4 receptors.

Costimulation or second signal involves ligand-receptor interactions at the surfaces of a responder lymphocyte and an "accessory" cell—antigen-presenting cells (APCs) for activation of T-cells, and helper T-cells for activation of B cells (**Fig 11.14**). Resting APCs express few or no B7 costimulatory molecules and fail to activate naive T-cells. Microbes and cytokines produced in response to microbes, activate APCs, and stimulate the expression of B7 costimulators. B7–CD28 interactions stimulate the expansion and differentiation of naive T-cells. Thus, costimulation makes the T-cell resistant to apoptosis. It upregulates growth factor receptors on the T-cell, thereby stimulating its proliferation. It also decreases the amount of time needed to trigger the T-cell.

## PATHOGEN ASSOCIATED MOLECULAR PATTERNS

Pathogen associated molecular patterns (PAMPs) are conserved molecules which do not evolve to interact with the immune system but perform essential physiological functions for bacteria.

- Peptidoglycan is a mesh-like exoskeleton that provides rigidity and shape to gram-positive bacteria, which induces the release of TNF-α from monocytes.
- Lipoteichoic acid is present only in gram-positive bacteria, which causes the release of TNF-α, IL-6.

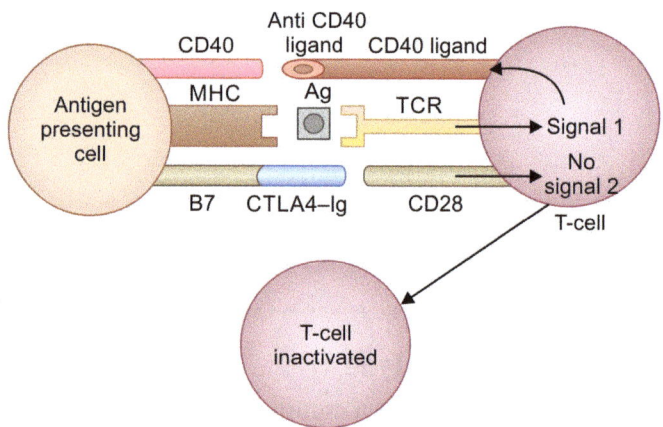

**Fig. 11.14:** Schematic representation showing costimulation.

- Lipopolysaccharides are present on the outer membrane of gram-negative bacteria. Structurally they are divided into three parts, i.e., O polysaccharides/O antigen, core polysaccharide, and lipid A. Major antigen is O antigen which stimulates macrophages through TLR-4 to produce IL-1β.
- Viral double-stranded or single-stranded RNA

## PATTERN RECOGNITION RECEPTORS

The innate immune system is well equipped with pattern recognition receptors (PRRs) specialized in initial sensing of infection. PRRs play an integral role in detecting invading pathogens as these receptors recognize PAMPs. They initiate intracellular signaling cascades and the expression of inflammatory mediators to get rid of the infected cells. The receptors are mainly expressed by antigen-presenting cells such as dendritic cells and macrophages. They are also expressed in other immune and nonimmune cells.[14]

Pattern recognition receptors are divided into four families, as follows:
1. Toll-like receptors (TLRs)
2. Nucleotide oligomerization receptors (NLRs)
3. C-type lectin receptors (CLRs)
4. RIG-1-like receptors (RLRs)

### Toll-like Receptors

Eleven members constitute them in mammals as a TLR-1 to TLR-11. They are specialized for sensing invading pathogens outside the cells in bacteria, viruses, fungi, and parasites.[15] Each TLR has a broad range of specificities:
- TLR-1, TLR-2, TLR-4 and TLR-6 recognize bacterial lipids
- TLR-3, TLR-7, and TLR-8 recognize viral RNA
- TLR-9 recognizes bacterial DNA

TLR-5 and TLR-10 recognize bacterial or parasite proteins. Toll-like receptors are type I transmembrane protein, which consists of an extracellular domain constituted by leucine-rich repeat (LRR). LRR is associated with the identification of microbial products, and a cytoplasmic TIR (Toll/Interleukin - 1 receptor) domain for recruiting different signaling molecules. This triggers the activation of the transcription of genes involved in inflammation and antimicrobial defenses. TLRs are found in different cellular compartments. TLR-1, TLR-2, TLR-4, TLR-5, TLR-6 are noted on the cell surface and TLR-3, TLR-7, TLR-8, and TLR-9 present in intracellular vesicles including endoplasmic reticulum.

The components induced upon TLR stimulation are as follows:
- Proinflammatory cytokines: IL-6, IL-12, TNF-α
- Anti-inflammatory cytokines: IL-10
- Type I interferons get involved in antiviral responses.
- Chemokines attract other immune cells at the site of infection.
- Chemokine receptors allow TLR-activated cells to migrate to lymph nodes.
- Antimicrobial molecules
- Costimulatory molecules, including CD80/86 and CD40, get involved in T-cell activation by antigen-presenting cells.
- Enhancement of antigen uptake and presentation.

> **Points to Ponder**
> - Pan-receptor defect: A reduction in all chemotaxin receptors characterizes this defect. It plays a significant role in localized aggressive periodontitis that is associated with a decrease in chemotactic responses to various chemotactic factors, such as C5a, FMLP (formyl peptide) and leukotriene B4.[16]
> - Clusters of differentiation (CD) system are the group of receptors that enable the cell to interact with each other molecules/cells.
> - Inflammatory actions of various chemical mediators
>
> | Chemical mediators | Actions |
> | --- | --- |
> | $PGI_2$, $PGE_1$, $PGE_2$, $PGD_2$, bradykinin | Vasodilatation |
> | Thromboxane $A_2$, leukotrienes $C_4$, $D_4$, $E_4$ | Vasoconstriction |
> | Leukotrienes, histamine, SRS-A, bradykinin | Increased permeability |
> | Leukotriene B4, HETE, lipoxin | Chemotaxis |
> | Bradykinin | Leukocyte adhesion |
> | α2-macroglobulin | Collagenase activity |

($PGI_2$: prostacyclin; $PGE_2$: prostaglandin $E_2$; $PGD_2$: prostaglandin $D_2$; SRS-A: slow-reacting substance of anaphylaxis; HETE: hydroxyeicosatetraenoic acid)

## REFERENCES

1. Kumar V, Abbas AK, Fausto N. Acute and chronic inflammation. In: Robbins & Cotran Pathologic Basis of Disease, 7th edition. Philadelphia, PA, USA: Elsevier-Saunders; 2005. pp. 47-86.
2. Abbas AK. Diseases of immunity. In: Kumar V, Abbas AK, Fausto N. Robbins & Cotran Pathologic Basis of Disease, 7th edition. Philadelphia, PA, USA: Elsevier-Saunders; 2005. pp. 193-268.
3. Ananthanarayan R, Paniker CK. Ananthanarayan & Paniker's Textbook of Microbiology, 8th edition. New Delhi, India: Orient Longman; 2009.
4. Malaviya R, Ikeda T, Ross E, Abraham SN. Mast cell modulation of neutrophil influx and bacterial clearance at sites of infection through TNF-alpha. Nature. 1996;381(6577):77-80.
5. Nisengard RC, Michael GN, Sanz M. Host response: basic concepts. In: Carranza FA, Newman MG, Takei HH (Eds). Carranza's Clinical Periodontology, 8th edition. Philadelphia, PA, USA: WB Saunders; 1996. pp. 111-120.
6. Kinane DF, Berglundh T, Lindhe J. Host-parasite interactions in periodontal disease. In: Lindhe J, Karring T, Lang NP (Eds). Clinical Periodontology and Implant Dentistry, 4th edition. Oxford, UK: Blackwell Munksgaard; 2003. pp. 150-78.
7. Tsoumis GS, Singh G, Dolby AE. Human antibody-dependent cellular cytotoxicity and natural killer cytotoxicity in periodontal disease. A preliminary report. J Periodontal Res. 1985;20(2):122-30.

## Section 3: Etiology

8. Nisengard RJ. The role of immunology in periodontal disease. J Periodontol. 1977;48(9):505-16.
9. Miyasaki KT, Nisengard RJ, Haake SK. Immunity and inflammation: basic concepts. In: Newman MG, Takei HH, Carranza FA (Eds). Carranza's Clinical Periodontology, 9th edition. Philadelphia, PA, USA: WB Saunders; 2003. pp. 113-31.
10. Meng H, Xu L, Li Q, Han J, Zhao Y. Determinants of host susceptibility in aggressive periodontitis. Periodontol 2000. 2007;43:133-59.
11. Graves D. Cytokines that promote periodontal tissue destruction. J Periodontol. 2008;79(8 Suppl):1585-91.
12. Gemmell E, Seymour GJ. Cytokine profiles of cells extracted from humans with periodontal diseases. J Dent Res. 1998;77(1):16-26.
13. Lamster IB. Inflammatory responses in periodontal diseases. In: Wilson TG, Kornman KS. Fundamentals of Periodontics, 2nd edition. Chicago, USA: Quintessence Publishing; 2003. pp. 159-68.
14. Mahanonda R, Pichyangkul S. Toll-like receptors and their role in periodontal health and disease. Periodontol 2000. 2007;43:41-55.
15. Medzhitov R, Preston-Hurlburt P, Janeway CA. A human homologue of the Drosophila Toll protein signals activation of adaptive immunity. Nature. 1997;388(6640):394-7.
16. Zadeh HH, Nichols FC, Miyasaki KT. The role of the cell-mediated immune response to *Actinobacillus actinomycetemcomitans* and *Porphyromonas gingivalis* in periodontitis. Periodontol. 2000. 1999;20:239-88.

### VIVA VOCE

**Q1. What is the fundamental difference between microphages and macrophages?**
**Ans.** Microphages are neutrophils that differentiate almost entirely within the bone marrow in 14 days and retain their small size of 10 μm when they exit from bone marrow. In contrast, macrophages are modified monocytes, which exits from bone marrow after two days and increase in size to about 22 μm.

**Q2. What is a pan-receptor defect?**
**Ans.** When all chemotaxin receptors are decreased, the defect is called a pan-receptor defect. It is seen in localized aggressive periodontitis. It is characterized by a decrease in chemotactic responses to a variety of chemotactic factors, including C5a, FMLP (formyl peptide), and leukotriene B4.

**Q3. What is a neutrophil extracellular trap (NET)?**
**Ans.** These are a network of extracellular fibers primarily composed of DNA from neutrophil, chromatin, and nucleosomes. Neutrophils can kill pathogens extracellularly by releasing neutrophil extracellular traps. It is considered as last resort by neutrophils to kill.

**Q4. What is ADCC?**
**Ans.** Antibody-dependent cell-mediated cytotoxicity is the non-phagocytic killing of an antibody-coated target cell by a cytotoxic effector cell. It is a process of cell-mediated immune defense and usually associated with the release of the content of cytotoxic granules or by the expression of cell death-inducing molecules.

**Q5. What are the types of T cells?**
**Ans.**
a. Helper T-cells
b. Cytotoxic T-cells
c. Memory T-cells
d. Regulatory T-cells earlier called as suppressor T-cells.

**Q6. What are Toll-like receptors?**
**Ans.** Toll-like receptors are transmembrane receptors that are expressed in sentinel cells such as macrophages, dendritic cells, etc. Nomura and colleagues first reported human toll-like receptors in 1994.

**Q7. Which immune response is considered as the first line of defense without antigenic specificity?**
**Ans.** Nonspecific/innate immune responses

**Q8. What are the cellular components of nonspecific immune responses?**
**Ans.** Neutrophils, macrophages, dendritic cells, and natural killer (NK) cells.

**Q9. What is the humoral component of nonspecific immune responses?**
**Ans.** Complement system.

**Q10. What are the cellular and the humoral component of specific immune responses?**
**Ans.** The cellular component is T-cells, and the humoral component consists of antibodies formed by B-cells.

# Chapter 12

# Pathogenesis and Host Response

*Shalu Bathla*

## Chapter Outline

- Microbiology and Immunology
- Stages of Pathogenesis
- Immunologic Aspects of the Microbial Interaction with the Host
- Concepts of Pathogenesis

## INTRODUCTION

Microorganisms trigger inflammatory host responses and determine the course and severity of periodontal diseases. Microorganism-induced pathogenic effects may involve direct tissue destruction or indirect modulation of the host responses. Microbial interaction mediates inflammatory host responses, usually determined by inherent characteristics of the host-like genetic factors. The host response is the protective body mechanism that prevents local infection from progressing to a systemic, life-threatening condition. Thus, the pathogenesis of periodontal destruction involves a complex interplay between bacterial pathogens and the host tissues.[1]

## MICROBIOLOGY AND IMMUNOLOGY

The gingival crevice harbors bacteria in both health and disease. In a clinically healthy periodontium, the microbial flora is primarily composed of gram-positive facultative microorganisms, predominately species, such as *Actinomyces* and *Streptococcus* sp. Gram-negative species and spirochetal forms also may be found, but they are considerably less prevalent and occur in much smaller numbers. Serum antibodies to microorganisms are usually in low titers, suggesting the minimal systemic antigenic stimulation by plaque during gingival health. The gingival tissues typically demonstrate some evidence of inflammation. Tissues are generally infiltrated with chronic inflammatory cells, generally lymphocytes.

Neutrophils are common within the junctional epithelium and in the gingival sulcus. The infiltration of inflammatory cells is thought to be a response to bacterial plaque. Host defense mechanisms in a healthy individual are effective in managing the bacterial challenge. Physical mechanisms of host defense are constituted by the integrity of the epithelial cell layer, shedding of epithelial cells, and the flow of crevicular fluid that may function to clear bacteria and their products from the subgingival environment. The complement, neutrophils and antibody production likely contributes to controlling the sulcular microbiota.[2]

## STAGES OF PATHOGENESIS

Stages in the pathogenesis of periodontal diseases are as follows:[1]
- Adhesion and colonization
- Host tissue invasion
- Bacterial evasion of host defense mechanisms
- Host tissue destruction
- Tissue healing

### Adhesion and Colonization

The periodontal environment consists of two fluid systems, i.e., saliva and gingival crevicular fluid (GCF), both are capable of flushing out the bacteria. Bacterial adhesion to a given substrate greatly enhances their ability to stay in the gingival sulcus and multiply.[3] The presence of adhesion in periopathogens is a 2-fold affair in that bacteria that can bind to host surfaces and also to other microorganisms. Thus, the surfaces available for attachment of microorganisms include the tooth, tissues, and pre-existing plaque mass.

### Attachment of Microorganisms to Tooth Surface

Bacteria that initially colonize the periodontal environment most likely attach to the pellicle or saliva-coated tooth surfaces. A relevant example is the adherence of *Actinomyces viscosus* through fimbriae on the bacterial surface to proline-rich proteins found on saliva-coated tooth surfaces.[4]

### *Attachment of Microorganisms to Tissues*

The bacterial adherence to host tissues plays a role in colonization and may be a critical step in the process of bacterial invasion. *Porphyromonas gingivalis* attaches through fimbriae to galactosyl residues of epithelial cells. *Treponema denticola* attaches through surface protein to galactosyl or mannose residues of fibroblasts. *A. viscosus,* and *A. naeslundii* attach through fimbriae to galactosyl residues of polymorphonuclear leukocytes (PMNL).[5]

### *Attachment of Microorganisms to Pre-existing Plaque Mass*

Bacterial attachment to the preexisting plaque is studied by examining the adherence between different bacterial strains (coaggregation). One of the best-characterized interactions is the adherence of *A. viscosus* through surface fimbriae to a polysaccharide receptor of *S. sanguinis*.[6]

## Host Tissue Invasion

The properties of a microorganism that enables it to cause disease are referred to as virulence factors. Thus, virulence properties can be broadly categorized into two groups:
1. Factors facilitating colonization and invasion of bacterial species into host tissues.
2. Factors enabling bacterial species to directly or indirectly cause host tissue damage.[1]

The bacteria or their products penetrate the connective tissue to a variable extent, even to the surface of the alveolar bone.[7] Capability of a microorganism to invade tissue has been proposed as a key factor in distinguishing pathogenic from nonpathogenic gram-negative species or strains. Tissue invasion makes it impossible to dislodge these bacteria by mechanical action.

The two means of tissue invasion are:
1. Bacteria may enter host tissues through ulcerations in the epithelium of the gingival sulcus or pocket and have been observed in intercellular spaces of the gingival tissues.
2. Another means of tissue invasion may involve the direct penetration of bacteria into host epithelial or connective tissue cells. *Aggregatibacter actinomycetemcomitans, P. gingivalis, Fusobacterium nucleatum,* and *T. denticola* can directly invade host tissue cells.

Examples of bacterial host tissue invasion in periodontal diseases are:
- Invasion of deep gingival connective tissue by viable *actinomycetemcomitans* in localized aggressive periodontitis
- Bacteria, particularly spirochetes invade the tissue in necrotizing ulcerative gingivitis (NUG)

Thus, the antigens, such as collagenase and toxins, enter gingival tissues where they trigger host responses and cause direct tissue destruction.

## Bacterial Evasion of Host Defense Mechanisms

Bacterial evasion helps the organisms to evade the host responses that attempt to eliminate them. Periodontal bacteria neutralize or evade host defenses via numerous other mechanisms.[8] The periodontium as a whole is endowed with both innate and acquired immune mechanisms to provide defense capabilities against the invading microorganisms. Innate immunity is conferred by the epithelial barrier and the cells of the innate mechanisms, i.e., dendritic cells, neutrophils, monocytes, and macrophages. Acquired immunity is provided by B and T lymphocytes.[9]

Following are the examples of host defense mechanisms evaded by bacterial species and bacterial properties:
- *Specific antibodies*: Immunoglobulins facilitate phagocytosis of bacteria by opsonization or block adherence by binding to the bacterial cell surface and restricting access to bacterial adhesins. The production of immunoglobulin-degrading proteases by specific microorganisms may counteract these host defenses.
- *Polymorphonuclear leukocytes (PMNL)*: Bacteria produce substances that suppress the activity of or kill PMNL normally involved in host defenses. An example of this is the production of two toxins (leukotoxin and cytolethal distending toxin) by *A. actinomycetemcomitans*, affecting leukocytes.
- *Lymphocytes*: *Tannerella forsythia* and *F. nucleatum* have been shown to induce apoptosis, a form of cellular suicide, in lymphocytes.
- *Interleukin-8 (IL-8)*: This is a proinflammatory chemokine that provides a signal for the recruitment of neutrophils (PMNL) to a local site. *P. gingivalis* can inhibit the production of IL-8 by epithelial cells which provide the microorganism with an advantage in evading PMNL-mediated killing.[8]

## Host Tissue Destruction

Periodontitis is characterized by remodeling of connective tissues resulting in a net loss of local soft tissues, bone, and the periodontal attachment apparatus. The process from gingivitis to periodontitis progresses from the loss of the soft tissue attachment to the tooth and the subsequent loss of alveolar bone.[10]

The tissue destructive mechanisms can be classified as follows:
- Direct mechanism
- Indirect mechanism

### *Direct Mechanism*

It results from the action of bacterial components that damage tissue directly. The bacterial metabolic byproducts, such as ammonia, volatile sulfur compounds, fatty acids, peptides, and indole, inhibit the growth or alter the metabolism of host tissue cells. Periodontal microorganisms also produce a variety of enzymes that are capable of degrading all host tissues and intercellular matrix molecules essentially. *P. gingivalis* produces collagenase, trypsin-like enzyme, keratinase, neuraminidase, and fibronectin-degrading enzymes **(Fig. 12.1)**.[11] Virulence factors of *A. actinomycetemcomitans* are collagenase, cytotoxin, leukotoxin, bacteriocin, endotoxin, Fc binding protein, invasins, immunosuppressive factors, adhesins, and chemotaxis inhibitor **(Fig. 12.2)**.

## Indirect Mechanism

It is through the destructive host responses triggered by the infecting microorganisms. Well-characterized interactions involve the release of interleukin-1 (IL-1), tumor necrosis factor (TNF), and prostaglandins from monocytes, macrophages, and PMNL exposed to bacterial endotoxin (lipopolysaccharide). These host-derived mediators have the potential to stimulate bone resorption and activate or inhibit other host immune cells. Inflammatory mediators contributing to tissue destruction are proteinases, prostaglandins, and cytokines.

*Proteinases*: Proteinases or proteases cleave proteins by hydrolyzing peptide bonds and may be classified into two major classes, endopeptidases and exopeptidases, depending on the location of activity of the enzyme on its substrate. Endopeptidases cleave bonds in their substrate within the polypeptide chain, whereas the exopeptidases cleave their substrate near the end of the polypeptide chain.

Matrix metalloproteinases: Matrix metalloproteinases (MMPs), also known as matrixins, are proteinases that degrade both matrix and non-matrix proteins.[12] They elicit periodontal tissue destruction by the degradation of the extracellular matrix (ECM) molecules. They are a family of homologous $Zn^{+2}$ endopeptidases that can hydrolyze most of the extracellular matrix constituents.

There are about 28 MMPs; some of them are mentioned in **Table 12.1**.

## Structure of MMPs

Typical MMPs consist of a catalytic domain formed by an active site with a $Zn^{+2}$ binding sequence. The catalytic domain is preceded by a propeptide consisting of 80 amino acids. It endows the enzyme with catalytic latency at the time of secretion. This is followed by a protein-rich hinge region suggesting conversion into the largest domain. A plexin-like COOH-terminal sequence of MMPs determines the substrate specificity **(Fig. 12.3)**. The two gelatinases, i.e., gelatinase-A and gelatinase-B, contain a gelatin-binding insert (fibronectin type II-like inserts) in the catalytic domain. Matrilysin, a smallest MMP (molecular weight = 28,000), lacks plexin-like domain.[13]

Activation: MMPs are secreted in the latent or inactive form. Enzyme activity in the tissues is partly controlled by activation of the latent enzyme and the level of enzyme inhibitors present. Proteases capable of activating MMPs

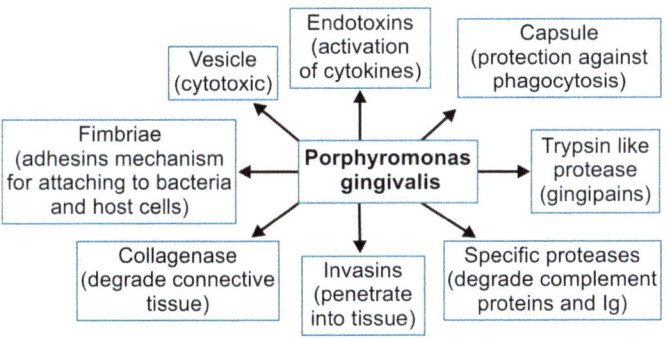

**Fig. 12.1:** Schematic representation showing virulence factors of *P. gingivalis*.

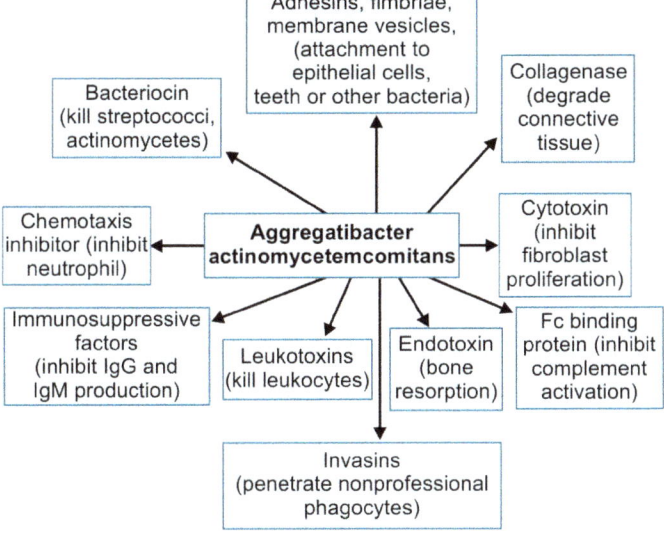

**Fig. 12.2:** Schematic representation showing virulence factors of *A. actinomycetemcomitans*.

**TABLE 12.1:** Matrix metalloproteinases (MMPs).

| Protease | MMP number | Matrix substrate |
| --- | --- | --- |
| Collagenase-1 | MMP-1 | Collagen |
| Collagenase-2 | MMP-8 | Collagen |
| Collagenase-3 | MMP-13 | Collagen |
| Collagenase-4 | MMP-18 | Collagen |
| Gelatinase-A | MMP-2 | Gelatin, elastin |
| Gelatinase-B | MMP-9 | Gelatin, elastin |
| Stromelysin-1 | MMP-3 | Laminin, fibronectin, non-triple helical region of collagen types II and III |
| Stromelysin-2 | MMP-10 | — |
| Stromelysin-3 | MMP-11 | Fibronectin |
| Matrilysin | MMP-7 (smallest) | Aggrecan, laminin |
| Enamelysin | MMP-20 | Amelogenin |

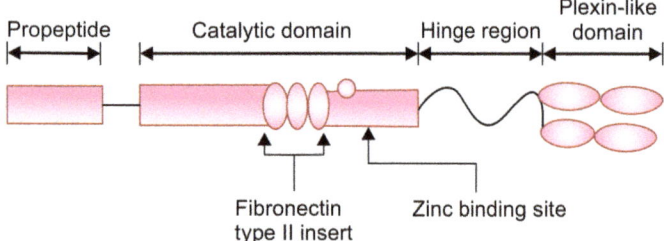

**Fig. 12.3:** Schematic representation showing the structure of matrix metalloproteinases (MMPs).

include bacterial enzymes, such as the chymotrypsin-like protease produced by *T. denticola*, as well as host cell enzymes, such as neutrophil cathepsin G.

The other activators are:
- Organomercurials, metal ions, thiol reagents, and oxidants
- Plasmins, trypsin, tryptase, kallikrein

Inhibition: MMPs are inactivated by α-macroglobulins that are found in serum and GCF.

The other inhibitors are:
- Tissue inhibitors of metalloproteinases: Locally produced tissue inhibitors
- Insulin-like growth factor (IGF), TNF-α, IL-1, transforming growth factor-beta (TGF-β), glucocorticoids, retinoic acid.

*Prostaglandins*: They are arachidonic acid derivatives synthesized under the action of cyclooxygenases [cyclooxygenase-1 (COX-1), cyclooxygenase-2 (COX-2)] isoenzymes. Arachidonic acid is a 20-carbon polyunsaturated omega-6 fatty acid present in most of the cellular plasma membrane.[14] In the periodontium, macrophages and fibroblasts are primarily responsible for prostaglandin $E_2$ ($PGE_2$) production. An increase in the concentration of $PGE_2$ in periodontal sites suggests initiation of inflammation and attachment loss. Induction of MMPs and osteoclastic bone resorption is induced by $PGE_2$.[12]

*Cytokines*: These are explained in "Chapter 11: Immunity and Inflammation".

## Tissue Healing

The healing stage is characterized by the resolution of inflammation and the healing of damaged periodontal tissues. Periods of remission are characterized by the reduction of inflammation, restoration of gingival tissues, and often gingival fibrosis. Changes in the alveolar bony contours, with remodeling, occur during remission suggests that healing has occurred. The chronic immune system plays an essential role in healing processes, which consist of regeneration and repair.

Regeneration involves the replacement of tissues with new, identical tissues that function as the original tissues. The repair involves replacing one tissue with another tissue, such as fibrous connective tissue, which may not function as the tissue is replaced. After the traumatic or surgical injury, healing is initiated as part of the immediate and acute inflammatory responses. The periodontal "healing" cycle during the pathogenesis of a periodontal disease is primarily postinflammatory, and cellular elements other than platelets provide important signals in this process. Periodontal repair occurs in overlapping phases of inflammation shutdown, angiogenesis, and fibrogenesis.

In the postinflammatory healing process, the shutdown of inflammatory processes and the initiation of post-inflammatory healing is orchestrated by leukocytes. Some of the essential anti-inflammatory signals generated by leukocytes include IL-1 receptor antagonist (IL-1ra) and TGF-β. In inflamed periodontal tissues, macrophages are a source of IL-1ra, whereas neutrophils, macrophages, and mast cells and lymphocytes produce TGF-β.[8]

Cytokines, such as IL-1β and TNF-β, help induce angiogenesis and fibrogenesis in inflammation and healing.[15] Platelet-derived growth factor (PDGF) activates fibroblasts and osteoblasts, resulting in the induction of protein synthesis. TGF-β is a multifunctional peptide responsible for the stimulation of osteoblasts and fibroblasts. It also leads to inhibition of osteoclasts, epithelial cells, and most immune cells.

The immune system can induce regenerative bone healing by preventing osteoclast formation and by activating osteoblasts.

## IMMUNOLOGIC ASPECTS OF THE MICROBIAL INTERACTION WITH THE HOST

Periodontal disease is dependent on bacteria, as discussed earlier, and bacteria may directly interact with the host tissues in mediating tissue destruction. Besides, many tissue changes associated with periodontal diseases appear to be well-orchestrated responses, suggesting the influence of host regulation. Among the orchestrated responses are the antimicrobial activities by acute inflammatory cells (neutrophils) and the adaptive activities brought about by monocytes/macrophages and lymphocytes. Adaptive responses include the epithelial alterations, angiogenesis, episodic remodeling of the underlying hard and soft connective tissues, and antigen-specific immune responses. Remodeling of the connective tissues appears to be episodic and occurs in cycles of destruction and reconstruction. Excessive destruction or inadequate reconstruction can result in periodontal disease.

The periodontal disease represents a well-regulated response to bacterial infection directed by the host immune system's inflammatory cells in the following manner.

### Innate Factors

Components of innate immunity, including complement, resident leukocytes, and mast cells, signal the endothelium to initiate inflammation. The bacterial infection triggers complement cascade resulting in the generation of the complement derived anaphylatoxins C3a and C5a. Anaphylatoxins indirectly stimulate vascular changes by causing degranulation of the resident leukocytes and mast cells. With an increase in gingival inflammation, degranulated mast cells also increase within the gingival connective tissue. Mast cells constitutively transcribe TNF-α, TGF-β, IL-4, and IL-6; when stimulated, they induce transcription of proinflammatory cytokines, such as IL-1, IL-6, IFN-α, and others. The stimulation of endothelial cells by C5a, IL-1β, TNF-α, and bacterial lipopolysaccharides results in the expression of selectins on the lumenal surface of the endothelial cells and the release of chemokines from the endothelial cells. These processes are central in transendothelial migration of leukocytes, which result in the movement of leukocytes into the local tissues.[8]

## Acute Inflammatory Cells

Neutrophils control the periodontal microbiota within the gingival crevice and junctional epithelium, thus protect the local tissue. Neutrophils induce phagocytosis and kill microbial agents and lead to local tissue changes by releasing tissue-degrading enzymes.

## Chronic Inflammatory Cells

Macrophages and lymphocytes avoid the transmission of local infection into the systemic and life-threatening condition and thus protect the entire host. These cells orchestrate connective tissue changes associated with both periodontal infection and periodontal repair and healing. They also function to assist the neutrophils in controlling bacterial infection by forming-specific opsonic antibodies. The host response in the connective tissues may result in local tissue destruction, which is evident as periodontal disease. In recent years, the potential systemic impact of periodontal disease has been increasingly recognized. However, the result of the periodontal host response is mostly successful for the host in preventing the progressive spread of the infection despite local tissue destruction.

## Resolution Molecules

In the late 20th century, Serhan CN reported the molecules playing a significant role in the resolution of inflammation as follows:
- Resolvins
- Lipoxins
- Protectins
- Maresins

These mediators are the topic of interest as they trigger pathways signaling the physiologic end of the acute inflammatory phase. Mediators possess strong pro-resolving actions to control cellular responses, regulate stages of inflammation and stimulate natural resolution.[16]

### Resolvins

Resolvins (Rvs) are lipid mediators generated endogenously from the precursor essential-3 polyunsaturated fatty acids: eicosapentaenoic acid (EPA) and docosahexaenoic acid (DHA) via Cyclooxygenase -2 /lipoxygenase (COX-2/ LOX) pathways. The two major groups of the resolvin family exhibit distinct chemical structures. E-series of Rvs is generated from EPA while D-series is derived from DHA.[17]

### Lipoxins

Lipoxins are natural pro-resolving molecules synthesized from endogenous fatty acids via COX-2/LOX pathways. Lipoxins (LXs) are LOX interaction product derivatives of arachidonic acid with potent anti-inflammatory and resolution actions. The two positional isomers lipoxin $A_4$ (LXA4) and lipoxin $B_4$ (LXB4) were found to inhibit PMNL infiltration and stimulate macrophages recruitment.[18]

### Protectins

Protectins are mediators generated from DHA via the lipoxygenase pathway as a response to oxidative stress. These mediators reduce neuropathic pain and protect retinal epithelial cells from apoptosis.

### Maresins

Maresins are mediators that are formed by lipoxygenation of DHA through lipoxygenase in macrophages and platelets. These are powerful regulators of inflammation, tissue regeneration, and pain resolution.

## CONCEPTS OF PATHOGENESIS

### Early Concept

In mid-1960, the concept of pathogenesis was that microorganisms cause periodontal disease. The model in **Figure 12.4** implicated deposition of bacterial plaque which acts as a primary and direct factor in the pathogenesis of periodontitis.[19,20]

### The 1980's Model

This model emphasized the central role of host immunoinflammatory response regulating the disease development and progression of periodontitis **(Fig. 12.5)**. Specific bacteria initiated the disease process by activating host responses, which were both protective and destructive.

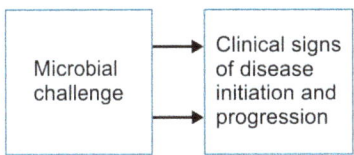

**Fig. 12.4:** Schematic representation showing early concept: Early linear model depicting the principal etiologic role of bacteria.

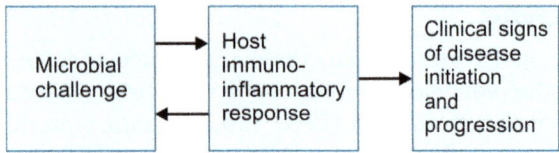

**Fig. 12.5:** Schematic representation showing the 1980's model emphasizing a central role of host immunoinflammatory response.

The actual destruction of connective tissue and bone resulted primarily from activated tissue mechanisms, such as MMPs, IL-1, and prostaglandins.[19,20]

## The 1997's Model

The primary conceptual change accepted the role of environmental and acquired risk factors as modifiers of the host immune response and changes in connective tissue and bone metabolism. The 1997's model was nonlinear, and this model implied a range of host responses and a range of clinical expressions of diseases that were primarily determined by genetic and environmental factors that modified the host response **(Fig. 12.6)**.[19,20]

### Points to Ponder

- Systemic diseases associated with neutrophil disorders and periodontal diseases are diabetes mellitus, Papillon–Lefevre syndrome, Down syndrome, Chédiak–Higashi syndrome, drug-induced agranulocytosis, cyclic neutropenia, and leukocyte-adhesion deficiency.
- Periodontal diseases with neutrophil disorders are NUG, localized aggressive periodontitis, and refractory periodontitis.
- Chemokine paralysis: *P. gingivalis* obstructs the transepithelial migration of neutrophils and inhibits IL-8 secretion from epithelial cells against bacterial challenge. Thus, *P. gingivalis* contributes to the virulence by interfering with the host immune response.[21]

## REFERENCES

1. Genco RJ. Pathogenesis and host responses in periodontal diseases. In: Genco RJ, Goldman HM, Cohen DW (Eds). Contemporary Periodontics. St. Louis: CV Mosby; 1990. pp. 184-93.
2. Ebersole JL. Immune responses in periodontal diseases. In: Wilson TG, Kornman KS (Eds). Fundamentals of Periodontics, 2nd edition. Chicago, USA: Quintessence Publishing; 2003. pp. 109-58.
3. Grant DA, Stern IB, Listgarten MA. Host response inflammation. In: Periodontics, 6th edition. St. Louis: CV Mosby; 1988. pp. 252-65.
4. Mergenhagen SE, Sandberg AL, Chassy BM, Brennan MJ, Yeung MK, Donkersloot JA, et al. Molecular basis of bacterial adhesion in the oral cavity. Rev Infect Dis. 1987;9(Suppl 5):S467-74.
5. Dickinson DP, Kubiniec MA, Yoshimura F, Genco RJ. Molecular cloning and sequencing of the gene encoding the fimbrial subunit protein of *Bacteroides gingivalis*. J Bacterial. 1988;170(4):1658-65.
6. McIntire FC, Bush CA, Wu SS, Li SC, Li YT, McNeil M, et al. Structure of a new hexasaccharide from the coaggregation polysaccharide of *Streptococcus sanguis*. Carbohydr Res. 1987;166(1):133-43.
7. Graves DT, Li J, Cochran DL. Inflammation and uncoupling as mechanisms of periodontal bone loss. J Dent Res. 2011;90(2):143-53.
8. Haake SK, Nisengard RJ, Newman MG, Miyasaki KT. Microbial interactions with the host in periodontal diseases. In: Newman MG, Takei HH, Carranza FA (Eds). Carranza's Clinical Periodontology, 9th edition. Philadelphia, PA, USA: WB Saunders; 2003. pp. 132-52.
9. Grant DA, Stern IB, Listgarten MA. Immunology of periodontal diseases. In: Periodontics, 6th edition. St. Louis: CV Mosby; 1988. pp. 266-92.
10. Eley BM, Manson JD. Host-parasite interaction. In: Periodontics, 5th edition. Edinburgh, UK: Wright; 2004. pp. 29-38.

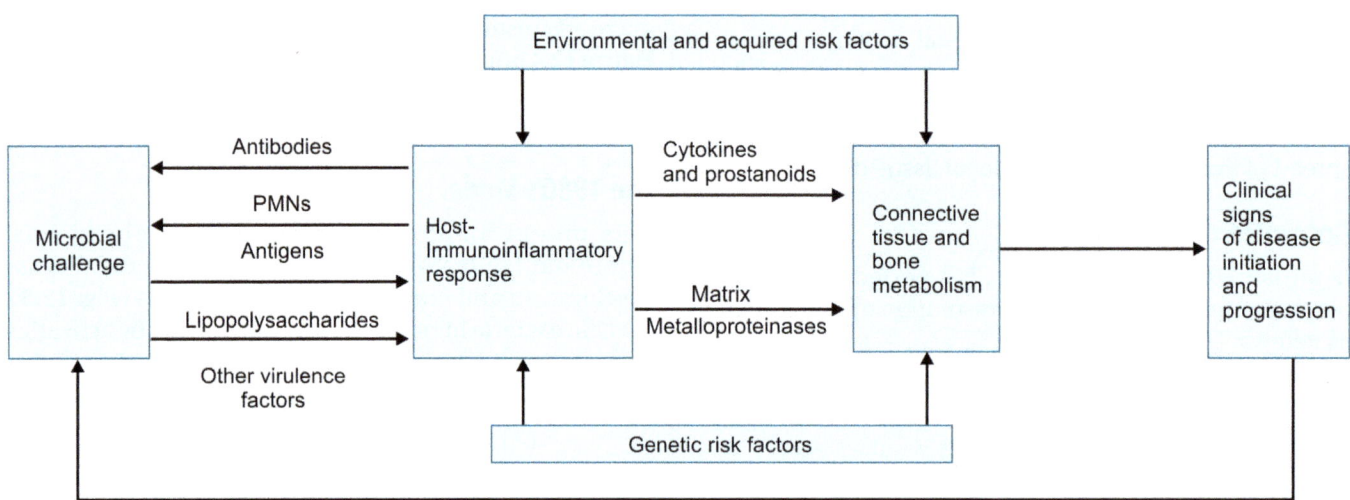

**Fig. 12.6:** Schematic representation showing the 1997's model demonstrating various factors contributing to the periodontal disease's pathogenesis.

## Chapter 12: Pathogenesis and Host Response

11. Holt SC, Kesavalu L, Walker S, Genco CA. Virulence factors of *Porphyromonas gingivalis*. Periodontol 2000. 1999;20:168-238.
12. Kinane DF, Berglundh T, Lindhe J. Host-parasite interactions in periodontal disease. In: Lindhe J, Karring T, Lang NP (Eds). Clinical Periodontology and Implant Dentistry, 4th edition. Oxford, UK: Blackwell Munksgaard; 2003. pp. 150-78.
13. Birkedal-Hansen H, Moore WG, Bodden MK, Windsor LJ, Birkedal-Hansen B, DeCarlo A, et al. Matrix metalloproteinases: a review. Crit Rev Oral Biol Med. 1993;4(2):197-250.
14. Gemmell E, Marshall RI, Seymour GJ. Cytokines and prostaglandins in immune homeostasis and tissue destruction in periodontal disease. Periodontol 2000. 1997;14:112-43.
15. Graves D. Cytokines that promote periodontal tissue destruction. J Periodontol. 2008;79(8 Suppl):1585-91.
16. Freire MO, Van Dyke TE. Natural resolution of inflammation. Periodontol 2000. 2013;63(1):149-64.
17. Van Dyke TE, Serhan CN. Resolution of inflammation: a new paradigm for the pathogenesis of periodontal diseases. J Dent Res. 2003;82(2):82-90.
18. Kirkwood KL, Cirelli JA, Rogers JE, and Giannobile WV. Novel host response therapeutic approaches to treat periodontal diseases. Periodontol 2000. 2007;43:294-315.
19. The pathogenesis of periodontal diseases. J Periodontol. 1999;70(4):457-70.
20. Kornman KS. Mapping the pathogenesis of periodontitis: a new look. J Periodontol. 2008;79(8 Suppl):1560-8.
21. Madianos PN, Bobetsis YA, Kinane DF. Generation of inflammatory stimuli: how bacteria set up inflammatory responses in the gingiva. J Clin Periodontol. 2005;32(Suppl 6):57-71.

## VIVA VOCE

**Q1. Which is the smallest MMP?**
Ans. Matrilysin is the smallest MMP.

**Q2. What are resolvins?**
Ans. Resolvins are lipid mediators that are induced endogenously during the resolution phase of inflammation. These are biosynthesized from the precursor essential-3 polyunsaturated fatty acids: eicosapentaenoic acid (EPA) and docosahexaenoic acid (DHA) derived from the diet.

**Q3. What are gingipains?**
Ans. They are trypsin-like proteases, which are virulence factors of *Porphyromonas gingivalis*.

**Q4. What is Chemokine paralysis?**
Ans. *Porphyromonas gingivalis* obstructs the transepithelial migration of neutrophils and inhibits IL-8 secretion from epithelial cells against bacterial challenge. Thus, *P.gingivalis* contributes to virulence by interfering with the host immune response.

**Q5. What is the periodontain?**
Ans. It is the cysteine proteinase produced by *Porphyromonas gingivalis* that is capable of inactivating the alpha-1 proteinase inhibitor, the primary endogenous regulator of human neutrophil elastase.

**Q6. How do the host tissue damages occur during host-microbial interaction?**
Ans. A. Through metabolic byproducts of microbes: Ammonia, fatty acid, peptides, and enzymes (collagenase, keratinase, trypsin-like enzyme, fibronectin-degrading enzyme).
B. Through the release of biologic mediators from host tissue cells: IL-1, tumor necrosis factor, and prostaglandins.

**Q7. What are the virulence factors?**
Ans. The properties of a microorganism that enables it to cause disease are referred to as virulence factors.

**Q8. What are the various virulence factors of *A. actinomycetemcomitans*?**
Ans. Collagenase, cytotoxin, leukotoxin, bacteriocin, endotoxin, Fc binding protein, invasins, immunosuppressive factors, adhesins, and chemotaxis inhibitor.

**Q9. What are prostaglandins?**
Ans. Prostaglandins are arachidonic acid derivatives synthesized under the action of cyclooxygenases [cyclooxygenase-1 (COX-1), cyclooxygenase-2 (COX-2)] isoenzymes.

**Q10. What are lipoxins?**
Ans. Lipoxins are the natural pro-resolving molecules synthesized from endogenous fatty acids via COX-2/ LOX pathways.

# Chapter 13: Genetic Basis of Periodontal Diseases

*Veenu M Hans, Shalu Bathla*

## Chapter Outline

- Genetic Variance
- Genetic Basis of Disease
- Methods of Genetic Analysis
- Disease and Polymorphism
- Associated Problems
- Clinical Implications
- Nutrigenomics

## INTRODUCTION

Periodontal disease is an inflammatory host response initiated by the deposition of plaque on the tooth surface. In certain susceptible individuals, this inflammatory process turned into a chronic destructive condition called "periodontitis." Regardless of the role of microbial and environmental factors in disease progression, specific genes are also found to increase the risk for and rate of periodontal diseases progression. Advanced knowledge of periodontal disease's genetic basis offers new insight into periodontitis diagnostic and therapeutic aspects.

## GENETIC VARIANCE

Subtle interpatient genetic variations are found in the same population of a species. Evolution in the human genome study supports the evidence that genes can present in various forms or status. Genetics reported the presence of different gene forms as allelic variants or alleles responsible for genetic variations. Allelic variants of the gene occur due to an alteration in normal nucleotide sequence. When a specific allele occurs in at least 1% of the population, the phenomenon is termed as "genetic polymorphism." On the other hand, when nucleotide changes are rare but permanent and present in exceptional individuals, the process is called "mutation." Genetic polymorphism is considered normal variation, but the mutation can lead to abnormal forms of genes. When a nucleotide change in codon does not significantly change the amino acids, the mutation is termed as silent. Though the single nucleotide polymorphisms (SNPs) in genes do not regularly change the protein products of the gene, they can affect the final gene product.

Phenotype = Environment + Genotype + Genotype × Environment

## GENETIC BASIS OF DISEASE

Phenotypic differences between individuals of the same population of the same species are mainly due to genetic variation and environmental exposure. The genetic component becomes the basic biological mechanism of many human diseases. The extent of this genetic contribution to disease can vary greatly for different diseases.[1]

Based on the pattern of gene transmission, genetic diseases can be divided into two main groups as simple Mendelian and complex genetic diseases.

### Simple Mendelian Diseases

Genetic diseases following simple and expected patterns of gene transmission are called as simple Mendelian diseases. The prevalence of these conditions is reported as only 0.1%. They follow one of the classical Mendelian patterns of inheritance as autosomal-dominant, autosomal-recessive or X-linked, e.g., Amelogenesis imperfecta, Crouzon syndrome.

### Complex Genetic Diseases

Contrary to simple Mendelian diseases, complex genetic disorders are more common. The frequency of disease occurrence is estimated to be more than 1% of the population. Complex diseases do not follow classical Mendelian patterns of inheritance with familial distribution or transmission. The occurrence of disease cannot be attributed to the presence of disease-associated alleles. This is because specific genetic alleles suspected of disease occurrence can be present in diseased patients and, at the same time, in unaffected individuals. Even some individuals with the disease may lack specific genetic alleles. Hence, the presence of disease-associated allele is not sufficient for the diagnosis of complex genetic diseases.[1]

## METHODS OF GENETIC ANALYSIS

### Familial Aggregation

Familial aggregation is the first step to find out the genetic cause of disease. This primary tool uses the phenotypic characteristics of the individual to determine the genetic etiology of the disease. The basis for familial aggregation is the trait shared by a family member that suggests the possibility of passing genes causing a particular disease. Apart from genetic inheritance, families also share other aspects of the environment like diet and nutrition, pollutants and behavior such as smoking. Moreover, families can get exposed to certain infectious agents at the same time. Hence, familial aggregation is also considered as a result of shared genes, environmental exposures, and similar socioeconomic influences. Previously conducted clinical reports favor the critical role of familial aggregation in aggressive periodontitis.

### Twin Study

The twin study, especially in monozygotic (MZ) twins arising from one fertilized egg, is a useful design to study the absolute and relative influence of genetic and environmental factors in disease occurrence. In MZ twins, differences in disease experience are usually related to environmental factors while in dizygotic twins it could be due to both genetic and ecological differences.[2]

### Segregation Analysis

Genes always show a predictable form of inheritance while passing from parents to offspring. According to Mendel's first law or Law of Segregation, genes segregate in families that determine the transmission of the trait or particular characteristics. Evaluation of this pattern of a trait transmission in families is done by the method called "segregation analysis." The segregation ratio determines the proportion of the offspring with a particular trait or phenotype. The methodology uses a sequential comparison of models with each other and identifies the model that best accounts for the observed transmission of a trait in the given population. Relevant genetic characteristics, such as the mode of transmission, penetration, and frequency of disease and nondisease alleles are evaluated. This method is more suitable to determine a best-fitting model when the dataset is available from many families.[3] However, segregation analysis has certain limitations like it does not always give a true model of transmission. Such limitations should be taken into consideration while determining the transmission of at least one form of early-onset periodontitis.

### Linkage Analysis

It is a wonderful technique to recognize the specific chromosomal location of genes involved in disease etiology. Genes that reside in close proximity on a chromosome inherited together during meiosis. As they are less likely to get separated, they get transmitted as a unit from generation to generation. This forms the basis of the linkage analysis technique. However, these genes violate Mendel's Law of Independent Assortment. A quantitative analysis can be used to detect the lack of independent assortment of genetic loci and map genes to specific chromosome locations. A linkage is known to follow a specific trait as it gets segregates through the family of interest. This specific trait is determined when it gets segregate with known genetic polymorphism localized to a specific chromosomal location. This helps to determine a trait that appears to segregate in a manner consistent with linkage and recognizes the known genetic marker.[2] Hence, the linkage is a powerful tool to identify the genetic basis of disease.

### Association Studies

Genetic association analysis mainly utilizes population- and family-based approaches. The population-based study uses a standard case-control design comparing allele frequency in between cases and control groups. Recently, genetic testing focuses more on the clinical use of disease-associated genetic polymorphism.

Presence of positive association suggests the following possible interpretations:
- The associated allele can be one of the predisposing alleles.
- The associated allele can exist in linkage disequilibrium forming actual disease predisposing locus.
- Association may be related to population stratification.
- Association can be a sampling or statistical artifact.

## DISEASE AND POLYMORPHISM

Following are the requirements for proving a disease and polymorphism association:
- Polymorphism should influence the gene product
- Biases in the study population should be identified as well as controlled.
- Confounders in the selected population should be controlled.
- Affected gene product should exist as a part of the disease etiopathology.[4]

## Syndromic Form of Periodontitis

Severe periodontitis, when associated with clinical monogenetic syndromes, gene mutation, and biochemical defects, represents a syndromic form of periodontitis. All these conditions follow simple Mendelian traits of transmission and exist due to alteration in single gene locus.

### Neutrophil Functional Disorder

- *Leukocyte adhesion deficiency syndrome*: Generalized form of aggressive periodontitis is an oral manifestation of leukocyte adhesion deficiency (LAD). It exists in two forms LAD I and LAD II and inherited as autosomal-recessive traits.
- *Chédiak–Higashi syndrome*: The syndrome is characterized by the abnormal functional capacity of the neutrophils, including chemotactic and bactericidal functions. The syndrome is inherited as an autosomal-recessive trait.[5]

### Deficiency in Neutrophil Number

- *Infantile genetic agranulocytosis*: This is a rare autosomal-recessive disease characterized by a lower number of neutrophil. This disease has shown to be related to aggressive periodontitis.
- *Cohen syndrome*: This disease is presented as mental retardation, obesity, dysmorphia, and neutropenia. This syndrome follows autosomal-recessive trait and associated with more frequent and extensive alveolar bone loss.

### Genetic Defects of Structural Components

- *Papillon–Lefevre syndrome*: It is a rare autosomal-recessive disorder presented as oral and dermatological manifestations. Oral manifestations are present in the form of aggressive periodontitis affecting both the primary dentition and the secondary dentition. Papillon–Lefevre syndrome (PLS) is the result of a mutation in the cathepsin C gene,[6] located on chromosome 11. Cathepsin C is a cysteine protease and functions in protein degradation and activation of proenzymes in immune and inflammatory cells, thus causing severe periodontal bone loss in affected patients.[7]
- *Haim–Munk syndrome*: It is a sporadic genetic condition and clinically slightly different from PLS. Both PLS and Haim-munk syndrome represents allelic variants of cathepsin C gene mutations. This syndrome is also associated with aggressive periodontitis.
- *Weary–Kindler syndrome*: Aggressive periodontitis is reported in Weary–Kindler syndrome, which is characterized by abnormalities in the basement membrane.

## Interleukin-1 and Tumor Necrosis Factor-α Gene Polymorphism

The genes encoding for interleukin-1 (IL-1) and tumor necrosis factor-alpha (TNF-α) are the ideal candidates for genetic studies due to following reasons:[7]

- IL-1α, IL-1β, and TNF-α endow proinflammatory properties that make them potent immunological mediators.
- IL-1β and TNF-α usually stimulate bone resorption and regulate fibroblast cell proliferation of both gingival and periodontal ligament origin.
- Previous studies favor the notion that polymorphism in the IL-1 cluster and TNF-α genes lead to an elevation in IL-1 and TNF-α protein levels.
- Inherent interindividual differences were noted for IL-1 and TNF-α production by blood leukocytes when isolated from individuals with or without periodontitis.

### Interleukin-1 Gene Polymorphism

The genes encoding for proteins IL-1α, IL-1β, and IL1-RA reside close to the IL-1 gene cluster on chromosome 2. For the first time in 1997, Kornman et al., reported polymorphism for the IL-1 gene in association with periodontitis. He evaluated gingival crevicular fluid (GCF) samples at baseline and three weeks of treatment they were analyzed by enzyme-linked immunosorbent assay (ELISA) for IL-1α. At baseline, IL-1β in GCF was 2.5 times higher inpatient with R-allele at IL-1α -889 and IL-1β +3954 (IL composite genotype) compared to those without composite genotype. After treatment, IL-1β levels in GCF were still 2.2 times higher for IL-1 composite genotype patients. However, the results are conflicting with other authors who did not notice a significant correlation between genotype and cytokine production.[8]

Considering the risk for periodontitis or severity of periodontal destruction in the general population, polymorphisms in the IL-1 gene cluster cannot be considered as a (putative) risk factor. In Caucasian patients, the IL-1 composite genotype seems to play a critical role in chronic periodontitis. However, the pieces of evidence are still not clear, and the results of many studies are conflicting and negative.[8]

### TNF-α Gene Polymorphism

Tumor necrosis factor-α gene is present on chromosome 6 within the major histocompatibility complex (MHC) gene cluster. SNP in gene encoding TNF-α has been studied in promoter regions -1031, -863, -367, -308, -238 and coding region +489. Among Japanese, SNPs at -1031 and -863 were reported in relation to chronic periodontitis.[9] Another study did not found an association of TNF-α gene polymorphism with aggressive periodontitis.[10] To date, few findings support the association between any reported TNF-α gene variation and periodontitis.

## Fc Gamma Receptor Gene Polymorphism

Leukocytes from myeloid and lymphoid lineage express receptors [Fc gamma receptor (FcγR)] for constant (Fc) region of IgG molecules. FcγR might involve in the pathogenesis of periodontitis as a connecting part of both cellular and humoral branches of the immune system. Microorganisms can be opsonized by antibodies and are phagocytosed via FcγR on neutrophils. A genetic polymorphism in FcγR genes compromised FcγR-mediated leukocyte functions and affect the susceptibility to and/or severity of periodontitis. FcγR genes, found on chromosome 1, encode mainly three main receptors classes:[11]
1. FcγR I (CD 64): Ia, Ib
2. FcγR II (CD 32): IIa, IIb, IIc
3. FcγR III (CD 16): IIIa, IIIb

Among these, genetic polymorphism has been identified for FcγRIIa, IIb, IIIa, and IIIb. Although many studies have been carried out to associate periodontitis with this polymorphism in many races, the results vary.[12] A recent meta-analysis of these studies focuses on the association between FcγRIIIb NA1/NA2 polymorphism with both chronic and aggressive periodontitis. In Asians, a weak association was reported between FcγRIIa H131R polymorphism and aggressive periodontitis. The same meta-analysis did not found any association between FcγRIIIa F158V and periodontal disease.

## CD14 Gene Polymorphism

R allele from the promoter region of CD14 at position-260 (-159) is known to increase the gene's transcriptional activity. Individuals who are homozygous for R allele show elevated levels of soluble CD14 (sCD14) and increased density of CD14 in monocytes. Elevated levels of serum sCD14 have found to be associated with periodontitis. Studies in Caucasians subjects on CD14-260 polymorphism, no association was found. In another study, polymorphism at -1359 (N/N genotypes) was reported in relation to severe periodontitis.

## TLR-2 and TLR-4 Gene Polymorphism

Toll-like receptor-2 (TLR-2) exhibits polymorphism at position 677 with the transition from arginine to threonine and at position 753 with the transition from arginine to glycine. These polymorphisms invalidate the capacity of TLR-2 to initiate host response against bacterial cell wall components. A similar polymorphism of TLR-4 at positions 299 and 399 with the transition from asparagine to glycine and threonine to isoleucine, respectively, affect the extracellular domain of TLR-4 protein, leading to an attenuated efficacy of lipopolysaccharide signaling and hamper the capacity to initiate inflammation. Few studies have been done on the association of polymorphism of these receptors with periodontitis, but despite the importance of these receptors, the relation with periodontitis has not been established.

## Interleukin-10 Gene Polymorphism

Gene encoding for IL-10 is presented on chromosome 1. Monocytes and macrophages initiate the production of IL-10 as a part of the inflammatory response. IL-10 is an anti-inflammatory cytokine and downregulates other pro-inflammatory cytokines, such as IL-1 and TNF-α. While few studies found no association between IL-10 polymorphism and chronic as well as aggressive periodontitis. A later study, associated IL-10 1087 polymorphism with susceptibility to periodontitis.[13]

## ASSOCIATED PROBLEMS

- Exposures, such as smoking or systemic disease modifiers, have large influences on phenotype expression, thus interfering with results.
- There are methodological problems also associated with these studies, e.g., deciding the study design.
- Publishing negative results can impose a tremendous impact on available literature on the subject.
- Results of many studies cannot be generalized, especially when they fail to report the sensitivity and specificity of tests and unable to describe associated environmental aspects.
- The number of cases and control are usually insufficient to prove an association between genetic polymorphism and the occurrence of disease.
- Racial and ethnic background differences in both cases and control will render the influence of genes questionable.
- It is not always sure whether the controls are truly not susceptible or are not exposed to environmental factors required for phenotypic expression.
- An allele may not always be active and may need an environment or other gene to be active. This is the phenomenon of penetrance.

## CLINICAL IMPLICATIONS

- Genetic tests may be developed and useful for identifying susceptibility of patients to a particular disease.
- Genetic risk in an individual, if known, can help the clinician in environment-based prevention and treatment to a patient susceptible to periodontal disease.

- The treatment outcome will become more predictable, and the maintenance schedule can vary according to the patient's genetic risk factor.

It should be remembered that periodontitis has a complex etiology, and all the risk factors contribute to the expression of disease. Thus, the identification of genetic risk factors does not mitigate the importance of recognizing other risk factors and controlling them.

## NUTRIGENOMICS

The term "nutrigenomics" refers to the effect of nutrients on gene expression. This branch deals with nutritional genomics and studies the interaction between nutrients and dietary bioactive with the gene at the molecular level. The understanding of nutrigenomics helps to select the dietary components suitable for the health of a specific individual.

### Applications of Nutrigenomics

Following are the applications of nutrigenomics:[14]

- Recognizing genes expression in both health and disease and try to modify them by nutrients.
- Identifying various beneficial or harmful genes, proteins, and metabolites that can be influenced by specific nutrients:
    - Identifying genes, proteins, and metabolites that get altered by dietary fats causing cardiovascular disease.
    - Identifying genes, proteins, and metabolites that change due to omega-3 fatty acids.
    - Identifying genetic variations are changing the nutrient- gene interactions in the first two applications.

### Points to Ponder

- The genotype is the genetic composition of an organism.
- Phenotype is the collection of traits or characteristics.
- Variations in nucleotide sequence at a locus are termed as "alleles."
- PST® genetic susceptibility test is the first genetic test used to analyze two IL-1 genes for variations and recognize an individual's susceptibility to overexpression of inflammation and risk for periodontal disease. This test employs user-friendly sample collection packets. Samples are collected using a soft brush inside the cheek, which is then sent to the laboratory for testing. This sample is tested for the presence of IL-1 composite genotype for recognizing test positivity.

## REFERENCES

1. Kinane DF, Hart TC. Genes and gene polymorphisms associated with periodontal disease. Crit Rev Oral Biol Med. 2003;14(6):430-49.
2. Michalowicz BS, Pihlstrom. Genetic factors associated with periodontal disease. In: Newman MG, Takei HH, Carranza FA (Eds). Carranza's Clinical Periodontology, 9th edition. Philadelphia, PA, USA: WB Saunders; 2003. pp. 168-81.
3. Diehl SR, Wang YF, Brooks CN, Burmeister JA, Califano JV, Wang S, et al. Linkage disequilibrium of interleukin-1 genetic polymorphisms with early-onset periodontitis. J Periodontol. 1999;70(4):418-30.
4. Laine ML, Crielaard W, Loos BG. Genetic susceptibility to periodontitis. Periodontol 2000. 2012;58(1):37-68.
5. Kinane DF, Peterson M, Stathopoulou PG. Environmental and other modifying factors of the periodontal diseases. Periodontol 2000. 2006;40:107-19.
6. Hart TC, Hart PS, Bowden DW, Michalec MD, Callison SA, Walker SJ, et al. Mutations of the cathepsin C gene are responsible for Papillon-Lefevre syndrome. J Med Genet. 1999;36(12):881-7.
7. Loos GB, Van der Velden U. Genetics in Relation to Periodontitis In: Lindhe J, Karring T, Lang NP (Eds). Clinical Periodontology and Implant Dentistry, 4th edition. Oxford, UK: Blackwell Munksgaard; 2003. pp. 387-403.
8. Kornman KS, Crane A, Wang HY, di Giovine FS, Newman MG, Pirk FW, et al. The interleukin-1 genotype as a severity factor in adult periodontal disease. J Clin Periodontol. 1997;24(1):72-7.
9. Suzuki A, Ji G, Numabe Y, Muramatsu M, Gomi K, Kanazashi M, et al. Single nucleotide polymorphisms associated with aggressive periodontitis and severe chronic periodontitis in Japanese. Biochem Biophys Res Commun. 2004;317(3):887-92.
10. Shapira L, Stabholz A, Rieckmann P, Kruse N. Genetic polymorphism of the tumor necrosis factor (TNF)-alpha promoter region in families with localized early-onset periodontitis. J Periodontal Res. 2001;36(3):183-6.
11. van der Pol WL, van de Winkel JG. IgG receptor polymorphisms: risk factors for disease. Immunogenetics. 1998;48(3):222-32.
12. Loos BG, Leppers-Van de Straat FG, Van de Winkel JG, Van der Velden U. Fc gamma receptor polymorphisms in relation to periodontitis. J Clin Periodontol. 2003;30(7):595-602.
13. Berglundh T, Donati M, Hahn-Zoric M, Hanson LA, Padyukov L. Association of the -1087 IL-10 gene polymorphism with severe chronic periodontitis in Swedish Caucasians. J Clin Periodontol. 2003;30(3):249-54.
14. Kornman KS, Martha PM, Duff GW. Genetic variations and inflammation: a practical nutrigenomics opportunity. Nutrition. 2004;20(1):44-9.

## Chapter 13: Genetic Basis of Periodontal Diseases

### VIVA VOCE

**Q1.** Which human leukocyte antigens (HLAs) are usually associated with aggressive periodontitis?
**Ans.** HLA-A9 and HLA-B15, are two antigens that appear to be associated with aggressive periodontitis.

**Q2.** On which chromosome, genes for the class I and II HLAs are located?
**Ans.** Genes for the class I and II HLAs are located on chromosome 6.

**Q3.** Who originally coined the term epigenetics?
**Ans.** Conrad Waddington originally coined the term epigenetics in 1937.

**Q4.** Name neutrophil functional disorders.
**Ans.** Leukocyte adhesion deficiency syndrome and Chédiak–Higashi syndrome.

**Q5.** In which disorders neutrophil number is deficient?
**Ans.** Infantile genetic agranulocytosis and Cohen syndrome.

**Q6.** What is genetic polymorphism?
**Ans.** When a specific allele occurs in at least 1% of the population, the phenomenon is termed as "genetic polymorphism."

**Q7.** Which is the first step to find out the genetic cause of disease using phenotypic characteristics of the individual for the determination of genetic etiology of disease?
**Ans.** Familial aggregation.

**Q8.** Name syndromes associated with aggressive periodontitis.
**Ans.** Weary–Kindler syndrome, Haim–Munk syndrome, Leukocyte adhesion deficiency syndrome.

**Q9.** Which study is useful to calculate the absolute and relative influence of genetic and environmental factors in disease occurrence?
**Ans.** The twin study, especially in monozygotic (MZ) twins.

**Q10.** What is nutrigenomics?
**Ans.** The term "nutrigenomics" refers to the effect of nutrients on gene expression.

# Chapter 14

# Systemic Factors and Periodontium

*Balaji Manohar, Shalu Bathla*

## Chapter Outline

- Hormonal Factors
- Hematological Disorders
- Immunodeficiency Disorders
- Effect of Nutrition
- Psychosomatic Disorders
- Other Systemic Conditions
- Drugs Induced Manifestations

## INTRODUCTION

The periodontium in health and disease can be affected by an intricate combination of systemic factors, such as debilitating systemic diseases, stress, medications, or malnutrition. These systemic factors may modify the neuroendocrine-immunologic mechanisms that compose host defenses and, thus, are called as systemic modifiers.

## HORMONAL FACTORS

Hormonal disturbances may directly affect the periodontal tissues by modifying the tissue response to plaque in gingival and periodontal disease and producing anatomic changes in the oral cavity that may favor plaque accumulation.

### Diabetes Mellitus

Diabetes mellitus is a chronic metabolic disease characterized by persistent high blood glucose levels or hyperglycemia (**Box 14.1**). In a diabetic individual, the progression of periodontal disease does not follow any peculiar pattern. Diabetic patients with poor oral hygiene often present with gingival inflammation, periodontal pockets, rapid bone loss, and periodontal abscesses (**Fig. 14.1**). Though diabetes does not directly contribute to gingivitis or periodontal pockets, it can modify the periodontal tissues' response to local factors. This hastens the bone loss and retards postsurgical healing of the periodontal tissues.[1]

### Effects on Microbiota

Uncontrolled diabetic patients with poor glycemic control present with an elevated percentage of spirochetes, motile rods, and decreased cocci levels in periodontal lesions. In type I diabetes patient with periodontitis, subgingival microbiota is mainly formed with wider an array of microbial species. The main pathogenic flora is composed of *Capnocytophaga*, *anaerobic vibrios*, *Actinomyces* species, *Porphyromonas gingivalis*, *Prevotella*

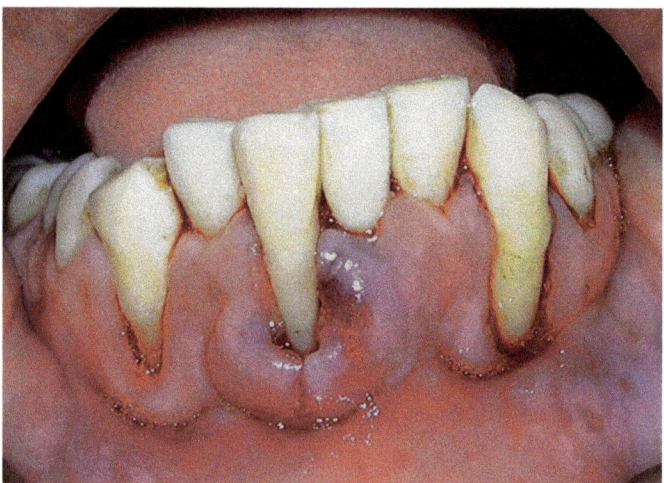

**Fig. 14.1:** Clinical picture showing gingival inflammation, periodontal pockets, attachment loss and periodontal abscesses in a diabetic patient.

**BOX 14.1:** Periodontal findings in diabetes mellitus.
- The propensity for enlarged gingiva
- Sessile or pedunculated gingival polyps
- Frequent periodontal abscesses

*intermedia,* and *Aggregatibacter actinomycetemcomitans.* Glucose-mediated advanced glycation end-product (AGE) accumulation inhibits the migration and phagocytic activity of inflammatory cells, leading to substantial pathogenic subgingival flora.[1]

### Effects on Host Response

- *Polymorphonuclear leukocytes*: Deficiencies of polymorphonuclear leukocytes (PMNs) in diabetic patients impair the protective immune mechanism of the body, including chemotaxis, phagocytosis, and adherence. This increases the susceptibility of diabetics to frequent infections.[2] Moreover, in chronic diabetes, AGEs augment the activity of the nicotinamide adenine dinucleotide phosphate (NADPH) oxidases and the respiratory burst of neutrophils. Neutrophils flare up the periodontal pathogenesis due to the extracellular release of their lysosomal contents that significantly enhance local tissue damage. Arachidonic acid plays an essential role in AGE-augmented neutrophil respiratory bursting and upregulating the neutrophil NADPH. This increases the local production of reactive oxygen species and further inflammation.[3]
- *Cytokines, monocytes, and macrophages*: Persistent hyperglycemia in diabetic patients stimulates the formation of nonenzymatic AGEs. AGEs are glucose-derived irreversible compounds form slowly over the period of time and are an indicator of blood glucose concentration. Macrophage carries high-affinity receptors for binding to AGE-modified proteins. This receptor protein binding, also known as RAGE (receptor for AGE), initiates cytokine upregulation and synthesis of tumor necrosis factor-alpha (TNF-α) and interleukin-1 (IL-1).[3] Synthesis and secretion of cytokines are increased triggering degradative cascade and lead to connective tissue degradation **(Flowchart 14.1)**.[4]

**Flowchart 14.1:** AGE-mediated tissue destruction in diabetes mellitus.

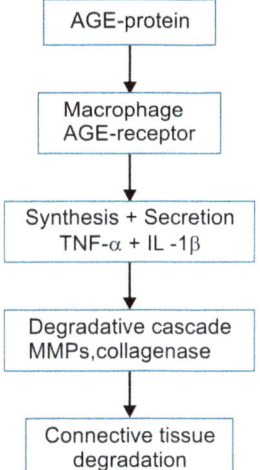

(TNF-α: tumor necrosis factor-alpha; AGE: advanced glycation end-product; IL-1β: interleukin-1β; MMPs: matrix metalloproteinases)

- *Altered collagen metabolism*: Usually, in diabetic patient collagenase activity is high, whereas collagen synthesis is considerably low. AGE stimulates the formation of cross-linked collagen, which is less soluble and less likely to be repairable or replaceable. Cellular migration through cross-linked collagen is hampered, and tissue integrity is also impaired. Hence, the collagen in the tissues of poorly controlled diabetics is aged and easily susceptible to breakdown.[1]
- *Altered bone metabolism*: Persistently high blood glucose level in a diabetic patient induces a significant impact on bone metabolism. Diabetes is associated with inhibition of the process of collagen matrix formation; changes in protein synthesis pathways; enhancement in time for mineralization of osteoid; reduction in bone turnover; and reduction in the number of osteoblasts and osteocalcin production.[1]

## Adrenal Insufficiency/Corticosteroid Hormones

The systemic administration of cortisone in experimental animals is reported to result in:

- Capillary dilation with hemorrhage in the periodontal ligament and gingival connective tissue.
- Degeneration and reduction in the number of collagen fibers of the periodontal ligament.
- Osteoporosis of alveolar bone.

The clinical finding of primary adrenal failure is hyperpigmentation of the gingiva which may appear as irregular spots that vary in color, ranging from pale brown to black.[5]

People with primary adrenal insufficiency have no adrenal reserve and, thus, have no means of increasing circulating cortisol levels for stressful situations other than by increasing exogenous steroid dosages. Physician consultation is valuable before treating patients with a history of recent or current steroid use to determine whether his/her dental needs and proposed treatment requires supplemental steroids.

## Pituitary Gland

In adults, hyperpituitarism results in acromegaly that is characterized by a disproportionate overgrowth of the facial bone and overdeveloped sinuses. The face is large, and the lips are greatly enlarged. An increase in the size of the dental arch results in significant overgrowth of the alveolar process. This subsequently causes spacing of the teeth and food impaction, which may affect the periodontium. Hypercementosis is usually seen in patients with hyperpituitarism.

Hypopituitarism results in decreased skeletal growth and leads to crowding and malposition of teeth. The periodontal tissues of experimental animals with artificially induced hypopituitarism show increased gingival inflammation, resorption of cementum in the molar furcation areas, reduced apposition of cementum, decreased osteogenesis in interdental areas, reduced vascularity of the periodontal ligament and cystic degeneration of the ligament and calcification of many of the epithelial rests.

## Thyroid Gland

The thyroid gland secretes three hormones: (1) thyroxine; triiodothyronine, and (3) calcitonin. Of these three, the bulk is made up of thyroxine. In the peripheral tissues, thyroxine is converted into its more active form, triiodothyronine. In animals with thiouracil-induced hypothyroidism, the apposition of alveolar bone is retarded, and the size of the Haversian system is reduced with no evidence of any periodontal disease. Myxedema develops hyperparakeratosis of the gingival epithelium, edema, and disorganization of the collagen bundles in the connective tissues, hydropic degeneration, and fragmentation of the fibers of periodontal ligament and osteoporosis of the alveolar bone.

## Parathyroid Glands

Hyperparathyroidism produces generalized demineralization of the skeleton, increased osteoclasis with the proliferation of the connective tissue in the enlarged marrow spaces, and formation of bone cysts and giant cell tumors. The disease is called *osteitis fibrosa cystica* or "Von Recklinghausen's bone disease." There is alveolar osteoporosis with loosely meshed trabeculae and widened periodontal ligament space. Loss of the lamina dura and giant cell tumors in the jaws are late but uncommon signs of hyperparathyroid bone disease.[6]

## Sex Hormones

This is explained in "Chapter 28: Sex Hormones and Periodontium."

## HEMATOLOGICAL DISORDERS

Blood cells contribute a vital role in the preservation of a healthy periodontium. Hence, hematological disorders involving diseases of the blood or blood-forming organs have a significant impact on the periodontium. Inflammatory cells, such as PMNs, lymphocytes, macrophages, and plasma cells, are key defensive cells to maintain adequate tissue responses and antigenic challenges from the subgingival plaque microbiota. Likewise, hematological components like the red blood cells (RBCs) support gaseous exchange and nutrient supply to the periodontium. Platelets preserve adequate hemostasis of well perfuse tissue, which otherwise becomes hyperemic and hemorrhagic during inflammation. Thus, hematological components act as a nondefensive mechanism of a healthy periodontium. Many different types of hematological conditions can have a profound effect on the periodontium. Hematological disorders take many different forms depending upon the types of blood components affected. The most common types of hematological disorders are hemostatic, red blood cells, and white blood cell disorders (WBCs). Out of this, leukocyte disorders affecting the WBCs are the important cause of ill-health of the periodontium. However, other hemostatic and RBC disorders may affect the integrity of the periodontium.[7]

## Leukemia

Leukemia is the proliferative disorder of WBCs forming tissues in the bone marrow. Abnormal proliferation of these tissues results in a marked increase in circulating immature or abnormal WBCs. These abnormal WBCs can infiltrate into different body organs and subsequently cause enlargement. Commonly affected organs are spleen, liver, and lymph nodes. Leukocytes from different stages, such as granulocytes (myeloid), monocytes, and lymphocytes, gets affected. The disorder can present in acute or chronic forms. The acute form is common in the patients who are usually under 20 years or over 55-year age and cell type commonly affected is a stem cell precursor or blast cell. Chronic leukemias, develop in people over 40 years of age and the cell type involved, are well differentiated.

All leukemias are characteristically present with anemia, infections, and thrombocytopenia.[7]

### Leukemic Gingival Enlargement

Likewise, other organ enlargements, gingival enlargement is noticeable in leukemic patients. This is due to the basic infiltration of the leukemic cells in the gingival corium that results in gingival pockets due to bacterial plaque accumulation and subsequent initiation of the secondary inflammatory lesions. In initial stages, the gingiva is bluish, red, and cyanotic, with rounding of the gingival margin (**Fig. 14.2**). Systemic management of the disease and practice of

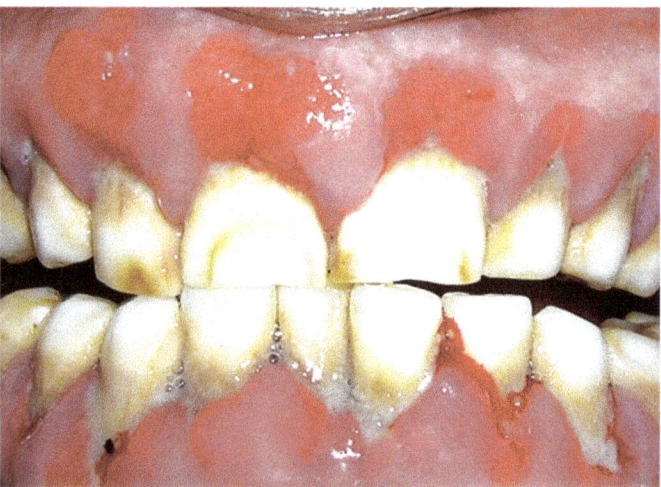

**Fig. 14.2:** Clinical picture showing gingival changes associated with leukemia: gingiva is inflamed, enlarged and edematous which bleeds spontaneously.

effective oral hygiene helps to control such enlargement to a larger extent.

### *Gingival Bleeding*

It is common in both the acute and chronic forms of leukemia. This is due to thrombocytopenia, a decrease in platelet count, associated with leukemia. It can also be related to the thin and atrophic gingival epithelium.

### *Oral Ulceration and Infection*

The granulocytopenia resulting from the replacement of bone marrow cells by leukemic cells which reduces the tissue resistance to opportunistic microorganisms and leads to ulcerations and infections.[1] Markedly altered and degenerated tissue is extremely susceptible to bacterial infection causing acute gingival necrosis and pseudomembrane formation.

Barrett in 1984 proposed the etiological classification for the gingival lesions in leukemic patients.[8] The classification system is based on the types of lesions produced as a direct effect of disease, treatment pattern, and lesions due to secondary effects, i.e., bone marrow and lymphoid tissue depression.

- *Category 1*: Lesions due to direct leukemic infiltration and includes gingival enlargement.
- *Category 2*: Lesions due to direct drug toxicity caused by chemotherapeutic agents. The common gingival changes noted are erosion and ulceration. Cyclosporine, an immunosuppressive agent, can also lead to gingival hyperplasia.
- *Category 3*: It is associated with the side effects of graft-versus-host reactions. It occurs due to the reaction between the transplanted lymphocytes against host antigens. Lichenoid striae, epithelial detachment, erosions, and ulceration are the common mucosal and useful markers of graft-versus-host activity.
- *Category 4*: The lesions develop as secondary effects of the marrow/lymphoid tissue depression associated with hemorrhage, neutropenic ulceration, and increased susceptibility to microbial infections.

The leukemic patient's treatment plan includes chemotherapy, radiation therapy, and bone marrow transplantation, each of which has the potential to produce a wide range of oral complications. Mucositis, xerostomia, and secondary infection with a variety of bacterial, viral, and fungal agents may occur. Candidiasis is almost universally seen in hospitalized leukemic patients undergoing chemotherapy. Absorbable gelatin sponge with topical thrombin or placement of microfibrillar collagen is used to stop gingival bleeding. Oral rinses of antifibrinolytic agents may also help in controlling bleeding.

## Red Blood Cell Disorders

Erythrocyte disorders, diseases of RBCs, do not hamper the periodontium significantly.

Acatalasia is a rare clinical entity associated with the lack of enzyme catalase in RBCs and WBCs. It is an inherited disorder. Typically, the enzyme catalase converts reactive hydrogen peroxide into water and oxygen. This neutralization process protects cells from harmful oxidizing agents. In the absence of enzyme catalase, the process of neutralization gets hampered, and reactive hydrogen peroxide denatures hemoglobin and produces local hypoxia and necrosis of the gingival tissues.

Aplastic anemia is a form of normocytic-normochromic anemia that results from a lack of bone marrow production of erythrocytes and other blood cells. The disorder may be genetic or acquired. The acquired form usually follows exposure to certain drugs, toxic chemicals, or ionizing radiation. Because all bone marrow-derived cells are affected, including the defensive leukocytes and platelets, hemorrhage, and infections are the major threats to patients with aplastic anemia. Oral manifestations include petechiae, gingival swelling and bleeding (often spontaneous), gingival overgrowth, and herpetic infections. Rapid bone loss has been reported, and periodontal infections have led to severe, life-threatening systemic infections.

## Thrombocytopenia

Thrombocytopenic purpura may be idiopathic, or it may occur secondary to some known etiologic factor responsible for reducing the number of circulating platelets. Such etiologic factors include aplasia of marrow and destruction of marrow by irradiation or drugs, such as benzene and arsenical agents.

Two forms of idiopathic thrombocytopenic purpura (ITP) are recognized: acute and chronic. Acute ITP is a self-limited disease that generally remits permanently without sequelae. The onset is usually sudden, with thrombocytopenia manifested by bruising, bleeding and petechiae occurring in a few days to several weeks after an otherwise uneventful viral illness. Conversely, chronic ITP is usually a disease of adults and can be sudden or insidious in onset. The oral manifestations of thrombocytopenia may be the first clinical sign of the disease. There is spontaneous gingival hemorrhage and prolonged bleeding after trauma and toothbrushing. Good oral hygiene and complete removal of plaque and calculus help to minimize gingival inflammation and reduce gingival bleeding associated with thrombocytopenia. Periodontal therapy should be limited unless platelet counts exceed a minimum of 50,000/mm$^3$, and surgery should be avoided until platelet counts are >80,000/mm$^3$. Drugs-like aspirin associated with the onset of thrombocytopenic episodes should be avoided.[9]

## Coagulation Disorders

Although hemostatic disorders do not cause periodontal disease, but can create a problem in nonsurgical and surgical periodontal therapy. In such patients, bleeding can occur during periodontal surgery. Hence, anticoagulant agents, platelet transfusions, or clotting factor supplements should be kept ready prior to surgery to avoid postsurgical inconvenience.

## IMMUNODEFICIENCY DISORDERS

### Leukocyte Disorders

#### Neutropenia

Neutropenia is a heterogeneous group of diseases affecting the circulating leukocytes. The characteristic feature involves either decrease or complete absence of circulating PMNs. Different forms of neutropenia are cyclic neutropenia, familial neutropenia, chronic idiopathic neutropenia, and agranulocytosis. Cyclic neutropenia is characterized by the periodic disappearance of circulating neutrophils, typically in 3 weeks. Familial neutropenia is an inherited autosomal-dominant trait.[10]

Inflamed gingiva, gingival ulceration, periodontal attachment, and bone loss are some of the common periodontal manifestations of neutropenia. A severe form of neutropenia is characterized by ulceration and necrosis of the marginal gingiva, which sometimes may involve attached gingiva.[10] These may be associated with gingival bleeding. Histological features of the affected gingival area show little or no PMNs infiltration. The affected gingiva exhibits edematous, hyperemic, and hyperplastic changes with areas of partial desquamation. Sometimes there is the formation of deep periodontal pockets and extensive generalized bone loss.

#### Agranulocytosis

This leukocytic disorder represents a reduction in the number of circulating granulocytes and results in severe infections, including ulcerative necrotizing lesions of the oral mucosa, skin, gastrointestinal, and genitourinary tracts. Drug idiosyncrasy is the most common cause of agranulocytosis. A striking feature is the absence of a notable inflammatory reaction due to a lack of granulocytes. Clinical features of agranulocytosis are gingival hemorrhage, necrosis, increased salivation, and fetid odor. The microscopic changes seen in the periodontium are hemorrhage into the periodontal ligament with the destruction of the principal fibers and small fragments of necrotic bone. Osteoporosis of the cancellous bone with osteoclastic resorption is there. There may be the formation of new bony trabeculae.

#### Papillon–Lefèvre Syndrome

Papillon and Lefèvre, in 1924, discovered this rare autosomal-recessive disorder syndrome. It is characterized by a mutation in the cathepsin C gene located on chromosome 11 (11q14-q21). Cathepsin C is a protease, normally found in high levels in the epithelium and immune cells, such as neutrophils, which act to degrade proteins and activate proenzymes in immune cells. Patients with Papillon–Lefèvre syndrome have little or no cathepsin C activity.[11] There are alterations in cementum. Collagenolytic activity in the periodontal ligament and osteoblastic activity of alveolar bone leads to the rapid generalized destruction of alveolar bone, affecting both the deciduous and permanent dentition. Systemic administration of retinoids, when combined with meticulous plaque control, debridement, topical antimicrobials along with systemic antibiotic therapy, may give the best chance for preventing the progression of periodontitis.

#### Chédiak–Higashi Syndrome

This syndrome was first reported by Chédiak in 1952 and later by Higashi in 1954.[12] It is an autosomal-recessive disease localized to chromosome 1q43. The formation of megabodies in neutrophils is the hallmark of this syndrome. These megabodies are formed due to the fusion of azurophil and specific granules into giant granules. The expected life expectancy in children with this syndrome is only six years, although some patients may live into early childhood. Ulcerations of the tongue and buccal mucosa, severe gingivitis and periodontitis are common oral manifestations. Bone loss is usually generalized and severe. Patients are resistant to periodontal therapy, and there is a premature loss of both deciduous and permanent dentitions. It is characterized by decreased chemotaxis, degranulation, and microbial activity. A mutation in the lysosomal trafficking regulator (LYST) gene is the identified mechanism for this syndrome. Bone marrow transplantation has good results for correcting neutrophil abnormalities.

#### Leukocyte Adhesion Deficiency

It is an autosomal-recessive disorder characterized by a deficiency in cell surface integrins. This avoids the adherence of neutrophils to the vessel wall at the site of an infection. The inability of neutrophils to move into the affected tissues sticks them within the vasculature only.
- *Leukocyte adhesion deficiency type I*: There is a deficiency of integrin β2 subunit (CD18) resulting in a leukocyte function impairment. This defect is usually associated with aggressive periodontitis.[13]
- *Leukocyte adhesion deficiency type II*: Neutrophils fail to express the ligand (CD15) for P and E selectins, resulting in impaired transendothelial migration in response to inflammation.

#### Lazy Leukocyte Syndrome

This rare disorder is associated with both quantitative and qualitative neutrophil defects. Deficiency in neutrophil chemotaxis combined with systemic neutropenia results in recurrent infections. There is rapidly progressive bone loss and tooth loss at an early age.

## Glycogen Storage Diseases

These diseases result due to enzymes abnormalities controlling glycogen synthesis and degradation. Patients with glycogen storage disease type 1b often have qualitative and quantitative neutrophil defects, leading to an increased susceptibility to infection. Gingivitis and periodontitis are common in patients with glycogen storage disease type 1b.

## Antibody Deficiency Disorders

### Agammaglobulinemia

B cells are deficient, whereas the T-cell function remains normal. It can be congenital (X-linked or Bruton's agammaglobulinemia) or acquired. The disease is characterized by recurrent infections, including destructive periodontitis in children.

### Acquired Immunodeficiency Syndrome

Infection with the human immunodeficiency virus (HIV) results in acquired immunodeficiency syndrome. This syndrome is characterized by the destruction of lymphocytes and enhances susceptibility to opportunistic infections. Periodontal manifestations in HIV individuals are linear gingival erythema, necrotizing ulcerative gingivitis (NUG), necrotizing ulcerative periodontitis (NUP), and severe destructive necrotizing ulcerative stomatitis (NUS). More about this is explained in "Chapter 26: AIDS and Periodontium."

## EFFECT OF NUTRITION

Periodontal health is determined by three factors and their interactions, namely the (1) host, (2) environment, and (3) bacterial factors. Though bacterial plaque is the prime cause of periodontitis, host susceptibility is also needed to initiate it. Nutrition is identified as the critical modifiable factors affecting both the host's immune response and the integrity of the oral tissues.[14] The diet containing different food (proteins, fats, carbohydrates, vitamins, and minerals) in such quantities and proportions that the need for energy is adequately met for maintaining health is called a balanced diet. Nutritional disorders are not only the result of inadequate dietary intake but also may be due to disturbances in absorption and utilization and self- imposed dietary restrictions. The components of host defense that may be adversely affected by inadequate nutrition include:
- Inflammatory and immune response
- Functional capacity of salivary glands and composition of saliva
- Gingival crevicular fluid production
- Responsiveness of the repair process
- The integrity of oral mucosa

The impact of nutrition on periodontal health is debatable because findings are derived mostly from laboratory or animal studies. The pieces of evidence are suggesting the role of nutrition in etiology of periodontitis lack in human.

## Vitamins

Vitamins have been defined as organic components in natural foods required in minute amounts for normal growth, maintenance, and reproduction. They are also called as "miracle workers." They are classified into two major groups as fat-soluble (A, D, E, and K) and water-soluble (B and C) vitamins. Fat-soluble vitamins are stored in the body, and water-soluble vitamins are not stored in the body.

### Vitamin A

Vitamin A is a fat-soluble vitamin and essential for the maintenance of normal vision. It is an important component of visual purple/rhodopsin and for the maturation of epithelial tissues. Retinoids, a form of preformed vitamin A is present in foods primarily animal fats and fish oils. Carotenoids are the precursors of vitamin A and function as a provitamin. β-carotene is the carotenoid present in foods, nontoxic at high doses, and function as an antioxidant. The recommended daily allowance (RDA) is 900 μg/day of retinol equivalents for men and 700 μg/day retinol equivalents for women.[15]

### Vitamin D

Vitamin D is a fat-soluble vitamin synthesized in the body in the presence of sunlight. This regulates the blood calcium levels and the metabolism of osseous tissues. This increases calcium absorption from the intestines. When blood calcium levels fall below an average, inadequate calcification of the osseous tissues leads to the development of rickets or osteomalacia. High doses of vitamin D can lead to toxicity. The adequate intake (AI) for adults <51 years old is 5 μg/day, 10 μg/day for those aged 51–70 years. Fortified milk acts as a good source of vitamin D.

### Vitamin E

Vitamin E is a fat-soluble vitamin that acts as an antioxidant. It is composed of eight related compounds called tocopherols or tocotrienols. The most active form of vitamin E is α-tocopherol present into the lipid membrane of cells and fight against free radicals. This function of vitamin E protects the fatty acids in the lipid bilayer. The RDA for vitamin E is 15 mg/day. It has a much greater margin of safety than that observed for vitamins A and D. Plant oils are the major source of the vitamin E in our diet. Systemic vitamin E appears to accelerate gingival wound healing.[16]

### Vitamin K

Vitamin K is an essential ingredient of the blood clotting system of the body. The word "K" comes from the Danish word "koagulation." Vitamin K is necessary for the carboxylation of glutamic acid that allows the synthesis of seven clotting factors produced in the liver. The drug warfarin (Coumadin) is a vitamin K antagonist and inhibits the production of the clotting factors. Vitamin K is also essential for the production of osteonectin and "matrix gla protein," which are necessary constituents of bone. The deficiency of vitamin K reduces bone density measurements. Diet is the main source of vitamin K, and intestinal bacteria also produce a significant amount. The AI for vitamin K is 90 µg/day for women and 120 µg/day for men.[15]

## Vitamin C

Ascorbic acid is synthesized by almost all plants and most of the animals. However, human beings cannot make ascorbic acid. The RDA for vitamin C for women is 75 mg/day and for men is 90 mg/day, with an additional 35 mg/day for smokers. The extra 35 mg/day for smokers is for balancing the oxidative effects of smoking.[17] The average body stores of vitamin C are 1–2 g.

## Minerals

Minerals constitute about 4% of the body weight. They are essential to carry out the vital function of the body. They assist in the formation of structure for bones and teeth. They also have a role in the maintenance of normal heart rhythm, muscle contraction, nerve conduction, and acid-base balance. Many minerals are required for the normal functioning of enzymes and hormones. Minerals are divided into two categories as major minerals with the nutritional need >100 mg/day and trace minerals with the nutritional need of <100 mg/day. Sodium, potassium, calcium, magnesium, phosphorus, and sulfur are the major minerals in the body. Iron, zinc, iodine, selenium, fluoride, copper, cobalt, chromium, manganese, and molybdenum are the trace elements in the body. The total amount of trace minerals in the body is about 15 g.

### Major Minerals

Following are the major minerals:[15]
- *Sodium*: It is the major cation in extracellular fluid. It acts as the key electrolyte and helps to maintain normal fluid balance in the body. It also plays an integral role in nerve conduction. Almost all dietary sodium is absorbed in the intestinal tract.
- *Potassium*: It is the major cation in intracellular fluid. It carries the same functions as sodium but acts intracellularly. It helps in reducing blood pressure and subsequent risk of stroke. A low-plasma potassium level is associated with muscle cramps, confusion, and an irregular heartbeat and can turn out life-threatening events.
- *Calcium*: It is another essential and major mineral in the body. The average body constitutes about 1,200 g of calcium, which is about 40% of the total body mineral, and 99% are in the skeleton. Most of the mineral is present as hydroxyapatite. Calcium is essential for nerve conduction and blood clotting. Calcium equilibrium is maintained between various parts of the body, including bone, extracellular water, and soft tissue. Calcium level is maintained by parathyroid hormone, calcitonin, and vitamin D. The AI for adults, is 1,000–1,200 mg/day.
- *Phosphorus*: It is present in almost every cell of plant and animal. On average, 600–900 g of phosphorus is found in bone in the form of hydroxyapatite. The RDA for phosphorus is 700 mg/day, and the daily value (DV) is 1,000 mg/day.
- *Magnesium*: It is found in all tissues and is the second most prominent intracellular cation after potassium. In a normal person, about 25 g of magnesium is found with most stored in bones, and rest 25% found in soft tissues. Magnesium is mainly concentrated in mitochondria and associated with energy transfer. The RDA for magnesium is 310 mg/day for women and 400 mg/day in men.
- *Sulfur*: It is the major constituent of proteins. It is commonly found in amino acids, including methionine and cysteine. The active sites of coenzyme A and glutathione contain sulfur residues. Sulfur is also found in heparin and chondroitin sulfate.

### Trace Minerals

- *Iron*: It is an integral functional component of hemoglobin and boosts the immune function of the body. A normal average human consists of about 4 g iron, mainly in the form of 2.5 g in hemoglobin, 0.3 g in myoglobin and cytochromes, and about 1 g in iron stores (ferritin). In the bone marrow, iron is commonly used to synthesize RBCs. Iron deficiency results in a clinical entity called anemia. Women are at the greatest risk of getting anemia during reproductive years. Iron deficiency is also common in children during the rapid growth period. Though average iron intake in a day is about 10 mg, only 10% of them get absorbed. Iron absorption increases in the presence of vitamin C. The RDA for iron is 18 mg/day for adult women and 8 mg/day for men.
- *Zinc*: It is an essential trace element and acts as a cofactor for over 50 enzymes (e.g., carbonic anhydrase, alkaline phosphatase, alcohol dehydrogenase, and superoxide dismutase). About 2 g of zinc is stored in the body most commonly inside the bone. Deficiency of zinc results in small stature, mild anemia, and impaired wound healing. Meats, whole grains, and legumes act as a good source of zinc. The RDA for zinc is 8 mg/day for women and 11 mg/day for men.
- *Fluoride*: It reduces the solubility of calcified tissues. The deposition of fluorapatite crystals on the tooth has found to increase resistance to decalcification. Some studies exhibited the role of fluoride in the enhancement of bone density and, hence, is sometimes used to treat

osteoporosis. The fluoride present in saliva accelerates the remineralization of enamel. The AI of fluoride is 3.1 mg/day for adult women and 3.8 mg/day for adult men.
- *Selenium*: It acts as an antioxidant and fights against free radical-induced oxidative damage. It is the functional part of the glutathione peroxidase system and reduces oxidative damage to lipid membranes with its antioxidant nature. This enzyme system keeps vitamin E as a reserve against free radical-induced injury. The RDA for selenium is 55 μg/day for adult men and women.
- *Copper and iron*: They both take part in the formation of hemoglobin. Copper is bound to store in ceruloplasmin. Ceruloplasmin is a copper-dependent ferroxidase that helps oxidize iron and is essential for ferritin's optimal use. Copper is found in two members of the superoxide dismutase family and assists in the neutralization of superoxide free radicals. The RDA for copper is 900 μg/day.
- *Chromium*: It is a mineral found in all body tissues in a small amount. The total body content of chromium is <6 mg. It regulates glucose metabolism by enhancing glucose uptake into cells through a chromium-binding protein, which upregulates insulin receptors. A chromium deficiency can lead to increased serum cholesterol levels and poor glucose tolerance.
- *Manganese*: It is a cofactor for enzymes associated with the synthesis of proteoglycans. Some manganese-containing enzymes are present in mitochondria. The AI of manganese is 1.8 mg/day for women and 2.3 mg/day for men.
- *Molybdenum*: It is a constituent of xanthine oxidase, aldehyde oxidase, and sulfite oxidase. No deficiency disorder has been recognized. The RDA for adults is 45 μg/day, and the DV is 75 μg/day.
- *Calcium*: It is the major mineral present in osseous tissues. Calcium deficiency is associated with a decrease in serum calcium levels and mobilization from host tissues. Calcium is essential for normal bone metabolism for maintaining the function of the osteoblasts, osteocytes, and osteoclasts. Calcium homeostasis is controlled by parathyroid hormone and calcitonin. Dietary calcium has a potential role in modulating periodontal disease.

## Nutritional Deficiencies

The nutritional deficiencies have known to produce significant changes in the oral cavity. These changes include alterations of the lips, oral mucosa, and periodontal tissues. These changes are considered to be periodontal or oral manifestations of nutritional diseases. However, nutritional deficiencies directly do not cause gingivitis or periodontal pockets.

### *Vitamin A Deficiency*

Vitamin A deficiency causes hyperplasia and hyperkeratinization of the gingival epithelium, along with the junctional epithelium's proliferation and prolongation of gingival wound healing. Very little is known about the effects of vitamin A deficiency on the oral structures in humans. Several epidemiological studies were unable to report a significant relationship between vitamin A and periodontal disease.

### *Vitamin B Complex Deficiency*

Oral changes common to vitamin B complex deficiencies are gingivitis, glossitis, glossodynia, angular cheilitis, and inflammation of the entire oral mucosa. The gingivitis in vitamin B deficiencies is nonspecific, as bacterial plaque rather than the deficiency causes it. The following oral changes may be seen due to thiamine deficiency: hypersensitivity and erosion of the oral mucosa, minute vesicles on the palate, or buccal mucosa. Changes observed in riboflavin-deficient animals include severe lesions of the gingiva, periodontal tissues, and oral mucosa (including noma). Oral manifestations of vitamin B complex and niacin deficiency in experimental animals include black tongue and gingival inflammation with destruction of the gingiva, periodontal ligament, and alveolar bone. Necrosis of the gingiva and other oral tissues and leukopenia are terminal features of niacin deficiency in experimental animals. Folic acid-deficient animals also demonstrate necrosis of the gingiva, periodontal ligament and alveolar bone without inflammation.[18]

### *Vitamin C (Ascorbic Acid) Deficiency*

Vitamin C plays an integral role in the formation of amino acids hydroxyproline and hydroxylysine, which are almost unique to collagen, the major protein of periodontium. Its deficiency causes scurvy, which is characterized by hemorrhagic diathesis and retardation of wound healing. There are defective formation and maintenance of collagen and increased capillary permeability.

Following are the possible etiologic relationships between vitamin C and periodontal diseases:[19]
- Low levels of vitamin C influence the metabolism of collagen within the periodontium, thereby affecting tissue ability to regenerate and repair itself.
- Its deficiency interferes with bone formation leading to loss of alveolar bone.
- Its deficiency increases the permeability of the oral mucosa to endotoxins and tritiated inulin and of normal human crevicular-epithelium to tritiated dextran.

Therefore, optimal levels of this vitamin would maintain the epithelium's barrier function to the various bacterial products.
- Increasing levels of vitamin C enhance both the chemotactic and the migratory action of leukocytes without influencing their phagocytic activity.
- An optimal level of vitamin C is required to maintain the integrity of the periodontal microvasculature.

- Vitamin C deficiency interferes with the ecologic equilibrium of bacteria in plaque and thus increases its pathogenicity.

### Vitamin D Deficiency

Vitamin D deficiency is characterized by generalized bone resorption in jaws, fibro-osteoid hemorrhage in the marrow spaces, and destruction of the periodontal ligament. The effect of such deficiency or imbalance on periodontal tissues results in osteoporosis of alveolar bone. Osteoid forms at a normal rate but remains uncalcified. Radiographically, there is generalized partial to complete loss of the lamina dura, and diminished density of the supporting bone, loss of trabeculae, increased radiolucency of the trabecular interstices, and increased prominence of the remaining trabeculae. Microscopic and radiographic changes in the periodontium are almost identical to those seen in experimentally induced hyperparathyroidism.

### Vitamin E Deficiency

No relationship has been demonstrated between vitamin E and oral disease deficiencies, but in experimental rats, systemic vitamin E appears to accelerate gingival wound healing.

### Protein Deficiency

Protein deprivation causes the following changes in the periodontium of experimental animals: degeneration of the connective tissue of the gingiva and periodontal ligament, osteoporosis of alveolar bone, retardation in the deposition of cementum and delayed wound healing.[20] Protein deficiency will retard growth, alter physiologic functions, and significantly reduce host defenses and wound healing. Protein deprivation adversely affects immunoglobulin A in saliva, PMN phagocytosis, and complement activation, and both cell-mediated and humoral immune responses. Severe protein deficiency (kwashiorkor) or general starvation (marasmus) has long been associated with glossitis, increased gingival inflammation, and alveolar bone loss.

## Antioxidants

In periodontal diseases, inflammatory cells, particularly PMNs release proteases. These proteases are known to contain free radicals, which may damage surrounding periodontal tissues.[21] Ongoing research is underway to determine whether or not antioxidants, nutritional supplements, namely β-carotene, retinol, ascorbic acid, α-carotene, and selenium, are of benefit in reducing the tissue destruction occurring in plaque-induced periodontal diseases.[22] The antioxidants showed promising results in the management of oral leukoplakia and even in oral cancer.

### Classification

- According to the mode of action:
  - Preventive: Superoxide dismutase enzymes (1, 2, 3), catalase, glutathione peroxidase, DNA repair enzyme, polymerase, albumin, lactoferrin, transferrin, haptoglobin, carotenoids, uric acid.
  - Scavenging (chain breaking): Vitamin C, carotenoids, uric acid, albumin, bilirubin, polyphenols, reduced glutathione.
- According to the location:
  - Intracellular: Superoxide dismutase enzymes 1 and 2, DNA repair enzyme.
  - Extracellular: Superoxide dismutase enzyme 3, lacto ferrin, transferrin, haptoglobin, carotenoids, uric acid
  - Membrane-associated: Alpha (α)-tocopherol.
- According to solubility:
  - Water-soluble: Haptoglobin, albumin, uric acid, ceruloplasmin.
  - Lipid soluble: α-tocopherol, carotenoids, bilirubin
- According to structures they protect:
  - DNA protective antioxidants: Superoxide dismutase enzymes 1 and 2, DNA repair enzyme, reduced glutathione, cysteine.
  - Protein protective antioxidants: Sequestration of transition metals by preventive antioxidants.
  - Lipid protective antioxidants: α-tocopherol, carotenoids, bilirubin, reduced glutathione.
- According to their origin:
  - Exogenous: Carotenoids, ascorbic acid, folic acid, cysteine, α-tocopherol.
  - Endogenous: Catalase, superoxide dismutase, transferrin, ceruloplasmin.
  - Synthetic: N-acetyl cysteine, tetracyclines, penicillamine.

## PSYCHOSOMATIC DISORDERS

In 1946, Selye coined the term "general adaptation syndrome (GAS)" as the systemic reactions that affect the body generally or produce an interrelated nonspecific tissue change resulting from continued exposure to stress. Selye considered GAS to be the basis of the pathogenesis of various diseases. The three stages of this syndrome are:
1. Stage I: Initial response (alarm reaction)
2. Stage II: Adaptation to a stress (resistant stage)
3. Stage III: Inability to maintain adaptation to stress in the final stage (exhaustion stage)

Stress is known to alter the immune response and increase the susceptibility to periodontal infection. The most commonly studied periodontal disease in relation to stress is NUG (Rest is explained in "Chapter 66: Periodontics-Psychiatry").

## OTHER SYSTEMIC CONDITIONS

### Metal Intoxication

Systemic absorption of certain heavy metals, such as mercury, lead, arsenic, and bismuth, can produce pigmentation or discoloration of gingival surfaces. These metals may come from environmental exposure or certain medications.[1]

#### *Bismuth Pigmentation*

It usually appears as a narrow, bluish-black discoloration of the gingival margin in pre-existing gingival inflammation areas. Such pigmentation results from the precipitation of particles of bismuth sulfide associated with vascular changes in gingival inflammation.

#### *Lead Pigmentation*

Lead is slowly absorbed, and toxic symptoms are not particularly definitive when they do occur. The pigmentation of the gingiva is linear (burtonian line), steel gray, and associated with local irritation.

#### *Mercury Pigmentation*

Gingival pigmentation in linear form results from the deposition of mercuric sulfide. The chemical also acts as an irritant, which accentuates the pre-existent inflammation and commonly leads to notable ulceration of the gingiva and adjacent mucosa and destruction of the underlying bone.

#### *Arsenic and Chromium*

It may cause necrosis of the alveolar bone with loosening and exfoliation of the teeth. Inflammation and ulceration of the gingiva are usually associated with the destruction of the underlying tissues.

## DRUGS INDUCED MANIFESTATIONS

Various medications are available to control chronic medical conditions and associated manifestations. However, in the long run, these medications can produce changes in the oral cavity due to toxic overdoses, side effects, allergic reactions, or sometimes as a consequence of the primary action of the drug.

Adverse effects of systemic medications on the periodontal tissues are discussed below:

### Drug-induced Xerostomia

It may result in increased plaque and calculus formation. Drugs with xerostomic potential include diuretics, antihypertensives, antipsychotics, and antidepressants.

### Leukoplakia

Drugs of abuse, such as cannabis and cocaine, can induce gingival leukoplakia and erythema.

### Agranulocytosis

Drug-induced agranulocytosis may result in severe gingival necrosis resembling generalized NUG. Drugs are implicated in agranulocytosis, including phenothiazines, sulfur derivatives, indomethacin, and antibiotics, such as penicillin, chloramphenicol, and co-trimoxazole.

### Gingival Enlargement

Drug-induced gingival enlargement is the most common adverse effect of systemic medications on the periodontal tissues. Intake of sex hormones such as estrogen and progesterone at therapeutic doses are known to induce gingival enlargement.

Three groups of drugs most often associated with gingival enlargement are: (1) anticonvulsants, (2) antihypertensives, and (3) immunosuppressants.

1. *Anticonvulsants*: Anticonvulsant drugs associated with gingival enlargement are phenytoin, phenobarbital, carbamazepine, sodium valproate, primidone, and felbamate. Phenytoin is a commonly prescribed anticonvulsant agent for the control of epileptic seizures. Almost half of the chronic epileptic individuals on long-term phenytoin regimen commonly develop gingival overgrowth. Gingival enlargement is frequent in teenagers and young adults of about 30 years of age compared to middle-aged or elderly persons. The anterior labial surfaces of the maxillary and mandibular gingiva are most commonly and severely affected **(Fig. 14.3)**. The earliest clinical signs of gingival changes may occur 2–3 weeks after phenytoin therapy is started. Gingival overgrowth is clinically detectable during the first 6–9 months of therapy. Overgrowth and extrusion of the interdental papillae results in the formation of the firm, mobile, and triangular tissue masses. They fuse mesially and distally to form a continuous curtain of the overgrown marginal gingiva.

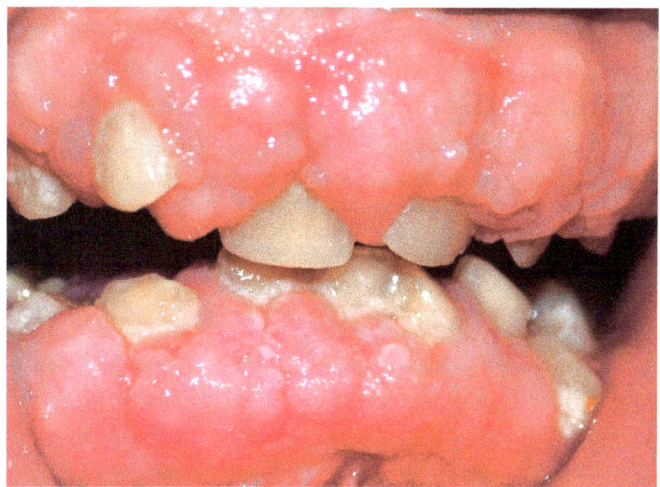

**Fig. 14.3:** Clinical picture showing phenytoin-induced gingival enlargement.

2. *Immunosuppressants*: Cyclosporine is an immunosuppressant drug widely prescribed to control the rejection of solid organ transplantation and autoimmune diseases. It exerts effect by selective suppression of specific subpopulations of T lymphocytes, interfering with the production of lymphokines, IL-1 and IL-2. The gingival lesions associated with cyclosporine are often identical, both clinically and histologically, to those produced by phenytoin. The clinical course is similar in that the lesions generally originate in the interdental area, and all dental arch segments may be affected. Dosage of cyclosporine greater than 500 mg/day induces gingival overgrowth.[23]
3. *Antihypertensives*: Antihypertensive drugs associated with gingival enlargement are: nifedipine, amlodipine, nimodipine, nicardipine, nitrendipine, diltiazem, felodipine, and bepridil. These antihypertensive drugs are mainly calcium-channel blockers group.

## Halitosis

Some of the psychiatric medications can cause halitosis, namely lorazepam, carbamazepine, amitriptyline, fluoxetine, and haloperidol.

## Abnormal Pigmentation

Several drugs may induce unusual pigmentation in the oral cavity. Implicated drugs include minocycline, zidovudine, phenothiazines, bismuth, gold salts, and anticancer drugs. Minocycline may produce a gray blue-black pigmentation of alveolar mucosa and attached gingiva.

### Points to Ponder

- Marasmus is a condition primarily caused by a deficiency in calories and energy, whereas kwashiorkor indicates an associated protein deficiency.
- Vitamin C is essential for collagen formation. Enzyme prolyl hydroxylase causes hydroxylation of proline in the presence of vitamin C (cofactor) during collagen formation.

## REFERENCES

1. Klokkevold PR, Mealey BL, Carranza FA. Influence of systemic disease and disorders on the periodontium. In: Newman MG, Takei HH, Carranza FA (Eds). Carranza's Clinical Periodontology, 9th edition. Philadelphia, PA, USA: WB Saunders; 2003. pp. 204-28.
2. Grossi SG, Genco RJ. Periodontal disease and diabetes mellitus: a two-way relationship. Ann Periodontol. 1998;3(1):51-61.
3. Preshaw PM, Foster N, Taylor JJ. Cross-susceptibility between periodontal disease and type 2 diabetes mellitus: an immunobiological perspective. Periodontol 2000. 2007;45:138-57.
4. Palmer R, Soory M. Modifying factors: diabetes, puberty, pregnancy, and menopause, and tobacco smoking. In: Lindhe J, Karring T, Lang NP (Eds). Clinical Periodontology and Implant Dentistry, 4th edition. Chicago, USA: Blackwell Munksgaard; 2003. pp. 179-97.
5. Mealey BL, Rees TD, Rose LF, Grossi SG. Systemic factors impacting the periodontium. In: Rose LF, Mealey BL, Genco RJ, Cohen DW (Eds). Periodontics: Medicine, Surgery, and Implants, 2nd illustrated edition. St. Louis: Elsevier-Mosby; 2004. pp. 235-45.
6. Silverman S, Gordan G, Grant T, Steinbach H, Eisenberg E, Manson R. The dental structures in primary hyperparathyroidism. Studies in forty-two consecutive patients. Oral Surg Oral Med Oral Pathol. 1962;15:426-36.
7. Kinane D. Blood and lymphoreticular disorders. Periodontol 2000. 1999;21:84-93.
8. Barrett AP. Gingival lesions in leukemia. A classification. J Periodontol. 1984;55(10):585-8.
9. Mealey LB, Klokkevold PR, Otomo-Corgel J. Periodontal treatment of medically compromised patients. In: Newman MG, Takei HH, Carranza FA (Eds). Carranza's Clinical Periodontology, 9th edition. Philadelphia, PA, USA: WB Saunders; 2003. pp. 527-50.
10. Kinane DF, Marshall GJ. Periodontal manifestations of systemic disease. Aust Dent J. 2001;46(1):2-12.
11. Hart TC, Hart PS, Bowden DW, Michalec MD, Callison SA, Walker SJ, et al. Mutations of the cathepsin C gene are responsible for Papillon-Lefèvre syndrome. J Med Genet. 1999;36(12):881-7.
12. Higashi O. Congenital gigantism of peroxidase granules; the first case ever reported of qualitative abnormality of peroxidase. Tohoku J Exp Med. 1954;59(3):315-32.
13. Meyle J. Leukocyte adhesion deficiency and prepubertal periodontitis. Periodontol 2000. 1994;6:26-36.
14. Grant DA, Stern IB, Listgarten MA. Diet and nutrition. In: Periodontics, 6th edition. St. Louis: CV Mosby; 1988. pp. 293-306.
15. Schifferle RE. Periodontal disease and nutrition: separating the evidence from current fads. Periodontol 2000. 2009;50:78-89.
16. Kim JE, Shklar G. The effect of vitamin E on the healing of gingival wounds in rats. J Periodontol. 1983;54(5):305-8.
17. Nishida M, Grossi SG, Dunford RG, Ho AW, Trevisan M, Genco RJ. Dietary vitamin C and the risk for periodontal disease. J Periodontol. 2000;71(8):1215-23.
18. Shaw JH. The relation of nutrition to periodontal disease. J Dent Res. 1962;41(Suppl 1):264.
19. Woolfe SN, Hume WR, Kenney EB. Ascorbic acid and periodontal disease: a review of the literature. J West Soc Periodontol Periodontal Abstr. 1980;28(2):44-56.
20. Carranza FA, Cabrini RL, Lopez Otero R, Stahl SS. Histometric analysis of inter radicular bone in protein-deficient animals. J Periodontal Res. 1969;4(4):292-5.
21. D'Aiuto F, Nibali L, Parkar M, Patel K, Suvan J, Donos N. Oxidative stress, systemic inflammation, and severe periodontitis. J Dent Res. 2010;89(11):1241-6.
22. Chapple IL, Matthews JB. The role of reactive oxygen and antioxidant species in periodontal tissue destruction. Periodontol 2000. 2007;43:160-232.
23. Daley TD, Wysocki GP, Day C. Clinical and pharmacologic correlations in cyclosporine-induced gingival hyperplasia. Oral Surg Oral Med Oral Pathol. 1986;62(4):417-21.

## Chapter 14: Systemic Factors and Periodontium

### VIVA VOCE

**Q1. What is the Burtonian line?**
**Ans.** It is a steel-gray linear gingival pigmentation seen in lead intoxication.

**Q2. What is the dosage of cyclosporine that induces gingival overgrowth?**
**Ans.** Dosage of cyclosporine >500 mg/day induces gingival overgrowth.

**Q3. What is the most common cause of agranulocytosis?**
**Ans.** Drug idiosyncrasy.

**Q4. What are the periodontal manifestations of hyperparathyroid bone disease?**
**Ans.** Loss of the lamina dura and giant cell tumors in the jaws.

**Q5. What is the hallmark of Chédiak–Higashi syndrome?**
**Ans.** Formation of megabodies in neutrophils.

**Q6. What is general adaptation syndrome (GAS)?**
**Ans.** The systemic reactions that affect the body generally or produce an interrelated nonspecific tissue change resulting from continued exposure to stress are called as general adaptation syndrome.

**Q7. Which drugs cause xerostomia?**
**Ans.** Diuretics, antihypertensives, antipsychotics, and antidepressants

**Q8. Which drugs cause gingival enlargements?**
**Ans.** Anticonvulsants, antihypertensives and immunosuppressants.

**Q9. Which vitamin is an essential ingredient of the blood clotting system of the body?**
**Ans.** Vitamin K.

**Q10. What are the different forms of neutropenia affecting periodontium?**
**Ans.** Cyclic neutropenia, familial neutropenia, chronic idiopathic neutropenia, and agranulocytosis.

# Chapter 15

# Periodontal Medicine

*Praveen Kudva, Sanjay Kalra*

## Chapter Outline

- Focal Infection Theory
- Bacterial Reservoir
- Effect on Cardiovascular System
- Effect on Endocrine System
- Effect on Reproductive System
- Effect on Respiratory System

## INTRODUCTION

Periodontal disease is a chronic infectious disease characterized by destruction and loss of supporting tissues of teeth. Periodontitis is multifactorial in origin associated with the involvement of various risk factors and systemic illness. In the ensuing period of the 1990s, the concept of periodontal disease has undergone an explicit change due to the addition of new findings. Tremendous advances in modern medicine strongly postulated periodontal health as an indication of systemic health. Thus, periodontal diseases are closely linked with systemic manifestations, such as cardiovascular disease, diabetes mellitus, osteoporosis, respiratory illness, and adverse pregnancy outcomes.

## FOCAL INFECTION THEORY

In the earlier part of the 1900s, Willoughby D Miller, a Philadelphia-based microbiologist, and William Hunter, a physician from London, introduced the concept of oral bacteria and sepsis. Both of them favored the opinion that oral bacteria and associated infection are the probable cause of various systemic illnesses in human beings.[1] According to Hunter, teeth were more susceptible to septic infection due to their structure and close proximity to the alveolar bone. He further specified that extent of systemic illness due to oral sepsis is determined by the virulence of oral bacterial infection and the degree of individual disease resistance. He also assumed that extraction of an infected tooth in order to remove underlying sepsis helps improve the person's systemic health. This could show the possible association between oral sepsis and the resulting systemic manifestations.[2] For the next 40 years, both physicians and dentists accepted the concept of infection, mainly originating in the mouth, as a reason for human suffering and systemic illness. The wholesale extraction of teeth could reduce the illness. This era was then popularly known as an "era of focal infection".[3]

However, extraction of teeth carried out from 1940 through 1950 often of the entire dentition failed to initiate or exacerbate the systemic illnesses which were supposedly due to infected dentition. Unfortunately, the "focal infection theory" proposed in the early 20th century has been discredited due to a lack of valid and scientific evidence. Recently, a combination of evidence-based medicine and dentistry provides an excellent environment to study the relationship between oral infection and systemic diseases.

## BACTERIAL RESERVOIR

In a patient with periodontitis, subgingival space acts as an ideal environment for the colonization of gram-negative bacteria. Subgingival microbiota of gram-negative bacteria imposes a continuous challenge to the host defense mechanism. These gram-negative bacteria, along with their lipopolysaccharides (LPS) products, disseminate systemically through the ulcerated and discontinued sulcular epithelium and periodontal tissues. More often the intended treatment failed to achieve complete eradication of these organisms resulting in rapid reemergence. In generalized moderate periodontitis, the total surface area of pocket epithelium usually exposes to subgingival bacteria, and their product is estimated as the size of the palm of an adult hand.[4] However, this area of contact is further increased in cases of more advanced periodontal destruction.

After mechanical periodontal therapy, bacteria are commonly detected in the blood. Bacteremia continuously noted even during daily function and oral hygiene procedures. This increases the risk of distant seeding of oral infection and subsequent systemic illness. In this way, periodontal biofilm infection initially leads to local inflammation followed by the destruction of a tooth's supporting structure and subsequently systemic illnesses.[3]

## EFFECT ON CARDIOVASCULAR SYSTEM

### Atherosclerosis

Atherosclerosis, also known as hardening of arteries, is a slow and progressive disease of blood vessels. It is characterized by deposition of fatty plaque on the inner wall of vessel lumen leading to obstruction of normal blood circulation.

Proposed mechanisms **(Flowchart 15.1)** suggesting the role of infections in atherosclerosis are as follows.

### Oral Pathogens

Host-bacterial interactions and virulence of oral bacteria play an important role in coronary thrombogenesis. It is also evident that oral bacteria activate platelets leading to localized thrombus formation. Moreover, some strains of *Streptococcus sanguinis* and *Porphyromonas gingivalis* express platelet aggregation-associated protein (PAAP) that contributes to platelet aggregation on the innermost layer of the vessel lumen. Platelet aggregation plays a crucial role in the pathogenesis of thrombogenesis and thromboembolism leading to acute myocardial infarction and stroke.[5]

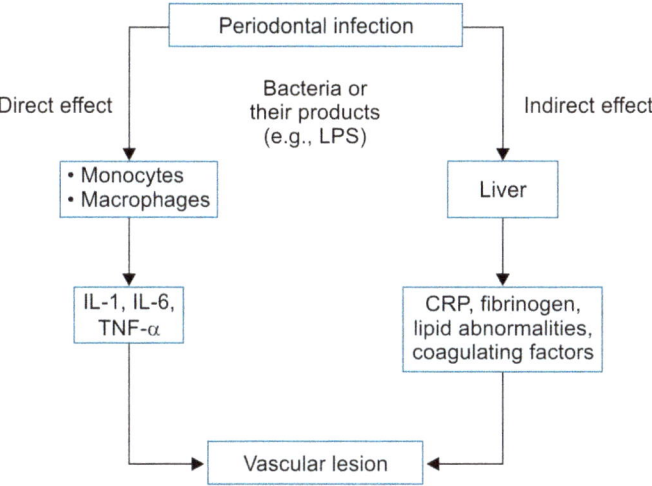

**Flowchart 15.1:** Systemic spread of periodontal infection.

(LPS: lipopolysaccharide; IL-1: interleukin-1; TNF-: tumor necrosis factor-; CRP: C-reactive protein)

### Host-mediated Effects

- *Acute-phase proteins*: Periodontitis is characterized by a local inflammatory response triggered by a bacterial infection. To some extent, acute-phase proteins are supposed to play a vital role in this inflammatory response. C-reactive protein (CRP) and fibrinogen are two important acute-phase proteins produced by the liver. Both are considered independent risk factors for coronary artery disease. Hence, periodontitis-induced elevation in the level of acute-phase proteins suggests the potential role of periodontal disease in cardiovascular disorders' pathogenesis.[6]
- *Heat shock proteins (HSPs)*: These proteins are the most immunogenic antigens of periopathogens *Bacteroides forsythias* and *P. gingivalis*. The extensive homology (~ 60%) between these periopathogens and human HSPs plays an essential role in the development and progression of atheroma. Antibodies to HSPs are usually detected in patients with periodontal disease. These HSP antibodies produced against periopathogens usually cross-react with HSPs antigens expressed on injured epithelium or atheromatous plaque leading to atheroma formation. Thus, HSP accelerates atheroma formation due to its autoimmune phenomena.[7]

### Common Genetic Predisposition

In light of genetic studies, a common genetic predisposition is predicted as one of the probable channels, suggesting the role of periodontitis and cardiovascular disease incidence. In this regard, a study by Beck J et al., executed a model of genetically determined hyperinflammatory macrophage phenotype in periodontal disease that eventually enhances the susceptibility of the individual for atherosclerotic lesions.[8]

### Common Risk Factors

Lifestyle, diabetes mellitus, and smoking are common risk factors shared by periodontitis and atherosclerosis. In this context, DeStefano et al., reported that periodontal disease and poor oral hygiene are a strong risk factor for coronary heart disease. As per DeStefano et al., oral hygiene is a marker for lifestyle with an influence on personal hygiene and health care. This further explains the link between periodontal diseases and cardiovascular diseases.[9]

### Role of Adhesion Molecules

The initial phase of atheroma formation involves the migration of inflammatory cells from circulation to the site of plaque formation. In this stage, adhesion molecules play a crucial role in adhesion of circulating monocyte to vascular endothelium. These adhesion molecules are usually expressed on vascular endothelium in response to inflammatory stimuli. Recruitment of inflammatory cells is mediated by some commonly expressed adhesion

## Section 3: Etiology

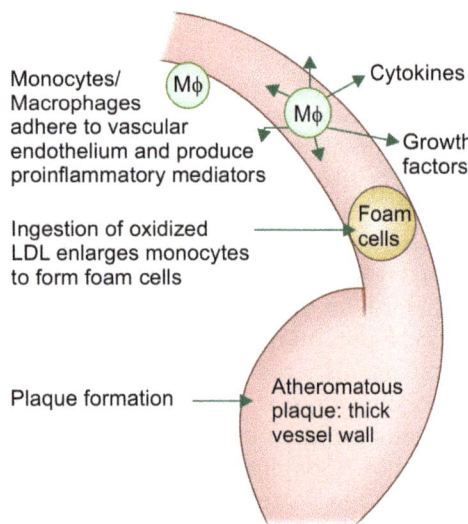

**Fig. 15.1:** Schematic representation showing pathogenesis of atherosclerosis.
(LDL: low-density lipoprotein)

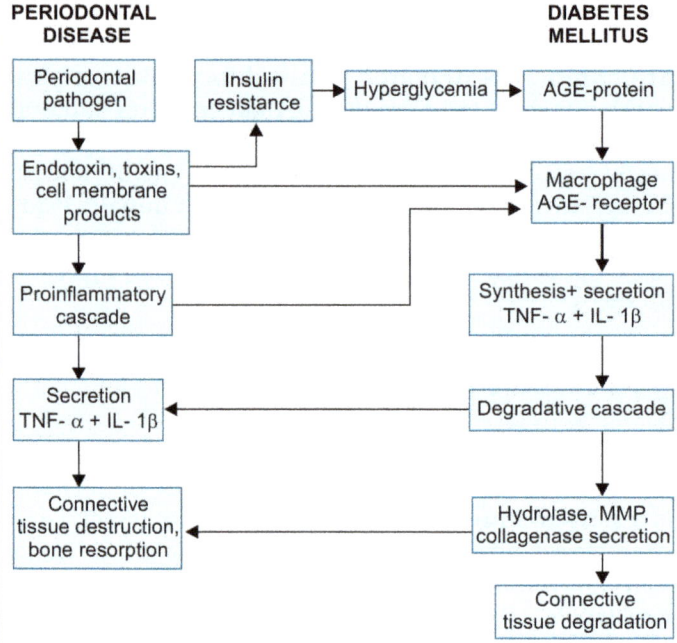

(AGE: advanced glycation end-product; IL-1: interleukin-1; TNF-α: tumor necrosis factor-α; MMP: matrix metalloproteinase)

molecules, such as intercellular adhesion molecules (ICAMs), endothelial leukocyte adhesion molecule 1 (ELAM-1) and vascular cell adhesion molecule 1 (VCAM-1). Bacterial LPS, prostaglandins, and proinflammatory cytokines upregulated these adhesion molecules. After binding to the endothelial cell lining, monocytes infiltrated the vascular endothelium and drifted under the arterial intima. The monocytes ingest circulating low-density lipoprotein (LDL) in its oxidized state and become engorged and form foam cells characteristic of atheromatous plaques **(Fig. 15.1)**. Once within the arterial media, monocytes also get transformed into macrophages. Additionally, proinflammatory cytokines and mitogenic factors further play a role in atheroma progression and thickening of the arterial wall.[10]

## EFFECT ON ENDOCRINE SYSTEM

### Diabetes Mellitus

Diabetes mellitus is a chronic metabolic disease characterized by persistently high blood glucose levels over a prolonged period. The preponderance of evidence suggests a two-way relationship between periodontal disease and diabetes.[11] Periodontitis is recognized as a potential aggravator of hyperglycemic state of diabetes mellitus. Periodontal infections increase tissue resistance to insulin, preventing glucose from entering target cells, causing elevated blood glucose levels, and requiring increased pancreatic insulin production to maintain a normal glucose level. In diabetes with significant insulin resistance, further tissue resistance to insulin-induced by periodontal infection exacerbates poor glycemic control.[12]

On the other hand, diabetes is found to enhance connective tissue destruction in periodontal diseases. This is due to the formation of advanced glycation end-products (AGEs). A persistent hyperglycemic environment in diabetes patients accelerates the nonenzymatic glycosylation of proteins and matrix molecules, resulting in AGEs. AGEs have a special affinity for receptors for advanced glycation (RAGE). In normal homeostasis, expression of RAGE is usually at low levels in many cell types like monocytes, endothelial cells, neurons, and smooth muscle cells. However, RAGE expression increases during perturbed states of the body, especially diabetes and inflammation. The subsequent interaction of AGEs with RAGE hampers the specific cellular functions and initiates a cycle of cytokine upregulation, mainly of interleukin-1 (IL-1) and tumor necrosis factor-α (TNF-α).[11] The synthesis and secretion of cytokines are increased, which triggers degradative cascade, resulting in connective tissue degradation, as explained in **Flowchart 15.2**.

## EFFECT ON REPRODUCTIVE SYSTEM

### Pregnancy Outcomes

It is well documented that periodontal diseases in women of childbearing age group (18–34 years) significantly affect the reproductive system. Periodontitis during pregnancy can be manifested as preterm birth (PTB). PTB infants are those infants who are born before the 37th week of gestation. Normal pregnancy usually lasts for about 40 weeks. PTB is a well-recognized cause for low birth weight (LBW). LBW infants are those born at term but weighing <2,500 g.

**Flowchart 15.3:** Effect of periodontal infection on pregnancy outcome.

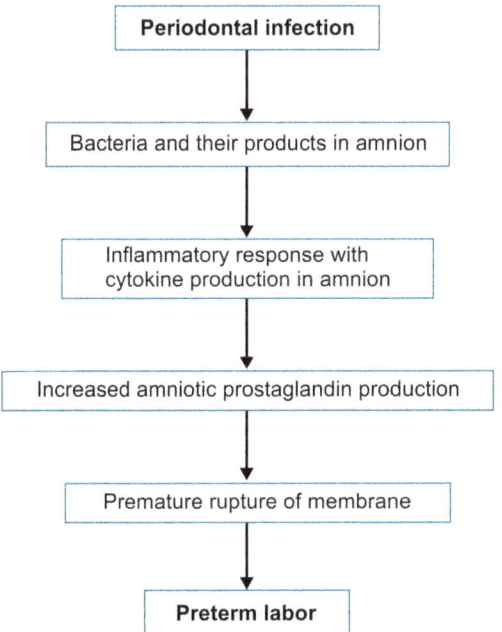

In recent years, subclinical and chronic infections such as periodontal disease have been proposed to play a role in premature birth and significantly increase the risk for both LBW and PTB.

The central role of periodontitis in PTB can be explained by transmitting gram-negative bacteria from the infected tooth into the uterine cavity via the bloodstream. Once inside the uterine cavity, these gram-negative bacteria start to produce endotoxins that stimulate an inflammatory cascade with the production of cytokines.[13] Cytokine cascade leads to an increase in the production of proinflammatory mediators, such as IL-1α and TNF-α, further stimulating prostaglandin synthesis. The high concentration of prostaglandins triggers uterine muscle contraction, cervical dilation and premature rupture of membranes leading to PTB **(Flowchart 15.3)**.[14]

## EFFECT ON RESPIRATORY SYSTEM

Likewise, other systemic manifestations, as described above, periodontal diseases have a modulating role in respiratory infections too. Specific invasive oral pathogens have a potential role in the pathogenesis of chronic obstructive pulmonary disease (COPD). COPD is an inflammatory disease of the respiratory system characterized by airflow obstruction.[15] It is commonly classified into two types as emphysema or chronic bronchitis. It is usually associated with enlargement of bronchial mucous glands and infiltration of inflammatory cells, including neutrophils and mononuclear inflammatory cells within the lung tissue. Both COPD and periodontal diseases are found to share similar pathogenic mechanisms. In both cases, a host inflammatory response is commonly triggered in response to the chronic challenge like a bacterial infection in periodontal disease while cigarette smoking in COPD.

Role of oral pathogens in the pathogenesis of respiratory infection can be explained by following three mechanisms:[16]

1. Aspiration of pathogens from oral lesions (*A. actinomycetemcomitans* and *P. gingivalis*) into the respiratory tract and lung tissues triggers the respiratory infection.
2. Periodontitis is commonly associated with the production of enzymes in saliva. These enzymes modify oral mucosal surfaces and favor adhesion as well as colonization of respiratory microbes. These microbes get further aspirated into the respiratory tract and lungs.
3. Cytokines-mediated alteration in respiratory epithelium promotes respiratory infection by respiratory pathogens. If periodontal disease is left unattended, continuous stimulation of cells of the periodontium by oral pathogens encourages the release of various cytokines and biologically active molecules. Epithelial and connective tissue cells of periodontium usually produce interleukin (IL) and TNF-α in response to bacterial infection, while stimulated peripheral mononuclear cells produce IL-1α and TNF-α. These cytokines lead to neutrophil influx and release of oxidative and hydrolytic enzymes that cause direct tissue destruction. In addition to this, monocytes and macrophages infiltration leads to further release of proinflammatory mediators.

> **Points to Ponder**
> - Periodontal medicine: It's a branch of periodontology that is concerned with periodontal disease's effect on various organ systems.
> - Willoughby D Miller and Willam Hunter originally proposed focal infection theory.
> - Periodontitis is considered the sixth complication of diabetes mellitus.

## REFERENCES

1. O'Reilly PG, Claffey NM. A history of oral sepsis as a cause of disease. Periodontology 2000. 2000; 23: 13-8.
2. Williams RC, David PD. Periodontitis as a risk for systemic disease. In: Lindhe J, Karring T, Lang NP (Eds). Clinical Periodontology and Implant Dentistry, 4th edition. Oxford, UK: Blackwell Munksgaard; 2003. pp. 366-86.
3. Mealey BL, Klokkevold PR. Periodontal medicine. In: Newman MG, Takei HH, Carranza FA (Eds). Carranza's Clinical Periodontology, 9th edition. Philadelphia, PA, USA: WB Saunders; 2003. pp. 229-44.
4. Waite DE, Bradley RE. Oral infections: Report of two cases. J Am Dent Assoc. 1965;71:587-92.
5. Mealey BL. Influence of periodontal infections on systemic health. Periodontol 2000. 1999;21:197-209.

6. Genco RJ, Offenbacher S, Beck J. Cardiovascular diseases and oral infections. In: Rose LF, Genco RJ, Mealey BL, Cohen DW (Eds). Periodontal Medicine, 1st edition. Toronto, Canada: BC Decker Publishers; 2000. pp. 63-82.
7. Leishman SJ, Ford PJ, Do HL, Palmer JE, Heng NC, West MJ, et al. Periodontal pathogen load and increased antibody response to heat shock protein 60 in patients with cardiovascular disease. J Clin Periodontol. 2012;39(10):923-30.
8. Beck J, Garcia R, Heiss G, Vokonas PS, Offenbacher S. Periodontal disease, and cardiovascular disease. J Periodontol. 1996;67(10 Suppl):1123-37.
9. DeStefano F, Anda RF, Kahn HS, Williamson DF, Russell CM. Dental disease and risk of coronary heart disease and mortality. BMJ. 1993;306(6879):688-91.
10. Kinane DF. Periodontal diseases' contributions to cardiovascular disease: an overview of potential mechanisms. Ann Periodontol. 1998;3(1):142-50.
11. Grossi SG, Genco RJ. Periodontal disease and diabetes mellitus: a two-way relationship. Ann Periodontol. 1998;3(1):51-61.
12. Mealey BL. Diabetes mellitus. In: Rose LF, Genco RJ, Mealey BL, Cohen DW (Eds). Periodontal Medicine, 1st edition. Toronto, Canada: BC Decker Publishing; 2000. pp. 121-50.
13. Corgel JO. Periodontal medicine and the female patient. In: Rose LF, Genco RJ, Mealey BL, Cohen DW (Eds). Periodontal Medicine, 1st edition. Toronto, Canada: BC Decker Publishing; 2000. pp. 151-66.
14. Offenbacher S, Jared HL, O'Reilly PG, Wells SR, Salvi GE, Lawrence HP, et al. Potential pathogenic mechanisms of periodontitis- associated pregnancy complications. Ann Periodontol. 1998;3(1):233-50.
15. Scannapieco FA, Bush RB, Paju S. Associations between periodontal disease and risk for nosocomial bacterial pneumonia and chronic obstructive pulmonary disease. A systematic review. Ann Periodontol. 2003;8(1): 54-69.
16. Scannapieco FA. Relationships between periodontal and respiratory diseases. In: Rose LF, Genco RJ, Mealey BL, Cohen DW (Eds). Periodontal Medicine, 1st edition. Toronto, Canada: BC Decker Publishers; 2000. pp. 83-98.

## VIVA VOCE

**Q1.** **What are the five classic complications of diabetes mellitus?**
**Ans.** The five classic complications of diabetes mellitus are:
1. Retinopathy
2. Nephropathy
3. Neuropathy
4. Macrovascular disease
5. Altered wound healing

**Q2.** **Which is the sixth complication of diabetes mellitus?**
**Ans.** Periodontal disease is the sixth complication of diabetes mellitus.

**Q3.** **Which of the antibiotic suppresses the glycation of proteins and reduces the activity of matrix metalloproteinase?**
**Ans.** Tetracyclines suppress the glycation of proteins and reduce the activity of matrix metalloproteinase.

**Q4.** **Name platelet aggregation-associated protein (PAAP) positive bacteria.**
**Ans.** Some strains of *S. sanguinis* and *P. gingivalis*.

**Q5.** **What are heat shock proteins?**
**Ans.** Heat shock proteins are the most immunogenic antigens of periopathogens *Bacteroides forsythus* and *P. gingivalis*.

**Q6.** **What is periodontal medicine?**
**Ans.** The branch of periodontology, concerned with the effect of periodontal disease on various organ systems.

**Q7.** **What are preterm birth (PTB) infants?**
**Ans.** Preterm birth infants are those infants who are born before the 37th week of gestation.

**Q8.** **What are low birth weight (LBW) infants?**
**Ans.** Low birth weight infants are those born at term but weighing <2,500 g.

**Q9.** **Name acute phase proteins produced by the liver.**
**Ans.** C-reactive protein (CRP) and fibrinogen.

**Q10.** **How is the advanced glycation end-product formed?**
**Ans.** A persistent hyperglycemic environment in diabetes patients accelerates the nonenzymatic glycosylation of proteins and matrix molecules, resulting in advanced glycation end products.

# Chapter 16

# Smoking and Periodontium

*Shalu Bathla*

## Chapter Outline

- Classifications
- Constituents of Tobacco Smoke
- Effects of Smoking
- Smoking Cessation

## INTRODUCTION

Smoking is a significant public health concern due to the detrimental effects of tobacco on various body systems. Cigarette smoking has both systemic and local side effects. Smoking is associated with a broad spectrum of diseases, including hypertension, atherosclerosis, cancer, chronic lung disease, ischemic heart disease, hypercoagulability, coronary artery disease, stroke, esophageal reflux, peripheral vascular disease, peptic ulcer disease, spontaneous abortion, prematurity, low birth weight and delayed wound healing.

Likewise, smoking is identified as an independent environmental risk factor for the development and progression of periodontal diseases. Smokeless tobacco use induces localized oral lesions in the form of leukoplakia and carcinoma. However, there are no generalized effects on periodontal disease progression, other than localized attachment loss and recession at the site of tobacco product placement. In 1947, Pindborg, for the first time, identified a potential causal relationship between smoking and periodontal disease. Tobacco smoking hampers the oral environment and ecology, the vasculature, the inflammatory, and immune responses and homeostasis and healing potential of the periodontal tissues. This favors the growth of periodontal pathogens and subsequent periodontal diseases.[1]

## CLASSIFICATIONS

- *According to the Centers for Disease Control and Prevention (CDC), smokers are classified as*:
    - *Current smokers*: Those that had smoked more than or equal to 100 cigarettes over their lifetime and smoked at the time of the interview.
    - *Former smokers*: Those that had smoked more than or equal to 100 cigarettes over their lifetime but were not currently smoking.
    - *Nonsmokers*: Those that had not smoked more than or equivalent to 100 cigarettes in their lifetime.
- *According to the number of cigarettes smoked/day, smokers can be classified as*:
    - *Heavy smokers*: Those that had smoked more than or equal to 20 cigarettes/day.
    - *Light smokers*: Those that had smoked less than or equal to 19 cigarettes/day.

## CONSTITUENTS OF TOBACCO SMOKE

Cigarette smoking is a very complex mixture of substances with over 4,000 known constituents.[2]

### Particulate Phase

It includes nicotine and cotinine. The patient's exposure to tobacco smoke is measured in various ways including interviewing the subject using a simple questionnaire and biochemical analysis. Cotinine is a metabolite of nicotine; its measurements are more reliable in determining a subject's exposure to tobacco smoke because its half-life is 14–20 hours compared with the shorter half-life of nicotine which is 2–3 hours.[3] Nicotine induces various effects, i.e., inhibits apoptosis in certain cell lines (e.g., fibroblasts, osteoclasts), exaggerates immune system activities, etc. Tar (compound of many chemicals), benzene, and benzo(a)pyrene are the other particulate constituents.

### Gas Phase

It includes carbon monoxide (declines the oxygen-carrying capacity of hemoglobin), ammonia, dimethyl-nitrosamine,

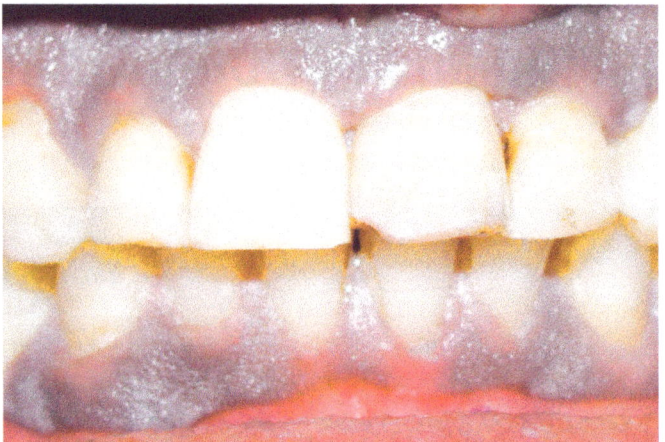

Fig. 16.1: Clinical picture showing effects of smoking on gingiva—decreased gingival inflammation and increased gingival pigmentation.

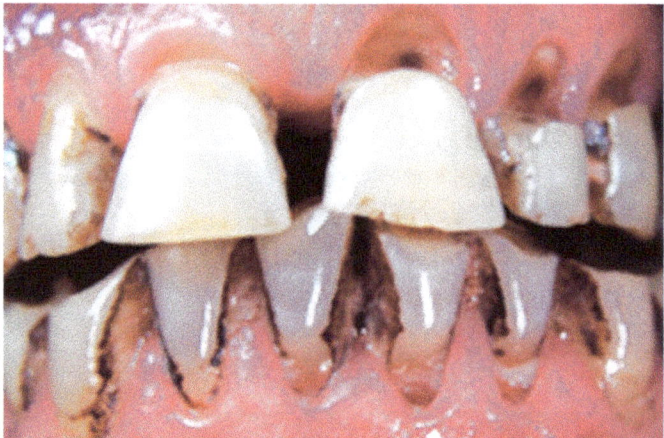

Fig. 16.2: Clinical picture showing the effects of smoking on periodontium—more attachment loss and bone loss.

formaldehyde, hydrogen cyanide (inhibits enzyme system necessary for oxidative metabolism) and acrolein.

# EFFECTS OF SMOKING

## Prevalence and Severity of Periodontal Disease

### Gingivitis

Effects of smoking on gingiva are as follows **(Fig. 16.1)**:[4]
- *Gingival inflammation*: Smoking causes a decrease in gingival inflammation.
- *Gingival blood flow*: Vasoconstrictive effect of nicotine reduces the blood flow to gingival tissues. Hence, smokers exhibit less bleeding on probing.
- *Oxygen tension*: Smokers do have lower oxygen saturation.
Less gingival redness, lower bleeding on probing, and fewer vessels visible clinically and histologically all suggest the suppressive effect of smoking on the gingival vasculature.

### Periodontitis

Effects of smoking on periodontal disease are as follows **(Fig. 16.2)**:
- Prevalence and severity of periodontal destruction increase with smoking.
- Pocket: There are deeper probing depths and a larger number of deep pockets in smokers.
- Attachment and bone loss: More attachment loss and bone loss are seen in smokers.
- In smokers, there is an increased rate of periodontal destruction and tooth loss.

## Etiology and Pathogenesis of Periodontal Disease

### Role of Smoking in the Pathogenesis of Periodontal Disease

Various mechanisms describe the role of smoking in the pathogenesis of the periodontal disease. The first mechanism suggests the effect of carbon monoxide on periodontal tissues. Carbon monoxide present in tobacco smoke is a strong reducing agent which produces a marked immediate reduction of redox potential at mucosal surfaces. It is likely a direct mechanism to promote the growth of anaerobes at superficial sites and progression of periodontitis. A second mechanism is an indirect microbiological effect of smoking that enhances the growth of bacteria, which supply growth factors for anaerobes at shallow sites. A third mechanism is the damaging of protective periodontal cells by the molecular byproducts of smoking. Smoking adversely affects the functioning of polymorphs. Leukocytic damage hinders the clearance of bacteria from the periodontal environment. Likewise, diabetes and smoking accelerate the production of advanced glycation end-products (AGEs), which have a role in the pathogenesis of periodontitis. AGE significantly damages the periodontal tissue vasculature and interferes with the functioning of polymorphs, proteins, and lactoferrin. These AGEs act as a predisposing factor for periodontal diseases.[5]

*Microbiology*: Smoking induces qualitative alteration in plaque microbes leading to altered microbial challenges.[6] It does not affect the rate of plaque accumulation, but there is an increase in the colonization of shallow periodontal pockets by periodontal pathogens. Smokers had 2.3 times more capacity to harbor *T. forsythia* than nonsmokers.[7]

*Physiology*: Smoking is associated with decreased gingival crevicular fluid (GCF) flow, blood flow, and bleeding on probing. Hence, the clinical signs of inflammation are less noticeable in smokers when compared with nonsmokers. Subgingival temperatures are lower in smokers than nonsmokers. Recovery from local anesthesia takes more time in smokers as compared to nonsmokers. This is due to prolongation in recovery from the vasoconstriction caused by local anesthetic administration in smokers.

*Immunology*: Smoking hampers the protective elements of the immune response that accelerates the extent and severity of periodontal destruction. In smokers, there is downregulation of the immune response to bacterial challenge **(Flowchart 16.1 and Box 16.1)**.[4]

- *Neutrophil function:*[1]
  - Neutrophils receptors: Neutrophils express various functional receptors for different components and metabolites of tobacco smoke including nicotine and cotinine (primarily the α3 β4 subtype of nicotinic receptors). In smokers, the expression of nicotinic receptors by neutrophils is high. Neutrophils also express receptors for endogenous factors, but their natural agonists get dysregulated in tobacco smokers.
  - Neutrophil migration and chemotaxis: In smokers, transmigration of neutrophils across the periodontal microvasculature is restricted. Neutrophil chemotaxis and phagocytosis also get altered due to smoking. The actin cytoskeleton plays a central role in neutrophil motility, which is essential for extravasation across the periodontal microvasculature and subsequent migration of neutrophils towards inflammatory stimuli. However, tobacco smoke exposure hinders the functioning of F-actin kinetics.
  - Neutrophil-derived degradative proteases: Smoking is associated with increased production of collagen-degrading enzymes, elastase, matrix metalloproteinases (MMP-1 and MMP-8), and decreases the levels of major endogenous MMP inhibitors (tissue inhibitors of MMP-1, alpha-1-antitrypsin and alpha-2-macroglobulin).
  - Neutrophil respiratory burst: This is the oxygen-dependent process that facilitates the phagocytic killing of bacterial cells by neutrophils with the formation of multiple reactive oxygen and reactive nitrogen species. Smoke components impede the respiratory burst of neutrophils. The gas-phase of cigarette smoke is associated with the suppression of neutrophil nicotinamide adenine dinucleotide phosphate (NADPH) oxidase.
- *T- and B-cell functions*: Smoking reduces the proliferative response to polyclonal B-cell activators (B-cell mitogens). Tobacco glycoprotein (a polyphenolic protein in tobacco) is a potent B-cell mitogen and stimulates the production of immunoglobulin classes (IgM, IgG, and IgA).
- *Osteoblasts*: Smoking suppresses cellular proliferation and alkaline phosphatase activity in osteoblasts and hence decreases the synthesis of bone matrix protein by interfering with oxygen levels in osteoblasts. Osteoclast cell remains longer, and the bone resorption phase continues long after their normal lifecycle.
- *Fibroblasts*: Nicotine significantly inhibits the proliferation of gingival fibroblasts at high concentrations. This reduces the production of type I collagen and fibronectin. Nicotine also inhibits periodontal fibroblast growth and attachment.

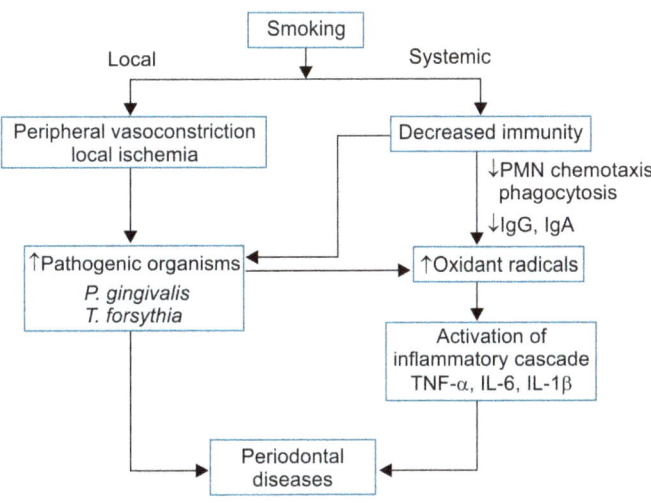

**Flowchart 16.1:** Relationship between smoking and periodontal diseases.

(PMN: polymorphonuclear leukocytes; IL-6: interleukin-6; TNF-α: tumor necrosis factor-α; IgG: immunoglobulin G)

**BOX 16.1:** Effects of smoking on the immune system.[4]
- Alters neutrophil, chemotaxis, and phagocytosis in smokers
- Increases TNF-α, $PGE_2$ in smoker's GCF
- Increases production of neutrophil, collagenase and elastase in smoker's GCF
- Nicotine suppresses osteoblast proliferation
- Nicotine adversely affects fibroblast functions

(TNF-α: tumor necrosis factor-α; $PGE_2$: prostaglandin $E_2$; GCF: gingival crevicular fluid)

## The Response of Periodontal Therapy

*Phase I: Nonsurgical Therapy*
- There is a decreased clinical response to scaling and root planing.
- Pocket depth reduction is less in smokers.
- There is less gain in clinical attachment level.

*Phase II: Surgical Therapy*
- There is less pocket depth reduction after surgery in smokers.
- There are greater chances of membrane exposure in smokers after the guided tissue regeneration (GTR) procedure.
- There is less gain in clinical attachment level and bone fill.[4]

*Phase III: Implant Surgery*
- Smoking addiction leads to poor outcomes in implant surgery. Tobacco use directly affects the osseointegration of root-form dental implants. Smoking along with plaque-induced inflammation greatly affects the bone loss around the implants.[8]

## Section 3: Etiology

*Phase IV: Maintenance Therapy*
- There is an increase in pocket depth during the maintenance phase in smokers.
- The gain in clinical attachment level is lesser in smokers as compared to nonsmokers.[4]

## SMOKING CESSATION

### Basic Steps of Smoking Cessation Program

Basic steps known as 5 A's for smoking cessation was first proposed by Marc Manley and Thomas Glynn of National Cancer Institute:
- *Ask*: Identify the tobacco use status of every patient. Fagerström test is used to estimate the nicotine dependency levels of the patient. It is a score-based test involving answers to questions such as the timing of the first cigarette smoked in the day, difficulty in not smoking in forbidden areas, most crucial cigarette during the day, number of cigarettes smoked/day, etc. Higher scores indicate more addicted smokers.[9]
- *Advice*: This increases the tobacco user's interest in quitting. The patients should be advised that smoking cessation would be beneficial.
- *Assess*: This step is about recognizing the patient's interest and readiness to attempt tobacco cessation.
- *Assist*: Help those who are ready with their problem-solving skills and with pharmacotherapy. Counseling should be brief and nonjudgmental. Motivational interviewing is the most popular behavior change counseling that helps patients explore and resolve ambivalence about changing behavior.[10]
- *Arrange*: Arrange follow-up support throughout the quitting process. During the first week of the cessation program, patients find difficulty in getting adjusted to smoking cessation. In such cases, the use of follow-up methods is beneficial. The methods of maintaining contact with the patient are usually appointments for office visits for monitoring and continued counseling and telephone calls and letters confirming quit dates.

### Treatment

- *Pharmacological intervention*:
  - Nicotine replacement therapy (NRT):
    - Nicotine gum: Releases nicotine via chewing and buccal absorption.
      Strength: 2 mg for < 25 cigarettes/day; 4 mg for > 25 cigarettes/day.
    - Nicotine patch: Patch is the most popular form of replacement for the patient who smokes pack approximately 20 cigarettes or less a day. 16 hours/24 hours patch; has to be administered each morning.
    - Nicotine inhaler
    - Nicotine nasal spray

**TABLE 16.1:** Pharmacotherapy for smoking cessation.

| Pharmacotherapy | Dosage | Duration |
|---|---|---|
| Nicotine gum | 1–24 cigs/day - 2 mg gum<br>25+ cigs/day - 4 mg gum | Up to 12 weeks |
| Nicotine patch | 22 mg/24 hours; 14 mg/24 hours; 7 mg/24 hours; 15 mg/16 hours | 4 weeks; then 2 weeks; then 2 weeks; 8 weeks |
| Nicotine inhaler | 6–16 cartridges/day | Up to 6 months |
| Nicotine nasal spray | 8–40 doses/day | 3–6 months |
| Bupropion | 150 mg every morning for three days, then 150 mg twice daily (begin treatment 1–2 weeks pre-cessation) | 7–12 weeks; maintenance up to 6 months |

(cigs: cigarettes)

  - Non-nicotine pharmacotherapy:
    - Bupropion: Bupropion-sustained release is the first-line pharmacotherapy for smoking cessation **(Table 16.1)**. It can be used alone or in combination with NRT. It is an antidepressant belonging to the class norepinephrine dopamine reuptake inhibitor (NDRI), enhancing the dopamine and norepinephrine levels.
      It decreases the craving and withdrawal symptoms.
    - Varenicline: It is a nicotine receptor partial agonist; it stimulates nicotine receptors more weakly than the nicotine itself.
      As a partial agonist, it reduces the craving for and decreases the pleasurable effects of cigarette smoking.
  - Alternative pharmacotherapies:
    - Nortriptyline
    - Clonidine
    - Nicotine vaccine
- *Nonpharmacological intervention*.

### Periodontal Effects of Smoking Cessation

Smoking cessation is good to reestablish periodontal health and improves periodontal treatment outcomes. Smoking cessation halts periodontal disease progression and restores the normal periodontal and microbial healing responses. The tissue healing response in an ex-smoker is almost similar to that of nonsmokers. Smoking has a great potential to affect the composition of subgingival microflora in patients with periodontitis. In such cases, antibiotic therapy and smoking cessation are the most effective treatment options for improving future outcomes.[11]

#### Points to Ponder

Relationship of smoking and vitamin C: Cigarette smoke contains various oxidative agents that are responsible for considerable periodontal tissue damage. $OH^-$ radical-induced tissue damage and accumulation of hydroperoxide disrupt membrane functions. Due to its potential antioxidant, vitamin C is a scavenger of $OH^-$ radicals and hypochlorous acid. These radicals are responsible for both neutrophil-derived and GCF collagenase. However, vitamin C neutralizes, such as oxidative activations.

## REFERENCES

1. Palmer RM, Wilson RF, Hasan AS, Scott DA. Mechanism of action of environmental factors—tobacco smoking. J Clin Periodontol. 2005;32(Suppl 6):180-95.
2. Lindhe J, Karring T, Lang NP. Modifying factors: diabetes, puberty, pregnancy, and the menopause and tobacco smoking. In: Clinical Periodontology and Implant Dentistry, 4th edition. Oxford, UK: Blackwell Munksgaard; 2003. pp. 179-97.
3. Jarvis MJ, Russell MA, Benowitz NL, Feyerabend C. Elimination of cotinine from body fluids: implications for noninvasive measurement of tobacco smoke exposure. Am J Public Health. 1988;78(6):696-8.
4. Novak MJ, Novak KF. Smoking and periodontal disease. In: Newman MG, Takei HH, Carranza FA (Eds). Carranza's Clinical Periodontology, 9th edition. Philadelphia, PA, USA: WB Saunders; 2003. pp. 245-53.
5. Eggert FM, McLeod MH, Flowerdew G. Effects of smoking and treatment status on periodontal bacteria: evidence that smoking influences control of periodontal bacteria at the mucosal surface of the gingival crevice. J Periodontol. 2001;72(9):1210-20.
6. Bergström J. Cigarette smoking as a risk factor in chronic periodontal disease. Community Dent Oral Epidemiol. 1989;17(5):245-7.
7. Zambon JJ, Grossi SG, Machtei EE, Ho AW, Dunford R, Genco RJ. Cigarette smoking increases the risk for subgingival infection with periodontal pathogens. J Periodontol. 1996;67(10 Suppl):1050-4.
8. Bain CA, Moy PK. The association between the failure of dental implants and cigarette smoking. Int J Oral Maxillofac Implants. 1993;8(6):609-15.
9. Heatherton TF, Kozlowski LT, Frecker RC, Fagerström KO. The Fagerström Test for Nicotine Dependence: a revision of the Fag- erström Tolerance Questionnaire. Br J Addict. 1991;86(9):1119-27.
10. Rollnick S, Miller WR. What is motivational interviewing? Behav Cogn Psychother. 1995;12:325-34.
11. Grossi SG, Zambon J, Machtie EE, Schifferle R, Andreana S, Genco RJ, et al. Effects of smoking and smoking cessation on healing after mechanical periodontal therapy. J Am Dent Assoc. 1997;128(5):599-607.

## VIVA VOCE

**Q1. What is gingivitis toxica?**
**Ans.** According to Pindborg, gingivitis toxica is a specific type of gingivitis in which there is the destruction of gingiva and the underlying bone due to the chewing of tobacco.

**Q2. How much time nicotine takes to reach the brain?**
**Ans.** Nicotine takes 10–19 seconds only to reach the brain.

**Q3. What is the half-life of nicotine and cotinine?**
**Ans.** The half-life of nicotine and cotinine is approximately 1–2 hours and 20 hours, respectively.

**Q4. What is the concentration of cotinine in saliva and urine?**
**Ans.** The concentration of cotinine in saliva and urine is 300 ng/mL and 1500 ng/mL, respectively.

**Q5. What are the effects of smoking on neutrophil?**
**Ans.** Smoking alters neutrophil's chemotaxis and phagocytosis.

**Q6. What are the basic steps of the smoking cessation program?**
**Ans.** Ask, Advise, Assess, Assist, and Arrange.

**Q7. What is the effect of smoking on advanced glycation end-products?**
**Ans.** Smoking accelerates the production of advanced glycation end-products.

**Q8. Which MMPs level increases with smoking?**
**Ans.** MMP-1 and MMP-8.

**Q9. What is the effect of smoking on osteoblasts?**
**Ans.** Smoking suppresses cellular proliferation and alkaline phosphatase activity in osteoblasts.

**Q10. Why recovery from local anesthesia takes more time in smokers as compared to nonsmokers?**
**Ans.** Due to prolongation in recovery from the vasoconstriction caused by local anesthetic administration in smokers.

# Pathology of Gingival and Periodontal Diseases

- Defense Mechanisms of Gingiva
- Gingival Inflammation
- Gingival Enlargement
- Acute Gingival Conditions
- Soft and Hard Tissue Lesions
- Periodontal Pocket
- Periodontal Abscess
- Bone Defects
- Periodontitis
- AIDS and Periodontium
- Trauma from Occlusion
- Sex Hormones and Periodontium

# Chapter 17

# Defense Mechanisms of Gingiva

*Shalu Bathla*

## Chapter Outline

- Junctional Epithelium
- Polymorphonuclear Leukocytes
- Saliva
- Gingival Crevicular Fluid

## INTRODUCTION

Mastication of food is the prime function of teeth, and hence supporting gingival tissues are persistently exposed to mechanical pressure. In addition to this, the oral cavity is the ideal place for microbial colonization. These two factors enhance the susceptibility of gingival tissues to different infections. However, the saliva, the epithelial surface, and the initial stages of the inflammatory response provide a great range of protection to gingival tissues against infections **(Box 17.1)**. In this chapter, the defensive role of the junctional epithelium (JE), polymorphonuclear leukocytes (PMNLs), saliva, and gingival crevicular fluid (GCF) are discussed.

## JUNCTIONAL EPITHELIUM

Junctional epithelium is the specialized gingival epithelium with unique structural and functional features, which make it an integral component of the periodontal defense mechanism. It exhibits potent antimicrobial mechanism by avoiding pathogenic microbial colonization in the subgingival tooth surface. As an epithelial component of a dentogingival unit, JE is firmly attached to the tooth surface, and it forms a strong epithelial barrier against the plaque bacteria. It permits the access of GCF, inflammatory cells, and the immunological host defense components to the gingival margin. Lastly, JE cells are inbuilt with a rapid turnover mechanism, which facilitates the host-parasite equilibrium and rapid repair of damaged tissue.[1] Thus, the specialized structural framework makes JE as an essential component of gingival defense mechanism **(Fig. 17.1)**.[2]

Junctional epithelial cells release chemokines interleukin-8 (IL-8) that attract and activate neutrophils and lymphocytes. Defensins and lysosomal enzymes and the active antimicrobial substances are also produced by junctional epithelial cells.[2]

**BOX 17.1:** Defense mechanisms of the oral cavity.

Defense mechanisms of the oral cavity are due to:
- Saliva
- Sulcular fluid
- Intact epithelial barrier: Junctional epithelium (JE)
- Presence of normal beneficial flora
- Local antibody production
- Migrating polymorphonuclear leukocytes (PMNLs) and other leukocytes

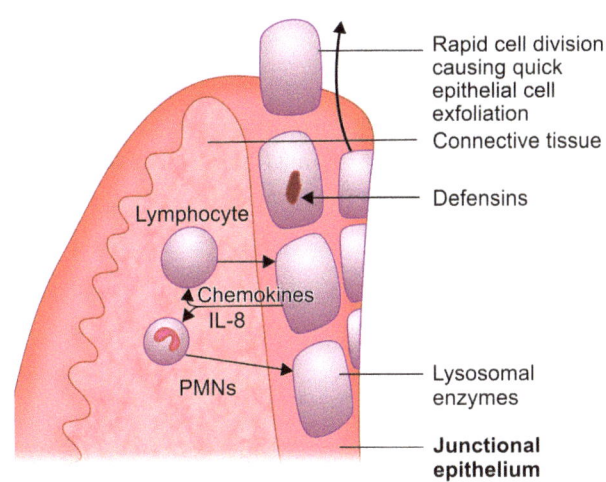

**Fig. 17.1:** Schematic representation showing antimicrobial mechanisms of the junctional epithelium (JE).
(PMNs: polymorphonuclear neutrophils)

# POLYMORPHONUCLEAR LEUKOCYTES

The role of PMNLs is primarily a defense mechanism against plaque bacteria at the gingival margin. On the gingival plaque, the PMNLs get degranulated and actively release lysosomal constituents. Discharge of lysosomal enzyme facilitates adherence to plaque bacteria and subsequent phagocytosis. By forming a protective wall against plaque, PMNLs act as a significant contributor to the host-parasite equilibrium. However, they have a limited capacity to reclaim any tooth surface once lost to the plaque bacteria. In the case of activated PMNLs, the tissue damage is mainly due to a variety of enzymes, oxygen metabolites, and other components that get release on degranulation during the battle against microbes.[1] (Rest is explained in "Chapter 11: Immunity and Inflammation").

# SALIVA

Saliva acts as the medium for biofilm suspension, having a great effect on plaque initiation, maturation, and metabolism. Salivary flow and composition determine the calculus formation, periodontal disease, and caries.[3] Xerostomia, a disease characterized by decreased salivary gland secretion, is associated with an increase in inflammatory gingival diseases, and rapid tooth destruction along with cervical or cemental caries. The normal and xerostomic values of stimulated saliva are approximately 1–2 mL/minute and <0.5 mL/minute, respectively. Xerostomia is produced as a component of a variety of diseases, including sialolithiasis, sarcoidosis, Sjögren's syndrome, Mikulicz's disease, irradiation and surgical removal of the salivary glands.[4] Salivary secretions maintain physiological equilibrium within the oral tissues and form a conditioning film on all oral surfaces. Saliva cleanses the exposed oral surfaces, neutralizes acids produced by bacteria, controls bacterial activity, and thus affects the plaque in a great way (Box 17.2).

## Composition of Saliva

Composition of saliva is as follows:[3]
- Electrolytes include potassium, sodium, chloride, bicarbonate, calcium, magnesium, and phosphorus.

---

**BOX 17.2:** Sialogogues and saliva substitutes.

Few sialogogues (increases salivary flow) are:
- ❑ Lemonade/acid drinks
- ❑ Xylitol chewing gums
- ❑ Pilocarpine

Few commercially available saliva substitutes are:
- ❑ *Saliva orthana (Nycomed)*: Oral spray containing porcine mucin
- ❑ *Luborant*: Lactose peroxidase
- ❑ *Salinum*: Water-soluble extract of linseed oil
- ❑ Salivix pastilles

---

- Organic:
  - Protein includes:
    - Acinar cell families include mucin, proline-rich proteins and glycoproteins, histatins, statherin, cystatins, amylase, peroxidases, and carbonic anhydrases.
    - Ductal and stromal products include lactoferrin, lysozyme, secretory immunoglobulin A (IgA), kallikrein, and fibronectin.
  - Lipids
  - Carbohydrates
  - Sulfates

## Role of Saliva

### In Oral Health

- Saliva provides physical protection via mucin and glycoprotein.
- It helps in lubrication via glycoprotein and mucin.
- Antibacterial action of saliva is because of the presence of IgA, salivary amylase, lactoferrin, salivary peroxidase, proline-rich protein, and lysozyme. Secretory IgA (sIgA) present in saliva provides the first line of defense via immunologic means in the oral cavity. sIgA binds to microbes, which inhibit their adherence to hard-tissue and soft-tissue surfaces, thus hindering microbial invasion into deeper host tissues. It plays an essential role in viral neutralization, viral growth attenuation, and replication on oral surfaces. It also neutralizes and disposes of toxins and food antigens. Lactoferrin acts against *Actinobacillus* and *Streptococcus*. Salivary lactothiocyanate peroxidase enzyme catalyzes the oxidation of thiocyanate ion (SCN) by hydrogen peroxide ($H_2O_2$), generating highly reactive, the oxidized form of thiocyanate ($OSCN^-$) and causing direct toxicity to *Streptococcus*. It neutralizes the deleterious effects of $H_2O_2$ produced by several oral microorganisms. Lysozyme causes lysis of cell wall of *Aggregatibacter actinomycetemcomitans* and *Veilonella*.[5]
- Saliva aids in tooth integrity via histatin, statherin, and cystatin.
- The cleansing action of saliva is due to its physical flow.
- Buffering action of saliva is due to the presence of urea and arginine-rich protein. Carbonic anhydrase causes the reversible hydration of carbon dioxide, leading to bicarbonate formation, which contributes to the buffering capacity.[6]
- Saliva provides data for diagnostic testing.
- Saliva hastens the blood coagulation and protects the wound from bacterial invasion due to the presence of some coagulating factors.
- Saliva helps in swallowing and formation of the food bolus.
- Saliva also helps in speech.

### In Oral Diseases
- Saliva helps in the formation of pellicle and thus, plaque deposition.
- It also aids in plaque mineralization to form calculus.
- It affects dental caries by cleansing mechanically and by direct antibacterial activity.

## GINGIVAL CREVICULAR FLUID

The gingival crevicular fluid is an inflammatory exudate present in the sulcus/periodontal pocket situated in between the tooth and marginal gingiva. This is mainly composed of a complex mixture of serum, inflammatory cells, connective tissue, epithelium, and microbial flora inhabiting in the gingival margin or the sulcus/pocket. In healthy sulcus, the volume of GCF is minimal.[1] Biochemical analysis of the GCF is a unique diagnostic marker for the assessment of periodontal conditions.

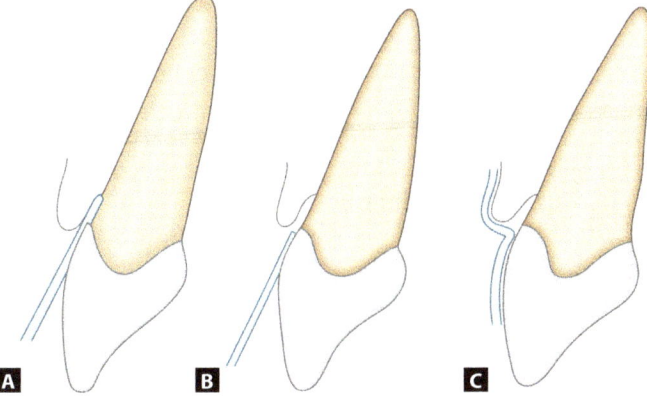

**Figs. 17.2A to C:** Schematic representation showing a collection of gingival crevicular fluid (GCF) through a filter strip. (A) Intracrevicular; (B and C) Extracrevicular.

### Methods of Collection
Important methods of collection of GCF are as follows:
- *Absorbing filter paper strips*[7] **(Figs. 17.2A to C)**:
  - *Intracrevicular*: This is the most frequently used method in which the strip is inserted into the gingival crevice.[8] It is further subdivided as to whether the strip is inserted just at the crevice's entrance or is inserted to the base of the pocket until resistance is encountered.
  - *Extracrevicular*: In order to avoid trauma, the strips are overlaid on the gingival crevice region to collect GCF.[9]
  
  The advantages of this method are:
    - It is quick and easy to use.
    - It can be applied to individual sites.
    - It is the least traumatic when used correctly.
  - *Preweighed twisted threads*: Weinstein et al., used the preweighed twisted threads to collect GCF. In this method, the threads are placed around the tooth in the gingival crevice.[10] The volume of collected fluid is measured by weighing the sample thread.
  - *Micropipettes or capillary tubing*: In this method, first, the ideal site is selected and dried. Capillary tubes of known internal diameter are inserted at the entrance of the gingival crevice. Under the influence of capillary action, GCF from the crevice migrates into the tube **(Fig. 17.3)**. The capillary's internal diameter is known; the volume of the collected fluid can be accurately determined by measuring the distance; the GCF has migrated. The technique provides an accurate assessment of the volume of the undiluted sample of native GCF. However, the technique involves holding the capillary tube at the gingival crevice's entrance for a prolonged period, and sometimes it is difficult to remove the complete sample from the tubing.

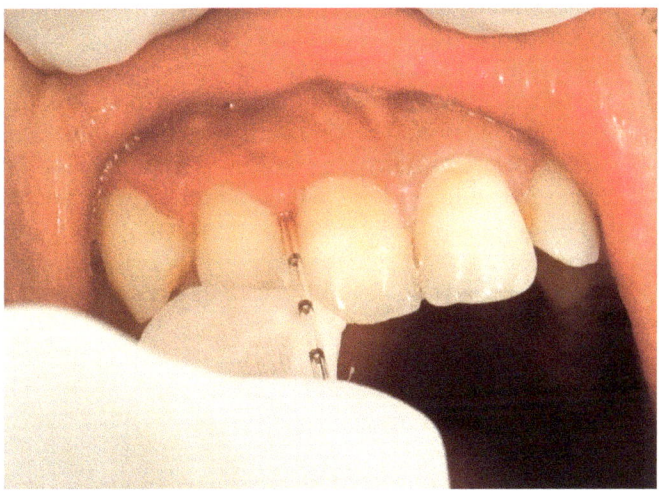

**Fig. 17.3:** Clinical picture showing gingival crevicular fluid (GCF) collection in a capillary tube.

- *Gingival washing methods*: Gingival sulcus is perfused with an isotonic solution of Hank's balanced salt of fixed volume. The method can be used in two ways. The first method involves the instillation and reaspiration of 10 µL of Hank's balanced salt solution at the interdental papilla. It is repeated 12 times to allow thorough mixing of transport solution and GCF. This is the simplest method to perform. The second method involves the construction of a customized acrylic stent used to isolate the gingival tissue from the rest of the mouth. The tissues are irrigated for 15 minutes with a saline solution, using a peristaltic pump, and the diluted GCF is removed.[11] This is a more complicated procedure.

  Limitations of this method are:[7]
  - Production of customized acrylic stents is complicated and technically demanding.
  - It has been useful only in the maxillary arch, due to the difficulties of producing a technically satisfactory appliance for the mandibular arch.
  - GCF from individual sites cannot be analyzed.

- All the fluid may not be recovered during the aspiration and reaspiration procedures.
- The precise dilution factor cannot be determined.
- Other strips, such as plastic strips or platinum loops, are placed along the tooth's long axis or inserted into the sulcus, and pressure is applied to collect the crevicular fluid.

## Measurement

The following ways measure the amount of GCF collected:
- *By direct viewing and staining*: Stain the strip with ninhydrin, especially at the area where GCF has accumulated. Staining produces a purple color. The disadvantage of this method is that it is not easily applied at the chairside.
- *By weighing*: Strip is weighed before and after collecting the GCF sample.
- *By electronic device Periotron®*: Sample strip paper (Periopaper) is inserted between the two jaws of Periotron. The wetness of the paper strip affects the flow of an electronic current and gives a digital readout on the screen. This rapidly conducted technique has no discernible effect upon the GCF sample. Three models of Periotron especially (1) the Periotron 600 (1976), (2) the Periotron 6000 (1983) and now (3) the Periotron 8000 (1995) are used to measure the volume of fluid collected on filter paper strips.[7]
- The amount of GCF is extremely less, i.e., 0.5–2.4 μL/day. The mean GCF volume in proximal spaces of anterior and molar teeth are 0.24–0.43 μL and 0.43–1.56 μL, respectively.[7,12]

Translation of Periotron values to clinical conditions and gingival index with which they are associated are explained in **Table 17.1**.[7]

Problems associated with GCF collection and data interpretation are as follows:[7]
- *Contamination*: The GCF sample is usually contaminated with blood, saliva, or plaque. Frank blood contamination is usually dealt with by discarding the sample and removing the data from analysis. Careful isolation should be performed in an effort to minimize the potential for saliva contamination.
- *Small sample size*: The amount of GCF collected is minimal.
- *Sampling time*: Prolonged sampling at the site results in protein concentrations approaching those of serum.

**TABLE 17.1:** Translation of Periotron values to clinical conditions and gingival index.

| Periotron reading | Level of gingival inflammation | Gingival index |
|---|---|---|
| 0–20 | Healthy | 0 |
| 21–40 | Mild | 1 |
| 41–80 | Moderate | 2 |
| 81–200 | Severe | 3 |

- *Volume determination*: Evaporation is a significant problem in the accurate volume determination of GCF samples.
- *Recovery of strips*: It depends on the type of paper, binding of GCF protein to the filter paper, and concentration of the original protein sample.

## Composition

The GCF constituents mainly depend on the relationship between the bacterial biofilm adherent to the tooth surfaces and the periodontal tissue cells.
- *Cellular elements*: The major cellular components of GCF are:
  - *Epithelial cells*: Desquamated epithelial cells originate from the oral, sulcular, and junctional epithelium.
  - *Leukocytes*: Neutrophils, monocytes, and lymphocytes present in GCF are derived from the gingival plexus of blood vessels **(Table 17.2)**.
  - *Bacteria*: The source of bacteria in GCF is adjacent to plaque mass.
  - *Erythrocytes*: The sources of erythrocytes are damaged small blood vessels and capillaries of gingival connective tissue.
- *Electrolytes*: Sodium, potassium, calcium, magnesium, fluoride.
- *Organic compounds*:
  - *Carbohydrates*: Hexuronic acid and glucose are the two major components in the GCF. The glucose concentration in GCF is approximately 3–4 times greater than that of serum.
  - *Proteins*: The total protein content of GCF is much <that of serum, and the major proteins present in GCF are immunoglobulins and complement components.
  - Lipids.
- *Metabolic and bacterial products*: Lactic acid, hydroxyproline, prostaglandins, urea, endotoxins, cytotoxic substances, and antibacterial factors.
- *Enzymes and enzyme inhibitors*: Acid phosphatase, alkaline phosphatase, pyrophosphatase, β-glucuronidase, lysozymes, hyaluronidase, proteolytic enzymes (mammalian proteinases, bacterial proteinases, serum proteinases inhibitors), lactic dehydrogenase, etc.

Fibroblasts or polymorphonuclear neutrophils (PMNs) are essential sources for collagenases. Bacteria can synthesize collagenases. Phospholipases are lysosomal and cytoplasmic enzymes, but microorganisms can also synthesize them. β-glucuronidase is a lysosomal enzyme, and lactic acid dehydrogenase is a cytoplasmic enzyme **(Box 17.3)**.

Methods used for the analysis of GCF components are:
- Enzyme-linked immunosorbent assay (ELISA) test to detect enzymes levels and IL-1β.[14]
- Fluorometry to detect metalloproteases.[15]

**TABLE 17.2:** Comparison of leukocyte components present between gingival crevicular fluid (GCF) and peripheral blood.[13]

| Parameters | GCF | Blood |
|---|---|---|
| Neutrophils | 95–97% | 60% |
| Monocytes | 2–3% | 5–10% |
| Lymphocytes | 1–2% | 20–30% |
| B-cells | 71% | 15–30% |
| T-cells | 29% | 50–75% |

**BOX 17.3:** Inflammatory mediators present in gingival crevicular fluid (GCF).[3]

Inflammatory mediators present in GCF at diseased sites:[18]
- Prostaglandin $E_2$
- Interleukin-1 (IL-1)
- Tumor necrosis factor
- Leukotriene $B_4$
- Thromboxane $B_2$
- T helper type 1: IL-2, interferon-γ
- T helper type 2 cytokines: IL-4, IL-6, IL-10 and IL-13
- Chemokines: IL-8
- Adhesion molecules: Selectins and soluble intercellular adhesion molecule
- Enzymes: Neutrophil elastase, neutrophil aspartate transaminase, neutrophil collagenase matrix metalloproteinase-8, and other collagenases: matrix metalloproteinase-3.

- Radioimmunoassay to detect cyclooxygenase derivatives.[16]
- High-pressure liquid chromatography (HPLC) to detect various drugs, such as timidazole.[17]
- Direct and indirect immunodots to detect acute-phase proteins.[18]

## Functions

- It cleans the sulcus and carries out shed epithelial cells, leukocytes, and microbes.
- It contains many antimicrobial agents.
- It provides neutrophils and macrophages for phagocytosing pathogenic bacteria.
- It carries immunoglobulins and immune factors to kill pathogenic microorganisms.
- The monitoring of GCF and quality of its contents is the diagnostic marker for accessing the severity of gingival inflammation, the effectiveness of oral hygiene, the response of tissues to periodontal therapy, and the effectiveness of chemotherapeutic agents.

## Clinical Significance

- *Inflammation*: GCF contributes to host defense and protects gingival tissues against inflammation. The GCF flow increases at the site of inflammation, and its composition becomes almost similar to that of inflammatory exudate. The GCF flow flushes out the bacterial colonies and their metabolites from the sulcus and prevents further penetration into the tissue. The amount of GCF at the site of inflammation is proportional to the severity of inflammation.[1]
- *Mechanical stimulation*: The production of GCF increases with toothbrushing and gingival massage.
- *Sex hormones*: Estrogen and progesterone increase the flow by increasing the permeability of gingival blood vessels. Pregnancy, ovulation, and hormonal contraceptives all increase gingival fluid production.
- *Periodontal therapy*: GCF production is increased during the healing period after periodontal surgery.
- *Smoking*: This produces an immediate transient increase in GCF flow.[19]
- *Circadian periodicity*: There is an increase in the GCF production from 6 AM to 10 PM and decreases afterward.[20]
- *Diagnostic marker*: New diagnostic tests for the detection of periodontal diseases are mainly based on GCF markers. The site-specific nature of the sample makes GCF as an ideal diagnostic marker, e.g., the concentration of prostaglandin $E_2$ increases during active phases of periodontal destruction. In contrast, levels are low in health in GCF. This allows laboratory investigations of GCF constituents to be linked to clinical assessments at the site of sample collection.[7]

### Points to Ponder

- Organulocytes are the living PMNs in saliva.
- Factors VIII, IX, X, plasma thromboplastin antecedent (PTA), and Hageman factor are the coagulation factors present in saliva.
- The drugs that cause xerostomia are anticholinergics, antipsychotics, anti-Parkinsonian, antidepressants, antihistamines, and antihypertensives.
- The 1: 3 ratio is the normal ratio of B-lymphocytes to T- lymphocytes in GCF.
- Various drugs excreted through GCF are tetracyclines, metronidazole, clindamycin, tinidazole, and erythromycin.

## REFERENCES

1. Pöllänen MT, Salonen JI, Uitto VJ. Structure and function of the tooth-epithelial interface in health and disease. Periodontol 2000. 2003;31:12-31.
2. Delima AJ, Van Dyke TE. Origin and function of the cellular components in gingival crevice fluid. Periodontol 2000. 2003;31:55-76.
3. Scannapieco FA, Levine MJ. Saliva and dental pellicles. In: Genco RJ, Goldman HM, Cohen DW (Eds). Contemporary Periodontics, 2nd edition. St. Louis: CV Mosby; 1990. pp. 117-25.
4. Bulkacz J, Carranza FA. Defense mechanisms of the gingiva. In: Newman MG, Takei HH, Carranza FA (Eds). Carranza's Clinical Periodontology, 9th edition. Philadelphia, PA, USA: WB Saunders; 2003. pp. 254-62.
5. Iacono VJ, Boldt PR, Mackay BJ, Cho MI, Pollock JJ. Lytic sensitivity of *Actinobacillus actinomycetemcomitans* Y4 to lysozyme. Infect Immun. 1983;40(2):773-84.

6. Mandel ID. Relation of saliva and plaque to caries. J Dent Res. 1974;53(2):246-66.
7. Griffiths GS. Formation, collection and significance of gingival crevice fluid. Periodontol 2000. 2003;31:32-42.
8. Brill N, Bronnestam R. Immunoelectrophoretic study of tissue fluid from gingival pockets. Acta Odontol Scand. 1960;18:95-100.
9. Loe H, Holm-Pedersen P. Absence and presence of fluid from normal and inflamed gingivae. Periodontics. 1965;3:171-7.
10. Weinstein E, Mandel ID, Salkind A, Oshrain HI, Pappas GD. Studies of gingival fluid. Periodontics. 1967;5:161-6.
11. Cimasoni G. Crevicular fluid updated. In: Myers HM (Ed). Monographs in Oral Science (Volume 12), 2nd edition. Basel, Switzerland: S Karger; 1983.
12. Goodson JM. Gingival crevice fluid flow. Periodontol 2000. 2003;31:43-54.
13. Ebersole JL. Humoral immune responses in gingival crevice fluid: local and systemic implications. Periodontol 2000. 2003;31:135-66.
14. Wilton JM, Bampton JL, Griffiths GS, Curtis MA, Life JS, Johnson NW, et al. Interleukin-1 beta (IL-1β) levels in gingival crevicular fluid from adults with previous evidence of destructive periodontitis. A cross-sectional study. J Clin Periodontol. 1992;19(1):53-7.
15. Egelberg J. Cellular elements in gingival pocket fluid. Acta Odontol Scand. 1963;21:283-7.
16. Offenbacher S, Williams RC, Jeffcoat MK, Howell TH, Odle BM, Smith MA, et al. Effects of NSAIDs on beagle crevicular cyclooxygenase metabolites and periodontal bone loss. J Periodontal Res. 1992;27(3):207-13.
17. Liew V, Mack G, Tseng P, Cvejic M, Hayden M, Buchanan N. Single- dose concentrations of tinidazole in gingival crevicular fluid, serum, and gingival tissue in adults with periodontitis. J Dent Res. 1991;70(5):910-2.
18. Champagne C, Buchanan W, Reddy MS, Preisser JS, Beck JD, Offenbacher S. Potential for gingival crevice fluid measures as predictors of risk for periodontal diseases. Periodontol 2000. 2003;31:167-80.
19. McLaughlin WS, Lovat FM, Macgregor ID, Kelly PJ. The immediate effects of smoking on gingival fluid flow. J Clin Periodontol. 1993;20(6):448-51.
20. Bissada NF, Schaffer EM, Haus E. Circadian periodicity of human crevicular fluid flow. J Periodontol. 1967;38(1):36-40.

## VIVA VOCE

**Q1.** Which stain is used to make the wetted area of gingival crevicular fluid (GCF) filter paper strip more visible?
**Ans.** Ninhydrin stain is used to make the wetted area of the GCF filter paper strip more visible.

**Q2.** Name the drugs which are excreted through GCF.
**Ans.** Tetracycline, metronidazole, and tinidazole are drugs that are excreted through GCF.

**Q3.** What is periopaper?
**Ans.** Periopaper is a kind of blotter paper on which GCF is collected.

**Q4.** What is periotron?
**Ans.** Periotron is the electronic machine used for measuring the amount of fluid or GCF collected on filter paper.

**Q5.** Name saliva substitutes.
**Ans.** Saliva substitutes are as follows:
- Xylitol chewing gum
- *Saliva orthana (Nycomed)*: Oral spray, which contains porcine mucin. It is available as lozenge.
- Sialogogues, such as pilocarpine, cevimeline, bethanechol.

**Q6.** What are defensins?
**Ans.** Defensins are active antimicrobial substances produced by junctional epithelial cells.

**Q7.** What are organulocytes?
**Ans.** Organulocytes are the living PMNs in saliva.

**Q8.** What is the effect of smoking on GCF flow?
**Ans.** Immediate transient increase.

**Q9.** Which immunoglobulin present in saliva provides the first line of defense in the oral cavity?
**Ans.** Secretory IgA (sIgA).

**Q10.** Name microbes that get affected by lactoferrin.
**Ans.** *Actinobacillus* and *Streptococcus*.

# Chapter 18

# Gingival Inflammation

*Sanjeev K Salaria*

## Chapter Outline

- Classifications
- Stages of Gingivitis
- Clinical Features

## INTRODUCTION

Inflammation of the gingiva is called gingivitis. This inflammation is the result of the development of adherent plaque on the tooth surface. Gingivitis is usually mild and does not destroy the attachment fibers and underlying bone. However, in a susceptible individual with poor dental hygiene, it may advance to deeper portions of the periodontium leading to tissue destruction and alveolar bone resorption. Thus, untreated gingivitis can progress to serious periodontal diseases. This chapter will describe the extent, duration, distribution, stages, clinical manifestations, and sequelae of gingival diseases induced by bacterial plaque.

## CLASSIFICATIONS

- *According to duration*:[1]
  - *Acute gingivitis*: It is sudden in onset, short in duration, and usually painful in nature.
  - *Chronic gingivitis*: It is slow in onset, long in duration and is mostly painless, unless complicated by acute or subacute exacerbations. It is the most common type of gingivitis.
- *According to distribution*:[1]
  - *Localized gingivitis*: Gingivitis when confined to the gingiva of a single tooth or group of teeth **(Fig. 18.1)**.
  - *Generalized gingivitis*: Gingivitis, which involves the entire gingiva of the mouth.
  - *Marginal gingivitis*: It involves the gingival margin and may include a portion of the contiguous attached gingiva **(Fig. 18.2)**.
  - *Papillary gingivitis*: Gingivitis which mainly involves the interdental papillae and may extend

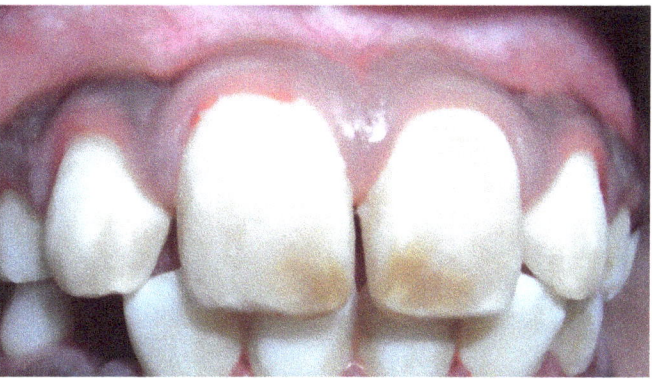

**Fig. 18.1:** Clinical picture showing localized gingivitis in left maxillary and mandibular anterior region.

**Fig. 18.2:** Clinical picture showing marginal gingivitis.

  into the adjacent portion of the gingival margin **(Fig. 18.3)**.
  - *Diffuse gingivitis*: It affects the gingival margin, interdental papillae, and attached gingiva.

Section 4: Pathology of Gingival and Periodontal Diseases

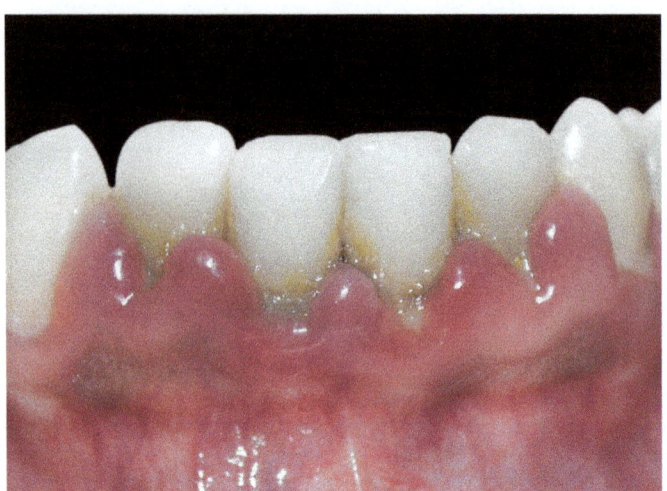

Fig. 18.3: Clinical picture showing papillary gingivitis.

## STAGES OF GINGIVITIS

Page and Schroeder categorized the periodontal inflammatory changes of periodontal diseases into four histopathological stages **(Table 18.1 and Fig. 18.4)**:[2]
1. Stage I: The initial lesion
2. Stage II: The early lesion
3. Stage III: The established lesion
4. Stage IV: An advanced lesion

**TABLE 18.1:** Stages of gingivitis.[2]

| Stages | Time | Immune cells | Clinical findings |
|---|---|---|---|
| I Initial lesion | 2–4 days | Polymorphonuclear neutrophils (PMNs) | Increase in gingival flow |
| II Early lesion | 4–7 days | Lymphocytes | Erythema, bleeding on probing |
| III Established lesion | 14–21 days | Plasma cells | Change in color, size, texture |

The initial and early lesions were considered as the histopathological changes in gingival tissues during the early stages of gingivitis. The established lesion was thought to be indicative of histopathological findings of gingival tissue in chronic gingivitis. The advanced lesion was known as the description of the histopathology of the advancement of gingivitis into periodontitis. Initially, the histopathological findings were gathered mainly from animal and human adolescent biopsies. However, currently, the interpretations based on such materials are considered as inappropriate with respect to the normal adult case.

Recently, healthy gingiva is classified into two types as per Kinane and Lindhe classification:[3]
1. Pristine or super-healthy state, which histologically has little or no inflammatory infiltrate.
2. Clinically healthy gingiva, which looks similar clinically, but histologically, has features of an inflammatory infiltrate.

During a routine clinical dental examination, only clinically healthy gingiva is visible. However, in some exceptional circumstances like in the clinical trial with professional assistance and supervised daily cleaning, one can see pristine gingiva.[4]

### Stage I: The Initial Lesion

Initial changes in the development of gingivitis occur after 2–4 days of plaque accumulation. The initial changes in gingival inflammation are characterized by vascular dilation of capillaries, arterioles, and venules of the dentogingival plexus and increased blood flow. The vascular changes enhance the permeability of the microvascular bed resulting in exudation of fluids and proteins into the tissues. As the lesion enlarges and gingival crevicular fluid flow increases,[5] noxious substances from microbes will be diluted both in the tissue and the crevice. The quantities of leukocytes, mainly polymorphonuclear neutrophils (PMNs) are increased in the junctional epithelium (JE), connective tissue, and gingival crevice. The recruitment of

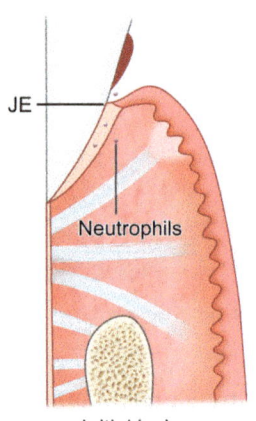
Initial lesion

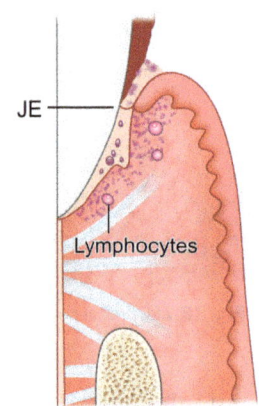
Early lesion

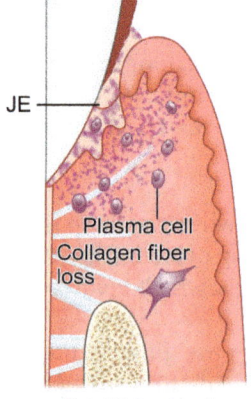
Established lesion

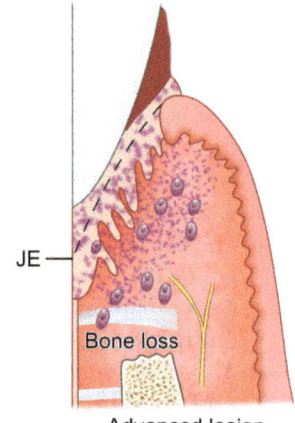
Advanced lesion (bone loss)

Fig. 18.4: Schematic representation showing stages of gingivitis.

| TABLE 18.2: Features of the initial lesion. | |
| --- | --- |
| Clinical features | ♦ This stage is called subclinical gingivitis as clinically no noticeable visible changes are seen except the presence of exudation of gingival fluid |
| Histological features | ♦ Widening of small capillaries or venules |
| | ♦ Neutrophils adherence to vessel walls (margination) and extravasations through the capillaries by migrating through the walls (diapedesis, emigration) |
| | ♦ Neutrophils quantities increase in the connective tissue, the junctional epithelium (JE) and gingival sulcus |
| | ♦ Exudation of fluid from the gingival sulcus |
| | ♦ Extravascular plasma proteins are present |

| TABLE 18.3: Features of the early lesion. | |
| --- | --- |
| Clinical features | ♦ Erythematous gingiva |
| | ♦ Bleeding on probing may also be evident |
| Histological features | ♦ The proliferation of capillaries and increased formation of capillary loops between rete pegs or ridges |
| | ♦ The predominance of lymphocytes (mainly T lymphocytes) and polymorphonuclear neutrophils (PMNs) and very few plasma cells are noted within the lesion |
| | ♦ Junctional epithelium develops widened intracellular spaces that are infiltrated mainly by neutrophils and small numbers of mononuclear cells, especially monocytes |
| | ♦ Circular and dentogingival fiber groups are mainly affected |

| TABLE 18.4: Features of established lesion. | |
| --- | --- |
| Clinical features | ♦ Moderately to severely inflamed gingiva |
| | ♦ Bluish hue on the reddened gingiva due to impaired venous return |
| Histological features[10] | ♦ The junctional epithelium (JE) develops rete pegs or ridges that protrude into the connective tissue |
| | ♦ Basal lamina destroys in some areas |
| | ♦ Preponderant inflammatory cell, i.e., plasma cells, invade JE and deep into the connective tissue around blood vessels and between bundles of collagen fibers |
| | ♦ The JE associated with widening of intercellular spaces filled with granular cellular debris. This also includes lysosomes derived from disrupted neutrophils, lymphocytes and monocytes |
| | ♦ The lysosomes contain acid hydrolases that can destroy tissue components |

leukocytes (predominantly PMNs) from the tissues to the crevice is due to the chemoattractant actions of the host systems (interleukin-8, C5a) and products derived from the biofilm (lipopolysaccharide). Thus, the increase in the migration of leukocytes and their accumulation within the gingival sulcus is correlated with an increase in gingival fluid flow into the sulcus. There is little or no proliferation of JE laterally (rete pegs).[6] Transudative and exudative fluids and plasma proteins arrive in the gingival sulcus **(Table 18.2)**.

## Stage II: The Early Lesion

The initial lesion may be transitory and may be quickly repaired after the removal of plaque. However, the clinical signs of inflammation appear within 4–7 days of plaque accumulation.[7] This is associated with capillaries proliferation and capillary loops formation between rete pegs or ridges and thus resulting in bleeding on probing. The stage is characterized by the predominance of lymphocytes (mainly T lymphocytes) and PMNs with very few plasma cells within the lesion. Around the cellular infiltrate, approximately 70% of the collagen is destroyed. Circular and dentogingival fiber assemblies are the fiber groups mainly affected. The JE develops widened intracellular spaces that are primarily infiltrated by neutrophils and small numbers of mononuclear cells, especially monocytes **(Table 18.3)**.

## Stage III: The Established Lesion

Engorged and congested blood vessels are responsible for the bluish hue of the gingiva.[8] Blood flow becomes sluggish due to the impairment of venous return. Extravasation of red blood cells into the connective tissue and breakdown of hemoglobin into its component pigments can also deepen the color of the chronically inflamed gingiva. This is associated with fluid exudation and leukocyte migration into the tissues and the gingival crevice. This lesion is dominated by plasma cells.[9] With the expansion in inflammatory cell infiltrate, collagen loss continues in both lateral and apical directions. This results in collagen depleted spaces extending deeper into the tissues available for further leukocytic infiltration. Continuous proliferation of the dentogingival epithelium along with the extension of rete pegs deeper into the connective tissue helps to maintain epithelial integrity and creates a barrier to microbial invasion. The JE is no longer closely attached to the tooth surface. There is no evidence of alveolar bone loss at this stage or of the apical migration of JE. Gingivitis develops within 2–4 weeks after the beginning of plaque accumulation.[7] Migrating leukocytes are found in the JE, within widened intercellular spaces **(Table 18.4)**.

## Stage IV: Advanced Lesion

This final stage of gingivitis is characterized by lateral and apical extension of inflammatory cell infiltrate into the connective tissue. The advanced lesion has all the features of the established lesion. However, advanced lesion differs as it is present with alveolar bone loss, extensive fiber damage,

## Section 4: Pathology of Gingival and Periodontal Diseases

**TABLE 18.5:** Features of the advanced lesion.

| | |
|---|---|
| Clinical features | • Formation of the periodontal pocket |
| | • Mobility |
| | • Suppuration |
| | • Eventually exfoliation |
| Histological features | • Neutrophils continue to dominate the junctional epithelium (JE) and gingival crevice |
| | • Infiltration of the inflammatory cell infiltrates laterally and further apically into the connective tissue |
| | • Plasma cells continue to dominate the connective tissue |
| | • Apical migration of JE from the cementoenamel junction (CEJ) |
| | • Extensive collagen fiber damage |
| | • Alveolar bone loss |

and JE's apical migration from the cementoenamel junction (CEJ). Plasma cells are found as the predominant cell type in the advanced lesion **(Table 18.5)**.[4]

## CLINICAL FEATURES

### Gingival Bleeding

Gingival bleeding is one of the earliest symptoms of gingival inflammation.[11] Duration, severity, and the ways of production of gingival bleeding differ from person-to-person.

### Pathogenesis of Gingival Bleeding

It is mainly due to the dilation and engorgement of capillaries. Degradation of intercellular cementing substances and the widening of intercellular spaces leads to an increase in the permeability of the sulcular epithelium. As the inflammation becomes chronic, ulceration of sulcular epithelium takes place. Because the capillaries are engorged and closer to the surface and epithelium being ulcerated and less protective, stimuli that are ordinally innocuous cause rupture of capillaries and gingival bleeding.[12]

### Etiological Factors of Gingival Bleeding

Factors responsible for gingival bleeding are:[12]
- *Local factors*:
  - *Acute bleeding*: It is the result of aggressive toothbrushing, sharp pieces of hard food, and gingival burns from chemicals or hot food. Spontaneous bleeding on slight provocation occurs in necrotizing ulcerative gingivitis (NUG).
  - *Chronic bleeding*: Chronic gingival inflammation.
- *Systemic factors*:
  - *Vascular abnormality*: Vitamin C deficiency and allergy-like Henoch–Schönlein purpura.
  - *Vitamin K deficiency*
  - *Platelet disorder*: Idiopathic thrombocytopenic purpura.
  - *Deficient platelet thromboplastic factors*: Uremia, multiple myeloma, and postrubella purpura.
  - *Coagulation defects*: Hemophilia, Christmas disease
  - *Malignancy*: Leukemia.
  - *Drugs*: Salicylates and anticoagulants (dicoumarol, heparin).

### Significance of Gingival Bleeding

Clinically, gingival bleeding can be easily noticed on probing. Hence, it is very significant for the early diagnosis and prevention of advanced gingivitis. It is a more objective sign and therefore requires less subjective estimation by the examiner.[12] It appears earlier than other visual signs of inflammation. Thus, several gingival indices have been developed based on this earliest sign. Gingival bleeding on probing helps to determine whether the lesion is an active or inactive.[13]

### Changes in Gingival Color

Normally, the gingiva is coral pink in color due to the vascular supply and modified by overlying the keratinized layer. With an increase in vascularization and reduction of keratinization, the gingiva turns into red. Gingival color changes depend mainly on the intensity of the inflammation.

Factors responsible for the change in gingival color are:
- *Color changes associated with local factors*:
  - *Acute gingivitis*:
    - *Necrotizing ulcerative gingivitis*: Marginal bright red erythema. In acute inflammation at its severe stage, the red color of gingival slowly turns into a dull, whitish-gray **(Fig. 18.5)**. The gray discoloration in NUG is due to tissue necrosis and is highlighted from the adjacent gingiva by sharply defined erythematous zone.
    - *Herpetic gingivostomatitis*: Diffuse.
    - *Chemical irritations*: Patch like/diffuse.
  - *Chronic gingivitis*: Chronic inflammation intensifies the red or bluish red color because of vascular proliferation and keratinization reduction due to epithelial compression by the inflamed tissue.
  - *Metallic pigmentation*: Systemically absorbed metals are responsible for gingival pigmentation. Perivascular precipitation of metallic sulfides in the subepithelial connective tissue gives rise to metallic pigmentation. Gingival pigmentation never indicates systemic toxicity. It is restricted in areas of inflammation only due to escape of the metal into the surrounding tissue associated with increased permeability of irritated blood vessels.[12]
    - *Bismuth pigmentation*: Black line.
    - *Arsenic pigmentation*: Black line.

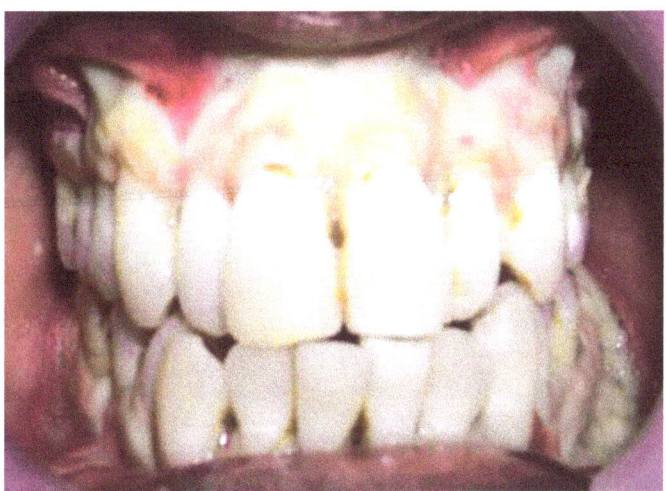

Fig. 18.5: Clinical picture showing necrotizing ulcerative gingivitis (NUG). (*Courtesy*: Dr. Ambika Gupta)

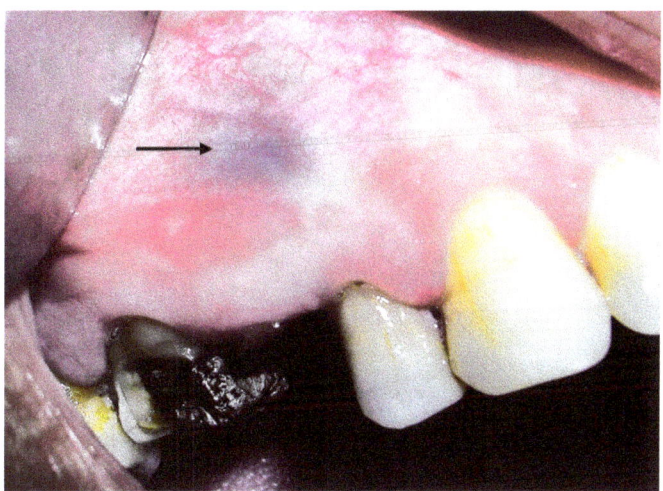

Fig. 18.6: Clinical picture showing amalgam tattoo. (*Courtesy*: Dr. Ambika Gupta)

- ♦ *Mercury pigmentation*: Black line.
- ♦ *Lead pigmentation*: Bluish red, deep blue, or gray (Burtonian line).
- ♦ *Silver pigmentation*: Violet marginal line.
- Color changes associated with systemic factors:
  - Endogenous factors:
    - ♦ *Addison's disease*: Increased melanin pigmentation
    - ♦ *Peutz-Jeghers syndrome*: Increased melanin pigmentation
    - ♦ *Albright's syndrome*: Increased melanin pigmentation
    - ♦ *Jaundice*: Yellowish color due to deposition of bilirubin
    - ♦ *Hemochromatosis*: Bluish gray due to deposition of iron
    - ♦ Diabetes
    - ♦ Pregnancy
    - ♦ Blood dyscrasias
    - ♦ Hyperthyroidism
    - ♦ *Drugs*: Chloroquine (slate grey), minocycline (brown), chlorpromazine, zidovudine, ketoconazole, methyldopa, and busulfan.
  - Exogenous factors:
    - ♦ *Tobacco/smoking*: Grayish color due to increased melanin pigmentation[14]
    - ♦ *Amalgam*: Localized bluish-black areas[15] (**Fig. 18.6**)
    - ♦ Coloring agents in food, lozenges and betel.

## Changes in Gingival Contour

Normally, the contour of marginal gingiva is scalloped and knife-edged. The interdental papilla is pointed and pyramidal in the anterior region, whereas in the posterior region, it is a tent-shaped, filling the area.

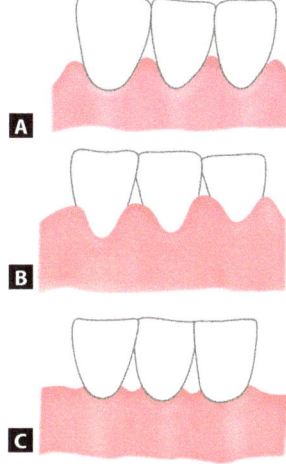

Figs. 18.7A to C: Schematic representation showing altered gingival contour. (A) Blunt papilla; (B) Bulbous papilla; (C) Cratered papilla.

Conditions in which gingival contour is altered are as follows:
- *Blunt/rolled*: Marginal gingiva may be rounded or rolled or blunt in case of acute and chronic gingivitis (**Fig. 18.7A**).
- *Bulbous papilla*: In gingival enlargement (**Fig. 18.7B**).
- *Cratered papilla*: In NUG (**Fig. 18.7C**).
- *Stillman's clefts*: These are apostrophe-shaped indentations, which extend from and into gingival margin along the root surface, most frequently on the labial or buccal surfaces. The margins of the cleft are rolled underneath the linear gap in the gingiva, and the remainder of the gingival margin is blunt instead of knife-edge (**Fig. 18.8**). It was initially described by Stillman, as a result of occlusal trauma. It may be simple-cleavage in a single direction or compound-cleavage in more than one direction.[16]

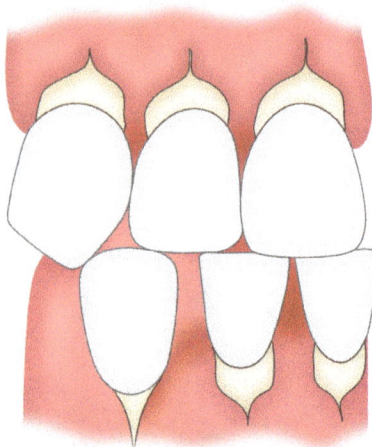

**Fig. 18.8:** Schematic representation showing Stillman's clefts.

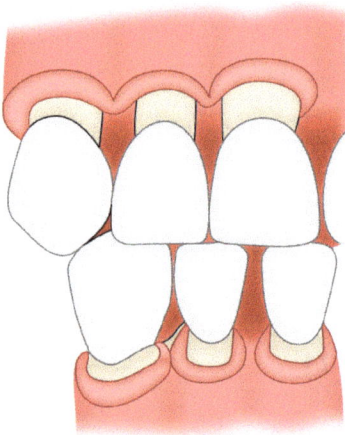

**Fig. 18.9:** Schematic representation showing McCall's festoons in relation to canine and premolars.

- *McCall's festoons*: These are enlargement of the marginal gingiva with the formation of "lifesaver" like gingival prominence in relation to canine and premolar facial surfaces mostly **(Figs. 18.9 and 18.10)**. These are semilunar enlargements named after John Opple McCall, who, along with Paul R Stillman, believed occlusal traumatism to be an etiologic factor.

## Changes in Gingival Consistency

In acute gingivitis, there is puffiness and softening of the gingiva. In chronic gingivitis, there is soggy puffiness that pits on pressure or firm, leathery consistency. In chronic gingivitis, the consistency of gingiva depends on the relative predominance of destructive or reparative changes. If destructive changes predominate, then consistency is edematous, and if reparative changes predominate, then it is fibrotic. The gingival lump is seen in the following conditions:
- Erupting 3rd molars
- Pregnancy gingivitis

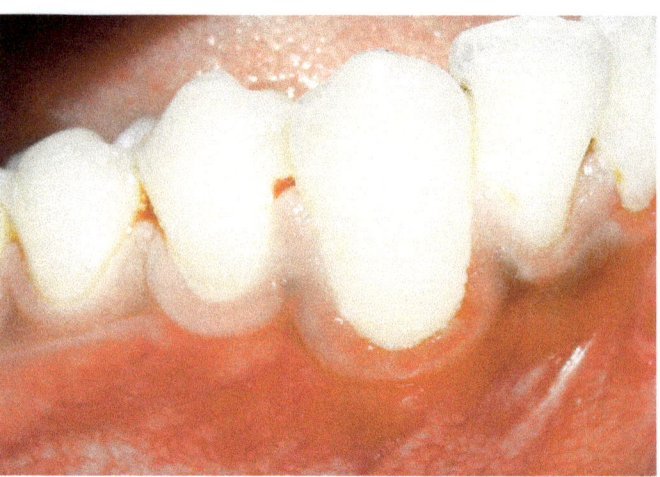

**Fig. 18.10:** Clinical picture showing McCall's festoons.

- Fibroepithelial polyp and malignant conditions (Kaposi's sarcoma, carcinoma, lymphoma).

## Changes in the Surface Texture of Gingiva

Normally, the surface texture of free gingiva is smooth, whereas of interdental and attached gingiva is stippled.

Following are the changes in the surface texture of gingiva in various gingival diseases and conditions:[12]
- Smooth, shiny surface due to loss of stippling, is seen in early gingivitis **(Fig. 18.11)** and chronic gingivitis when the dominant changes are exudative.
- Firm and nodular surface in chronic gingivitis is seen when the dominant changes are fibrotic.
- Smooth surface due to epithelial atrophy is seen in atrophic gingivitis.
- Smooth surface due to excoriation of the surface in chronic desquamative gingivitis.
- The leathery texture is seen in hyperkeratosis.
- The nodular surface is seen in drug-induced gingival overgrowth **(Fig. 18.12)**.

## Changes in the Position of the Gingiva

In a fully erupted tooth, the gingival margin position is 1–2 mm above CEJ at or slightly below the enamel contour. The junctional epithelium is at the CEJ. The actual position corresponds to the level of the epithelial attachment on the tooth, while the apparent position is the level of the crest of the gingival margin, which is seen by direct observation. The actual position is not directly visible but can be determined by probing.
- *Enlargement*: When the gingiva enlarges, the gingival margin may be high on the enamel, partly or nearly covering the anatomic crown **(Fig. 18.13)**.
- *Recession*: Apical shift in the marginal gingiva position gives full exposure of the root surface **(Fig. 18.14)**. The severity of the gingival recession depends on the gingiva's actual position and not on its apparent position.

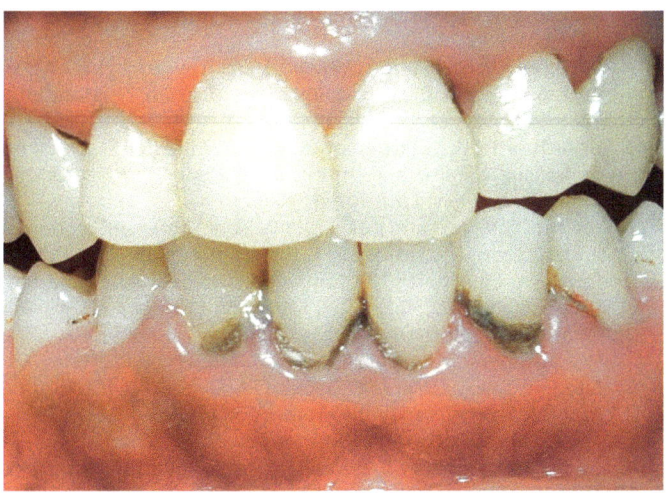

**Fig. 18.11:** Clinical picture showing loss of stippling (smooth, shiny gingival surface).

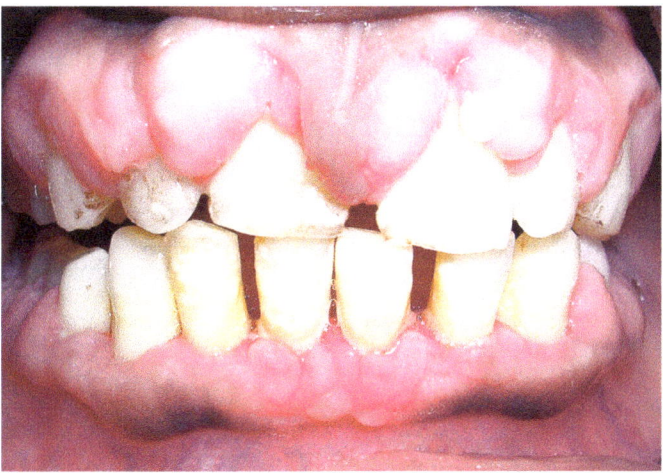

**Fig. 18.12:** Clinical picture showing the nodular surface in drug-induced gingival enlargement.

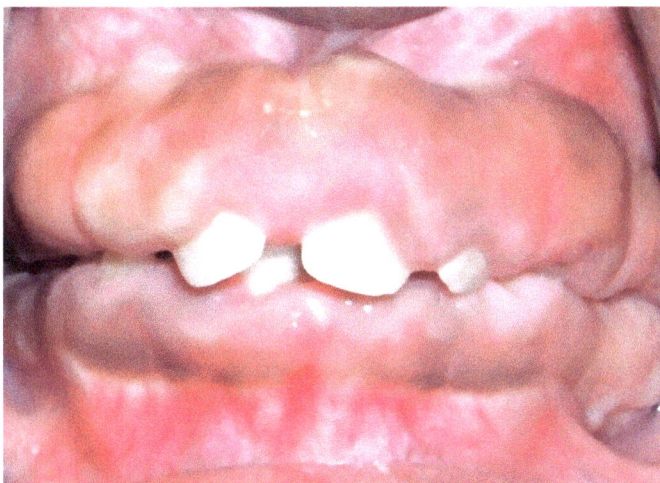

**Fig. 18.13:** Clinical picture showing idiopathic hyperplastic gingival enlargement.

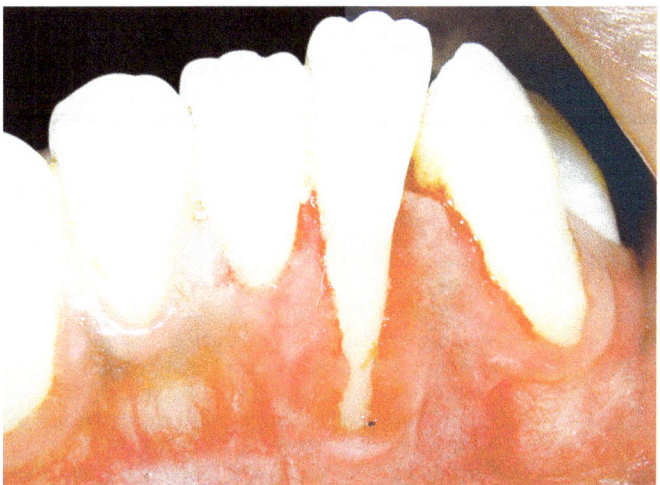

**Fig. 18.14:** Clinical picture showing localized recession around malposed incisor and canine.

There are two types of gingival recession. The first is visible and clinically observable, and the second is hidden, which is covered by gingiva and measured only by inserting a probe to the level of the epithelial attachment. Recession may affect one tooth or a group of teeth and stay localized, or it may spread throughout the mouth and become generalized.[12]

The characteristics of plaque-induced gingivitis are as follows:[17]

- Plaque present in relation to the gingival margin
- The disease originates at the gingival margin
- Bleeding upon provocation
- Change in gingival color
- Change in gingival contour
- Change in sulcular temperature
- Increased gingival exudates
- Absence of clinical attachment and bone loss
- Histological changes including an inflammatory lesion
- Reversible with plaque removal

### Points to Ponder

- ❏ Gingival conditions/diseases that mainly involve interdental papilla and gingival margin are gingival abscesses, NUG, linear gingival erythema, and drug-induced gingival enlargement.
- ❏ Gingival ulcers are usually seen in NUG, herpes simplex virus stomatitis, aphthae, self-injury, malignant neoplasms, drugs, dermatoses, systemic diseases (hematological disorders, tuberculosis, syphilis, herpes virus, human immunodeficiency virus).
- ❏ Gingival changes seen in mouth-breathers are erythema, edema, enlargement, diffuse smooth and shiny surface in the exposed gingival area affecting the mainly maxillary anterior region.
- ❏ Gingival red lesions are usually seen in erythroplasia, desquamative gingivitis, hemangiomas, orofacial granulomatosis, Crohn's disease, Wegener's granulomatosis, sarcoidosis, and Kaposi's sarcoma.

## REFERENCES

1. Carranza FA, Rapley JW. Clinical features of gingivitis. In: Newman MG, Takei HH, Carranza FA (Eds). Carranza's Clinical Periodontology, 9th edition. Philadelphia, PA, USA: WB Saunders; 2003. pp. 269-78.
2. Page RC, Schroeder HE. Pathogenic mechanisms. In: Schluger S, Youdelis R, Page RC, Johnson RH (Eds). Periodontal Diseases: Basic Phenomena, Clinical Management, Occlusal, and Restorative Interrelationships, 2nd sub-edition. Philadelphia, PA, USA: Lea & Febiger; 1989.
3. Kinane DF, Berglundh T, Lindhe J. Host-parasite interactions in periodontal disease. In: Lindhe J, Karring T, Lang NP (Eds). Clinical Periodontology and Implant Dentistry, 4th edition. Chicago, USA: Blackwell Munksgaard; 2003. pp. 151-78.
4. Kinane DF. Causation and pathogenesis of the periodontal disease. Periodontol 2000. 2001;25:8-20.
5. Attström R, Egelberg J. Emigration of blood neutrophils and monocytes into the gingival crevices. J Periodontal Res. 1970;5(1):48-55.
6. Grant DA, Stern IB, Listgarten MA. Gingivitis. In: Periodontics, 6th edition. St. Louis: CV Mosby; 1988. pp. 315-47.
7. Payne WA, Page RC, Ogilvie AL, Hall WB. Histopathologic features of the initial and early stages of experimental gingivitis in man. J Periodontal Res. 1975;10(2):51-64.
8. Hanioka T, Shizukuishi S, Tsunemitsu A. Changes in haemoglobin concentration and oxygen saturation in human gingiva with decreasing inflammation. J Periodontol. 1991;62(6):366-9.
9. Seymour GJ, Powell RN, Aitken JF. Experimental gingivitis in humans. A clinical and histologic investigation. J Periodontol. 1983;54(9):522-8.
10. Freedman HL, Listgarten MA, Taichman NS. Electron microscopic features of chronically inflamed human gingiva. J Periodontal Res. 1968;3(4):313-27.
11. Meitner SW, Zander H, Iker HP, Polson AM. Identification of inflamed gingival surfaces. J Clin Periodontol. 1979;6(2):93-7.
12. Carranza FA, Rapley JW, Haake SK. Gingival inflammation. In: Newman MG, Takei HH, Carranza FA (Eds). Carranza's Clinical Periodontology, 9th edition. Philadelphia, PA, USA: WB Saunders; 2003. pp. 263-8.
13. Lang NP, Joss A, Orsanic T, Gusberti FA, Siegrist BE. Bleeding on probing. A predictor for the progression of periodontal disease. J Clin Periodontol. 1986;13(6): 590-6.
14. Buchner A, Hansen LA. Amalgam pigmentation (amalgam tattoo) of the oral mucosa. A clinicopathologic study of 268 cases. Oral Surg Oral Med Oral Pathol. 1980;49(2):139-47.
15. Neville BW, Damm DD, Allen CM, Chi AC. Oral and Maxillofacial Pathology, 4th edition. Philadelphia, PA, USA: Elsevier-Saunders; 2016.
16. Stillman PR. Early clinical evidence of disease in the gingiva and pericementum. J Dent Res. 1921;3:25-31.
17. Mariotti A. Dental plaque-induced gingival diseases. Ann Periodontol. 1999;4(1):7-19.

## VIVA VOCE

**Q1.** In which stage of gingivitis plasma cells predominate?
**Ans.** Plasma cells predominate in "Stage III: The Established Stage" of gingivitis.

**Q2.** Name various conditions in which there is a change in the surface texture of gingiva.
**Ans.** The surface texture of gingiva changes under the following conditions:
- *Smooth surface texture (loss of stippling)*: Chronic gingivitis, atrophic gingivitis, chronic desquamative gingivitis
- *Leathery texture*: Hyperkeratosis
- *Nodular surface*: Drug-induced gingival overgrowth

**Q3.** Name conditions in which gingival contour is changed.
**Ans.** Gingival contour is changed under the following conditions:
- Acute and chronic gingivitis
- NUG
- Stillman's clefts and
- McCall's festoons

**Q4.** What is pristine gingiva?
**Ans.** Histologically perfect gingiva is called pristine gingiva.

**Q5.** What is "eruption gingivitis"?
**Ans.** Gingivitis associated with tooth eruption is called "eruption gingivitis."

**Q6.** Which metals cause intoxication?
**Ans.** Bismuth, lead, mercury, phosphorous, arsenic, and chromium.

**Q7.** How are Stillman's clefts classified?
**Ans.** Simple cleft: Occurs in a single direction—most common type
Compound cleft: Occurs in more than one direction.

**Q8.** In which stage of gingivitis polymorphonuclear neutrophils (PMNs) predominate?
**Ans.** Stage I: Initial lesion of gingivitis.

**Q9.** In which stage of gingivitis bleeding on probing is usually found?
**Ans.** Stage II: Early lesion of gingivitis.

**Q10.** Which fiber groups are mainly affected in Stage II early lesion of gingivitis?
**Ans.** Circular and dentogingival fiber groups.

# Chapter 19: Gingival Enlargement

*Md. Jalaluddin, Shalu Bathla*

## Chapter Outline

- Classifications
- Scoring
- Inflammatory Enlargement
- Drug-induced Enlargement
- Enlargement Associated with Systemic Diseases
- Neoplastic Enlargement
- False Enlargement

## INTRODUCTION

Gingival enlargement may be viewed as a spectrum extending from idiopathic gingival hyperplasia (fibromatosis), in which inflammatory elements are absent, to phenytoin hyperplasia, where inflammatory elements may be present, to hyperplastic inflammation, seen in mouth-breathers, to hormonally conditioned gingivitis in pregnancy.

## CLASSIFICATIONS

Gingival enlargement can be classified as:[1]
- *According to the etiologic factors and pathologic factors*:
    - Inflammatory enlargement:
        - Acute
        - Chronic
    - Drug-induced gingival enlargement
    - Idiopathic gingival fibromatosis
    - Enlargements associated with the systemic disease:
        - Conditioned enlargement:
            - Puberty
            - Pregnancy
            - Plasma cell gingivitis
            - Vitamin C deficiency
            - Nonspecific conditioned enlargement
        - Systemic diseases causing gingival enlargement:
            - Leukemia
            - Granulomatous diseases (Wegener's granulomatosis, sarcoidosis, and so on)
    - Neoplastic enlargement:
        - Benign neoplasm
        - Malignant neoplasm
    - False enlargement
- *According to location and distribution*:[1]
    - *Localized*: When the enlargement is limited to the gingiva adjacent to a single tooth or a group of teeth.
    - *Generalized*: Enlargement involving the gingiva throughout the mouth.
    - *Marginal*: Confined to the marginal gingiva.
    - *Papillary*: Confined to the interdental papilla.
    - *Diffuse*: Enlargement involving all the parts of the gingiva, i.e., marginal, interdental papilla, and attached.
    - *Discrete*: An isolated sessile or pedunculated enlargement.

## SCORING

Gingival enlargement can be scored in the following grades:[2]
- *Grade 0*: No signs of gingival enlargement.
- *Grade I*: Enlargement confined to interdental papilla only.
- *Grade II*: Enlargement that involves both papilla and marginal gingiva.
- *Grade III*: Enlargement that covers three quarters or more of the crown.

## INFLAMMATORY ENLARGEMENT

### Acute Inflammatory Enlargement

#### Gingival Abscess

A gingival abscess is a localized collection of pus involving marginal gingiva or interdental papilla. It is sudden in onset and painful condition due to associated inflammation.

An abscess develops due to penetration of bacteria into deep gingival tissues associated with aggressive injury to gingiva with a foreign substance, such as a toothbrush bristle, a piece of an apple core, or a lobster shell fragment. In initial stages, abscess develops as a red swelling with a smooth and shiny surface. Within 24–48 hours, the lesion usually becomes fluctuant and pointed with a surface orifice, which gives way to the purulent exudate.

### Histopathologic Features

In connective tissue, purulent foci are surrounded by diffuse infiltration of polymorphonuclear neutrophils (PMNs) and vascular engorgement. Intra- and extracellular edemas are present in the epithelium. Sometimes epithelium is ulcerated and invaded by leukocytes.

## Chronic Inflammatory Enlargement

Prolonged exposure to dental plaque associated with poor oral hygiene is the leading cause of chronic inflammatory enlargement of the gingiva.[3] Anatomic abnormalities, irritation by improper restorative and orthodontic appliances also contribute to this condition to some extent.

### Clinical Features

- It is presented in the form of slight ballooning of the interdental papilla and/or the marginal gingiva to the bulge covering most of the crown **(Figs. 19.1 and 19.2)**.
- Usually, it is painless in nature and progresses slowly over the period of time.
- The enlargement may be localized or generalized.
- It may occur as a discrete sessile or pedunculated mass on the interproximal or marginal or attached gingiva.

### Histopathological Features

There is a preponderance of inflammatory cells and fluid with vascular engorgement. There is an abundance of fibroblasts, collagen fibers, and new capillaries in the connective tissue.

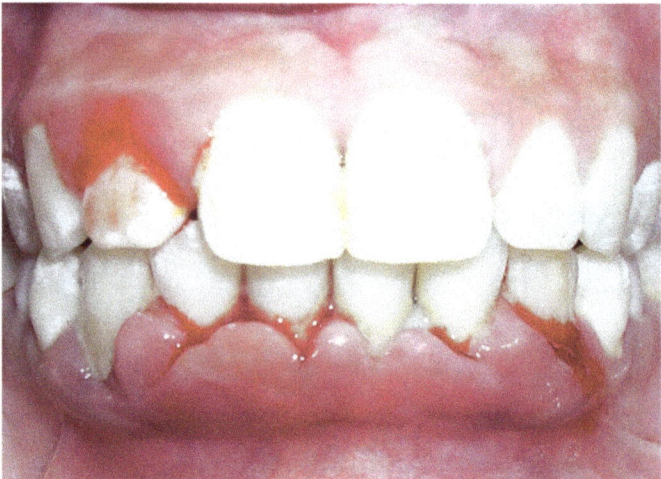

**Fig. 19.1:** Clinical picture showing chronic inflammatory gingival enlargement.

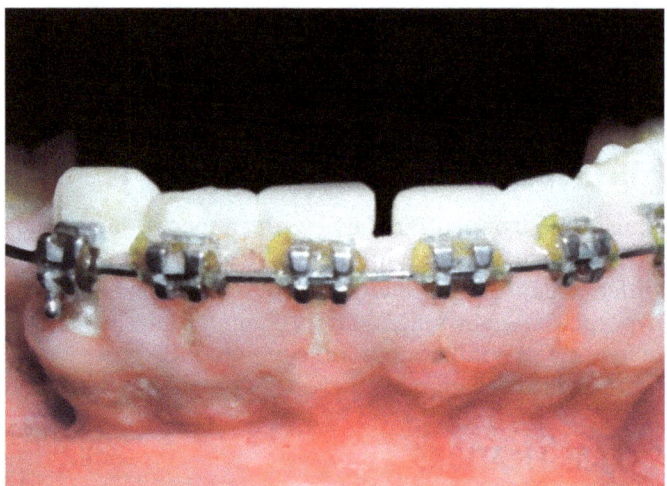

**Fig. 19.2:** Clinical picture showing chronic gingival enlargement around the orthodontic appliance.

## DRUG-INDUCED ENLARGEMENT

Medication-induced gingival enlargement occurs in prolong therapy with anticonvulsants, immunosuppressants, and antihypertensives. Anticonvulsant drugs associated with gingival enlargement are phenytoin, phenobarbital, carbamazepine, sodium valproate, primidone, and felbamate. Antihypertensive drugs associated with gingival enlargement are nifedipine, amlodipine, nimodipine, nicardipine, nitrendipine, diltiazem, felodipine and bepridil.

### Clinical Features

- In the early stages, the growth is firm and nontender. A bead-like enlargement of the interdental papilla get extends towards the facial and lingual gingival margins **(Fig. 19.3)**.
- Marginal and papillary enlargements sometimes completely cover the teeth' crowns and interfere with tooth eruption and alignment.
- The lesion is mulberry shaped, firm in consistency, pale pink in color, and resilient with no tendency to bleed when uncomplicated by inflammation **(Fig. 19.4)**.
- Common and severe in maxillary and mandibular anterior regions.
- Gingival enlargement is usually chronic in nature and slowly increases in size **(Box 19.1)**.[4-6]

### Pathogenesis

Pathogenesis of drug-induced gingival enlargement has a multifactorial etiology:[4]

## Chapter 19: Gingival Enlargement

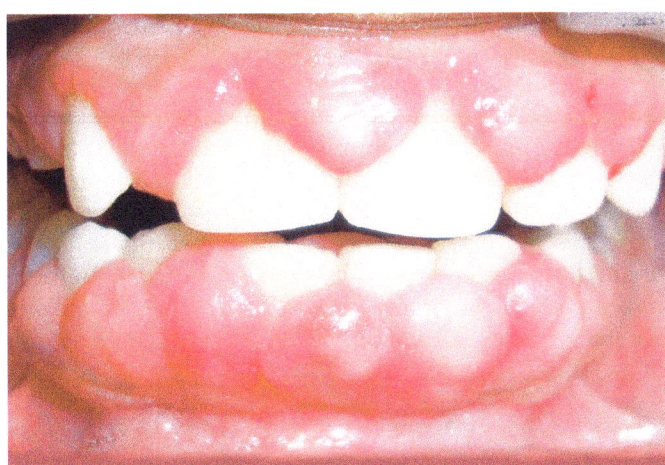

**Fig. 19.3:** Clinical picture showing phenytoin-induced gingival enlargement.

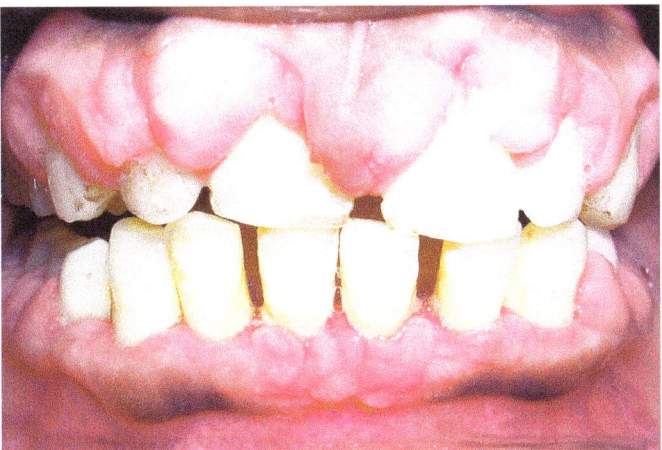

**Fig. 19.4:** Clinical picture showing cyclosporine-induced gingival enlargement.

**BOX 19.1:** Occurrence of gingival overgrowth.

Gingival overgrowth occurs in:
- About 50% of patients taking phenytoin[4]
- About 30% of patients taking cyclosporine[5]
- About 20% of patients taking nifedipine[6]

## Role of Fibroblasts

These medications are known to modify fibroblast function, either directly or indirectly, by altering cytokine/matrix metalloproteinase (MMP) activity within the tissue. Analogs of phenytoin that stimulate proliferation of fibroblast-like cells are 1-allyl-5-phenylhydantoinate and 5-methyl-5-phenylhydantoin.[7] Fibroblasts from phenytoin-induced gingival overgrowth show increased synthesis of sulfated glycosaminoglycans. Phenytoin may induce a decrease in collagen degradation due to the production of an inactive fibroblast collagenase. Phenytoin-activated fibroblasts produce large amounts of interleukins (ILs), such as IL-6, IL-1, and IL-8.

## Role of Noncollagenous Matrix

Patients on prolonged phenytoin therapy have significantly higher volume density of noncollagenous matrix with raised levels of hexosamine and uronic acid[8] compared to collagenous matrix.[9]

## Role of Inflammatory Cytokines

Phenytoin-activated fibroblasts produce large amounts of interleukins, such as IL-6, IL-1, and IL-8. Such mediators activate T cells' proliferation and the recruitment of neutrophils to the involved tissues, establishing a direct interaction between the immune system and the connective tissue. This interaction seems to be highly associated with fibrotic diseases.

## Role of Growth Factors

Epithelial-mesenchymal transition (EMT) is a biological process in which polarized epithelial cells transdifferentiate into fibroblast-like cells with various biochemical changes. Transforming growth factor-$\beta 1$ (TGF-$\beta 1$) is the prime inducer of EMT in multiple tissues. Connective tissue growth factor (CTGF) expression is increased in cells undergoing EMT.[10]

## Role of Matrix Metalloproteinase Synthesis and Function

Phenytoin inhibits the $Ca^{2+}$ influx, decreasing folic acid uptake and, subsequently, the production of active collagenase.[11] Human gingival fibroblasts managed with specific cyclosporine-A (CsA) significantly reduce MMP-1 and MMP-3 secretion levels and contribute to the accumulation of extracellular matrix components.[12]

## Role of Genetics

Phenytoin-induced gingival overgrowth is reported only in some susceptible individuals. This highlights that other factors, including genetic factors, may have a substantial role in the pathogenesis of phenytoin-induced gingival overgrowth. A genetic propensity greatly affects the other etiological factors in the drug-plaque-induced inflammation.

Phenytoin and its major metabolite 5-(p-hydroxyphenyl)-5-phenylhydantoin (pHPPH),[13] cyclosporine, and its major metabolite OL-17[14] react with a phenotypically distinct subpopulation of gingival fibroblast and cause an increase in protein synthesis and cell proliferation rate.

## Age

Phenytoin and cyclosporine drug-induced gingival overgrowth is more common in children and adolescents compared to adult counterparts.[15] Gingival fibroblasts are capable of metabolizing testosterone into active metabolite 5$\alpha$-dihydrotestosterone. Phenytoin enhances this rate of metabolite formation.[16] Drug-induced increase in gingival fibroblast androgen metabolism is identified as the main culprit in the pathogenesis of drug-induced gingival overgrowth. These active androgen metabolites usually attack the subpopulations of gingival fibroblasts. This favors either enhancement in collagen synthesis or reduction in collagenase activity leading to unwanted gingival outcomes in children and adolescents.

## Histological Features

There is acanthosis of epithelium and elongation of rete pegs. In connective tissue, there are foci of chronic inflammatory cells, particularly plasma cells, and a large number of fibroblasts and new blood vessels.

### Treatment

Where overgrowth is already present, the following measures may be taken:
- *Drug substitution*: Substitution of drugs or the reduction of dosage of phenytoin should be considered by the physician.
- *Oral hygiene*: Rigid oral hygiene practices are instituted.
- With good oral hygiene, the extent of overgrowth can be minimized or avoided.
- *Antibiotic*: Azithromycin decreases the severity of cyclosporine-induced gingival enlargement.[17]
- *Supplementation*: Folic acid supplementation significantly reduces the incidence of gingival overgrowth.[18]
- *Surgery*: Hyperplastic tissues are most often removed surgically by gingivectomy or undisplaced flap.

## Idiopathic Gingival Fibromatosis

Idiopathic gingival fibromatosis is a rare hereditary condition characterized by hereditary gingival hyperplasia, congenital familial fibromatosis, and elephantiasis.[19] The condition is usually idiopathic and inherited as either autosomal-recessive or autosomal-dominant form. The incidence is reported as 1: 350,000. It may exist as an isolated disease entity or as a part of a syndrome. The familial variation may occur with several inherited syndromes, e.g., Zimmerman Laband syndrome, Murray–Puretic–Drescher (juvenile hyaline fibromatosis), Rutherford syndrome, Cross syndrome, Cowden syndrome, multiple hamartomas, and tuberous sclerosis. It is commonly reported in tuberous sclerosis, a condition characterized by the triad of epilepsy, mental retardation, and cutaneous angiofibromas.

Autosomal-dominant forms of gingival fibromatosis are usually nonsyndromic, have been genetically linked to the chromosome 2p21-p22 and 5q13-q22.[20]

Mutation in the *son of sevenless-1 (SOS-1)* gene is also reported as one of the cause for isolated (nonsyndromic) gingival fibromatosis.[21]

### Clinical Features

The condition involves an overgrowth of the gingival margin, interdental papilla, and attached gingiva of the facial and lingual surfaces of the mandible and maxilla. The gingival overgrowth is usually in the form of a large mass of firm, dense, resilient, insensitive fibrous tissue expanding over the alveolar ridges and the teeth. Color is generally normal but turns erythematous on inflammation. It commonly presents at the time of permanent dentition eruption but can develop with the eruption of primary dentition. If the enlargement is present before tooth eruption, dense fibrous tissue may interfere with or prevent the eruption. Bulbous enlargement of the gingiva leads to distortion of the jaw, and the patient complains of functional and esthetic problems **(Figs. 19.5 and 19.6)**.

### Histological Features

There is moderate hyperplasia of a slightly hyperkeratotic epithelium with acanthosis and elongated rete pegs. There is a bulbous increase in the amount of connective tissue due to a dense collagen bundle that is relatively avascular.

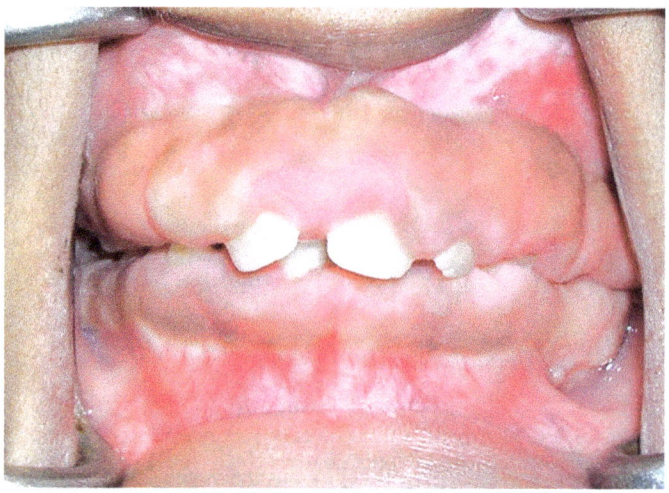

**Fig. 19.5:** Clinical picture showing idiopathic gingival fibromatosis: advanced gingival enlargement covering most of the crown portion.

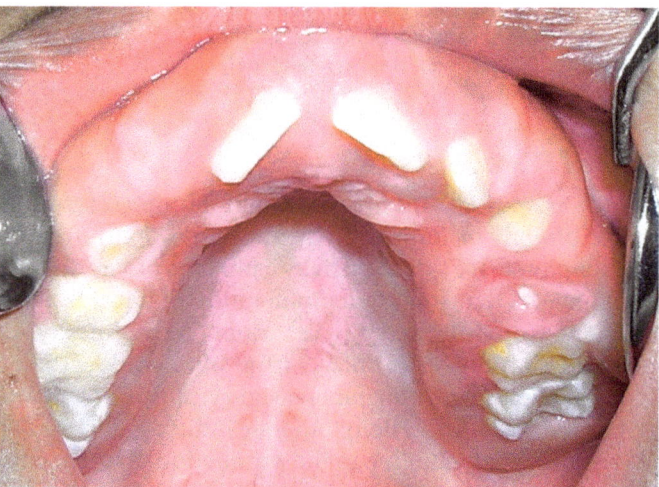

**Fig. 19.6:** Clinical picture showing idiopathic gingival fibromatosis (occlusal view).

## Differential Diagnosis

Idiopathic gingival fibromatosis is different from phenytoin-induced hyperplasia. Idiopathic gingival fibromatosis involves gingival margin, interdental papilla, and attached gingiva, whereas, in phenytoin-induced hyperplasia, only gingival margin and interdental papilla are involved. Histological examination may facilitate the differential diagnosis from another genetically determined gingival enlargement, such as Fabry disease, is characterized by telangiectasia.

Treatment involves surgical removal by a series of gingivectomies. If the volume of the overgrowth is extensive, repositioned flap surgery is done.

## ENLARGEMENT ASSOCIATED WITH SYSTEMIC DISEASES

Certain systemic conditions in the patient aggravate the gingival response to dental plaque. These are called conditioned enlargement. Although bacterial plaque is the primary etiological factor for the initiation of this type of enlargement but is not the sole determinant of the nature of enlargement. The various types of conditioned gingival enlargement are hormonal (pregnancy, puberty), nutritional (associated with vitamin C deficiency), and allergic.

## Conditioned Gingival Enlargement

### Specific Conditioned Gingival Enlargement

#### Enlargement in Pregnancy

Gingival enlargement during pregnancy is caused by hormonal changes that induce vascular permeability and increase in *Prevotella intermedia*. This results in gingival edema and an increased inflammatory response to dental plaque. Gingival enlargement during pregnancy may be marginal and generalized or may occur as single or multiple tumor-like masses.

*Marginal enlargement*: Bacterial plaque is an essential requirement for gingival enlargement. The marginal enlargement usually involves interproximal surfaces. The affected gingiva is bright red in color, soft and friable with a smooth, shiny surface (**Fig. 19.7**). Slight touch triggers bleeding in such cases.

*Tumor-like gingival enlargement*: Such gingival overgrowth commonly develops after the 3rd month of pregnancy. It appears as dark red or magenta, with a smooth, glistening surface that often exhibits numerous deep red, pinpoint markings (**Fig. 19.8**). The lesion appears as a soft, friable, discrete, mushroom-like, flattened spherical mass that protrudes from the gingival margin or, more commonly, from the interproximal space and is attached by a sessile or pedunculated base.

Although the spontaneous reduction in the size of gingival enlargement commonly follows the termination

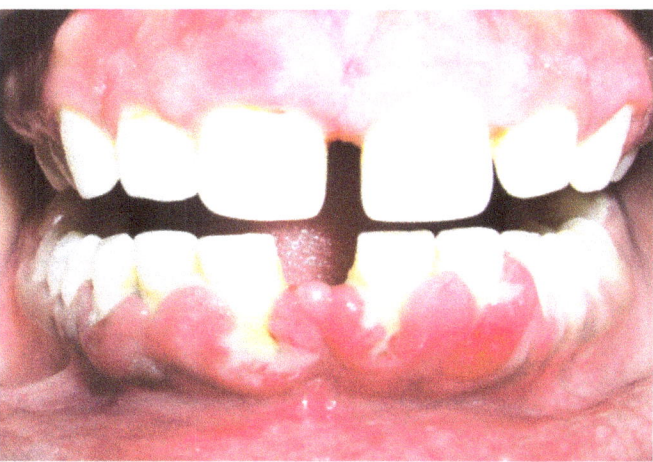

**Fig. 19.7:** Clinical picture showing conditioned gingival enlargement—pregnancy gingivitis.

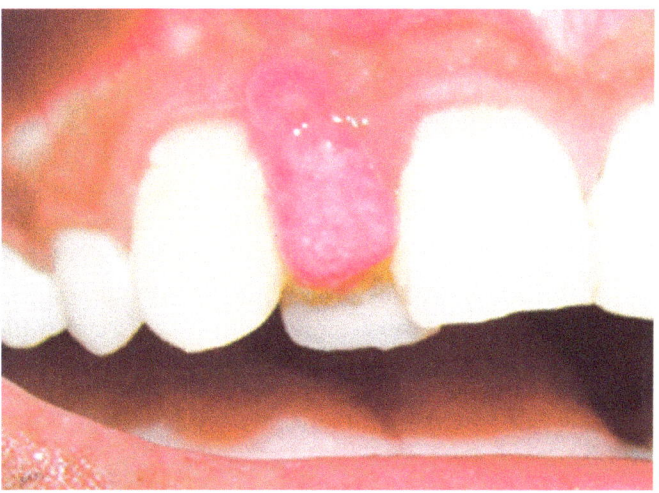

**Fig. 19.8:** Clinical picture showing pregnancy tumor.

of pregnancy, complete elimination of the residual inflammatory lesion requires the removal of all plaque deposits and factors that favor its accumulation.

#### Enlargement in Puberty

Enlargement of the gingiva is sometimes seen in both male and female adolescents and appears in areas of plaque accumulation. It is characterized by prominent bulbous interproximal papilla. Gingival enlargement during puberty has all the clinical features generally associated with the chronic inflammatory gingival disease. It is the degree of enlargement and the tendency to develop massive recurrence in the presence of relatively scanty plaque deposits that distinguish pubertal gingival enlargement from uncomplicated chronic inflammatory gingival enlargement (**Fig. 19.9**).

After puberty, there is a spontaneous reduction of enlargement, but it does not disappear until plaque and calculus are removed.

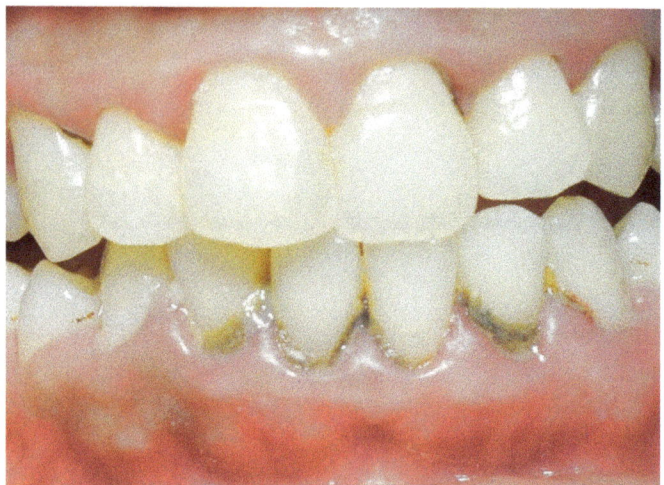

**Fig. 19.9:** Clinical picture showing conditioned gingival enlargement—puberty gingivitis.

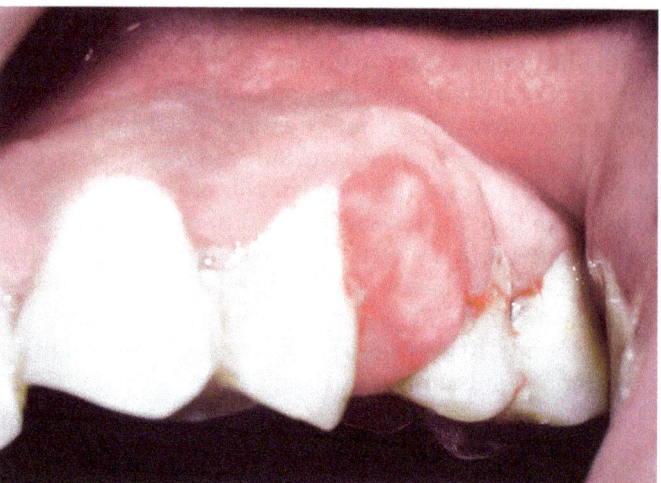

**Fig. 19.10:** Clinical picture showing pyogenic granuloma.

### Enlargement in Vitamin C Deficiency (Scurvy)

It is essentially a conditioned response to bacterial plaque. Acute vitamin C deficiency, as such, does not cause gingival inflammation, but it does cause collagen degeneration, hemorrhage, and edema of the gingival connective tissue. These changes modify the gingiva response to the plaque to the extent that the normal defensive delimiting reaction is inhibited, and the extent of the inflammation is exaggerated.

*Clinical features*: This is present as a marginal gingival enlargement in the form of bluish-red, soft and friable with a smooth, shiny surface. There is spontaneous bleeding or bleeding on slight provocation. There may be surface necrosis with pseudomembrane formation.

*Histological features*: Gingiva shows chronic inflammatory cellular infiltration with a separate area of hemorrhage and engorged capillaries. Marked diffuse edema with collagen degeneration and scarcity of collagen and fibroblasts are prominent features of this gingival enlargement.

### Plasma Cell Gingivitis

It is also called as atypical gingivitis and plasma cell gingivostomatitis. Plasma cell granuloma, a localized lesion, is present in the oral aspects of the attached gingiva and therefore differs from plaque-induced gingivitis.

Plasma cell gingivitis is suspected as an allergic in nature due to the presence of components of chewing gum, dentifrices, or various diet components. There is a mild marginal gingival enlargement that extends to the attached gingiva. The gingiva appears red, friable, and sometimes granular, which bleeds easily.

*Histological features*: Oral epithelium shows spongiosis and infiltration of inflammatory cells with the damaged spinous and basal layer. The underlying connective tissue contains dense infiltrate of plasma cells.

*Treatment*: Cessation of exposure to the allergen helps to resolve the lesion of such gingivitis.

### Nonspecific Conditioned Enlargement (Pyogenic Granuloma)

Pyogenic granuloma, also termed as granuloma pyogenicum, is the term introduced by Hartzell in 1904.[22] The condition is also known by other names, such as Crocker and Hartzell's disease; hemangiomatous granuloma; granuloma telangiectacticum. Pyogenic granuloma is a tumor-like overgrowth of gingival tissue that occurs due to exaggerated conditioned response to minor trauma.

*Etiology*: The role of systemic conditioning factor as a causative agent is still not well understood. Chronic low-grade trauma, physical trauma, hormonal factors, bacteria, viruses, and certain drugs have been reported as etiological factors in the pathogenesis of pyogenic granulomas. Other precipitating factors for this condition are local irritants, such as calculus, foreign material in the gingiva, and poor oral hygiene.

*Clinical features*: The lesion exhibits great variation in the form of discrete spherical, tumor-like mass with a pedunculated attachment to a flattened, keloid-like enlargement with a broad base **(Fig. 19.10)**. It is reddish or bluish, sometimes lobulated, and may be sessile or pedunculated with surface ulceration and purulent exudation. It may develop rapidly, and the size varies considerably. Bleeding from the ulcerated lesion is common, but typically it is not painful. Teeth may become separated due to the interdental growth of the lesion. Due to its red color, which may sometimes turn to a cyanotic hue, pyogenic granuloma may be mistaken for giant cell granuloma.

Pyogenic granuloma is similar in clinical and microscopic appearance to the conditioned gingival enlargement seen in pregnancy. The differential diagnosis depends on the patient's history.

*Histological features*: They are composed of granulation tissue mass with neutrophil and chronic inflammatory cellular infiltration. Numerous proliferating endothelial tissue and vascular spaces are the striking features of pyogenic granuloma. Surface ulceration and exudation are also present.

*Treatment:* The condition responds to the surgical excision and the elimination of irritating local factors.

## Systemic Diseases Causing Gingival Enlargement

### Leukemia

Gingival enlargement in leukemia is diffused or marginal, localized or generalized. The diffuse gingival enlargement is associated with overgrowth of the gingival mucosa with an oversized extension of the marginal gingiva or a discrete tumor-like interproximal mass. The affected gingiva is mostly bluish red with a shiny surface. It is moderately firm with a tendency towards friability. Hemorrhage occurs either spontaneously or on slight irritation **(Fig. 19.11)**. Patients with leukemia may also have a simple chronic inflammation without the involvement of leukemic cells and may present with the same clinical and microscopic features seen in patients without the disease. Most cases reveal features of both simple chronic inflammation and a leukemic infiltrate.

#### Granulomatous Diseases

*Wegener's granulomatosis* (WG): WG is a rare disease characterized by acute granulomatous necrotizing lesions of the respiratory tract, including nasal and oral defects. Renal lesions develop, and acute necrotizing vasculitis affects the blood vessels. The initial manifestations of Wegener's granulomatosis may involve the orofacial region and include oral mucosal ulceration, gingival enlargement, abnormal tooth mobility, exfoliation of teeth, and delayed healing response.[23] The cause of Wegener's granulomatosis is unknown. Still, the condition is considered as an immunologically mediated tissue injury. The granulomatous papillary enlargement is reddish-purple and bleeds easily on stimulation.

*Sarcoidosis*: Sarcoidosis is a granulomatous disease that starts in individuals in their 20s or 30s and predominantly affects blacks. Gingival enlargement may be red, smooth, and painless. The cause of sarcoidosis is unknown.

## NEOPLASTIC ENLARGEMENT

### Benign Tumors of the Gingiva

Epulis is a nonspecific term commonly used to designate all discrete tumors and tumor-like masses of the gingiva. This term refers to the location of the tumor but not with the description. The lesions describe under epulis are mostly inflammatory in nature rather than neoplastic.[24]

### Gingival Fibroma

Gingival fibroma usually originates from the gingival connective tissue or from the periodontal ligament.

*Clinical features:* They are slow-growing, spherical tumors. Consistency of fibroma is either firm and nodular or soft and vascular. Fibromas are usually pedunculated.

*Histopathological features*: There is hyperkeratinization of the epithelium. It consists of scattered angular and multinucleated cells of different appearance and nature than the giant cells in giant-cell granulomas. Connective tissue consists of a poor cell and hyperplastic collagenous tissue.

*Treatment:* It is managed by complete surgical excision, including superficial periodontal ligament fibers from where fibroma originate.

### Papilloma

Papillomas are benign proliferations of surface epithelium due to infection with the human papillomavirus (HPV).[1] They are mainly seen in the 3rd to 5th decade.

*Clinical features*: Gingival papillomas appear as reddish/normal or whitish/gray color, solitary, wart-like, or cauliflower-like protuberances **(Fig. 19.12)**. They may be small and discrete or broad, hard elevations with minutely irregular surfaces.

*Histopathological features*: The epithelium is hyperkeratotic stratified squamous with irregular rete ridges. Connective tissue is fibrovascular.

*Treatment:* Treatment involves the surgical excision along with the base of the lesion.

### Peripheral Giant-cell Granuloma

These lesions, however, occur as a response to local injury. The prefix "peripheral" is needed to differentiate them

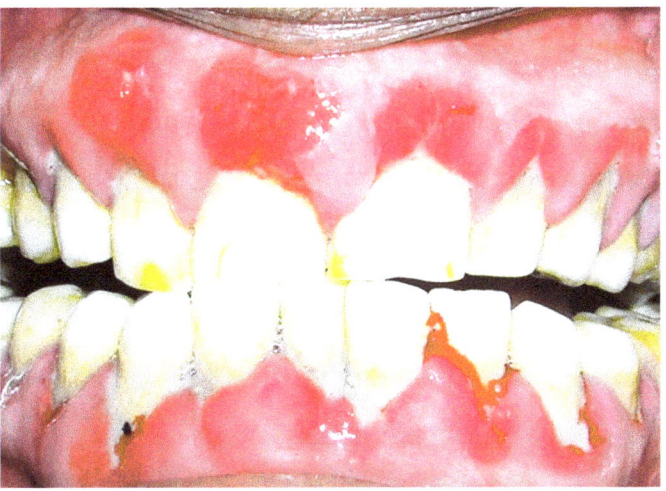

**Fig. 19.11:** Clinical photograph showing leukemic gingival enlargement.

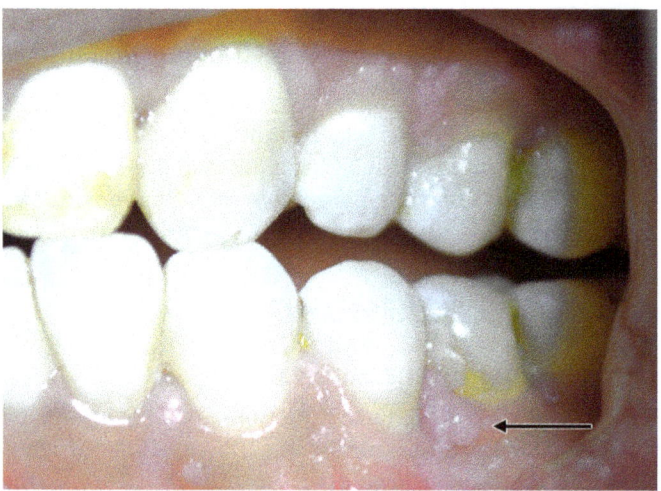

**Fig. 19.12:** Clinical photograph showing gingival papilloma.

from comparable lesions that originate within the jaw bone (central giant-cell granulomas). It is common in women compared to men, and the mandible is more often affected than the maxilla.

*Clinical features*: Granuloma develops on interdental or the gingival margin as red or purple ulcers. The lesions are pedunculated or sessile or maybe firm or spongy. Local irritation or trauma appears to be essential for these lesions to occur. They cause separation of teeth due to the pressure exerted by the growth. The granuloma can vary from smooth, regularly outlined masses to irregularly shaped, multilobulated protuberances with surface indentations. Ulceration of the margin is rare. The lesions are usually nontender with an extension over several teeth and pink to deep red or purplish-blue in color. In some instances, the giant-cell granuloma of the gingiva is locally invasive and destroys the underlying bone.

*Histopathological features*: There is hyperplasia of the epithelium with ulceration at the base. The granuloma lesion involves focal collections of multinucleated osteoclast-like giant cells enrich with cellular and vascular stroma separated by collagenous septa.

*Treatment:* The lesions are not encapsulated. However, they are well delimited and readily excised.

### Central Giant-cell Granuloma

These lesions arise within the jaws and produce central cavitation. They occasionally create a deformity of the jaw that makes the gingiva appear enlarged. Mixed tumors, salivary gland type tumors, and plasmacytomas of the gingiva have also been described but are not often seen.

### Leukoplakia

World Health Organization defined leukoplakia as a white patch or plaque that does not rub off and cannot be diagnosed as any other disease. The cause of leukoplakia remains obscure, although it is associated with tobacco use (smoke or smokeless). Other probable factors are *Candida albicans*, HPV-16, HPV-18, and trauma.[1]

*Clinical features*: Leukoplakia presents as solitary or multiple grayish-white patches or plaques. These patches have distinct and sharply demarcated borders. Patches are usually thickened and smooth or wrinkled and fissured or sometimes present as raised, corrugated, verrucous plaques.

*Histopathological features*: Hyperkeratosis varies in thickness, may show parakeratosis or orthokeratosis hyperplastic oral epithelium. Epithelium may show acanthosis. Rete pegs are usually drop/tear-shaped.

*Treatment:* Treatment of leukoplakia may include administration of vitamin A, B complex, surgical excision, and topical chemotherapy.

### Gingival Cysts

These cysts are of developmental origin. They occur in the mandibular canine and premolar areas, most often on the lingual surface.

*Clinical features*: Gingival cyst appears as localized enlargements that may involve the marginal and attached gingiva. They are painless, but with expansion, they may cause erosion of the alveolar bone's surface. The cysts develop from odontogenic epithelium or from the surface or sulcular epithelium traumatically implanted in the area.

*Histopathological features*: The gingival cysts are lined by stratified squamous epithelium with a parakeratotic surface and flat palisading basal cells. The cyst lumen is filled with keratin. The gingival cyst of adults is lined with a thin, nonkeratinized squamous epithelium, sometimes exhibiting focal thickenings of the epithelial lining.

*Treatment:* Gingival cysts of adults are treated by local surgical excision, and usually, there is no tendency to recur.

## Malignant Tumors of the Gingiva

### Squamous Cell Carcinoma

Squamous cell carcinoma is the well-known malignant tumor of the gingiva. It may be exophytic, presenting as an irregular outgrowth, or ulcerative, which appears as flat, erosive lesion. It is often symptom-free, often going unnoticed until complicated by inflammatory changes that may mask the neoplasm but cause pain and loosening of teeth. It is locally invasive, involving the underlying bone and periodontal ligament of adjoining teeth and the adjacent mucosa. Metastasis is usually confined to the region above the clavicle; however, more extensive involvement may include the lung, liver, or bone.

*Histopathological features*: Islands and cords of malignant epithelial cells are seen infiltrating the underlying tissues. Varying amounts of "horn pearls" are formed, and usually, a strong inflammatory reaction is found in the stroma.

*Treatment:* Gingival squamous cell carcinomas are usually treated by surgery, irradiation, or a combination of these.

### Malignant Melanoma

It usually occurs in the hard palate and maxillary gingiva of older persons.[25] It is often darkly pigmented, which is preceded by the occurrence of localized pigmentation. It may appear as flat or nodular growth. It is characterized by rapid growth and early metastasis. It originates from melanoblasts in the gingiva, cheek, or palate. Infiltration into the underlying bone and metastasis to cervical and axillary lymph nodes is common.

### Malignant Lymphoma

It presents as a diffuse swelling, which is usually ulcerated. The diagnosis may be quite challenging to arrive at as the first manifestations may resemble nonspecific periodontitis, pyogenic granuloma, or pericoronitis. In human immunodeficiency virus (HIV)-infected patients, non-Hodgkin's lymphomas occur with increased frequency. Occasionally, a gingival tumor may be the first manifestation of a non-Hodgkin's lymphoma in an HIV-infected patient.

Histomorphologic features, immunologic and genetic markers are used to diagnose and classify malignant lymphomas. The lesions contain lymphocytic-appearing cells; in low-grade tumors, the cells are well-differentiated small lymphocytes, whereas high-grade tumors contain less differentiated cells. Common to all lymphomas are infiltrative growth as characteristically seen in all malignant tumors.

Depending on the extension and spread of the tumor, surgical removal, irradiation, cytostatics, and combinations of these may be the treatment of choice.

### Kaposi's Sarcoma

Kaposi's sarcoma often occurs in the oral cavity of patients with acquired immunodeficiency syndrome (AIDS), particularly in the palate and the gingiva. It usually manifests first as skin lesions followed by oral lesions.

They may represent single or multiple blue, violet, or red, slightly raised lesions.

*Histopathological features*: The typical features are a lesion with bundles of spindle-shaped cells and many thin-walled vascular luminae, often lined by plump endothelial cells. There are usually a number of mitotic figures, of which some are atypical.

*Treatment:* There is no curative treatment, but palliative treatment includes both cytostatics and irradiation.

## FALSE ENLARGEMENT

False enlargements are the gingival enlargement that occurs due to an increase in the size of the underlying osseous or dental tissues **(Fig. 19.13)**. These are not the actual or real enlargements of the gingival tissues. The massive increase in the size of the gingival area is the only identifiable feature of false enlargement. No other clinical abnormalities are detected in this condition.

### Underlying Osseous Lesions

Enlargement of the bone subjacent to the gingival area occurs in tori, exostosis **(Figs. 19.14 and 19.15)**, fibrous dysplasia, cherubism, central giant-cell granuloma, ameloblastoma, osteoma, and osteosarcoma. The gingival tissue appears either normal or with discrete inflammatory changes.

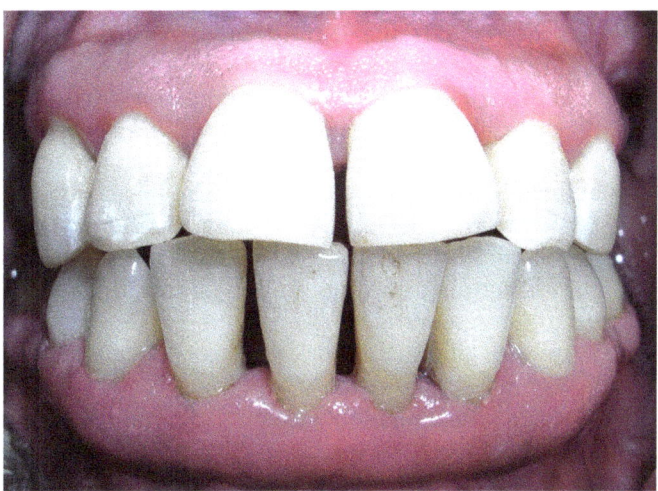

**Fig. 19.13:** Clinical picture showing false enlargement.

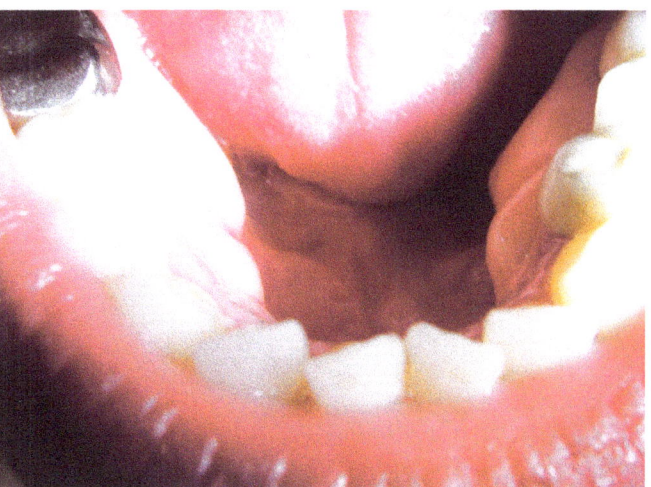

**Fig. 19.14:** Clinical picture showing enlargement due to the presence of bilateral mandibular exostosis.
(*Courtesy*: Dr SK Salaria)

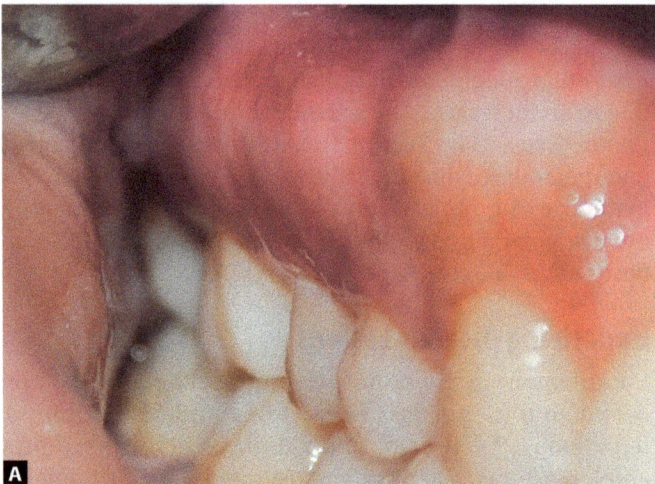 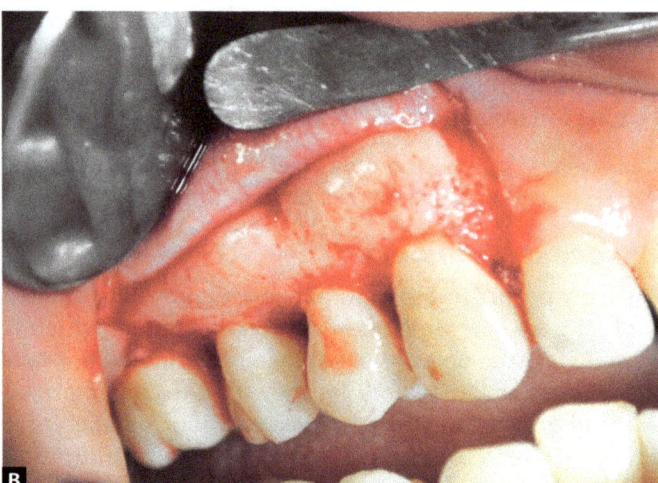

**Figs. 19.15A and B:** Clinical picture showing maxillary exostosis.

## Underlying Dental Tissues

Developmental gingival enlargement in the form of abnormal gingival overgrowth is noted during the different stages of tooth eruption. During the primary dentition eruption, the labial gingiva exhibits the bulbous marginal distortion due to the overlapping of the bulk of the gingiva on the normal prominence of the enamel in the gingival half of the crown. This enlargement has been termed as "developmental enlargement" (**Fig. 19.16**) and continues until the junctional epithelium has migrated from the enamel to the cementoenamel junction. In a strict sense, developmental gingival enlargements are physiologic and ordinarily present no problems.

However, when such enlargement is complicated by marginal inflammation, the composite picture gives the impression of extensive gingival enlargement.

Treatment to alleviate the marginal inflammation rather than resection of the enlargement is sufficient in these cases.

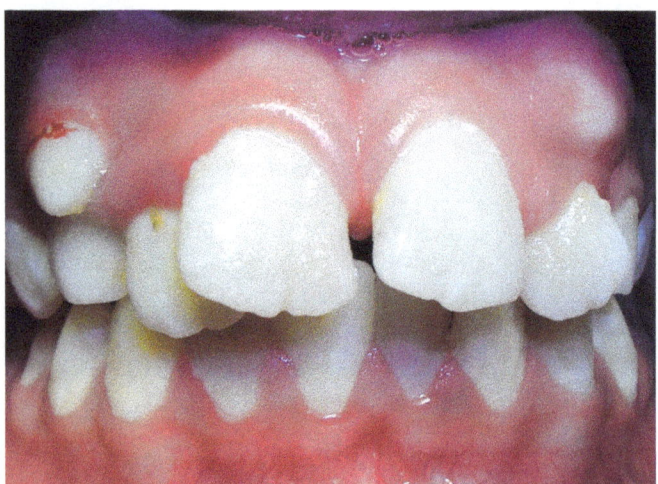

**Fig. 19.16:** Clinical picture showing developmental gingival enlargement.

### Points to Ponder

- Hypertrophy is an increase in the size of cells, causing an increase in the tissues' size.
- Hyperplasia is an increase in the number of cells in a tissue, thus, contributing to an overall increase in the size. Gingival hyperplasia is caused mainly by an increase in the number of local cellular elements and intercellular fibers.
- The clinical features of phenytoin-induced hyperplasia are different from that of idiopathic fibrous hyperplasia. The administration of phenytoin often leads to the overgrowth of the papillae, leaving the attached gingiva, whereas, in idiopathic fibrous hyperplasia, there is the involvement of all marginal, interdental and attached gingiva.
- The allergens associated with plasma cell gingivitis are cinnamaldehyde and cinnamon used as flavoring agents in chewing gums and dentifrices.
- Pyogenic granuloma is not associated with pus, and histologically it resembles angiomatous lesion rather than granulomatous lesion, indicating that the term "pyogenic granuloma" is a misnomer.

### REFERENCES

1. Carranza FA, Hogan EL. Gingival enlargement. In: Newman MG, Takei HH, Carranza FA (Eds). Carranza's Clinical Periodontology, 9th edition. Philadelphia, PA, USA: WB Saunders; 2003. pp. 279-96.
2. Bökenkamp A, Bohnhorst B, Beier C, Albers N, Offner G, Brodehl J. Nifedipine aggravates cyclosporine A-induced hyperplasia. Pediatr Nephrol. 1994;8(2):181-5.
3. Hirschfeld I. Hypertrophic gingivitis; its clinical aspect. J Am Dent Assoc. 1932;19: 799.
4. Seymour RA, Thomason JM, Ellis JS. The pathogenesis of drug-induced gingival overgrowth. J Clin Periodontol. 1996;23(3 Pt 1):165-75.
5. Seymour RA, Smith DG, Rogers SR. The comparative effects of azathioprine and cyclosporine on some gingival health parameters of renal transplant patients. A longitudinal study. J Clin Periodontol. 1987;14(10):610-3.
6. Barclay S, Thomason JM, Idle JR, Seymour RA. The incidence and severity of nifedipine-induced gingival overgrowth. J Clin Periodontol. 1992;19(5):311-4.

7. Shafer WG. Effect of dilantin sodium on various cell lines in tissue culture. Proc Soc Exp Biol Med. 1961;108:694-6.
8. Goultschin J, Sofer B, Shoshan S. The effect of prolonged phenytoin administration on non-collagenous components of gingival tissue. Int J Tissue React. 1983;5(2):227-30.
9. Dahllöf G, Reinholt FP, Hjerpe A, Modeer T. A quantitative analysis of connective tissue components in phenytoin-induced gingival overgrowth in children. A stereological study. J Periodontal Res. 1984;19(4):401-7.
10. Sume SS, Kantarci A, Lee A, Hasturk H, Trackman PC. Epithelial to mesenchymal transition in gingival overgrowth. Am J Pathol. 2010;177(1):208-18.
11. Hassell TM. Evidence for production of an inactive collagenase by fibroblasts from phenytoin-enlarged human gingivae. J Oral Pathol. 1982;11(4):310-7.
12. Bolzani G, Della Coletta R, Martelli Junior H, Martelli Junior H, Graner E. Cyclosporin A inhibits production and activity of matrix metalloproteinases by gingival fibroblasts. J Periodontal Res. 2000;35(1):51-8.
13. Hassell TM, Gilbert GH. Phenytoin sensitivity of fibroblasts as the basis for susceptibility to gingival enlargement. Am J Pathol. 1983;112(2):218-23.
14. Jacobs D, Buchanan J, Cuchens M, Hassell TM. The effect of cyclosporine metabolite OL-17 on gingival fibroblast subpopulations. J Dent Res. 1990;69: 221.
15. Hefti AF, Eshenaur AE, Hassell TM, Stone C. Gingival overgrowth in cyclosporine A treated multiple sclerosis patients. J Periodontol. 1994;65(8):744-9.
16. Sooriyamoorthy M, Harvey W, Gower DB. The use of human gingival fibroblasts in culture for studying the effects of phenytoin on testosterone metabolism. Arch Oral Biol. 1988;33(5):353-9.
17. Strachan D, Burton I, Pearson GJ. Is oral azithromycin effective for the treatment of cyclosporine-induced gingival hyperplasia in cardiac transplant recipients? J Clin Pharm Ther. 2003;28(4):329-38.
18. Poppell TD, Keeling SD, Collins JF, Hassell TM. Effect of folic acid on recurrence of phenytoin-induced gingival overgrowth following gingivectomy. J Clin Periodontol. 1991;18(2):134-9.
19. Holmstrup P, Reibel J. Differential diagnoses: periodontal tumors and cysts. In: Lindhe J, Karring T, Lang NP (Eds). Clinical Periodontology and Implant Dentistry, 4th edition. Chicago, USA: Blackwell Munksgaard; 2003. pp. 298-317.
20. Hart TC, Pallos D, Bowden DW, Bolyard J, Pettenati MJ, Cortelli JR. Genetic linkage of hereditary gingival fibromatosis to chromosome 2p21. Am J Hum Genet. 1998;62(4):876-83.
21. Hart TC, Zhang Y, Gorry MC, Hart PS, Cooper M, Marazita ML, et al. A mutation in the SOS1 gene causes hereditary gingival fibromatosis type 1. Am J Hum Genet. 2002;70(4):943-54.
22. Hartzell MB. Granuloma pyogenicum. J Cuttan Dis Syph. 1904;22:520-5.
23. Buckley DJ, Barrett AP, Bilous AM, et al. Wegener's granulomatosis-are gingival lesions pathognomonic? J Oral Med. 1987;42: 169.
24. Eley BM, Soory M, Manson JD. Epulides and tumours of the gingivae and oral mucosa. In: Periodontics, 5th edition. Philadelphia, PA, USA: Churchill Livingstone; 2004. pp. 380-2.
25. Neville BW, Damm DD, Allen CM, Chi A. In: Oral and Maxillofacial Pathology, 4th edition. Philadelphia, PA, USA: WB Saunders; 2015.
26. Hassell TM, Page RC, Lindhe J. Histological evidence for impaired growth control in diphenylhydantoin gingival overgrowth in man. Arch Oral Biol. 1978;23(5):381-4.

## VIVA VOCE

**Q1. What are hypertrophy and hyperplasia?**
**Ans.** *Hypertrophy*: It is an increase in the size of cells, causing an increase in the size of the tissues.
*Hyperplasia*: It is an increase in the number of cells in a tissue, thus contributing to an overall increase in the size.

**Q2. Why the term gingival hyperplasia/hypertrophy was replaced with the condition gingival enlargement/ overgrowth?**
**Ans.** The term gingival hyperplasia/hypertrophy was replaced with term gingival enlargement/overgrowth. The histological analysis of gingiva did not accurately reflect an increase in the size/number of fibroblasts, but the accumulation of extracellular matrix within the gingival connective tissue. Hence, the term accepted is gingival overgrowth.[26]

**Q3. How is idiopathic gingival fibromatosis different from phenytoin-induced hyperplasia clinically?**
**Ans.** Idiopathic gingival fibromatosis involves gingival margin, interdental papillae, and attached gingiva, whereas, in phenytoin-induced hyperplasia, only gingival margin and interdental papillae are involved.

**Q4. Strawberry gums are seen in which type of gingival disease?**
**Ans.** Wegener's granulomatosis.

**Q5. What are false enlargements?**
**Ans.** These are gingival enlargement that occurs due to the increase in the size of the underlying osseous or dental tissues.

**Q6. Which antibiotic decreases the severity of cyclosporine-induced gingival enlargement?**
**Ans.** Azithromycin.

**Q7. Why "pyogenic granuloma" is a misnomer?**
**Ans.** Pyogenic granuloma is not associated with pus, and histologically it resembles angiomatous lesion.

**Q8. In which tumors of the gingiva horn pearls are present.**
**Ans.** Squamous cell carcinoma.

**Q9. What is a gingival abscess?**
**Ans.** A gingival abscess is a localized collection of pus involving marginal gingiva or interdental papilla.

**Q10. What are papillomas?**
**Ans.** Papillomas are benign proliferations of surface epithelium due to infection with the human papillomavirus.

# Chapter 20

# Acute Gingival Conditions

Subash C Raj, Shalu Bathla

## Chapter Outline

- Necrotizing Ulcerative Gingivitis
- Primary Herpetic Gingivostomatitis
- Pericoronitis

## INTRODUCTION

Acute infections are painful, occur with sudden onset, and are of short duration. Acute gingival lesion includes gingival abscess, necrotizing ulcerative gingivitis, herpangina, herpes zoster, primary herpetic gingivostomatitis, and pericoronitis. In this chapter, necrotizing ulcerative gingivitis, primary herpetic gingivostomatitis, and pericoronitis are only discussed.

## NECROTIZING ULCERATIVE GINGIVITIS

### Historical Perspective

In the 4th BC, Xenophon identified necrotizing ulcerative gingivitis (NUG) in Greek soldiers who developed oral lesions in the form of sore, ulcerated, and foul-smelling mouths. Afterward, in 1778, John Hunter, for the first time, clinically differentiated NUG, scurvy, and chronic periodontitis. In the 19th century, NUG developed in the epidemic form. In 1886, Hersch described that increased salivation, enlarged lymph nodes, fever, and malaise were characteristically associated with NUG. According to the 1999 American Academy of Periodontology classification system, acute NUG (ANUG) is classified under the category of *necrotizing periodontal disease*. ANUG is a distinct and specific clinical entity associated with rapidly progressive ulceration, especially commencing at the tip of the interdental papilla, spreads along the gingival margins leading to acute destruction of the periodontal tissue.

Synonyms of NUG are trench mouth, Vincent's gingivostomatitis, Vincent's gingivitis, ulceromembranous gingivitis, ANUG, and fusospirochetal gingivitis. "Trench mouth" is also termed Vincent's stomatitis or Vincent's angina by French Bacteriologist Jean Hyacinth Vincent (1862–1950). The term "trench mouth" originated in World War I, when many soldiers were stuck in the trenches and developed these peculiar ulcerative oral lesions due to improper care of mouth and teeth.[1]

### Clinical Features

The characteristic features of NUG are:[2]
- *Rapid onset of gingival pain*: The NUG lesions are extremely tender. The presence of constantly radiating, gnawing pain intensified by eating hot and spicy foods is characteristic of NUG pain.
- *Interdental gingival necrosis*: Lesions of NUG are usually punched out, and crater-like depressions located at the crest of the interdental papillae. These lesions further get spread to the marginal gingiva and occasionally to the attached gingiva and oral mucosa. The ulcers are covered by a yellowish-white or grayish slough, which has been termed as "pseudomembrane," demarcated from the remainder of the gingival mucosa by pronounced linear erythema. However, the sloughed material has no coherence and bears little resemblance to a membrane (**Fig. 20.1**). It consists primarily of fibrin and necrotic tissue with leukocytes, erythrocytes, and masses of bacteria. Removal of the sloughed material results in bleeding and exposure of underlying ulcerated tissue.
- *Bleeding*: NUG lesions are touch-sensitive and exhibited spontaneous gingival hemorrhage or pronounced bleeding on the slightest stimulation. This is attributed to the acute inflammation and necrosis of the underlying connective tissue.

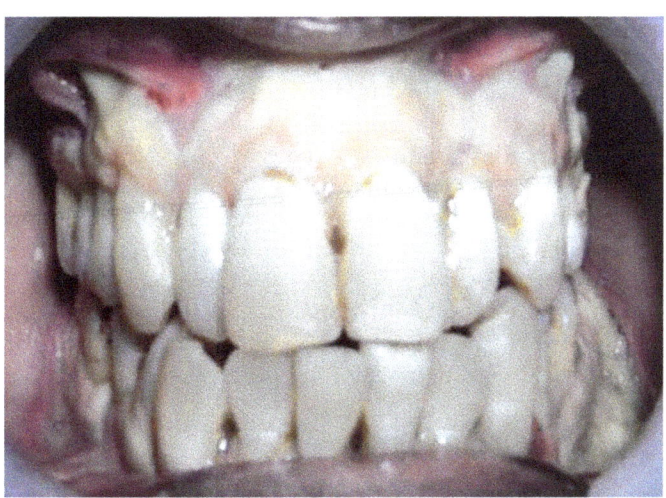

**Fig. 20.1:** Clinical picture showing necrotizing ulcerative gingivitis. (*Courtesy*: Dr. Ambika Gupta)

Other clinical features are:
- *Fetid odor*: A characteristic and pronounced *fetor ex ore* is often associated with NUG, but can vary in intensity.
- *Increased salivation*: Metallic foul taste imparts a constant feeling of an excessive amount of "pasty" saliva.
- *Site and extent of involvement*: The interdental cols and tips of the interdental papillae are characteristically affected first, although the disease may involve the gingival margins. The distribution of the disease does not follow any consistent pattern and may differ from person-to-person.[3] The reasons for necrotic lesions appearing at the interdental papilla are 2-fold:
  - The papilla has relatively less vascularity, with the tip being supplied by a single vessel arising from the papillary plexus. If the vascularity arising from this vessel is cut off for some reason, the resultant lack of oxygenation leads to the death of tissues.
  - There is an extensive infiltration of spirochetes into the tissues of the gingiva. Among the other vessels, the papillary plexus is affected as well by spirochetal infiltration. The lack of an alternate supply with the blockage of the existing one leads to tissue necrosis. This manifests clinically as the characteristic punched- out crater-like lesions at the crest of the papilla.
- *Relation of necrotizing ulcerative periodontal (NUP) disease to pocket*: This condition is otherwise termed as atypical periodontitis. The pockets that are a characteristic clinical sign associated with periodontitis are absent in this condition. Pocket formation necessitates apical migration of junctional epithelium, and this requires viable epithelial cells. Necrosis of the epithelial cells results in an epithelium that is unable to exhibit any proliferation or migration. Therefore, in necrotizing gingival inflammation, the spread of inflammation does not result in pocket formation.

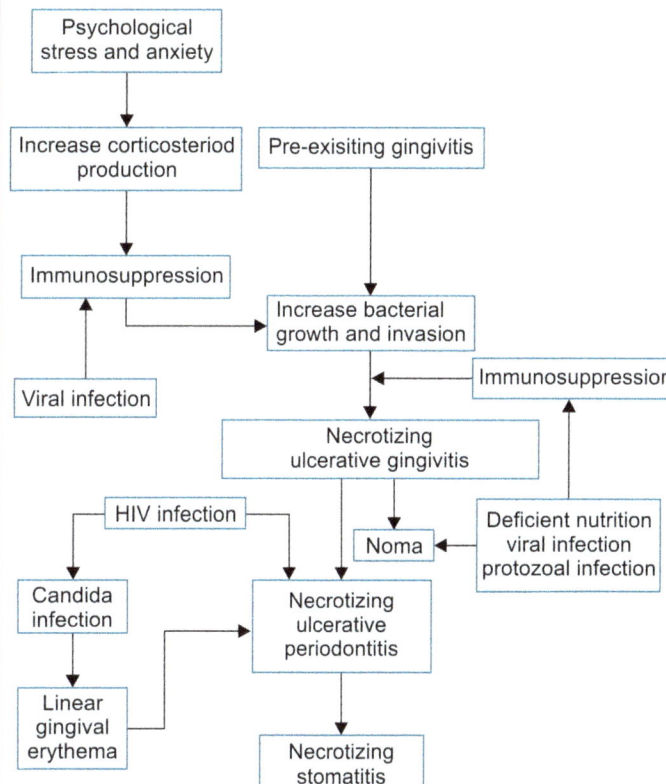

**Flowchart 20.1:** Necrotizing ulcerative gingivitis (NUG): Possible mechanisms and sequelae.

Extraoral clinical features are the presence of local lymphadenopathy, slight elevation in temperature to high fever, high pulse rate, leukocytosis, loss of appetite, and general lassitude.

## Etiology

The possible etiological and predisposing factors are explained in **Flowchart 20.1**.

### Etiological Factors

*Bacterial flora*: NUG is considered as an infectious disease with the significant role of microbial flora in its causation and progression. Reduce the microbial plaque with antibiotic therapy, mechanical debridement, or both bring dramatic resolution to NUG's signs and symptoms. The bacterial flora, as a causative agent of NUG, suggests the significant role of primary bacterial etiology in the periodontal disease. Plaut[4] in 1894 and Vincent[5] in 1896 proposed the concept of bacterial etiology in the periodontal disease. In an independent experiment, both demonstrated the role of fusiform-spirochete bacterial flora in the lesions of NUG.

### Predisposing Factors

- *Psychological stress*: Emotional stress usually precipitates the lesions of NUG.[6] Such form of stress is common among military cadets, in harsh physical conditions, in drug addicts during periods of drug withdrawal, in

college students during the examination and in stressful living endemic contagious diseases, especially measles.
- Synergistic association between malnutrition and measles (a viral infection) accelerates the secondary infection with resident oral microorganisms and promotes the rapid spreads of NUG. Stress is reported to cause NUG by different mechanisms, such as an elevation in adrenocortical secretion and the release of substance P. This peptide hormone suppresses both specific and nonspecific immunities. Stress significantly affects mood, which severely affects the patient's oral hygiene and nutrition.
- Other predisposing factors are immunosuppression, malnutrition, tobacco smoking, pre-existing gingivitis, and trauma.[7]

## Stages

Pindborg and colleagues have described the following stages in the progression of NUG:[8]
- *Stage I*: Only the tip of the interdental papilla is affected.
- *Stage II*: The lesion extends to marginal gingiva and causes punched-out papilla.
- *Stage III*: The attached gingiva is also affected.
- *Stage IV*: The bone is exposed.

Horning and Cohen extended the staging of these oral necrotizing diseases as follows:[9]
- *Stage 1*: Necrosis of the tip of the interdental papilla (93%)—NUG.
- *Stage 2*: Necrosis of the entire papilla (19%)—either NUG or NUP.
- *Stage 3*: Necrosis extending to the gingival margin (21%)—NUP.
- *Stage 4*: Necrosis also extending to the attached gingiva (1%)—NUP.
- *Stage 5*: Necrosis extending into buccal or labial mucosa (6%)—Necrotizing stomatitis.
- *Stage 6*: Necrosis exposing alveolar bone (1%)—Necrotizing stomatitis.
- *Stage 7*: Necrosis perforating skin of cheek (0%)—Noma.

## Histopathology

The microscopic picture of NUG exhibited the presence of an acute inflammatory process with surface ulceration and formation of the pseudomembrane. Damaged epithelium gets replaced with a meshwork of fibrin, necrotic epithelial cells, polymorphonuclear neutrophils (PMNs), and microorganisms. This is the zone that appears clinically as pseudomembrane. The connective tissue has numerous engorged capillaries and dense infiltration of PMNs.[10]

In 1965, Listgarten provided an electron microscopic data of NUG lesions. The data reported the invasion of large and intermediate-sized spirochetes into the non-necrotic gingiva. This invasion in the ulcerated lesions by spirochetes is further demarcated into four zones of increasing depth from the tissue surface:[11]
1. *Zone 1*: Bacterial zone, the most superficial, consists of varied bacteria, including a few spirochetes of the small, medium, and large types.
2. *Zone 2*: Neutrophil-rich zone contains numerous leukocytes, mainly neutrophils with bacteria, including many spirochetes of various types between the leukocytes.
3. *Zone 3*: Necrotic zone consists of disintegrated tissue cells, fibrillar material, remnants of collagen fibers, and numerous spirochetes of the medium and large types with few other organisms.
4. *Zone 4*: Zone of spirochetal infiltration consists of well-preserved tissue infiltrated with medium and large spirochetes without other organisms.

## Diagnosis

Gingival pain, ulceration, and bleeding, all are the diagnostic features of NUG. Microscopic examination of a biopsy specimen can be used to differentiate NUG from specific infections, such as tuberculosis or neoplastic. However, it does not differentiate between NUG and other necrotizing conditions of nonspecific origin, such as those produced by trauma or caustic medications. Moreover, microscopic findings are not sufficient to diagnose NUG.[10] Thus, it is essential to take history to determine the underlying predisposing factors responsible for the disease.[12]

## Differential Diagnosis

Other conditions resembling with NUG in some respects are herpetic gingivostomatitis, chronic periodontitis, desquamative gingivitis, streptococcal gingivostomatitis, aphthous stomatitis, diphtheritic and syphilitic lesions, tuberculous gingival lesion, candidiasis, agranulocytosis, pemphigus, erythema multiforme and lichen planus. Perhaps the most important differential diagnosis of NUG is that from primary herpetic gingivostomatitis.

The differentiating features of NUG and acute herpetic gingivostomatitis (AHG) are presented in **Table 20.1**.

## Treatment

Treatment of NUG should follow an orderly sequence, which is divided mainly into two stages:[3]
1. *Control of acute phase*:
    - Alleviation of the acute inflammation plus treatment of chronic disease, either underlying the acute involvement or elsewhere in the oral cavity.
    - Relief from generalized toxic symptoms, including fever and malaise.
2. *Management of the residual condition*:
    - Elimination of predisposing factors
    - Correction of tissue deformities by surgery

**TABLE 20.1:** Differences between NUG and AHG.

| Parameters | NUG | AHG |
|---|---|---|
| Site of ulcers | Interdental papilla, marginal gingiva | Gingiva, no predilection for interdental papilla, entire oral mucosa |
| Character of ulcers | ◆ Punched-out crater-like depression covered by yellow/white/gray slough<br>◆ Bleed readily/spontaneously<br>◆ Painful on stimulation | ◆ Multiple vesicles that coalesce and form shallow fibrin-covered regular-shaped ulcers<br>◆ No marked tendency to bleed<br>◆ Nontender |
| Fever | Doubtful/slight only | 38°C (or more) |
| Symptoms | Painful gums/dead feeling teeth | Sore mouth |
| Duration of ulcers and discomfort | Short-lived (1–3 days) with appropriate therapy | >1 week, even with therapy |
| Etiology | Interaction between host and bacteria, most probably fusospirochetes | Specific viral etiology |
| Age | Uncommon in children | More frequent in children |
| Contagious | Noncontagious | Contagious |
| Immunity | No demonstrated immunity | An acute episode results in some degree of immunity |

(NUG: necrotizing ulcerative gingivitis; AHG: acute herpetic gingivostomatitis)

## Control of Acute Phase

First visit treatment mainly targets the acutely affected areas:
- *Isolation*: The affected site is isolated with cotton rolls and dried.
- *Removal of surface debris*: Under the effect of local anesthesia (LA), the affected areas are gently swabbed with a cotton pellet to remove the pseudomembrane and nonattached surface debris. For each small area, a separate cotton pellet is used and discarded after completion. Use of a single pellet with sweeping motions over large areas is contraindicated.[13]
- *Ultrasonic scaling*: The affected area is cleansed with warm water, and ultrasonic scaling is used to remove superficial calculus. Subgingival scaling and curettage at this stage enhance the possibility of extending the infection to deeper tissues and subsequent bacteremia. Hence, these procedures are not usually recommended.

Following instructions are given to the patient:
- *Do's*:
  - Rinse mouth with a glassful of an equal mixture of 3% hydrogen peroxide ($H_2O_2$) and warm water every 2 hours and/or twice daily with 0.12% chlorhexidine solution.
  - Pursue usual activities.
  - Patients with moderate or severe NUG and local lymphadenopathy, penicillin 500 mg orally every six hours, and for penicillin-sensitive patients, erythromycin is prescribed. Metronidazole (400 mg TID for seven days) is also effective. Antibiotics are continued until the systemic complications, or the local lymphadenopathy has subsided.
- *Do not's*:
  - Avoid frequent use of tobacco and alcohol.
  - Avoid excessive physical exertion.
  - Avoid prolonged exposure to the sun, especially in golf, tennis, swimming, or sunbathing.
  - Avoid harsh toothbrushing and the excessive use of dental floss or interdental cleaners.

*Second visit*: At the second visit, 1–2 days later, the patient's condition is improved, then scaling is performed, if sensitivity permits. The instructions to the patient are the same as those given during the first visit.

*Third visit*: At the next visit, 1–2 days after the second visit, the patient's condition should be improved significantly. Scaling and root planing should be done frequently to improve treatment outcomes. The patient is instructed to discontinue $H_2O_2$ rinses. However, chlorhexidine rinses should be advised to continue for further 2 or 3 weeks.

## Management of the Residual Condition

*Elimination of predisposing factors*: In further visits, the tooth surfaces in the affected areas are scaled and smoothed regularly as per the requirement. The adoption of plaque control methods by the patient is checked and corrected. Patients without gingival disease other than the treated acute involvement are dismissed for one week. If the condition is satisfactory at that time, the patient is dismissed for one month, at which time the schedule for subsequent recall visits is determined according to the patient's needs. However, if the chronic gingivitis, periodontal pockets, and pericoronal flaps are present, then appointments are scheduled for their treatment and elimination of all forms of local irritation.

Patients with toxic systemic complications or local lymphadenopathy need systemic administration of antibiotics for adequate control of infection.

*Nutritional supplements*: It may be indicated in rare instances when NUG patients suffer such severe pain that the ingestion of a normal diet is difficult. Thus, difficulty in chewing raw fruits and vegetables in such painful conditions could lead to the selection of a diet inadequate in vitamins B and C. Standard multivitamin preparation combined with a therapeutic dose of vitamins B and C is recommended, which may be discontinued after two months.

Supportive systemic treatments, including bed rest, copious fluid consumption, and analgesics for relief of pain, are prescribed.

*Correction of gingival tissue deformities by surgery*: Remaining gingival interproximal craters increase plaque retention. Such defects are eliminated by reshaping gingiva surgically or with electrosurgery to establish and maintain the normal interproximal gingival contour. If the defects are more severe, flap surgery or periodontal plastic surgery may be required. Surgery should not be attempted until the local etiologic factors have been eliminated, and inflammation has resolved.

Treatment of NUG includes:[14]
- Oral hygiene instructions
- Mechanical debridement of the teeth
- Systemic antimicrobial therapy
- Surgical correction of gingival contour

## PRIMARY HERPETIC GINGIVOSTOMATITIS

Primary herpetic gingivostomatitis is the most common viral infection of the gingiva caused by the herpes simplex virus type 1 (HSV-1).[15] Both males and females get affected equally with this viral condition. Infants and children younger than six years of age are the frequent victims of primary herpetic gingivostomatitis.[16] However, it is also noted in adolescents and adults. The course of the disease is limited to 7–10 days. In most persons, however, the primary infection is asymptomatic. Once the primary infection gets over, the virus ascends through sensory and autonomic nerves and stays in neuronal ganglia that innervate the site as latent HSV. The virus may be reactivated by various stimuli, including ultraviolet light, trauma, fever, stress, or immunosuppression. Herpes labialis, herpes genitalis, ocular herpes, and herpetic encephalitis are some of the common secondary manifestations of HSV-1 infection.

## Oral Manifestations

### Signs

Oral lesions affect both oral mucosa and gingiva. Lesions are diffuse, erythematous with shiny involvement of the gingiva and the adjacent oral mucosa with varying edema degrees. Gingival bleeding is common. Herpetic lesions are characteristically discrete, spherical gray vesicles occupying the area of the gingiva, labial and buccal mucosa, soft palate, pharynx, sublingual mucosa, and tongue. Subsequently, the vesicles get rupture to form painful, small ulcers with a red, elevated, halo-like margin and a depressed, yellowish, or greyish-white central portion **(Fig. 20.2)**. Occasionally, primary herpetic gingivitis lacks overt vesiculation. Diffuse, erythematous, shiny discoloration, and edematous enlargement of the gingiva with a tendency towards bleeding are the peculiar features. Though the ulcerative lesions healed, the diffuse gingival erythema and edema persist for several days. Scarring is absent in the areas of healed ulcerations.[17]

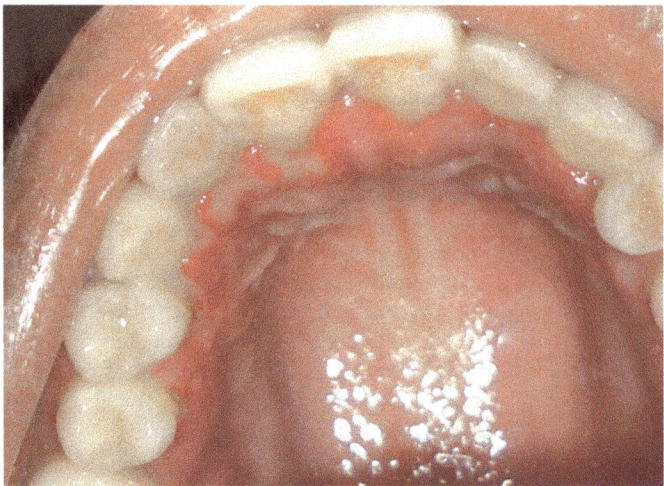

**Fig. 20.2:** Clinical picture showing herpetic gingivostomatitis. (*Courtesy*: Dr. Gayathri Rao)

### Symptoms

Generalized soreness of the oral cavity interferes with normal eating and drinking. The ruptured vesicles are extremely painful and sensitive to touch, thermal changes, foods such as condiments and fruit juices, and the action of coarse foods. Infants with this condition are irritable and refuse to take food.

Cervical adenitis, fever as high as 101–105°F (38.3–40.6°C), and generalized malaise are common systemic signs and symptoms.

## Histopathology

The virus targets the epithelial cells causing acantholysis and nuclear clearing resulting in the formation of Tzanck cells. Intraepithelial vesicles are formed, which contain fluid, degenerating cells, and herpes virus. Discrete ulcerations exhibit a central portion of acute inflammation with the varying degree of purulent exudates and surrounding zone of engorged blood vessels.

## Diagnosis

The diagnosis is usually established from the patient's history and the clinical findings. The confirmatory diagnosis depends on one or more of the following laboratory tests:
- *Inoculation of the virus from a suspected site to tissue culture*: This technique takes 3–6 days; the virus can be distinguished as type 1 and 2.
- *Fluorescent monoclonal antibody testing of scraping*: This technique requires 15–20 minutes.
- Serologic studies

## Differential Diagnosis

Primary herpetic gingivostomatitis should be differentiated from the following conditions:

- *Herpangia* is the result of group A coxsackievirus. The lesions in herpes simplex are located predominantly in the anterior portion of the mouth, whereas those resulting from coxsackievirus are seen in the posterior oral pharynx. Furthermore, the duration of illness is longer with the herpes simplex virus
- *Erythema multiforme* can be differentiated because the vesicles in erythema multiforme are generally more extensive than those in primary herpetic gingivostomatitis and on rupture demonstrate a tendency towards pseudomembrane formation.
- *Stevens–Johnson syndrome* is a comparatively rare form of erythema multiforme, characterized by vesicular hemorrhagic lesions in the oral cavity, hemorrhagic ocular lesions, and bullous skin lesions.
- *Bullous lichen planus* is very rare and painful condition. It is characterized by large blisters on the tongue and cheek that rupture and undergo ulceration; it runs a prolonged, indefinite course. Patches of linear, gray, lace-like lesions of lichen planus are often interspersed among the bullous eruptions. Lichen planus involvement of the skin may coexist with the oral lesions and facilitate differential diagnosis.
- *Aphthous ulcer* is usually manifested as single ulceration with an erythematous halo surrounding a yellowish fibrinopurulent membrane **(Fig. 20.3)**.

## Treatment

- *Supportive treatment*: Palliative measures make the patient comfortable until the disease runs its course. It runs a 7–10 days course and heals without a scar. Bland foods and liquid supplements are recommended.[17] If the patient is experiencing the pain of longer duration, aspirin or a nonsteroidal anti-inflammatory agent can be given systemically. Plaque, food debris, and superficial calculus are removed to reduce gingival inflammation, which complicates the acute herpetic involvement. Extensive periodontal therapy should be postponed until the acute symptoms subside to avoid the possibility of exacerbation.
- *Mucosal ointments*: Mucosal ointments (orabase) can be applied to lesions with cotton swabs for temporary relief. Especially before meals, topical local anesthetic, such as lidocaine hydrochloride viscous solution, can be applied to the affected areas.
- *Antiviral chemotherapy*: Herpes virus-specific drugs, such as acyclovir ointment (apply five times daily for five days) are used to lessen the spread and severity of recurrent herpes virus infection. Systemic administration of acyclovir has not demonstrated to alter the clinical course of primary herpes. Still, it may reduce the duration of viral shedding during which the patient is potentially infectious. Acyclovir blocks the replication of the virus by inhibiting viral DNA polymerase activity.[18] Systemically administered acyclovir (200 mg 5 times daily for five days) may be beneficial for an immunocompromised patient.

## PERICORONITIS

### Definition

Pericoronitis refers to inflammation of the gingiva in relation to the crown of an incompletely erupted tooth. It may be acute, subacute or chronic. It commonly affects the partially erupted or impacted mandibular third molar. Food debris gets accumulated in the space between the crown of the tooth and the overlying gingival flap. This favors bacterial growth and inflammation in the respective space **(Fig. 20.4)**. Chronic inflammation of the gingival flap and varying degrees of ulceration along its inner surface are common findings. Such findings are present even when the

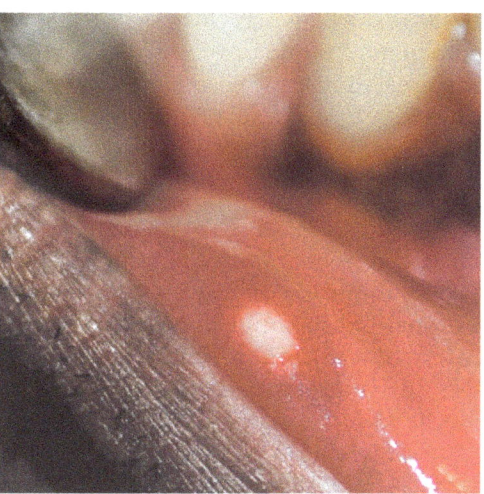

**Fig. 20.3:** Clinical picture showing aphthous ulcer.

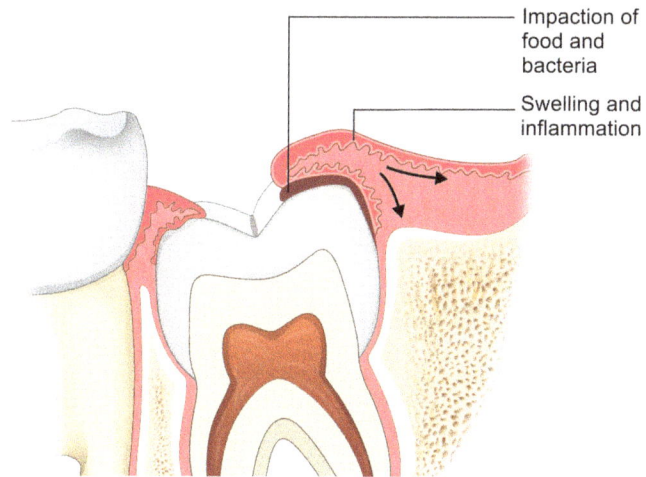

**Fig. 20.4:** Schematic representation showing pericoronitis.

patient is without clinical features. Acute pericoronitis is identified by varying degrees of inflammatory involvement of the pericoronal flap and adjacent structures along with systemic complications. The inflammatory fluid and cellular exudates increase the bulk of the flap. A bulky flap usually interferes with the jaws' closure and is injured by contact with the opposing jaw. This enhances further the inflammatory reactions.[19]

## Clinical Features

A patient with pericoronitis usually exhibit the following clinical features:

### Symptoms

- *Pain*: Pain is usually mild. However, a quite intense pain gets radiate to the external neck, throat, ear, or oral floor.
- *Trismus*: Inability of the patient to open the jaw more than a few millimeters represents the tenderness and extreme pain.[20]
- A bad taste in the mouth is due to oozing of pus from beneath the flap.
- Swelling in the neck or the area of the affected tooth.
- Fever

### Signs

- A partially erupted tooth.
- Markedly red, swollen, and suppurating lesion around a partially erupted tooth (**Fig. 20.5**).
- Pus oozing from under an overlaying tissue flap.
- A painful reaction when finger pressure is applied.
- Swelling of the cheek (in the region of the angle of the jaw).
- Cervical lymphadenopathy
- Signs of toxic systemic complications, such as elevated temperature, leukocytosis, malaise, and ipsilateral tonsillitis or upper respiratory infection.

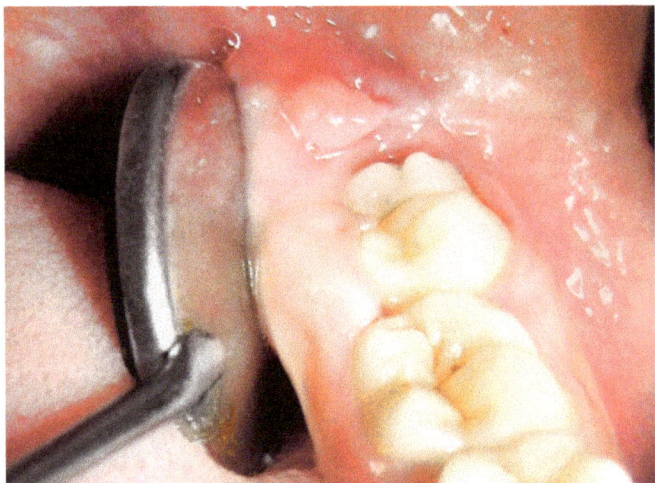

**Fig. 20.5:** Clinical picture showing pericoronitis the third molar partially covered by an infected flap.

## Complications

Common complications associated with pericoronitis are as follows:
- Pericoronal abscess
- *Lymphadenopathy*: Submaxillary, posterior cervical, deep cervical, and retropharyngeal lymph nodes are involved. However, lymph node involvement depends on the extent and severity of the infection.
- Peritonsillar abscess formation, cellulitis, and Ludwig's angina are infrequent sequelae of acute pericoronitis.

## Treatment

Following emergency procedures are recommended in the treatment of pericoronitis.

### Nonsurgical Therapy

Debris and exudates from the affected area are removed by flushing warm water and $H_2O_2$. After elevating the flap gently from the tooth with a scaler, the area is swabbed with antiseptic. The underlying debris is removed, and the area is again flushed with warm water. If the patient is febrile or with palpable lymph nodes, appropriate antibiotics (amoxicillin and metronidazole combination) are advised.

### Surgical Therapy

With the recovery from acute symptoms, a further plan of action is decided about retaining or extracting the tooth. The decision as to whether to save the tooth or to extract it depends on various factors like its position, opposing tooth, chances of the eruption to proper occlusion and periodontal status.

*Operculectomy*: If it is decided to save the tooth, an operculectomy is done. LA is given (usually inferior alveolar nerve block) for a mandibular molar. Periodontal knives or electrosurgery is used to remove the pericoronal flap. The incision is given anterior to the anterior border of ramus and brought downwards and forward to the distal surface of the crown as close as possible to the level of cementoenamel junction (CEJ), which will detach a wedge-shaped tissue. It is necessary to remove the tissue distal to the tooth, as well as the flap on the occlusal surface (**Figs. 20.6A and B**). Incising only the occlusal portion of the flap leaves a deep distal pocket. This can enhance the recurrence of acute pericoronal involvement.

*Extraction*: It is best to extract the tooth after acute symptoms subside if the tooth is not going to serve any purpose. All pericoronal flaps should be viewed with suspicion. Persistent symptom-free pericoronal flaps should be removed as a preventive measure against subsequent acute involvement. With the extraction of partially or entirely impacted third molars, bone loss on the distal surface of the second molars is a common complication. The problem is significantly greater if third molars are extracted after the

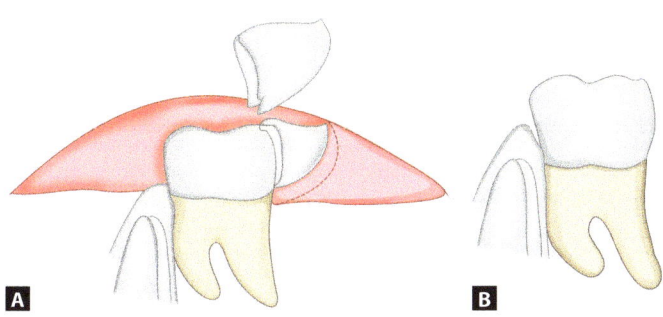

**Figs. 20.6A and B:** Schematic representation showing operculectomy: (A) Removal of operculum distal to the 3rd molar; and (B) Appearance of healed area.

roots are formed or in patients older than their early 20s. To reduce the risk of bone loss around second molars, partially or entirely impacted third molars should be extracted as early as possible in their development.

> **Points to Ponder**
>
> ❏ Necrotizing ulcerative gingivitis is a tender and infectious gingival disease involving mainly the interdental and marginal gingiva.
> ❏ In NUG, the zone between the marginal necrosis and the relatively unaffected gingiva usually exhibits a well-demarcated narrow erythematous zone, sometimes referred to as the linear erythema. Patients with pericoronitis are extremely uncomfortable due to foul taste in the mouth and an inability to close the jaws completely. Moreover, the condition is very painful.
> ❏ While removing pseudomembrane in NUG patients, the use of a single pellet with a sweeping motion over large areas is contraindicated. Each cotton pellet is used in a small area and is then discarded.

## REFERENCES

1. Cogen RB. Acute necrotizing ulcerative gingivitis. In: Genco RJ, Goldman HM, Cohen DW (Eds). Contemporary Periodontics. St. Louis: CV Mosby; 1990. pp. 459-65.
2. Carranza FA, Klokkevold PR. Acute gingival infections. In: Newman MG, Takei HH, Carranza FA (Eds). Carranza's Clinical Periodontology, 9th edition. Philadelphia, PA, USA: WB Saunders; 2003. pp. 297-307.
3. Grant DA, Stern IB, Listgarten MA. Necrotizing ulcerative gingivitis. In: Periodontics, 6th edition. St. Louis: CV Mosby; 1988. pp. 398-12.
4. Plaut HC. Bacterial diagnostic studies of diphtheria and oral diseases. Dtsch Med Wochenschr. 1894;20:920-3.
5. Vincent H. The etiology and the histopathology of hospital rot. Ann de l'Insti Pasteur. 1896;10:488-510.
6. Eley BM, Soory M, Manson JD. Acute necrotizing ulcerative gingivitis. In: Periodontics, 5th edition. Philadelphia, PA, USA: Churchill Livingstone; 2004. pp. 354-57.
7. Folayan MO. The epidemiology, etiology, and pathophysiology of acute necrotizing ulcerative gingivitis associated with malnutrition. J Contemp Dent Pract. 2004;5(3):28-41.
8. Pindborg JJ, Bhat M, Devanath KR, Narayana HR, Ramachandra S. Occurrence of acute necrotizing gingivitis in South Indian children. J Periodontol. 1966;37(1):14-9.
9. Horning GM, Cohen ME. Necrotizing ulcerative gingivitis, periodontitis, and stomatitis: clinical staging and predisposing factors. J Periodontol. 1995;66(11):990-8.
10. Holmstrup P, Westergaard J. Necrotizing periodontal disease. In: Lindhe J, Karring T, Lang NP (Eds). Clinical Periodontology and Implant Dentistry, 4th edition. Chicago, USA: Blackwell Munksgaard; 2003. pp. 243-59.
11. Listgarten MA. Electron microscopic observations on the bacterial flora of acute necrotizing ulcerative gingivitis. J Periodontol. 1965;36:328-39.
12. Rowland RW. Necrotizing ulcerative gingivitis. Ann Periodontol. 1999;4(1):65-73.
13. Klokkevold PR, Takei HH. Treatment of acute gingival disease. In: Newman MG, Takei HH, Carranza FA (Eds). Carranza's Clinical Periodontology, 9th edition. Philadelphia, PA, USA: WB Saunders; 2003. pp. 622-8.
14. Johnson BD, Engel D. Acute necrotizing ulcerative gingivitis. A review of diagnosis, etiology and treatment. J Periodontol. 1986;57(3):141-50.
15. Scott TF, Steigman AJ, Convey JH. Acute infectious gingivostomatitis: etiology, epidemiology, and clinical pictures of a common disorders caused by the virus of herpes simplex. JAMA. 1941;117:999-1005.
16. McNair ST. Herpetic stomatitis. J Dent Res. 1950;29:647.
17. Grant DA, Stern IB, Listgarten MA. Viral infections. In: Periodontics, 6th edition. St. Louis: CV Mosby; 1988. pp. 413-20.
18. Rose LF. Infective forms of gingivostomatitis. In: Genco RJ, Goldman HM, Cohen DW (Eds). Contemporary Periodontics. St. Louis: CV Mosby; 1990. pp. 243-50.
19. Genco RJ. Periodontal diagnosis, prognosis, and treatment planning. In: Genco RJ, Goldman HM, Cohen DW (Eds). Contemporary Periodontics. St. Louis: CV Mosby; 1990. pp. 348-59.
20. Grant DA, Stern IB, Listgarten MA. Pericoronitis. In: Periodontics, 6th edition. St. Louis: CV Mosby; 1988. pp. 421-4.

## VIVA VOCE

**Q1. Name various acute periodontal diseases.**
**Ans.** Acute periodontal diseases are gingival abscess, periodontal abscess, necrotizing ulcerative gingivitis, acute herpetic gingivostomatitis, pericoronal abscess (pericoronitis) and combined endodontic- periodontal lesions.

**Q2. Why was necrotizing ulcerative gingivitis called a trench mouth?**
**Ans.** Necrotizing ulcerative gingivitis was called a trench mouth because it was frequently found among soldiers in the frontline trenches during World War I.

**Q3. Which mouthwash is usually recommended for necrotizing ulcerative gingivitis patients?**
**Ans.** Mouthwash 3% hydrogen peroxide ($H_2O_2$) is usually recommended for necrotizing ulcerative gingivitis patients. The patient is asked to rinse with a glassful of an equal mixture of 3% $H_2O_2$ and warm water every 2 hours. A twice-daily rinse with 0.12% chlorhexidine is also very effective.

**Section 4:** Pathology of Gingival and Periodontal Diseases

**Q4. What is the course of acute herpetic gingivostomatitis?**
**Ans.** The course of acute herpetic gingivostomatitis is usually limited to 7–10 days. Ulcers heal without scars.

**Q5. Why is trismus associated with pericoronitis?**
**Ans.** Superficial and deep head of masseter muscle gets inserted to the lower one-fourth of the mandibular ramus. It functions synergistically with the medial pterygoid muscle in forming a sling that pulls the mandible upward and forward. The deep belly origins of the masseter muscle intermingle with the superficial fibers of the temporalis muscle along the mandible's external oblique ridge. Irritation of these muscle fibers attributable to pericoronal inflammation in the mandibular molars commonly causes myospasm and trismus.

**Q6. What are the clinical findings of NUG?**
**Ans.**
- Constantly radiating and gnawing gingival pain. Ulceration: Punched-out crater-like depression at the crest of the interdental papilla.
- Spontaneous gingival bleeding.[14]

**Q7. What are the synonyms of NUG?**
**Ans.** Trench mouth, Vincent's gingivostomatitis, Vincent's gingivitis, ulceromembranous gingivitis, ANUG, and fusospirochetal gingivitis.

**Q8. Why there is no pocket formation in NUG?**
**Ans.** Necrosis of the epithelial cells results in an epithelium that is unable to exhibit any proliferation or migration. Therefore, there is no pocket formation.

**Q9. What are the secondary manifestations of HSV-1 infection?**
**Ans.** Herpes labialis, herpes genitalis, ocular herpes, and herpetic encephalitis.

**Q10. What are the common complications associated with pericoronitis?**
**Ans.** Pericoronal abscess, lymphadenopathy, peritonsillar abscess formation, cellulitis, and Ludwig's angina.

# Chapter 21

# Soft and Hard Tissue Lesions

*Shailja Chatterjee, Shalu Bathla*

## Chapter Outline

- Desquamative Gingivitis
- Metastatic Tumors of the Jaws
- Malignant Lesions of Gingiva
- Reactive Lesions of Gingiva
- Peripheral Odontogenic Lesions
- Granulomatous Gingivitis
- Benign Neoplasms
- Malignant Neoplasms

## INTRODUCTION

Some hard and soft pathological conditions may affect various parts of the body, including the oral cavity. These lesions are widespread and may affect the periodontium. Some of these lesions involving gingiva and other periodontal tissues are summarized in this chapter.

## DESQUAMATIVE GINGIVITIS

Prinz, in 1932, coined the term "chronic desquamative gingivitis," which describes the various gingival conditions presenting with peculiar features of intense erythema, desquamation, and ulceration.[1] In 1960, McCarthy reported desquamative gingivitis as a gingival response to several other associated diseases. It was not a specific disease entity affecting gingiva as it was thought before. Still, it found as clinical manifestations of other disorders.[2] It was reported that 75% of desquamative gingivitis cases have a dermatologic origin.

## Diagnosis

Desquamative gingivitis is a clinical manifestation of other diseases that characteristically describe the gingival condition and not a diagnosis. Hence, it requires a series of laboratory procedures to arrive at a final diagnosis.[3]

- *Clinical history*: A thorough clinical case history is needed to begin the assessment of desquamative gingivitis.
- *Clinical examination*: Pattern of distribution of the lesions, i.e., focal or multifocal, with or without the involvement of skin provides leading information to begin the formulation of a differential diagnosis.
- *Biopsy*: An incisional biopsy is the best alternative to begin the microscopic and immunological evaluation. For conventional hematoxylin and eosin (H&E) evaluation, buffered formalin (10%) should be used to fix the tissue. For immunofluorescent assessment, Michell's buffer (ammonium sulfate buffer, pH 7.0) is used as a transport solution.
- *Microscopic examination*: Formalin-fixed sections of approximately 5 μm, paraffin-embedded, tissue stained with conventional H&E are obtained for light microscopy examination.
- *Immunofluorescence*: They are of two types: (1) direct immunofluorescence and (2) indirect immunofluorescence. Immunofluorescence tests are positive if a fluorescent signal is seen either in the epithelium, basement membrane, or in connective tissue.

### Lichen Planus

Lichen planus is a common mucocutaneous disease with unknown etiology. Most of the patients with oral lichen planus are middle-aged and particularly affect older women (2:1 ratio of female-to-male). The condition is rare in children.

### *Clinical Features*

Clinically, oral lesions of lichen planus consist of asymptomatic, chronic bilateral interlacing white lines (Wickham's striae) occupying the area of the posterior buccal mucosa (90% cases), tongue (30%) or alveolar ridge/

gingiva (13%).[4] Clinical manifestations may include white lacy slightly elevated patterns, plaque-type, and atrophic, ulcerative or bullous presentations.

The gingival lesions of lichen planus fall into one or more of the following categories:[5]

- *Keratotic lesions*: These are small-raised, round white papules of pinhead size with a flattened surface and usually present on the attached gingiva. The keratotic lesions are further classified as papular, plaque-like, linear, reticular (**Fig. 21.1**), or annular.
- *Vesiculobullous lesions*: These raised, fluid-filled lesions are uncommon and short-lived on the gingiva. They quickly rupture and leave ulcerations. These uncommon lesions make diagnosis difficult.
- *Atrophic lesions*: Atrophy of the gingival tissues with ensuing epithelial thinning results in erythema confined to the gingiva. It is the most common type of gingival lichen planus producing desquamative gingivitis.
- *Erosive lesions/ulcerative lesions*: Erosive form may appear as desquamative gingivitis (**Fig. 21.2**).

These extensive erythematous areas with a patchy distribution may present as focal or diffuse hemorrhagic areas exacerbated by slight trauma (e.g., toothbrushing).

### Histopathological Features

Hyperkeratosis, hydropic degeneration of the basal layer, the saw-tooth configuration of the rete ridges, and a dense band-like infiltrate primarily of T lymphocytes in the lamina propria are observed. Colloid bodies (civatte bodies) may be seen at the epithelium connective tissue interface.[6]

### Treatment

- *Steroids (topical steroids)*: The erosive, bullous, or ulcerative lesions of oral lichen planus are treated with high-potency topical steroids 0.05% fluocinonide ointment TID. Intralesional injections of 10–20 mg triamcinolone are effective in treating lesions that are nonresponsive to topical or systemic steroids.[7]
- *Antifungals*: Secondary candidiasis, which develops after constant use of topical steroids, can be treated by antifungals. Nystatin oral pastilles (100,000 IU) BID for a month. Other antifungals are nystatin ointment, ketoconazole tablets, clotrimazole oral troches and griseofulvin.[7]
- *Topical and systemic retinoids*: These are synthetically derived vitamin A analogues that affect keratinization and thus beneficial for treating lichen planus.[7]
- *Cyclosporine*: This immunosuppressant drug suppresses the T helper cell and inhibits the lymphocytic infiltrate in lichen planus. However, drug-associated side effects and high cost restricts its use in severe and resistant cases only.[7]
- *Free gingival grafts*: They are usually beneficial to treat an erosive form of lichen planus.[8]

## Cicatricial Pemphigoid (Mucous Membrane Pemphigoid)

It is also known as mucous membrane pemphigoid (MMP). It is a chronic vesiculobullous autoimmune disorder. It is closely related to bullous pemphigoid (BP), but there are no circulating antibodies, unlike BP. MMP predominantly affects women in their 5th decade of life, and occasionally young children. The target antigens identified in MMP include the BP antigens 1 and 2 (BPAg 1 and BPAg 2), type VII collagen, β4 integrin subunit, and laminins 5 and 6.

*Clinical features*: Lesions are vesiculobullous in nature. The gingiva manifests persistent erythema for weeks after the original erosions have healed. These oral lesions rarely scar.

*Histopathological features*: Subepithelial clefting occurs with separation of the epithelium from the underlying lamina propria, leaving an intact basal layer. A mixed inflammatory infiltrates consisting of lymphocytes, plasma

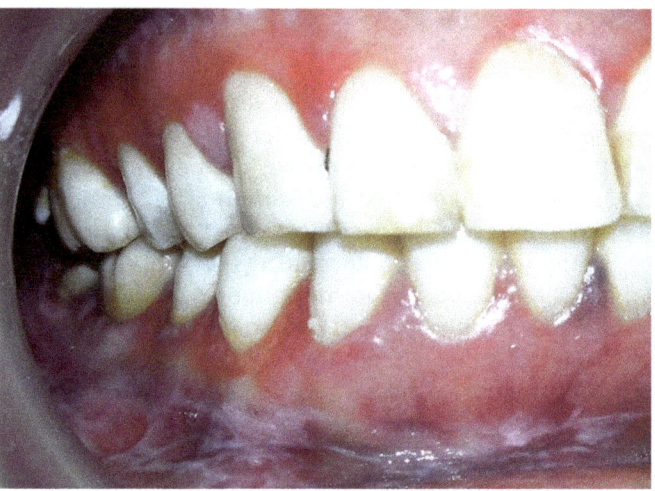

**Fig. 21.1:** Clinical picture showing reticular lichen planus.

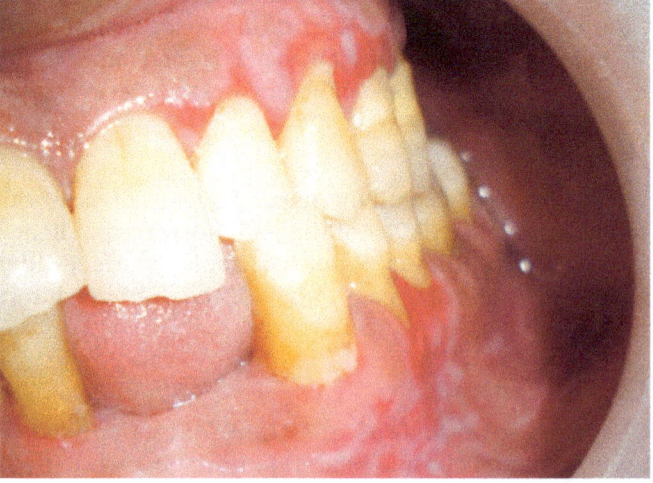

**Fig. 21.2:** Clinical photograph showing erosive lichen planus.
(*Courtesy*: Dr Gayathri Rao)

cells, neutrophils, and scarce eosinophils is observed in the stroma. Direct immunofluorescence reveals deposits of immunoglobulin G (IgG) and complement components (C3) restricted to the basement membrane.

*Treatment:* Topical corticosteroid therapy using fluocinonide (0.05%) and clobetasol propionate (0.05%) in an adhesive vehicle, which can be used three times a day for up to 6 months. When lesions do not respond to steroids, systemic dapsone is given.

## Pemphigus

Pemphigus is a group of rare autoimmune mucocutaneous disorders presented with epithelial blistering of cutaneous and/or mucosal surfaces. These are serious conditions and turn out as potentially life-threatening events. The term "pemphigus' is derived from the Greek word "Pemphix," meaning "bubble or blister." A linkage to human leukocyte antigen (HLA) class II alleles suggests a strong genetic potential for pemphigus inheritance.[9]

### Pemphigus Vulgaris

Pemphigus vulgaris (PV) is the most common type of pemphigus. It is a blistering autoimmune disease mediated by circulating autoantibodies, especially IgG antibodies, against the cadherin-type adhesion molecules: Desmoglein 1 (Dsg1) and desmoglein 3 (Dsg3).[10] The condition is potentially life-threatening, with a significant mortality rate.

*Clinical features*: Oral lesions are the first sign of the disease in approximately 60% of patients and may present one year or more before the cutaneous lesions. Virtually, any region of the oral cavity can be involved, but multiple lesions often develop at sites of irritation or trauma. The soft palate is more frequently involved (80%), followed by the buccal mucosa (46%), ventral aspect or dorsum of the tongue (20%), and lower labial mucosa (10%). The gingiva is not a major intraoral site; however, when gingival lesions occur, they are desquamative. These are initially vesiculobullous but readily rupture with ulcer formation.

*Diagnosis*: The Nikolsky sign is positive in PV. This clinical test is performed using either an air syringe to blow air on the perilesional tissue or gently rubbing the perilesional tissue with a finger. If the mucosa surface layer separates from the underlying tissue, the patient is said to exhibit a positive Nikolsky sign. Diagnosis mainly depends on histological and immunostaining examination of biopsy material of perilesional tissue. Serum autoantibodies to either Dsg1 or Dsg3 are detected by indirect immunofluorescence technique employing monkeyoesophagus or by enzyme-linked immunosorbent assay.

*Histopathological features*: PV lesions demonstrate a characteristic intraepithelial clefting or vesiculation above the basal cell layer with a characteristic "tombstone"

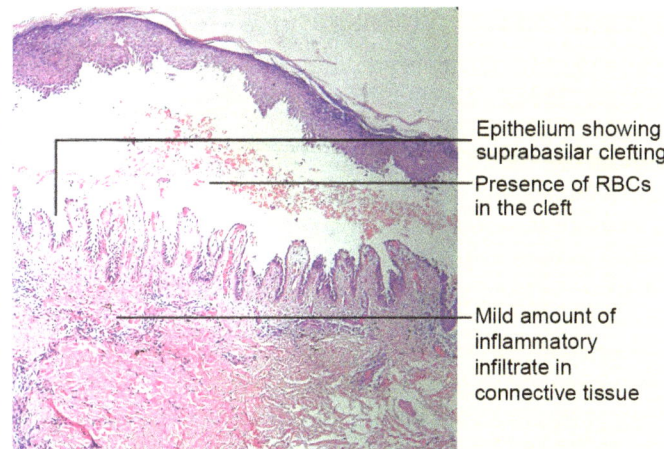

**Fig. 21.3:** Histological representation showing pemphigus.

appearance. Rounded acantholytic Tzanck cells are visible in the cleft. The subjacent stroma usually exhibits a mild-to-moderate chronic inflammatory cells infiltrate **(Fig. 21.3)**.[9]

### Paraneoplastic Pemphigus

The other important variant of pemphigus affecting the oral cavity is paraneoplastic pemphigus, which is usually associated with lymphoproliferative disease. Sometimes, oral lesions might be the only manifestation. The autoantibodies are IgG or IgA type and are directed against Desmoplakin 1, Desmoplakin 2 and BP230 (bullous pemphigoid antigen 1).[11]

*Treatment:* Current treatment is largely based on systemic corticosteroids with or without immunosuppressive agents and tacrolimus. Previously only steroids were administered to control the disease. However, high initial and maintenance doses of steroids were necessary to control the disease. If the patient responds well to corticosteroids, the dosage can be gradually reduced, but a low-maintenance dosage is usually necessary to prevent or minimize the recurrence of lesions. In patients not responsive to corticosteroids or who gradually adapt to them, steroid-sparing therapies are used. They consist of combinations of steroids plus other medications, such as azathioprine, cyclosporine, dapsone, gold, and methotrexate. Topical antifungal medication may be needed to eliminate iatrogenic *candidiasis*, which often arises when topical steroids are used intraorally. Intravenous administration of immunoglobulins has found to be safe and with a good outcome in steroid-resistant PV. Plasmapheresis, sometimes with cyclosporin or cyclophosphamide, has also been reported to be of benefit.

Meticulous oral hygiene and periodontal care are essential for the overall management of patients with pemphigus.[12] Patients in the maintenance phase may require prednisolone before professional oral prophylaxis and periodontal surgery.

## Systemic Lupus Erythematosus

The systemic lupus erythematosus (SLE) or lupus is a chronic inflammatory disease with multiorgan system involvement. It is an autoimmune disease involving connective tissue with various clinical manifestations and characteristically following relapsing and remitting pattern. It is more prevalent in young women, compared to men with a female-to-male ratio as 9:1. In women, the peak age of disease onset is between late teens and early 40s.

Systemic lupus erythematosus can turn out potentially life-threatening disorders. Although the exact etiology is still unknown, a complex genetic involvement has a significant role in disease causation. Sunlight and drugs are well-identified precipitating factors for disease progression, and antichromatin, anti-DNA, and antihistone antibodies are the identified underlying pathogenic causes. Circulating autoantibodies may be present for many years before and there may be an increase in numbers of these antibodies before clinical manifestations.[13]

Oral manifestations are prevalent in 7–52% in patients with SLE. However, most of the oral lesions are asymptomatic.

*Clinical features:* Clinical presentations of SLE are of three types: (1) discoid, (2) erythematous, and (3) ulcerations. Discoid lesions present with central areas of erythema with white spots and surrounding radiating white striae and telangiectasia at its periphery. Erythematous lesions are often present with edema and petechial reddening. Ulcers are shallow, 1–2 cm in diameter, and usually appear in crops.

*Histopathological features:* There are hyperkeratosis, keratotic plugging, and liquefactive degeneration of the basal layer of epithelium. Lamina propria shows chronic inflammatory perivascular infiltrates (lymphohistiocytic) **(Fig. 21.4)**. Direct immunofluorescence shows immunoglobulin M (IgM), IgG, complement, and fibrinogen deposits along the dermal-epidermal junction.

*Treatment:* Management of SLE is mostly based on disease severity and its extent. Cutaneous rashes are treated with topical steroids, sunscreens, and hydroxychloroquine. For severe systemic organ involvement, moderate-to-high doses of prednisolone are effective. For severe SLE cases or when side effects to prednisolone develop, immunosuppressive drugs, such as cytotoxic drugs (cyclophosphamide and azathioprine) and plasmapheresis alone or in conjunction with steroids are useful.

## Erythema Multiforme

Erythema multiforme is an acute, self-limiting inflammatory disorder of the skin and mucous membranes with a the tendency for recurrence and distinctive clinical appearance. It is considered as a hypersensitivity reaction to a variety of precipitating agents, including drugs, neoplasms, and infections.

Circulating immune complexes play an essential role in the pathogenesis of erythema multiforme. Direct immunofluorescence studies show granular deposits of C3 and IgM in the superficial dermal vessels or at the dermal-epidermal junction.[14]

*Clinical features:* Cutaneous involvement exhibits as erythematous papules. Target lesions are distributed symmetrically over the extensor surfaces. Mucosal involvement is in the form of ulcerations or papules, as in Stevens–Johnson's syndrome. There are multiple, large, shallow, painful ulcers with an erythematous border. They may affect the entire oral mucosa in approximately 20% of erythema multiforme patients. The lesions commonly affect the buccal mucosa and tongue, followed by the labial mucosa with hemorrhagic crusting of the lips. Less commonly affected are the floor of the mouth, hard and soft palate, and the gingiva. Chewing and swallowing are impaired.

*Histopathological features:* Microvascular proliferation is seen in the papillary dermis/lamina propria juxta-epithelial. Perivasculitis is evident.

*Treatment:* There is no specific treatment for erythema multiforme. Some cases may even resolve spontaneously, and erythematous lesions may require no treatment. For mild symptoms, systemic and local antihistamine coupled with topical anesthetics and debridement of lesions with an oxygenating agent is adequate. In patients with severe symptoms, corticosteroids are prescribed.

## METASTATIC TUMORS OF THE JAWS

The majority of metastasis to the oral region is intraosseous. The gingiva (including the alveolar mucosa) is most often the seat of soft-tissue metastasis in the mouth. In the oral regions, soft-tissue metastasis from lung cancer is encountered most frequently in men, while metastasis from breast cancer accounts for most soft-

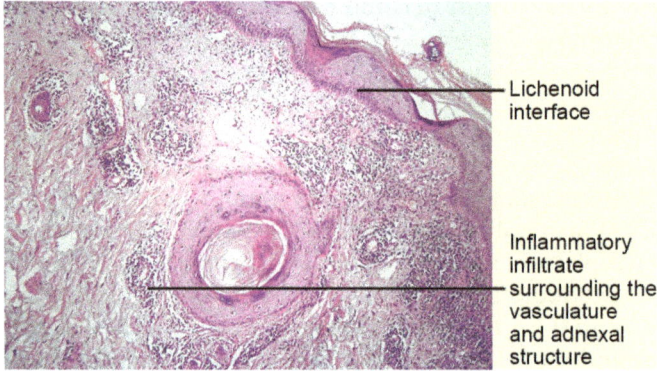

**Fig. 21.4:** Histological representation showing systemic lupus erythematosus (SLE).

tissue metastasis in women. About 20% of oral soft-tissue metastasis was manifested before the primary tumor was diagnosed. Furthermore, in 90% of the cases, the clinical manifestation resembled a hyperplastic or reactive lesion. These observations emphasize the need for a histological examination of all such tumors. The histopathology resembles the tumor of origin. Most cases are carcinomas whereas, sarcomas rarely metastasize to the oral region.

Poorly differentiated histopathological appearance of metastatic jaw disease imposes difficulties in determining the primary site of the lesion.

Radiologically, lesions appear as well to poorly circumscribed radiolucencies. An extension into the alveolar bone may be mistakenly considered as a periodontal disease when the metastatic disease of the jaws spread into the overlying soft tissues gives the impression of a dental or periodontal infection. Metastasis may occur directly in the soft tissues, including the gingiva.

Pyogenic granuloma, peripheral giant cell granuloma, peripheral ossifying fibroma, or fibroma are the important differential diagnoses of metastatic peripheral lesions on the gingiva or alveolar ridge excluded before diagnosis.[15]

## MALIGNANT LESIONS OF GINGIVA

### Proliferative Verrucous Leukoplakia

The term "proliferative verrucous leukoplakia (PVL)" was based upon its clinical appearance resembling an expanding verrucal white growth. The early lesions of PVL appear as a deceptive solitary homogenous leukoplakia. Despite its innocuous appearance, the leukoplakia recurs and rapidly spreads over time, resulting in a diffuse, multifocal, and exophytic or verrucous type of oral lesions.

*Clinical features*: The most common site is buccal mucosa, followed by the gingiva and the tongue. However, gingival lesions exhibit the greatest malignant transformation rate, usually seven years after the initial diagnosis.

*Histopathological features*: Varying grades of epithelial dysplasia can be seen with superficial surface showing verrucal exophytic growth **(Fig. 21.5)**.

*Treatment*: Surgical eradication and laser vaporization of the lesions is difficult due to the widespread nature of the condition with disappointing results of repeated recurrences.

### Squamous Cell Carcinoma

Squamous cell carcinoma is the most common malignancy of the oral cavity and oropharynx. The gingival involvement represents about 15–25% for oral epithelial malignancies. Gingiva is reported as the third most common site for squamous cell carcinoma. Mandibular gingival squamous cell carcinoma is more common compared to the maxillary counterparts in a 2: 1 ratio.

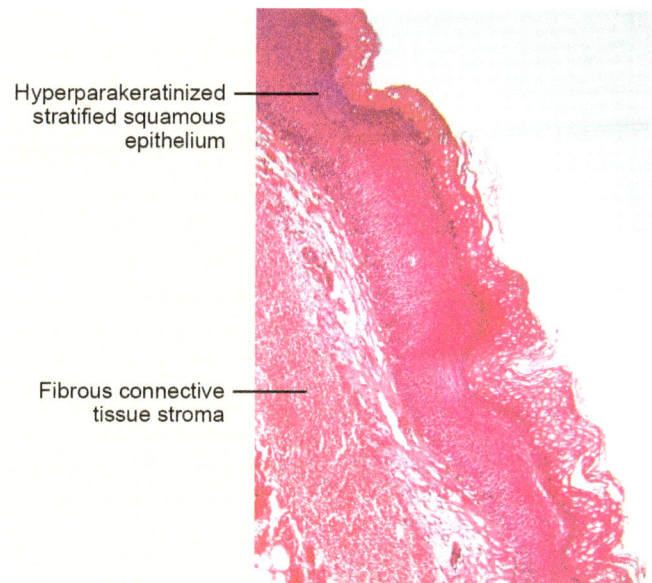

**Fig. 21.5:** Histological representation showing proliferative verrucous leukoplakia (PVL).

*Clinical features*: Clinical manifestations of gingival squamous cell carcinoma vary from exophytic irregular outgrowth, ulcerative to flat, erosive lesions. It sometimes deceptively mimics innocuous inflammatory conditions. These are locally invasive, involving the underlying bone and periodontal ligament of adjoining teeth and the adjacent mucosa. Metastasis is usually confined to the region above the clavicle, but extensive involvement may include the lung or liver.

*Histopathological features*: Microscopically, infiltrative cords, islands, and sheets of malignant keratinocytes invade the connective tissue and exhibit cellular pleomorphism, hyperchromatism, and aberrant mitosis. The well-differentiated squamous cell carcinomas show keratin pearl formation that facilitates their identification. In contrast, the poorly differentiated carcinomas may have to be subjected to immunocytochemical examination to be diagnosed appropriately.

*Treatment*: Gingival squamous cell carcinoma is usually treated by surgery, radiotherapy, or combinations of these. When irradiation therapy is required, the extraction of involved teeth is necessary before irradiation is instituted if the teeth suffer from severe periodontitis. This is due to an increased risk of osteoradionecrosis after the extraction of teeth situated in the irradiated bone as the result of permanently reduced vascularization.

### Malignant Melanoma

Melanoma originates from two types of neural crest cells—melanocytes and nevus cells. Melanocytes are dendrites cells that reside in the epithelium and show contact inhibition. In contrast, nevus cells reside in the subjacent connective tissue and tend to aggregate in clusters.

Although the most common site for melanoma is the palate (40%), gingival melanomas represent close to one-third of these tumors.

*Clinical features:* Oral melanoma may exhibit three presentations: (1) a pigmented macula, (2) a pigmented nodule with or without areas of ulceration, and (3) a nodule with a similar color to the surrounding oral mucosa (amelanotic melanoma). It may appear de novo as a rapidly growing mass, although the presence of pigmentation in a rapidly growing mass is an ominous sign suggestive of melanoma requiring biopsy without delay.

*Histopathological features:* Microscopically, the pigmented nodular type of melanoma is the most common, consisting of proliferating atypical, pleomorphic, spindle-shaped, or epithelioid tumor cells containing melanin with frequent mitotic figures.

*Treatment:* The treatment of choice for oral melanoma is surgical excision with adequate negative margins. Radiotherapy and chemotherapy are palliative interventions that may be used in addition to the surgical excision.

## Sarcomas

Intraoral soft-tissue sarcomas (STS) are extremely rare, and periodontal tissues are affected the least. Usually, STS are diagnosed in patients older than 20 years with no sex predilection.

*Clinical features:* Oral STS are exophytic, infiltrative masses that may exhibit rapid growth and may or may not be painful. STS initially produces a bulging of the mucosa without destroying it but may grow rapidly, causing destruction.

The prognosis of a malignant tumor is mainly dependent on early diagnosis.

## REACTIVE LESIONS OF GINGIVA

### Pyogenic Granuloma

Pyogenic granuloma is a painless condition occurring mainly in women during the second and fifth decades of life. The so-called pregnancy tumor is a clinical term used to identify a pyogenic granuloma that occurs in pregnant women.

*Clinical features:* Pyogenic granuloma is a nodular, purple to red, hemorrhagic circumscribed friable polypoid lesion that bleeds easily and is often ulcerated. Microtrauma from toothbrushing and local irritants, such as dental plaque and calculus, seems to be the etiologic factor of this condition. The usual site is the anterior mandibular or maxillary gingiva.

*Histopathological features:* Microscopically, this lesion exhibits ulceration of the surface epithelium and, characteristically, there is fibroendothelial proliferation of

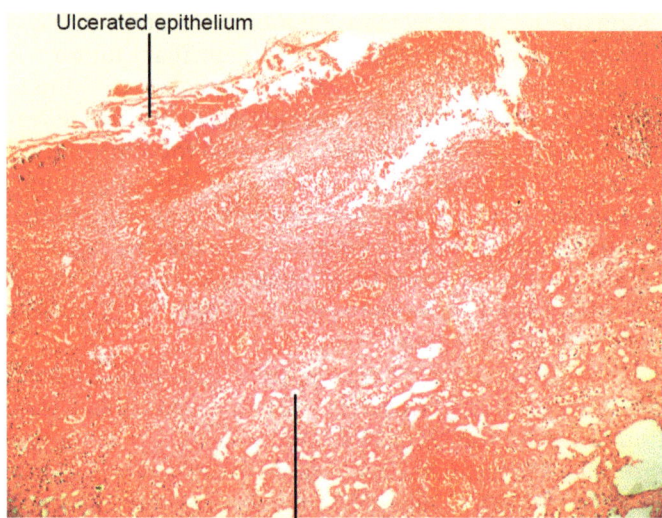

**Fig. 21.6:** Histological representation showing pyogenic granuloma.

the stroma surrounded by acute and chronic inflammatory cells **(Fig. 21.6)**.

*Treatment:* Surgical excision, along with the removal of local irritants to prevent a recurrence, is the ideal treatment of choice. During pregnancy, a conservative approach is preferred for safety purposes. The lesion usually resolves after parturition. Hence, excision is not recommended during pregnancy, especially in the absence of significant aesthetic or functional problems. Removal of local irritants, such as plaque and calculus, is an integral part of treatment. Surgical excision is recommended when lesions fail to resolve with adequate management. Follow-up of the patient is essential as pyogenic granuloma can recur in most of the cases.

### Peripheral Fibroma

*Clinical features:* Peripheral fibroma is typically an asymptomatic, dome-shaped nodule. True fibromas are very less in incidence. The usual site of occurrence is an interdental region. These lesions can be sessile as well as pedunculated.

*Histopathological features:* Microscopically, the peripheral fibroma is surfaced by parakeratinized stratified squamous epithelium with or without focal hyperkeratinization. The main feature is the presence of hyperplastic collagen fibers arranged in intersecting fascicles with a varied amount of blood capillaries and, occasionally, inflammatory cells **(Fig. 21.7)**.

*Treatment:* This lesion is managed by surgical excision and has an excellent prognosis with a low recurrence rate.

### Peripheral Ossifying Fibroma

Peripheral ossifying fibroma may appear from the first to sixth decades of life with a peak incidence in the second decade of life.

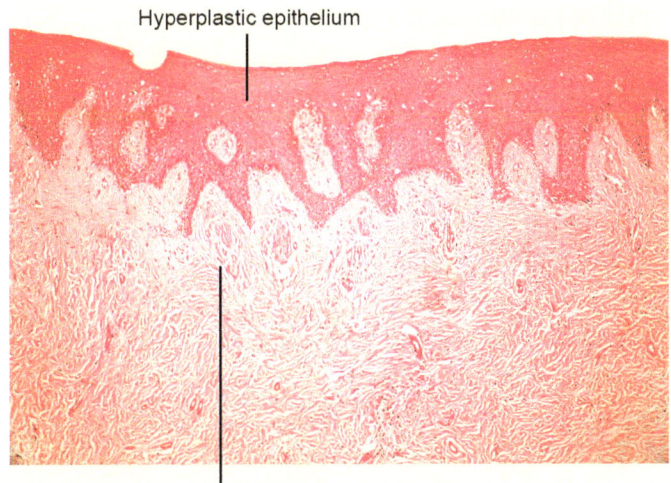

**Fig. 21.7:** Histological representation showing peripheral fibroma.

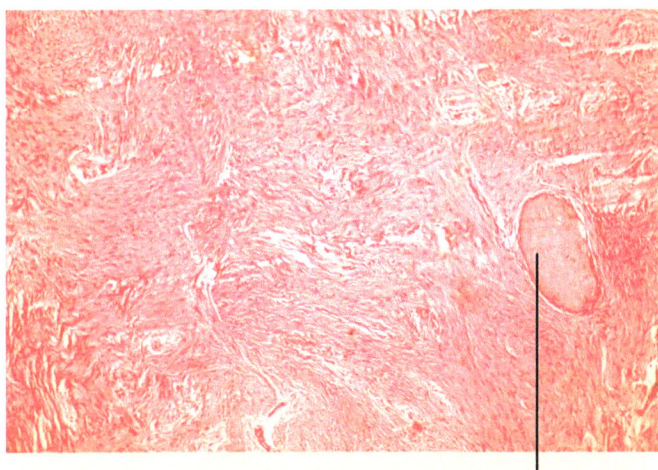

**Fig. 21.9:** Histological representation showing peripheral ossifying fibroma.

*Treatment*: Treatment includes deep surgical excision up to the periosteum and periodontal ligament with thorough root planing.

## Peripheral Giant Cell Tumor

These have been reported to occur from the first to the eighth decades of life with a mean age of 35 years with a female-to-male ratio of 2: 1. Local etiologic factors, such as plaque, calculus, ill-fitting restorations or prosthesis, and trauma, play a significant role in developing peripheral giant cell tumors.

*Clinical features*: Peripheral giant cell tumor presents as a gingival nodule with a sessile base and a red to purple discoloration that may sometime produce a displacement of the teeth.

*Histopathological features*: Microscopically, the surface epithelium may or may not show areas of ulceration. The underlying fibrous connective tissue exhibits the presence of conspicuous, distinct nodules of multinucleated giant cells between spindle mesenchymal cells, and numerous vascular channels. Hemosiderin granules, hemorrhage, and on some occasions, dystrophic calcifications, osteoid, and even frank bone metaplasia may also be observed. In those cases, the presence of multinucleated giant cells may be absent or present only in small numbers.

*Treatment*: Surgical excision is the treatment of choice for peripheral giant cell lesions.

## PERIPHERAL ODONTOGENIC LESIONS

### Gingival Cyst

The gingival cyst of adults is a rare odontogenic lesion with a slight predilection for men in their fifth to sixth decades of life. Almost 75% of these lesions are present on the labial

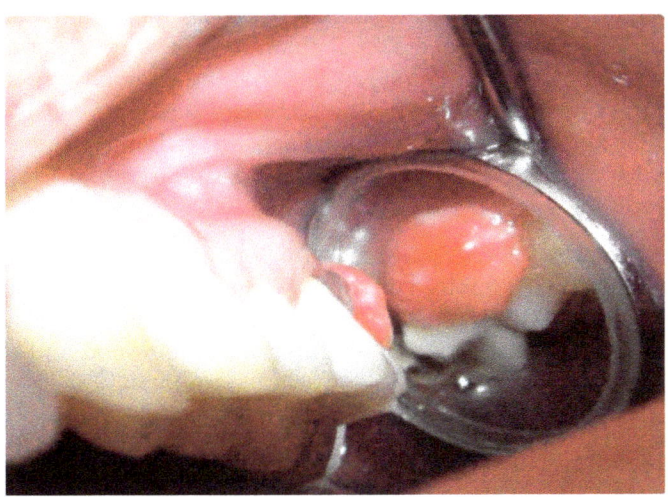

**Fig. 21.8:** Clinical picture showing peripheral ossifying fibroma.

*Clinical features*: Peripheral ossifying fibroma usually presents as a polypoid, pink mass in the interdental papilla (**Fig. 21.8**).

*Diagnosis*: This lesion may be impossible to distinguish from a pyogenic granuloma. In some cases, the clinician may make a clinical diagnosis of peripheral ossifying fibroma by taking a periapical film of the suspicious area that reveals the presence of radiopacities in the gingival lesion. However, calcifications within the lesions may not always be visible radiographically.

*Histopathological features*: Microscopically, the surface epithelium may or may not be ulcerated, but in the presence of ulceration, associated granulation tissue is observed.

The main microscopic feature is the presence of either bone metaplasia or dystrophic calcification in the fibrous connective tissue stroma of the lesion (**Fig. 21.9**).

aspect of the attached or free gingiva of the mandible in the premolar-canine-incisor area.

*Clinical features*: Clinically, a single, small-raised lesion reminiscent of a vesicle shows a bluish discoloration (**Fig. 21.10**). Interestingly this bluish discoloration with fluid content is suggestive of mucocele. However, gingival tissues do generally do not contain minor salivary glands, and only rarely are ectopic gingival salivary glands observed. On rare occasions, multiple unilateral or bilateral gingival cysts may be present.

*Histopathological features*: Microscopically, the gingival cyst is typically lined by a thin epithelium with or without focal intraluminal budding and a noninflamed cyst wall (**Fig. 21.11**).

*Treatment*: Surgical excision is the preferred treatment, and, in some cases, superficial saucerization of the alveolar bone may be seen during surgery. If incompletely excised, the recurrence of the lesion is feasible.

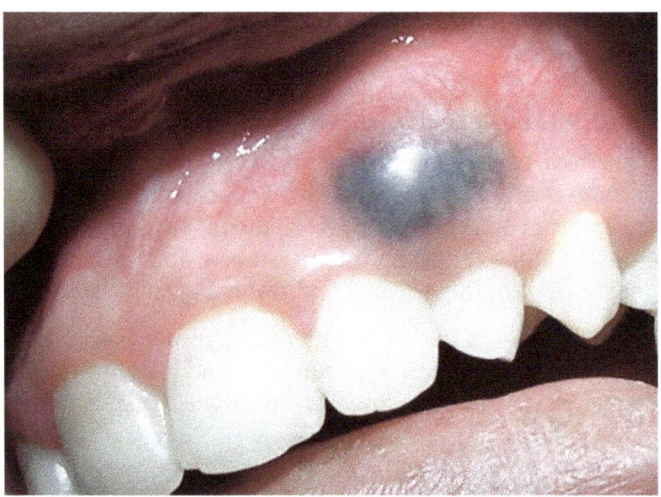

**Fig. 21.10:** Clinical picture showing gingival cyst.

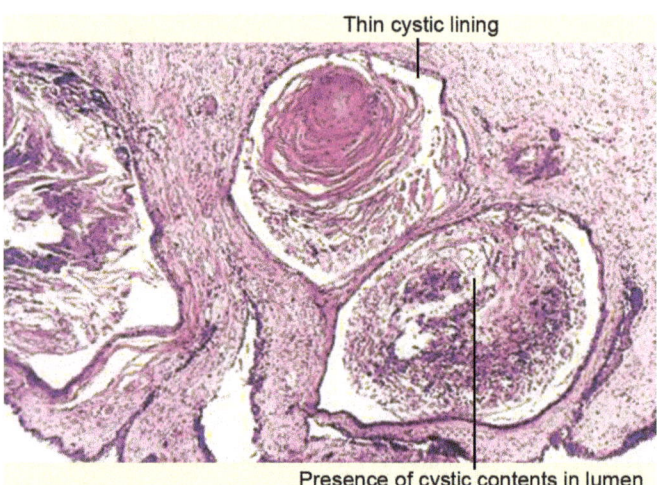

**Fig. 21.11:** Histological representation showing the gingival cyst.[3]

## Peripheral Ameloblastoma

Peripheral ameloblastoma is a painless, sessile growth with a firm consistency.

*Clinical features*: The surface is usually smooth and similar in color to the surrounding mucosa, but in some cases, it has been described as erythematous, papillary, or even warty. On rare occasions, the lesion is ulcerative rather than exophytic.

*Histopathological features*: The microscopic features of peripheral ameloblastoma are identical to those seen in the central ameloblastoma. The most common histologic patterns are the follicular and acanthomatous patterns.

*Treatment*: Surgical excision with adequate margins is the treatment of choice. Recurrence is thought to be caused by incomplete removal.

## Peripheral Odontogenic Keratocysts

*Clinical features*: Keratocysts may occur at any age, and they are most frequent in males. The common location of this is the mandibular 3rd molar region but may occur anywhere in the jaws, including the alveolar bone.[16] Radiographically, they may appear as small, round or ovoid, radiolucent areas with a smooth periphery or scalloped margins or even multilocular.[17]

*Histopathological features*: Characteristically, 7–8 layered cystic lining exhibits a tombstone appearance in the basal cell layer with parakeratinized surface corrugation. The epithelial-connective tissue interface is flattened and is highly friable.

*Treatment*: A high recurrence rate has been reported; therefore, conservative surgical treatment is advised.

## GRANULOMATOUS GINGIVITIS

### Orofacial Granulomatosis

Orofacial granulomatosis (OFG) is an uncommon clinical entity in which the patient presents with persistent swelling of the facial and/or oral tissues. Histological findings of OFG suggest the presence of noncaseating granulomatous inflammation. OFG class includes idiopathic disorders, such as Melkersson-Rosenthal syndrome, Miescher chronic granulomatous cheilitis, localized orofacial presentations of Crohn's disease, and sarcoidosis. Granulomatous gingivitis may occur in 21–26% of patients.

Crohn's disease, also termed as regional enteritis or granulomatous enteritis, is a chronic granulomatous inflammatory disease that is characteristically involved in the gastrointestinal tract, particularly the terminal ileum. It was first described by Crohn and his colleagues in 1932. Almost 6–20% of patients with Crohn's disease present with oral lesions. These lesions are more prominent when

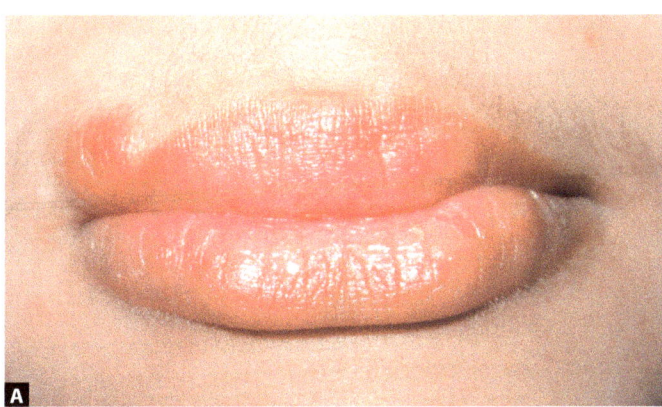 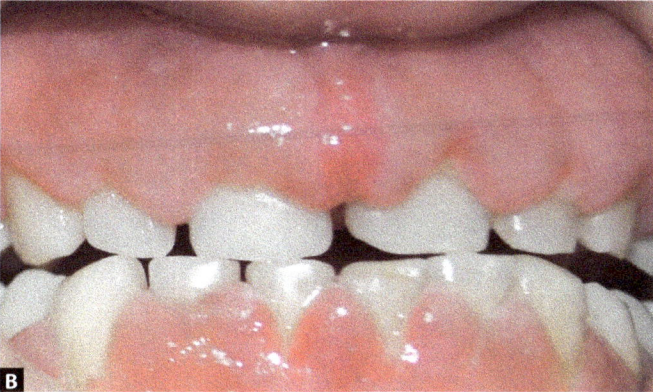

**Figs. 21.12A and B:** Clinical picture showing orofacial granulomatosis (OFG): (A) Swelling of lips; and (B) Gingival overgrowth.

Crohn's disease precedes the intestinal symptoms in up to 60% of cases.

*Clinical features*: Hypertrophy and swelling of lips (**Fig. 21.12A**), gingival swelling[18] (**Fig. 21.12B**), cobblestone appearance of buccal mucosa and palate, and deep ulcers are the common presenting symptoms.

*Diagnosis*: Orofacial granulomatosis may be the associated symptom of sarcoidosis. However, the lack of clinical features of sarcoidosis, a normal chest radiograph, and normal levels of serum angiotensin-converting enzymes exclude the diagnosis of sarcoidosis. Tuberculosis and leprosy are the other possibilities in patients presenting with features of OFG. This required, proper examination to confirm the final diagnosis.

*Histopathologic features*: Microscopic examination reveals an ulcerated, edematous epithelium infiltrated with aggregates of neutrophils and lymphocytes. It also reveals the presence of numerous granulomas with epithelioid histiocytes intermixed with lymphocytes and Langerhan's giant cells in the subjacent connective tissue.

*Treatment*: Treatment for oral lesions is the application of medium-to-high potency steroids (clobetasol propionate 0.05% mixed with benzocaine). Systemic treatment protocols include drugs like cyclosporine, thalidomide and steroid-sparing agents such as azathioprine, methotrexate, and hydroxychloroquine and fully human immunoglobulin G1 antitumor necrosis factor agents and humanized anti-α4-integrin IgG4 antibody.[19]

## BENIGN NEOPLASMS

### Ameloblastoma

Ameloblastoma is the second most common odontogenic tumor originating from any sort of odontogenic epithelium, including dental lamina rests, epithelial rests of Malassez, reduced enamel epithelium, and cystic epithelial lining. It occurs commonly between ages 20 years and 40 years and exhibits no sex predilection.

*Clinical features*: Most frequent location is the molar region of the mandible.[20] Tumors grow slowly and are usually asymptomatic. Ameloblastoma may lead to the expansion of cortical bone and the displacement of teeth. They are discovered during a routine radiographic examination or the exploration of a painless jaw swelling. Radiographically, ameloblastoma demonstrates well-circumscribed unilocular or multilocular radiolucency.

*Histopathologic features*: There is palisading and nuclear hyperchromatism with reverse polarization and vacuolization of basal cells.

*Treatment*: Surgical excision with margins free of the tumor is the treatment of choice—application of conservative treatments, such as enucleation and curettage results in high recurrence rates.

## MALIGNANT NEOPLASMS

### Osteosarcoma

Osteosarcoma is the most common primary malignant tumor of bone. It is a malignant tumor characterized by the direct formation of bone or osteoid tissue by the tumor cells. The rapidly growing firm or hard tumor may cause loosening and migration of the teeth. Osteosarcoma of the jaws can appear throughout a wide age spectrum, but it is usually diagnosed during the third to fourth decades of life. Men are affected more commonly than women. The maxilla and mandible are affected with equal frequency.

*Clinical features*: Common signs and symptoms of osteosarcoma are swelling, pain, mobile teeth, nasal obstruction, and paresthesia.

*Diagnosis*: Radiographically, the neoplasm demonstrates a variety of patterns ranging from radiolucent to radiopaque changes.

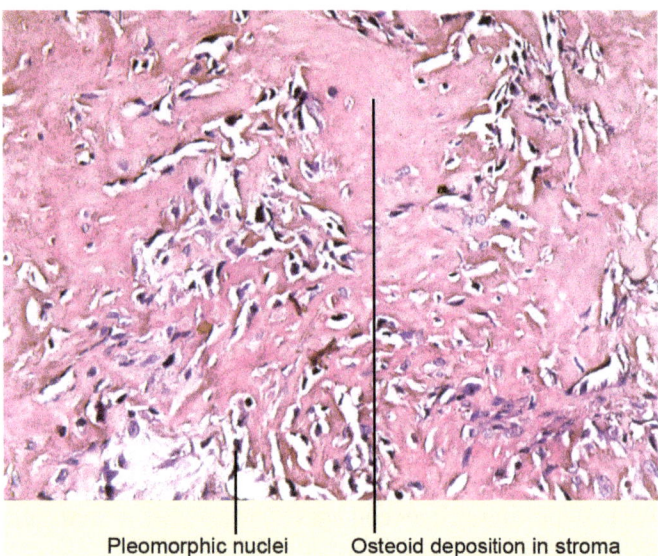

**Fig. 21.13:** Histological representation showing Osteosarcoma.

*Histopathologic features*: Microscopically, osteosarcoma is composed of malignant stromal cells that form osteoid or primitive bone **(Fig. 21.13)**. Sometimes the formation of bony trabeculae results in a sunray appearance in a direction perpendicular to the outer surface called "sunburst" appearance. Asymmetric widening of the periodontal ligament space is a significant feature of osteosarcoma.

*Treatment*: Resection of involved and surrounding bone is the common treatment. Sometimes supplementary chemotherapy and/or radiotherapy are used.

### Points to Ponder

- Wickham striae: Interlacing white lines are the hallmark of reticular oral lichen planus.
- Nikolsky's sign is the hallmark of pemphigus vulgaris.
- Target or iris lesions with central clearing are the hallmark of erythema multiforme.

## REFERENCES

1. Prinz H. Chronic diffuse desquamative gingivitis. Dent Cosmos. 1932;74:331-33.
2. McCarthy FP, McCarthy PL, Shklar G. Chronic desquamative gingivitis: a reconsideration. Oral Surg. 1960;13:1300-13.
3. Aguirre A, Neiders MF, Nisengard R. Desquamative gingivitis. In: Newman MG, Takei HH, Carranza FA (Eds). Clinical Periodontology, 9th edition. Philadelphia, PA, USA: WB Saunders; 2003. pp. 314-35.
4. Scully C, Beyli M, Ferreiro MC, Ficarra G, Gill Y, Griffiths M, et al. Update on oral lichen planus: etiopathogenesis and management. Crit Rev Oral Biol Med. 1998;9(1):86-122.
5. Scully C, el-Kom M. Lichen planus: review and update on pathogenesis. J Oral Pathol. 1985;14(6):431-58.
6. Shafers WG, Hine MK, Levy BM. Diseases of the skin. In: A Textbook of Oral Pathology, 4th edition. Philadelphia, PA, USA: WB Saunders; 1983. pp. 806-53.
7. Nisengard RJ. Periodontal implications: mucocutaneous disorders. Ann Periodontol. 1996;1(1):401-38.
8. Chaikin BS. A treatment of desquamative gingivitis by the use of free gingival grafts. Quintessence Int. 1980;9:105-9.
9. Scully C, Challacombe SJ. Pemphigus Vulgaris: update on etiopathogenesis, oral manifestations, and management. Crit Rev Oral Biol Med. 2002;13(5):397-408.
10. Ahmed AR, Graham J, Jordon RE, Prevost TT. Pemphigus: current concepts. Ann Intern Med. 1980;92(3):396-405.
11. Anhalt GJ, Kim SC, Stanley JR, Korman NJ, Jabs DA, Kory M, et al. Paraneoplastic pemphigus. A mucocutaneous autoimmune disease associated with neoplasia. N Engl J Med. 1990;323(25):1729-35.
12. Aguirre A, Tapia JL. Selected soft and hard tissue lesions with periodontal relevance. In: Rose LF, Mealey BL, Genco RJ, Cohen DW (Eds). Periodontics: Medicine, Surgery, and Implants, 2nd revised edition. Philadelphia, PA, USA: Elsevier Mosby; 2004. pp. 879-911.
13. Simon JA, Cabiedes J, Ortiz E, Alcocer-Varela J, Sanchez-Guerrero J. Anti-nucleosome antibodies in patients with systemic lupus erythematosus of recent onset. Potential utility as a diagnostic tool and disease activity marker. Rheumatology (Oxford). 2004;43(2):220-4.
14. Lozada F, Spitter L, Silverman S. Results of immunologic testing in patients with erythema multiforme. J Dent Res. 1980;59(3):567-72.
15. Holmstrup P, Reibel J. Differential diagnoses: periodontal tumours and cysts. In: Lindhe J, Karring T, Lang NP (Eds). Clinical Periodontology and Implant Dentistry, 4th edition. Chicago, USA: Blackwell Munksgaard; 2003. pp. 298-317.
16. Faustino SE, Pereira MC, Rossetto AC, Oliveira DT. Recurrent peripheral odontogenic keratocyst: a case report. Dentomaxillofac Radiol. 2008;37(7):412-4.
17. Shear M, Speight P. Cysts of the Oral and Maxillofacial Regions, 4th edition. Oxford, UK: Blackwell Munksgaard; 2007.
18. Chandna S, Mahendra A, Kaur R. Gingival manifestations of Orofacial Granulomatosis: A rare finding. Clin Adv Periodontics. 2017; 7(2): 57-62.
19. Leão JC, Hodgson T, Scully C, Porter S. Review article: orofacial granulomatosis. Aliment Pharmacol Ther. 2004;20(10):1019-27.
20. Reichart PA, Philipsen HP, Sonner S. Ameloblastoma: biological profile of 3677 cases. Euro J Cancer B Oral Oncol. 1995;31B(2):86-99.

### VIVA VOCE

**Q1. In which conditions red gingival lesion is seen?**
**Ans.** Desquamative gingivitis; Erythroplasia; Hemangiomas; Orofacial granulomatosis; Crohn's diseases; Sarcoidosis; Wegener's granulomatosis and Kaposi's sarcoma.

**Q2. What is the configuration of rete ridges in lichen planus?**
**Ans.** In lichen planus saw tooth configuration of rete ridges are observed.

**Q3. In which mucocutaneous disorders Nikolsky sign is seen?**
**Ans.** Pemphigus vulgaris.

**Q4. Which autoantibodies are seen in pemphigus vulgaris?**
**Ans.** Serum Ig G autoantibodies against Desmoglein ($Dsg_1$) and Desmoglein ($Dsg_3$) are seen in Pemphigus vulgaris.

**Q5. In which chronic granulomatous disease lip swelling is common?**
**Ans.** Lip swelling is common in orofacial granulomatous.

**Q6. Who coined the term "chronic desquamative gingivitis"?**
**Ans.** Prinz in 1932

**Q7. What are the clinical presentations of systemic lupus erythematosus?**
**Ans.** Three types: Discoid, erythematous, and ulcerations.

**Q8. What are the sources of ameloblastoma origin?**
**Ans.** Dental lamina rests, epithelial rests of Malassez, reduced enamel epithelium and cystic epithelial lining.

**Q9. What are the common symptoms of orofacial granulomatosis?**
**Ans.** Hypertrophy and swelling of lips, gingival swelling, cobblestone appearance of buccal mucosa and palate, and deep ulcers.

**Q10. What are the treatment modalities for lichen planus?**
**Ans.** Steroids, antifungals, topical and systemic retinoids, and cyclosporine.

# Chapter 22: Periodontal Pocket

*Sanjeev Jain*

## Chapter Outline

- Definition
- Classifications
- Clinical Features
- Pathogenesis
- Histopathology
- Clinical Assessment

## INTRODUCTION

A periodontal pocket is one of the most important clinical features of periodontal disease. The histopathologic features, mechanisms of tissue destruction, and the healing mechanism of periodontal pocket are almost the same in all types of periodontitis.

## DEFINITION

A periodontal pocket is pathologically deepened gingival sulcus.[1] It is formed due to an increase in original sulcular depth and apical migration of junctional epithelium (JE). Hence, it has the JE at its base with tooth border on one side and ulcerated epithelium on the other side. The area is usually inaccessible for plaque removal and eventually results in the subsequent plaque buildup due to following feedback mechanism:

Plaque → gingival inflammation → periodontal inflammation → periodontal pocket formation → more plaque buildup

## CLASSIFICATIONS

- *Depending on morphology*:[1]
  - Gingival pocket/pseudopocket: Deepening of the gingival sulcus, mainly owing to an increase in the size of the gingiva, without any considerable loss of the underlying tissues or apical migration of the junctional epithelium. It is also called a false pocket or relative pocket.
  - Periodontal pocket **(Figs. 22.1A to C)**: It is also called a true pocket or absolute pocket.
    - Suprabony pocket: The base of the pocket is coronal to the crest of the alveolar bone. Bone loss is horizontal.
    - Infrabony pocket: The base of the pocket is apical to the crest of the alveolar bone. Bone loss is vertical.
  - Combined pocket
- *Depending on the number of surfaces involved* **(Figs. 22.2A to C)**:
  - Simple pocket: It involves one tooth surface.
  - Compound pocket: This type of pocket involves two or more tooth surfaces. The base of the pocket is in direct communication with the gingival margin along each of the involved surface.

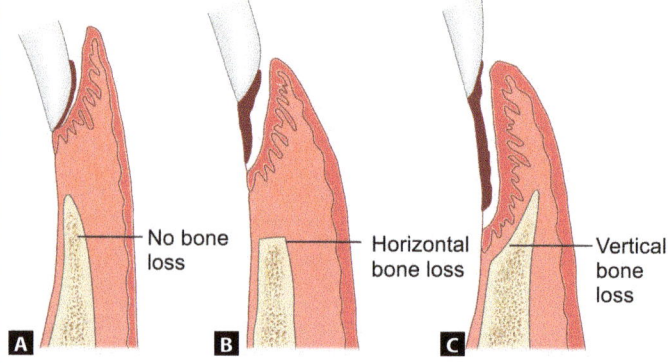

**Figs. 22.1A to C:** Schematic representation showing different types of pocket: (A) Gingival pocket—no bone loss; (B) Suprabony pocket—horizontal bone loss and (C) Infrabony pocket—vertical bone loss.

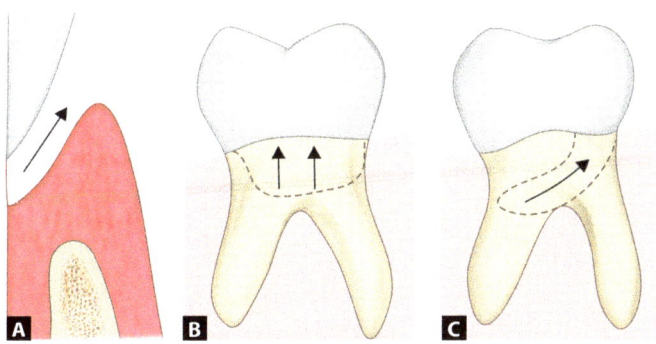

**Figs. 22.2A to C:** Schematic representation showing the classification of pocket according to involved tooth surface: (A) Simple pocket; (B) Compound pocket: and (C) Complex/spiral pocket (tortuous).

- Complex/spiral pocket (tortuous): This type of pocket originates on one tooth surface and twists around the tooth to involve one or more additional surfaces. The only communication with the gingival margin is at the surface where the pocket originates.[1] It is more common in the furcation areas.
- *Depending on disease activity*:
  - Active pocket: It consists of more of the inflammatory content and is marked by spontaneous bleeding or bleeding on slight provocation.
  - Inactive pocket: It contains less inflammatory contents and shows no signs of attachment loss or bone loss.
- *Depending on the nature of the soft-tissue wall*:
  - Edematous: It contains more cellular exudates, and inflammatory infiltrates, and the pocket wall appears bluish-red, soft, friable with a smooth, shiny surface.
  - Fibrotic: It contains more connective tissue fibers and the pocket wall appears pink and relatively firm.
- *Depending on the lateral wall of the pocket* **(Fig. 22.3 and Table 22.1)**:
  - Suprabony (S): It consists of soft tissue alone.
  - Infrabony (I): It consists of both soft tissue and bone. The alveolar bone becomes a part of the pocket wall.

## CLINICAL FEATURES

### Symptoms

Following are the symptoms which are suggestive of the presence of periodontal pocket:
- Localized pain or pressure sensation, especially after eating, which gradually diminishes in intensity.
- Radiating pain deep in the bone.
- A foul taste in localized areas.
- A gnawing feeling or feeling of itching in the gingiva.
- Urge to dig with a pointed instrument into the gingiva.
- A tendency to suck material from the interproximal spaces.
- Enhance sensitivity to heat and cold and the presence of toothache even in the absence of dental caries.

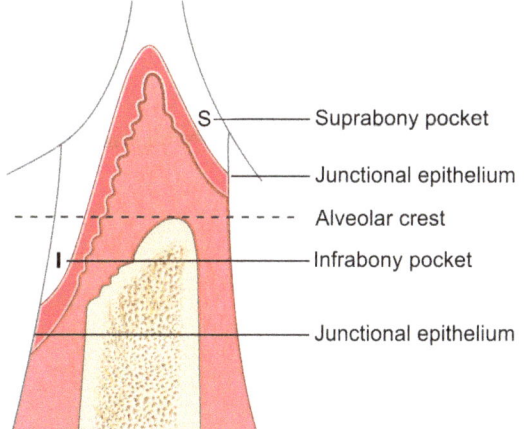

**Fig. 22.3:** Schematic representation showing (S) suprabony and (I) infrabony pockets.

**TABLE 22.1:** Differences between suprabony and infrabony pocket.

| Parameters | Suprabony pocket | Infrabony pocket |
| --- | --- | --- |
| Relationship of the soft-tissue wall of the pocket to the alveolar bone | The base of the pocket is coronal to the level alveolar bone | The base of the pocket is apical to the crest of the alveolar bone |
| The pattern of bone destruction | Horizontal | Vertical |
| The direction of transseptal fibers interproximally | Horizontal | Oblique |
| The direction of the periodontal ligament, on facial and lingual surfaces | Normal horizontal-oblique course between the tooth and the bone | Follows the angular pattern of the adjacent bone. They extend from the cementum beneath the base of the pocket along the bone and over the crest to join with the outer periosteum |

### Clinical Signs

Following are the clinical signs which are suggestive of the presence of periodontal pocket:
- Enlarged, bluish-red thickened marginal gingiva with a rolled edge separated from the tooth surface.
- Bluish-red color vertical zone extending from the gingival margin to the alveolar mucosa.
- A break in the faciolingual continuity of the interdental gingiva.
- Shiny, discolored, and puffy gingiva associated with the exposed root surfaces.
- Gingival bleeding and suppuration from the gingival margin.
- Extrusion, mobility, diastema, and migration of teeth **(Fig. 22.4)**.

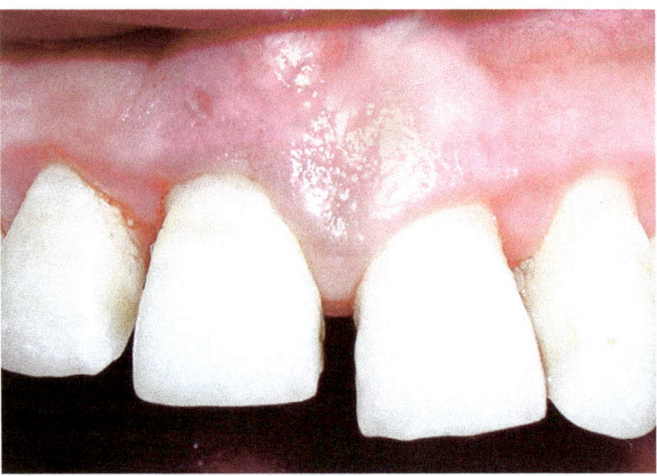

**Fig. 22.4:** Clinical picture showing extrusion and diastema associated with periodontal pocket.

## PATHOGENESIS

The following old theories related to the pathogenesis of periodontal pocket are presented as useful background for the interpretation of current and future concepts:[2]
- Destruction of gingival fibers is a prerequisite for the initiation of pocket formation—*Fish (1946)*.
- The initial change in pocket formation occurs in cementum—*Gottlieb (1948)*.
- Stimulation of the epithelial attachment by inflammation rather than the destruction of gingival fibers is the prerequisite for the initiation of periodontal pocket—*Aisenberg (1948)*.
- Pathologic destruction of the epithelial attachment due to infection or trauma is the initial histologic changes in pocket formation—*Skillen (1930)*.
- The invasion of bacteria initiates the periodontal pocket at the base of the sulcus or the absorption of bacterial toxins through the epithelial lining of the sulcus—*Box (1941)*.
- The pocket formation is initiated as a defect in sulcus—*Becks*.
- The proliferation of the epithelium of the lateral wall, rather than epithelium at the base of the sulcus, is the initial change in the formation of periodontal pocket—*Wilkinson (1935)*.
- Two-stage pocket formation—*James and Counsell*
  - The proliferation of the subgingival epithelium (epithelial attachment).
  - Loss of superficial layers of proliferated epithelium, which produces space or pocket.
- Inflammation is the initial change in the formation of periodontal pocket—*J Nuckolls (1950)*.
- Pathologic epithelial proliferation occurs secondary to noninflammatory degenerative changes in periodontal membranes.

The most accepted recent concept is that the apical migration of apical cells of junctional epithelium and the detachment of the coronal portion of junctional epithelium

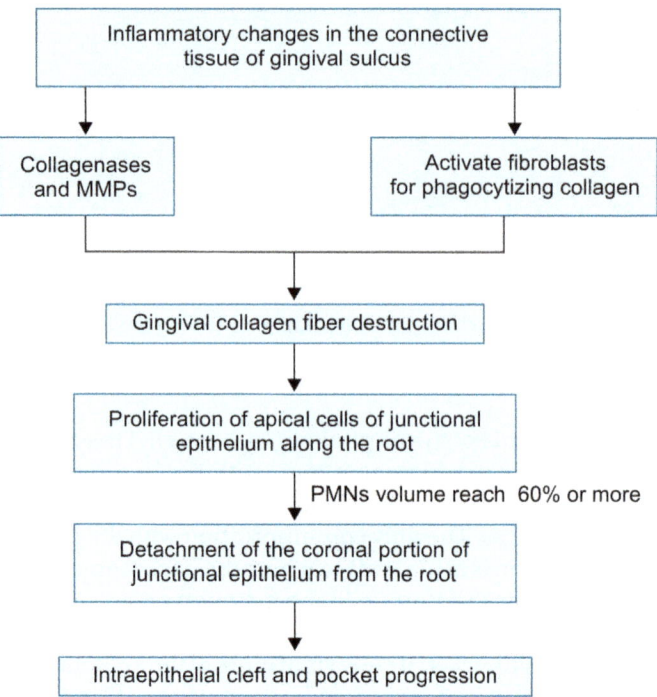

**Flowchart 22.1:** Pathogenesis of periodontal pocket.

(MMPs: matrix metalloproteinases; PMNs: polymorphonuclear leukocytes)

leading to intraepithelial cleft[3,4] and pocket formation and deepening. The loosening of the (directly attached to the tooth (DAT) cells from the tooth surface leads to loss of cellular cohesion in the coronal most sections of the junctional epithelium.[5,6]

An increased number of inflammatory cells, including mononuclear leukocytes (T and B lymphocytes and monocytes) and polymorphonuclear leukocytes (PMNs) are reported to provide an additional role in the junctional epithelium's focal disintegration. **Flowchart 22.1** clearly shows how the periodontal pocket is formed.

## HISTOPATHOLOGY

*The periodontal pocket's soft-tissue wall presents the following microscopic features*: the epithelium of the lateral wall of the pocket presents striking proliferative and degenerative changes. The most characteristic feature is the protrusion of epithelium buds or interlacing cords of epithelial cells from the lateral wall of the pocket into the adjacent inflamed connective tissue. These epithelial projections and rest of the lateral epithelium are densely infiltrated by leukocytes and edema from the inflamed connective tissue. Epithelial cells undergo vacuolar degeneration and rupture to form vesicles. Progressive degeneration and necrosis of the epithelium lead to ulceration of the lateral wall and exposure of underlying connective tissue.

The base of the pocket is formed by junctional epithelium, and it is almost shorter than that of the normal sulcus. The corono-apical length of junctional epithelium

**Chapter 22: Periodontal Pocket**

**TABLE 22.2:** Correlation of clinical and histopathologic features of the periodontal pocket.

| Parameters | Clinical features | Histopathologic features |
|---|---|---|
| Color | The gingival wall of the periodontal pocket is usually bluish-red | The discoloration is caused by circulatory stagnation |
| Surface texture | The smooth, shiny surface which pits on pressure | The smooth, shiny surface is due to the atrophy of the epithelium and edema; the pitting on pressure is because of edema and degeneration |
| Consistency | Usually flaccid but less frequently, the gingival wall may be pink and firm | Flaccidity is due to destruction of the gingival fibers and surrounding tissues but is firm when fibrotic changes predominate over exudation and degeneration |
| Bleeding | It is elicited by gently probing the soft-tissue wall of the pocket | Ease of bleeding results from increased vascularity, thinning and degeneration of the epithelium, and the proximity of the engorged vessels to the inner surface |
| Pain | When explored with a probe, the inner aspect of the periodontal pocket is generally painful | Pain on tactile stimulation is due to ulceration of the inner aspect of the pocket wall |
| Pus | Sometimes pus may be expressed by applying digital pressure | Pus occurs in pockets with suppurative inflammation of the inner wall |

is reduced to only 50–100 μm.[7] The epithelium lining the gingival crest of a periodontal pocket is usually intact and thickened and with the presence of prominent rete pegs.

The connective tissue is edematous and densely infiltrated, with approximately 80% of plasma cells,[8] lymphocytes, and PMNs. The normal vasculature is tortuous and engorged with an increased number of vessels. The connective tissue presents a proliferation of the endothelial cells with newly formed capillaries, fibroblasts, and collagen fibers **(Table 22.2)**.

Some bacteria may invade the intracellular space and are found between deeper epithelial cells and accumulate on the basement lamina. *Porphyromonas gingivalis*, *Prevotella intermedius*, and *Aggregatibacter actinomycetemcomitans* traverse the basement lamina and invade the subepithelial connective tissue.

## Microtopography of the Gingival Wall of the Pocket

Different areas are showing the different type of activity in the soft-tissue wall of the pocket due to the host-microbial interactions:[9]

- Areas of relative quiescence, showing flatten surface along with minor depressions and mounds and occasional shedding of cells.
- Areas of bacterial accumulation, presenting as epithelial surface depressions along with abundant debris and bacterial clumps invading into the enlarged intercellular spaces. These bacteria are mainly cocci, rods, and filaments with a few spirochetes.
- Areas of the emergence of leukocytes, where leukocytes appear in the pocket wall through holes located in the intercellular spaces.
- Areas of leukocyte-bacteria interaction, where numerous leukocytes are present and covered with bacteria in an apparent process of phagocytosis. Bacterial plaque associated with the epithelium is seen either as an organized matrix covered by a fibrin-like material along with a cell surface or as bacteria invading into the intercellular spaces.
- Areas of intense epithelial desquamation consist of semi-attached and folded epithelial squames, which are sometimes partially covered with bacteria.
- Areas of ulceration with exposed connective tissue.
- Areas of hemorrhage with numerous erythrocytes.

## Periodontal Pockets as Healing Lesions

They are chronic inflammatory lesions and are constantly undergoing repair. Complete healing does not occur because of the persistence of local irritants. The balance between destructive and constructive changes determines clinical features, such as color, consistency/surface texture of the pocket wall.

- If a destructive phase predominates, the pocket wall is bluish-red, soft, spongy, friable, smooth, and shiny (edematous pocket wall).
- If a constructive phase predominates, the pocket wall is firmer and pink (fibrotic pocket wall).

The most severe degenerative changes occur adjacent to the tooth surface and subgingival plaque (i.e., internally).

### Pocket Contents

Periodontal pockets are composed of microbial colonies and their products (enzymes, endotoxins, and other metabolic products), gingival crevicular fluid, salivary mucin, food debris, desquamated epithelial cells, and leukocytes. Purulent exudate consists of living, degenerated and necrotic leukocytes, living and dead bacteria, serum and fibrin.[10]

### Root Surface Wall Changes

The root surface wall of periodontal pockets often undergoes significant changes because they may perpetuate periodontal infection, cause pain, and complicate periodontal treatment. Root surface walls may undergo structural, chemical, and cytotoxic changes.

*Structural changes*: It includes the presence of pathologic granules,[11] which represent the area of collagen degradation. There may be areas of hypermineralization or demineralization, causing root caries.

*Chemical changes*: The mineral content of exposed cementum is increased. Exposed cementum absorbs calcium, phosphorus, and fluorides from its local environment, making it possible to develop a highly calcified layer that appears to be highly resistant to decay. This ability of cementum to absorb from its environment, on the other hand, maybe detrimental if these absorbed materials are toxic to the surrounding tissues.

*Cytotoxic changes*: Endotoxins are found in the cementum of periodontally involved teeth. Endotoxin limits the proliferation and attachment of fibroblasts to the diseased root surfaces.[12]

## CLINICAL ASSESSMENT

A careful examination of the gingival margin along each tooth surface with a periodontal probe gives the exact location and extent of the periodontal pocket. The probe is usually inserted parallel to the tooth's vertical axis **(Fig. 22.5)** and moved circumferentially around each tooth's surface to identify periodontal pocket depth. Probe tip penetrates the most coronal intact fibers of the connective tissue's attachment and goes about 0.3 mm apical to the junctional epithelium in the periodontal pocket.[13] Patients usually well tolerate the probing forces of about 0.75 N.[14] Probe reading that falls between two calibrated marks on the probe should be rounded upwards to the next highest millimeter, e.g., if the probe penetrates far enough to cover the 4 mm mark, it should be recorded as five mm.[15]

Gutta-percha points or calibrated silver points generally are used with radiographs to determine the level of attachment of periodontal pockets.

## Periodontal Pocket and Attachment Loss

Attachment loss is measured from the cementoenamel junction (CEJ) (fixed point) or from the occlusal stent to the pocket's sulcus or base. Pocket depth is measured from the gingival crest/gingival margin (position not fixed) to the pocket base. The location of the base of the pocket on the root surface determines the degree of attachment loss **(Fig. 22.6)**.

Attachment loss versus pocket formation in two different situations:
1. *Different pocket depths with the same amount of attachment loss*: The distance between the base of the pocket and the CEJ remains the same despite different probing pocket depths **(Fig. 22.7)**.
2. *Same pocket depths with different amounts of attachment loss*: The distance between the gingival margin and the base of the pocket remains the same despite different attachment loss **(Fig. 22.8)**.

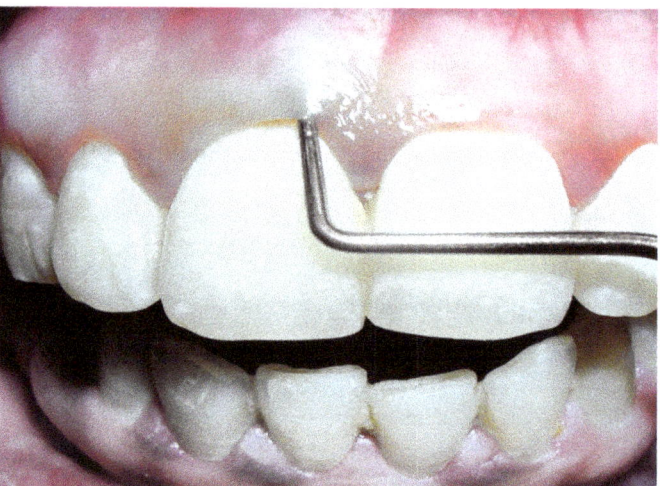

**Fig. 22.5:** Clinical picture showing pocket probing: the probe is inserted parallel to the vertical axis of the tooth.

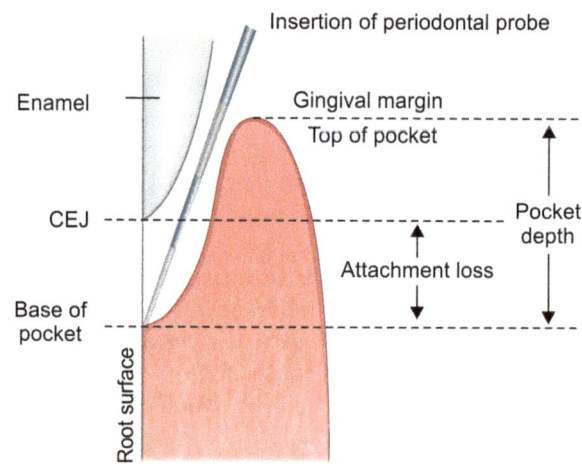

**Fig. 22.6:** Schematic representation showing the relationship between the periodontal pocket and attachment loss.
(CEJ: cementoenamel junction)

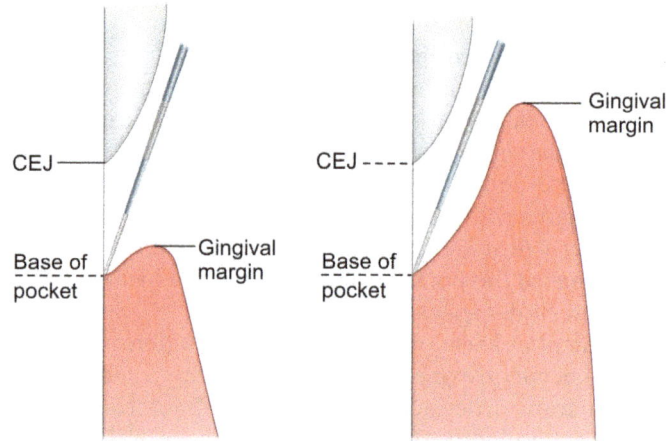

**Fig. 22.7:** Schematic representation showing different pocket depths with same attachment loss.
(CEJ: cementoenamel junction)

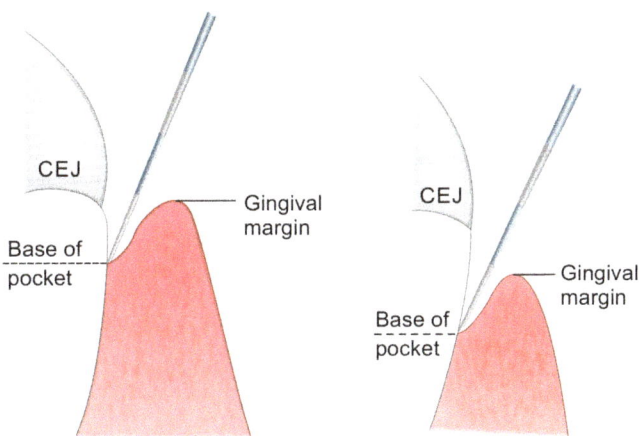

**Fig. 22.8:** Schematic representation showing same pocket depths with different attachment loss.
(CEJ: cementoenamel junction)

## Periodontal Pocket and Bone Loss

The inflammatory, proliferative and degenerative changes in infrabony and suprabony pockets are the same and associated with the damage of the supporting periodontal tissues.

In the suprabony pocket, the base of the pocket is coronal to the alveolar bone's crest. Suprabony pocket is usually associated with a horizontal pattern of bone loss **(Fig. 22.1B)**.

In infrabony pocket, the base of the pocket is apical to the crest of the alveolar bone, and the pocket wall lies between the tooth and the bone. Infrabony pockets most often occur interproximally but may be located on the facial and lingual tooth surfaces. In infrabony pockets, the morphology of the alveolar crest changes completely with the formation of angular bony defects as a result of vertical bone loss **(Fig. 22.1C)**.

### Points to Ponder

- A periodontal pocket is a soft-tissue change, thus cannot be detected during radiographic examination.
- Biologic/histologic depth is the distance between the gingival margin and the base of the pocket (coronal end of the junctional epithelium).
- Clinical/probing depth is the distance between the gingival margins to the base of the probeable crevice up to which probe penetrates the pocket.

- Classification of periodontal pocket:
  - Can be pseudopocket or true pocket.
  - Can be a simple, compound, or complex pocket.
  - Can be suprabony or infrabony pocket.

## REFERENCES

1. Carranza FA, Camargo PM. The periodontal pocket. In: Newman MG, Takei HH, Carranza FA (Eds). Carranza's Clinical Periodontology, 9th edition. Philadelphia, PA, USA: WB Saunders; 2003. pp. 336-53.
2. Glickman I. Clinical Periodontology: Recognition, Diagnosis, and Treatment of Periodontal Disease in the Practice of General Dentistry, 3rd edition. Philadelphia, PA, USA: WB Saunders; 1964.
3. Schluger S, Youdelis RA, Page RC, Johnson RH (Eds). Periodontal Diseases: Basic Phenomena, Clinical Management, and Occlusal and Restorative Interrelationships, 2nd sub-edition. Philadelphia, PA, USA: Lea & Febiger; 1989.
4. Schroeder HE. Histopathology of the gingival sulcus. In: Lehner T, Cimasoni G (Eds). The Borderland Between Caries and Periodontal Disease II. London, UK: Academic Press; 1977. pp. 43-78.
5. Takata T, Donath K. The mechanism of pocket formation. A light microscopic study on undecalcified human material. J Periodontol. 1988;59(4):215-21.
6. Bosshardt DD, Lang NP. The junctional epithelium: from health to disease. J Dent Res. 2005;84(1):9-20.
7. Carranza FA. Histometric evaluation of periodontal pathology. A review of recent studies. J Periodontol. 1967;38(6 Suppl):741-50.
8. Wittwer JW, Dickler EH, Toto PD. Comparative frequencies of plasma cells and lymphocytes in gingivitis. J Periodontol. 1969;40(5):274-5.
9. Saglie FR, Carranza FA, Newman MG, Pattison GA. Scanning electron microscopy of the gingival wall of deep periodontal pockets in humans. J Periodontal Res. 1982;17(3):284-93.
10. McMillan L, Burrill DY, Fosdick LS. An electron microscope study of particulates in periodontal exudate (Abstract). J Dent Res. 1958;37:51.
11. Aleo JJ, Vandersall DC. Cementum. Recent concepts related to periodontal disease therapy. Dent Clin North Am. 1980;24(4):627-50.
12. Aleo JJ, De Renzis FA, Farber PA, Varboncoeur AP. The presence and biologic activity of cementum-bound endotoxin. J Periodontol. 1974;45(9):672-5.
13. Listgarten MA, Mao R, Robinson PJ. Periodontal probing and the relationship of the probe tip to periodontal tissues. J Periodontol. 1976;47(9):511-3.
14. van der Velden U. Probing force and the relationship of the probe tip to the periodontal tissues. J Clin Periodontol. 1979;6(2):106-14.
15. Parr RW, Green E, Ratcliff PA, et al. Recognizing Periodontal Diseases, 2nd edition. San Francisco, USA: Praxis Publishing Company; 1978.

## VIVA VOCE

**Q1.** How can the infrabony pocket be differentiated clinically from a suprabony pocket?

**Ans.** Infrabony pocket can be differentiated clinically from the suprabony pocket by inserting the probe parallel to the long axis of the tooth and pulling it towards the gingiva. If bony resistance is felt the pocket is said to be infrabony. Bony resistance felt is the bony wall of the infrabony pocket, as the base of the pocket is apical to the alveolar crest.

**Section 4:** Pathology of Gingival and Periodontal Diseases

**Q2. Which types of pockets are found in furcation defects?**
**Ans.** Spiral/complex pockets are found in furcation defects.

**Q3. What is the relative volume of PMNs, when junctional epithelium loses its cohesiveness and detaches from the tooth surface?**
**Ans.** The relative volume of PMNs is approximately 60% or more when the junctional epithelium loses its cohesiveness and detaches from the tooth surface.

**Q4. What is the most reliable clinical method to detect a periodontal pocket?**
**Ans.** The most reliable clinical method to detect a periodontal pocket is by using a periodontal probe.

**Q5. What is the significance of pus in the pocket?**
**Ans.** It is the characteristic feature of periodontal disease but is only a secondary sign. It reflects the nature of inflammatory changes in the pocket wall. It is not an indication of the depth of pocket or severity of the destruction of supporting tissues.

**Q6. What is the basic difference between an active and an inactive pocket?**
**Ans.** Active pocket consists of more of the inflammatory content and is marked by spontaneous bleeding or bleeding on slight provocation. The inactive pocket contains less inflammatory contents and shows no signs of attachment loss or bone loss.

**Q7. What kind of bone loss is found in the suprabony pocket?**
**Ans.** Horizontal bone loss.

**Q8. What kind of bone loss is found in the infrabony pocket?**
**Ans.** Vertical bone loss.

**Q9. What are the contents of periodontal pockets?**
**Ans.** Microbial colonies and their products (enzymes, endotoxins and other metabolic products), gingival crevicular fluid, salivary mucin, food debris, desquamated epithelial cells, and leukocytes.

**Q10. What is probing depth?**
**Ans.** It is the distance between the gingival margin to the base of the probeable crevice up to which probe penetrates the pocket.

# Chapter 23: Periodontal Abscess

Harpreet S Grover, Shalu Bathla

## Chapter Outline

- Definition
- Classifications
- Clinical Features
- Microbiology
- Pathogenesis and Histopathology
- Diagnosis
- Differential Diagnosis
- Treatment
- Complications

## INTRODUCTION

A periodontal abscess is a localized purulent infection of periodontal tissues, which can be a common clinical finding among patients with moderate to advanced periodontitis. This chapter focuses on the classification of periodontal abscesses, etiology, clinical characteristics, and their management.

## DEFINITION

The periodontal abscess is defined as a suppurative lesion associated with periodontal breakdown and localized accumulation of pus within the gingival wall of a periodontal pocket.

The periodontal abscess has also been defined as a lesion with an expressed periodontal breakdown. It occurs during a limited time and with easily detectable clinical symptoms, with the localized accumulation of pus, located within the gingival wall of the periodontal pocket.

## CLASSIFICATIONS

- *Depending on the location of the lesion*:[1]
  - Periapical abscess
  - Periodontal abscess
  - Pericoronal abscess
- *Depending on the course of lesion*:
  - Acute abscess
  - Chronic abscess
- *Depending on the tissue involved*:
  - Gingival abscess
  - Periodontal abscess
  - Pericoronal abscess
- *Depending on the cause of the acute infectious process, two types of the periodontal abscess may occur*:[2]
  - Periodontitis-related abscess
  - Non-periodontitis related abscess
- *Depending on the number of abscesses*:
  - Single
  - Multiple

## CLINICAL FEATURES

### Intraoral

Following are the signs and symptoms of periodontal abscess:[3,4]

- The pain of acute periodontal abscess is throbbing and radiating, whereas, in the chronic periodontal abscess, pain is dull and gnawing **(Table 23.1)**.

**TABLE 23.1:** Acute and chronic periodontal abscesses.

| The acute periodontal abscess is associated with: | Pain |
| --- | --- |
| | Tenderness |
| | Sensitivity to palpation |
| | Suppuration upon gentle pressure |
| The chronic periodontal abscess is associated with: | Asymptomatic |
| | Sinus tract |

### Section 4: Pathology of Gingival and Periodontal Diseases

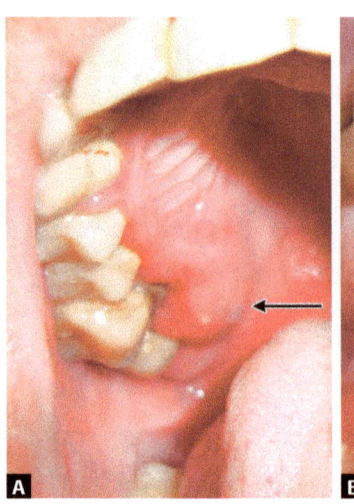 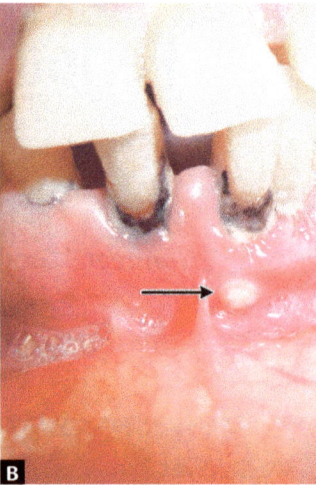

**Figs. 23.1A and B:** Clinical picture showing periodontal abscess associated with; (A) Palatal surface of the maxillary molar, (B) Labial surface of the mandibular central incisor.

(*Courtesy*: Dr Vikrender Yadav)

- Gingiva is swollen, red in color, with a smooth and shiny surface and ovoid elevation (**Fig. 23.1A**).
- Suppuration is either spontaneous or due to pressure on the outer surface of the gingiva.
- Swelling
- Sensitivity to the percussion of the affected tooth
- Tooth elevation
- During the periodontal examination, the abscess frequently lies at a site with a deep periodontal pocket.
- Bleeding on probing
- Pinpoint orifice of sinus may be present. Sinus is usually enclosed with a small, pink, bead-like mass of granulation tissue (**Fig. 23.1B**).

## Extraoral

In some patients, a periodontal abscess is present with following additional clinical features:
- Elevated body temperature
- Malaise
- Regional lymphadenopathy

## MICROBIOLOGY

The periodontal abscess is the destructive process in the periodontium constituted with complex microflora. Polymicrobial flora of periodontal abscess consists of gram-negative, strict anaerobe rods similar to the microbiota of chronic periodontitis lesions. gram-negative anaerobic species are non-fermentative and display moderate-to-strong proteolytic activity mainly. *Porphyromonas gingivalis, Prevotella intermedia*. In periodontal abscesses, strict anaerobic Gram-positive bacterial species mainly includes *Peptostreptococcus micros* and *Actinomyces* sp.[5]

## PATHOGENESIS AND HISTOPATHOLOGY

Following are the factors that may provoke the formation of an abscess:[3]
- Obstruction to the opening of a deep pocket, frequently one which is tortuous or associated with furcation defect.
- Gingival injury with a foreign body, e.g., toothbrush bristles or wood stick, which carries bacteria into the tissues. Careless subgingival scaling may also take microorganisms into the damaged tissue, as can powerful irrigation of a pocket.
- Incomplete removal of plaque and subgingival calculus from the depths of a pocket. Frequently after scaling, there is a tightening of the gingival cuff which occludes pocket containing bacteria.[6]
- Infection of tissues damaged by excessive occlusal stress, which may be produced by:
  - Bruxism
  - Excessive orthodontic forces
- As a consequence of pulp disease:
  - Where a periapical lesion spreads up to the lateral surface of a tooth.
  - Where a lateral pulp canal links with the periodontal ligament. This is especially common in the furcation.
  - Perforation of the lateral wall of a tooth during endodontics.
- Altered host response as in diabetes

The periodontal abscess formation takes place with the bacterial invasion of the soft-tissue wall of the pocket and further multiplication. Infiltration of inflammatory cells in the periodontal tissues initiates the destruction of the connective tissue. This favors the encapsulation of the bacterial mass and process of pus formation. The disease's progression is determined by microbial virulence, host resistance, and the number of bacteria present in the lesion. The extracellular enzymes and inflammatory cells facilitate the periodontal tissue destruction. An acidic environment will favor the activity of lysosomal enzymes and promote tissue destruction.

Periodontal abscess contains bacteria, bacterial products, inflammatory cells, tissue breakdown products, and serum. The central area of the abscess is mainly constituted with neutrophils and close to soft-tissue debris (**Fig. 23.2**). At a later stage, macrophages and neutrophils get organized to form a pyogenic membrane.[7]

## DIAGNOSIS

A periodontal abscess diagnosis is established with understanding the patient's chief complaint, overall clinical evaluation, and the assessment of clinical and radiographic findings. Careful probing of the suspected area along the gingival margin in association with each tooth surface helps to identify a tract from the marginal area to deeper

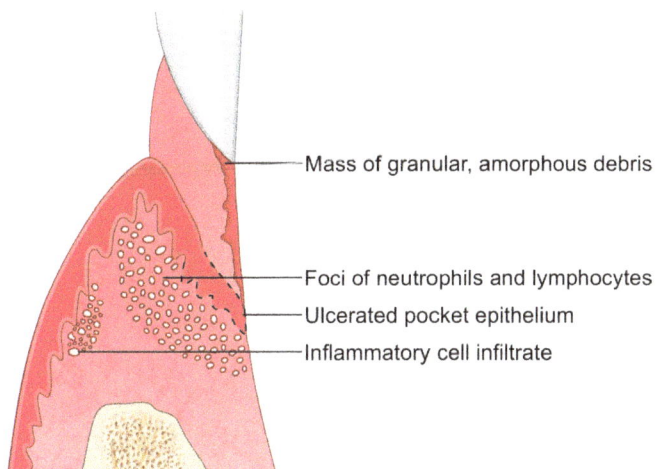

**Fig. 23.2:** Schematic representation showing histopathology of periodontal abscess.

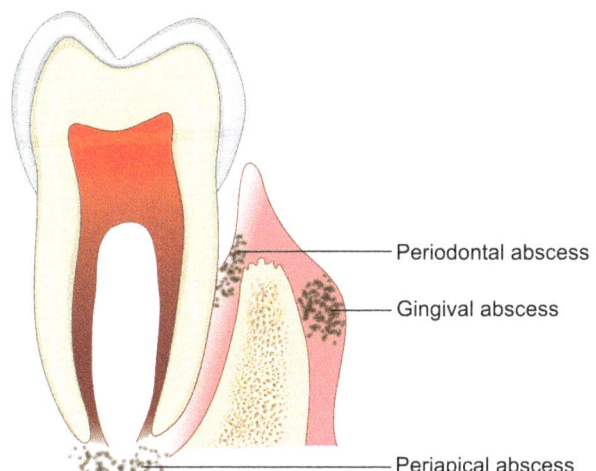

**Fig. 23.3:** Schematic representation showing various abscesses that occur in the oral cavity.

periodontal tissues. Radiographically, the interdental bone is either normal or associated with some bone loss. Bone loss usually extends from a widening of the periodontal ligament space to bone loss involving most of the affected tooth. Radiographs taken in the earliest stage of periodontal abscess provide little useful information, but once the lesion is established, its position can be identified. The radiolucent area along the lateral surface of the root suggests the presence of a periodontal abscess. A radiograph taken with Gutta-percha point inserted gently into the suspected pocket can help define the abscess's origin.

## DIFFERENTIAL DIAGNOSIS

The periodontal abscess needs to be differentiated from other abscesses occurring in the oral cavity. Gingival abscess, periapical abscess, endoperiodontal abscess **(Fig. 23.3)**, lateral periapical cysts, and vertical root fractures may have a similar appearance. A gingival abscess is usually sudden in onset, localized, tender, and rapidly spreading lesion. It is generally restricted to the marginal gingiva or interdental papilla. Signs such as lack of pulp vitality, the presence of deep carious lesions, the presence of a sinus tract and findings made in the radiographic the examination will aid in the distinction between abscesses **(Table 23.2)** of different etiologies.[2]

## TREATMENT

Treatment of periodontal abscess depends upon the stage of abscess development, the amount of bone loss, and the possibility of involvement of pulp pathology.

### Gingival Abscess

After topical anesthesia is applied, the lesion's fluctuant area is incised with a Bard–Parker handle and surgical blade, and the incision is gently widened to permit drainage. The area is cleansed with warm water and covered with a gauze pad. After bleeding stops, the patient is dismissed for 24 hours and instructed to rinse every 2 hours with a glassful of warm water.[8]

**TABLE 23.2:** Differences between periodontal and periapical abscesses.

| Parameters | Periodontal abscesses | Periapical abscesses |
|---|---|---|
| History | Periodontal disease | Caries, fracture, tooth-wear |
| | Periodontal treatment | Restorative and endodontic treatment |
| Clinical findings | Vital pulp responses | Questionable/nonresponsive pulp tests |
| | Periodontal probing release pus | Narrow probing defect (maybe isolated vision) |
| | Periodontal disease evident | Advanced caries, advanced tooth wear, large restoration |
| | Swelling is generalized and located around the involved tooth and gingival margin. Seldom with a fistulous tract | Swelling is localized often with a fistulous opening in the apical area |
| | Pain is usually dull, constant, and less severe than in a periapical abscess. Pain is localized, and the patient usually can locate the offending tooth | Pain is usually severe, throbbing and patient may not be able to locate the offending tooth |
| Radiographic findings | Alveolar crest bone loss, angular bone defects, furcation involvements | Apical radiolucency **(Fig. 23.4)** Endodontic or post-perforations |
| Response to treatment | Responds dramatically to the release of pus, subgingival debridement | Responds poorly, or not at all to periodontal treatment |

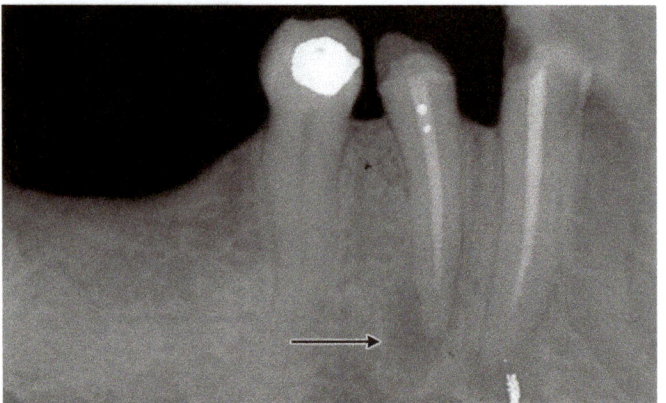

**Fig. 23.4:** Radiographic image of periapical abscess.

## Acute Periodontal Abscess (Incision and Drainage)

### Drainage through the Pocket

After the application of topical anesthesia, a flat instrument or a probe is carefully introduced into the pocket in an attempt to distend the pocket wall. A small curette or a Morse scaler can then be gently used to penetrate the tissue and establish drainage.

### Drainage through an External Incision

After local anesthesia is given, with a Bard–Parker handle and blade number 11, a vertical incision is made in the most fluctuant part of the lesion, extending from the mucogingival fold to the gingival margin **(Fig. 23.5)**. If swelling is on the lingual surface, the incision is started just apical to the swelling extending through the gingival margin. The blade should penetrate to firm tissue to be sure of reaching deep, purulent areas. After initial extravasation of blood and pus, irrigate the area with warm water and gently spread the incision to facilitate drainage. Postoperative instructions are given to rinse hourly with a solution of a teaspoon of salt in a glass of warm water. Antibiotics penicillin and metronidazole are prescribed for a patient with systemic complications.[2,9]

## Chronic Periodontal Abscess

### Treatment by Flap Operation

All deposits are scaled from the teeth, and the root surfaces are planed with scalers and smoothened with curettes. Systemic antibiotics amoxicillin and metronidazole are prescribed. To locate the abscess area, probing is done around the gingival margin, following tortuous pockets to their termination. If a sinus is present, the abscess may be probed through it.
- *Anesthetize*: The area is anesthetized with local infiltration.
- *Incision*: Two vertical incisions are made from the gingival margin to the mucobuccal fold, outlining the field of operation. If the lingual approach is used, the

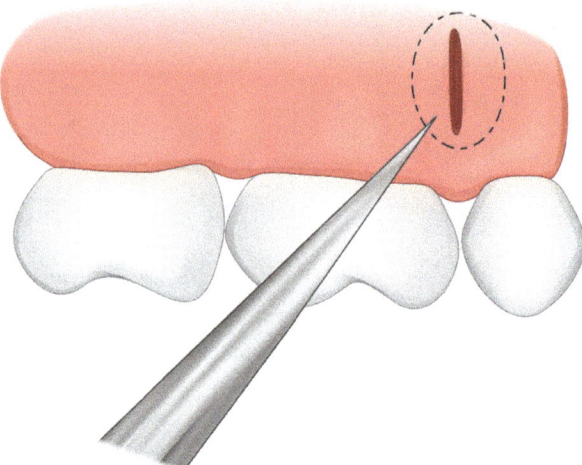

**Fig. 23.5:** Schematic representation showing vertical incision.

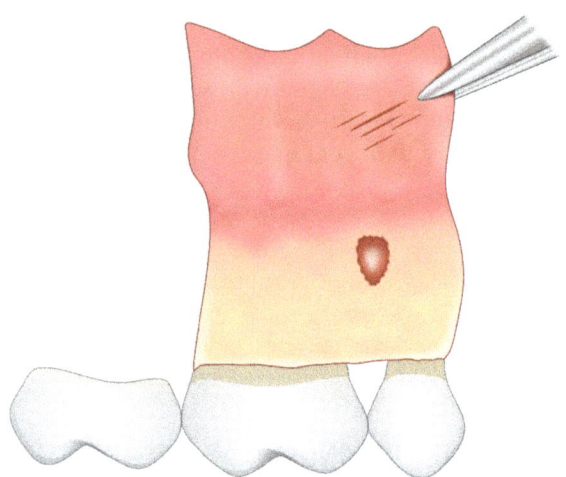

**Fig. 23.6:** Schematic representation showing a full-thickness flap (raised to facilitate removal of granulation tissue).

incisions are made from the gingival margin to the level of the root apices. After the vertical incisions are made, a mesiodistal incision is made across the interdental papilla with a knife to facilitate the detachment of the flap **(Fig. 23.6)**.
- *Reflect the flap*: A full-thickness flap is raised with a periosteal elevator and held in the position with a retractor.
- *Remove granulation tissue*: The granulation tissue is removed with curettes to provide a clear view of the root. If a sinus is present, it is explored and curetted.
- *Control bleeding*: The facial and lingual surfaces are covered with a U-shaped gauze, held in position until the bleeding stops.
- *Suture*: The gauze is then removed, and the flap is sutured and covered with a periodontal pack.

### Sorrin's Operation

It is a surgical technique, a type of flap approach, in the treatment of a periodontal abscess. The procedure is suitable when the marginal gingiva is healthy and there is no access to the abscess area. The method involved making a semilunar incision underneath the involved area in the attached gingiva and leaving the gingival margin undisturbed. A flap is raised to enter in the abscessed area for curettage.

## COMPLICATIONS

### Tooth Loss

Periodontal abscesses are identified as one of the causative agents for tooth extraction in the process of supportive periodontal therapy.[10]

### Dissemination of the Infection

Cellulitis, subcutaneous infection, phlegmon, and mediastinitis can result from odontogenic infections but are very uncommon with periodontal abscess. Mechanical management of a periodontal abscess may result in bacteremia, which in patients with endoprosthesis or immunocompromised states can result in nonoral infections. Occasional dissemination of periodontal bacteria can result in brain abscess also.

### Points to Ponder

- Multiple periodontal abscesses are seen in diabetes mellitus.
- *Periodontitis associated abscess*: It is the result of acute infection emerging from a biofilm present in a deepened periodontal pocket.
- *Postscaling periodontal abscess*: This type of abscess develops due to the migration of small fragments of calculus into the deep and previously noninflamed portion of the periodontal tissues.
- *Postsurgery periodontal abscess*: Such type of abscess occurs due to incomplete removal of subgingival calculus or to the presence of foreign bodies in the periodontal tissues, such as sutures, regenerative devices, or periodontal pack.
- *Postantibiotic periodontal abscess*: In patients with advanced periodontitis, the administration of systemic antibiotics without subgingival debridement may lead to abscess formation.

## REFERENCES

1. Meng HX. Periodontal abscess. Ann Periodontol. 1999;4(1):79-83.
2. Sanz M, Herrera D, Winkelhoff AJ. The Periodontal Abscess. In: Lindhe J, Karring T, Lang NP (Eds). Clinical Periodontology and Implant Dentistry, 4th edition. Chicago, USA: Blackwell Munksgaard; 2003. pp. 260-68.
3. Eley BM, Manson JD. The periodontal abscess. In: Periodontics, 5th edition. Edinburgh, Scotland: Wright Publishing; 2004. pp. 328-31.
4. Herrera D, Roldan S, Sanz M. The periodontal abscess: a review. J Clin Periodontol. 2000;27(6):377-86.
5. Herrera D, Roldan S, González I, Sanz M. The periodontal abscess (I). Clinical and microbiological findings. J Clin Periodontol. 2000;27(6):387-94.
6. Dello Russo NM. The post-prophylaxis periodontal abscess: etiology and treatment. Int J Periodontics Restorative Dent. 1985;5(1):28-37.
7. DeWitt GV, Cobb CM, Killoy WJ. The acute periodontal abscess: microbial penetration of the soft tissue wall. Int J Periodontics Restorative Dent. 1985;5(1):38-51.
8. Takei HH. Treatment of the periodontal abscess. In: Newman MG, Takei HH, Carranza FA (Eds). Carranza's Clinical Periodontology, 9th edition. Philadelphia, PA, USA: WB Saunders; 2003. pp. 629-30.
9. Siqueira JF, Rôças IN. Microbiology and treatment of acute apical abscesses. Clin Microbiol Rev. 2013;26(2):255-73.
10. Chace RJ, Low SB. Survival characteristics of periodontally-involved teeth: a 40-year study. J Periodontol. 1993;64(8):701-5.

## VIVA VOCE

**Q1. Name the drugs of choice for periodontal abscess.**
Ans. Antibiotics-amoxicillin and metronidazole, are the drugs of choice for periodontal abscess.

**Q2. What is gingival abscess and its etiology?**
Ans. A gingival abscess is a localized, painful, rapidly expanding lesion usually of sudden onset. It is generally limited to the marginal gingiva or interdental papilla.
*Etiology*: Irritation from foreign substances, toothbrush bristle; apple core; lobster shell forcefully embedding into the gingiva.

**Q3. In which systemic disease, multiple periodontal abscesses are seen?**
Ans. Diabetes mellitus.

**Q4. Why incomplete removal of subgingival plaque and calculus from the depths of pocket leads to abscess formation?**
Ans. Frequently after scaling, there is a tightening of the gingival cuff, which occludes pocket containing bacteria, which leads to abscess formation.

**Q5. What is the nature of the pain of periodontal abscess?**
Ans. In acute periodontal abscess, the pain is throbbing and radiating, whereas in chronic periodontal abscess, pain is dull and gnawing.

**Q6. What are the various complications of a periodontal abscess?**
Ans. Tooth loss, cellulitis, subcutaneous infection, phlegmon, and mediastinitis

**Q7. What is the nature of pain of periapical abscess?**
Ans. Severe and throbbing pain.

**Q8. Name the microorganisms mainly present in periodontal abscesses?**
Ans. Gram-positive bacterial species mainly *Peptostreptococcus micros* and *Actinomyces* sp.

**Q9. What is the radiographic feature of a periapical abscess?**
Ans. Apical radiolucency.

**Q10. What is the radiographic feature of a chronic periodontal abscess?**
Ans. Lateral radiolucency with alveolar crest bone loss, angular bone defects, and furcation involvement.

# Chapter 24

# Bone Defects

*Sanjeev K Salaria*

## Chapter Outline

- Factors Determining Bone Morphology
- Etiology
- Bone Defects
- Diagnosis

## INTRODUCTION

Alveolar bone loss is one of the most important and distinct features of periodontal disease. The height and density of the alveolar bone are normally maintained by an equilibrium regulated by local and systemic factors between bone formation and bone resorption. When resorption exceeds formation, bone height, density, or both are reduced. The variation is seen in bone loss patterns between individuals and different sites in the same mouth and even on different aspects of the same tooth.

## FACTORS DETERMINING BONE MORPHOLOGY

- *Normal variation in alveolar bone*: Various anatomic features that influence destructive bone pattern in periodontal disease are: thickness, width and crestal angulation of the interdental septa, the thickness of facial and lingual alveolar plates, presence of fenestration and dehiscence, alignment of teeth, proximity with another tooth surfaces, root and root trunk anatomy and root position within alveolar bone.[1]
- *Exostosis*: These are outgrowths of the bone of varied size and shape. They can occur as small nodules, large nodules, sharp ridges, spike-like projections, or any combination of these.[2]
- *Trauma from occlusion*: It may be a factor in determining the dimension and shape of bone deformities. It may cause a thickening of the cervical margin of the alveolar bone or a change in the morphology of the angular bone defects and buttressing bone.[3]
- *Buttressing bone formation*: Bone formation sometimes occurs in an attempt to buttress bony trabeculae weakened by resorption. When it occurs within the jaw, it is termed as "central buttressing bone formation." When it occurs on the external surface, it is referred to as "peripheral buttressing bone formation." The latter may cause bulging of the bone contour, termed lipping, which sometimes accompanies the production of osseous craters and angular defects.[4]
- *Food impaction*: Interdental bone defects often occur where proximal contact is abnormal or absent. Pressure from food impaction contributes to the inverted bone architecture.[1]
- *Aggressive periodontitis*: A vertical or angular pattern of alveolar bone destruction is found around the first molars in aggressive periodontitis.

## ETIOLOGY

The various causes of alveolar bone loss are:
- Extension of gingival inflammation
- Trauma from occlusion
- Systemic disorders

### Extension of Gingival Inflammation

The most common cause of bone destruction in periodontal disease is the extension of inflammation from the marginal gingiva into the deeper periodontal tissues. The inflammatory invasion of the bone surface and the initial bone loss mark the transition from gingivitis to periodontitis.[1]

#### Histopathology

Interproximally, gingival inflammation spreads to the loose connective tissue around the blood vessels,[5] through the fibers and into the bone through vessel channels that perforate the interdental septum's crest. The inflammation may sometimes spread from the gingiva directly into the periodontal ligament and from there into the interdental septum (**Flowchart 24.1 and Fig. 24.1A**).

Facially and lingually, inflammation from the gingiva spreads along the outer periosteal surface of the bone and penetrates the marrow spaces through vessels' channel in the outer cortex (**Fig. 24.1B**). The gingival and transseptal fibers are destroyed meanwhile. Once the inflammation reaches the bone, it spreads into marrow spaces and replaces the marrow with a leukocytic and fluid exudate, new blood vessels, and the proliferating fibroblasts. Bone surfaces are lined with multinucleated osteoclasts and Howship's lacunae.

In the marrow spaces, resorption proceeds from within, causing a thinning of the surrounding bony trabeculae and enlargement of marrow spaces. This destroys bone and reduction in bone height.

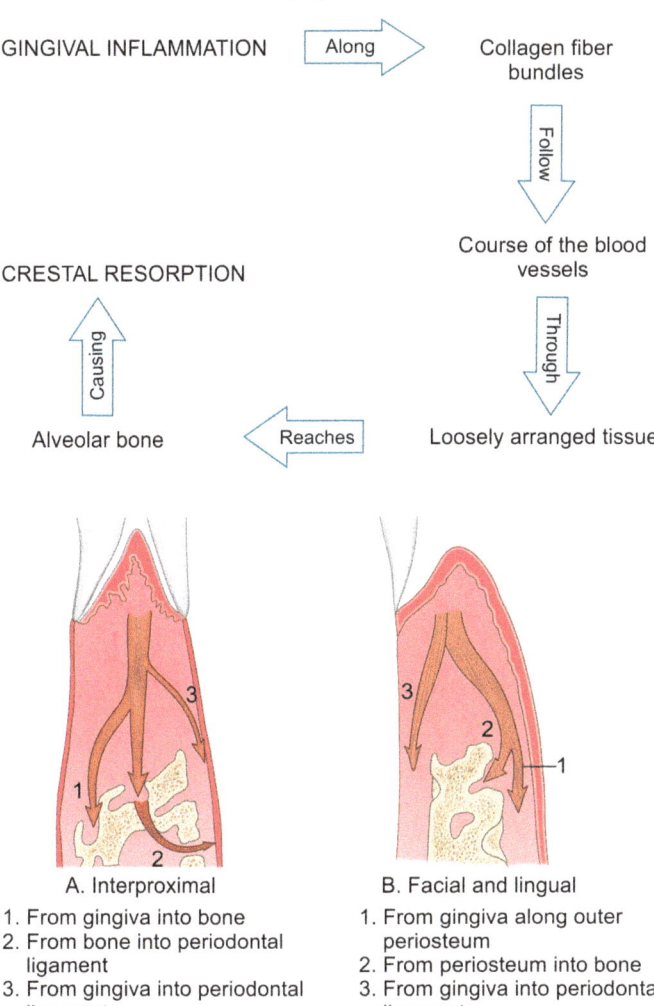

**Flowchart 24.1:** Extension of gingival inflammation to alveolar bone.

A. Interproximal
1. From gingiva into bone
2. From bone into periodontal ligament
3. From gingiva into periodontal ligament

B. Facial and lingual
1. From gingiva along outer periosteum
2. From periosteum into bone
3. From gingiva into periodontal ligament

**Figs. 24.1A and B:** Schematic representation showing pathways of inflammation from gingiva to periodontal tissues in periodontitis: (A) Interproximal; and (B) Facial and lingual.

## Radius of Action

Garant and Cho were the first to point out that bone resorption stimulators produced by microbial plaque have a finite radius of action.[6] Page and Schroeder postulated a range of effectiveness of about 1.5–2.5 mm within which bacterial plaque can cause bone destruction.[7] Waerhaug applied this principle to human periodontium by making measurements on radiographs, histological sections and extracted teeth to determine the distance between microbial plaque and the bone surface. Waerhaug has shown that the bone margin is never located closer than 0.5 mm to plaque and not farther than 1.5–2.5 mm from plaque.

## Rate of Bone Loss

Rate of bone loss depends upon the type of disease present and tooth surface: an average of 0.2 mm/year on facial surfaces and 0.3 mm/year on proximal surfaces.

Three subgroups were distinguished according to attachment loss:[8]
1. About 8% population had rapid progression (RP) of periodontal disease, loss of attachment of 0.1–1.0 mm yearly.
2. About 81% had moderately progressive (MP) periodontal disease, loss of attachment of 0.05–0.5 mm yearly.
3. About 11% had minimal or no progression (NP) of periodontal disease, loss of attachment of 0.05–0.09 mm yearly.

## Mechanisms of Bone Destruction

Bone resorption occurs in the presence of both osteoblasts and osteoclasts. Stimulators of bone resorption are interleukin-1 (IL-1), IL-6, parathyroid hormone (PTH), parathyroid hormone-related peptide (PTHrP), prostaglandin $E_2$ ($PGE_2$), receptor activator of nuclear factor kappa B (RANK), RANK ligand (RANKL) and vitamin D. Inhibitors of bone resorption are interferon-alpha (IFN-α), osteoprotegerin (OPG), calcitonin, estrogen, and androgen. Systemic and local bone-resorbing factors exert their influence by stimulating the osteoblast, and this osteoblast is involved in the regulation of osteoclast function at several levels. Osteoblasts stimulated by these factors mediate their response through a series of intracellular secondary messenger systems; one pathway involves cyclic adenosine monophosphate (AMP). The second involves membrane phospholipids and protein kinase C. Both of these mechanisms are stimulated by $PGE_2$, prostacyclin ($PGI_2$), and thrombin.

According to Hausmann, the following are the possible pathways of alveolar bone loss in periodontal diseases:[9]
- The direct action of plaque products on bone progenitor cells induces the differentiation of these cells into osteoclasts.
- Plaque products act directly on bone, destroying it through a noncellular mechanism.

- Plaque products stimulate gingival cells, causing them to release mediators, which in turn induce bone progenitor cells to differentiate into osteoclasts.
- Plaque products cause gingival cells to release agents that can act as cofactors in bone resorption.
- Plaque products cause gingival cells to release agents that destroy bone by direct chemical action, without osteoclasts.

The sequence of events in the bone resorptive process are:[10]

- *Formation of osteoclast*: Osteoclasts are multinucleated giant cells of 50–100 μm size derived from circulating blood cells monocytes **(Fig. 24.2)**. Osteoclasts are found in bay-like depression in the bone called Howship's lacunae. The part of the cell in contact with bone shows convoluted surface and is called ruffled border.[11]
- *Osteoblast-osteoclast coupling*: The development of osteoclasts is controlled by the stromal cells through the RANK/RANKL/OPG axis. RANK is activated through its ligand RANKL. RANKL is produced from the osteoblasts/stromal cells. Upon RANK/RANKL binding, the activation of osteoclasts occurs, which subsequently leads to bone resorption. OPG acts as a soluble decoy receptor of RANKL and thus prevents osteoclastogenesis **(Fig. 24.3 and Flowchart 24.2)**.
- *Attachment of osteoclasts to the mineralized surface of bone*: The part of the osteoclast in contact with bone shows a convoluted surface. The ruffled border is the site of significant activity due to ion transport protein secretion. The ruffled border is surrounded by a clear zone that has no organelles but only fine granular cytoplasm with microfilaments. The peripheral region of the apical membrane is tightly juxtaposed to the matrix, which is called a sealing zone. Clear zone and sealing zone are responsible for the attachment of osteoclast to the bone matrix. This contains podosomes, which are specialized protrusions of the osteoclast's ventral membrane, which adhere directly to the bone surface being broken down.
- *Creation of a sealed acidic environment through action of the proton pump, which demineralizes bone and exposes the organic matrix*: The mineral is dissolved by acid secretion, which is brought about by an electrogenic hydrogen ion transporting system. This is an ATP driven proton pump. Intracellular pH regulation is achieved by carbonic anhydrase, which is abundant in the osteoclast cytoplasm. Bicarbonate generated by the carbonic anhydrase appears to be secreted from the basal outer membrane. The hydrogen ions are released in the functional extracellular lysosomal compartment, and there they dissolve the mineral and expose the organic matrix **(Fig. 24.4)**.
- *Degradation of the exposed organic matrix to its constituent amino acids*: Stimulated osteoblast also secretes procollagenase and plasminogen activator, which generates plasmin from plasminogen, and this activates procollagenase for removing the nonmineralized collagenase surface layer **(Flowchart 24.3)**.
- Sequestering of mineral ions and amino acids within the osteoclast **(Flowchart 24.4)**.

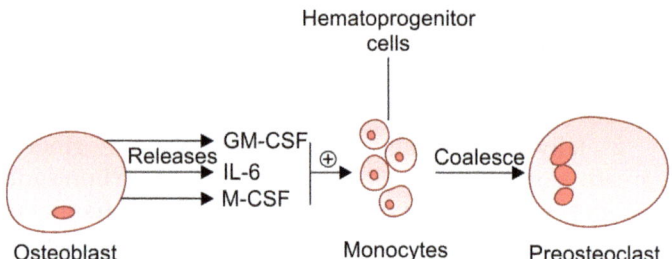

**Fig. 24.2:** Schematic representation showing the pre-osteoclast formation.
(GM-CSF: granulocyte-macrophage colony-stimulating factor; M-CSF, macrophage colony-stimulating factor; IL-6: interleukin-6)

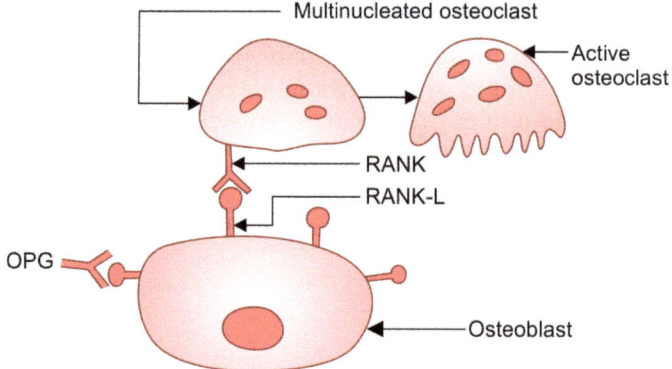

RANK-L is a cell surface protein on osteoblast
RANK is present on osteoclast
OPG block the action of RANK-L by acting as decoy receptor

**Fig. 24.3:** Schematic representation showing activation of osteoclast through RANK/RANKL/OPG axis.
(RANK: receptor activator of nuclear factor kappa B; RANKL: receptor activator of nuclear factor kappa B ligand; OPG: osteoprotegerin)

**Flowchart 24.2:** RANKL/OPG ratio determine whether bone resorption or bone formation will occur.

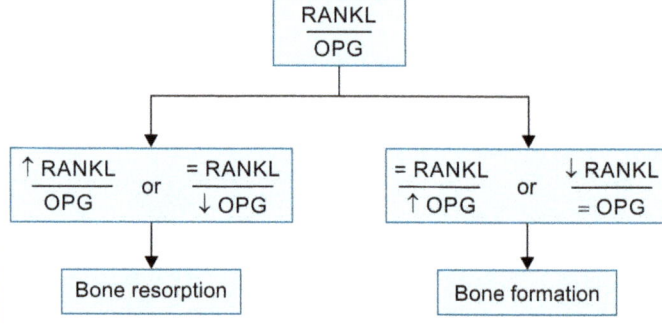

(RANKL: receptor activator of nuclear factor kappa B ligand; OPG: osteoprotegerin)

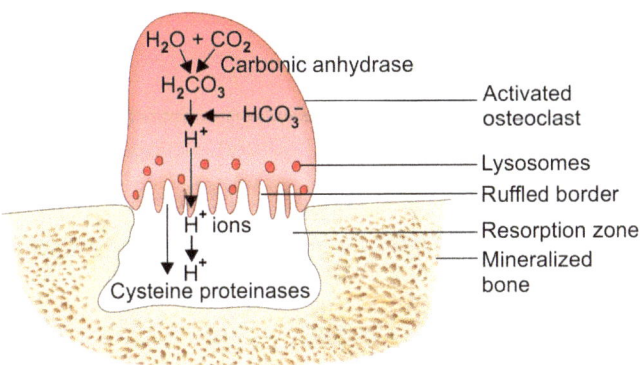

**Fig. 24.4:** Schematic representation showing activated osteoclast causing resorption of mineralized bone matrix.
($H_2CO_3$: carbonic acid; $HCO_3^-$: bicarbonate ion)

**Flowchart 24.3:** Osteoblast causing degradation of nonmineralized bone matrix.

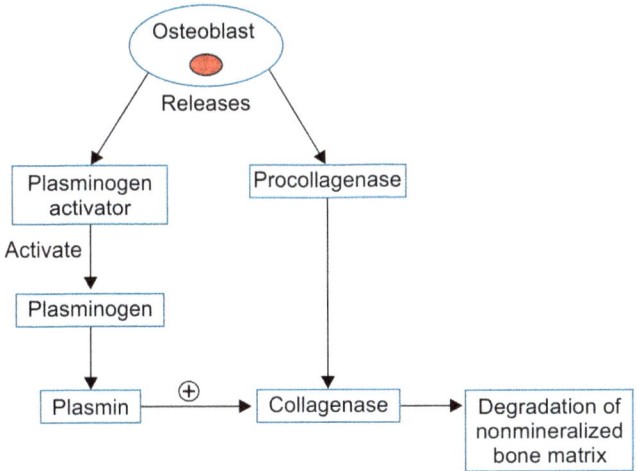

**Flowchart 24.4:** Bone resorption sequence.

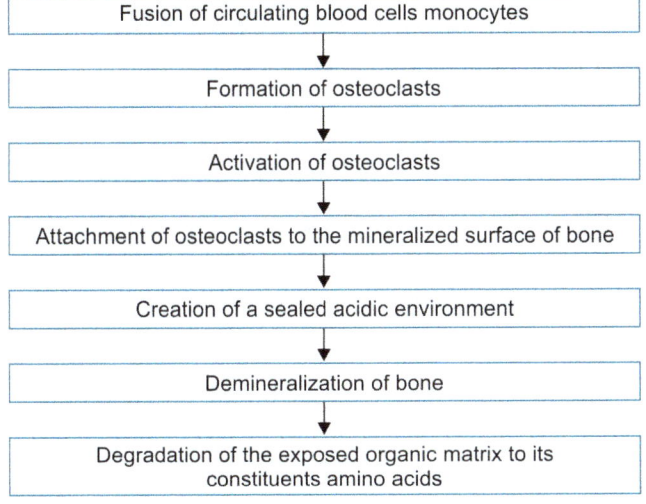

## Trauma from Occlusion

Trauma from occlusion can produce bone destruction either in the absence or presence of inflammation. In the absence of inflammation, the changes caused by trauma from occlusion vary from increased compression and tension of the periodontal ligament and increased osteoclasis of alveolar bone, to necrosis of the periodontal ligament and bone and resorption of bone and tooth structure. These changes are reversible in that they can be repaired if the offending forces are removed. However, persistent trauma from occlusion results in funnel-shaped widening of the crestal portion of the periodontal ligament, with resorption of the adjacent bone. These changes, which may cause the bony crest to have an angular shape, represent an adaptation of the periodontal tissues aimed at cushioning increased occlusal forces, but the modified bone shape may weaken tooth support and cause tooth mobility. When combined with inflammation, trauma from occlusion aggravates the bone destruction caused by the inflammation and causes bizarre bone patterns.[3]

## Systemic Disorders

Periodontal bone loss may also occur in generalized skeletal disturbances, such as hyperparathyroidism, leukemia, or Langerhan's cell histiocytosis.[12] Irving Glickman gave the concept of a bone factor in the early 1950s. This concept presents a clinical guide for determining the diagnosis and prognosis of periodontal disease based upon the response of alveolar bone to local injurious factors. The systemic regulatory influence on the response of alveolar bone is termed a bone factor in periodontal disease. The individual bone factor affects the severity of bone loss associated with local destructive factors in periodontal disease. The destructive effect of inflammation and trauma from occlusion varies with the status of individual bone factor. It is less severe in a healthy individual in the presence of positive bone factor.[13]

## BONE DEFECTS

The variety of bone defect is infinite, but for description, they have been classified according to their morphology as marginal defects, intra-alveolar defects, perforation, and furcation defects **(Box 24.1)**. These are very rough groupings with considerable overlap.[14]

**BOX 24.1:** Various bone destructive patterns.

- Horizontal bone loss
- Vertical or angular defects
- Interdental osseous craters
- Bulbous bone contours
- Reversed architecture
- Ledges
- Furcation involvement
- Fenestration and dehiscence
- Marginal gutter
- Irregular bony margins

## Horizontal

When the bone loss occurs on a plane that is parallel to a line drawn from the cementoenamel junction (CEJ) of a tooth to that of an adjacent tooth, it is called horizontal bone loss. It is one of the common patterns of bone loss in periodontal disease. The bone margin remains roughly perpendicular to the tooth surface **(Fig. 24.5)**.

## Vertical

Vertical or angular defects are those that occur in an oblique direction, leaving a hollowed-out trough in the bone alongside the root; the base of the defect is located apical to the surrounding bone **(Fig. 24.6)**. When there is sufficient volume of the bone surrounding the roots of teeth, resorptive bone patterns may take a vertical or funnel-form, resulting in the formation of intrabony defects **(Fig. 24.7)**. Vertical bone loss usually consists of one or many infrabony pockets, because the base of the pocket is usually located apical to the crest of the surrounding bone. Goldman and Cohen classified angular defects based on the number of osseous walls remaining **(Figs. 24.8A to C)**.[15]

One-walled osseous defects where only one wall (1W) is present. The one walled vertical defect is called as hemiseptum. Two-walled osseous defects where two walls (2W) are present. Three-walled osseous defects where three walls (3W) are present. In combined osseous defects, the number of walls in the apical portion of the defect is often greater than that in its occlusal portion.

Interproximal vertical defects can often be detected radiographically, whereas radicular surface vertical defects are not readily visible.

## Osseous Craters

Interdental osseous craters are concavities in the crest of the alveolar septa centered under adjacent teeth' contact point. Thus, it can be described as a cup or bowl-shaped

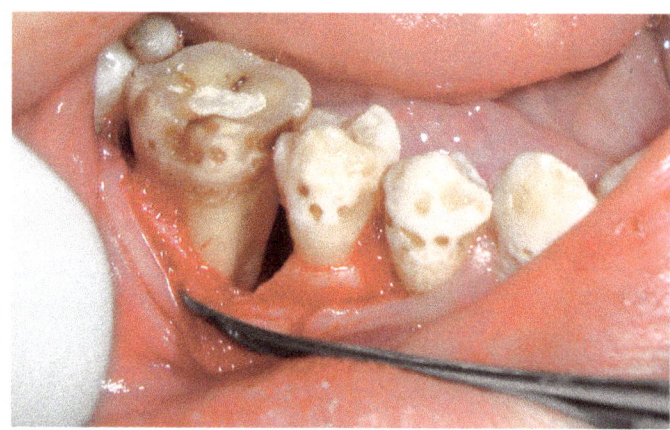

**Fig. 24.7:** Clinical picture showing intrabony defect.

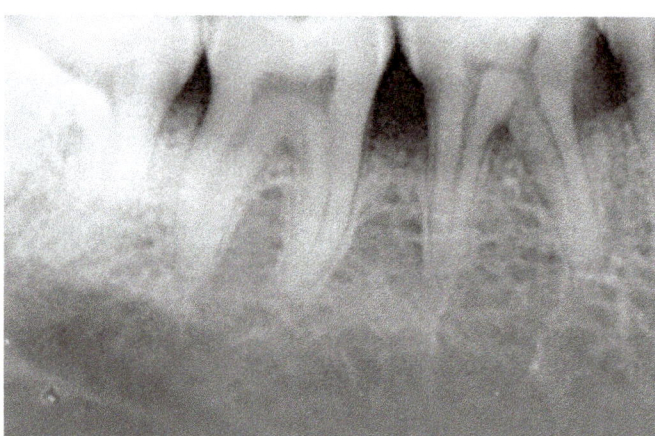

**Fig. 24.5:** Radiographic image showing horizontal bone loss.

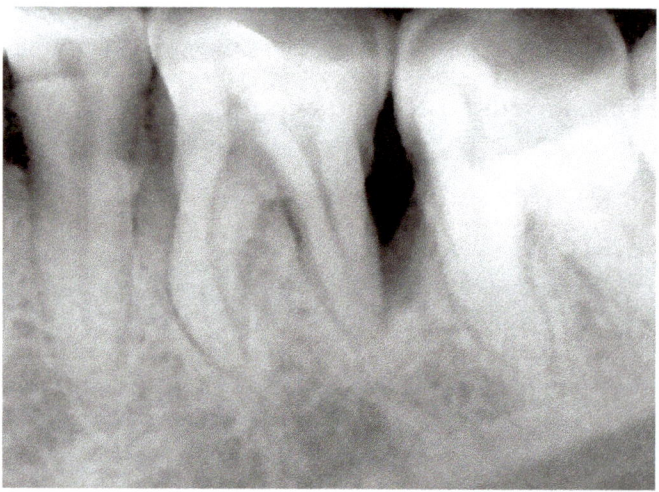

**Fig. 24.6:** Radiographic image showing vertical bone loss.

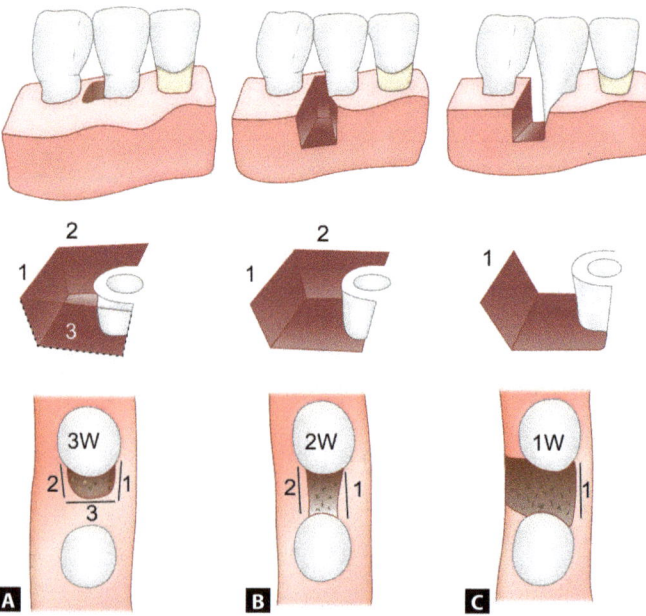

**Figs. 24.8A to C:** Schematic representation showing various vertical osseous defects: (A) Three-wall (3W) bony defect; (B) Two-wall (2W) bony defect and (C) One-wall (1W) bony defect.

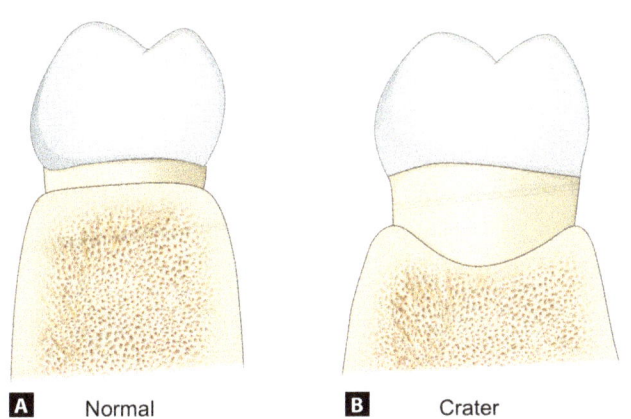

**Figs. 24.9A and B:** Schematic representation showing faciolingual longitudinal section (A) Normal bone contour and (B) Osseous crater.

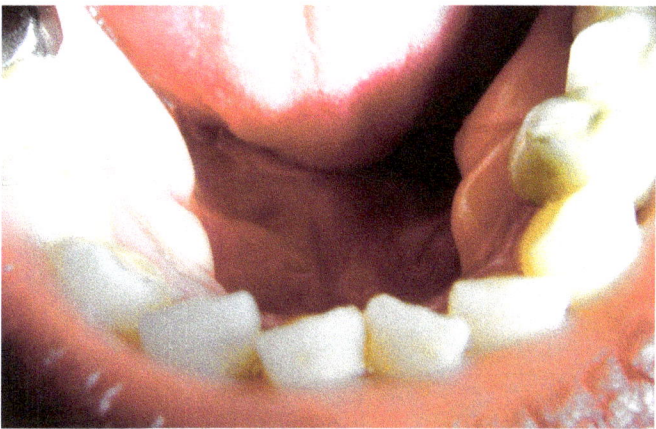

**Fig. 24.10:** Clinical picture showing bilateral lingual exostosis.

defect in the interdental alveolar bone **(Figs. 24.9A and B)**.[16] As cancellous bone is more vascular and less dense than cortical bone it is likely that, the central cancellous part of a broad alveolar septum will resorb more rapidly than the lateral parts made up of cortical bone forming an interdental crater. Craters have been found to make up about one-third (35.2%) of all maxillary defects and about two-thirds (62%) of all mandibular defects.[17] They are twice as common in posterior segments as in anterior segments as the interproximal bone is sufficient to result in such kind of defects. Ochsenbein divided bony craters into three basic types: (1) shallow (1–2 mm), (2) medium (3–4 mm), and (3) deep (5 mm and more).[18] Following are the reasons for the high frequency of interdental craters:

- The interdental area collects plaque and is difficult to clean.[19]
- The normal flat or even concave faciolingual shape of the interdental septum in lower molars may favor crater formation.[20]
- Vascular patterns from the gingiva to the center of the crest may provide a pathway for inflammation.

## Bulbous Bone Contours

Bulbous bone contours are bony enlargements caused by exostosis adaptation to function, or buttressing bone formation, which is found frequently in the maxilla than mandible. Exostosis is a localized harmless idiopathic thickening of bony tissue; whose cause is unknown **(Figs. 24.10 and 24.11)**. Depending on their location in the jaws, they are identified as torus mandibularis[21] (lingual mandibular plate) or torus palatinus (hard palate). Sometimes, several bony overgrowths occur on the vestibular alveolar bone and are simply called multiple exostosis. A peculiar condition consisting of bone exostosis has been reported to occur in some patients after undergoing either a skin graft vestibuloplasty or an autogenous free gingival graft. A slowly growing exostosis develops at the recipient site of the gingival graft. A definitive

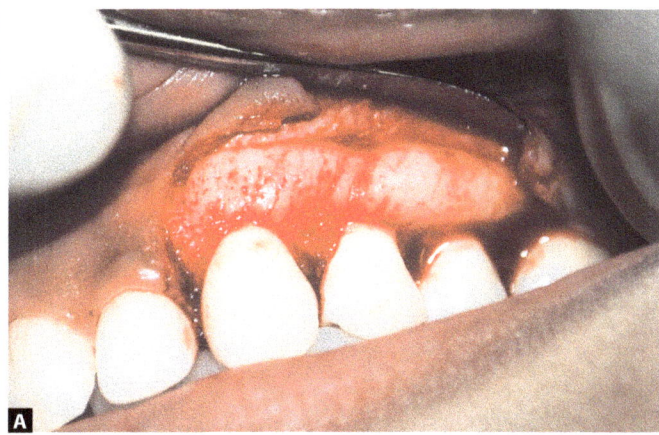

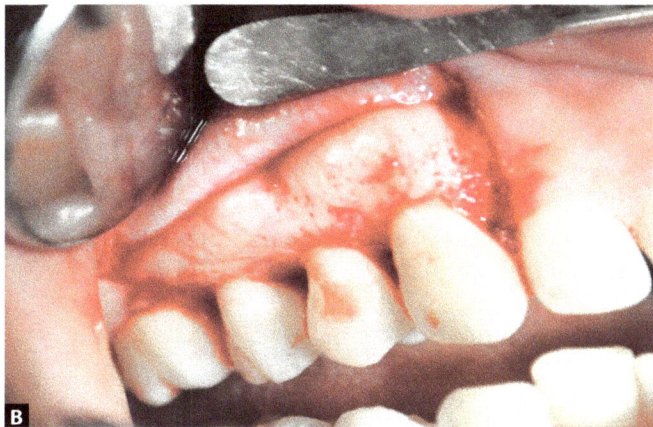

**Figs. 24.11A and B:** Clinical picture showing bilateral maxillary exostosis after flap reflection.

female sex predilection is characteristic of this condition, which usually presents in the canine premolar area of the mandible or maxilla.

## Reversed Architecture

Reversed architecture forms when the interdental septum resorbs more rapidly than radicular bone **(Fig. 24.12)**.

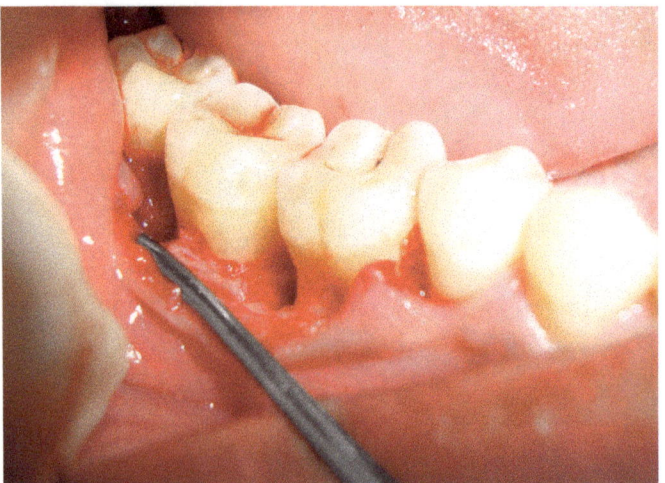

**Fig. 24.12:** Clinical picture showing the reversed bony architecture.

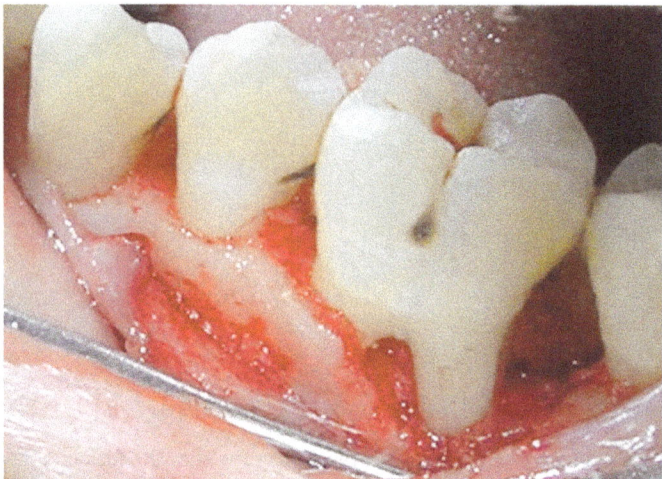

**Fig. 24.14:** Clinical photograph showing furcation defect.

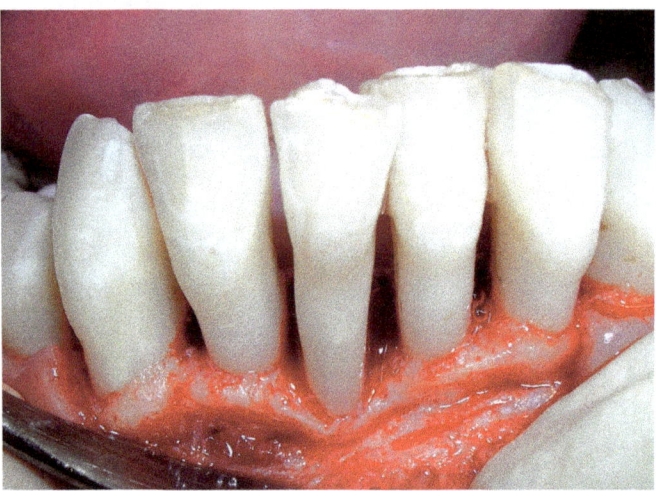

**Fig. 24.13:** Clinical picture showing ledge.

## Ledges

Ledges are plateau-like bone margins caused by resorption of thickened bony plates **(Fig. 24.13)**.

## Furcation Involvement

Furcation involvement refers to the invasion of the bifurcation and trifurcation of multirooted teeth by periodontal disease **(Fig. 24.14)**.

### Glickman Classification

Glickman classified furcation defect into four grades:[22]
1. *Grade I*: It is the incipient stage of furcation involvement, but radiographically changes are not usually found.
2. *Grade II*: The furcation lesion is a *cul-de-sac* with a definite horizontal component. Radiographs may or may not depict the furcation involvement.
3. *Grade III*: The bone is not attached to the dome of the furcation.
4. *Grade IV*: The interdental bone is destroyed, and soft tissues have receded apically so that the furcation opening is clinically visible.

## Fenestration and Dehiscence

Fenestrations are the isolated areas in which root is denuded of bone, and the marginal bone is intact. Dehiscences are the denuded areas that extend through the marginal bone.

### Location

Dehiscence and fenestration are both associated with an extreme buccal or lingual version of teeth. It occurs in 20% of all teeth. These are more frequent over anterior than posterior teeth. The root in such defects is covered only by periodontal ligament and the overlying gingiva. According to Elliot and Bowers, dehiscences were more prevalent in the mandible, whereas fenestrations are more common in the maxilla.[23]

### Clinical Significance

- The defects are significant clinically because where they occur, the root is covered only by the periosteum and overlying gingiva **(Figs. 24.15A and B)**. These areas become crucial if the periodontal disease occurs or if gingival recession takes place since they may complicate therapy and adversely affect the area's prognosis.
- Before any mucogingival surgical procedure, especially lateral pedicle existence of osseous dehiscence or fenestration should be ruled out.
- In the case of gingival grafting procedure, if the receptor site has fenestration defect, soft tissue is capable of reattaching to the exposed surface with higher predictability than dehiscence.
- If the abutment tooth has dehiscence or fenestration, the partial denture will damage the abutment and abutment loss will occur in a short period.

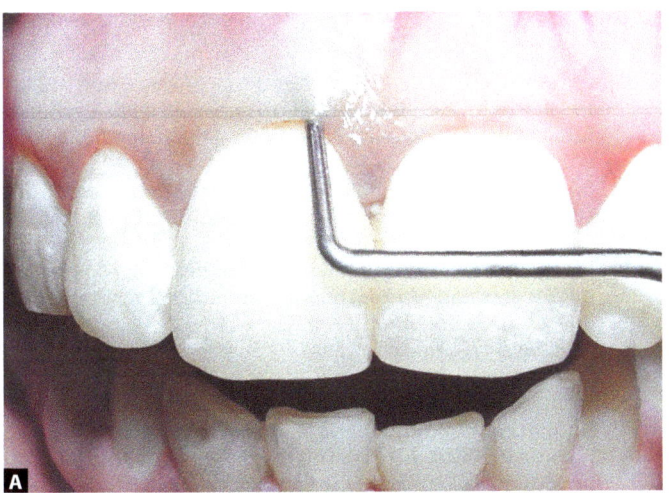
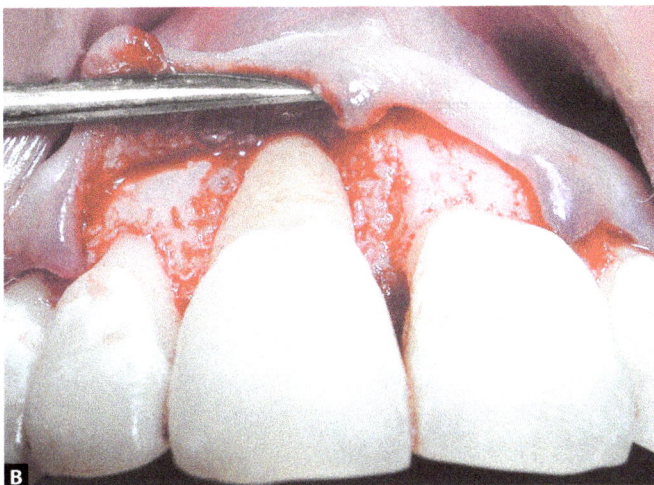

**Figs. 24.15A and B:** Clinical picture showing: (A) Probe in the pocket ; and (B) Dehiscence after flap reflection.

## Marginal Gutter

The marginal gutter is a shallow linear defect between the marginal bone of the radical cortical plate or interdental crest. It extends the length of one or more root surfaces, usually formed by resorption of the plate's socket side and deposition of the facial surface.

## Irregular Bony Margins

Irregular bony margins are the abrupt irregularities in the scalloped level of marginal bone and interdental septa.

## DIAGNOSIS

- *Probing*: Probing to determine the presence of these destructive patterns must be done horizontally and vertically around each involved root and in the crater area to establish the depth of the vertical component. The diagnosis of furcation involvement is made by clinical examination and careful probing with one of the specially designed Naber's probe **(Fig. 24.16)**
- *Bone sounding*: It is done by anaesthetizing the tissue locally and inserting probe horizontally and walking along with the tissue tooth interface so that the operator can feel the bony topography. It is also called as transgingival probing **(Fig. 24.17)**.
- *Radiographic examination*: Radiographic examination of the area is helpful, but furcation lesions can be obscured by angulation of the beam and the radiopacity of neighboring structures **(Fig. 24.18)**[16,24,25]
- *Surgical exposure*: Surgical exposure of bone defect through full-thickness flap is the best way to determine the bone defect pattern **(Fig. 24.19)**.[22]

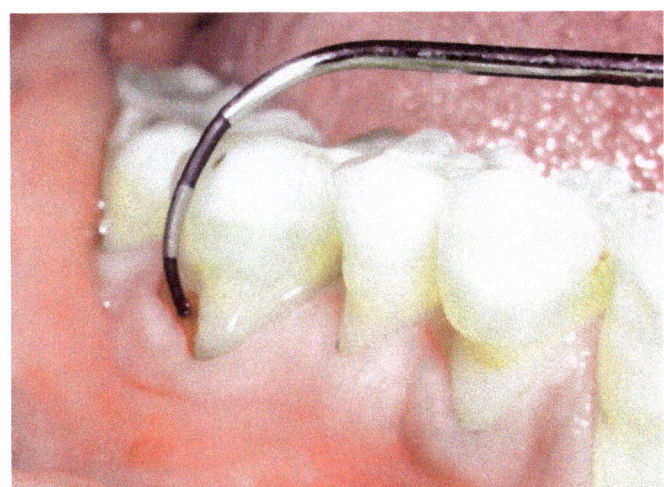

**Fig. 24.16:** Clinical picture showing probing of furcation defect with Naber's probe.

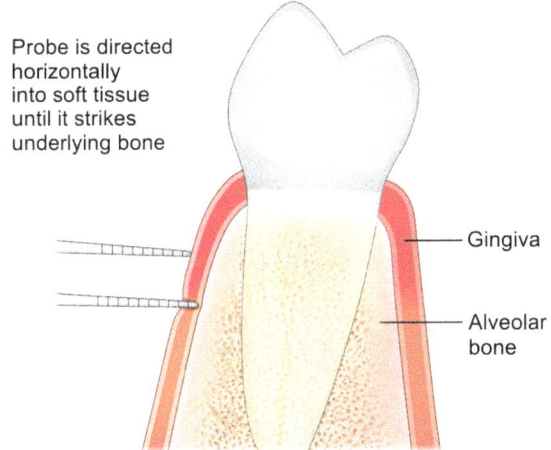

**Fig. 24.17:** Schematic representation showing bone sounding.

## Section 4: Pathology of Gingival and Periodontal Diseases

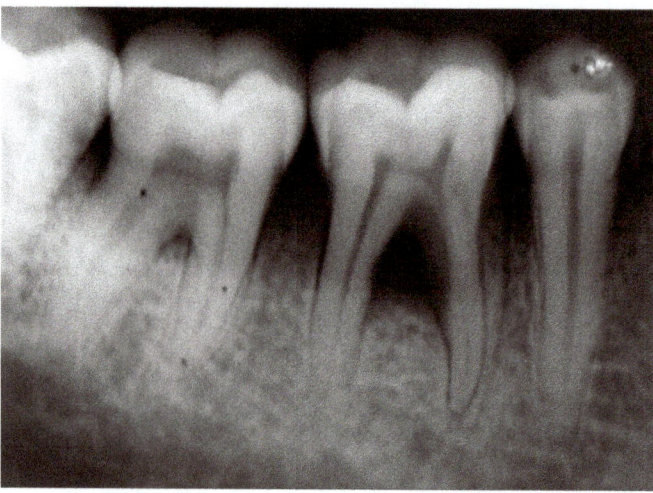

**Fig. 24.18:** Radiographic image showing furcation defect.

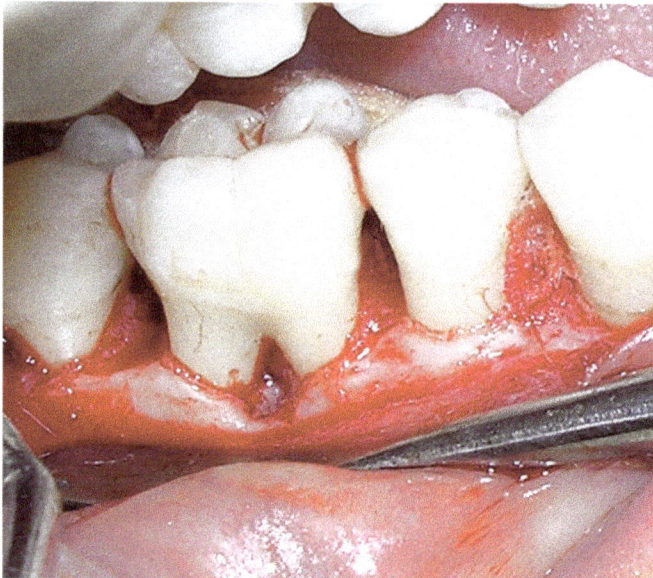

**Fig. 24.19:** Clinical picture showing surgical exposure of furcation defect—the only sure way to diagnose a bony defect.

### Points to Ponder

- 1.97 mm ± 33.16% is the distance between the apical extent of calculus and alveolar crest.
- 0.5–2.7 mm is the distance between the attached plaque and alveolar bone.
- The rate of bone loss depends upon the type of disease present and tooth surface. An average of 0.2 mm/year on facial surfaces and 0.3 mm/year on proximal surfaces.
- The most common bony lesion described, and encountered in periodontal disease is the interdental crater.
- Approximately 1.5–2 mm is the radius of action of bacterial plaque that can induce bone loss.
- In osteoclastic bone resorption, first, there is the solubilization of the mineral content of bone and then is the dissolution of the organic matrix.

### REFERENCES

1. Carranza FA. Bone loss and patterns of bone destruction. In: Newman MG, Takei HH, Carranza FA (Eds). Carranza's Clinical Periodontology, 9th edition. Philadelphia, PA, USA: WB Saunders; 2003;354-70.
2. Jainkittivong A, Langlais RP. Buccal and palatal exostosis: prevalence and concurrence with tori. Oral Surg Oral Med Oral Pathol Oral Radiol Endod. 2000;90(1):48-53.
3. Lindhe J, Svanberg G. Influence of trauma from occlusion on the progression of experimental periodontitis in the beagle dog. J Clin Periodontol. 1974;1(1):3-14.
4. Glickman I, Smulow JB. Buttressing bone formation in the periodontium. J Periodontol. 1965;36(5):365-70.
5. Weinmann JP. Progress of gingival inflammation into the supporting structures of the teeth. J Periodontol. 1941;12:71.
6. Garant PR, Cho MI. Histopathogenesis of spontaneous periodontal disease in conventional rats. I. Histometric and histologic study. J Periodontal Res. 1979;14(4):297-309.
7. Page RC, Schroeder HE. Periodontitis in Man and Other Animals: A Comparative Review. Basel, Switzerland: Karger; 1982.
8. Löe H, Anerud H, Boysen H, Morrison E. Natural history of periodontal disease in man. Rapid, moderate and no loss of attachment in Sri Lankan laborers 14 to 46 years of age. J Clin Periodontol. 1986;13(5):431-45.
9. Hausmann E. Potential pathways for bone resorption in human periodontal disease. J Periodontol. 1974;45(5): 338-43.
10. Schwartz Z, Goultschin J, Dean DD, Boyan BD. Mechanisms of alveolar bone destruction in periodontitis. Periodontol 2000. 1997;14:158-72.
11. Bar-Shavit Z. The osteoclast: a multinucleated, hematopoietic-origin, bone-resorbing osteoimmune cell. J Cell Biochem. 2007;102(5):1130-9.
12. Shafers WG, Hine MK, Levy BM. A Textbook of Oral Pathology, 4th edition. Philadelphia, PA, USA: WB Saunders; 1983.
13. Glickman I. The experimental basis for the bone factor concept in periodontal disease. J Periodontol. 1949;20(1): 7-22.
14. Manson JD. Bone morphology and bone loss in periodontal disease. J Clin Periodontol. 1976;3(1):14-22.
15. Goldman HM, Cohen DW. The infrabony pocket: classification and treatment. J Periodontol. 1958;29:272.
16. Manson JD, Nicholson K. The distribution of bone defects in chronic periodontitis. J Periodontol. 1974;45(2):88-92.
17. Prichard JF. The aetiology, diagnosis, and treatment of the intrabony defect. J Periodontol. 1967;38(6):455-65.
18. Ochsenbein C. A primer for osseous surgery. Int J Periodontics Restorative Dent. 1986;6(1):8-47.
19. Cohen B. Morphological factors in the pathogenesis of the periodontal disease. Brit Dent J. 1959;107:31-9.
20. O'Connor TW, Biggs NL. Interproximal bony contours. J Periodontol. 1964;35:326-30.
21. Pynn BR, Kurys-Kos NS, Walker DA, Mayhall JT. Tori mandibularis: a case report and review of the literature. J Can Dent Assoc. 1995;61(12):1057-8, 1063-6.
22. Glickman I, Carranza FA. Glickman's Clinical Periodontology. Philadelphia, PA, USA: WB Saunders; 1958.
23. Carranza FA. Bone loss and patterns of bone destruction. In: Newman MG, Takei HH, Carranza FA (Eds). Carranza's Clinical Periodontology, 9th edition. Philadelphia, PA, USA: WB Saunders; 2003. pp. 354-70.
24. Elliot JR, Bowers GM. Alveolar dehiscence and fenestration. Periodontics. 1963;1:245.
25. Papapanou PN, Tonetti MS. Diagnosis and epidemiology of periodontal osseous lesions. Periodontol 2000. 2000;22: 8-31.

## VIVA VOCE

**Q1. What is the radius of action of bacterial plaque that can induce bone loss?**
Ans. The radius of action of bacterial plaque that can induce bone loss is 1.5–2.5 mm approximately.

**Q2. What is the yearly rate of bone loss when periodontal disease is allowed to progress untreated?**
Ans. Rate of bone loss depends upon the type of disease present: an average of 0.2 mm/year on facial surfaces and 0.3 mm/year on proximal surfaces.

**Q3. What is hemiseptum?**
Ans. The one-wall (1W) vertical defect is called as hemiseptum.

**Q4. What is a moat?**
Ans. When crater-like bone loss involves all the four surfaces of the same tooth, it is called a moat.

**Q5. What is RANKL?**
Ans. Receptor activator of nuclear factor-kappa β ligand (RANKL) is a cytokine essential for osteoclastogenesis, which is expressed by osteoblast. Osteoclast precursor express RANK (a receptor of RANKL) and recognizes RANKL expressed by osteoblasts through cell-to-cell interaction and differentiate into osteoclasts in the presence of macrophage colony-stimulating factor (CSF).

**Q6. What is osteoprotegerin?**
Ans. It is a soluble decoy receptor for RANKL, produced mainly by osteoblasts. It blocks osteoclastogenesis by inhibiting RANKL-RANK interaction.

**Q7. What are interdental osseous craters?**
Ans. Interdental osseous craters are concavities in the crest of the alveolar septa centered under the contact point of adjacent teeth.

**Q8. What are the various types of craters?**
Ans. Ochsenbein divided bony craters into three basic types: (1) shallow (1–2 mm); (2) medium (3–4 mm) and (3) deep (5 mm and more).

**Q9. What are ledges?**
Ans. Ledges are plateau-like bone margins caused by resorption of thickened bony plates.

**Q10. Which is the best way to determine the bone defect pattern?**
Ans. Surgical exposure of bone defect through the full-thickness flap.

# Chapter 25: Periodontitis

*Shalu Bathla*

## Chapter Outline

- Status of Periodontitis in 1999 Classification
- Chronic Periodontitis
- Aggressive Periodontitis
- Status of Periodontitis in 2017 Classification

## STATUS OF PERIODONTITIS IN 1999 CLASSIFICATION

According to the 1999 classification periodontitis was further subdivided as follows:
- Chronic periodontitis, representing the forms of destructive periodontal disease that are generally characterized by slow progression.
- Aggressive periodontitis, a diverse group of highly destructive forms of periodontitis affecting primarily young individuals, including conditions formerly classified as "early-onset periodontitis" and "rapidly progressing periodontitis."
- Periodontitis as a manifestation of systemic disease, a heterogeneous group of systemic pathological conditions that include periodontitis as a manifestation.
- Necrotizing periodontal diseases, a group of conditions that share a characteristic phenotype where necrosis of the gingival or periodontal tissues is a prominent feature.

In this chapter, chronic and aggressive periodontitits are explained in detail as per the 1999 classification.

## CHRONIC PERIODONTITIS

Chronic periodontitis is defined as an infectious disease resulting in inflammation within the supporting tissues of the teeth leading to progressive attachment and bone loss.[1] It is also characterized by pocket formation and/or gingival recession. It is recognized as the most frequently occurring form of periodontitis. The presence of accumulated bacterial plaque and host defense mechanism plays a crucial role in the pathogenesis of chronic periodontitis.[2] Repeated clinical examinations help identify the disease's progressive nature.

### Classification

Chronic periodontal diseases are classified by disease extent and severity. Extent is the number of sites involved and can be described as localized or generalized.[1]
- *Localized*: If less than or equal to 30% of the sites are affected **(Fig. 25.1)**.
- *Generalized*: If more than 30% of the sites are affected **(Fig. 25.2)**.

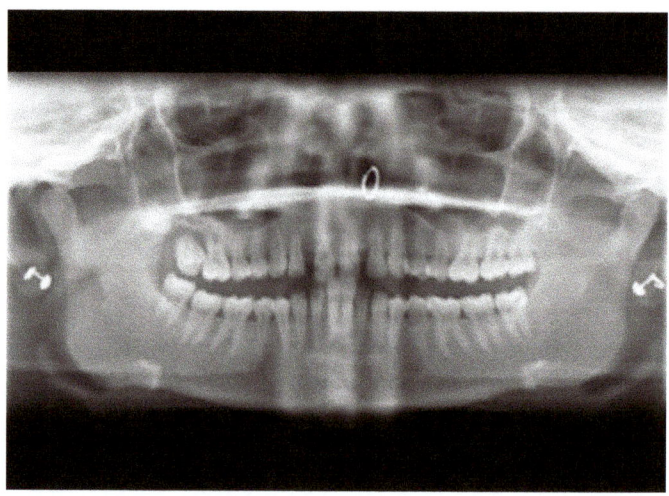

**Fig. 25.1:** Radiographic image showing the localized bone loss in localized chronic periodontitis.

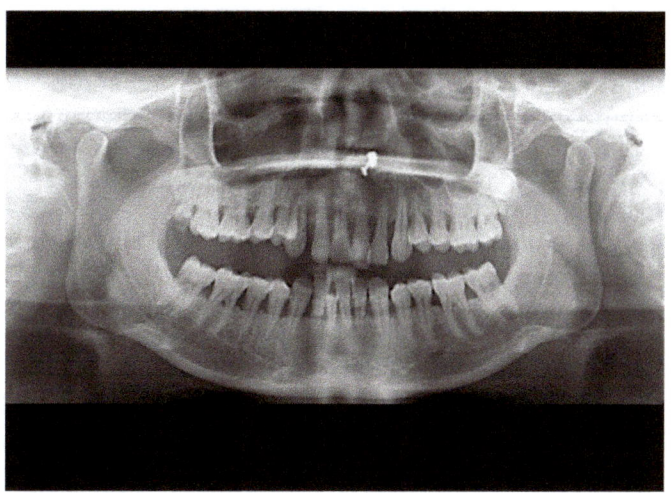

**Fig. 25.2:** Radiographic image showing the generalized bone loss in generalized chronic periodontitis.

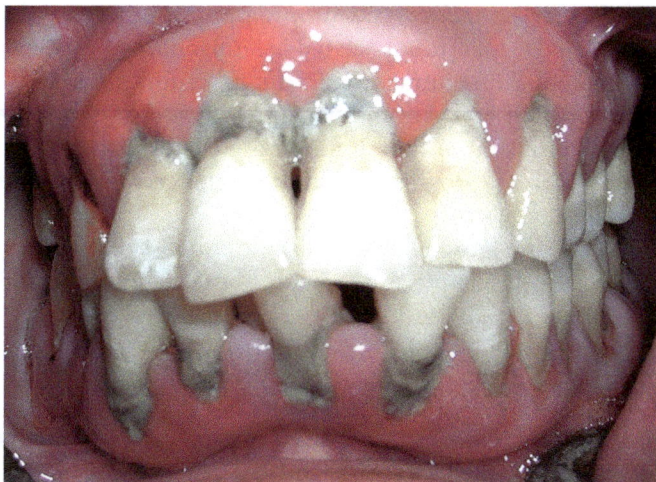

**Fig. 25.3:** Clinical picture showing an increased amount of calculus and plaque associated with chronic periodontitis.

Severity can be described for the entire dentition or individual teeth and sites. As a general guide, severity can be categorized based on the amount of CAL as follows:[3]
- Slight/mild = 1–2 mm CAL
- Moderate = 3–4 mm CAL
- Severe ≥5 mm CAL

## Clinical Features

- *Amount of destruction is consistent with the presence of local factors*: Patients with chronic periodontitis classically presents with supragingival and subgingival plaque accumulation that is mainly related to subgingival calculus formation **(Fig. 25.3)**.
- *Gingival inflammation*: The infected gingiva is mild to moderately swollen and presents alterations in color, ranging from pale red to magenta. Loss of gingival stippling blunted or rolled gingival margins and flattened or cratered papillae are common clinical examination findings. Frequent gingival bleeding occurs either spontaneously or with simple touching. Inflammation-related exudates are found in crevicular fluid **(Fig. 25.4)**.[4]
- *Periodontal pocket formation*: Pocket depths are variable, and suppuration from the pocket can be found.
- *Loss of periodontal attachment*: Chronic periodontitis usually, it exhibits slight-to-moderate loss of periodontal supporting tissues, which is either localized or generalized **(Fig. 25.5)**.
- *Loss of alveolar bone*: Resorption of alveolar bone in the form of both horizontal and vertical bone loss can be seen. There is considerable variation in the form, pattern, and rate of alveolar bone resorption.
- *Mobility*: In advanced cases, the presence of tooth mobility suggests considerable bone loss.

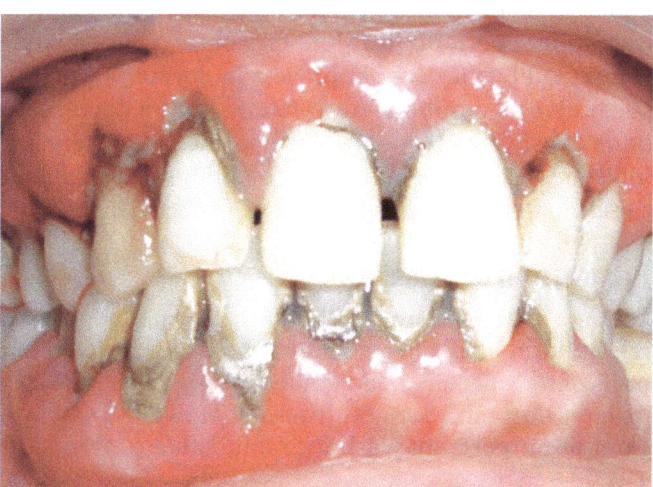

**Fig. 25.4:** Clinical picture showing gingival inflammation associated with chronic periodontitis.

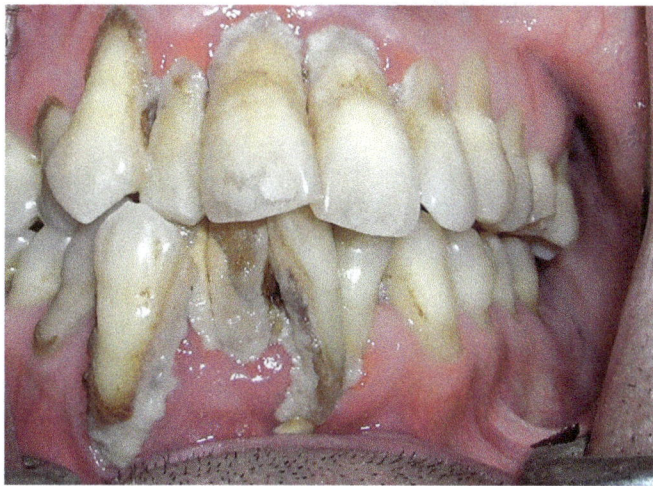

**Fig. 25.5:** Clinical picture showing generalized loss of attachment.

## Section 4: Pathology of Gingival and Periodontal Diseases

- *Predisposing factors*: Chronic periodontitis may be related to local tooth-related or iatrogenic predisposing factors. The course of chronic periodontitis may be modified by systemic diseases, including diabetes mellitus and human immunodeficiency virus (HIV). The disease progression is also affected by smoking and emotional stress.[5]
- *Rate of progression*: Rate of disease progression is usually slow-to-moderate and sometimes associated with rapid progression period.

## Radiographic Features

Radiographic examination is an essential part of periodontal diagnosis. With certain limitations, radiographic examination provides evidence of the alveolar bone height, extent, form of bone destruction, and the density of cancellous trabeculation. Various bone loss patterns can be seen in chronic periodontitis patients **(Fig. 25.6)** and are explained in "Chapter 24: Bone Defects". In a case of marginal periodontitis, the loss of the dense margin (presented by the alveolar process in normal) is the first suggestive sign of bone destruction. With a decrease in bone density, the bone margins become radiolucent and indistinct. As the bone resorption continues, the height of the alveolar bone gets reduced.

## Progression of Disease

The rate of disease progression in chronic periodontitis is not uniform in all affected areas of the oral cavity. Some parts of the affected area do not show significant disease progression for a longer duration. However, diseases from other parts may exhibit remarkable progression. Rapidly progressive lesions are common in interproximal areas. Also, they are mainly related to areas of greater plaque accumulation and areas inaccessible to plaque control measures (furcation areas, overhanging margins, malpositioned teeth).

Following are the models that describe the rate of disease progression:[6]
- Continuous/linear disease model
- Random/episodic burst disease model
- Stochastic disease model

### Continuous/Linear Disease Model

In this model, loss of attachment has commenced and proceeds continuously and slowly until tooth loss eventually results. Linear correlation between age and loss of attachment supports this concept of gradual destruction **(Fig. 25.7)**.

### Random/Episodic Burst Disease Model

In 1982, Goodson et al., challenged the continuous disease model and proposed that destruction occurs during periods of exacerbation, interjected with remission intervals. Breakdown occurs in recurrent acute episodes/bursts of activity over a short period, interspersed with periods of quiescence **(Fig. 25.8)**.

### Stochastic Disease Model

In 1989, Manji and Nagelkerke proposed a stochastic model for the periodontal breakdown that essentially combines both of the above models. They suggested that as well as an underlying slow continuous breakdown (the progression rate of which depends on host and sites), some sites of some individuals are also undergoing random bursts of activity as a result of a combination of biological events.[7]

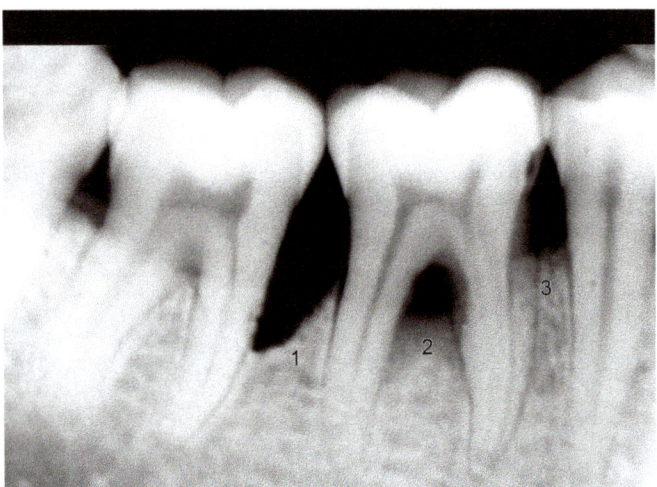

**Fig. 25.6:** Radiographic image showing various patterns of bone loss: 1. Vertical bone loss, 2. Furcation defect, 3. Horizontal bone loss in chronic periodontitis.

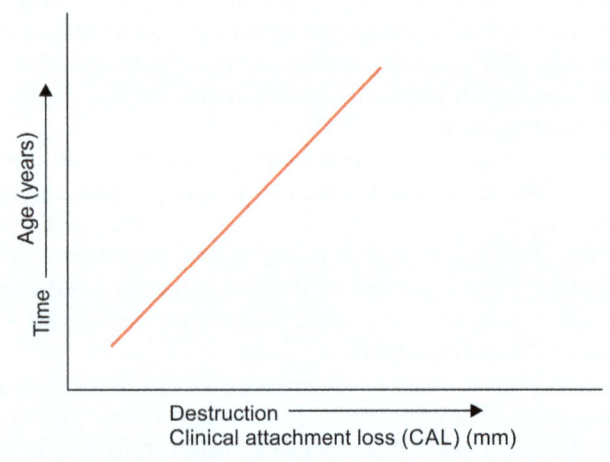

**Fig. 25.7:** Schematic representation showing continuous disease model.

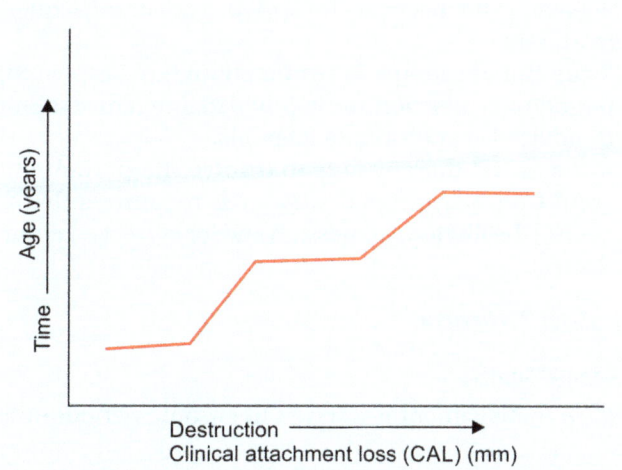

**Fig. 25.8:** Schematic representation showing random burst disease model.

## Risk Factors

### Prior History of Periodontitis

The previous history of periodontitis enhances the risk of further loss of tooth attachment and bone destruction due to bacterial plaque accumulation. Though it is not a true risk factor for disease development but acts as a disease predictor, this means that patients with pocket, attachment and bone loss will continue to lose periodontal support if not successfully treated.

### Bacterial Risk Factors

Plaque accumulation on the tooth and gingival surfaces at the dentogingival junction is considered the primary initiating agent in chronic periodontitis etiology. Specific microorganisms have been identified as potential periodontal pathogens. However, only the presence of periodontal pathogens is not sufficient to propagate disease activity.[8] Microbial plaque (biofilm) is an important factor in initiating inflammation of the periodontal tissues. Additionally, the progression of gingivitis to periodontitis is mainly induced by host-based risk factors. Microbial biofilms of particular compositions will initiate chronic periodontitis in certain individuals whose host response and cumulative risk factors predispose them to periodontal destruction rather than to gingivitis.

### Contributing Local Factors

Plaque retentive factors are important contributing factors for the development and progression of periodontal disease. Rest is explained in Chapter 10: "Dental Calculus."

### Systemic Factors

The rate of progression of plaque-induced chronic periodontitis is generally considered to be slow. However, when chronic periodontitis occurs in a patient who also suffers from a systemic disease that influences the host response's effectiveness, the rate of periodontal destruction may be significantly increased. Diabetes is a systemic condition that can increase the severity and extent of periodontal disease in an affected patient.

### Age

The prevalence of periodontal disease enhances with age. However, becoming older does not significantly increase susceptibility to periodontal disease. It is more likely that the cumulative effects of disease over a lifetime, i.e., deposits of plaque and calculus, and the increased number of sites capable of harboring such deposits, as well as attachment and bone loss experience, possibly increase the prevalence of the disease in older people.

### Smoking

It is not only the risk of developing the disease that is enhanced by smoking, but the response to periodontal therapy is also impaired in smokers. Clinical features of both gingivitis and chronic periodontitis, such as gingival redness and bleeding on probing, are obscured due to the dampening of inflammation.

### Stress

Stress and other psychosomatic conditions induce direct anti-inflammatory, anti-immune effects, and behavior-mediated effects on the body's defenses.

### Genetics

There is convincing evidence from twin studies for a genetic predisposition to periodontal diseases. The twin studies have indicated that the risk of chronic periodontitis has a high inherited component. Chronic periodontitis likely involves many genes, the composition of which may vary across individuals and races. Much attention has been focused on polymorphisms associated with the genes involved in cytokine production. Such polymorphisms have been linked to an increased risk for chronic periodontitis, but these findings have yet to be corroborated.

## Treatment

The periodontal therapy aims at eradicating the microbial flora responsible for periodontal infection. This also includes controlling other risk factors causing periodontitis. This helps to halt the disease progression and prevents the recurrence of periodontitis. Appropriate periodontal therapy is needed to maintain healthy dentition, which should be comfortable, and function with appropriate esthetics. Additionally, the regeneration of the periodontal attachment apparatus is considered if indicated. Clinical judgment is a crucial part of deciding suitable periodontal therapy. The process of making decisions for the appropriate therapy(ies) and the expected therapeutic outcomes depends on several factors. Systemic health, age, compliance, therapeutic preferences, and patient's ability to control plaque are some of the integral patient-oriented factors. While other identified factors are the clinician's skills to get rid of subgingival deposits, restorative and prosthetic demands, and the presence and treatment of teeth with more advanced chronic periodontitis.[9]

Treatment options for patients with slight-to-moderate loss of periodontal attachment apparatus are discussed below.

### Nonsurgical Therapy

- Instruction, motivation, and reinforcement of the patient for adopting adequate plaque control should be attempted.[10]
- *Plaque control*:[10]
  - Personal mechanical plaque control daily.
  - Scaling and root planing: Supragingival and subgingival scaling and root planing should be attempted to get rid of microbial plaque and calculus.
- *Removal of other contributing factors*:
  - Removal or reshaping of restorative overhangs and overcontoured crowns
  - Correction of ill-fitting prosthetic appliances
  - Restoration of carious lesions
  - Odontoplasty
  - Tooth movement
  - Restoration of open contacts which have resulted in food impaction
  - Treatment of occlusal trauma
- *Antimicrobial agents*: These agents may have an adjunctive role in the management of chronic periodontitis.[11] Depending on the administration route to diseased sites, antimicrobial therapies are categorized as either systemic or local drug delivery.
- Systemic risk factors exhibit a significant impact on treatment and therapeutic outcomes for chronic periodontitis. Commonly affecting systemic illness are diabetes, smoking, certain periodontal bacteria, aging, gender, genetic predisposition, systemic diseases and conditions (immunosuppression), stress, nutrition, pregnancy, HIV infection, substance abuse, and medications. Elimination, alteration, or control of systemic risk factors contributing to chronic periodontitis with the physician's consultation is useful to control disease progression.

### Evaluation

- Assessment of the initial therapy's outcomes is recommended after a period of resolution of inflammation and tissue repair. Comparing the initial clinical findings with re-evaluated findings help to identify the outcomes of initial therapy. This also aids to determine the necessity for and the type of subsequent treatment.
- If the initial therapy is strong enough to resolve the periodontal infection, periodontal maintenance should be advised at appropriate intervals.
- If the initial therapy fails to resolve the periodontal condition, periodontal surgery is recommended to control the disease progression and/or correct anatomic defects.

### Surgical Therapy

#### Periodontal Surgery

Surgical management is advised in chronic periodontitis for:
- Allocating good access for eradicating causative agents, e.g., flap procedures (Modified Widman flap)
- Reducing deep probing depths, e.g., apically displaced flap
- Regenerating or reconstructing lost periodontal tissues,[12-14] e.g., regenerative osseous surgery: bone replacement grafting, guided tissue regeneration, and combined regenerative techniques.

### Desired Outcome

Both nonsurgical and surgical periodontal therapy for chronic periodontitis should be associated with expected outcomes, such as elimination of clinical signs of gingival inflammation; reduction of probing depths; stabilization, or gain of clinical attachment apparatus and reduction of clinically detectable plaque suitable for adequate gingival health.

## AGGRESSIVE PERIODONTITIS

Aggressive periodontitis is a relatively rare form of periodontitis characterized by a pattern of rapid alveolar bone loss around the permanent first molars and incisors. Rapidity and severity of the destruction are not proportional to the mass of plaque and calculus.

## Historical Perspective

Various terms have been implicated in describing a type of periodontal disease with peculiar features of deep pocket formation and advanced alveolar bone loss in young children, adolescents, and adults, in an otherwise systemically healthy individual.[15] In 1923, Gottlieb defined a term of "diffuse atrophy of the alveolar bone" marked with significant destruction of collagen fibers in the periodontal ligament and their substitution with loose connective tissue and extensive bone resorption leading to distended periodontal ligament space. However, this terminology had undergone a series of changes over the period. In 1928, Gottlieb termed deep cementopathia hypothesizing inhibition of continuous cementum formation.[16] In 1938,

Wannenmacher described it as parodontitis marginalis progressiva. In 1942, Orban and Weinmann introduced the term "periodontosis" and described the disease's development in three stages. In 1966, the World Workshop in Periodontics introduced the concept of periodontosis. In 1967, Chaput and colleagues and in 1969 Butler proposed the term "juvenile periodontitis".[17] In 1971, Butler defined it as "a disease of the periodontium occurring in an otherwise healthy adolescent which is characterized by a rapid loss of alveolar bone about more than one tooth of the permanent dentition. The amount of destruction manifested is not commensurate with the amount of local irritants".[18] Page and Baab in 1985, suggested that all forms of the disease be designated as early-onset periodontitis (EOP). In 1989, World Workshop in Clinical Periodontics categorized this disease as localized juvenile periodontitis (LJP), a subset of the broad classification of EOP. At the 1999 International Classification Workshop, the different forms of periodontitis were reclassified into chronic, aggressive periodontitis and periodontitis as a manifestation of systemic diseases. It was finally renamed as aggressive periodontitis.

## Definition

Aggressive periodontitis can be defined as a disease of the periodontium occurring, in an otherwise healthy adolescent, which is characterized by a rapid loss of alveolar bone around more than one tooth of the permanent dentition.[18]

Definition of aggressive periodontitis is based on its multifactorial features of disease described as follows (Lang, et al., 1999):[19]

- Insignificant medical history or otherwise healthy individuals with the absence of systemic diseases.
- The progressive loss of periodontal attachment apparatus along with rapid bone destruction.
- Familial aggregation of cases suggestive of the involvement of the familial component.

Secondary features that are generally present but not universally found are:

- Amount of microbial deposits normally discordant with the severity of periodontal tissue destruction (**Fig. 25.9**).
- An increased amount of *Aggregatibacter actinomycetemcomitans*
- Phagocyte abnormality
- Hyperresponsive macrophage phenotype leading to increased production of prostaglandin E2 ($PGE_2$) and interleukin1β (IL-1 β)
- Progression of attachment loss and bone loss may be self-arresting.

Aggressive periodontitis is of two types: Localized aggressive periodontitis and generalized aggressive periodontitis (**Table 25.1**).

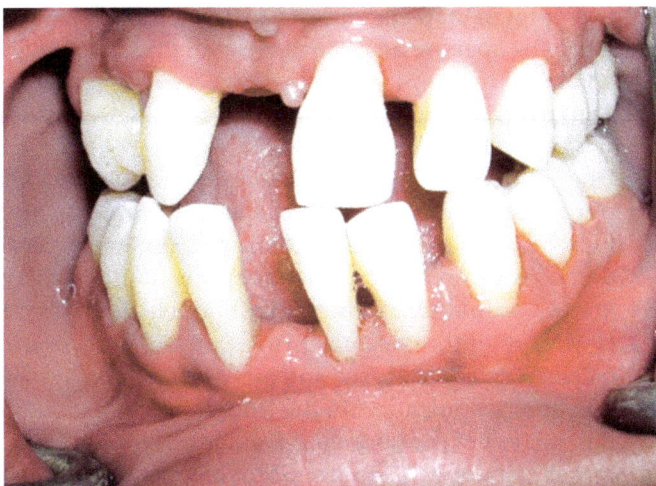

**Fig. 25.9:** Clinical picture showing generalized aggressive periodontitis (GAP): the amount of plaque is inconsistent with the amount of periodontal destruction.

**TABLE 25.1:** Comparison between chronic periodontitis, localized aggressive periodontitis (LAP) and generalized aggressive periodontitis (GAP).

| Chronic periodontitis | LAP | GAP |
|---|---|---|
| Most prevalent in adults although it can occur in children | Usually occur in adolescents | Usually affects people under 30 years of age, but patients may be older |
| Slow-to-moderate rate of progression | The rapid rate of progression | The rapid rate of progression (pronounced episodic periods of progression) |
| Amount of microbial deposits consistent with the severity of destruction | Amount of microbial deposits not consistent with the severity of destruction | Amount of microbial deposits sometimes consistent with the severity of destruction |
| The variable distribution of periodontal destruction; no discernible pattern | Periodontal destruction localized to permanent 1st molars and incisors | Periodontal destruction in addition to 1st molars and incisors |
| No marked familial aggregation | Familial aggregation | Marked familial aggregation |
| The frequent presence of subgingival calculus | Subgingival calculus usually absent | Subgingival calculus may or may not be present |

## Localized Aggressive Periodontitis

### Characteristics Features

- The typical circumpubertal pattern of onset.
- Robust serum antibody response to invading pathogens.
- Localized involvement of first molar/incisor with characteristic interproximal attachment loss on at least

two permanent teeth, one of which is a first molar and involving no more than two teeth other than first molars and incisors.

The involvement of periodontal areas of only certain teeth is due to following reasons:[20]

- Once initial microbial colonization on the first erupting permanent dentition takes place (1st molars and incisors), *A. actinomycetemcomitans* hampers the host defenses by an array of mechanisms. Some of them are the production of polymorphonuclear leukocyte (PMN) chemotaxis-inhibiting factors, endotoxin, collagenases, leukotoxin, and other factors that initiate bacterial colonization in the pocket and subsequent destruction of the periodontal tissues. Once the initial attack gets over, the immune mechanism plays its role by producing opsonic antibodies to increase the clearance and phagocytosis of penetrating bacteria and neutralize leukotoxic activity. This prevents the microbial colonization of other sites in oral cavity.[21] development of a strong antibody response to infectious agents is the peculiar feature of localized aggressive periodontitis (LAP).
- Antagonistic bacteria to *A. actinomycetemcomitans* may colonize the periodontal tissues and hamper the activity of *A. actinomycetemcomitans* and localize actinomycetemcomitans infection and tissue destruction to the particular site.
- Once *A. actinomycetemcomitans* loses its leukotoxin producing ability for unknown reasons, the disease progression comes to a halt, and bacterial colonization on new periodontal sites are avoided.
- The defect in cementum formation may enhance the possibility of localization of the lesion.

### *Radiographic Findings*

Vertical loss of alveolar bone around the 1st molars and incisors giving an impression of arc-shaped radiolucency, commencing at puberty in otherwise healthy teenagers, is a classical diagnostic feature of LAP. This alveolar bone loss extends from the distal surface of the 2nd premolar to the mesial surface of the 2nd molar (**Fig. 25.10**). It is usually bilaterally symmetrical in both the 1st molars of each jaw.

### *Generalized Aggressive Periodontitis*

Clinically, generalized aggressive periodontitis (GAP) is characterized by "generalized interproximal attachment loss affecting at least three permanent teeth other than 1st molars and incisors".
- Prevalent in person under 30 years of age, but may involve older patients.[19]
- Generalized interproximal attachment loss affecting at least three permanent teeth other than first molars and incisors.

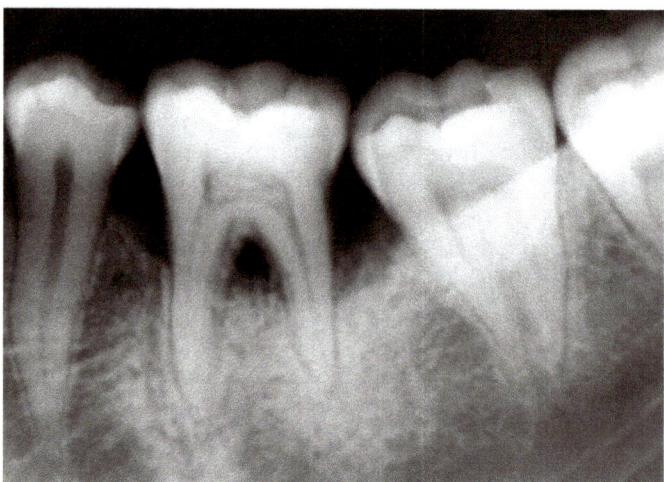

**Fig. 25.10:** Radiographic image showing arc-shaped bone loss around mandibular 1st molar.

- Episodic nature of the loss of attachment apparatus and alveolar bone destruction.
- Poor serum antibody response to invading pathogens.

## Risk Factors

Aggressive periodontitis is thought to be multifactorial in origin developing due to complex interactions between specific host genes and the environment (**Fig. 25.11**). The development of disease requires both inheritances of disease and environmental exposure to potential pathogens endowed with specific virulence factors. Host inability to effectively deal with bacterial aggression and to avoid inflammatory tissue damage usually results in the initiation of the disease process. Interactions between the disease process and environmental (e.g., cigarette smoking) and genetically controlled [e.g., immunoglobulin G2 response to *A. actinomycetemcomitans*] modifying factors are thought to contribute to determining the specific clinical manifestation of disease.[22]

### *Microbiological Factors*

*A. actinomycetemcomitans* is the principal causative agent for LAP.[23] However, other specific microorganisms commonly detected in patients with LAP are *A. actinomycetemcomitans*, *Eikenella corrodens*, *Prevotella intermedia*, and *Campylobacter rectus*.

### *Immunological Factors*

Immunological factors play a significant role in the pathogenesis of aggressive periodontitis. The human leukocyte antigens (HLAs) act as a potential marker for aggressive periodontitis due to their role in mediating regulation of immune responses. Patients with aggressive periodontitis presented with functional defects of PMNs, monocytes, or both. Patients with LAP exhibit a

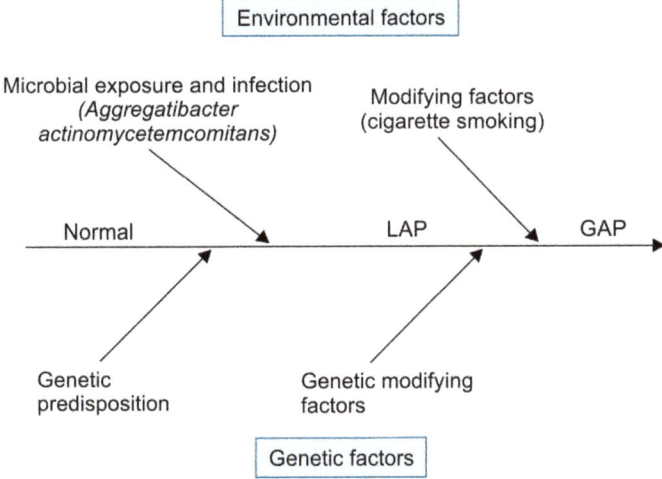

**Fig. 25.11:** Schematic representation showing risk factors associated with aggressive periodontitis.
(LAP: localized aggressive periodontitis; GAP: generalized aggressive periodontitis)

PMN chemotactic defect and depressed phagocytosis in peripheral blood. Neutrophil migration into the gingival crevice is slower. In a classic form of LAP, neutrophils characteristically present with a decrease in chemotactic responses to a variety of chemotactic factors, including C5a, FMLP (a formyl peptide), and leukotriene B4.[24] The neutrophil dysfunction is associated with a functional decrease in chemotaxin receptors on the polymorphonuclear neutrophil surface. The defect is known as a pan-receptor defect due to a reduction in all chemotaxin receptors.[25]

Neutrophil defects associated with aggressive periodontitis are:
- Abnormalities in adherence: Leukocyte adhesion deficiency-I (LAD-I), LAD-II
- Abnormalities in chemotaxis:
  - Decreased number of several receptors for chemotactic factors: Pan-receptor defect
  - Papillon–Lefevre syndrome
  - Chédiak–Higashi syndrome
- Abnormalities in phagocytosis and intercellular killing.

Monocytes show hyperresponsiveness with respect to their production of PGE2 in response to lipopolysaccharide (LPS).[26] This hyperresponsive phenotype may be associated with excessive production of the catabolic factors and enhanced connective tissue or bone loss.

## Genetic Factors

Susceptibility to aggressive periodontitis varies among individuals. Specific genes responsible for these diseases are still not identified. However, some segregational analysis and linkage analysis of families with a genetic predisposition suggest that LAP is inherited as an autosomal-dominant mode.[27]

## Environmental Factors

Smoking is considered to be an important environmental risk factor for aggressive periodontitis.[28] Smoker with GAP exhibited more affected teeth and more loss of clinical attachment apparatus compared to their nonsmoker counterparts.

## Prognosis

The prognosis for patients with aggressive periodontitis is determined by various factors, including whether the disease is generalized or localized; the degree of destruction present at the time of examination, and the ability to control future progression. When associated with systemic involvement, the generalized forms exhibit a bad prognosis compared to the localized forms. GAP rarely undergoes spontaneous remission, whereas the localized form of the disease has been known to arrest spontaneously due to burning out phenomenon.

### Treatment Modalities for Localized Aggressive Periodontitis

#### Past Treatment Modalities

Past treatment modalities for LAP are:[29,30]
- *Extraction*: The affected teeth (the 1st molars) are usually extracted. Substitution of the sockets of previously extracted 1st molars with developing 3rd molars is also attempted.
- *Standard periodontal therapy*: It included scaling and root planing, curettage, flap surgery with and without bone grafts, root amputations and hemisections.
- *Antibiotic therapy*: Genco and colleagues recommended treatment of LAP with scaling and root planing plus systemic administration of tetracycline (250 mg 4 times daily for 14 days every eight weeks) for good outcomes.

#### Current Treatment Modalities

Current treatment modalities for LAP:[31] Successful treatment of aggressive periodontitis is considered to be dependent on:
- *Early detection*: It is a crucial part of the management of aggressive periodontitis because prevention of tissue destruction is always beneficial rather than attempting to regenerate the lost supporting structures.
- *Education*: Educate the patient about the disease, including the cause and risk factors for disease and the patient's role in the success of treatment. Educate family members, especially younger siblings, because it is known to have familial aggregation.
- Efforts to control factors that affect the composition and the quantity of the subgingival microbiota.
- Providing an environment conducive to long-term maintenance.

Different treatment approaches are as follows:

### Nonsurgical Therapy

- *Conventional periodontal therapy*: It consists of patient education, oral hygiene instruction, scaling and root planing, and regular recall maintenance. The response to conventional periodontal therapy alone has been limited and unpredictable.
- *Full mouth disinfection*: Treatment of aggressive periodontitis includes full mouth disinfection, which was proposed by Quirynen et al.[32] It was observed that *A. actinomycetemcomitans* could translocate from one person to another and from site to site. It involves two settings of full mouth debridement completed within 24 hours. In addition to scaling and root planing, the tongue is brushed with chlorhexidine (CHX) gel (1%) for 1 minute, mouth rinsed with CHX solution (0.2%) for 2 minutes, and periodontal pockets are irrigated with CHX solution (1%).
- *Antimicrobial therapy*: Systemic antibiotics should only be administered as an adjunct to mechanical debridement because, in undisturbed subgingival plaque, the target organisms are effectively protected from the antibiotic agent due to the biofilm effect. Antibiotics have been used in essentially two ways for the treatment:
    - In combination with intensive instrumentation over a short period of time after the achievement of adequate plaque control in a pretreatment motivation period; or
    - As a staged approach after completion of the initial therapy.
- Administration of systemic tetracycline (250 mg of tetracycline hydrochloride four times daily for at least one week) along with local mechanical therapy is the beneficial treatment option for improved outcomes. In the case of surgical approach, the administration of systemic tetracycline approximately 1 hour before surgery is advised. Doxycycline, 100 mg/day may also be used. CHX rinses should also be prescribed and continued for several weeks.
- *Local delivery*: The significant advantage of local therapy is the delivery of a smaller total dosage of topical agents inside the pocket to prevent systemic antibacterial agents' side effects. Additionally, direct delivery enhances the exposure of the target microorganism to higher concentrations and subsequently gives more therapeutic outcomes. The various local delivery agents have been formulated in the form of solutions, gels, chips, and fibers.
- *Host modulation*: Modulation in the host immune response with the modulating agents in a specified way in the treatment of aggressive periodontitis. The various host modulatory agents used are subantimicrobial dose doxycycline (SDD), flurbiprofen, indomethacin, and naproxen.
- *Occlusal adjustment*: Migration of incisors is a late characteristic of aggressive periodontitis, but orthodontic treatment is usually contraindicated. If teeth which are to remain have drifted into premature contact, these should be treated by selective grinding.

### Surgical Therapy

The resective and regenerative periodontal therapy can be effective in reducing or eliminating pocket depth. Regenerative procedures, such as open flap debridement, root conditioning, and regenerative materials, including bone grafts, barrier membranes, and growth factors, have been successfully demonstrated in a patient with LAP.

Recent advances in regenerative therapy, i.e., enamel matrix protein (Emdogain®, Biora AB, Malmö, Sweden), have been advocated to aid in the regeneration of cementum and new attachment in periodontal defects.

### Periodontal Maintenance

Recurrence of disease is an indication for a repetition of microbiologic tests, for the re-evaluation of the host immune response, and reassessment of the local and systemic modifying factors. In refractory cases, tetracycline-resistant Actinobacillus species are suspected, and a combination of amoxicillin and metronidazole can be tried.

With the completion of therapy, microbiologic testing should be conducted after 1–3 months to clarify the complete eradication or significant suppression of causative pathogens. With the resolution of the periodontal infection, an individually tailored maintenance care program is attempted, including continuous evaluation of the occurrence and the risk of disease progression.

Regular maintenance visit is one of the important steps in the control of disease and the success of treatment. Each maintenance visit should consist of medical history review, inquiry about any recent periodontal problems, comprehensive periodontal examination, thorough scaling and root planing, followed by oral hygiene instruction. The duration between these recall visits is usually short during the first period after the patient completes therapy generally no longer than a 3-month interval. Active monitoring as frequently as every 3–4 weeks is necessary when the disease is thought to be active. Since the rate of disease progression is faster in younger patients, therefore, such patients are more frequently monitored. Over time, the recall maintenance interval can be adjusted according to the patient's level of oral hygiene and control of disease, as determined by each examination.

## Treatment Modalities for Generalized Aggressive Periodontitis

The therapeutic approaches for the management of generalized forms of aggressive periodontitis are identical to the management of refractory forms of the disease.

## STATUS OF PERIODONTITIS IN 2017 CLASSIFICATION

There is no evidence of a specific pathophysiology that enables the differentiation of cases as "aggressive" or "chronic" periodontitis or provides guidance for different kinds of intervention. There is little consistent evidence that aggressive and chronic periodontitis are different diseases. The forms of the disease previously described as "chronic" and "aggressive" are now described under the single category of "periodontitis." Three forms of periodontitis have been identified: (1) Periodontitis; (2) Necrotizing periodontitis; (3) Periodontitis as a direct manifestation of systemic diseases.[33]

1. Necrotizing periodontal diseases
   a. Necrotizing gingivitis
   b. Necrotizing periodontitis
   c. Necrotizing stomatitis
2. Periodontitis as manifestation of systemic diseases: Based on the primary systemic diseases according to the International Statistical Classification of Diseases and Related Health Problems (ICD) codes
3. Periodontitis
   a. Stages: Based on severity and complexity of management
      ♦ Stage I: Initial periodontitis
      ♦ Stage II: Moderate periodontitis
      ♦ Stage III: Severe periodontitis with potential for additional tooth loss
      ♦ Stage IV: Severe periodontitis with potential for loss of the dentition
   b. Extent and distribution: Localized, generalized, molar–incisor distribution
   c. Evidence or risk of rapid progression
      Grades: anticipated treatment response
      i. Grade A: Slow rate of progression
      ii. Grade B: Moderate rate of progression
      iii. Grade C: Rapid rate of progression

A multidimensional system of stages and grades has been devised further to describe the different manifestations of periodontitis in individual cases. Stages describe the severity and the extent of the disease; grades describe the likely rate of progression. Staging involves four categories (stages 1 through 4) and is determined after considering several variables including clinical attachment loss, amount and percentage of bone loss, probing depth, presence and extent of angular bony defects and furcation involvement, tooth mobility, and tooth loss due to periodontitis. Grading includes three levels (grade A – low risk, grade B – moderate risk, grade C – high risk for progression) and encompasses, in addition to aspects related to periodontitis progression, general health status, and other exposures, such as smoking or level of metabolic control in diabetes. Thus, grading allows the clinician to incorporate individual patient factors into the diagnosis, which are crucial to comprehensive case management.[34]

## REFERENCES

1. Nagy RJ, Novak MJ. Chronic periodontitis. In: Newman MG, Takei HH, Carranza FA (Eds). Carranza's Clinical Periodontology, 9th edition. Philadelphia, PA, USA: WB Saunders; 2003. pp. 398-402.
2. Flemmig TF. Periodontitis. Ann Periodontol. 1999;4(1):32-8.
3. Kinane DF, Lindhe J. Chronic periodontitis. In: Lindhe J, Karring T, Lang NP (Eds). Clinical Periodontology and Implant Dentistry, 4th edition. Chicago, USA: Blackwell Munksgaard; 2003. pp. 209-15.
4. Manson JD, Eley BM. Chronic periodontitis. In: Outline of Periodontics, 4th edition. Oxford, UK: Butterworth-Heinemann; 1980. pp. 97-117.
5. Grant DA, Stern IB, Listgarten MA. Periodontitis. In: Periodontics, 6th edition. St. Louis: CV Mosby; 1988. pp. 348-75.
6. Socransky SS, Haffajee AD, Goodson JM, Lindhe J. New concepts of destructive periodontal disease. J Clin Periodontol. 1984;11(1):21-32.
7. Manji F, Nagelkerke N. A stochastic model for the periodontal breakdown. J Periodontal Res. 1989;24(4):279-81.
8. Nishihara T, Koseki T. Microbial etiology of periodontitis. Periodontol 2000. 2004;36:14-26.
9. Papapanou PN. Risk assessment in the diagnosis and treatment of periodontal diseases. J Dent Educ. 1998;62(10):822-39.
10. Hujoel PP, Cunha-Cruz J, Loesche WJ, Robertson PB. Personal oral hygiene and chronic periodontitis: a systematic review. Periodontol 2000. 2005;37:29-34.
11. Drisko CH. Nonsurgical pocket therapy: pharmacotherapeutics. Ann Periodontol. 1996;1(1):491-566.
12. Consensus report: Surgical pocket therapy. Ann Periodontol. 1996;1(1):618-20.
13. Consensus report: Periodontal regeneration around natural teeth. Ann Periodontol. 1996;1(1):667-70.
14. Consensus report: Mucogingival therapy. Ann Periodontol. 1996;1(1):702-6.
15. Carranza FA. Prepubertal and juvenile periodontitis. In: Newman MG, Takei HH, Carranza FA (Eds). Carranza's Clinical Periodontology, 8th edition. Philadelphia, PA, USA: WB Saunders; 1996. pp. 336-42.
16. Gottlieb B. The formation of the pocket: Diffuse atrophy of alveolar bone. J Am Dent Assoc. 1928;15:462.
17. Butler JH. A familial pattern of juvenile periodontitis (periodontosis). J Periodontol. 1969;40(2):115-8.
18. Baer PN. The case for periodontosis as a clinical entity. J Periodontol. 1971;42(8):516-20.
19. Lang NP, Bartold PM, Cullinan M, Jeffcoat M, Mombelli A. Consensus report: aggressive periodontitis. Ann Periodontol. 1999;4:53.
20. Nagy RJ, Novak KF. Aggressive periodontitis. In: Newman MG, Takei HH, Carranza FA (Eds). Carranza's Clinical Periodontology, 9th edition. Philadelphia, PA, USA: WB Saunders; 2000. pp. 409-14.
21. Zambon JJ, Christersson LA, Slots J. Actinobacillus actinomycetemcomitans in human periodontal disease. Prevalence in patient groups and distribution of biotypes and serotypes within families. J Periodontol. 1983;54(12):707-11.
22. Lindhe Tonetti MS, Mombelli A. Aggressive periodontitis. In: Lindhe J, Karring T, Lang NP (Eds). Clinical Periodontology

and Implant Dentistry, 4th edition. Chicago, USA: Blackwell Munksgaard; 2003. pp. 216-42.
23. Tonetti MS, Mombelli A. Early-onset periodontitis. Ann Periodontol. 1999;4(1):39-53.
24. Miyasaki KT. Altered leukocyte function and periodontal disease. In: Newman MG, Takei HH, Carranza FA (Eds). Carranza's Clinical Periodontology, 8th edition. Philadelphia, PA, USA: WB Saunders; 1996. pp. 132-50.
25. Van Dyke TE, Schweinebraten M, Cinaciola LJ, Offenbacher S, Genco RJ. Neutrophil chemotaxis in families with localized juvenile periodontitis. J Periodontal Res. 1985;20(5):503-14.
26. Shapira L, Soskolone WA, Van Dyke TE. Prostaglandin E2 secretion, cell maturation, and CD14 expression by monocyte-derived macrophages from localised juvenile periodontitis patients. J Periodontol. 1996;67(3):224-8.
27. Vieira AR, Albandar JM. Role of genetic factors in the pathogenesis of aggressive periodontitis. Periodontol 2000. 2014;65(1):92-106.
28. Haber J, Wattles J, Crowley M, Mandell R, Joshipura K, Kent RL. Evidence for cigarette smoking as a major risk factor for periodontitis. J Periodontol. 1993;64(1):16-23.
29. Nagy RJ, Newman MG. Treatment of refractory periodontitis, aggressive periodontitis, necrotising ulcerative periodontitis, and periodontitis associated with systemic diseases. In: Newman MG, Takei HH, Carranza FA (Eds). Carranza's Clinical Periodontology, 9th edition. Philadelphia, PA, USA: WB Saunders; 2003. pp. 558-66.
30. Wilson TG, Kornman KS. Treating aggressive forms of periodontal disease. In: Fundamentals of Periodontics. IL, USA: Quintessence Publishing Company; 1996. pp. 389-422.
31. Teughels W, Dhondt R, Dekeyser C, Quirynen M. Treatment of aggressive periodontitis. Periodontol 2000. 2014;65(1):107-33.
32. Quirynen M, Bollen CM, Vandekerckhove BN, Dekeyser C, Papaioannou W, Eyssen H. Full- vs. partial-mouth disinfection in the treatment of periodontal infections: short-term clinical and microbiological observations. J Dent Res. 1995;74(8):1459-67.
33. Papapanou PN, Sanz M, et al. Periodontitis: Consensus report of Workgroup 2 of the 2017 World Workshop on the Classification of Periodontal and Peri-Implant Diseases and Conditions. J Clin Periodontol. 2018;45(Suppl 20):S173-S182.
34. Tonetti MS, Greenwell H, Kornman KS. Staging and grading of Periodontitis: Framework and proposal of a new classification and case definition. J Periodontal. 2018; 89 (Suppl 1): S159-S172.

## VIVA VOCE

**Q1.** How periodontitis is clinically distinguished from gingivitis?
**Ans.** Periodontitis is clinically distinguished from gingivitis by the presence of:
- Clinical attachment loss (CAL)
- Alveolar bone loss

**Q2.** Who proposed a random/ episodic burst disease model?
**Ans.** In 1982, Goodson.

**Q3.** What is burnout phenomenon?
**Ans.** Sometimes a sudden and unexplainable decrease in the rate of bone destruction occurs, generally when the patient is in the middle and late 20s. Arrests of this kind have been referred to as "burnout." These sudden remissions in the course of the disease may represent an altered host-parasite interaction.

**Q4.** What is the rate of bone loss in aggressive periodontitis as compared to chronic periodontitis?
**Ans.** The rate of bone loss is 3 or 4 times higher in aggressive periodontitis than the rate of progression of chronic periodontitis.

**Q5.** What is a panreceptor defect?
**Ans.** When all chemotaxin receptors are decreased, the defect is called a pan-receptor defect. It is seen in LAP. It is characterized by a decrease in chemotactic responses to a variety of chemotactic factors, including C5a, FMLP, and leukotriene B4.

**Q6.** Who gave the termed deep cementopathia?
**Ans.** In 1928, Gottlieb.

**Q7.** Who introduced the term periodontosis?
**Ans.** In 1942, Orban and Weinmann.

**Q8.** Who proposed full mouth disinfection?
**Ans.** Marc Quirynen et al.

**Q9.** Which different forms of periodontitis are recognized in the present revised classification system?
**Ans.** Based on pathophysiology, three clearly different forms of periodontitis have been identified: (A) Necrotizing periodontitis; (B) Periodontitis as a direct manifestation of systemic diseases; (C) Periodontitis.

**Q10.** Do the acute periodontal lesions have distinct features when compared with other forms of periodontitis?
**Ans.** Periodontal abscesses, lesions from necrotizing periodontal diseases and acute presentations of endo-periodontal lesions, share the following features that differentiate them from periodontitis lesions: (1) rapid-onset nature, (2) rapid destruction of periodontal tissues, and (3) pain or discomfort.

# Chapter 26: AIDS and Periodontium

*Shalu Bathla*

## Chapter Outline

- Structure of HIV
- Pathogenesis
- Periodontal Diseases in AIDS
- Periodontal Pathologies
- Diagnosis
- Treatment

## INTRODUCTION

The acquired immunodeficiency syndrome (AIDS) is a major global public health problem that can turn out as a life-threatening event if not treated adequately. It is caused by the human immunodeficiency virus (HIV), which characteristically leads to immunosuppression and enhances host susceptibility to opportunistic infections, neurologic manifestations, and secondary neoplasms. In 1981, the Centers for Disease Control and Prevention (CDC) identified the first AIDS case in young homosexual men. Subsequently, further cases were recognized in injecting drug users and persons with hemophilia. The virus was first identified in 1983. In 1984, in France, Montagnier and his colleague fully recognized HIV virus.[1] Fortunately, in the same year, Gallo et al., from the USA called this virus as the human T-cell leukemia/lymphoma virus (HTLV- III). Oral lesions in the form of oral candidiasis and oral hairy leukoplakia are the common presenting symptoms of HIV/AIDS infection. However, the clinical features of periodontal involvement in HIV-infected people were initially detected in 1986. In 1987, for the first time, Winkler and Murray described distinctive form of gingivitis developing in HIV seropositive individuals in the form of the distinct erythematous band at the marginal gingiva and was associated with petechiae.[2]

HIV can be transmitted through three major routes, namely: (1) unprotected sexual contact, (2) parenteral inoculation, and (3) passage of the virus from infected mothers to her newborns. Sexual transmission accounting for over 75% of all cases and is a predominant mode of HIV transmission. Parenteral transmission occurs in intravenous drug abusers, hemophiliacs, and blood recipients. Parenteral inoculation, in the form of intravenous drug users, is the largest group of HIV-infected populations. This mainly occurs due to the sharing of needles and syringes contaminated with HIV containing blood.

Previously studied clinical periodontal parameters and microbiological assessment on periodontopathogens reported moderate deterioration of periodontal health in the HIV-positive patients compared to their healthy counterparts. The periodontal destruction in HIV positive patients is related, to some extent, to atypical microbial infections of the periodontium and altered host response.

## STRUCTURE OF HIV

HIV belongs to the retrovirus family of viruses. HIV virion is typically spherical with the presence of electron-dense, cone-shaped core and surrounding lipid envelope derived from the host cell membrane (Fig. 26.1).

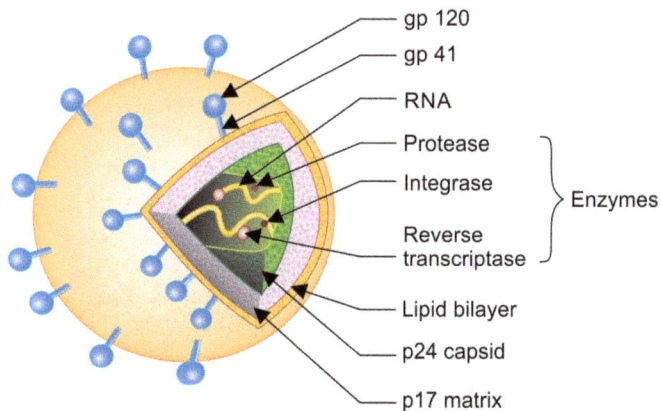

**Fig. 26.1:** Schematic representation showing the structure of the human immunodeficiency virus (HIV).

The virus core is constituted with single-stranded ribonucleic acid (RNA), the major capsid protein p24, and enzymes, namely protease, reverse transcriptase, and integrase. p24 is the most easily detected viral antigen and a common target for the antibodies used for the diagnosis of HIV infection in the widely used enzyme-linked immunosorbent assay.

The viral envelope consists of two viral glycoproteins, external glycoprotein gp120, and transmembrane protein gp4l, which plays an integral role in the HIV infection of cells. The HIV-1 RNA genome contains the *gag, pol,* and *env* genes, which code for various viral proteins. The other accessory genes, including *tat, rev, vif, nef, vpr,* and *vpu,* regulate the synthesis and assembly of infectious viral particles.[3,4]

## PATHOGENESIS

Binding of the gp120 envelope glycoprotein to CD4 molecules initiate the process of HIV infection. Glycoprotein gp120 receptors show a high affinity for CD4 receptors present on T cells. This binding results in a conformational change leading to the formation of a new recognition site on gp120 for the coreceptors CCR5 (C-C chemokine receptor type 5) or CXCR-4 (C-X-C chemokine receptor type 4). Subsequently, a conformational change in gp4l results in the insertion of a fusion peptide at the tip of gp4l into the cell membrane of T cells or macrophages. After fusion, the virus core containing the HIV genome and viral enzymes enter the host cell's cytoplasm. The entry of RNA inside the cytoplasm leads to activation of reverse transcriptase, which converts RNA into cDNA (complementary deoxyribonucleic acid) followed by integration of this proviral genome into the host genome. cDNA is then integrated into the host genome with the help of enzyme integrase. Integrated viral DNA is replicated and transcribed into mRNA (messenger RNA), giving rise to a new virion. This new virion infects other healthy cells.[5]

The HIV virus commonly enters the body through mucosal tissues and blood. Initially, it infects T cells along with dendritic cells and macrophages. With the establishment of infection in lymphoid tissues, the virus stays latent for long periods. Active viral replication constituted more infection of cells and progression to AIDS **(Flowchart 26.1)**.[3,5]

General oral manifestations in the form of oral candidiasis and oral hairy leukoplakia are prominent features of HIV infection known since a long time. However, apart from this, HIV infection is strongly related to the development of specific periodontal manifestations. Periodontitis is multifactorial in origin with the significant role of environmental, genetic, and systemic conditions along with altered host response and associated microbial challenge. Risk factors for the development of periodontitis in seropositive patients are age, smoking, viral load,

**Flowchart 26.1:** Pathogenesis of HIV infection.

```
Primary infection of cells in blood, fluids
(CD4 T cell, dendritic cell, macrophages)
            │
Drainage to lymph nodes, spleen
            ▼
Infection established in lymphoid tissue (lymph node)
            │
         Viremia
    Acute HIV syndrome
            ▼
Spread of infection throughout the body
            │
    Immune response
            ▼
Anti-HIV antibodies; partial control of viral replication
    Clinical latency
            ▼
        Latent infection
Other microbial infections
    Cytokines (TNF)
            ▼
Extensive viral replication; CD4 cell lysis
           AIDS
            ▼
Destruction of lymphoid tissue; Depletion of CD4 T cells
```

(HIV: human immunodeficiency virus; AIDS: acquired immunodeficiency syndrome; TNF: tumor necrosis factor)

microorganisms (viz. *Fusobacterium nucleatum, Prevotella intermedia, Aggregatibacter actinomycetemcomitans*) and enzymes [viz. gingival crevicular fluid (GCF) neutrophil elastase and beta glucuronidase].

Advancement in the stages of HIV infection is characteristically associated with enhanced severity of the systemic illnesses and decrease in numbers of CD4+ lymphocytes in peripheral blood, leading to marked immunosuppression. At these stages, the risk of occurrence of periodontal disease may enhance. Immunosuppression facilitated colonization and overgrowth of atypical pathogenic species that lead to gingival inflammation. However, the loss of attachment apparatus in HIV-positive patients can be due to lifestyle factors, such as smoking habits and poor oral hygiene rather than HIV infection alone. It is commonly noted that periodontitis progression is more rapid in HIV-positive patients compared to HIV-negative patients and this may be due to marked immunosuppression in the seropositive patient. However, periodontopathogens remains the same in both HIV-positive and HIV-negative patients.

Depression in local host response can lead to the progression of chronic periodontitis in HIV-positive patients. Both local and systemic host inflammatory and humoral immune responses in HIV infection lead to an acceleration of periodontal diseases.

The HIV-positive patients, lesions of chronic periodontitis are associated with an increased number of plasma cells, mast cells, macrophages and neutrophils that release proinflammatory cytokines and other mediators resulting in a considerable periodontal loss.

## PERIODONTAL DISEASES IN AIDS

Severe forms of periodontal diseases have long been known to be associated with immune system defects. Different HIV-related periodontal disease classifications have been presented.[6]

According to the CDC Surveillance Case Classification (1993), AIDS patients have been grouped as follows **(Table 26.1)**:[7]

Laboratory categories:
- *Category 1*: More than or equal to 500 CD4 lymphocytes/mm$^3$
- *Category 2*: 200–499 CD4 lymphocytes/mm$^3$
- *Category 3*: Less than 200 CD4 lymphocytes/mm.$^3$

The HIV-associated periodontal diseases are categorized as follows:
- HIV-associated gingivitis (HIV-G)
- HIV-associated periodontitis (HIV-P)
- Necrotizing ulcerative gingivitis (NUG)
- Necrotizing stomatitis (NS)

In a later classification, the term HIV has been dropped as any of those conditions could also be found in non-HIV-infected subjects. The HIV-associated periodontal lesions accepted by the EC Clearing house 1993 include:
- Linear gingival erythema (LGE), non-plaque-induced gingivitis exhibiting a distinct erythematous band of the marginal gingiva, which either diffuses or punctuates erythema of the attached gingiva.
- Necrotizing periodontal diseases, which are subclassified as NUG, necrotizing ulcerative periodontitis (NUP), and NS. NUG involves the destruction of one or more interdental papillae and is limited to the marginal gingiva. NUP extends beyond the papillae and marginal gingiva, causing loss of periodontal attachment, possibly exposing bone. When the necrosis extends beyond the periodontium into the mucosa and osseous tissue, it results in NS. These three conditions appear to be different stages of the same disease. The only distinction appears to be their severity.

## PERIODONTAL PATHOLOGIES

Periodontal pathologies usually found in HIV-infected patients are discussed below.[4,8,9]

### Linear Gingival Erythema

Linear gingival erythema is defined as a gingival manifestation of immunosuppressed patients, which is characterized by distinct linear erythema limited to the free gingival margin. The LGE in HIV-infected patients is refractory to conventional periodontal therapy, including plaque control, scaling, and root planing.

This forms an ideal diagnostic feature of LGE in a seropositive patient. Another critical feature of LGE is its association with *Candida* infection (*Candida dubliniensis*). LGE usually is present as a bright red band along the gingival margin.

In some cases, LGE may be associated with bleeding and discomfort. It is characteristically noted in association with anterior teeth. The microbiological findings are consistent with that of conventional periodontitis rather than gingivitis. It is a potential clinical marker of HIV infection. The proportion of T-cells and macrophages decreases whereas the number of polymorphonuclear leukocytes, immunoglobulin G and plasma cells increases in HIV-positive patients.[10]

### Necrotizing Ulcerative Gingivitis

Necrotizing ulcerative gingivitis is presented with ulcerated, necrotic papilla and gingival margins that are covered by pseudomembrane and associated with intense pain and spontaneous gingival bleeding. It may or may not be associated with depressed CD4 T-cell count.

### Necrotizing Ulcerative Periodontitis

Necrotizing ulcerative periodontitis is presented with peculiar features of sharp pain, loosening of teeth, bleeding, fetid odor, ulcerated gingival papilla, and rapid and extensive loss of bone and soft tissue.[11] It is an indication of severe immunosuppression. Patients often refer to the pain

**TABLE 26.1:** Centers for Disease Control and Prevention (CDC) surveillance case classification.

| *Category A patients have* | *Category B patients have* | *Category C patients have* |
|---|---|---|
| ◆ Asymptomatic HIV-1 infection | ◆ Oropharyngeal candidiasis | ◆ Full-blown disseminated life-threatening bacterial, viral and protozoal infections |
| ◆ Persistent generalized lymphadenopathy | ◆ Oral hairy leukoplakia | ◆ Malignancy |
| ◆ Acute (primary) HIV-1 infection or history of acute HIV-1 infection | ◆ Idiopathic thrombocytopenia | ◆ CD4$^+$ T lymphocytes level <200/mm$^3$ |
| | ◆ Constitutional symptoms of fever, diarrhea and weight loss | |
| | During all this period (category A+B): The patients are HIV positive infected but not yet got AIDS | |

(HIV: human immunodeficiency virus; AIDS: acquired immunodeficiency syndrome)

as deep jaw pain. Other features include lymphadenopathy, fever, and malaise. The microbial flora is similar to that of chronic periodontitis; it has the same pathogens but at a higher level. There is evidence of the increased prevalence of *Candida*. NUP is a predictive marker for CD4+ lymphocyte count less than 200/mm$^3$.

## Necrotizing Ulcerative Stomatitis

Necrotizing ulcerative stomatitis (NUS) is an acutely tender and extremely destructive pathology. It is occasionally reported in HIV-positive patients. Condition is peculiarly present with necrosis of significant areas of oral soft tissue and underlying bone. It may occur separately or as an extension of NUP and is commonly associated with severe depression of CD4 immune cells. The condition appears to be identical to cancrum oris (noma), a rare destructive process reported in nutritionally deprived individuals, especially those in Africa.

## DIAGNOSIS

Patient's medical and dental history in combination with oral examination findings helps to reach the diagnosis of periodontitis in HIV patients. The presence of disease-associated peculiar signs and symptoms should be taken into consideration. The clinical features of periodontitis in HIV patients are due to associated inflammation and related pathological changes. Inflammation-mediated injury is the result of the inability of the host to resolve the inflammation. The altered immune response in HIV-positive patients is only a varied presentation of the normal but is not in itself diagnostic. There are not any specific criteria to distinguish periodontal diseases in HIV-positive from those in HIV-negative patients. Also, it is identified that the lesions of NUP are commonly observed in individuals with systemic conditions, severe malnutrition, and immunosuppression and not only limited to HIV infection.

Following are the various diagnostic serological, molecular, confirmatory tests with their advantages and disadvantages **(Table 26.2)**.

## TREATMENT

*Goals of periodontal disease treatment in HIV-positive patients are*:
- To reduce dental morbidity and overall mortality and improve the quality of life
- To restore and preserve adequate immunocompetence
- To suppress viral load maximally and durably

*Chemotherapeutic agents used in the treatment of HIV*:[4] Since the mid-1990s HAART (highly active antiretroviral therapy) is a widely recognized and highly acceptable treatment approach for HIV infection management. It is a combination of various drugs that significantly modify the course of HIV infection, slow down the disease progression, and improves survival rate. The drugs commonly used as a part of HAART are as follows:
- Nucleoside reverse transcriptase inhibitors (NRTI): Azidothymidine (AZT), zalcitabine (ddC), lamivudine (3TC), stavudine (d4T).
- Non-nucleoside reverse transcriptase inhibitors (NNRTI): Delavirdine and nevirapine.
- Protease inhibitors (PIs): Saquinavir, indinavir, ritonavir, nelfinavir.
- Entry (fusion) inhibitors

These drugs act at various stages in the lifecycle of the virus. The drug administration is hugely helpful in reducing the viral load to undetectable levels and allows effective immune restoration. HAART significantly increases absolute CD4+ lymphocyte counts, reduces HIV viral load and improves patient survival even when absolute CD4+ lymphocyte counts decreases.[12,13]

Primary care consultation is essential to rule out associated systemic opportunistic infections. The painful

**TABLE 26.2:** Available diagnostic tests.[5]

| Parameters | Advantages | Disadvantages |
|---|---|---|
| **Serological assays** | | |
| ELISA | Screens large sample size; easy to perform | Many false-positive results |
| Home HIV test | Simple, does not require to expertize to evaluate | Expensive |
| Rapid test | Lesser time required to produce results | High range of false-positive results |
| Rapid latex agglutination | Simple, require minimum equipment | Non-specific results |
| Dot blot assay | Simple to perform | High range of false-positive results |
| **Molecular assays** | | |
| PCR | The rapid procedure detects approximately within 4 hours | Prone to false-positive results due to cross contamination |
| P24 antigen assay | Highly specific | Susceptible to false-positive results |
| **Confirmatory tests** | | |
| Western assay | Detects viral antibodies; highly specific to HIV proteins | Expensive and needs expertize to interpret the results |
| Indirect immunofluorescence | Detects virus antigen and antibodies | Requires fluorescence microscope as well as a trained technician |

(ELISA: enzyme-linked immunosorbent assay; HIV: human immunodeficiency virus; PCR, polymerase chain reaction)

nature of periodontal lesions usually restricts food intake, and hence proper nutritional care is important in such patients. Optimization of oral hygiene, the establishment of regular review periods, and screening and management for HIV-related oral lesions is necessary for better treatment outcome.

## Linear Gingival Erythema

Following are the treatment for linear gingival erythema:[14]
- Meticulous oral hygiene instructions.
- Scaling, subgingival irrigation with chlorhexidine.
- Chlorhexidine digluconate 0.12% mouthwash.
- If persists, evaluate for candidiasis and retreat if necessary.

## Necrotizing Ulcerative Gingivitis

Following are the treatment for necrotizing ulcerative gingivitis:[15]
- Debridement of the necrotic lesion and light scaling
- Scaling and root planing
- Chlorhexidine digluconate 0.12% mouthwash
- Meticulous oral hygiene
- Antibiotic: Metronidazole 400 mg BID for 5–7 days

## Necrotizing Ulcerative Periodontitis

Following are the treatment for necrotizing ulcerative periodontitis:
- Scaling, root planing and subgingival irrigation
- Removal of necrotic soft tissues utilizing a 0.12% chlorhexidine digluconate or 10% povidone-iodine lavage.
- *Antibiotic*: Metronidazole 400 mg BID for a week
- Prophylactic systemic antifungal agent
- Frequent follow-up visits

### Points to Ponder

- The human immunodeficiency virus is a lentivirus of the retrovirus family.
- In HIV infection, B lymphocytes are not infected primarily. However, the altered function of infected T lymphocytes secondarily results in B-cell dysregulation.
- Seven oral cardinal lesions strongly associated with HIV infection are oral candidiasis, Hairy leukoplakia, Kaposi's sarcoma, linear gingival erythema, necrotizing ulcerative gingivitis, necrotizing ulcerative periodontitis, non-Hodgkin's lymphoma.

## REFERENCES

1. Broder S. Pathogenic human retroviruses. N Engl J Med. 1988;318(4):243-5.
2. Winkler JR, Murray PA. Periodontal disease. A potential intraoral expression of AIDS may be rapidly progressive periodontitis. CDA J. 1987;15(1):20-4.
3. Abbas AK. Diseases of immunity. In: Kumar V, Fausto N, Abbas AK (Eds). Robbins and Cotran Pathologic Basis of Disease, 7th edition. Philadelphia, PA, USA: Elsevier-Saunders; 2004. pp. 193-268.
4. Yin MT, Dobkin JF, Grbic JT. Epidemiology, pathogenesis, and management of human immunodeficiency virus infection in patients with periodontal disease. Periodontol 2000. 2007;44:55-81.
5. Arya S, Lal P, Singh P, Kumar A. Recent advances in diagnosis of HIV and future prospects. Indian J Biotechnol. 2015;14:9-18.
6. Wilkins EM, Romano JE. Infection control: Transmissible diseases. In: Wilkins EM (Ed). Clinical Practice of the Dental Hygienist, 8th edition. Philadelphia, PA, USA: Lippincott Williams & Wilkins; 1999. pp. 13-41.
7. 1993 revised classification system for HIV infection and expanded surveillance case definition for AIDS among adolescents and adults. MMWR Recomm Rep. 1992;41(RR-17):1-19.
8. Rees TD. AIDS and the periodontium. In: Newman MG, Takei HH, Carranza FA (Eds). Carranza's Clinical Periodontology, 9th edition. Philadelphia, PA, USA: WB Saunders; 2003. pp. 415-31.
9. Velegraki A, Nicolatou O, Theodoridou M, Mostrou G, Legakis NJ. Paediatric AIDS-related linear gingival erythema: a form of erythematous candidiasis? J Oral Pathol Med. 1999;28(4):178-82.
10. Gomez RS, de Costa JE, Loyola AM, de Araújo NS, de Araújo VC. Immunohistochemical study of linear gingival erythema from HIV-positive patients. J Periodontal Res. 1995;30(5):355-9.
11. Rees TD, Mealey BL. Periodontal treatment of the medically compromised patient. In: Rose LF, Mealey BL, Genco RJ, Cohen DW (Eds). Periodontics: Medicine, Surgery, and Implants, 2nd revised edition. Philadelphia, PA, USA: Elsevier Mosby; 2004.
12. Ryder MI. An update on HIV and periodontal disease. J Periodontol. 2002;73(9):1071-8.
13. Ryder MI, Nittayananta W, Coogan M, Greenspan D, Greenspan JS. Periodontal disease in HIV/AIDS. Periodontol 2000. 2012;60(1):78-97.
14. Rees TD. Periodontal management of HIV-infected patients. In: Newman MG, Takei HH, Carranza FA (Eds). Carranza's Clinical Periodontology, 9th edition. Philadelphia, PA, USA: WB Saunders; 2003. pp. 688-96.
15. Ryder MI. Periodontal management of HIV-infected patients. Periodontol 2000. 2000;23:85-93.

### VIVA VOCE

**Q1. Name the cells that are primarily affected by HIV.**
**Ans.** HIV primarily affects T lymphocytes, which carry CD4 cell surface receptors. It also affects the macrophages, monocytes, langerhan cells, and glial cells.

**Q2. What is OraQuick?**
**Ans.** OraQuick is an over-the-counter test for HIV by OraSure technologies. This test detects HIV antibodies in oral fluids with the help of oral swabs within 30 minutes. One red line indicates a negative result, and two red lines indicate a positive result.

**Section 4:** Pathology of Gingival and Periodontal Diseases

**Q3. What are highly active antiretroviral therapy (HAART) drugs?**
**Ans.** The drugs which combine three or more drugs from at least two different classes used to suppress the viral replication are known as HAART drugs.

**Q4. What is Orasure?**
**Ans.** It is a commercially available kit for the collection of HIV 1 antibodies in which an oral specimen collecting device is placed between the buccal mucosa and buccal gingiva for 2 to 5 minutes. This does not collect saliva; instead, a sample called oral mucosal transudate.

**Q5. Which opportunistic infection is usually associated with linear gingival erythema?**
**Ans.** Candida infection.

**Q6. What is linear gingival erythema?**
**Ans.** Linear gingival erythema is non-plaque-induced gingivitis exhibiting a distinct erythematous band of the marginal gingiva, which either diffuses or punctuates erythema of the attached gingiva.

**Q7. Name various genes present in the HIV-1 RNA genome.**
**Ans.** Genes are gag, pol, and env, which code for various viral proteins.

**Q8. What initiates the process of HIV infection?**
**Ans.** Binding of the gp120 envelope glycoprotein to CD4 molecules initiate the process of HIV infection.

**Q9. How HIV virus enters the body?**
**Ans.** The HIV virus commonly enters the body through mucosal tissues and blood.

**Q10. What are the common presenting oral lesions of HIV/AIDS infection?**
**Ans.** Oral candidiasis and oral hairy leukoplakia.

# Chapter 27: Trauma from Occlusion

*Sumidha R Bansal, Shaili Pradhan*

## Chapter Outline

- Definitions
- Types
- Concepts
- Tissue Response
- Clinical Features
- Radiographic Features
- Role of Occlusal Trauma
- Treatment
- Effect of Trauma on Implants
- Pathologic Tooth Migration

## INTRODUCTION

Harmonious relationships of teeth, jaw, occlusion, and temporomandibular joint (TMJ) contribute to the periodontium's health. Conversely, when this interrelationship is disturbed, periodontal disease will occur. In this chapter, the precise role of occlusion, along with trauma from occlusion and pathologic tooth migration, are discussed.

## DEFINITIONS

When occlusal forces exceed the adaptive capacity of the tissues, it results in tissue injury. The resultant injury is termed as trauma from occlusion.[1] Thus, trauma from occlusion refers to tissue injury, not the occlusal force. This term is generally used in relation with injury to the periodontium rather than injury to the temporomandibular joint, tooth structure, or masticatory musculature. Other terms, which also denote this, are occlusal trauma or traumatism.

Trauma from occlusion refers to tissue injury rather than occlusal force. An occlusion that produces such an injury is called a traumatic occlusion.[2] The magnitude, direction, duration, and frequency of occlusal forces affect the periodontium.

Stillman in 1917 defined trauma from occlusion as a condition where injury results to the supporting structures of the teeth by the act of bringing the jaws into a closed position.[3]

The World Health Organization (WHO) in 1978 defined trauma from occlusion as damage in the periodontium caused by stress on the teeth produced directly or indirectly by teeth of the opposing jaw.

In Glossary of Periodontal Terms [The American Academy of Periodontology (AAP) 1986], occlusal trauma was defined as an injury to the attachment apparatus as a result of excessive occlusal forces.[4]

In Glossary of Periodontal Terms (AAP 1992), occlusal trauma refers to a response or effect and is defined as an injury to the attachment or tooth as a result of excessive occlusal forces.[5]

According to the 2017 classification, excessive occlusal force is renamed as traumatic occlusal force. Traumatic occlusal force is defined as any occlusal force resulting in injury of the teeth and/or the periodontal attachment apparatus.[6]

## TYPES

### Primary Trauma from Occlusion

When trauma from occlusion is the result of alterations in occlusal forces, it is called primary trauma from occlusion. Periodontal tissue injury occurs when excessive occlusal forces are applied to the tooth/teeth in nonfunctional activities.[7] The muscular contraction is isometric, and force is large up to 250 lb/sq inch.[8] Examples are: (i) placement of a high restoration, (ii) insertion of a fixed bridge or partial denture that places excessive force on the abutment teeth, and (iii) the drifting movement or extrusion of teeth into spaces created by unreplaced missing teeth. Primary trauma from occlusion occurs if trauma from occlusion is considered the primary etiologic factor in periodontal

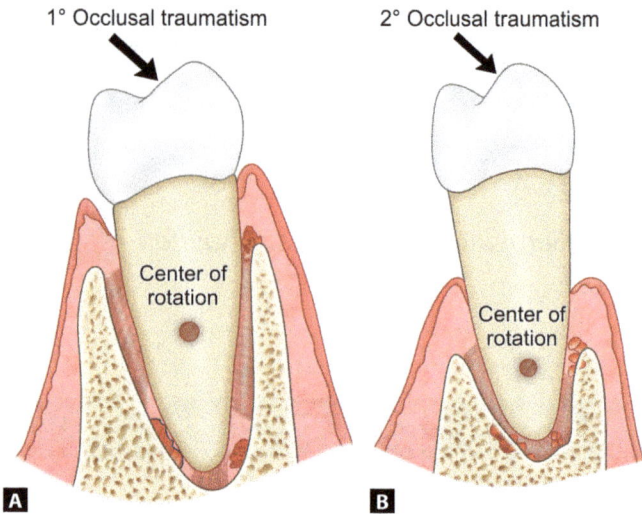
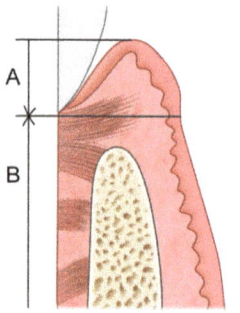
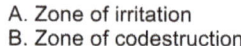
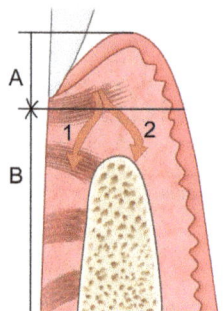

**Figs. 27.1A and B:** Schematic representation showing primary and secondary trauma from occlusion.

**Fig. 27.2:** Schematic representation showing Glickman's concept.

destruction and if the only local alteration to which a tooth is subjected is from occlusion **(Fig. 27.1A)**. Thus, it occurs in the presence of—(1) normal bone level, (2) normal attachment level, and (3) excessive occlusal force.

## Secondary Trauma from Occlusion

When trauma from occlusion results from the reduced ability of the tissues to resist the occlusal forces, it is known as secondary trauma from occlusion. Such injury occurs when the tissues' adaptive capacity to withstand normal occlusal forces is reduced due to bone loss resulting from marginal inflammation **(Fig. 27.1B)**.[7] The muscular contraction is isotonic, and force is physiologic, i.e., 2–15 lb/sq inch.[8] The periodontium becomes more vulnerable to injury, and previously well-tolerated occlusal forces become traumatic. Thus, it occurs in the presence of— bone loss, (2) attachment loss, and (3) normal/excessive occlusal force.

## CONCEPTS

### Glickman's Concept

According to Glickman (1965), the pathway of the spread of a plaque-associated gingival lesion can be changed if forces of an abnormal magnitude are acting on teeth harboring subgingival plaque.[9]

According to Glickman's concept, the periodontal structures can be divided into two zones based on the effect of trauma from occlusion on the spread of the plaque-associated lesion:
1. The zone of irritation
2. The zone of codestruction

### The Zone of Irritation

This includes marginal and interdental gingiva. The soft tissue of this zone is bordered by hard tissue (the tooth) only on one side and is not affected by occlusion forces. This means that gingival inflammation cannot be induced by trauma from occlusion but is the result of irritation from microbial plaque. The plaque-associated lesion at a nontraumatized tooth propagates in apical direction by first involving the alveolar bone and later the periodontal ligament area. The progression of this lesion results in an even (horizontal) bone destruction **(Fig. 27.2)**.

### The Zone of Codestruction

This includes the periodontal ligament, the root cementum, and the alveolar bone and is coronally demarcated by the transseptal (interdental) and the dentoalveolar collagen fiber bundles. The tissue in this zone may become the seat of a lesion caused by trauma from occlusion. The spread of the inflammatory lesion from the zone of irritation directly down into the periodontal ligament (i.e., not via the interdental bone) may hereby be facilitated. This alteration of the normal pathway of the spread of the plaque-associated inflammatory lesion results in the development of angular bony defects. According to a review paper by Glickman (1967), trauma from occlusion is the significant causative agent (codestructive factor) in situations where angular bony defects combined with infrabony pockets are found at one or several teeth.

### Waerhaug's Concept

According to Waerhaug, the loss of connective tissue attachment and the resorption of bone around teeth are exclusively the result of inflammatory lesions associated with subgingival plaque. Waerhaug concluded that angular bony defects and infrabony pockets occur when the subgingival plaque of one tooth has reached a more apical level than the microbiota on the neighboring tooth and when the volume of the alveolar bone surrounding the roots is comparatively large.[10]

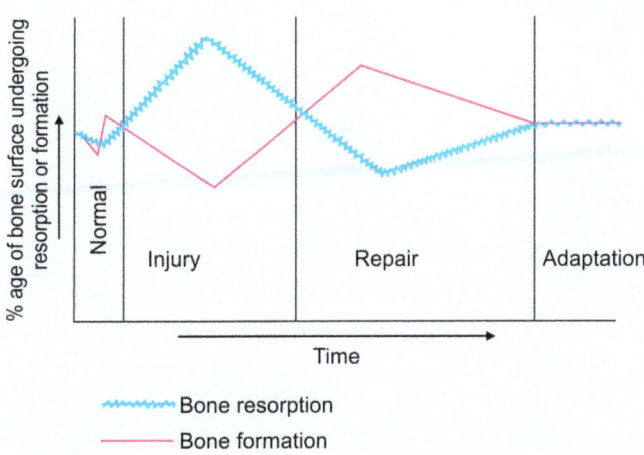

**Fig. 27.3:** Schematic representation showing stages of tissue response due to increased occlusal forces.

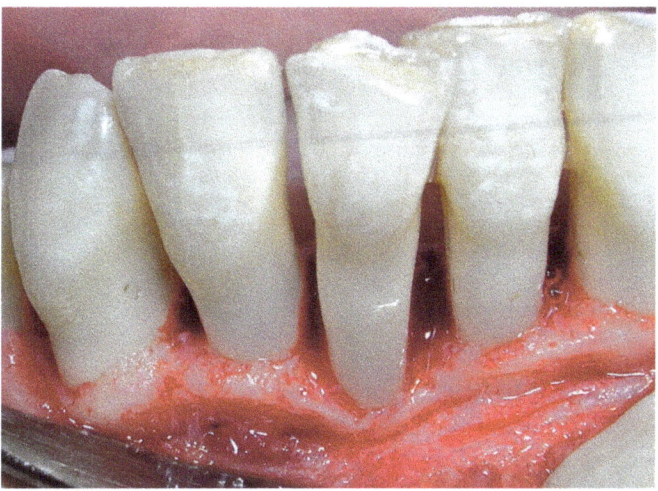

**Fig. 27.4:** Clinical picture showing lipping of alveolar bone.

Glickman's conclusion was suggestive that trauma from occlusion aggravates the periodontal tissue destruction. At the same time, Waerhaug's concept exhibited no relationship between occlusal trauma and the degree of periodontal tissue destruction.

## TISSUE RESPONSE

Tissue response occurs in three stages: (1) injury, (2) repair, and (3) adaptive remodeling of the periodontium **(Fig. 27.3 and Table 27.1)**.[11]

## Stage I: Injury

Slightly excessive pressure initiates alveolar bone resorption and results in the widening of the periodontal ligament space. However, slightly excessive tension causes elongation of the periodontal ligament fibers and the apposition of alveolar bone. Greater pressure produces compression of periodontal fibers, which produces an area of hyalinization and increased resorption of alveolar bone and tooth surface. In contrast, severe tension causes widening and tearing of periodontal ligament fibers and increased resorption of alveolar bone. The areas of the periodontium most susceptible to injury from excessive occlusal forces are the furcations.

## Stage II: Repair

During the process of bone resorption due to excessive occlusal forces, the body tries to strengthen the thinned bony trabeculae with new bone formation. This process is termed as buttressing bone formation, and it is an attempt to compensate for the lost bone. It is a characteristic feature of the reparative process associated with trauma from occlusion. Buttressing bone formation peculiarly takes place within the jaw, i.e., central buttressing and on the bone surface, i.e., peripheral buttressing. Central buttressing involves the deposition of new bone by endosteal cells associated with restoration of the bony trabeculae with a reduction of the size of the marrow spaces. Peripheral buttressing usually takes place on the facial and lingual surfaces of the alveolar plate. Depending on its severity, peripheral buttressing can result in a shelf-like thickening of the alveolar margin called lipping **(Fig. 27.4)**, or prominent bulge in the contour of the facial and lingual bone.[12]

## Stage III: Adaptive Remodeling of the Periodontium

If the repair process cannot keep pace with the destruction caused by the occlusion, the periodontium is remodeled to create a structural relationship in which the forces are no longer harmful to the tissues. This results in a thickened periodontal ligament, which is funnel-shaped at the crest, and angular defects in the bone, with no pocket formation. The involved teeth become mobile.

## CLINICAL FEATURES

### Increased Tooth Mobility

In the injury stage of trauma from occlusion, the destruction of periodontal fibers occurs, increasing the tooth's mobility. In the final stage, the periodontium accommodation to increased forces entails a widening of the periodontal ligament, which also leads to increased tooth mobility. Although this tooth mobility is greater than the so-called normal mobility, it cannot be considered pathologic

| **TABLE 27.1:** Tissue response to increased occlusal forces. | |
|---|---|
| Injury phase | Increased resorption and decreased bone formation |
| Repair phase | Decreased resorption and increased bone formation |
| Adaptive remodeling phase | Bone resorption and formation return to normal |

## Section 4: Pathology of Gingival and Periodontal Diseases

**BOX 27.1:** Clinical and radiographic indicators of occlusal trauma.

Indicators of occlusal trauma include the following:
- Mobility
- Fremitus
- Premature occlusal contacts
- Wear facets
- Fractured teeth
- Tooth migration
- Widened periodontal ligament space
- Bone loss
- Root resorption

because it is an adaptation and not a disease process. When it becomes progressively worse, it can be regarded as pathologic[13] **(Box 27.1)**.

### Increasing Tooth Mobility

Diagnosis of trauma from occlusion can be made in situations where progressive mobility is seen. Progressive increasing tooth mobility is usually recognized with a series of repeated tooth mobility measurements conducted over several days or weeks.[14]

### RADIOGRAPHIC FEATURES

- Increased width of the periodontal space, often with thickening of the lamina dura along the lateral aspect of the root, in the apical region, and bifurcation areas **(Fig. 27.5)**.
- Usually, there is vertical rather than horizontal bone loss.
- Radiolucency and condensation of the alveolar bone with root resorption are sometimes seen **(Fig. 27.6 and Box 27.1)**.

### ROLE OF OCCLUSAL TRAUMA

Excessive occlusal forces result in the widening of periodontal ligament space with loss of alveolar volume. Maximum compressive stress occurs just apical to alveolar crest, at the rim of the socket, leading to the development of an angular bony defect on a radiograph.

In the absence of periodontal inflammation, this happens without the occurrence of pocket as there is no loss of connective tissue attachment, probably due to structural and functional independence of periodontal and gingival blood circulation. In such a situation, the base of the sulcus remains in the same position, and there is an increase in the supracrestal connective tissue area. This lesion is reversible once the occlusal stress is removed. Hence, a tooth free of periodontal infection but widened ligament and alveolar crestal bone loss caused by occlusal forces is not more susceptible to plaque-induced inflammation and attachment loss.

Teeth with a reduced but healthy periodontium (treated case), respond to occlusal forces in the same way as teeth

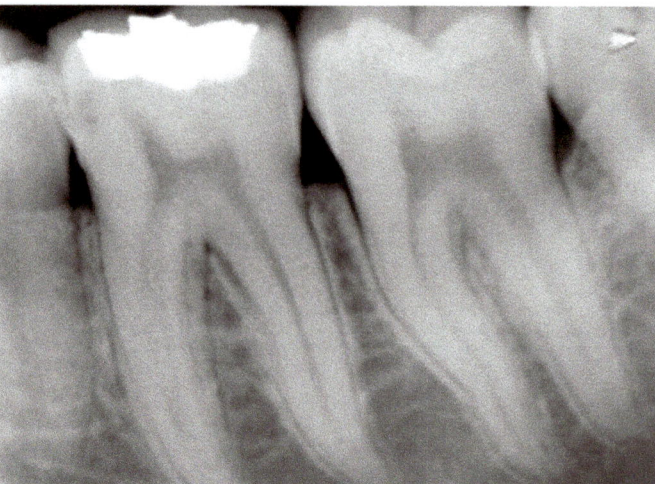

**Fig. 27.5:** Radiographic image showing features of trauma from occlusion (discontinuity and thickening of lamina dura).

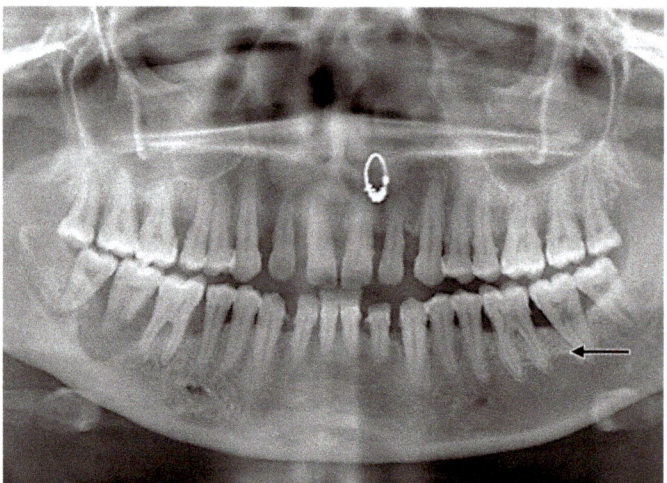

**Fig. 27.6:** Radiographic image showing features of trauma from occlusion.

with normal support. This means that physiologic adaptation may result in the widened periodontal ligament, mobility, and crestal bone loss but no further loss of attachment.

Thus, there is no evidence regarding the role of occlusal trauma in initiating periodontal destruction. However, its role in the progression of periodontal disease cannot be excluded.

### TREATMENT

The decision to treat occlusal trauma present is not made promptly in one appointment. It requires reevaluation after a sequence of initial therapeutic procedures. Mobility should be evaluated so that differentiation can be made between increased mobility and progressively increasing mobility.

### Primary Trauma from Occlusion

The reason is determined, and defective restorations/prostheses are/is corrected. If, however, it has occurred

due to orthodontic tooth movement in functionally unacceptable position or drifting of teeth in edentulous spaces, occlusal treatment consists of:
- Use of bite appliance
- Adjusting occlusion by altering the occlusal relationship between teeth, which can be done by orthodontic therapy or selective grinding. This will create a permanent change in the distribution of forces and hence, needs to be done with proper technique and skill.[15]
- Occlusal treatment is considered if the patient is symptomatic (sensitivity to temperature or pain on chewing, mobility, wear facets are present). If a patient is asymptomatic, treatment of occlusion is not indicated even if significant discrepancies are present.

## Secondary Trauma from Occlusion

Occlusal treatment should be considered after inflammation has subsided through nonsurgical periodontal treatment as that would reduce mobility and induce occlusal stability. In case the patient has difficulty or pain in chewing that appears directly due to occlusal trauma, occlusal treatment would precede periodontal treatment. Surgical periodontal therapy should be avoided in the early stages of a treatment plan if occlusal trauma is suspected as that would remove tissues just coronal to crest of resorbed bone, which, after removal of excessive forces, might have osteogenic potential.

## EFFECT OF TRAUMA ON IMPLANTS

Effect of occlusal trauma on osseointegrated implants is controversial. Implant studies in monkeys have supported a significant loss of osseointegration due to occlusal overload even in the absence of inflammation and no loss of osseointegration in the presence of heavy plaque and no occlusal overload.[16] On the contrary, other studies on the same model failed to show notable peri-implant bone loss solely with prolonged excessive supraocclusal force (without peri-implant inflammation).[17] Previous literature published in cellular biomechanics, engineering principles, bone loss differences related to bone density, animal studies, and clinical reports favor an important role of occlusal overload as an etiological agent in peri-implant bone loss.[18] Methods to decrease occlusal stress to the implant prosthesis should be undertaken.

## PATHOLOGIC TOOTH MIGRATION

### Definition

Pathologic tooth migration (PTM) is defined as a change in tooth position that occurs when there is the disruption of forces that maintain teeth in a normal relationship.[19] The tooth displacement in PTM is mainly due to disturbance in the balance between the factors that maintain a physiologic tooth position. This disturbance occurs in the advanced form of chronic periodontitis. Pathologic migration is relatively common and may be an early sign of disease, or it may occur in association with gingival inflammation and pocket formation as the disease progresses.

## Etiology

Various factors maintain a normal tooth position, and hence many possible etiologic factors play a significant role in PTM. Thus, PTM is multifactorial in origin with complex etiology. The various reasons for incisor flaring highlight the complexity of differential diagnosis. The tooth position is commonly affected by factors, namely tissues of the periodontium; soft tissue pressures of the cheek, tongue, and lips; and a variety of oral habits (Fig. 27.7).

Periodontal inflammation and eruptive forces influence tooth position and can result in total tooth displacement.[20]

### Destruction of Periodontal Supporting Tissues

Destruction of periodontal tissues plays a significant role in the etiology of PTM. The destruction of transseptal fibers is identified as one of the critical causes of PTM. Transseptal fibers form a chain from tooth to tooth and hold the adjacent teeth throughout the arch. If the continuity of this chain is broken or weakened in the case of periodontal disease, they can disturb the balance of forces and result in tooth displacement. It is considered that the contractile force within the transseptal fiber gets originate from gingival fibroblasts, which are known to produce collagen contraction.

### Occlusal Factors

Occlusal factors responsible for PTM are posterior bite collapse from loss of posterior teeth, class II malocclusion, occlusal interferences, the anterior component of force, protrusive functional patterns of mastication, bruxism and

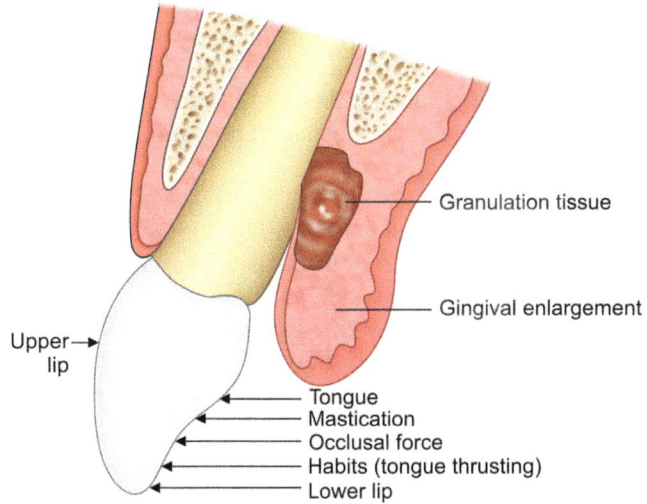

**Fig. 27.7:** Schematic representation showing factors influencing tooth position.

shortened dental arches. Posterior bite collapse is a pattern of unfavorable occlusal change that commonly occurs after 1st molar teeth are lost and not replaced.

Following are the consequences of failure to replace 1st molars:
- The 2nd and 3rd molars tilt, resulting in a decrease in the vertical dimension.
- The premolars move distally, and the mandibular incisors tilt or drift lingually.
- Anterior overbite is increased.
- The mandibular incisors strike the maxillary incisors near the gingiva and traumatize the gingiva.
- The maxillary incisors are pushed labially and laterally.
- The anterior teeth extrude because the incisal apposition has largely disappeared.
- The separation of the anterior teeth creates diastema.

Closely related to posterior bite collapse is arch integrity. Interproximal contacts help to maintain occlusal forces pertaining to teeth in the arch. Once the interproximal contacts get damaged, tooth displacement takes place. Common factors damaging the interproximal contacts are tooth loss, dental caries, faulty restorations, and severe attrition.

### Soft Tissue Pressure of the Tongue, Cheek, and Lips

Previously conducted orthodontic studies reported that soft tissue forces of the tongue, cheek, and lips play a crucial role to move teeth, especially after the loss of periodontal attachment. A long duration of these light forces makes them significant over the relatively short duration of occlusal contacts during the speech, swallowing and mastication.

### Periodontal and Periapical Inflammation

In 1933, Hirschfeld reported a pathologic drifting of the teeth due to excessive pressure exerted by inflammatory tissue in periodontal pockets. Recently conducted animal research focused more light on this observation, concluding that inflamed gingiva enhances interstitial fluid pressure due to an increase in capillary filtration. The extravasation of fluid into the interstitial tissue causes a rise in interstitial hydraulic pressure. When gingival inflammation is controlled then; there is a spontaneous correction of migration.

### Habits

Oral habits of patients usually affect tooth position and result in PTM. Lip and tongue thrusting habits (**Fig. 27.8**), fingernail biting, thumb-sucking, pipe-smoking, bruxism, and playing wind instruments are some to enumerate. The duration of force in tooth movement is more important than force magnitude. Longer the duration of the habit, the greater is the ability to move teeth.

### Treatment

Treatment of pathological tooth migration depends on involved etiological factors and the severity of tooth

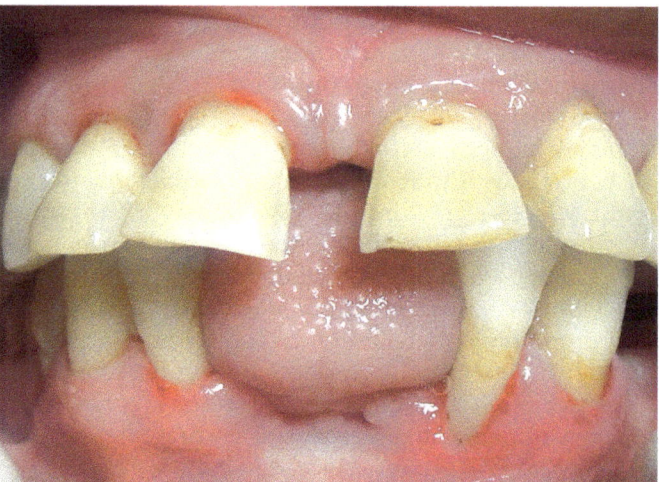

**Fig. 27.8:** Clinical picture showing pathologic migration associated with tongue thrusting habit.

displacement. It usually constitutes orthodontic therapy that is preceded by nonsurgical and surgical periodontal therapy and prosthodontic treatment. Selecting an appropriate method to treat PTM is usually based on an interdisciplinary approach.

Correction of PTM is usually categorized as follows:
- Spontaneous correction of the early stages of PTM following periodontal therapy.
- Limited or adjunctive orthodontic therapy.
- Conventional orthodontic treatment.
- Extraction and replacement of migrated teeth in cases of very severe migration.

Apart from this, patient factors should be taken into consideration before deciding the appropriate treatment approach for PTM. Such factors include patient compliance and cooperation, motivation to keep the natural teeth, skeletal factors, economic factors, availability for treatment, systemic health, and acceptance of surgical periodontal treatment, if necessary. Literature mentioned a few cases of reactive positioning or spontaneous correction of pathologic migration following periodontal treatment only. Occasionally migrated teeth repositioned to their normal location after nonsurgical periodontal treatment alone or when combined with surgical methods in some cases.

### Points to Ponder

- Physiologic occlusion was defined by Goldman and Cohen as one that operates in harmony and presents no pathologic manifestations in the supporting structures of the teeth. A physiologic occlusion is one that may be anatomic malocclusion but free of any occlusal-induced disease.[21]
- A pathologic occlusion is one that requires therapeutic alteration of present occlusion as it shows evidence of disease owing to occlusal activity.
- Drifting differs from PTM in that it does not result from the destruction of periodontal tissues.

## REFERENCES

1. Carranza FA, Camargo PM. Periodontal response to external forces. In: Newman MG, Takei HH, Carranza FA (Eds). Carranza's Clinical Periodontology, 9th edition. Philadelphia, PA, USA: WB Saunders; 2003. pp. 371-83.
2. Bhaskar SN, Orban B. Experimental occlusal trauma. J Periodontol. 1955;26:270.
3. Stillman PR. The management of pyorrhea. Dental Cosmos. 1917;59:405-14.
4. Glossary of Periodontal Terms, 2nd edition. Chicago, IL, USA: The American Academy of Periodontology; 1986.
5. Glossary of Periodontal Terms, 3rd edition. Chicago, IL, USA: The American Academy of Periodontology; 1992.
6. Jepsen S, Caton JG, et al. Periodontal manifestations of systemic diseases and developmental and acquired conditions: Consensus report of workgroup 3 of the 2017 World Workshop on the Classification of Periodontal and Peri-Implant Diseases and Conditions. J Periodontol. 2018;89(Suppl 1):S237–S248.
7. Prichard JF. Advanced Periodontal Disease: Surgical and Prosthetic Management, 2nd edition. Philadelphia, PA, USA: WB Saunders; 1972. p. 29.
8. Amsterdam M. Periodontal prosthesis. Twenty-five years in retrospect. Alpha Omegan. 1974;67(3):8-52.
9. Glickman I, Smulow JB. Effect of excessive occlusal forces upon the pathway of gingival inflammation in humans. J Periodontol. 1965;36:141-7.
10. Waerhaug J. The infrabony pocket and its relationship to trauma from occlusion and subgingival plaque. J Periodontol. 1979;50(7):355-65.
11. Carranza FA. Histometric evaluation of periodontal pathology. A review of recent studies. J Periodontol. 1970;38(6 Suppl):741-50.
12. Glickman I, Smulow JB. Buttressing bone formation in the periodontium. J Periodontol. 1965;36(5):365-70.
13. Lindhe J, Nyman S, Ericsson I. Trauma from occlusion. In: Lindhe J, Karring T, Lang NP (Eds). Clinical Periodontology and Implant Dentistry, 4th edition. Chicago, USA: Blackwell Munksgaard; 2003. pp. 352-65.
14. Lindhe J, Nyman S. Occlusal therapy. In: Lindhe J, Karring T, Lang NP (Eds). Clinical Periodontology and Implant Dentistry, 4th edition. Chicago, USA: Blackwell Munksgaard; 2003. pp. 731-43.
15. Solberg W, Seligman D. Coronoplasty in periodontal therapy. In: Carranza FA, Takei HH, Newman MG (Eds). Carranza's Clinical Periodontology, 8th edition. Philadelphia, PA, USA: WB Saunders; 1996. pp. 537-58.
16. Isidor F. Loss of osseointegration caused by the occlusal load of oral implants. A clinical and radiographic study in monkeys. Clin Oral Imp Res. 1996;7(2):143-52.
17. Miyata T, Kobayashi Y, Araki H, Motomura Y, Shin K. The influence of controlled occlusal overload on peri-implant tissue: a histologic study in monkeys. Int J Oral Maxillofac Implants. 1998;13(5):677-83.
18. Misch CE, Suzuki JB, Misch-Dietsh FM, Bidez MW. A positive correlation between occlusal trauma and peri-implant bone loss: literature support. Implant Dent. 2005;14(2):108-16.
19. Chasens AI. Periodontal disease, pathologic tooth migration, and adult orthodontics. N Y J Dent. 1979;49(2):40-3.
20. Brunsvold MA. Pathologic tooth migration. J Periodontol. 2005;76(6):859-66.
21. Goldman HM, Cohen DW. Periodontal Therapy, 6th edition. St. Louis: Mosby; 1980.

## VIVA VOCE

**Q1. What is Karolyi effect?**
Ans. Karolyi effect is an effect named after Moritz Karolyi, a Viennese dentist, who described the possible role of hyperfunction of the masticatory muscles in eliciting traumatic occlusion as a cause of periodontitis. He recommended its correction by grinding the occlusal surfaces and the use of bite planes at night. He introduced the current concept of bruxism but never used the term.

**Q2. What is the difference between trauma from occlusion and traumatic occlusion?**
Ans. When occlusal forces exceed the tissues' adaptive capacity, tissue injury results, and this resultant injury is termed as trauma from occlusion. Trauma from occlusion refers to tissue injury and not the occlusal force. An occlusion that produces such an injury is called a traumatic occlusion.

**Q3. What is the sequence of periodontal tissue response to increased occlusal forces?**
Ans. • Injury • Repair • Adaptive remodeling.

**Q4. What are the radiographic features of trauma from occlusion?**
Ans.
- Thickening of lamina dura
- Angular bone loss
- Increase in the width of the periodontal ligament space

**Q5. What is tongue thrusting?**
Ans. Tongue thrusting is the persistent, forceful wedging of the tongue against the teeth, especially in the anterior region. It is a habit in which the patient, instead of placing the dorsum of the tongue against the palate with the tip behind the maxillary teeth during swallowing, the tongue is thrust forward against the mandibular anterior teeth, which tilt and also spread laterally.

**Q6. What is the effect of tongue thrusting on dentition?**
Ans.
- Pathologic migration
- Spreading and tilting of the anterior teeth
- Open bite, anteriorly, and posteriorly

**Q7. What is the zone of irritation?**
Ans. The zone of irritation includes the marginal and interdental gingiva. The soft tissue of this zone is bordered by hard tissue (the tooth) only on one side and is not affected by occlusion forces.

**Q8. What is central buttressing bone formation?**
Ans. It involves the deposition of new bone by endosteal cells associated with restoration of the bony trabeculae with a reduction of the size of the marrow spaces.

**Q9. Where usually peripheral buttressing bone formation takes place?**
Ans. On the facial and lingual surfaces of the alveolar plate.

**Q10. What is pathologic tooth migration?**
Ans. It is defined as a change in tooth position that occurs when there is the disruption of forces that maintain teeth in a normal relationship.

# Chapter 28: Sex Hormones and Periodontium

*Shalu Bathla*

## Chapter Outline

- Effects on Periodontium
- Puberty
- Menstrual Cycle
- Pregnancy
- Oral Contraceptives
- Menopause
- Effects on Wound Healing

## INTRODUCTION

Sex hormones appear to have a significant effect on periodontal tissues, bone turnover rate, wound healing process, and periodontal disease progression. Increased concentrations of female sex hormones in the circulation during phases of puberty, pregnancy, and menstrual cycle commonly lead to gingival inflammation and hyperplasia. In periodontics, the impact of hormonal concentration during the prime phases of a woman's lifecycle should be taken into consideration while determining therapeutic approaches.

## EFFECTS ON PERIODONTIUM

Sex hormones, namely estrogen, progesterone, and testosterone, are steroid hormones, which are derivatives of cholesterol. They consist of a combination of three rings of six carbon atoms each and one ring of five carbon atoms.[1] These steroid sex hormones have profound effects on the periodontium and have been linked with the pathogenesis of periodontal diseases **(Fig. 28.1)**.[2]

### Estrogen

Estrogen is a vital, steroid sex hormone in females. It produces significant physiological changes in women during the specific phase of their lifecycle commencing from the puberty. Estradiol, an estrogen sex hormone, levels may reach as high as 30 times in the plasma during the reproductive cycle. Apart from the reproductive system, estrogen receptors are also found on dental structures, namely periosteal fibroblasts, periodontal ligament fibroblasts, and osteoblasts. Hence, estrogen has a considerable potential to affect periodontal tissues.

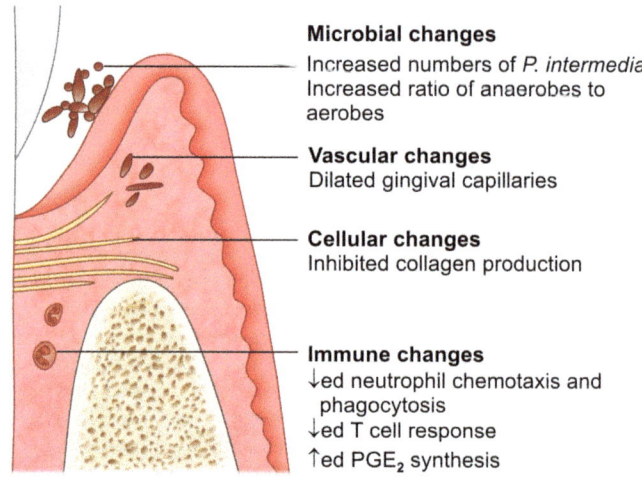

**Fig. 28.1:** Schematic representation showing the effects of increased sex hormones on the periodontium.
(PGE: prostaglandin E)

Commonly noted effects of estrogen on periodontal tissues are as follows:
- The stimulatory effect of estrogen enhances the metabolism of collagen and angiogenesis.[3]
- Estrogen usually activates autocrine or paracrine polypeptide growth factor signalling pathways.
- Estrogens influence the cytodifferentiation of stratified squamous epithelium and the synthesis and maintenance of fibrous collagen.

## Progesterone

Progesterone is another vital steroid sex hormone in the female after estrogen. It is mainly secreted by the placenta, corpus luteum, and adrenal cortex. It plays an active role in the metabolism of bone and significantly modulates the process of coupling of bone resorption and formation.[1]

During pregnancy, progesterone levels reach as high as 100 ng/mL, i.e., about ten times the peak level in the luteal phase of the menstrual cycle. Progesterone shows a significant impact on the gingival vascular system, causing increased exudation, as well as affecting the integrity of the capillary endothelial cells.

### Effects of Progesterone on the Periodontal Tissues

Estrogen and progesterone both in association with interaction with inflammatory mediators modulate vascular responses and connective tissue turnover in the periodontium.[4]

## Androgens (Testosterone)

Androgens are primarily male sex hormones responsible for the masculinization. Androgen hormone, mainly testosterone receptors, are located in the periodontal tissues and fibroblast. Testosterone is also associated with bone metabolism.

### Effects of Androgens on the Periodontal Tissue

- Stimulate matrix synthesis by osteoblasts and periodontal ligament fibroblasts[5]
- Inhibit prostaglandin secretion[6]
- Reduce interleukin-6 (IL-6) production during inflammation[7,8]
- Stimulate osteoblast proliferation and differentiation[9]

## PUBERTY

Puberty is a complex developmental process that involves sexual maturation of an individual for the effective reproduction. Puberty is responsible for significant physical and behavior changes due to increased levels of the steroid sex hormones, namely testosterone in males and estrogens in females. In girl child, puberty occurs at the average age of 11–14 years. The levels after that remain relatively constant throughout the remaining phase of the reproductive cycle. During puberty, periodontal tissues may exhibit an exaggerated response to local factors.[10]

## Periodontal Manifestations

### Gingivitis

The inflamed tissues of the gingiva become erythematous, lobulated, and retractable (**Fig. 28.2**). Bleeding on probing is very commonly noted.

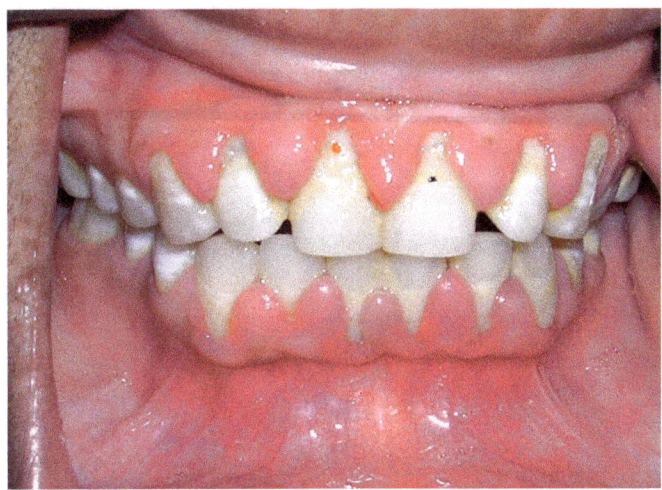

**Fig. 28.2:** Clinical picture showing puberty gingivitis.

### Subgingival Microflora

Puberty is usually associated with higher bacterial counts, especially of *Prevotella intermedia*. Kornman and Loesche have postulated that the anaerobic organism may use ovarian hormone as a substitute for vitamin K growth factor.[11]

### Perimolysis

It is a smooth erosion of the enamel and dentin due to eating disorders, bulimia and anorexia nervosa which occur commonly on the lingual surfaces of maxillary anterior teeth.[12]

### Management

Puberty-related gingival problems need preventive care that includes a vigorous program of oral hygiene. During puberty, oral health education is given to the parents also. A mild form of gingivitis can be managed with only scaling and root planing along with the reinforcement of frequent oral hygiene. Antimicrobial mouthwashes, local site drug delivery or antibiotic therapy improves the treatment outcomes in severe cases of gingivitis.

## MENSTRUAL CYCLE

During the normal menstrual cycle, under the influence of FSH (follicle-stimulating hormone) and LH (luteinizing hormone), the ovaries produce estrogen and progesterone. During the menstrual cycle, the progesterone level increases from the 2nd week and reaches its peaks on approximately ten days, and after that, it dramatically drops down before menstruation. Premenstrual syndrome (PMS) may also occur during the peak level of progesterone, i.e., about 7–10 days before menstruation.[10]

## Periodontal Manifestations

- Gingival bleeding: Imbalance and/or increase in sex hormones levels usually aggravate the process of gingival inflammation.

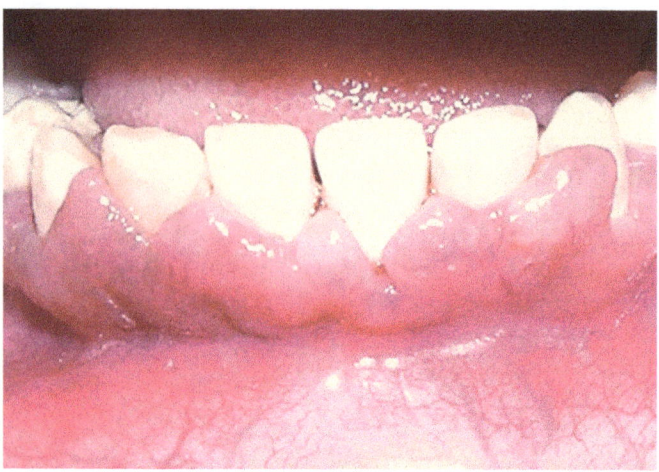

**Fig. 28.3:** Clinical picture showing gingivitis during the menstrual cycle.

- Preceding the onset of menses, the gingival tissues appear to be more edematous and erythematous in some individuals. There is an increased production of gingival exudates **(Fig. 28.3)**.
- There is an alteration in the production rate and pattern of gingival collagen.
- A minor increase in tooth mobility is associated with the menstrual period occasionally.[13]
- Postextraction osteitis incidence has also been reported to be higher during the initiation of menses.
- In some women, intraoral recurrent aphthous ulcers, herpes labialis lesions, and candida infections occur in a cyclic pattern.

## Management

Management of periodontal manifestations during the menstrual cycle mainly emphasizes the practice of oral hygiene. An antimicrobial mouth rinse may be indicated before the cyclic inflammation. The gingival and oral mucosal tissues need gentle treatment. Careful retraction of the oral mucosa, cheeks, and lips is necessary for both the aphthous and herpetic prone patients. Avoid prescribing nonsteroidal anti-inflammatory medications and high alcohol content mouthwashes. Acidic foods exacerbate gastroesophageal reflux disease (GERD). Management of PMS involves the administration of selective serotonin reuptake inhibitors (SSRI) and antidepressants.

## PREGNANCY

Pregnancy is a noteworthy phase during the reproductive period of women's lifecycle. During pregnancy, both progesterone and estrogen are continuously secreted by the corpus luteum. This leads to increased levels of these hormones in blood circulation. During the reproductive process, hormonal influences change periodontal and oral tissue responses to local factors and produce diagnostic and therapeutic dilemmas.

## Maternal Immunoresponse

Effects of elevated estrogen on the periodontium during pregnancy:[10]
- Decreases keratinization with an increase in epithelial glycogen
- Increases cellular proliferation in blood vessels
- Inhibits pro-inflammatory cytokines release
- Inhibits polymorphonuclear leukocyte (PMN) chemotaxis

Effects of increased progesterone level on the periodontium during pregnancy:[10]
- Increases production of prostaglandins
- Increases PMN and $PGE_2$ in the gingival crevicular fluid (GCF)
- Reduces glucocorticoid anti-inflammatory effect
- Increases vascular permeability
- Alters collagen and noncollagenous protein synthesis
- Alters periodontal fibroblast metabolism

In pregnancy, there is decreased neutrophil chemotaxis, phagocytosis, and depressed antibody production. Elevated sex hormones-induced gingival mast cells destruction increases the release of histamine and protcolytic enzymes that contribute to the exaggerated an inflammatory response to local factors. There is an increased number of periodontopathogens, especially *Porphyromonas gingivalis* and *P. intermedia* because these microbes use estrogen and progesterone as a substitute for menadione (vitamin K growth factor). $PGE_2$ synthesis is increased during pregnancy.

## Periodontal Manifestations

### Pregnancy Gingivitis

Pregnancy-induced gingivitis is a common entity. It is seen in approximately 30–100% of all pregnant women. The severity of gingivitis enhances by the 8th month and reduces during the 9th month. Marginal gingiva and interdental papilla get commonly affected by pregnancy gingivitis and characteristically present as erythema, edema, and hyperplasia **(Fig. 28.4)**. Bleeding occurs spontaneously or on slight provocation. The gingiva appears smooth and shiny, giving a raspberry-like appearance **(Flowchart 28.1)**. Pregnancy is also associated with enhanced tooth mobility, pocket depth, and gingival fluid.

The microscopic examination of gingival disease in pregnancy exhibits the presence of inflammation—nonspecific, vascularizing, and proliferative. In the gingival epithelium and connective tissue of the diseased tissue, there is marked inflammatory cellular infiltration along with edema and degeneration.

The gingival epithelium is hyperplastic with the presence of accentuated rete pegs and reduced surface keratinization. Intra- and extracellular edemas of varying degrees and leukocyte infiltration are commonly observed. Newly formed engorged capillaries are present in abundance.

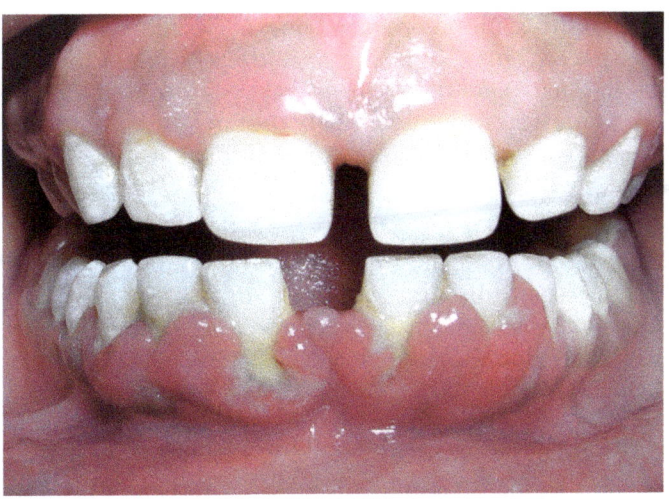

**Fig. 28.4:** Clinical picture showing pregnancy gingivitis in mandibular anterior teeth.

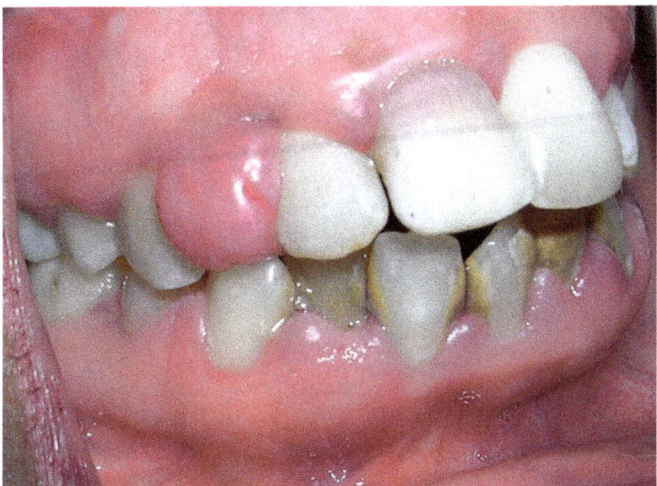

**Fig. 28.5:** Clinical picture showing pregnancy tumor in between right maxillary lateral incisor and canine.

**Flowchart 28.1:** Gingival changes were seen during pregnancy.

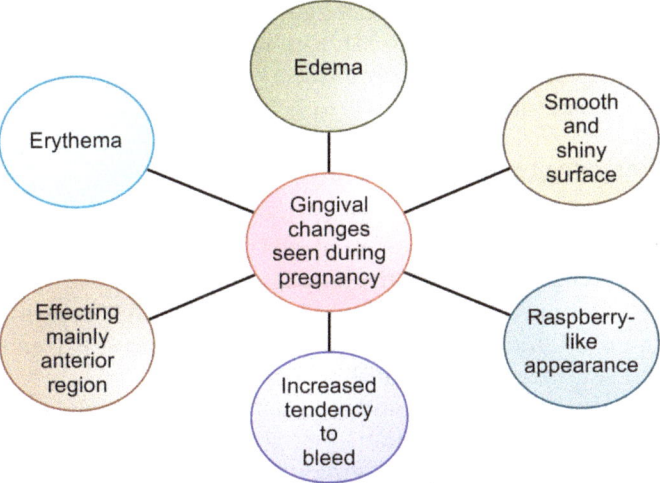

## Pregnancy Tumors

Usually appears during the 2nd trimester in the interproximal areas of anterior teeth.[14] The lesion appears as an isolated, hyperplastic, protruding, bright red growth with a mulberry-like surface. It is a superficial lesion that does not invade the underlying bone. The consistency varies from semifirm to soft and friable. Gingiva bleeds on the slightest provocation **(Fig. 28.5)**. The tissue growth may cause migration and increased mobility of the adjacent teeth.

## Management

Following precautions should be taken during the treatment of a pregnant patient:[15,16]

- Setting frequent appointments in series because the patient easily feels weak and fatigue during pregnancy.
- Adjusting the chair properly (gentle lowering and straightening) for the pregnant patient because of genuine awkwardness due to new shape and weight gain.
- Placing the patient on her left lateral position or elevate the right hip 5-6 inches by placing a pillow or blanket roll underneath. The supine position allows the weight of developing fetus to bear down directly on vena cava, aorta, and major vessels. The reduction in cardiac return reduces blood supply resulting in supine hypotensive syndrome with decreased placental perfusion.
- Advice nonalcoholic mouthwash and neutral sodium fluoride rinse.
- Nausea and vomiting are common symptoms observed in the first trimester (also known as hyperemesis gravidarum). So, advise the patient not to brush right after vomiting as this may cause erosion.
- It is advisable to recommend dentifrices that are less strong in flavor, because of the adverse reaction to strong smells and flavor to the pregnant females.
- A small toothbrush is always recommended; precaution must also be taken while using instruments and also while placing radiographic film to prevent gagging.
- Ideally, no medications should be prescribed because of toxic or teratogenic effects of therapy on the fetus.
- The use of dental radiographs during pregnancy should be kept to a minimum. If the radiographs are immensely required during pregnancy, take certain precautions, such as covering the patient with a lead apron, thyroid collar, and use of a second apron for the back. This will avoid secondary radiations from reaching the abdomen.
- In breastfeeding mothers, the prescribed drugs should be administered approximately 4 hours before nursing to reduce the drug concentration in breast milk.
- *Plaque control*: During pregnancy state, the adequate achievement of the healthy oral environment is the primary objective to avoid plaque formation. To achieve this objective, advising a preventive periodontal program that involves nutritional counseling and the rigorous plaque control measures in the dental office and at home might prove beneficial. Scaling, polishing,

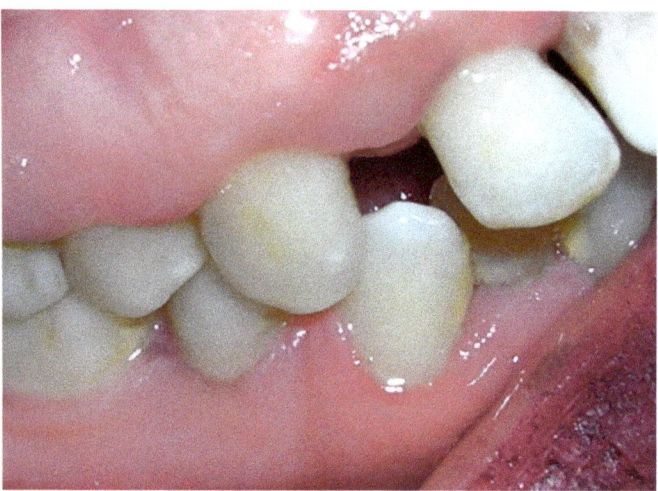

**Fig. 28.6:** Clinical picture showing the excised area of pregnancy tumor.

and root planing should be performed as required throughout the pregnancy.
- Generally, pregnancy tumors might regress up to some extent during the postpartum period, but surgical excision is often required for the complete resolution of the tumor **(Fig. 28.6)**. The tumor is surgically removed in pregnancy only if it is being traumatized by opposing teeth or restoration, causing bleeding.

## ORAL CONTRACEPTIVES

Oral contraceptives (OCs) are the hormonal preparations that induce a hormonal condition very similar to a state of pregnancy and avoid ovulation by the use of gestational hormones. Synthetic hormones that mimic the effects of the endogenous female hormones are used as OCs. These hormonal OCs contain progesterone, often combined with estrogen. As pregnancy hormonal level changes, do not affect healthy tissues in a clean mouth, but exaggerate preexisting gingivitis and is secondary to bacterial plaque, the same is with OCs.

### Periodontal Manifestations
- *Gingival inflammation*: There is an increased prevalence of gingivitis in females taking OCs. Gingival involvement may vary from mild inflammation with edema and erythema to severe inflammation with hemorrhagic or hyperplastic gingival tissues. The degree of inflammation seems to be related to the length of time the woman is taking the pill.
- There is an increase in the amount of gingival exudates.
- Higher gingival index scores.
- More loss of attachment apparatus.
- *Subgingival microflora*: *Bacteroides* species enhance almost by 16-fold in the OC group versus the nonpregnant group.[17] Increased female sex hormones substitute the naphthoquinone requirement of certain *Bacteroides* species. This may be the possible reason for the increase in *Bacteroides* species in OC takers.
- Sometimes, the use of OC therapy causes gingival melanosis in light complexion individuals.

### Management
The dental management of patients taking OC should include establishing a plaque control program and eliminating all local predisposing factors. Antibiotics, such as tetracycline should be avoided, as these antibiotics may lead to failure of the OC therapy.

## MENOPAUSE

Menopausal gingivostomatitis occurs during menopause or in the postmenopausal period. When women reach menopausal age, the levels of estrogen reduce, especially during the late follicular and luteal phases of the menstrual cycle. The reduced level of estrogen decreases the anti-inflammatory effect of this hormone on the periodontium. Osteopenia and osteoporosis have been associated with the menopausal patient.[18]

### Periodontal Manifestations
- The gingiva appears dry, varies in color from abnormal paleness to redness and bleeds easily.
- Fissuring occurs in the mucobuccal fold.
- The patient complains of a dry, burning sensation throughout the oral cavity, associated with extreme sensitivity to thermal changes.
- Alveolar bone loss and alveolar ridge resorption.
- Altered taste sensation.

Microscopically, the gingiva exhibits atrophy of the germinal and prickle cell layers of the epithelium and, in some instances, areas of ulceration.

### Management
Advise the patient to use extra-soft toothbrush and dentifrices with minimal abrasive particles. Mouthrinses should have low alcohol concentration. Debridement of the root surfaces should be done gently to cause minimal soft-tissue trauma. Hormone replacement therapy (HRT) or estrogen replacement therapy (ERT) should be advised. If the patient is osteoporotic, advice bisphosphonates or selective estrogen receptor modulators after consulting physician.[10,19]

## EFFECTS ON WOUND HEALING

Sex hormones impart regulatory effect on growth factors, including keratinocytes growth factor and stimulate wound healing. These growth factors cause stimulation, proliferation, and morphogenesis of pluripotent cells. Lack of sex hormones usually reduces bone density. Osteoporosis is considered a risk factor for implant success.[2]

> **Points to Ponder**
>
> *P. intermedia* is increased in puberty and pregnancy gingivitis because it uses estrogen and progesterone as a substitute for menadione (vitamin K growth factor), which increases with an increased level of gonadotropic hormone in puberty and pregnancy.

## REFERENCES

1. Mariotti A. Sex steroid hormones and cell dynamics in the periodontium. Crit Rev Oral Biol Med. 1994;5(1):27-53.
2. Mascarenhas P, Gapski R, Al-Shammari K, Wang HL. Influence of sex hormones on the periodontium. J Clin Periodontol. 2003;30(8):671-81.
3. Sultan C, Loire C, Kern P, Fenard O, Terraza A. [Collagen and steroid hormones]. Ann Biol Clin (Paris). 1986;44(3):285-8.
4. Soory M. Targets for steroid hormone-mediated actions of periodontal pathogens, cytokines and therapeutic agents: some implications on tissue turnover in the periodontium. Curr Drug Targets. 2000;1(4):309-25.
5. Kasperk CH, Wergedal JE, Farley JR, Linkhart TA, Turner RT, Baylink DJ. Androgens directly stimulate proliferation of bone cells in vitro. Endocrinology. 1989;124(3):1576-8.
6. ElAttar TM, Lin HS, Tira DE. Testosterone inhibits prostaglandin formation by human gingival connective tissue: relationship to 14C-arachidonic acid metabolism. Prostaglandins Leukot Med. 1982;9:25-34.
7. Parkar M, Tabona P, Newman H, Olsen I. IL-6 expression by oral fibroblasts is regulated by androgen. Cytokine. 1998;10(8):613-9.
8. Gornstein RA, Lapp CA, Bustos-Valdes SM, Zamorano P. Androgens modulate interleukin-6 production by gingival fibroblasts in vitro. J Periodontol. 1999;70(6):604-9.
9. Morley JE. Testosterone. In: Morley JE, Berg LV (Eds). Contemporary Endocrinology: Endocrinology of Aging, 1st edition. New Jersey, USA: Humana Press Incorporation; 1999. pp. 127-49.
10. Corgel JO. Periodontal therapy in the female patient (puberty, menses, pregnancy, menopause). In: Newman MG, Takei HH, Carranza FA (Eds). Carranza's Clinical Periodontology, 9th edition. Philadelphia, PA, USA: WB Saunders; 2003. pp. 513-26.
11. Kornman KS, Loesche WJ. The subgingival microbial flora during pregnancy. J Periodontal Res. 1980;15(2):111-22.
12. Brown S, Bonifazi DZ. An overview of anorexia and bulimia nervosa, and the impact of eating disorders on the oral cavity. Compendium. 1993;14(12):1594, 1596-602.
13. Grant D, Stern J, Listgarten M. The epidemiology, etiology and public health aspects of periodontal disease. In: Periodontics. St. Louis: Mosby; 1988.
14. Rose LF. Sex hormonal imbalances, oral manifestations and dental treatment. In: Genco RJ, Goldman HM, Cohen DW. Contemporary Periodontics, 1st edition. St. Louis: CV Mosby; 1990. pp. 221-27.
15. Mealey BL, Klokkevold PR, Corgel JO. Periodontal treatment of medically compromised patients. In: Newman MG, Takei HH, Carranza FA (Eds). Carranza's Clinical Periodontology, 9th edition. Philadelphia, PA, USA: WB Saunders; 2003. pp. 527-50.
16. Otomo-Corgel J. Dental management of the female patient. Periodontol 2000. 2013;61(1):219-31.
17. Jensen J, Liljemark W, Bloomquist C. The effect of female sex hormones on the subgingival plaque. J Periodontol. 1981;52(10):599-602.
18. Palmer R, Soory M. Modifying factors: diabetes, puberty, pregnancy and the menopause and tobacco smoking. In: Lindhe J, Karring T, Lang NP (Eds). Clinical Periodontology and Implant Dentistry, 4th edition. Chicago, USA: Blackwell Munksgaard; 2003. pp. 179-97.
19. Friedlander AH. The physiology, medical management and oral implications of menopause. J Am Dent Assoc. 2002;133(1):73-81.

## VIVA VOCE

**Q1. Why does mobility increases in pregnancy?**
**Ans.** Mobility increases in pregnancy due to the extravasation of fluid from the engorged blood vessels.

**Q2. What is the role of *P. intermedia* in puberty and pregnancy gingivitis?**
**Ans.** *P. intermedia* uses estrogen and progesterone as a substitute for menadione vitamin K growth factor, which increases with an increased level of gonadotropic hormone in puberty and pregnancy.

**Q3. What is perimolysis?**
**Ans.** It is a smooth erosion of the enamel and dentin due to eating disorders, bulimia, and anorexia nervosa. It is usually seen on the lingual surfaces of anterior maxillary teeth.

**Q4. What is the appearance of gingiva in pregnancy gingivitis?**
**Ans.** The gingiva appears smooth and shiny, giving a raspberry-like appearance.

**Q5. In which trimester, pregnancy tumors appear?**
**Ans.** Usually appears during the second trimester.

**Q6. What is the effect of increased progesterone level on the collagen during pregnancy?**
**Ans.** Alters collagen and noncollagenous protein synthesis.

**Q7. What is the effect of increased progesterone levels on the production of prostaglandins during pregnancy?**
**Ans.** Increases the production of prostaglandins.

**Q8. What is the effect of increased progesterone level on the fibroblasts during pregnancy?**
**Ans.** Alters periodontal fibroblast metabolism.

**Q9. What is the effect of increased progesterone level on vascular permeability during pregnancy?**
**Ans.** Increases vascular permeability.

**Q10. What are the effects of menopause on the alveolar bone?**
**Ans.** Osteopenia and osteoporosis.

# Section 5

# Diagnosis

- ❖ Clinical Diagnosis
- ❖ Radiographic Diagnostic Aids
- ❖ Microbiological Diagnostic Aids
- ❖ Clinical Risk Assessment
- ❖ Prognosis

# Chapter 29

# Clinical Diagnosis

*Shalu Bathla*

## Chapter Outline

- Definition
- Types
- Key Stages
- History Taking
- Clinical Examination
- Investigations
- Diagnosis
- Treatment Plan

## INTRODUCTION

Periodontal diagnosis should first determine whether a disease is present; then identify its type, extent, distribution, and severity; and, finally, provide an understanding of the underlying pathologic processes and its cause.[1] Accurate diagnosis is essential for treating and managing periodontal patients efficiently.

## DEFINITION

Diagnosis may be defined as an identifying disease from an evaluation of the history, signs and symptoms, laboratory tests, and procedures.

The best pathway to reach an accurate diagnosis involves a thorough evaluation of systematically collected data by various procedures. These procedures primarily include:
- Patient's detail history taking
- Medical consultation as indicated
- Clinical periodontal evaluation
- Radiographic findings
- Laboratory tests as needed

From this information, the clinician has to distinguish between normal and abnormal findings.

## TYPES

- *Provisional diagnosis*: It is the diagnosis made before investigations. It is also called a working or probable diagnosis.
- *Differential diagnosis*: The diagnosis, which differentiates between two or more conditions and shares similar signs and symptoms, is called differential diagnosis.
- *Final diagnosis*: It is the diagnosis made after getting the results of investigations.

## KEY STAGES

Periodontal patients can be well managed and treated after taking a proper history, clinical examination, diagnosis, and investigations **(Flowchart 29.1)**.

## HISTORY TAKING

History taking is the first and most crucial step of clinical diagnosis in dentistry. It includes the patient's interview

**Flowchart 29.1:** Key stages of management of periodontal patient.

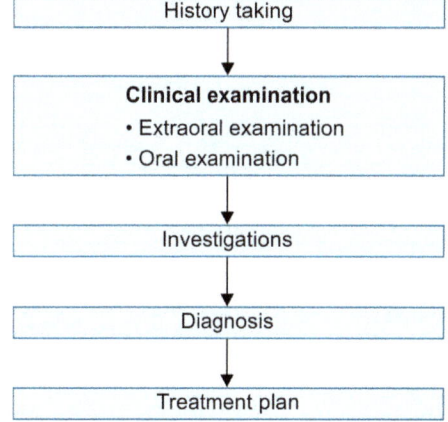

in detail regarding the source of referral, chief complaints experienced by a patient, associated symptoms, and previous medical and dental history. The referral source became an essential parameter of diagnosis when another dentist or physician referred the patient (**Flowchart 29.2**).

## Patient's Interview

Vital statistics include the patient's name, age, sex, home, and business address, phone number, marital and family status, and occupation. These are all significant because of the following reasons:[2]

- *Importance of name*: Name is mandatory for identification purposes and also aids in establishing rapport with the patient.
- *Importance of age*: Certain diseases have a predilection at specific age-groups, e.g., herpetic gingivostomatitis is common in children below six years. Age also affects dental procedures and personal care.
- *Importance of sex*: Certain diseases are common in either males or females, e.g., desquamative gingivitis is more common in females; pregnancy tumor presents only in females.
- *Importance of address*: Various conditions are endemic to certain areas. The address tells about the presence of fluoride in drinking water.
- *Importance of telephone number*: The telephone number is required for any change of appointment. Immediate consultation may be needed so that urgent treatment may proceed.
- *Importance of occupation*: It may be a factor in the etiology of certain occupational diseases like a professional wine taster is prone to erosion; thread biting by tailors and holding of nails between teeth by carpenters causes abrasion of teeth.
- *Economic and social status*: People who are under stress are more likely to suffer from psychosomatic diseases like lichen planus and acute necrotizing ulcerative gingivitis (ANUG).

## Medical and Dental History

### Objectives

Following are the objectives of medical history:[3]

- To identify systemic factors that may help to account for the periodontal condition. Debilitating diseases like diabetes can influence periodontal health.
- To note the existence of systemic conditions for which special precautions, e.g., antibiotic prophylaxis, are required to safeguard the patient during periodontal therapy.
- To note the existence of any transmissible disease which may present a hazard to the clinician, dental staff, or other patients.

The dental history should include the reference to the frequency, date of the most recent visit, nature of the treatment, and oral prophylaxis by a dentist. The patient's oral hygiene regimen should be noted, including toothbrushing frequency, time of day, method, type of toothbrush and dentifrice, and the interval at which brushes are replaced. Previous periodontal problems, if any, should be identified regarding its nature and severity. Furthermore, note down the previously offered treatment for overcoming the periodontal problems and approximate period of its termination.[4]

## CLINICAL EXAMINATION

Subjective sensations resulting from the disease that is reported by the patient are called symptoms. Signs of illness are objective findings that are observed by the clinician. The clinical evaluation should consist of an examination of the extraoral, parafunctional habits, and intraoral tissues, including teeth, gingiva, and the periodontal tissues (**Flowchart 29.3**). Abnormal clinical findings should be taken into consideration to reach a definitive diagnosis or further investigation by referral or biopsy.

## Extraoral Examination

Observe the patient during reception and seating to note physical characteristics and abnormalities and make an overall appraisal.

- The inspection includes evaluating bilateral symmetry and comparing the anatomy of one side of the head, face, and neck to the opposite side.
- Palpation is used to determine the texture, size, and consistency by the sense of touch. Palpation may be accomplished by using both hands, comparing one side

**Flowchart 29.2:** Key stages in history taking for periodontal patient.

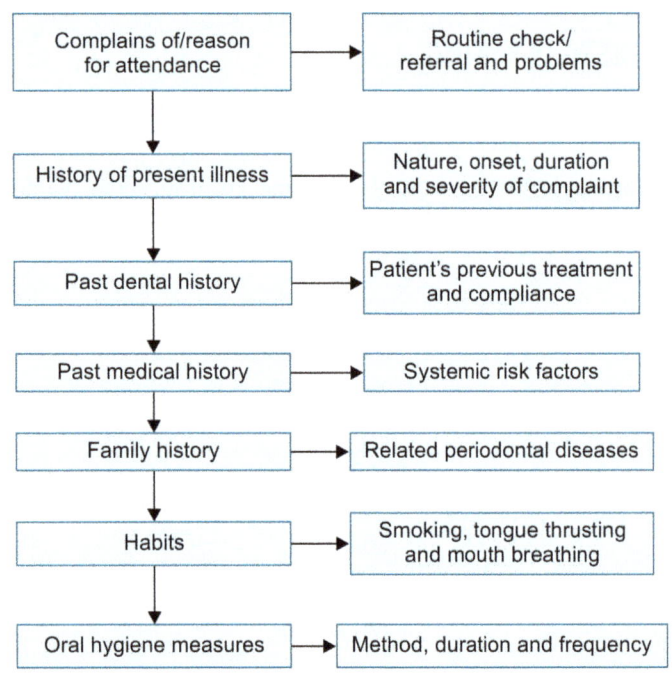

**Chapter 29:** Clinical Diagnosis

**Flowchart 29.3:** Clinical examination.

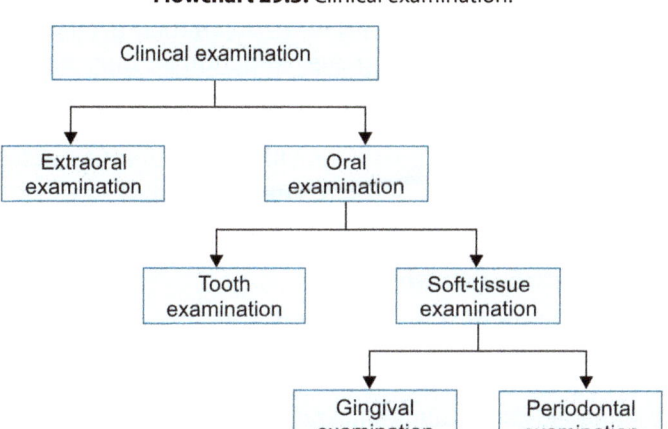

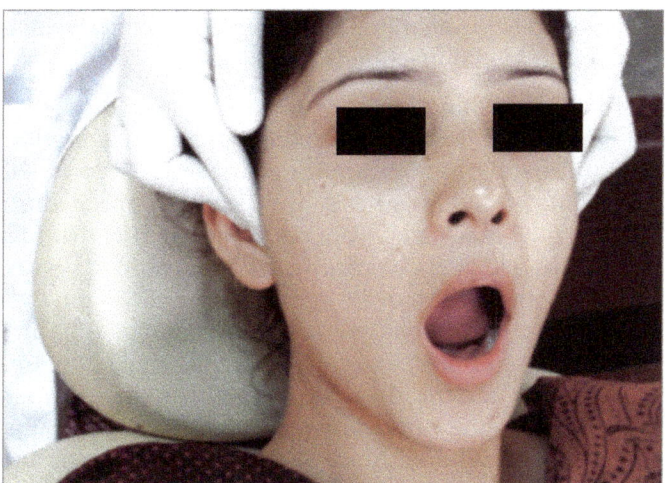

**Fig. 29.1:** Clinical picture showing palpation of temporomandibular joint.

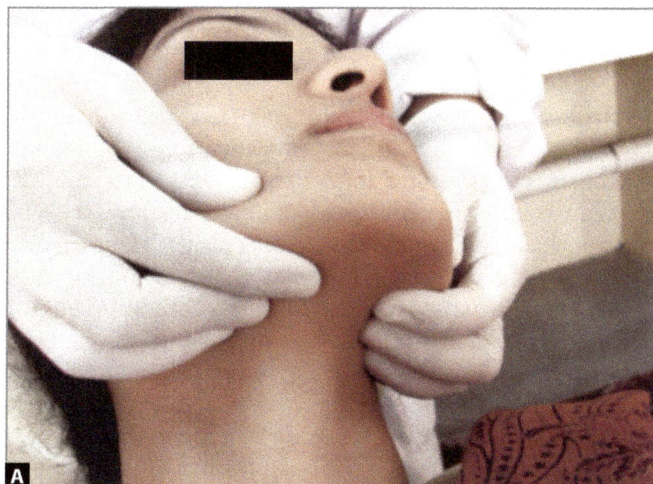

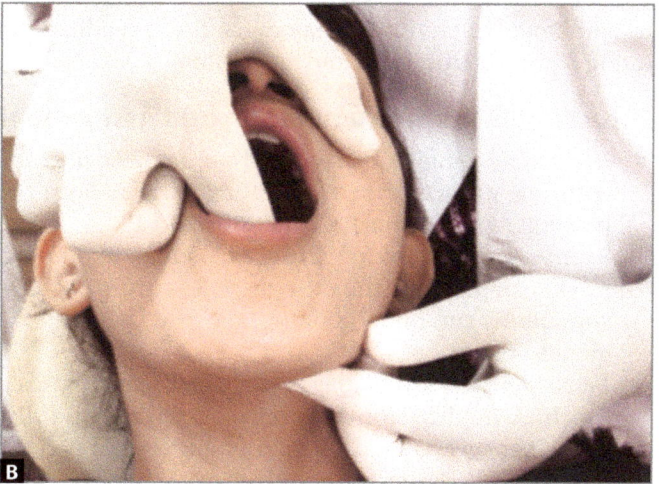

**Figs. 29.2A and B:** Clinical picture showing palpation of the submandibular gland and lymph nodes.

of the head, face, and neck with the other side. This is called bimanual palpation. The clinician may palpate the structures of the neck, lymph nodes, and salivary glands.

- The temporomandibular joint (TMJ) is found just in front of the ear. The TMJ may be examined by palpation and auscultation. Palpating with the index and middle finger over the head of the condyle or a finger just inside the external auditory meatus allows the clinician to evaluate TMJ's function **(Fig. 29.1)**.[5]
- Lymph nodes may become enlarged in certain gingival and periodontal diseases like necrotizing ulcerative gingivitis, primary herpetic gingivostomatitis, and acute periodontal abscesses. Submandibular gland and lymph nodes can be palpated by either of the two methods: (1) Resting the thumbs of each hand near the inferior mandibular border while pressing the fingertips inferior and medial to the mandibular border **(Fig. 29.2A)**; (2) Clinician palpates under the chin and along the mandible. With one digit compressing the floor of the mouth and another digit placed medially to the mandible's inferior border **(Fig. 29.2B)**.

- Auscultation for joint sounds may be accomplished by listening with the unaided ear or a stethoscope placed over the TMJ.[4,5]

## Intraoral Examination (Teeth, Gingiva, and Periodontium)

It includes both the hard-tissue examination and soft-tissue examination.

The oral cavity should be adequately examined for cleanliness in the form of accumulation of food debris, the presence of detectable plaque, materia alba, and tooth surface stains. For undetectable plaque, use a disclosing solution for better identification.

Halitosis is foul or offensive odor originating from the oral cavity. Most of the time, mouth odors hold diagnostic significance and suggest oral or extraoral pathologies. Rest is explained in "Chapter 35: Halitosis".

Parafunctional habits mean abnormal, altered, or deviated functions. It can be classified according to the cause in three ways:
1. Tooth to tooth function, e.g., bruxism.

2. Tooth to soft tissue, e.g., thumb-sucking.
3. Tooth to a foreign object, e.g., chewing of pens and pencils.

Bruxism means a constant or intermittent occlusal contact of the teeth aside from mastication, swallowing/speech. It is the term for abnormal grinding of the teeth. It may cause excessive tooth wear characterized by facets on tooth surfaces and widening of the occlusal surfaces. It may also lead to a reduction in the vertical dimension.

Tongue thrusting is the persistent, forceful wedging of the tongue against the teeth, especially in the anterior region. It is a habit in which the patient, instead of placing the dorsum of the tongue against the palate with the tip behind the maxillary teeth during swallowing, the tongue is thrust forward against the mandibular anterior teeth. Tongue thrusting causes excessive lateral pressure leading to pathologic migration. It may cause the spreading and tilting of the anterior teeth and open bite.

## Tools for Intraoral Examination and Assessment

- *Inspection*: Gingiva is examined for changes in color, contour, surface texture, and size. It tells about the position of frenal attachment **(Table 29.1)**.
- *Exploration*: It helps to diagnose bleeding on probing, pocket depth, whether the pocket is true/pseudo, suprabony/infrabony, about subgingival calculus, and gingival recession.
- *Percussion*: It helps to diagnose a healthy or ankylosed tooth. A healthy tooth percussed with a metallic instrument gives metallic sound, while teeth embedded in inflamed tissue gives dull sound. In periapical abscess, the tooth will be tender.
- *Palpation*: It helps to diagnose whether gingiva is normal, i.e., firm and resilient or fibrosed or edematous.

It also helps to test the degree of mobility. Gentle pressure with the finger can elicit tenderness in inflamed areas. It helps to diagnose exudation or suppuration present or absent. Certain gingival or periodontal disease, in which lymph nodes are enlarged, can be diagnosed through palpation like necrotizing ulcerative gingivitis, primary herpetic gingivostomatitis, and acute periodontal abscesses.

## Hard-tissue Examination

The teeth are examined for caries, failing restorations, evidence of food impaction, wasting diseases, hypersensitivity, mobility, trauma from occlusion, pathologic tooth migration, and occlusal relationships.

*Caries*: Carious lesions provide a rough surface for plaque and food debris retention. They leave open contact areas that permit food impaction **(Fig. 29.3)**.

*Restorations*: Characteristics of restorations that leave an effect on periodontium are the margin of restoration, contour, overhang, material, occlusion, design of the removable partial prosthesis, and restorative procedure. Overhanging margin contributes to periodontal diseases by providing ideal niches for the accumulation of plaque and by changing the ecological balance of the gingival sulcus from gram-positive facultative species to gram-negative anaerobic species. Overhanging make the area inaccessible for the direct application of toothbrush and other plaque removal interdental aids. Overhangs catch and tear dental floss. Overcontoured crown and restorations contribute to periodontal diseases by providing ideal locations for the accumulation of plaque and by preventing self-cleansing mechanisms of adjacent cheek, lips, and tongue.

*Proximal contact relations*: Slightly open contacts allow food impaction. Clinical observation and dental floss help to identify the tightness of contacts.

*Food impaction*: It is the forceful wedging of food into the periodontium by occlusal forces.

**TABLE 29.1:** Various intraoral examination tools.

| Assessment of tissue | Tool used |
|---|---|
| Gingiva: Color | Visual inspection |
| Gingiva: Surface texture | Visual inspection |
| Gingiva: Consistency | Side of the periodontal probe |
| Gingiva: Position (recession) | Calibrated periodontal probe |
| Bleeding on probing | Periodontal probe |
| Frenal attachment | Tension test |
| Plaque | Disclosing agent |
| Calculus | Explorer |
| Calculus | Compressed air |
| Pocket depth | Calibrated periodontal probe |
| Clinical attachment level | Calibrated periodontal probe |
| Alveolar bone loss | Bone sounding: Periodontal probe; radiographs |
| Mobility | Instrument handle |
| Furcation defects | Naber's probe |
| Trauma from occlusion | Fremitus test: Dampened index finger |

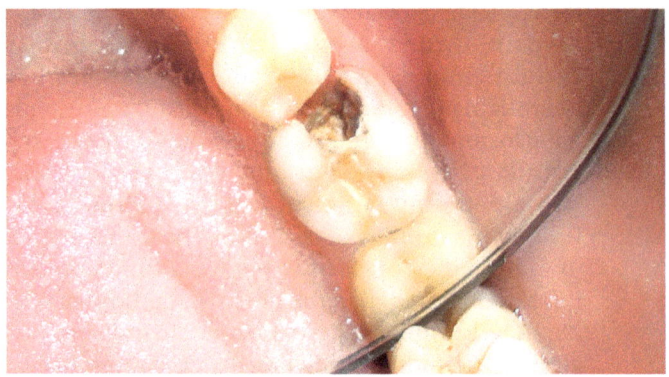

**Fig. 29.3:** Clinical picture showing dental caries acting as plaque retentive area.

Hirschfeld in 1930 classified vertical food impaction relative to etiologic factors as:[6]
- Class I: Occlusal wear
- Class II: Loss of proximal support
- Class III: Extrusion of a tooth beyond the occlusal plane
- Class IV: Congenital morphologic abnormalities
- Class V: Improperly constructed restorations.

Plunger cusps are the cusps that tend to forcibly wedge food into interproximal embrasures of opposing teeth **(Fig. 29.4)**. Distolingual cusps of maxillary molars are the most common plunger cusp. Plunger cusp effect may occur with wear, or it may be the result of a shift in tooth positions following the failure to replace a missing tooth.

*Wasting diseases*: Wasting disease of a tooth is defined as any gradual loss of tooth substance characterized by the formation of smooth, polished surfaces, without regard to the possible mechanism of this loss. The various forms of wasting diseases are attrition, erosion, abrasion, and abfraction.
- *Attrition*: It is occlusal wear resulting from functional contacts with opposing teeth. Flat occlusal or incisal surfaces/facets with accurate interdigitation of upper and lower teeth are found in attrition **(Fig. 29.5)**. There is hypertrophy of masseter muscle.

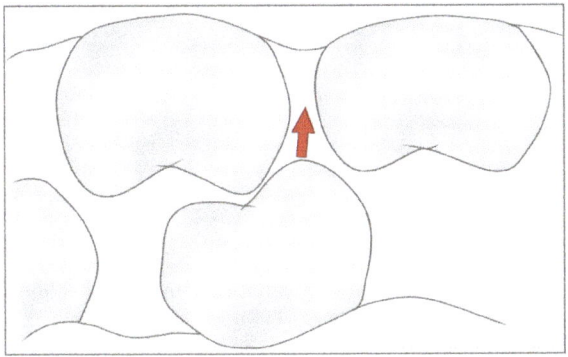

**Fig. 29.4:** Schematic representation showing plunger cusp.

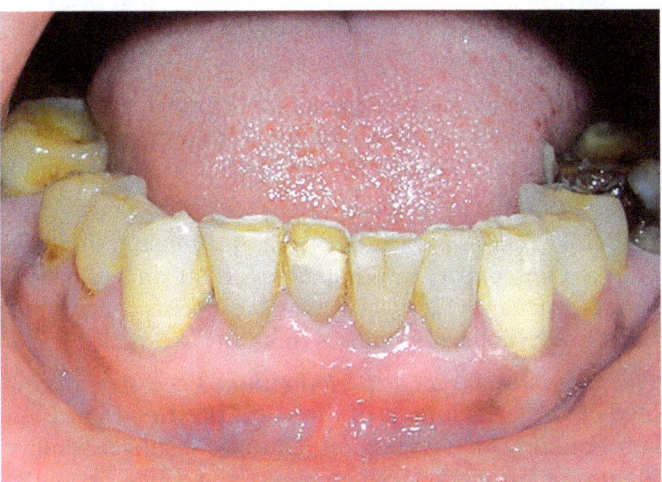

**Fig. 29.5:** Clinical picture showing attrition on the incisal edges of incisors.

- *Erosion*: Dental erosion is the loss of the nonoccluding tooth surfaces present in the form of sharp, defined wedge-shaped depression in the cervical area of the facial tooth surface.[7] Usually, the long-axis of the eroded area runs perpendicular to the vertical axis. Buccal and lingual surfaces of anterior teeth are affected by erosion resulting in smooth and shiny surfaces with a generated loss of anatomy. In the case of upper incisors, the palatal surface of the exposed dentin is smooth, presenting with a halo of enamel surrounding the lesion.

Causes of erosion:
- Eating disorders, such as anorexia nervosa, bulimia nervosa, and rumination, present with continuous vomiting.
- Reflux or chronic regurgitation associated with gastrointestinal problems.
- Regular and high intake of acidic medication (chewable acetylsalicylic acid tablets).
- Regular intake of chewable vitamin C tablets
- High consumption of acidic drinks and foods.
- Professional wine tasting
- Field of occupation: Acid battery worker
- Pregnancy

Smooth, clean surfaces and the presence of dentin hypersensitivity suggest that the process of erosion is active, whereas stained teeth suggest its inactivity. When the erosion affects the tooth with the restoration, the tooth gets gradually dissolved, but the restoration remains unaffected as it is resistant to acid. A comparison between the dated study casts with the clinical teeth condition over time also helps to identify whether the erosion lesion is active or inactive.

The following measures can prevent erosion:
- Reduce the frequency and amount of consumption of acidic drinks and food, especially at bedtime.
- If soft drinks are consumed, it should be chilled and consumed in one sitting at mealtime.
- Avoid sipping the acidic drink or swishing it around the mouth before swallowing.
- Consume neutralizing food such as cheese after the intake of an acidic drink or food.
- Encourage the consumption of water and nutritious beverages such as milk.

The occurrence of erosion and attrition leads to cupping or undermining of occlusal surfaces. The dentin is less mineralized than enamel, and that is why wear preferentially results in occlusal cupping **(Fig. 29.6)**.
- *Abrasion*: It is the loss of tooth substance due to mechanical wear and not associated with the process of mastication **(Fig. 29.7)**. It may manifest as rounded blunted or worn flat cusp tip/incisal edge exposing the dentin, causing a "scooped out" appearance that is softer and more porous than enamel. Foreign substances usually cause them.

**Section 5:** Diagnosis

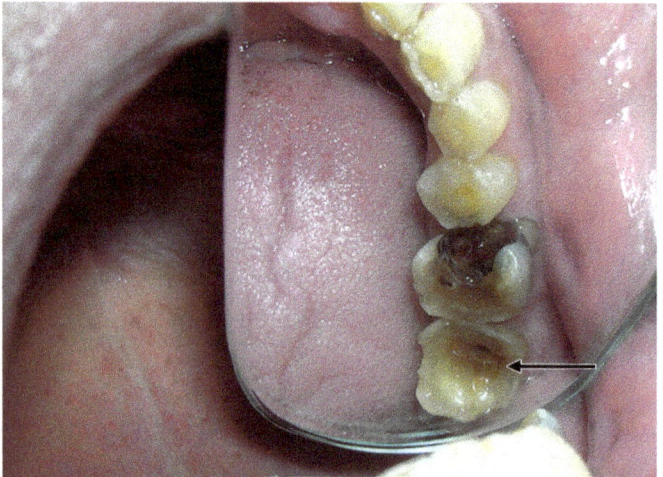

**Fig. 29.6:** Clinical picture showing both attrition and erosion causing occlusal cupping of molar.

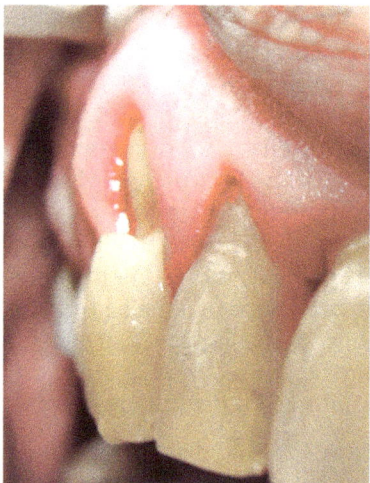

**Fig. 29.8:** Clinical picture showing abrasion due to horizontal toothbrushing.

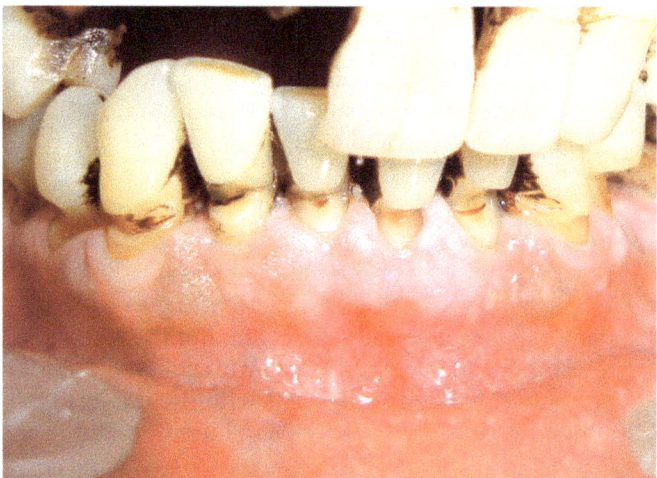

**Fig. 29.7:** Clinical picture showing abrasion due to aggressive toothbrushing (V-shaped notches).

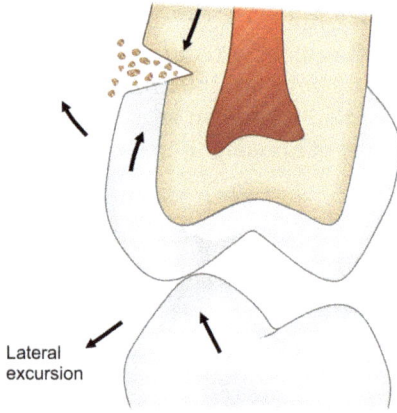

**Fig. 29.9:** Schematic representation showing abfraction.

Causes of abrasion are:
- Hard-bristle toothbrush
- Coarse-abrasive tooth powder
- Horizontal toothbrushing technique at right angles to the vertical axis of teeth **(Fig. 29.8)**
- Action of clasps
- Abrasion of incisal edges due to habits, such as opening bobby pins, nails held by carpenters, pins by dressmakers.
- Pipe held between teeth

- *Abfraction*: It is the flexure of a tooth under heavy lateral load, which may lead to displacement/fracture of enamel rods at the cementoenamel junction (CEJ). The lost enamel exposes more dentin, in which the same stresses may crush dentinal tubules and more readily demineralize **(Fig. 29.9)**.
- *Frictional ablation/dentoalveolar ablation*: It is the process caused by the juxtaposition of natural and artificial dental surfaces and hyper functional oral soft tissues.[8] It is caused by the action of soft tissues and saliva against the dentition due to vestibular pressures of suction, swallowing, tongue motions, and the intervening forced flow of saliva.

*Dental stains:* These are pigmented deposits located on the tooth surfaces. A careful examination of dental stain should be carried out to determine their origin. Rest is explained in "Chapter 9: Dental Plaque."

*Occlusal relationship*: The occlusion relationship should be checked for centric, working, nonworking and protrusive interferences. Evidence of possible occlusal trauma is ideally recorded with fremitus (mobility in function).

*Effect of malocclusion on periodontium*: Excessive overbite leads to encroachment of the teeth on the gingiva and subsequently food impaction. This also results in gingival inflammation, gingival enlargement, and pocket formation **(Fig. 29.10)**. Open bite reduces mechanical cleansing by the passage of food and results in debris accumulation,

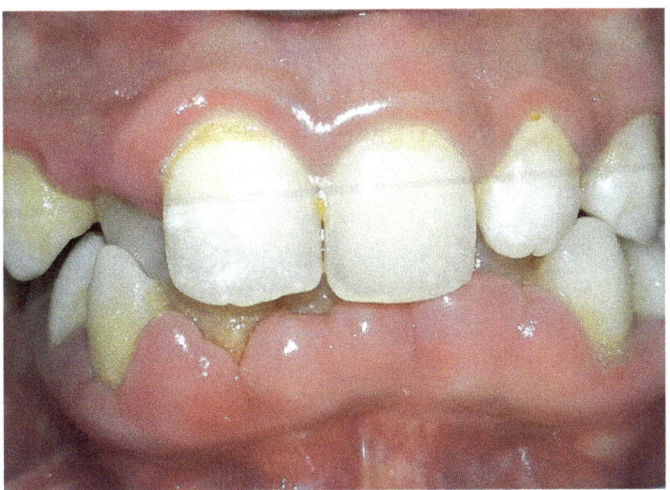

**Fig. 29.10:** Clinical picture showing deep bite causing impingement of maxillary teeth on mandibular gingiva.

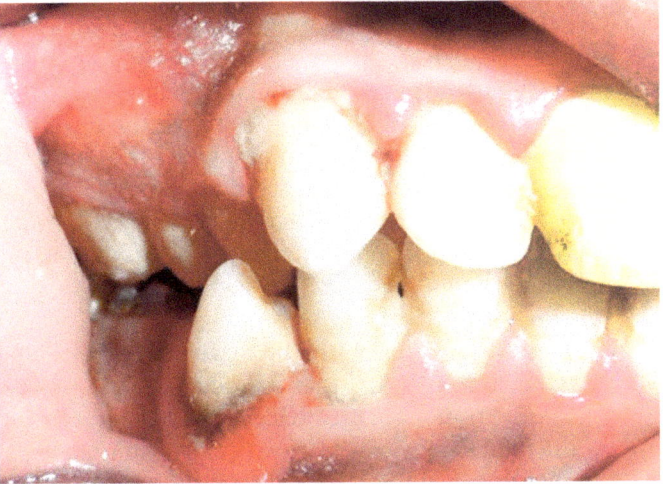

**Fig. 29.11:** Clinical picture showing crossbite.

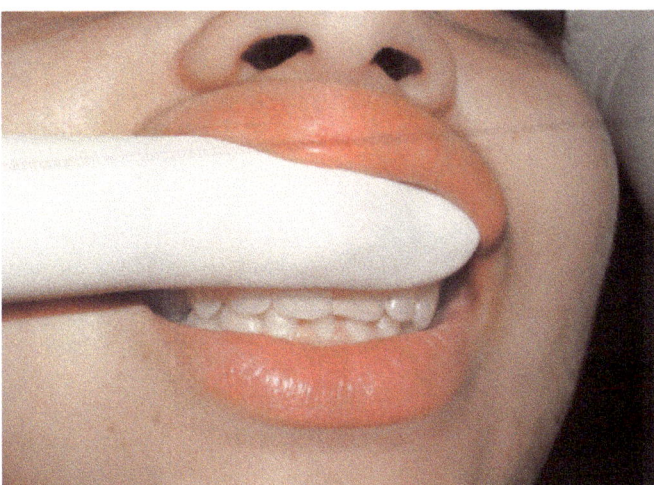

**Fig. 29.12:** Clinical photograph showing fremitus test.

calculus formation, and extrusion of teeth. Crossbite leads to trauma from occlusion, food impaction, and spreading of mandibular teeth **(Fig. 29.11)**.

*Trauma from occlusion*: When occlusal forces exceed the adaptive capacity of the tissues, it results in tissue injury, and this resultant injury is termed as trauma from occlusion. An occlusion producing such injury is called traumatic occlusion. Trauma from occlusion refers to tissue injury and not the occlusal force. The main clinical finding associated with trauma from occlusion is progressively increasing tooth mobility. Rest is explained in "Chapter 27: Trauma from Occlusion".

*Fremitus test*: Dampen index finger and place along the buccal and labial surfaces of maxillary teeth. The patient is then asked to tap the teeth together in the maximum intercuspation and to do lateral and protrusive movements **(Fig. 29.12)**.

- *Class I*: Mild vibration detected; the first degree is recorded as "+."
- *Class II*: Easily palpable vibration, recorded as "++."
- *Class III*: Movements visible with the naked eye, recorded as "+++."

It is a test used to diagnose a case of trauma from occlusion by measuring the vibratory pattern of teeth when teeth are placed in contacting positions.

*The rationale behind the fremitus test*: When an individual experiences trauma from occlusion, periodontal fremitus takes place in either of the alveolar bones. It usually occurs in teeth displaying slight mobility rubbing against the adjacent walls of their sockets. The socket volume enhances slightly over time due to inflammatory responses, bone resorption, or both. The test is used to identify the the severity of the periodontal disease. A patient is asked to close his or her mouth into maximum intercuspation and is told to grind his or her teeth. Placing a finger in the labial vestibule against the alveolar bone helps to detect fremitus. Fremitus is tooth displacement, which is created by the patient's occlusal force. Therefore, the amount of force varies greatly from patient-to-patient, whereas in mobility, the force with which it is measured tends to be the same for each examiner. Fremitus is a guide to the ability of the patient to displace and traumatize the teeth.

*Pathologic tooth migration*: It can be recognized by noting alterations in tooth position, especially regarding a view towards identifying abnormal forces, tongue thrusting habit, or other habits that may be the contributing factors **(Fig. 29.13)**. Pathologic anterior teeth migration may be seen in localized aggressive periodontitis.

### Soft-tissue Examination

*Examination of gingiva*: Before starting the gingival examination, it should be dried well enough for accurate observations. Light reflection from moist gingiva usually masks detail. Start the gingival examination by noting the architecture of the gingiva. It should be noted for changes in the normal knife-edged appearance of the free gingival

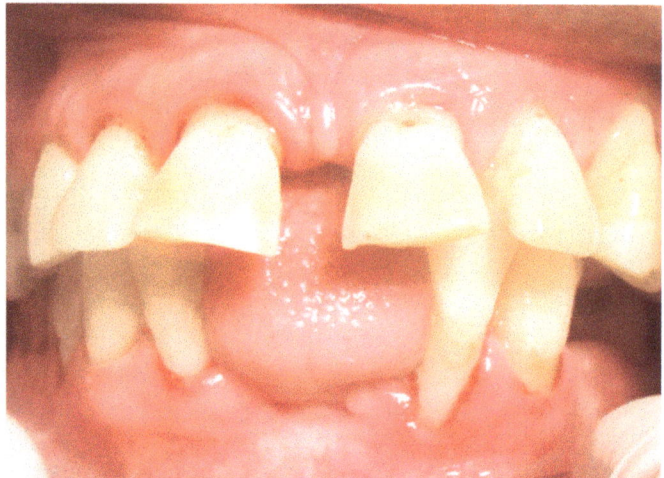

**Fig. 29.13:** Clinical picture showing pathologic migration associated with tongue thrusting habit.

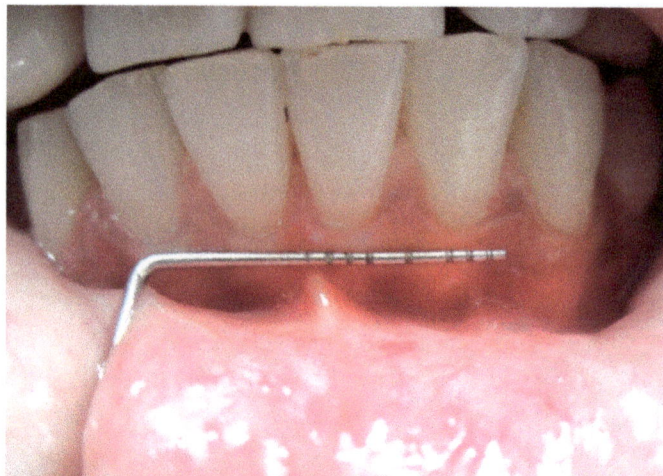

**Fig. 29.14:** Clinical picture showing the evaluation of the consistency of gingiva with the side of a periodontal probe.

margin and interdental papilla as it meets the teeth. Any swelling or an enlarged appearance of the marginal gingiva is indicative of inflammation provided that it is produced in the absence of systemic disease or not related to drug-associated gingival enlargement.

Any significant lack of attached gingiva, especially if it is associated with gingival recession or a high frenum attachment, should be noted and recorded in the dental record. The presence of previous interdental cratering should be noted, particularly when it is associated with the necrosis of the gingiva with or without exposure of the underlying bone. Interdental necrosis is suggestive of necrotizing ulcerative gingivitis or necrotizing ulcerative periodontitis. It also represents a clinical sign of immunocompromised status in patients with acquired immunodeficiency syndrome (AIDS). The various mucogingival problems are inadequate width of attached gingiva, abnormal frenum attachment, gingival recession, decreased vestibular depth, pockets extending up to the mucogingival junction, gingival excess (pseudopocket), inconsistent gingival margin, excessive gingival display and abnormal color of the gingiva.

- *Gingival stippling*: Gingival stippling, is best viewed by drying the gingiva and switching off the chair light. As light reflection from moist gingiva obscure detail.
- *Gingival consistency*: Any gingival enlargement should be checked for its consistency with the side of a periodontal probe to note whether it is edematous or fibrotic **(Fig. 29.14)**.
- Edematous gingiva appears as smooth, shiny, glossy red whereas fibrotic gingiva appears as opaque, firm, stippled, and thicker.
- *Width of attached gingiva*: Inadequate attached gingiva zone can accelerate subgingival plaque formation due to improper closure of the pocket leading to movability of the marginal tissue and favor attachment loss and soft-tissue recession due to the less resistance of the tissue. It would also facilitate the accumulation of food particles during mastication and impede proper oral hygiene measures.

Measurement of the width of the attached gingiva:
- *Anatomically*: Ask the patient to stretch the lip/cheek to identify the mucogingival line while the pocket is being probed. Measure the total width of the gingiva (gingival margin to the mucogingival line) and subtract the sulcus/pocket depth from it to get the width of the attached gingiva.
- *Functionally*:
  - *Tension test*: Stretch the lip or cheek outward and forward to demarcate the mucogingival line and see for any free gingival margin movement. Measure the total width of the gingiva (gingival margin to the mucogingival line) and subtract the sulcus/pocket depth from it to determine the width of the attached gingiva.
  - *Roll test*: Push the adjacent mucosa coronally with a dull instrument to mark a mucogingival line. Measure the total width of the gingiva (gingival margin to the mucogingival line) and subtract the sulcus/pocket depth from it to determine the attached gingiva's width.
- *Histochemically*:
  - *Staining test*: Paint the gingiva and oral mucosa with Schiller's or Lugol's solution (iodine and potassium iodide solution). The alveolar mucosa takes on a brown color due to its glycogen content, and the attached gingiva stays unstained as it is glycogen free. Measure the total width of the unstained gingiva and subtract the sulcus/pocket depth from it to determine a width of an attached gingiva.[4]

*Measurement of thickness of gingiva*: Earlier the thickness of the gingiva was measured using traumatic techniques, such as probes and injection needle. But now it can be measured without inducing trauma by using the newer ultrasonic

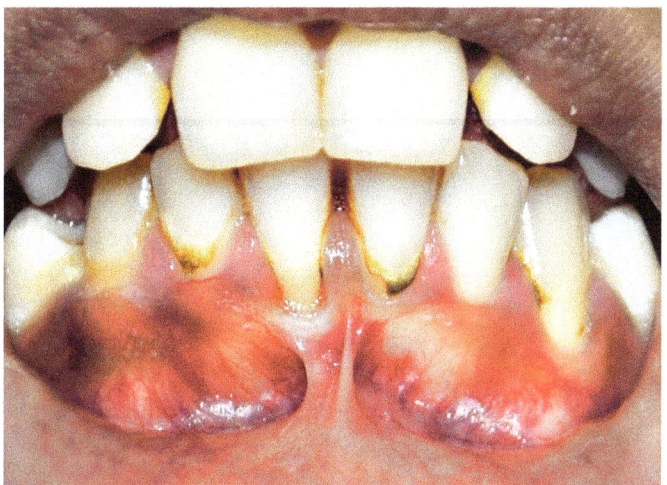

**Fig. 29.15:** Clinical picture showing abnormal frenum (broad).

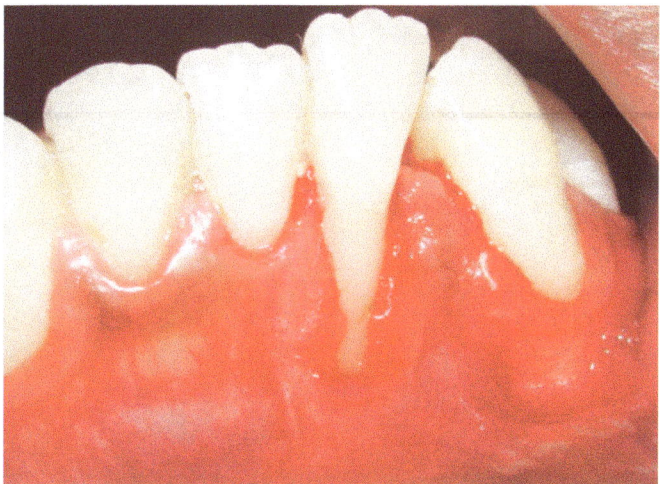

**Fig. 29.17:** Clinical picture showing localized recession on malposed teeth

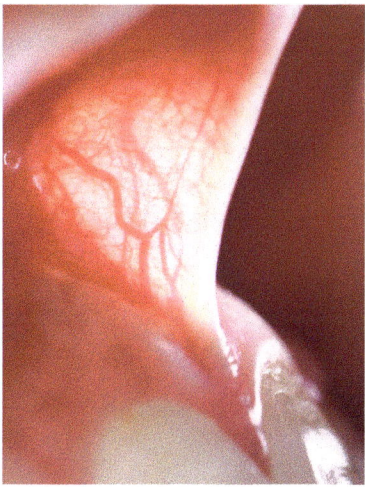

**Fig. 29.16:** Clinical picture showing papillary frenum.

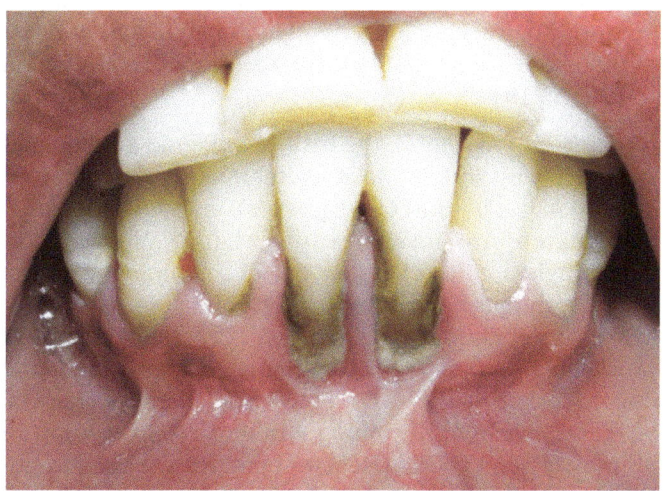

**Fig. 29.18:** Clinical picture showing grade III marginal tissue recession.

device called "Krupp SDM." This device uses a pulse-echo principle. A pulse generator at a measurement frequency of 5 MHz allowed a piezo crystal to oscillate. Ultrasonic pulses get transmitted at an interval through the sound permeable gingiva. When it reaches the bone or tooth surface, it starts being reflected due to the difference in acoustic impedance. A transducer probe of a 4 mm diameter is moistened with saliva and applied to the measurement site with slight pressure to produce acoustic coupling. By timing, the received echo with respect to the transmission of pulse, the thickness of mucosa is determined within seconds and is digitally displayed with a resolution of 0.1 mm.

*Abnormal frenum*: Abnormal frenum jeopardizes gingival health as it interferes with proper placement of a toothbrush and open gingival crevice by muscle pull. The frenum is judged abnormal when the frenum is unusually broad, or there is no apparent attached gingival in the midline or interdental papilla moves by stretching the frenum **(Figs. 29.15 and 29.16)**. A tension test is done to detect any abnormal frenum attachment (explained earlier in this chapter).

*Measurement of gingival recession*: Gingival recession can be seen on malposed teeth **(Fig. 29.17)**. It can be calculated during periodontal probing as the distance of the free gingival margin to the CEJ.

In 1985, Miller classified marginal tissue recession into four classes:[9]

1. *Class I*: Marginal tissue recession not extending to the mucogingival junction. No loss of interdental bone/soft tissue.
2. *Class II*: Marginal tissue recession extends to or beyond the mucogingival junction. No loss of interdental bone/ soft tissue.
3. *Class III*: Marginal tissue recession extends to or beyond the mucogingival junction. Loss of interdental bone/soft tissue or malpositioning of the tooth **(Fig. 29.18)**.

**Section 5:** Diagnosis

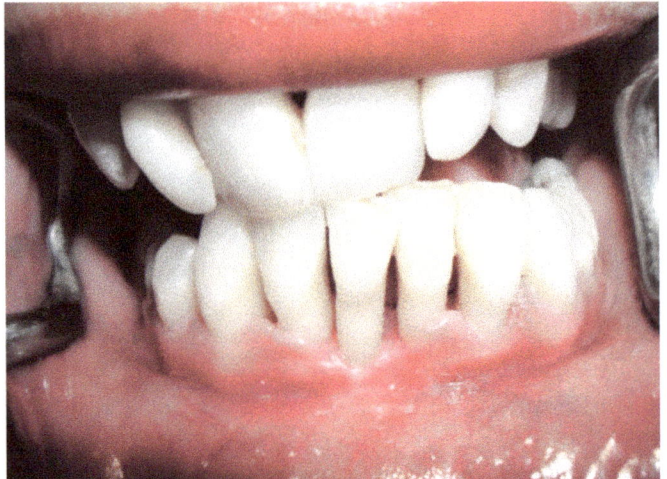

**Fig. 29.19:** Clinical picture showing grade IV marginal tissue recession.

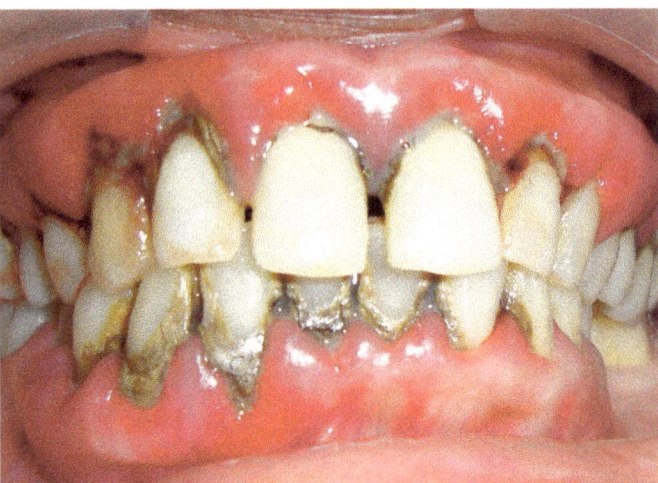

**Fig. 29.20:** Clinical picture showing pus discharge.

4. *Class IV*: Marginal tissue recession extends beyond the mucogingival junction. Loss of interdental bone and soft tissue loss interdentally and/or severe tooth malposition **(Fig. 29.19)**.

*Bleeding on probing*: In the case of inflamed gingiva and atrophic or ulcerated pocket epithelium, the insertion of a probe to the bottom of the pocket can induce bleeding. Bleeding on probing is an earlier sign of inflammation than gingival color changes. For checking bleeding on probing, the probe is introduced carefully to the bottom of the pocket and moved gently laterally along the pocket wall. Bleeding may appear immediately after removal of the probe or delayed by few seconds. Bleeding is checked after 30–60 seconds of probing. As a single test, bleeding on probing is not a good indicator of progressive attachment loss; however, its absence is suggestive of good periodontal stability.[4]

*Suppuration*: For clinical detection of pus in a periodontal pocket, the ball of the index finger is placed along the lateral aspect of the marginal gingiva, and pressure is applied in a rolling motion towards the crown. Visual examination without digital pressure is not enough **(Fig. 29.20)**.

### Examination of Periodontal Tissues

Examination of periodontal tissues is a routine part of all oral examinations. It usually consists of a visual inspection of the gingiva, dental plaque and calculus deposition, assessment of mobility, periodontal pocket depth, level of attachment, alveolar bone loss, furcation lesion, and abscesses **(Table 29.2)**.

*Plaque and calculus*: Several methods are available for assessing plaque and calculus accumulation. Plaque can be detected by using a disclosing solution or tablet **(Fig. 29.21)**. Supragingival calculus can be detected directly by a calibrated probe, which helps to measure the amount. Subgingival calculus is detected by deflecting the pocket wall through a periodontal probe **(Fig. 29.22)**. The ball end of the CPITN probe can also be used with a light touch to detect the subgingival calculus. Compressed air is commonly used to deflect the gingiva and to get the complete visualization of the calculus. Sometimes the radiograph reveals the presence of massive calculus deposits interproximally.

**TABLE 29.2:** Various tests used during a periodontal examination.

| Tests | Assessment of tissue |
|---|---|
| Tension test is used to detect | Abnormal frenum |
| Fremitus test is used to detect | Trauma from occlusion |
| Transgingival probing is used to determine | Alveolar bone loss |

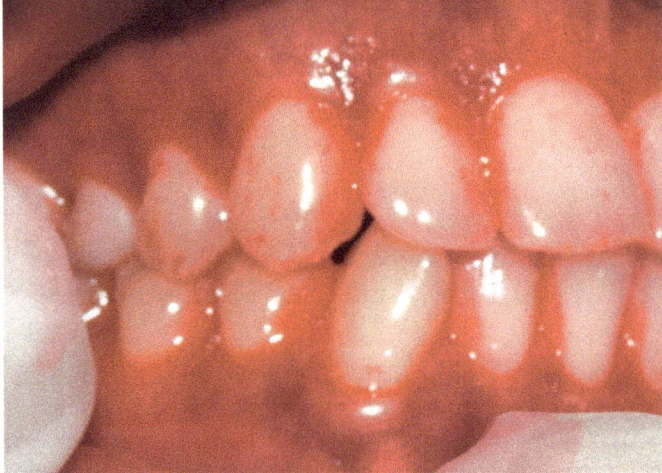

**Fig. 29.21:** Clinical picture showing plaque visible through the use of disclosing agent.

*Mobility*: Mobile teeth usually exhibit poorer prognosis and increased attachment loss. Hence, measurement of tooth mobility is an important part of periodontal disease diagnosis. The tooth movements when extending beyond the physiologic range becomes abnormal or pathologic.

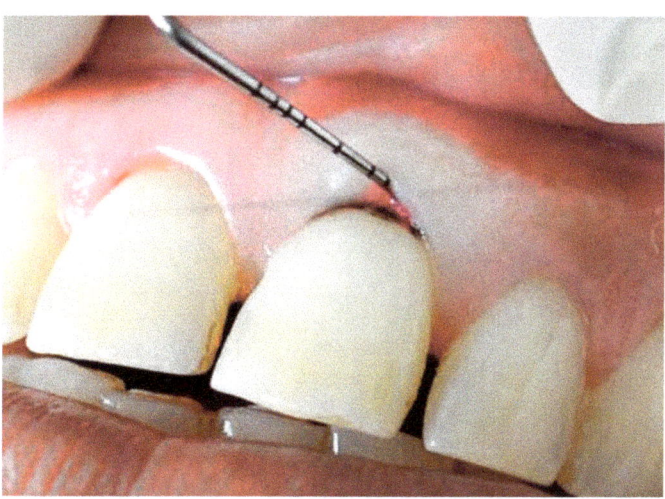

**Fig. 29.22:** Clinical picture showing subgingival calculus, revealed by deflecting pocket wall through the periodontal probe.

- *Etiology*: One or more of the following factors affects tooth mobility:
  - *Local factors*: Bone loss or loss of tooth support, trauma from occlusion, hypofunction, periapical pathology, after periodontal surgery, parafunctional habits, pathology of jaws, such as tumors, traumatic injuries to the dentoalveolar unit.
  - *Systemic factors*: Menstrual cycle, oral contraceptives, pregnancy, systemic diseases (Papillon-Lefèvre syndrome, Down's syndrome, neutropenia, Chédiak-Higashi syndrome, hypophosphatasia, hyperparathyroidism, acute leukemia, and Paget's disease).
- *Measurement*: Mobility is measured by moving the teeth in a buccolingual and occlusal-apical direction between the blunt handle end of two instruments or between the finger and instrument handle **(Figs. 29.23A to C)**. But the method of detecting mobility with an instrument and finger is not reliable. The degree of movement is observed by comparison with adjacent teeth that are not being moved.

The degree of movement is indicated on an arbitrary scale 0–3 in Miller index:[10]
- Score 0: No detectable movement when force is applied
- Score 1: Mobility greater than normal (physiologic)
- Score 2: Mobility up to 1 mm in buccolingual directions
- Score 3: Mobility more than 1 mm in buccolingual directions combined with the ability to depress the tooth.

Carranza proposed the following grades:[11]
- Grade 0: Normal
- Grade I: Slightly more than normal
- Grade II: Moderately more than normal
- Grade III: Severe mobility faciolingually and/or mesiodistally, combined with vertical displacement.

These classifications are highly subjective and depend on individual evaluation. The various instruments used to measure mobility are macroperiodontometer, microperiodontometer, and periotest.

*Periodontal pocket depth*: Periodontal pockets examination should involve the following parameters—the presence of periodontal pocket, distribution on each tooth surface, pocket depth, level of attachment on the root, and type of pocket (suprabony or infrabony). A careful exploration of a periodontal pocket with a periodontal probe helps detect and measure periodontal pockets accurately. Periodontal probing should be conducted on all surfaces of every tooth in the dentition. Radiographic examination is not suitable to identify the pockets. The periodontal pocket is a soft-tissue change, and radiographs may indicate areas of bone loss where pockets are suspected. They do not show pocket presence or depth. Gutta-percha points or calibrated silver points can be used with the radiograph to assist in determining the level of attachment of periodontal pockets.

To detect the areas of deepest penetration, the probe should be inserted parallel to the vertical axis of the tooth and "walked" circumferentially around each tooth's surface without taking out the probe completely from the gingival sulcus **(Fig. 29.24)**.[12] For the interproximal pocket, it is

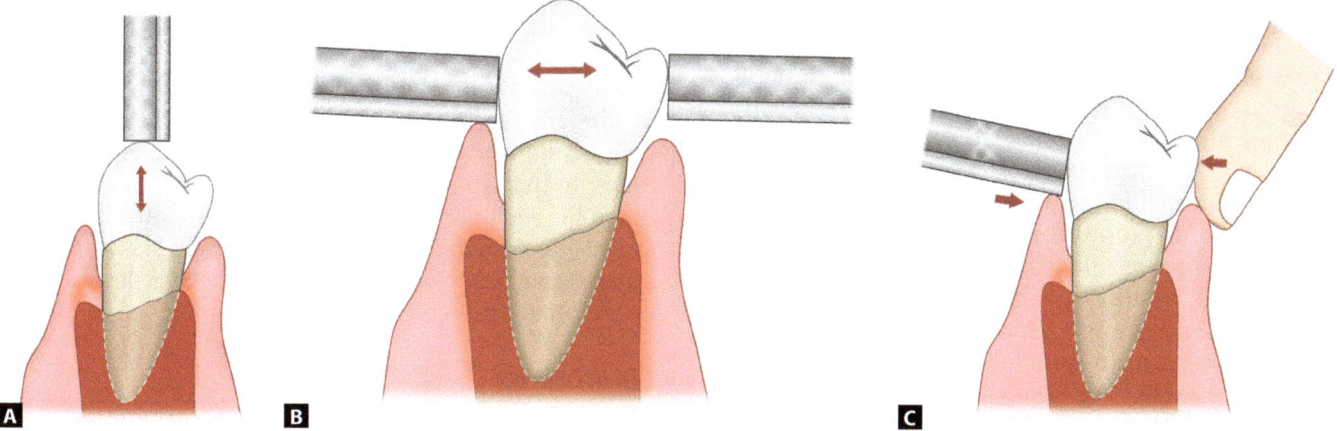

**Figs. 29.23A to C:** Schematic representation showing tooth mobility which is checked with: (A) One instrument in the vertical direction; (B) Two instruments in buccolingual directions; (C) One metal instrument and one finger in buccolingual direction (not reliable method).

**Section 5:** Diagnosis

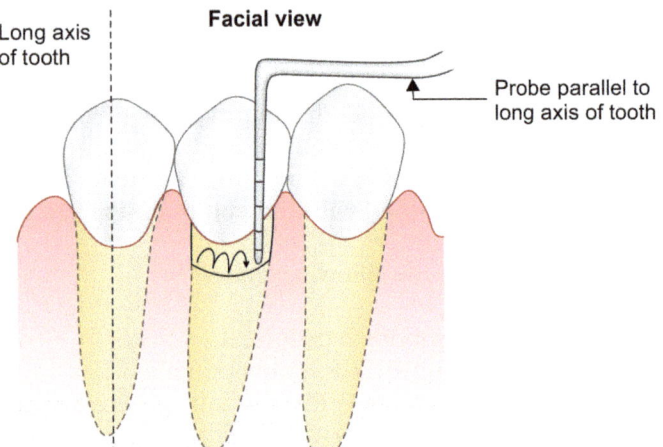

**Fig. 29.24:** Schematic representation showing walking stroke.

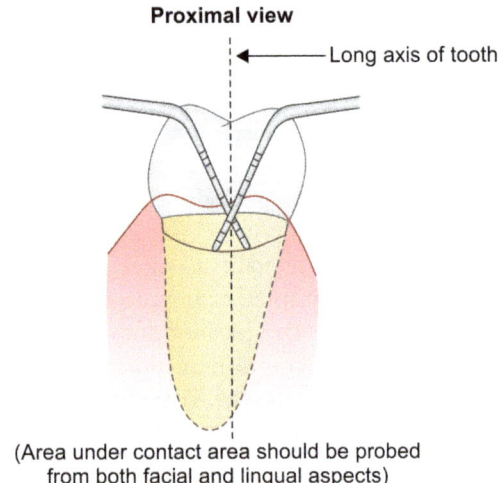

**Fig. 29.25:** Schematic illustration showing probing in interproximal area.

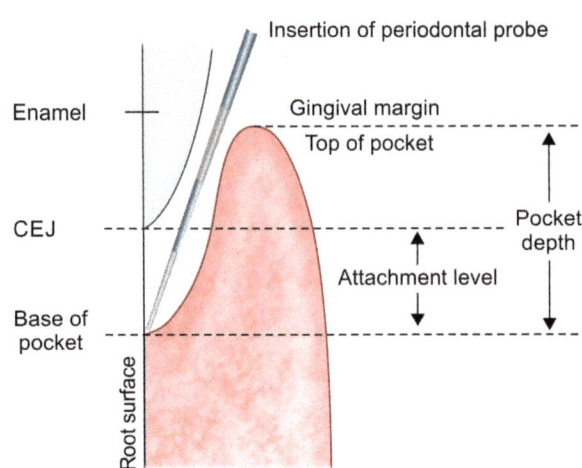

**Fig. 29.26:** Schematic representation showing clinical attachment level. (CEJ: cementoenamel junction)

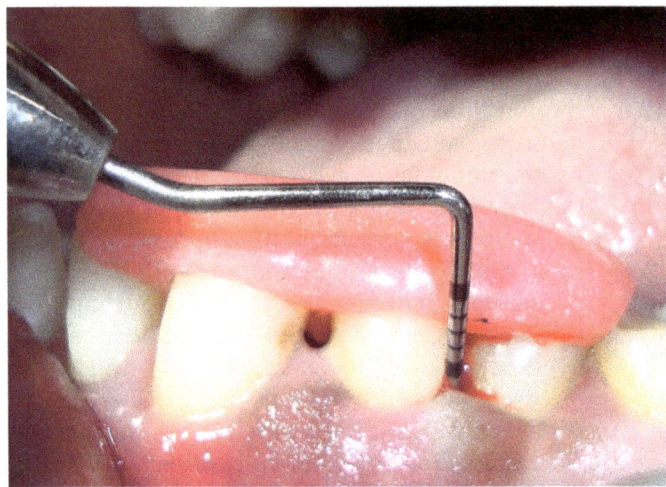

**Fig. 29.27:** Clinical picture showing template/splint to determine relative attachment level (Groove acrylic stent to standardize the direction of the probe).
(*Courtesy*: Dr Nitika Narula)

necessary to angulate the probe beneath the contact area from both the facial and the lingual areas **(Fig. 29.25)**.

Probing of pockets is conducted at various phases of disease activity ranging from diagnosis to monitoring the course of treatment and maintenance. The initial probing of moderate or advanced cases is usually hampered by the presence of heavy inflammation and abundant calculus and cannot be done very accurately. Initial probing, along with the clinical and radiographic examinations, is useful to determine the tooth condition either to save or need extraction. Once the patient has performed an adequate plaque and calculus control, the major inflammatory changes disappear, and a more accurate probing of the pockets can be performed. This second probing is to accurately establish the level of attachment and degree of involvement of roots and furcations.

Various periodontal probes are available to measure pocket depth around natural dentition. The plastic periodontal probes should be used to prevent scratching of the implant surface, instead of the usual steel probes used for the natural dentition.

*Level of attachment*: It is the distance between the base of the pocket and the fixed reference point such as CEJ on the crown **(Fig. 29.26)**, the margin of a permanent restoration; for animal research, a notch made in the tooth; in human research studies template/splint may be made for each patient **(Fig. 29.27)**. There may be gain or loss of attachment. The clinical attachment loss reveals the approximate extent of the root surface that is devoid of the periodontal ligament.

### Limitations

- The parameter is useful as an indicator of the amount of periodontal support at a specific location on the tooth. However, the measurement fails to provide an accurate

## Chapter 29: Clinical Diagnosis

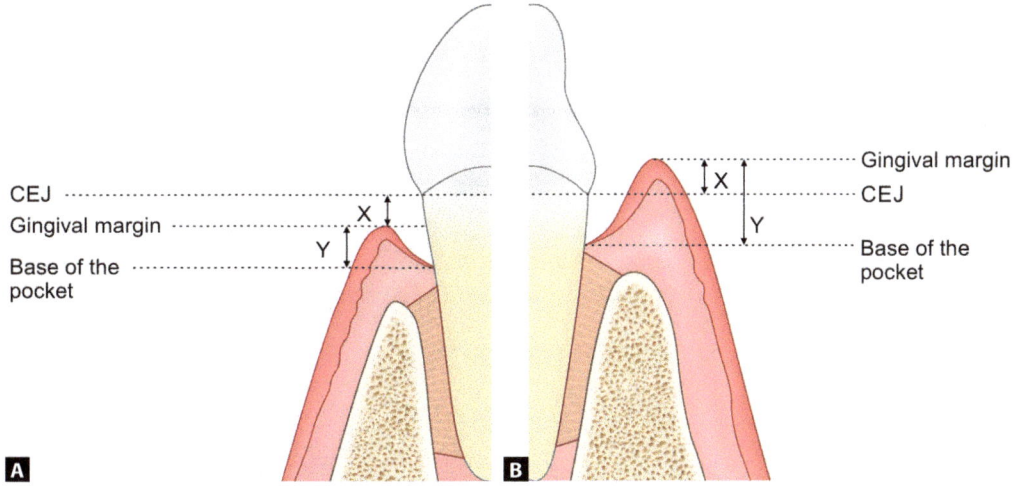

**Figs. 29.28A and B:** Schematic representation showing CAL's calculation in different situations: (A) When gingival margin is below CEJ (clinical gingival recession). Clinical attachment loss is calculated by adding the probing depth (Y) to the distance between CEJ and gingival margin (X); (B) When gingival margin covers the CEJ, located on the anatomic crown, clinical attachment loss is calculated by subtracting the probing depth (Y) to the distance between CEJ and gingival margin (X).

(CAL: clinical attachment level; CEJ: cementoenamel junction)

- assessment of support in terms of three dimensions/root surface area.
- Degree of inflammation, probing force, probe tip thickness, angulation, and position of probing and root anatomy, particularly in furcation areas, ideally determined the apical extent of periodontal probe penetration and depth.
- Another limitation is intra- and interexaminer reliability[13] and probe marking accuracy.[14]

*Determining the level of attachment* **(Figs. 29.28A and B)**: If the gingival margin is present on the anatomic crown; the level of attachment is measured by subtracting the distance from the gingival margin to the CEJ to the depth of the pocket. If both are the same, the loss of attachment is zero. When the gingival margin coincides with the CEJ, the loss of attachment equals the pocket depth.[15,16]

If the gingival margin is present apical to the CEJ, the level of attachment is usually more than the pocket depth. Hence, the distance between the CEJ and the gingival margin should be added to the pocket depth.

*Alveolar bone loss*: Both clinical and radiographic examinations are needed to determine the alveolar bone loss. Bone sounding is done by anesthetizing the tissue locally and inserting the probe horizontally and walking along with the tissue tooth interface so that the operator can feel the bony topography.[17] It gives three-dimensional information regarding bone contour. It is also called as transgingival probing. It helps to determine the height and contour of facial and lingual bone; the architecture of the interdental bone; the extent and configuration of the intrabony component of the pocket **(Fig. 29.29)**.

*Furcation defects*: Cowhorn explorer or Naber's probe can determine the furcation lesions. The probe is directed

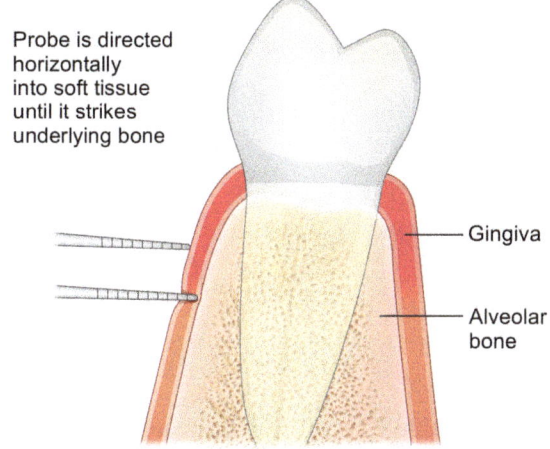

**Fig. 29.29:** Schematic representation showing transgingival probing/bone sounding.

beneath the gingival margin. When a probe reaches the bottom of the pocket, rotate its tip towards the tooth to fit it into the opening of the furcation **(Fig. 29.30)**. The terminal shank of Naber's probe holds parallel to the long axis of the tooth surface that is being examined.

Distal furcation of maxillary molar can be probed from either buccal or palatal aspects, but mesial furcation of maxillary molar is easily probed from the palatal aspect. Radiographs are useful in assessing root morphology and apicocoronal position of the furcation but do not allow the clinician to determine attachment loss in the furcation. It appears that radiographs alone do not detect the furcation lesion with any predictable accuracy and that probing the furcation areas is necessary to confirm the presence and severity of the furcation defect.

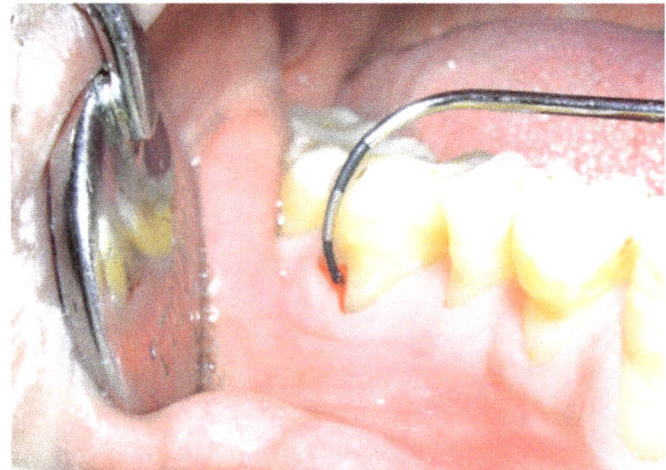

**Fig. 29.30:** Clinical picture showing grade II furcation defect (*cul-de-sac*).

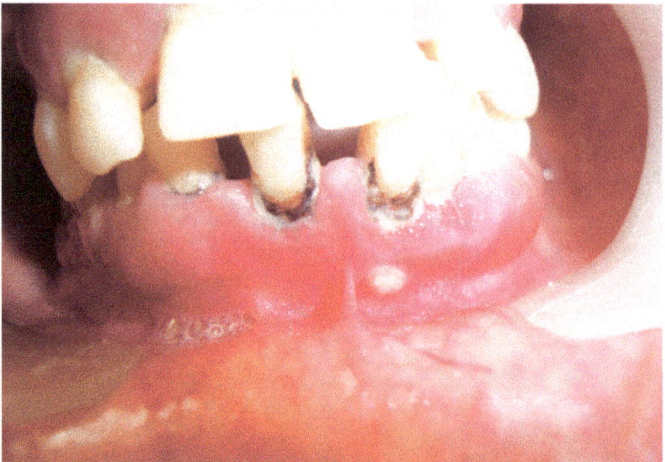

**Fig. 29.32:** Clinical picture showing periodontal abscess.

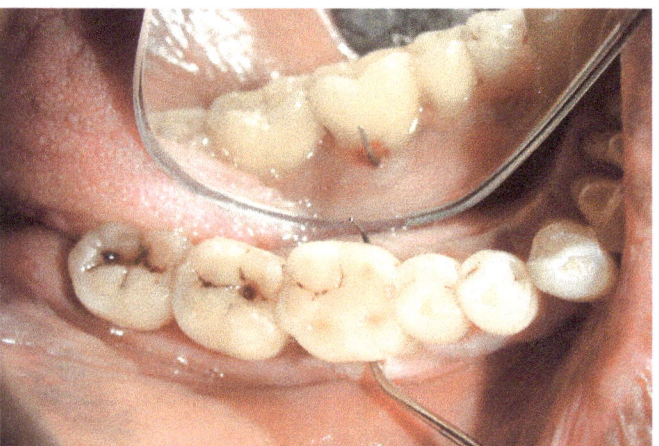

**Fig. 29.31:** Clinical picture showing grade III furcation defect (through and through).

Glickman classified furcation defects into four grades:[18]
- *Grade I*: It is the incipient stage of furcation involvement, but radiographically changes are not usually found.
- *Grade II*: The furcation lesion is a *cul-de-sac* with a definite horizontal component. Radiographs may or may not depict the furcation involvement **(Fig. 29.30)**.
- *Grade III*: The bone is not attached to the dome of the furcation. This furcation displays the defect as a radiolucent area in the crotch of the tooth **(Fig. 29.31)**.
- *Grade IV*: The interdental bone is destroyed, and soft tissues have receded apically so that the furcation opening is clinically visible.

*Determination of disease activity*: The determination of pocket depth or attachment levels is usually insufficient to identify whether the lesion is in an active or inactive state.
- *Inactive lesion*: There are little or no bleeding and minimal amounts of gingival fluid. It is characterized by a higher number of coccoid cells and intact pocket epithelium.
- *Active lesion*: Readily bleed on probing, and a large amount of gingival fluid and exudate is present. It is characterized by a higher number of spirochetes and motile bacteria. The pocket epithelium is ulcerated and infiltrated mainly by plasma cells and polymorphonuclear leukocytes.

*Gingival abscesses*: Gingival abscess is a localized, painful, rapidly expanding lesion usually of sudden onset. It is generally limited to the marginal gingiva or interdental papilla. It may be due to irritation from foreign substances, toothbrush bristle, apple core, or lobster shell forcefully embedded into the gingiva.

Several characteristics can be used as guidelines in differentiating a periodontal abscess from a periapical abscess. If the tooth is nonvital, the lesion is most likely periapical. When the apex and lateral surface of a root are involved by a single lesion that can be probed directly from the gingival margin, the lesion is more likely to have originated in a periodontal abscess **(Fig. 29.32)**. Rest is explained in "Chapter 23: Periodontal Abscess".

## INVESTIGATIONS

### Radiographic Examination

Radiographs are essential adjuncts to other means of assessment when planning the complete care program for the patient. The radiographic survey of full mouth should consist of a minimum of 14 intraoral films and four posterior bitewing films. Rest is explained in "Chapter 30: Radiographic Diagnostic Aids".

### Laboratory Investigations

Laboratory tests are advised to get more information about the patient's medical status. The tests are also helpful to the dentist to determine the cause or prognosis of periodontal disease.

#### Blood Investigations

Testing of blood smears for red and white blood cell counts, white blood cell differential counts, and erythrocyte sedimentation rates are useful to determine the presence of diseases, such as blood dyscrasias and generalized infections. Determination of coagulation time, bleeding time, clot retraction time, prothrombin time, capillary fragility test, and international normalized ratio (INR) may be required at times.

### Other Tests

Other tests, such as urine tests, blood smears, and biopsies, are indicated to identify the systemic factors that might affect or modify periodontal treatment.

*Microbiological tests*: Microbiological evaluations are not usually conducted in the majority of periodontal patients. However, it is helpful to the dentist to define the accurate cause of periodontal disease and determine specific treatment modalities for particular patients. In such patients, it is immensely needed to know whether the organisms are sensitive to specific antibiotics. Thus, microbiological testing is helpful to control or treat disease by combining mechanical debridement with appropriate antimicrobial chemotherapy. Various methods of microbiological testing are available to assess the bacterial flora of patients with periodontal disease. For such evaluations, plaque samples are collected with a curette or a paper point and analyzed using phase-contrast or dark-field microscopy, bacterial enzyme analysis, immunoassay, deoxyribonucleic acid (DNA) probes, polymerase chain reaction or traditional microbiological culturing and sensitivity. Rest is explained in "Chapter 31: Microbiological Diagnostic Aids".

*Casts*: These are indicative of the position of the gingival margins and the position and inclination of the teeth, proximal contact relationships, wasting diseases **(Fig. 29.33)**, food impaction areas, and lingual-cusp relationships. Casts also function as visual aids while discussing the disease problem with the patient. They are useful for pre- and post-treatment comparisons, as well as for reference at check-up visits.

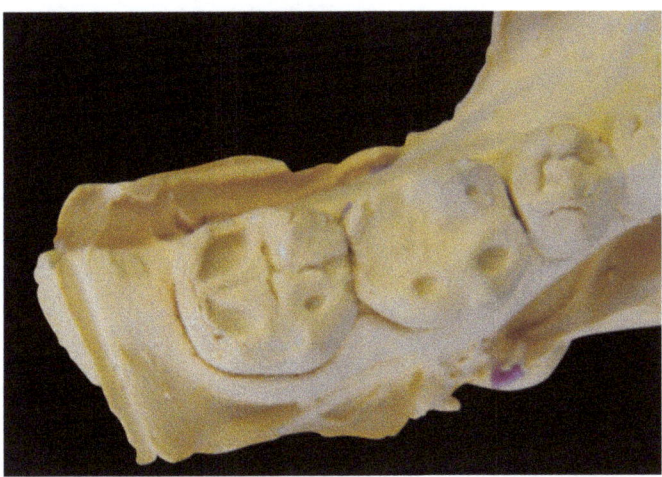

**Fig. 29.33:** Clinical picture showing cast with attrition (wear facets).

*Color photographs*: They are useful for noting the appearance of the tissue before and after conducting treatment.

## DIAGNOSIS

Periodontal diagnosis should first determine whether the disease is present, then identify its type, extent, distribution, and severity.

## TREATMENT PLAN

The treatment plan is divided into an emergency and four basic phases that are:
- Emergency/preliminary phase
- Phase I: Etiotropic phase
- Phase II: Surgical phase
- Phase III: Restorative phase
- Phase IV: Maintenance phase.
  Rest is explained in "Chapter 34: Treatment Plan".

### Points to Ponder

- Gingivitis toxica is a specific type of gingivitis in which there is the destruction of gingiva and the underlying bone due to the chewing of tobacco.
- Infrabony pocket can be differentiated clinically from the suprabony pocket by inserting the probe parallel to the long axis of the tooth and pulling it towards the gingiva. If bony resistance is felt the pocket is said to be infrabony. Bony resistance felt is the bony wall of the infrabony pocket, as the base of the pocket is apical to the alveolar crest.
- The international normalized ratio is usually 0.9–1.3 for a healthy person. An INR of 2.0–3.0 is recommended for people on warfarin therapy except for prosthetic mechanical heart valves and prophylaxis of recurrent myocardial infarction (MI), for which higher intensity warfarin therapy (INR 2.5–3.5) is suggested.

## REFERENCES

1. Pihlstrom BL. Periodontal risk assessment, diagnosis, and treatment planning. Periodontol 2000. 2001;25:37-58.
2. Rhodus NL, Taybos GM. Physical and extraoral examination. In: Daniel SJ, Harfst SA, Wilder R (Eds). Mosby's Dental Hygiene: Concepts, Cases, and Competencies, 2nd edition. St. Louis: Mosby; 2004. pp. 214-27.
3. Wilkins EM. Examination procedures. In: Clinical Practice of the Dental Hygienists, 11th edition. Philadelphia, PA, USA: Lippincott Williams & Wilkins; 2012. pp. 201-23.
4. Carranza FA. Clinical diagnosis. In: Newman MG, Takei HH, Carranza FA (Eds). Carranza's Clinical Periodontology, 9th edition. Philadelphia, PA, USA: WB Saunders; 2003. pp. 432-53.
5. Wilkins EM. Extraoral and intraoral examination. In: Clinical Practice of the Dental Hygienist, 11th edition. Philadelphia, PA, USA: Lippincott Williams & Wilkins; 2012. pp. 116-33.
6. Hirschfeld I. Food impaction. J Am Dent Assoc. 1930;17:1504-11.
7. Robinson HB. Abrasion, attrition, and erosion of teeth. Health Center J Ohio State Univ. 1949;3:21.

8. Sognnaes RF. Periodontal significance of intraoral frictional ablation. J West Soc Periodontol Periodontal Abstr. 1977;25(3):112-21.
9. Miller PD. A classification of marginal tissue recession. Int J Periodontics Restorative Dent. 1985;5(2):8-13.
10. Miller SC. Textbook of Periodontia, 3rd edition. Philadelphia, PA, USA: The Blakeston Corporation; 1950.
11. Carranza FA. Glickman's Clinical Periodontology, 7th edition. Philadelphia, PA, USA: WB Saunders; 1996.
12. Armitage GC. Clinical periodontal examination. In: Genco RJ, Goldman HM, Cohen DW (Eds). Contemporary Periodontics, 1st edition. St. Louis: CV Mosby; 1990. pp. 339-47.
13. Hassell TM, Germann MA, Saxer UP. Periodontal probing: inter investigator discrepancies and correlations between probing force and recorded depth. Helv Odontol Acta. 1973;17(1):38-42.
14. van der Velden U. Errors in the assessment of pocket depth in vitro. J Clin Periodontol. 1978;5(3):182-7.
15. Genco RJ. Periodontal diagnosis, prognosis, and treatment planning. In: Genco RJ, Goldman HM, Cohen DW (Eds). Contemporary Periodontics, 1st edition. St. Louis: CV Mosby; 1990. pp. 348-60.
16. Armitage GC. Clinical periodontal examination. In: Rose LF, Mealey BL, Genco RJ, Cohen DW (Eds). Periodontics, Medicine, Surgery, and Implants, 1st edition. Philadelphia, PA, USA: Elsevier- Mosby; 2004. pp. 134-45.
17. Lindhe J, Karring T, Lang NP. Examination of patients with periodontal disease. In: Clinical Periodontology and Implant Dentistry, 4th edition. Chicago, USA: Blackwell Munksgaard; 2003. pp. 403-13.
18. Glickman I, Carranza FA. Glickman's Clinical Periodontology, 7th edition. Philadelphia, PA, USA: WB Saunders; 1990.

## VIVA VOCE

**Q1. What is the method to assess the proximal contact relationship?**
**Ans.** The tightness of proximal contact is checked by means of clinical observation and with dental floss.

**Q2. Which is the most common plunger cusp?**
**Ans.** Distolingual cusp of maxillary molars is the most common plunger cusp.

**Q3. In which gingival or periodontal diseases, lymph node enlargement is seen?**
**Ans.**
- Necrotizing ulcerative gingivitis
- Primary herpetic gingivostomatitis
- Acute periodontal abscesses.

**Q4. When is a frenum judged abnormal?**
**Ans.** A frenum is judged abnormal under the following conditions:
- When interdental papilla moves by stretching the frenum
- When the frenum is unusually broad
- When there is no apparent attached gingiva in the frenal area.

**Q5. What is the basic difference between mobility and fremitus test?**
**Ans.** Fremitus is tooth displacement, which is created by the patient's occlusal force. Therefore, the amount of force varies greatly from patient-to-patient, whereas in mobility, the force with which it is measured tends to be the same for each examiner. Fremitus is a guide to the ability of the patient to displace and traumatize the teeth.

**Q6. What is the ideal probing force?**
**Ans.** The ideal probing force is 25 grams.

**Q7. Which tool is used to assess BOP?**
**Ans.** Periodontal probe.

**Q8. What is attrition?**
**Ans.** Attrition is occlusal wear resulting from functional contacts with opposing teeth.

**Q9. In which position, gingival stippling is best viewed.**
**Ans.** Gingival stippling is best viewed by drying the gingiva and switching off the chair light.

**Q10. Name the device used to measure the thickness of gingiva without inducing trauma.**
**Ans.** An ultrasonic device called "Krupp SDM" is used.

# Chapter 30

# Radiographic Diagnostic Aids

*Amit Aggarwal, Rachna V Prabhu*

## Chapter Outline

- Ideal Requisites
- Radiographic Techniques
- Normal Radiographic Features
- Pathologic Radiographic Changes
- Limitations
- Advanced Radiographic Aids

## INTRODUCTION

Radiological examination is an essential part of a periodontal assessment in patients presenting with clinical manifestations of periodontal destruction. The advent of improved current approaches to diagnosing periodontal diseases associated with the existing classification system suggests the integral role of radiographs in the diagnosis of various periodontal conditions. Assessment of both clinical and radiographic data is useful in diagnosing the presence and extent of periodontal disease.

Radiographs are useful tools in the diagnosis of periodontal diseases in association with clinical examination. They provide information about the bony tissues wrapped by the gingiva, which are undetectable by clinical inspection alone **(Fig. 30.1)**. Radiographic image formation is based on the principle of projecting a three-dimensional (3D) object onto a two-dimensional (2D) image plane, and therefore this technique also has limitations. In principle, the radiographic image lacks information about the third dimension, at least in a way that is easily perceptible by the human visual system.

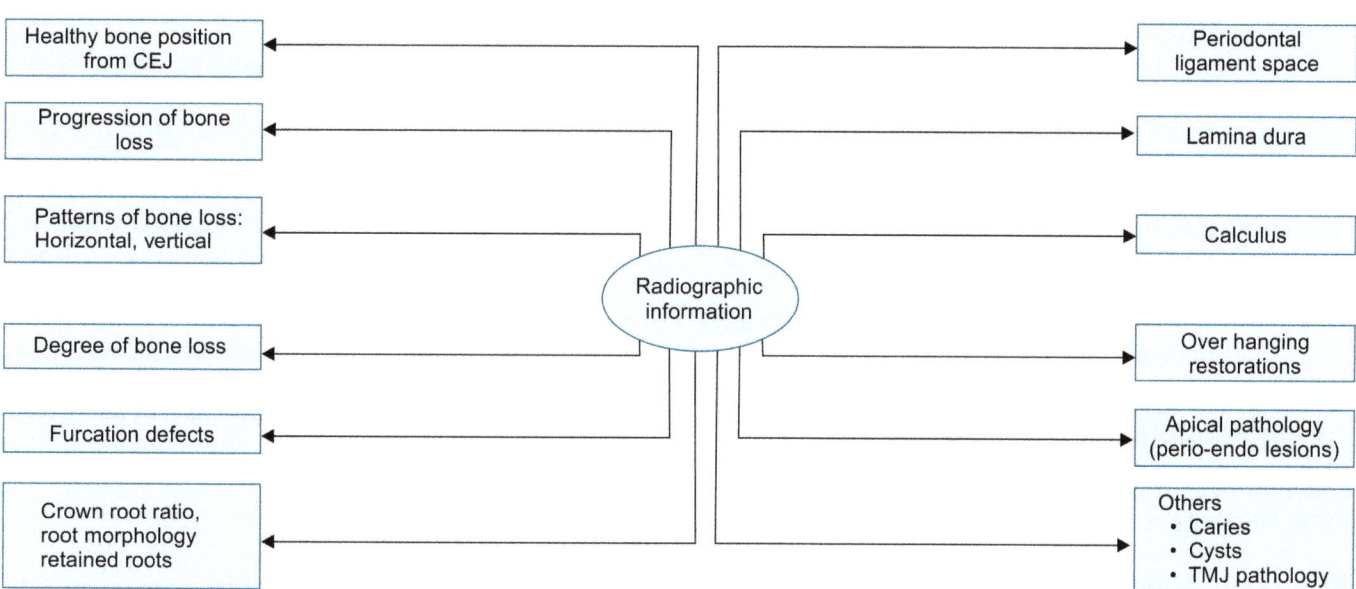

**Fig. 30.1:** Schematic representation showing key aspects of a radiographic periodontal assessment.
(CEJ: cementoenamel junction; TMJ: temporomandibular joint)

## IDEAL REQUISITES

The attention to radiation exposure by following the fundamental principle of choosing exposures "As Low As Reasonably Achievable" (ALARA) for diagnostic radiology is imperative; no diagnostic exposure is justifiable without a valid clinical indication.

For achieving appropriate radiographs, a proper exposure technique factors suitable for the patient's size and the condition is selected. It is usually conceptualized on a planned exposure system, which helps to get adequate image quality for diagnosis. It also includes:
- Use of the fastest image receptor compatible with the diagnostic task.
- Collimation of the beam to the size of the receptor whenever feasible.
- Proper film exposure and processing techniques.
- Use of lead aprons and thyroid collars.

The radiograph thus taken should be ideal. To be useful for diagnosis, radiographs have to satisfy the requirements of standardization and reproducibility. The ideal radiographic procedure should also facilitate the collection of quantitative data with regard to the condition of lesion areas and should provide sufficient information about the shape and the extent of the lesion in three dimensions. These requirements are even more critical in the radiographic diagnosis of periodontal disease.[1] Following points should also be kept in mind:
- Radiographs should only be considered following a full clinical examination.
- A provisional diagnosis should be made with radiographs' choice based on the type, severity, and distribution of disease.
- Radiographs were taken for reasons other than the periodontal disease (e.g., horizontal bitewings for caries diagnosis) will often provide useful information and should be examined before further radiographs are requested.
- Prichard established the following four criteria to determine the adequate angulation of periapical radiographs:[2]
    - The radiographs should show the tips of molar cusps with little or none of the occlusal surface.
    - Enamel caps and pulp chambers should be distinct.
    - Interproximal spaces should be open.
    - Proximal contacts should not overlap unless teeth are out of line anatomically.

## RADIOGRAPHIC TECHNIQUES

Different radiographic exposure types are helpful in the formulation of periodontal treatment plans **(Table 30.1)**.[3-5]

### Panoramic Radiographs

Panoramic oral radiographs/orthopantomogram (OPG) are useful in getting a general view of the oral structures and in

**TABLE 30.1:** Types of radiographs required in various periodontal diseases.

| | | | |
|---|---|---|---|
| Gingivitis | | | No radiographs are indicated |
| Localized periodontitis | Posterior teeth | Mild | Radiographs not usually indicated |
| | | Moderate | Bitewings or periapical if furcation involvement |
| | | Severe | Periapical of affected teeth or panoramic ± periapical |
| | Anterior teeth | Mild | Radiographs not usually indicated |
| | | Moderate and severe | Periapical radiographs |
| Generalized periodontitis | | Mild | Radiographs not usually indicated |
| | | Moderate | Panoramic + periapical or bitewings of specific areas |
| | | Severe | Panoramic or periapical of standing teeth |

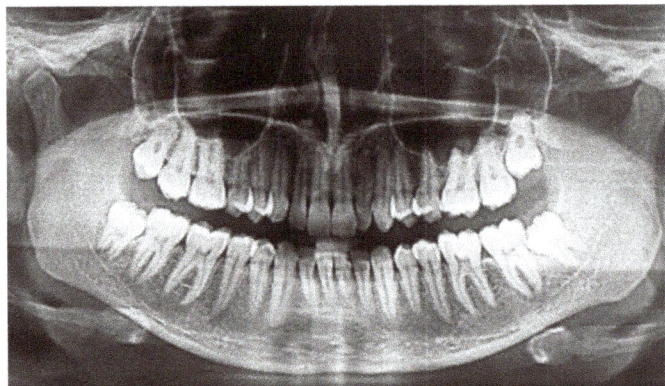

**Fig. 30.2:** Radiographic image showing a panoramic view of normal bone height.

screening bone height in general **(Fig. 30.2)**. Well, tolerance by patients, minimal exposure time compared to intraoral radiographs, wide anatomical coverage, and relatively low patient doses are some of the important advantages of panoramic radiographs. The main disadvantage of panoramic images is poor resolution compared to intraoral films. Also, they are inappropriate for assessing the degree of bone loss in individual teeth because of severe distortion and unclear outline of the bone margin produced by the superimposition of intervening structures. The panoramic view is useful when assessing generalized periodontitis **(Fig. 30.3)**, where large areas of jaws have to be viewed. Panoramic oral radiographs may also need additional intraoral views.

### Periapical Radiographs

Periapical radiographs are commonly used for getting the differential diagnosis of the patient's presenting symptoms. They are also useful in screening for undetected pathological

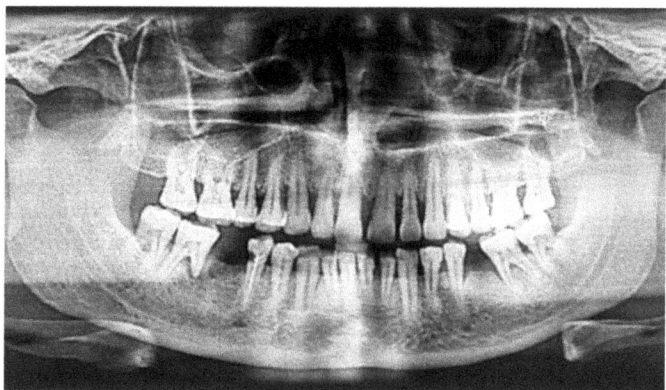

**Fig. 30.3:** Radiographic image showing a panoramic view of generalized bone loss.

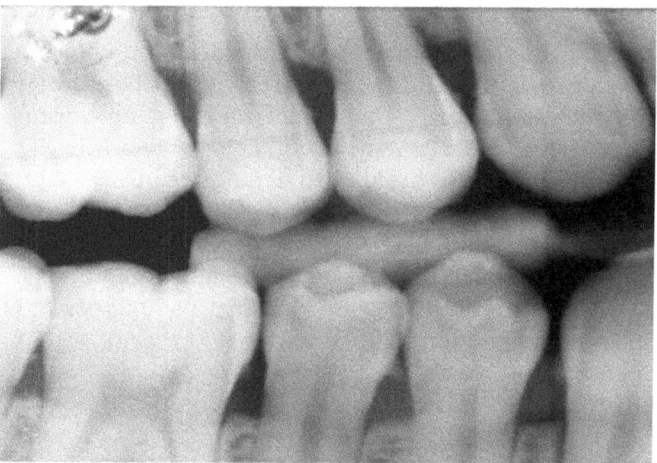

**Fig. 30.5:** Radiographic image showing bitewing radiograph.

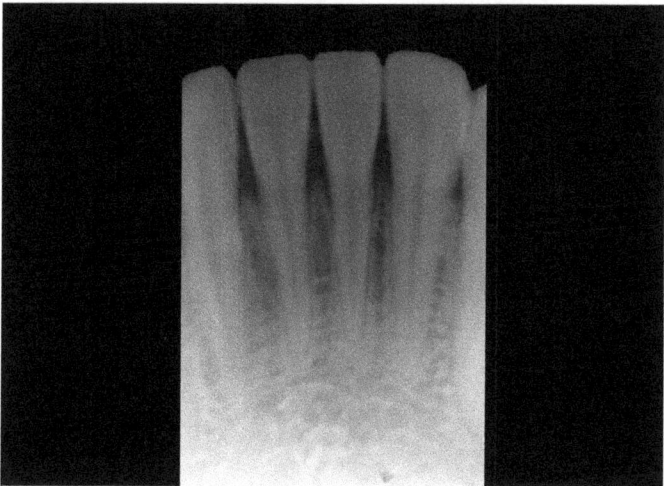

**Fig. 30.4:** Radiographic image showing ideal intraoral periapical radiograph.

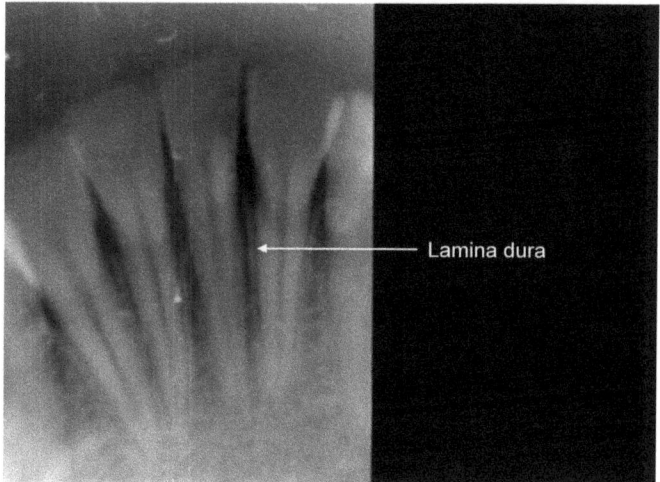

**Fig. 30.6:** Radiographic image showing lamina dura.

processes of the teeth and surrounding alveolar bone. In the process of periodontal disease diagnosis, periapical radiographs are useful in collecting information, which is difficult to obtain through the examination of the tissues alone **(Fig. 30.4)**.

## Bitewing Radiographs

These are useful in examining the teeth' proximal surfaces and the crest of the alveolar bone of both the maxilla and the mandible on the same film **(Fig. 30.5)**. They are mainly suitable for detecting interproximal decay and providing valuable information on the patient's periodontal status. The height of the interproximal alveolar bone margin in relation to the cementoenamel junction (CEJ) can be measured. Interproximal deposits of subgingival calculus can also be detected. The importance of bitewing radiographs in the diagnosis of periodontal diseases is restricted due to the fact that only the coronal sections of the roots of the teeth are detected, and the approach is limited to the molar-premolar regions. The posterior bitewing projection gives both optimal geometry and detail of intraoral radiography in patients with small amounts of uniform bone loss.

## NORMAL RADIOGRAPHIC FEATURES

### Alveolar Bone

In an individual, the dense cortical alveolar bone forming the wall of the tooth's socket appears radiographically as a distinct, opaque, uninterrupted, white line parallel to the tooth root. This is known as the lamina dura **(Fig. 30.6)**. The lamina dura is a continuation of the jawbone cortex, and it covers the root in a socket of cortical bone.[3]

Radiographically a normal, healthy alveolar bone exhibits a characteristic appearance. The alveolar crest in a young individual is close to the CEJ. The alveolar crests are positioned approximately 2–3 mm apical to the CEJ of the teeth, and its shape varies from rounded to flat.

The alveolar crest is usually pointed in between incisors. In between premolar and molar teeth, the alveolar crest appears parallel to a line between the adjacent CEJs, where the enamel becomes thins and disappears. The alveolar crest will be continuous with the lamina dura of the adjacent teeth. On examining the lamina dura and the periodontal ligament, only the interproximal portions are noticeable.

However, the buccal and lingual areas are unnoticeable in the radiograph. Widening of the periodontal ligament space and loss of lamina dura suggests resorption of the alveolar bone. The trabecular pattern of interdental bone is distinct and fills the interradicular space.

Although these are the usual features of the healthy periodontium, they are not always evident. Their absence from radiographs does not necessarily mean that periodontal disease is present. Failure to see these features may be due to technical error, overexposure, or normal anatomic variation in alveolar bone shape and density.

## Interdental Septa

The interdental septum, or septal bone, is present between the roots of adjacent teeth. It is noticeable compared to the bone situated on the buccal or lingual aspect of the tooth (the latter being partially obscured by the superimposed image of the root). The shape of the interdental septum suggests the function of the morphology of the contiguous teeth.

## Periodontal Ligament Space

Radiographically, the periodontal ligament present as a fine, black, radiolucent line adjacent to the root surface as it is composed of connective tissue. The radiolucent image between the lamina dura and tooth is the periodontal space known radiographically as the lamina lucida. With disease, the periodontal ligament space may appear at varying thicknesses. A widened periodontal space is considered to be a sign of chronic inflammation. Commonly, the periodontal ligament space is found to change in width from patient to patient and from tooth to tooth in the individual and even from location to location around one tooth.[6,7]

## PATHOLOGIC RADIOGRAPHIC CHANGES

## Osseous Defects

### Horizontal Bone Loss

Usually, horizontal bone loss is found in the suprabony pocket during a clinical examination. Radiographically, horizontal bone loss is present as a reduced alveolar marginal bone around adjacent teeth. The crestal bone is positioned 1-2 mm apical to the CEJ in a normal healthy oral cavity. However, with horizontal bone loss resorption, both the buccal and lingual bone and interdental bone plates occur. When the epithelial attachment is coronal to the bony defect, the remaining bone margin appears roughly perpendicular to the long axis of the tooth **(Fig. 30.7)**.

### Vertical Bone Loss

Contrary to horizontal bone loss, vertical bone loss is commonly seen in an infrabony pocket. It produces when the walls of the pocket lie within a bony housing. Radiographically, vertical bone defects appear as V-shaped with sharp outlines **(Fig. 30.8)**.

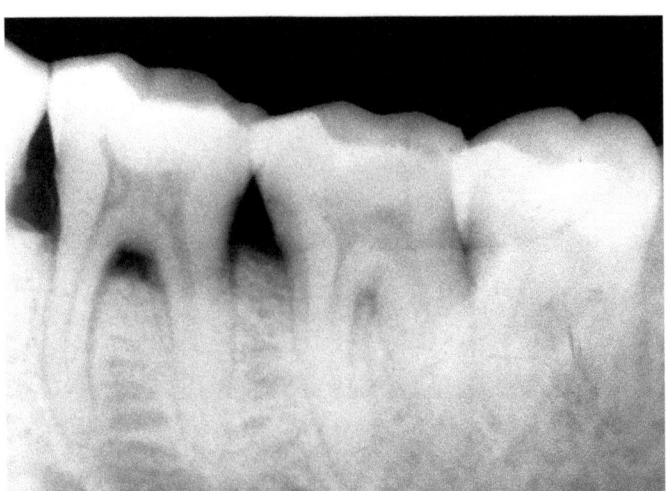

**Fig. 30.7:** Radiographic image showing horizontal bone loss and furcation defect.

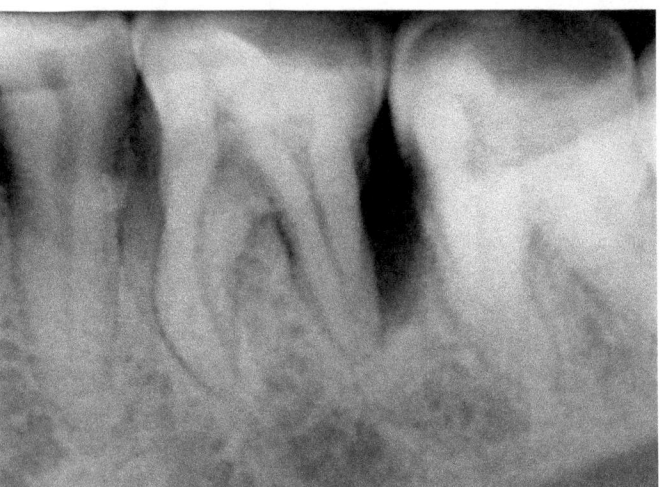

**Fig. 30.8:** Radiographic image showing vertical bone loss.

### Defect Angle

If X is considered as the CEJ at a tooth with a vertical defect, Z represents the most apical or the bottom of the bony defect, and Y exhibits the most coronal position of the crest adjacent to the vertical defect, the angle between the two lines XZ and YZ is termed as the defect angle. The defect angle is one of the diagnostic radiographic parameters. During periodontal regenerative surgery narrow periodontal defects less than or equal to 22° heal better than defects more than or equal to 36°.[8]

### Furcation Defects

The furcation represents a multiple tooth roots division at the trunk of the tooth. The furcation is considered as a normal structure commonly filled with bone. Furcation exposure results from intra-radicular bone loss due to advanced periodontal disease. In class I (incipient) furcation involvement, bone density gets reduced at the furcation. Bone loss at the furcation may or may not

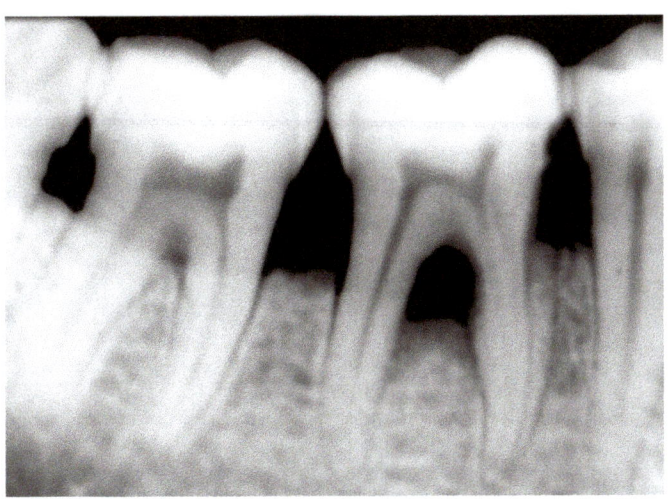

**Fig. 30.9:** Radiographic image showing furcation involvement of mandibular 1st molar.

be seen in class II furcation defect. Class III furcation involvement (through and through) presents a visible area of complete bone loss on radiological examination. Advanced furcation exposures characterized by resorption of cortical plates are easy to recognize on radiographs **(Fig. 30.9)**. Early change in furcation areas of maxillary molars is more challenging to assess because of the presence of three roots. Occasionally, radiological examinations can detect bone loss in facial furcation. However, the superimposition of the palatal root imposes difficulties in such detections. Radiological examination quickly detects defects present between the mesiobuccal and palatal roots and between the distobuccal and palatal roots. The presence of furcation "arrows" commonly presents lesions involving these mesial and distal furcations. The slightest radiographic change in the furcation area should be investigated clinically, especially if there is bone loss on adjacent roots. Diminished radiodensity in the furcation area in which outlines of bony trabeculae are visible suggests furcation involvement. Whenever there is marked bone loss in relation to a single molar root, it may be assumed that the furcation is also involved.

### *Interdental Craters*

Interdental craters are visualized as irregular areas of decreased radiopacity on the alveolar bone crests. They are poorly demarcated from the rest of the alveolar bone and get blend gradually with the same bone. Radiographs fail to show exact morphology or depth of interdental craters, and occasionally it appears as a vertical defect. The defect is usually difficult to visualize on the radiograph like the two-walled crater. This is because the buccal and lingual walls remain intact and hide the radiographic image of the defect.[9]

## Chronic Periodontitis

Following is the sequence of radiographic changes in periodontitis and the tissue changes that produce them:

- There are fuzziness and a break in the lamina dura's continuity at the mesial or distal aspect of the crest of the interdental septum. These result from the extension of gingival inflammation into the bone causing a widening of the vessel channels and a reduction in calcified tissue at the septal margin.[1]
- *Triangulation (funneling)*: Triangulation is the widening of the periodontal ligament space by the resorption of bone along either the mesial or distal aspect of the interdental (interseptal) crestal bone. The alveolar bone and root surfaces form the sides of the triangle, the base is towards the tooth crown, and the apex of the triangle is pointed towards the root. This is an early sign of bone degeneration and necessitates a search for possible etiologic factors, such as plaque, calculus, gingivitis, or food impaction.
- The destructive process extends across the crest of the interdental septum, and the height is reduced. Finger-like radiolucent projections extend from the crest into the septum. The radiolucent projections into the interdental septum result from the deeper extension of the inflammation into the bone.
- The height of the interdental septum gets gradually reduced due to the extension of inflammation and the resorption of bone.

## Aggressive Periodontitis

The radiographic appearance of aggressive periodontitis is characterized by the presence of deep vertical bone loss peculiarly affecting the 1st molar and incisor regions and relative sparing of other segments of the dentition. Radiologically, it is present as an arc-shaped loss of alveolar bone running from the distal surface of the 2nd premolar to the mesial surface of the 2nd molar **(Fig. 30.10)**. It is usually bilaterally symmetrical in both the 1st molars of each jaw.

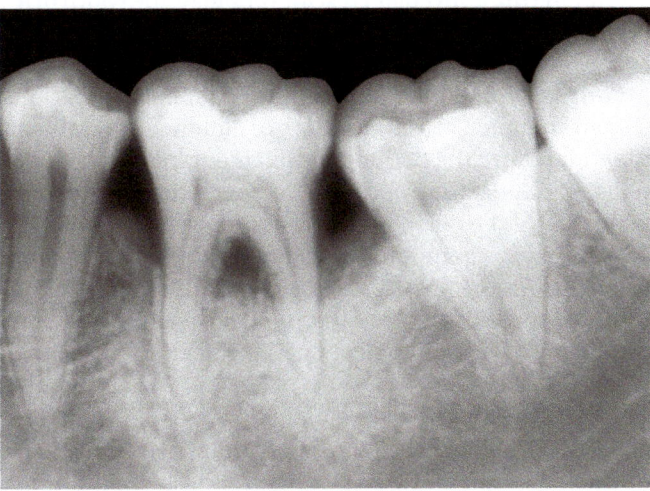

**Fig. 30.10:** Radiographic image showing arc-shaped bone loss around mandibular 1st molar in localized aggressive periodontitis.

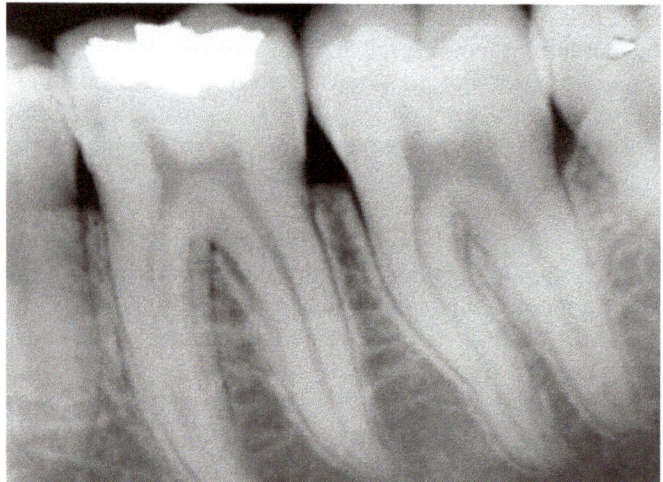

**Fig. 30.11:** Radiographic image showing radiographic features of trauma from occlusion (discontinuity and thickening of lamina dura).

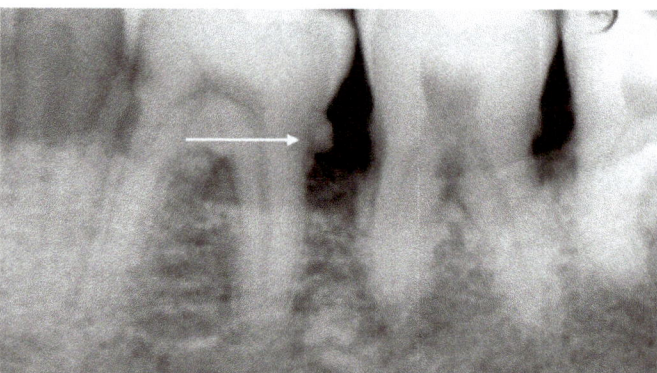

**Fig. 30.12:** Radiographic image showing subgingival calculus around mandibular 1st molar.

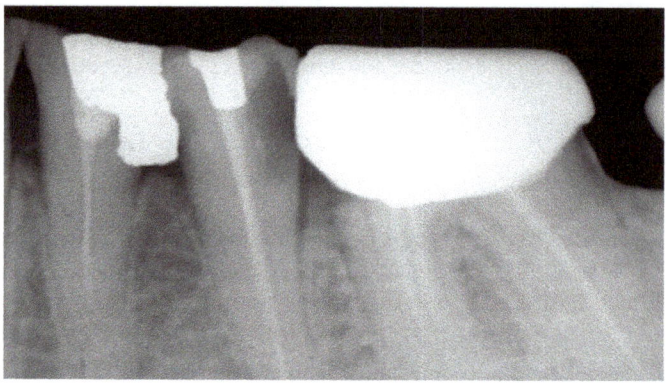

**Fig. 30.13:** Radiographic image showing overhanging restorations in mandibular 1st premolar and molar.

## Periodontal Abscesses

Radiologically, the periodontal abscess is present as a discrete area of radiolucency along the root's lateral aspect. However, the radiographic appearance can show variations, and hence it cannot be considered a clear finding for the diagnosis of a periodontal abscess.

## Conditions Associated with Periodontal Diseases

Various changes in teeth and its supporting structures are associated with periodontal diseases. These include occlusal trauma and local irritants.

### Trauma from Occlusion

Traumatic occlusion by itself does not cause periodontitis. Still, it can result in some traumatic lesion in response to occlusal pressures, which are greater than the physiological tolerances of the tooth's supporting structures. Radiographically trauma from occlusion presents noticeable changes in the lamina dura, alveolar crest morphology, the width of the periodontal ligament space, and density of the surrounding cancellous bone. The injury phase of trauma from occlusion produces a loss of the lamina dura at apices, furcations, and/or marginal areas—this loss of lamina dura results in the widening of the periodontal ligament space. The repair phase of trauma from occlusion radiographically shows the widening of the periodontal ligament space **(Fig. 30.11)**, which may be generalized or localized. More advanced traumatic lesions may result in deep angular bone loss. In terminal stages, these lesions extend around the root apex, producing a wide radiolucent periapical image.

### Local Irritating Factors

Many local factors contribute to periodontal disease. Some of these factors can be visualized on the radiographs. These include calculus deposits **(Fig. 30.12)**, overhanging restorations **(Fig. 30.13)**, lack of local contact points, malposed teeth, partial dentures, faulty restorations, and caries. Most of the subgingival calculus deposits are undetectable on a radiograph. Hence, the clinician should not consider the absence of calculus on the radiographic image as an indication of an absence of calculus clinically.

## Skeletal Disturbances Manifested in the Jaws

Skeletal disturbances sometimes produce changes in the jaws that affect the interpretation of radiographs from the periodontal perspective.[10]

In scleroderma, the periodontal ligament is uniformly widened at the cost of the surrounding alveolar bone **(Figs. 30.14 and 30.15)**.

In osteitis fibrosa cystica (von Recklinghausen's disease of bone), there is osteoclastic resorption of bone, creating a mass known as a brown tumor. There is generalized disappearance of the lamina dura.

In Paget's disease, the normal trabecular pattern is replaced by a hazy, diffuse meshwork of closely knit, fine trabecular markings. The lamina dura is absent in it.

In fibrous dysplasia, there is a small radiolucent area at a root apex or an extensive radiolucent area with irregularly arranged trabecular markings. There may be enlargement of the cancellous spaces, distortion of the normal trabecular pattern giving a ground-glass appearance, and obliteration of the lamina dura.

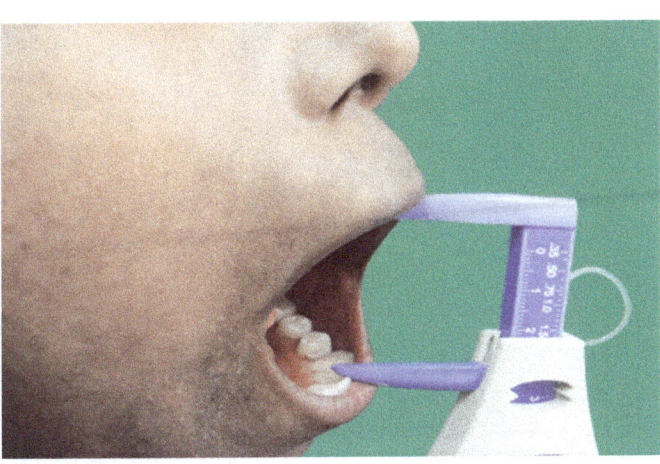

**Fig. 30.14:** Clinical picture of scleroderma patient showing restricted mouth opening.
(*Courtesy*: Dr Aneet Mahendra)

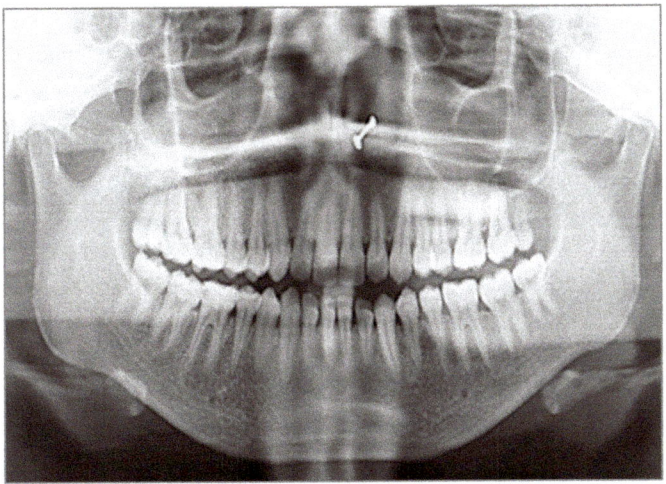

**Fig. 30.15:** Panoramic image of scleroderma showing widening of periodontal ligament and lamina dura.
(*Courtesy*: Dr Sanjeev Gupta)

In osteopetrosis, the outlines of the roots may be obscured by diffuse radiopacity of the jaws.

## LIMITATIONS

- A 2D image of complex 3D anatomy produced by conventional radiographs results in the following problems in periodontal assessment:
    - Difficult to differentiate between buccal and lingual crestal bone levels.
    - One-wall defects may obscure the rest of the defects.
    - Tooth or restoration shadows may obscure bone defects and resorption in the furcation area.
- Superimposition results in loss of the details of the bony architecture.
- Radiographs usually failed to identify the incipient disease because apparent radiographic changes require a minimum of 55–60% demineralization.
- Radiographs commonly fail to demonstrate soft-tissue contours and are unable to detect changes in the periodontium's soft tissues.
- Technique variations can affect the appearance of the periodontal tissues.
- Overexposure may lead to false interpretations—the "burn-out" phenomenon.
- Panoramic radiographs cannot be completely relied upon, although they provide a reasonable overview of the periodontal status.

## ADVANCED RADIOGRAPHIC AIDS

In a conventional system, more than 30% of the bone mass at the alveolar crest must be lost for a change in bone height in order to be recognized on radiographs. Hence, conventional radiographs are very specific but lack sensitivity.[11-13] Nowadays, many clinicians are switching to digital X-ray systems over conventional film-based images. Periodontal bone changes are usually indefinite, and hence digital subtraction radiography (DSR) technique (software algorithms) is developed to overcome shortcomings of conventional radiography.

Digital radiography permits the use of computerized images. Hence, it is easy to store, manipulate, and correct radiological images for under- and overexposures. There is an important dose reduction obtained with this technique (between one-third to half of the dose reduction compared with conventional radiographs). Two digital radiography systems rely on the sensor—the direct and indirect methods. The direct method uses a charge-coupled device (CCD) sensor linked with a fiberoptic or other wire to the computer system. This method is useful for obtaining a real-time image and helps both the clinician and the patient get an improved visualization of the periodontium by image manipulation and comparison with previously stored images. The indirect method (DIGORA system) uses a phosphor luminescence plate. This plate is a flexible film-like radiation energy sensor placed intraorally and exposed to conventional X-ray tubes. A laser scanner is used to read the exposed plates offline and unfold the digital image data, which can be enhanced, stored and compared with previous images.[12]

## Digital Subtraction Radiography

This technique uses the concept of conversion of serial radiographs into digital images. The serially obtained digital images can then be superimposed and the resultant composite viewed on a video screen. Changes in bone density and/or volume are recognized as lighter areas (bone gain) or dark areas (bone loss). In the DSR technique, a second image is taken at some point after the initial image. Both images are compared after normalization and image alignment. The unchanged elements are subtracted from the two images, and the remaining image information is displayed. Using pseudocolorization techniques, only the areas that change are visible to the dentist.

## Computer-assisted Densitometric Image Analysis System

Computer-assisted densitometric image analysis (CADIA) system uses a video camera to measure the light transmitted through a radiograph. The signals from the camera are converted into gray-scale images. The camera is interfaced with an image processor and a computer that help to store and do mathematical manipulation of the images.

## Cone-beam Computed Tomography

There are four important 3D views: (1) axial, (2) transversal or sagittal, (3) panoramic or coronal, and (4) the 3D reconstructions. The panoramic image reconstructed from the data set of cone-beam computed tomography (CBCT) differs substantially from that produced in the conventional panoramic radiograph. It can be viewed through software for the evaluation of the most comprehensive aspects of the arch. CBCT enables the planning in virtual 3D software. CBCT uses a radiation dose significantly lower than conventional computed tomography (CT). This technique enables a reduction in the radiation absorbed by the patient because it utilizes a single 360° rotation and a cone beam. At the same time, spiral CT comprises several rotations and a fan beam. The radiation dose in CBCT is about 40% smaller compared to conventional CT. However, it is still 3–7 times higher compared to that of the panoramic radiographic examinations. For an intraoral status of the entire dentition, an effective dose ranging from 33 to 84 µSv is required. Like any other diagnostic procedure involving ionizing radiation, their use should involve clinical judgment rather than routine practice. Research comparing the use of 3D volumetric images and 2D images in artificial bone defects reported 80–100% sensitivity of CBCT in the detection and classification of bone defects compared to 63–67% sensitivity of intraoral radiographs. CBCT provides high-resolution images that can be used to gather diagnostic and quantitative information on periodontal bone health. The 3D images are ideal for evaluating the infrabony defects and assessing the treatment outcomes **(Figs. 30.16A and B)**. Compared to 2D imaging, CBCT is costly and has an effective radiation dose but has lower resolution and lack of availability. The presence of metal artifacts, i.e., image flaws that are unrelated to the scanned object, is caused by metal and amalgam restorations, and, to a lesser extent, root-canal filling material implants is a major limitation of CBCT imaging. Such artifacts include streaks around materials and the presence of dark zones that affect the overall quality of the image.[14-16]

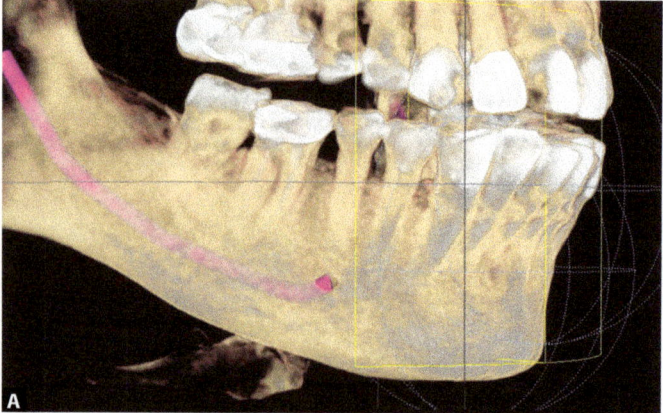
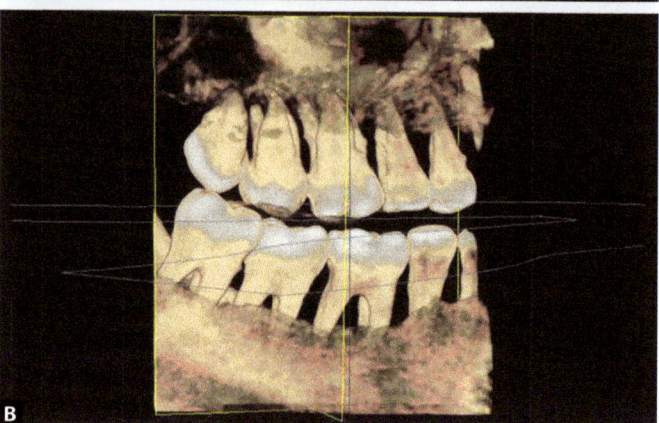

**Figs. 30.16A and B:** Radiographic image showing images of cone-beam computed tomography (CBCT): (A) Interproximal bone loss; and (B) Furcation defects.
(*Courtesy*: Dr Avani Dixit)

## Soft-tissue Cone-beam Computed Tomography

This is helpful in the measurement of gingival tissue and the dimensions of the dentogingival unit. This method uses a novel soft-tissue CBCT (ST-CBCT) technology to visualize and precisely measure distances corresponding to the hard and soft tissues of the periodontium and dentogingival attachment apparatus. This simple and non-invasive technique helps the clinicians to determine the relationships between:

- Gingival margin and the facial bone crest
- Gingival margin and the CEJ
- CEJ and facial bone crest

However, ST-CBCT images are unable to detect the differences between the epithelial, fat, and connective tissues.

### Points to Ponder

- Radiographs are useful for assessing the width of the periodontal ligament, amount of bone present, condition of the alveolar crest, and bone loss in the furcation areas.
- Furcation arrow is a small triangular radiographic shadow noted in the radiographs of maxillary molars over an either mesial or distal root in the proximal Class II or III furcation defects.
- The defect angle is one of the diagnostic radiographic parameters. During periodontal regenerative surgery, narrow periodontal defects ≤22° heal better than defects ≥36°.

## REFERENCES

1. Carranza FA, Takei HH. Radiographic aids in the diagnosis of periodontal disease. In: Newman MG, Takei HH, Carranza FA (Eds). Carranza's Clinical Periodontology, 9th edition. Philadelphia, PA, USA: WB Saunders; 2003. pp. 454-68.
2. Prichard JF. Advanced Periodontal Disease: Surgical and Prosthetic Management, 2nd edition. Philadelphia, PA, USA: Saunders; 1972.
3. Karjodkar FR. Periodontal tissues and periodontal diseases. In: Textbook of Dental and Maxillofacial Radiology, 2nd edition. New Delhi, India: Jaypee Brothers Medical Publishers; 2009. pp. 419-32.
4. Whaites E, Drage N. Periodontal tissues, and periodontal diseases. In: Essentials of Dental Radiography and Radiology, 3rd edition. Philadelphia, PA, USA: Churchill Livingstone; 2003. pp. 241-52.
5. Miles DA, Thomas MV. Radiography for the periodontal examination. In: Rose LF, Mealey BL, Genco RJ, Cohen DW (Eds). Periodontics, Medicine, Surgery, and Implants, 1st edition. Philadelphia, PA, USA: Elsevier Mosby; 2004. pp. 146-61.
6. White SC, Pharoah MJ. Periodontal tissues and periodontal diseases. In: Oral Radiology: Principles and Interpretation, 5th edition. St. Louis: Mosby; 2000. pp. 314-29.
7. Reddy MS. Radiographic methods in the evaluation of periodontal therapy. J Periodontol. 1992;63(12 Suppl):1078-84.
8. Tsitoura E, Tucker R, Suvan J, Luarell L, Cortellini P, Tonetti M. Baseline radiographic defect angle of the intrabony defect as a prognostic indicator in regenerative periodontal surgery with enamel matrix derivative. J Clin Periodontol. 2004:31(8):643-7.
9. Rees TD, Biggs NL, Collings CK. Radiographic interpretation of periodontal osseous lesions. Oral Surg Oral Med Oral Pathol. 1971;32(1):141-53.
10. Shafer WG, Hine MG, Levy BM. Diseases of bone and joints. In: A Textbook of Oral Pathology, 4th edition. Philadelphia, PA, USA: WB Saunders; 1983. pp. 674-718.
11. Khocht A, Janal M, Harasty L, Chang KM. Comparison of direct digital and conventional intraoral radiographs in detecting alveolar bone loss. J Am Dent Assoc. 2003;134(11):1468-75.
12. Sanz M, Newman MG. Advanced diagnostic techniques. In: Newman MG, Takei HH, Carranza FA (Eds). Carranza's Clinical Periodontology, 9th edition. Philadelphia, PA, USA: WB Saunders; 2003. pp. 487-502.
13. Mol A. Imaging methods in periodontology. Periodontol 2000. 2004;34:34-48.
14. Aljehani YA. Diagnostic applications of cone-beam CT for periodontal diseases. Int J Dent. 2014;2014:865079.
15. Acar B, Kamburoğlu K. Use of cone-beam computed tomography in periodontology. World J Radiol. 2014;6(5):139-47.
16. Tyndall DA, Rathore S. Cone-beam CT diagnostic applications: caries, periodontal bone assessment, and endodontic applications. Dent Clin North Am. 2008;52(4):825-41.

## VIVA VOCE

**Q1.** Name various ways to improve the reproducibility and accuracy of dental radiographs.
**Ans.** Various ways to improve the reproducibility and accuracy of dental radiographs are:
- The use of film holders
- The paralleling technique
- A low-dosage technique combining E-speed film and rectangular collimation.

**Q2.** Which radiographic technique produces the idealistic image of the level of alveolar bone?
**Ans.** The long cone paralleling technique produces the idealistic image of the level of alveolar bone.

**Q3.** What is the minimum number of intraoral periapical (IOPA) radiographs that should be taken for a radiographic survey of complete periodontium?
**Ans.** The minimum number of IOPA radiographs that should be taken for the radiographic survey of the complete periodontium is 14.

**Q4.** What is the difference range between the actual alveolar crestal height and radiographic alveolar crestal height?
**Ans.** The difference range between the actual alveolar crestal height and radiographic alveolar crestal height is 0–1.6 mm.

**Q5.** What are the disadvantages associated with CBCT?
**Ans.** The disadvantages associated with CBCT are machine cost, complexity, high radiation, and relatively low resolution.

**Q6.** Write the radiation dosage of various radiographs.
**Ans.**

| Types of radiograph | Radiation dosage |
| --- | --- |
| Full mouth radiographs with F-speed film with rectangular collimation | 34.9 µSv |
| Four-image posterior bitewings with The F-speed film with rectangular collimation | 5.0 µSv |
| Panoramic oral radiographs (orthopantomograph) | 14.2 µSv |
| Cone-beam computed tomography | 33–1,073 µSv |

**Q7.** Which radiograph is used for severe generalized periodontitis?
**Ans.** Panoramic or periapical radiograph of standing teeth.

**Q8.** What radiograph is useful in examining the teeth' proximal surfaces and the crest of the alveolar bone of both the maxilla and the mandible on the same film?
**Ans.** Bitewing radiograph.

**Q9.** Name important 3D views of CBCT.
**Ans.** Axial; transversal or sagittal; panoramic or coronal and 3D reconstructions.

**Q10.** Which irritating local factors are visualized on a radiograph?
**Ans.** Calculus deposits, overhanging restorations, lack of local contact points, malposed teeth, partial dentures, faulty restorations, and caries.

# Microbiological Diagnostic Aids

*Vishakha Grover, Shalu Bathla*

## Chapter Outline

- Indications
- Biomarkers
- Candidates for Biomarkers
- Limitations

## INTRODUCTION

Subgingival oral bacteria are the main initiating agents in the development of periodontal diseases; thus, it is logical to look for specific bacteria through the various microbiological methods. These microbiologic tests have potential relevance to both diagnosis and treatment because current clinical diagnostic methods are not precisely accurate and only allow retrospective diagnosis of attachment and bone loss. Thus, diagnostic tests would need to be predictive of disease activity rather than just correlate with its occurrence.

## INDICATIONS

Following are the indications of microbiologic assays:
- *During diagnosis and treatment planning*: Some chronic periodontitis patients do not exhibit good responses to local mechanical and chemical periodontal therapy. These patients include those with refractory periodontitis, recurrent periodontitis, and aggressive periodontitis. Microbiological assays are often indicated in these patients as an adjunct to the usual clinical and radiographic examinations in the formulation of an etiology-based diagnosis.[1]
- *To monitor treatment efficacy*: Microbiologic assays can tell the clinician if the mechanical, surgical and chemotherapeutic approach has been effective in eliminating the microbial etiology identified initially.
- *To select an appropriate recall interval*: After periodontal therapy has been completed, microbiologic tests using pooled plaque samples can be useful in determining the rate of reinfection, if any, by periodontal pathogens as an additional parameter to be assessed in determining an individual patient's optimum recall interval.
- *To determine sites of "active" tissue destruction*: Appropriate samples for analysis of site-specific tissue destruction include subgingival plaque from the site or tooth in question, and these can be analyzed by rapid tests targeted to specific periodontal pathogens.
- To identify antibiotic susceptibility of infecting organisms colonizing diseased sites.
- For the prevention of periodontitis in persons "at-risk" for either the initial onset of periodontal disease or recurrent disease.

## BIOMARKERS

A biomarker is a substance that is measured objectively and evaluated as an indicator of normal biologic processes, pathogenic processes, or pharmacological responses to a therapeutic intervention.[2]

### Sources of Biomarkers

Various potential sources of biomarkers are:
- Blood
- Gingival crevicular fluid (GCF)
- *Saliva*: Salivary biomarker analysis provides some advantages over GCF. Collecting saliva sample is very easy, noninvasive, and rapid. Also, it requires less manpower and fewer materials as compared to the analysis of GCF.
- Plaque biofilm

### Methods of Sampling

Subgingival plaque is considered as the ideal plaque sample for analysis. It is located near the gingiva and epithelial attachment and is found to carry higher numbers

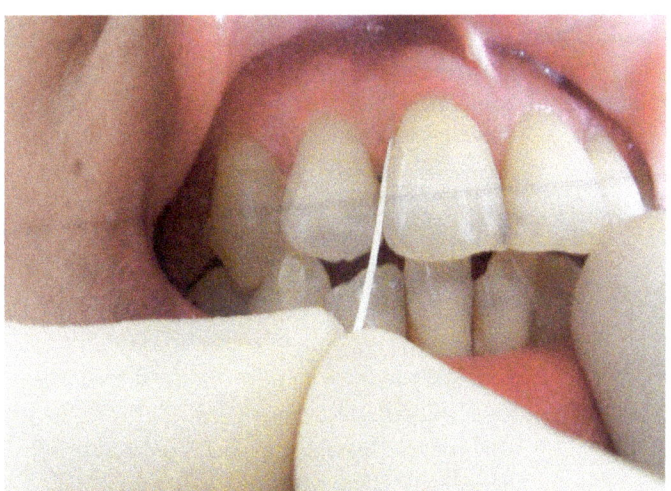

**Fig. 31.1:** Clinical picture showing a sampling of the subgingival plaque using paper point.

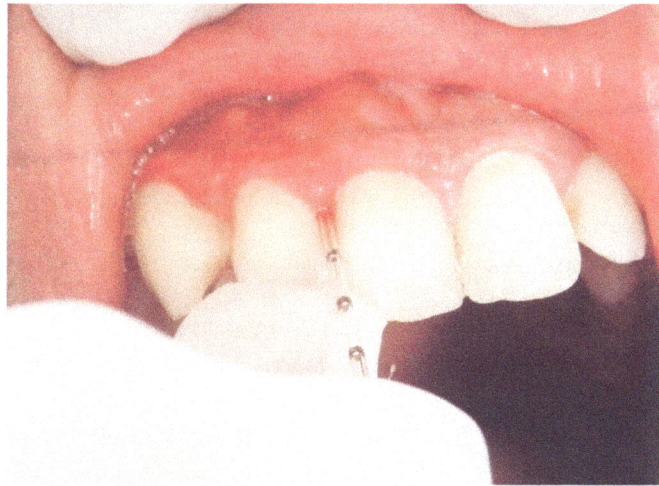

**Fig. 31.2:** Clinical picture showing a sampling of the gingival crevicular fluid using a micropipette.
(*Courtesy*: Dr Harsh Kapil)

and proportions of pathogenic microorganisms than supragingival plaque.

Subgingival dental plaque can be sampled in several ways. A one expeditious and noninvasive method for sampling subgingival dental plaque involves using sterile endodontic paper points **(Fig. 31.1)**. In this method, an appropriate site or site of interest is chosen and delineated with cotton rolls to avoid contamination of the sample with bacteria in saliva and then allow for air dry. Supragingival plaque is removed using either a sterile cotton pellet or a sterile curette. The instrument is moved in a coronal direction to avoid pushing supragingival plaque into subgingival space. Subgingival plaque can also, be sampled using a sterile curette. Again, after the sample site has been isolated and the supragingival dental plaque removed as described above, a curette is placed to the depth of the gingival sulcus/periodontal pocket and moved coronally with firm lateral pressure against the root surface. The material is then dislodged from the curette tip into the transport medium, sterilized in a salt sterilizer, and then used to sample the next site. Some investigators advocate using nickel-plated curettes to avoid oxidation within the sample and the death of oxygen intolerant anaerobic microorganisms.

### *Gingival Crevicular Fluid*

The various GCF collection methods are absorbing filter paper strips, pre-weighed twisted threads, and micropipettes **(Fig. 31.2)**. Rest is explained in "Chapter 17: Defense Mechanisms of Gingiva."

## CANDIDATES FOR BIOMARKERS

The leading candidates in the search for biomarkers are:[3]
- Microorganisms (bacteria)
- Bacterial products (enzymes)
- Inflammatory and immune products
- Host derived enzymes
- Enzymes released from dead cells
- Connective-tissue degradation products
- Products of bone resorption and formation

These are procured from the patients/sites undergoing the progression of periodontitis.[4]

## Microorganisms (Bacteria)

The bacterial plaque has a potential role in the initiation and progression of periodontal diseases. Still, the composition of the subgingival flora is complex and may vary from patient to patient and site to site. Samples from the oral mucosa or saliva are obtained with sterile paper points or swabs and then transferred directly into an appropriate anaerobic transport medium.

The various diagnostic aids **(Table 31.1)** for detecting bacteria are:
- Culture techniques
- Dark-field microscopy
- Immunodiagnostic methods
- Deoxyribonucleic acid (DNA) probes
- Polymerase chain reaction (PCR)

### *Culture Techniques*

Culture techniques are helpful to identify and characterize the composition of the subgingival microflora. Until now, they are selected as the reference method (gold standard) for determining the performance of new microbial diagnostic methods.[5]

*Advantages:*
- It gives both relative and absolute count of the cultured species.
- It can assess for antibiotic susceptibility of microbes.

**Section 5:** Diagnosis

**TABLE 31.1:** Various microbiological aids.

| Method | Usage/Principle | Disadvantage |
| --- | --- | --- |
| Culture techniques | Culturing of oral specimens on a medium to detect viable bacteria<br>Antibiotic sensitivity | Some bacteria are fastidious and difficult to culture<br>Require strict sampling and transport conditions<br>Require experienced personnel |
| Dark-field microscopy | Directly assess the morphology and motility of bacteria in the sample | Detects only motile bacteria |
| Enzymatic methods | Measurement of enzymatic activities produced by periopathogens<br>Commercial kits are available | Cannot identify bacterial species |
| Immunodiagnostic methods | Detection of specific bacteria using antibodies<br>Available for specific bacteria | Cannot discriminate between living and dead cells<br>Requires special techniques |
| PCR | Detection of bacteria by DNA amplification<br>Highly sensitive | Cannot discriminate between viable and dead bacteria<br>Requires a thermal cycler |

(PCR: polymerase chain reaction; DNA: deoxyribonucleic acid)

*Disadvantages:*
- Putative pathogens, such as *Treponemas* and *Tannerella forsythia,* are fastidious and difficult to culture.
- Strict sampling and transport conditions are essential.
- Time-consuming and expensive.
- Sophisticated types of equipment and experienced personnel are required.
- It can only grow live bacteria.

### Dark-field Microscopy

Dark-field or phase-contrast microscopy has been suggested as an alternative to culture methods based on its ability to directly and rapidly assess the morphology and motility of bacteria in a plaque sample.

*Advantages:*
- Through it, motile spirochetes are seen.
- Assessment can be done during progression and treatment.

*Disadvantages:*
- Unable to identify nonmotile species.
- Unable to recognize the various species of Treponema.
- Inability to determine their relative susceptibility to an antimicrobial agent.

### Immunodiagnostic Methods

Immunologic assays are based on the concept of using antibodies to identify specific bacterial antigens to detect target microorganisms. The various immunodiagnostic procedures are direct and indirect immunofluorescent microscopy assays (IFA), flow cytometry, and latex agglutination.
- *IFA*: Direct IFA uses both monoclonal and polyclonal antibodies conjugated to a fluorescein marker. These antibodies get bind with the bacterial antigen and lead to the formation of fluorescent immune-complex, which is detectable under a microscope. Indirect IFA uses a secondary fluorescein-conjugated antibody, which interacts with the primary antigen-antibody complex. Both direct and indirect immunofluorescence assays are helpful to recognize the causative pathogen and directly quantify the percentage of the pathogen with the use of plaque smear **(Fig. 31.3)**.
- *Flow cytometry*: It is another useful diagnostic method, which contains labelling of bacterial cells from a patient plaque sample with both species-specific antibody and a second fluorescein-conjugated antibody. The suspension is poured into the flow cytometer. With the use of the laminar flow technique, passing through a narrow tube flow cytometer easily separates the bacterial cells into an almost single-cell suspension. The disadvantages associated with it is the sophistication and procedure cost.
- *Latex agglutination*: It involves binding the protein to latex, where latex beads are coated with the

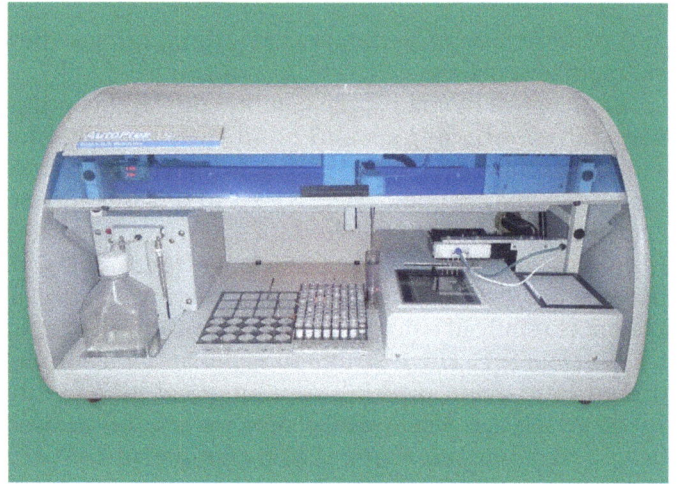

**Fig. 31.3:** Photograph showing autoplex enzyme-linked immunosorbent assays and chemiluminescence immunoassay (CLIA).
(*Courtesy*: Dr Swantika Chaudhry)

species-specific antibody. When these beads come in proximity with the microbial cell surface, antigens or antigen extracts lead to cross-linking formation. Such agglutination or clumping is usually visible in 2–5 minutes.

*Commercial diagnostic test kit*: Evalusite is a chairside kit consisting of enzyme-linked immunosorbent assays (ELISA) that uses antibodies to antigens detection. It is used to detect *Aggregatibacter actinomycetemcomitans*, *Porphyromonas gingivalis,* and *Prevotella intermedius*.

*Advantages:* Identify dead target cells, thus not requiring stringent sampling and transport methodology.

*Disadvantages:*
- Local sampling cannot be done, so site-specific disease parameters cannot be assessed.
- Immunoassays cannot be used to determine bacterial virulence.
- It cannot be used to determine antibiotic susceptibility.

### Deoxyribonucleic Acid Probes

Deoxyribonucleic acid probes are useful in recognizing nucleotide sequences that are specific for bacteria. Because of this property, it holds important diagnostic significance in identifying suspected periodontal pathogens. DNA probes involve segments of single-stranded nucleic acid, which are labeled with an enzyme or radioisotope. They identify and bind to their complementary nucleic acid sequences with low cross-reactivity to nontarget organisms. DNA probe can target whole genomic DNA or individual genes. To prepare the probe, specific pathogens used as marker organisms are lysed to remove their DNA. Their double-helix is denatured, creating single strands that are individually labeled with a radioactive isotope. Subsequently, when a plaque sample is sent for analysis, it undergoes lysis and denaturation. Single strands are chemically treated, attached to a special filter paper, and then exposed to the DNA library. If complementary base pairs hybridize (cross-link), the radiolabeled strands will also be fixed to the filter paper. After the filter is washed to remove any unhybridized strands, it is covered with a radiographic plate. The radioactive labels create spots on the film, which are read with a densitometer. The darkness and size of the spots indicate the concentration of the organisms present in the given plaque sample. The assay can rapidly test for multiple bacteria, including *A. actinomycetemcomitans, P. gingivalis, B. intermedius, Campylobacter rectus, Eikenella corrodens, Fusobacterium nucleatum,* and *Treponema denticola* in multiple clinical plaque samples. The probes can detect as few as $10^2$ to $10^4$ bacteria.

*Commercial diagnostic test kit*: OmniGene is a commercially available DNA probe system for detecting the number of subgingival bacteria. The procedure involves placing a paper point sample of subgingival plaque in the provided container and mailing off to the company for assay. Microorganisms detected through DNA probe are *A. actinomycetemcomitans, P. gingivalis, B. intermedius, C. rectus, E. corrodens, T. denticola,* and *F. nucleatum*.[6,7]

### Polymerase Chain Reaction

Kary Mullis first conceptualized the process of PCR in 1985. There is amplification by exponential multiplication of specific fragments of DNA during successive cycles. PCR cycle has three phases which are carried in an instrument called thermocycler at different temperatures (**Fig. 31.4**):

1. *Denaturation (strand separation)*: This phase is carried at 94–96°C for 20–30 seconds, the double-helical arrangement of the sample template DNA is denatured yielding a single-stranded DNA molecule.
2. *Annealing (primer-binding)*: This phase allows annealing of primers to the single-stranded DNA template at a lower temperature of 68°C for 20–40 seconds.
3. *The extension (new DNA synthesis)*: This final phase of the cycle occurs at 72°C; the Taq DNA polymerase enzyme is added to the reaction mixture to make the primer extend along the length of the DNA strand. At the end of this phase, a complementary strand is formed for each DNA strand of the sample DNA that was denatured.

A standard amplification usually consists of 25–35 cycles resulting in the formation of billion copies of the original sample DNA, which can then be visualized.[8] The existence of the specific amplification product is usually suggestive of the presence of the target microorganism. Hence, this method is useful to recognize the number of periodontopathic bacteria at periodontal sites quantitatively. This property makes the procedure valuable in the evaluation of therapeutic efficacy.

Various types of PCR are simplex, nested, multiplex, and real-time PCR.

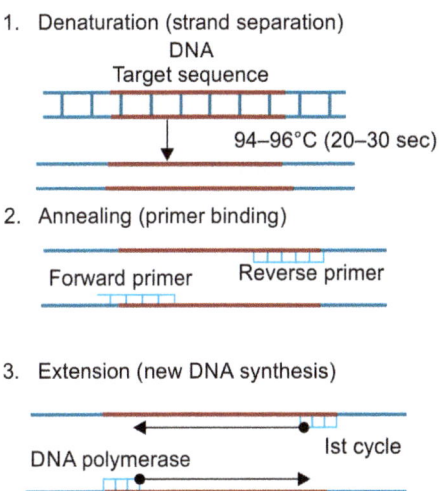

**Fig. 31.4:** Schematic representation showing polymerase chain reaction.
(DNA: deoxyribonucleic acid)

*Advantages:*
- *Specific*: It helps to identify specific bacteria.
- *Relatively sensitive*: Single-molecule of DNA in the sample can be detected. The procedure has significant potential to produce millions to billions of copies of a specific product for sequencing, cloning, and analysis.
- *Rapid*: The process may take just a few hours to a day.
- A variety of samples from different sources can be tested simultaneously.
- It can detect and identify even when no viable organisms present in the sample and the organisms that are difficult to cultivate.

*Disadvantages:*
- It cannot discriminate between viable and dead bacteria.
- Not useful for sensitivity tests guiding for the selection of antibiotics.
- Since small samples are used for the amplification process, if this small quantity of the plaque sample does not contain the targeted microorganism, the assay will not detect it.
- Subgingival plaque contains enzymes that can alter the amplification process.
- Require thermocycler, specific primers, and reagents.
- Expensive.
- Require experienced personnel.

*Commercial diagnostic test kit*: Commercially, a PCR-based diagnostic method is available for the detection of periodontopathic species in subgingival plaque samples (MicroDent test), which is quick, easy to use, and more sensitive compared to culture methods.

## Bacterial Products (Enzyme)

*Enzymatic method of bacterial identification (BANA test):* A trypsin-like enzyme is produced by *Tannerella forsythia, P. gingivalis,* the small spirochete *T. denticola,* and *Capnocytophaga* species. The activity of trypsin is usually measured with the hydrolysis of the colorless substrate N-benzoyl-DL-arginine-2-naphthylamide hydrochloride (BANA). During hydrolysis, it produces the chromophore, β-naphthylamide. This product turns into orange-red color on adding a drop of fast garnet to the solution. Positive BANA test is the indication of the presence of *T. denticola, P. gingivalis* at the sampled sites and thus risk indicator for periodontal attachment loss.[9]

*Disadvantages:*
- Nonavailability of quantitative data.
- It fails to identify which of the three bacteria is responsible for enzyme production.
- BANA system does not include inhibitors of host proteinases, which could cleave this substrate and could also contaminate the bacterial sample tested.
- It cannot identify the presence of other pathogens that do not produce trypsin-like enzymes.

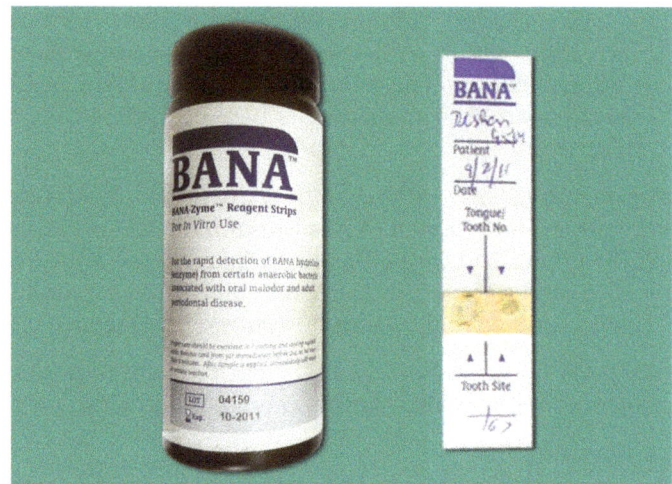

**Fig. 31.5:** Photograph showing BANA (N-benzoyl-DL-arginine-β-naphthylamide hydrochloride) chairside kit.
(*Courtesy*: Dr Harveen)

*Commercial diagnostic test kit*: Perioscan is a chairside diagnostic test kit system that utilizes the BANA test to detect bacteria producing trypsin-like proteases (**Fig. 31.5**). The bacteria detected through Perioscan are *T. denticola, P. gingivalis, T. forsythia,* and *Capnocytophaga*.

## Volatile Sulfur Compounds

Gram-negative bacteria *P. gingivalis, Prevotella intermedia, Prevotella melaninogenica, T. forsythia, T. denticola,* and *F. nucleatum* have been shown to be capable of producing hydrogen sulfide ($H_2S$), methyl mercaptan ($CH_3SH$), dimethyl disulfide [$(CH_3)_2S_2$] through their metabolic pathways.

*Commercial diagnostic test kit*: The diamond probe is a recently developed instrument, which combines the features of a periodontal probe with the silver sulfide sensor for the detection of volatile sulfur compounds.

## Inflammatory and Immune Products

The microorganisms also trigger inflammatory and immune host responses, which, along with the direct effects of the bacteria, cause most of the tissue destruction. Several substances are released from inflammatory and immune cells into the tissues, and many of these pass into GCF and are thus, easily available for analysis. Samples of these substances can usually be obtained from GCF through paper strips.

### Immune Response

Patients with various forms of periodontal disease produce antibodies to antigens from periodontopathogens. These antibodies, total immunoglobulin G (IgG) and IgG subgroups and complement component, can be detected in serum, saliva, gingival tissue, and GCF.

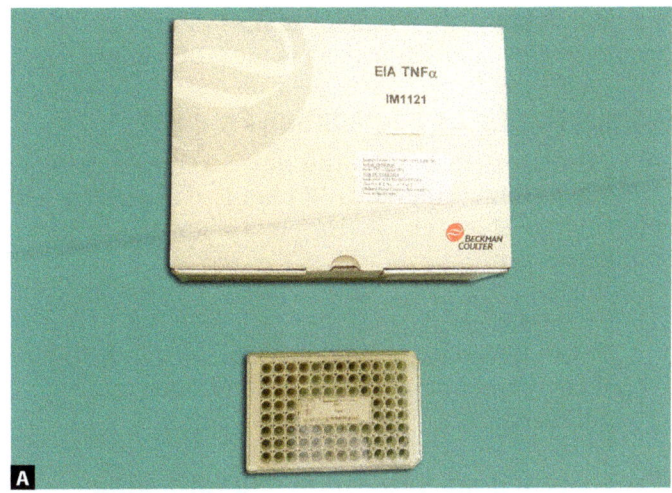 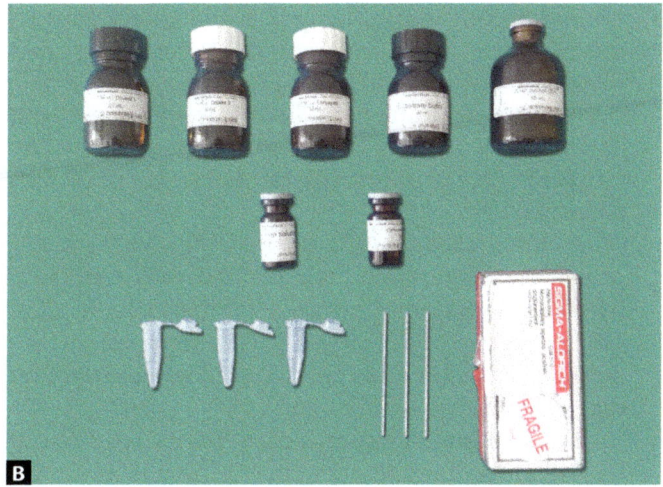

**Figs. 31.6A and B:** Photograph showing (A) Tumor necrosis factor-alpha (TNF-α) estimation kit; (B) TNF-α estimation kit components and 0–5 μL microcapillary tubes.
(*Courtesy*: Dr Swantika Chaudhry)

## Inflammatory Mediators

*Arachidonic acid derivatives*: Prostaglandin $E_2$ is a product of the cyclooxygenase pathway of the metabolism of arachidonic acid. It is a potent mediator of inflammation and induces bone resorption. The concentration of prostaglandin $E_2$ found in GCF is increased during active phases of periodontal destruction, whereas levels are low in health.

*Cytokines*: These are best described as cell-to-cell messengers or local hormones. They are all small proteins or peptides which are produced and released by one cell type so they can link onto a specific receptor on the cell membrane of another cell(s) of either the same type or another type(s). The best-known examples of cytokines are the interleukins (ILs), which pass messages between the leukocytes. IL-α and IL-β are present in inflamed gingiva. They are also present in GCF of patients with periodontitis with extremely low concentrations at healthy sites. IL-8 is secreted by monocytes, macrophages, and vascular endothelial cells and mediates chemotaxis and neutrophils activation. Their levels are reduced in periodontal destruction.

Commercial diagnostic test kits:
- *Periocheck* detects the presence of neutral proteinase, such as collagenase in GCF. The GCF sample is collected by paper strip and is placed in contact with a collagen gel to which a blue dye has been covalently bonded. It is then incubated at 43°C. If the neutral proteinase is present in the sample, then they will attack the collagen gel and release the blue dye producing the blue color in the strip. The intensity of the color is proportional to the amount of enzyme present in the sample. The intensity and the blue color area are then scored on a scale of 0–2 by comparing it with three standards on a color card, which is provided with the test kit.
- A chairside kit consisting of ELISA is used to detect tumor necrosis factor-alpha (TNF-α) **(Figs. 31.6A and B)**.

## Host-derived Enzymes

Various enzymes are released from host cells during the initiation and progression of periodontal disease. The enzymes, which are used as markers of active periodontal destruction, are aspartate aminotransferase (AST), elastase, β-glucuronidase, alkaline phosphatase, arylsulfatase, neutral proteases, cathepsins, lactate dehydrogenase (LDH), matrix metalloproteinases (MMPs) and myeloperoxidase (MPO).

- *Cathepsins*: They are a group of acidic lysosomal enzymes playing a significant role in the degradation of the intracellular protein.
- *Alkaline phosphatase*: It is a membrane-bound enzyme. It is a glycoprotein in nature and presents in most of the body tissues, including the liver, bone, and intestine. Many cells, such as fibroblasts, osteoblasts, and osteoclasts, produce alkaline phosphatase. However, the important source of its production is neutrophils found in gingival crevice fluid. At alkaline pH, it hydrolyzes monophosphate ester bonds and enhances local concentrations of phosphate ions. An alkaline phosphatase level in gingival crevice fluid is also increased by bacteria present in the sulcus or pocket. Hence, a significant increase in alkaline phosphatase level in gingival crevice fluid is considered as a potential diagnostic marker for periodontitis.[10] Occasionally high levels of alkaline phosphatase have been noted in naturally occurring and experimental gingivitis.
- *β-glucuronidase*: Primary granules of neutrophil produces β-glucuronidase. It is a lysosomal enzyme and mainly hydrolyze the glycosyl bonds of intercellular ground substance.

- *Cathepsin B*: It is a proteolytic enzyme belonging to the class of cysteine proteinases. It is considered that in gingival crevice fluid macrophages possibly secrete, cathepsin-B. Chronic periodontitis is associated with cathepsin-B activity in GCF. Cathepsin-B activity enhances in periodontitis but is not increased in gingivitis.
- *Matrix metalloproteinases*: These are primary proteinases involved in periodontal tissue destruction by the degradation of extracellular matrix molecules. MMPs levels, especially MMP-8, increase at the periodontitis sites and thus are used as a method for detecting destructive periodontitis.[11]
- *Myeloperoxidase*: It is a peroxidase enzyme synthesized by polymorphonuclear leukocytes. It acts as potent antibacterial enzyme and salivary myeloperoxidase levels significantly enhance in untreated chronic periodontitis patients compared with healthy counterparts.
- *Lysozyme*: It is an antibacterial enzyme, particularly present in body secretions. Their levels are reduced in chronic periodontitis patients.
- *Elastase*: Neutrophil elastase is the serine proteinase in nature and released abundantly from the azurophilic granules of neutrophils. It is also termed as granulocyte elastase and acts as an indicator of neutrophil activity. Neutrophil elastase plays an essential role in the degradation of microbiological components, which may occur with or without phagocytosis. It can degrade host intercellular matrix components, including elastin, fibronectin, and collagen. Macrophage elastase, also called MMP-12, may exhibit the same activities as neutrophil elastase. In periodontitis patients, elastase levels are found to increase in GCF.

## Enzymes Released by Dead Cells

Enzymes released from dead cells are aspartate aminotransferase and lactate dehydrogenase.

### Aspartate Aminotransferase

This is an enzyme released from dead cells from a variety of tissues throughout the body, including the heart after myocardial infarction and the liver during hepatitis. The level of AST in GCF elevates at sites with gingival inflammation and progressive attachment loss.[12]

*Commercial diagnostic test kits*: *Periogard* is a rapid chairside test kit for AST. The test includes a collection of GCF with a filter paper strip, which is then placed in the tromethamine hydrochloride buffer. A substrate reaction mixture containing L-aspartic and α-ketoglutaric acids are added and allowed to react for 10 minutes. In the presence of AST, the aspartate and α-glutarate are catalyzed to oxaloacetate and glutamate. The addition of a dye, such as fast red, results in a color product, the intensity of which is proportional to the AST activity in the GCF sample.

## Connective Tissue Degradation Products

In periodontitis, there is the destruction of collagen and extracellular matrix. GCF obtained from sites with periodontitis shows elevated levels of following breakdown products:
- Collagen (hydroxyproline, collagen cross-links, and N-peptide).
- Proteoglycans [glycosaminoglycans (GAGs), heparin sulfate, chondroitin 6 sulfate, chondroitin 4 sulfate].
- Fibronectin.

## Products of Bone Resorption and Formation

Few markers suggestive of bone resorption and subsequently periodontal disease activity are pyridinium cross-link collagen peptide fragment, tartrate-resistant acid phosphatase (TRAP), galactosyl hydroxylysine (GHYL), hydroxyproline, N-terminal osteocalcin fragment, and GAGs. Pyridinoline cross-links of the carboxy-terminal telopeptide of type I collagen is identified as a good marker of bone collagen degradation. This degradation product of bone was initially recognized as a GCF marker for the progression of periodontitis. Bone formation markers are type I procollagen propeptide, alkaline phosphatase, osteocalcin, and bone Gla protein (BGP) mineralization.

## LIMITATIONS

The various limitations and inconsistency of microbiologic aids are due to:
- *Technical problems*: It includes difficulties in processing and collecting samples. It also includes challenges in the cultivation of plaque microorganisms and identification of isolates.[13]
- *Conceptual problems*: There is the complexity of the periodontal microbiota. Periodontal infections are mixed infections, in which it is difficult to distinguish secondary invaders from true pathogens.
- *Problems associated with the nature of periodontal diseases*: Differentiation between active and inactive sites for sampling is difficult as periodontal diseases appear to be episodic.

### Points to Ponder

- The DNA probe is not an instrument but an agent that binds directly to a predefined sequence of nucleic acids. These are synthesized in the laboratory, with a sequence complementary to the target DNA sequence.
- Enzymatic methods do not identify specific bacteria and thus are not helpful in the selection of antibiotics.
- Enzymatic and PCR methods are used for the qualitative examination of periopathogens.

## REFERENCES

1. Zambon JJ. Microbial diagnosis in periodontal therapy. In: Genco RJ, Goldman HM, Cohen DW (EDs). Contemporary Periodontics, 1st edition. St. Louis: CV Mosby; 1990. pp. 449-58.
2. Taba M, Kinney J, Kim AS, Giannobile WV. Diagnostic biomarkers for oral and periodontal diseases. Dent Clin North Am. 2005;49(3):551-71.
3. Eley BM, Manson JD. Diagnostic tests of periodontal disease activity. In: Periodontics, 5th edition. Edinburgh, Scotland: Wright Publishing; 2004. pp. 161-88.
4. Armitage GC. Research, Science, and Therapy Committee of the American Academy of Periodontology. Diagnosis of periodontal diseases. J Periodontol. 2003;74(8):1237-47.
5. Sanz M, Newman MG. Advanced diagnostic techniques. In: Newman MG, Takei HH, Carranza FA (Eds). Carranza's Clinical Periodontology, 9th edition. WB Saunders; 2003. pp. 487-502.
6. Yoshida A, Nagashima S, Ansai T, Tachibana M, Kato H, Watari H, et al. Loop-mediated isothermal amplification method for rapid detection of the periodontopathic bacteria Porphyromonas gingivalis, Tannerella forsythia, and Treponema denticola. J Clin Microbiol. 2005;43(5):2418-24.
7. Osawa R, Yoshida A, Masakiyo Y, Nagashima S, Ansai T, Watari H, et al. Rapid detection of *Actinobacillus actinomycetemcomitans* using a loop-mediated isothermal amplification method. Oral Microbiol Immunol. 2007;22(4):252-9.
8. Ananthanarayan R, Paniker CK. Recent advance in diagnostic techniques in clinical microbiology. In: Ananthanarayan and Paniker's Textbook of Microbiology, 8th edition. New Delhi, India: Universities Press; 2009. pp. 686-700.
9. Loesche WJ. The identification of bacteria associated with periodontal disease and dental caries by enzymatic methods. Oral Microbiol Immunol. 1986;1(1):65-72.
10. Lamster IB, Oshrain RL, Harper DS, Celenti RS, Hovliaras CA, Gordon JM. Enzyme activity in crevicular fluid for the detection and prediction of clinical attachment loss in patients with chronic adult periodontitis. Six-month results. J Periodontol. 1988;59(8):516-23.
11. Sorsa T, Golup LM, Lee HM, Ryan ME, Kallis GB, Lundquist C, et al. The anti-collagenolytic effect of low-dose doxycycline (LDD) regimen in adult human periodontitis from gingival crevicular fluid (GCF) can be monitored by the immunological test for neutrophil collagenase (MMP-8). J Dent Res. 1998;77:647.
12. Persson GR, Page RC. Diagnostic characteristics of crevicular fluid aspartate aminotransferase (AST) levels associated with periodontal disease activity. J Clin Periodontol. 1992;19(1):43-8.
13. Listgarten MA. Microbiological testing in the diagnosis of periodontal diseases. J Periodontol 1992;63(4 Suppl):332-7.

## VIVA VOCE

**Q1. What is LAMP?**
**Ans.** Loop-mediated isothermal amplification (LAMP) is a modification of the PCR, which was developed by Eiken Chemical Corporation Limited, Japan. This is one of the most rapid bacterial diagnostic methods that takes around 1 hour and requires no special detection equipment; thus, it can be observed through the naked eye only. It rapidly detects *P. gingivalis, T. forsythia, T. denticola* and *A. actinomycetemcomitans*.[6,7]

**Q2. What is the difference between BAPNA and BANA test?**
**Ans.** In the BANA test, the peptide substrate is N-Benzoyl DL- arginine-2-naphthylamide. In this test, an additional color developer, i.e., fast garnet, is added.
In the BAPNA test, the peptide substrate is Benzoyl DL- arginine-p-nitroanilide. In this test, there is no need for an additional color developer as this peptide substrate forms a color when it hydrolyzes.

**Q3. What are the various types of DNA probe?**
**Ans.**
- Closed DNA probe
- Randomly cloned probe
- Whole genomic DNA probe
- Synthetic oligonucleotide probe

**Q4. Which microscope is used to visualize spirochetes?**
**Ans.** Dark Field microscopy.

**Q5. Name various commercial diagnostic kits.**
**Ans.**
- *Perioscan*—BANA (N-benzoyl-DL-arginine-2- naphthylamide hydrochloride) test kit
- *OmniGene*—DNA (deoxyribonucleic acid) probe system
- *Periogard*—Aspartate aminotransferase (AST) kit
- *Evalusite*—ELISA (enzyme-linked immunosorbent assays) kit.

**Q6. What are the various potential sources of biomarkers?**
**Ans.** Blood; GCF; saliva and plaque biofilm.

**Q7. What is evalusite?**
**Ans.** Evalusite is a chairside kit consisting of enzyme-linked immunosorbent assays (ELISA) that uses antibodies to detect antigens. It is used to detect *Aggregatibacter actinomycetemcomitans, Porphyromonas gingivalis,* and *Prevotella intermedius*.

**Q8. What is the use of periocheck?**
**Ans.** Periocheck detects the presence of neutral proteinase, such as collagenase in GCF.

**Q9. Which bacteria can be detected through perioscan?**
**Ans.** *T. denticola, P. gingivalis, T. forsythia* and *Capnocytophaga*.

**Q10. What are the three phases of polymerase chain reaction?**
**Ans.** Denaturation (strand separation); annealing (primer binding); extension (new DNA synthesis).

# Chapter 32

# Clinical Risk Assessment

*Deepika Bali, Shalu Bathla*

## Chapter Outline

- Definitions
- Risk Factors
- Risk Determinants
- Risk Indicators
- Risk Markers
- Risk Assessment

## INTRODUCTION

Infectious agents induced tissue loss is the hallmark of chronic inflammatory disease. However, destructive periodontal disease differs from other chronic inflammatory diseases as infectious agents' presence does not necessarily lead to the development of periodontal tissue loss. Moreover, it is identified that only a subset of individuals and a limited percentage of sites in these affected individuals will exhibit severe periodontal tissue loss. Such findings arouse interest in identifying susceptible individuals and associated risk factors that make the individual prone to develop these diseases. Cross-sectional studies are significantly beneficial in the identification of risk indicators or markers.

## DEFINITIONS

*Risk*: It is defined as the probability that an event will occur in the future or the probability that an individual develops a given disease or experiences a change in health status during a specified time interval. Risk factors may be defined as distinctive characteristics or exposures that increase the probability of developing periodontitis or lead to a measurable change in the status of periodontal supporting tissues. A periodontal risk group can be defined as a subgroup (of a larger population) whose members, on average, have a higher probability of developing periodontitis and for loss of periodontal support, within a given time, than the remaining population.[1]

*Risk factors*: Risk factors are identified through longitudinal studies of patients with the disease of interest. These may be environmental, behavioral, or biological factors. These are tobacco smoking, diabetes, pathogenic bacteria, and microbial tooth deposits.

*Risk determinants*: The term risk determinant/ background characteristics are those risk factors that cannot be modified. These are genetic factors, age, gender, socio-economic status, and stress.

*Risk indicators*: These are probable or putative risk factors that have been identified in cross-sectional studies only. These are HIV/AIDS, osteoporosis, and infrequent dental visits.

*Risk predictors/markers*: These are, although associated with increased risk for disease, do not cause the disease and are identified in cross-sectional, longitudinal studies. These are the previous history of periodontal diseases and bleeding on probing.

*Risk assessment*: American Academy of Periodontology defines risk assessment as the process by which qualitative or quantitative assessments are made of the likelihood for adverse events to occur as a result of exposure to specified health hazards or by the absence of beneficial influences.[2]

Among the main measures used to express health risk are as follows:
- Absolute risk (RR)
- Relative risk (RR)
- Odds ratio (OR)
- Attributable risk

*Absolute risk:* It is the probability that an individual will develop the disease over a specified period of time (**Fig. 32.1**).

*Relative risk:* It is the comparison of the health risk between two populations. This measure is commonplace in

| EXPOSURE \ OUTCOME | + | – | |
|---|---|---|---|
| + | a | b | a + b |
| – | c | d | c + d |
| | a + c | b + d | |

Risk of outcome in exposed (absolute risk of exposed) $= \frac{a}{a+b}$

Risk of outcome in unexposed (absolute risk of nonexposed) $= \frac{c}{c+d}$

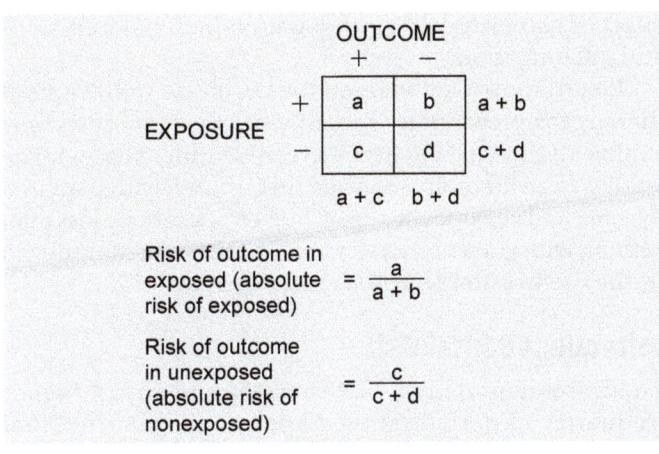

**Fig. 32.1:** Risk assessment parameters.

$$\text{Relative risk} = \frac{\frac{a}{a+b}}{\frac{c}{c+d}}$$

$$\text{Attributable risk} = \frac{a}{a+b} - \frac{c}{c+d}$$

$$\text{Exposure odds ratio} = \frac{\frac{a}{c}}{\frac{b}{d}} = \frac{ad}{bc}$$

**Fig. 32.2:** Risk assessment parameters (relative risk, attributable risk, odds ratio).

perspective and cohort studies. It should be noted that RR can be measured only when the outcome is dichotomous **(Fig. 32.2)**.

*Odds ratio:* It is commonly used to express risk. It provides a fairly good estimate of the true RR of exposure in the target population, provided that the outcome is rare[3] **(Fig. 32.2)**.

*Attributed risk:* It is also a comparison of the health risk between two populations. However, in contrast to the RR, the AR is assessed as the difference in the incidence rates (risk ratios or probabilities) of occurrence of disease between exposed and unexposed individuals (or populations) **(Fig. 32.2)**.

*Population-attribution risk:* (Also called AR fraction or etiologic fraction). It is an additional measure sometimes used to express the impact of exposure on the outcome (or disease occurrence) in the target population from which the study sample derives. It measures the proportion of all cases of outcome in the target population that is attributed to exposure, or the proportion of cases of outcome that would disappear (change to normal) if exposure in the target population were eliminated.

*Prevalence rate ratio:* In cross-sectional studies, the selection of groups is by exposure, and the outcome is measured as prevalence rather than incidence. In these studies, the prevalence rate ratio is often used as an approximation of the RR. It is assessed as the ratio of the disease prevalence in the two populations.

## RISK FACTORS

### Tobacco Smoking

Several studies reported an association between smoking and the development of periodontal disease. These studies suggested that smoking reduces immunity and negatively affects immunoglobulin levels, thereby increasing susceptibility to periodontal disease. Moreover, studies comparing the response to periodontal therapy in smokers, former smokers, and non-smokers reported reduced response to treatment in smokers. The risk of development of periodontal disease enhances with number of cigarettes smoked per day.[4]

### Diabetes

Periodontitis is considered as the sixth complication of diabetes mellitus. The epidemiological studies have reported the increased risk of development and severity of periodontitis in diabetic patients.[5]

Chronic gram-negative infections in periodontal diseases worsen glycemic control by increasing insulin tissue resistance. However, in well-controlled diabetic patients, the susceptibility to periodontal infections is similar to nondiabetic patients.

### Pathogenic Bacteria/Microbial Teeth Deposits

The cross-sectional and longitudinal studies have demonstrated a causal relationship between bacterial plaque accumulation and gingival inflammation. The quality of plaque is a significant risk factor for periodontal disease. *Aggregatibacter actinomycetemcomitans, P. gingivalis, T. forsythia, C. rectus, E. nodatum, P. intermedia, T. denticola* have been isolated from diseased sites as compared to healthy sites. Anatomic factors (furcation, developmental grooves, CEP, enamel pearls) and restorative factors are known to accelerate plaque accumulation, increasing the chances of the susceptibility of periodontitis for specific teeth. However, both anatomic and restorative factors are not clearly defined as risk factors for periodontitis.[6]

## RISK DETERMINANTS

### Genetic Risk Factors

Gene polymorphisms are now identified as candidates for use as markers of increased susceptibility for the development of periodontal diseases. In defined populations, the composite IL-1 genotype is associated with severe periodontitis. However, its usefulness as a genetic marker for periodontitis in the general population is limited. $IgG_2$ antibody response to *Aggregatibacter actinomycetemcomitans* in patients with aggressive periodontitis is also regulated by genetics. Decreased neutrophil chemotaxis, monocytic hyperresponsiveness, alterations of receptors on the $F_c$ portion of the antibody has also been regulated by genetics.[7]

## Age

Both the prevalence and severity of the periodontal disease increase with age. Loe and Brown reported age as a significant risk indicator for the occurrence of aggressive periodontitis. However, the weak association has been found between the development of chronic periodontitis and age. Age-associated loss of attachment and alveolar bone mainly depends on the presence of plaque and calculus.[8]

## Gender

Men have poorer oral hygiene than women, as evidenced by higher levels of plaque and calculus. NHANES III survey also found poorer oral hygiene levels in males compared to females. Along with this hormonal and other physiological and behavioral differences between two gender groups can enhance the risk for periodontal disease in males compared to females.[5]

## Socioeconomic Status

The studies have suggested that socioeconomic status (SES), i.e., income, urban status, and educational levels, is are fairly good risk indicator for periodontal diseases. In the low SES group, the increased risk level may be related to behavioral and environmental factors.[5] This may be due to decreased dental visits because of decreased dental awareness and financial problems.

## Stress

Previously conducted studies demonstrated that in adult psychosocial measures of stress associated with financial strain significantly increases the risk for severe periodontal diseases. Psychological stress is associated with more acute forms of gingival diseases like ANUG. Psychological stress may reduce favorable response to periodontal therapy.[9]

## RISK INDICATORS

### Osteoporosis

Osteoporosis is a disease characterized by an imbalance between bone formation and resorption, which favors bone resorption and enhances the demineralization of bone. Osteoporosis usually leads to a reduction in alveolar bone density, which is further susceptible to resorption due to the effect of associated or subsequent periodontal infections and inflammation.

Postmenopausal women on hormone replacement therapy for prevention or treatment of osteoporosis may exhibit additional benefit of increased tooth retention. The studies from literature reported that women with poor oral hygiene and osteoporosis are at higher risk of bone loss than women with good oral hygiene. This risk is usually reduced by the use of estrogen replacement therapy.[10,11]

### Infrequent Dental Visit

The infrequent dental visit is associated with a higher frequency of periodontitis. Lopez et al., reported that persons who had visited a dentist 6–12 months ago, more than 1 year ago or had never seen a dentist before were 1.2, 1.7 and 2.1 times more susceptible to developing chronic periodontitis than those visited less than 6 months ago.[12]

*HIV infection*: Cross-sectional studies measuring clinical attachment loss or radiographic alveolar bone loss reported a strong association between HIV infection and risk of periodontal disease.[4]

## RISK MARKERS

### Previous History

Patients with the previous severe attachment and bone loss are at the greatest risk for future loss also. On the other hand, patients who are free of periodontitis have a decreased risk of developing the disease in the future.

### Bleeding on Probing

Bleeding on probing (BOP) represents an objective inflammatory parameter for the evaluation of periodontal conditions. Individuals with low mean BOP% may be considered as patients with a low risk for recurrent diseases.

## RISK ASSESSMENT

Risk assessment represents an innovative approach to manage periodontal disease. AAP has defined risk assessment as the process by which qualitative or quantitative assessments are made of the likelihood for adverse events to occur as a result of exposure to specified health hazards or by the absence of beneficial influences. Risk assessment is commonly related to the diagnosis and management of the disease. It helps the clinician to develop a risk profile of each patient. Various risk models have been formulated to determine the risk.[13-15]

## Risk Models/Risk Calculators

American Academy of Periodontology has developed a risk calculator to identify specific risk factors for predicting clinical outcomes in a given patient. Similarly, Framingham calculators are available for measuring several other cardiovascular outcomes (CHD, stroke, etc.).

## Risk Model: Previser Risk Calculator

In 2002, Page et al., developed the previser risk calculator (PRC) risk model to yield simple results. An individual is assigned an ordinal risk score from 1 (lower risk) to 5 (high risk) compared to AAP tool that yields risk into three categories as low, medium and high risk.[16]

*Risk variables*: It includes 11 key factors/parameters which are recorded at the onset of treatment. The calculation is based on mathematically derived algorithms which assign relative weight to following risk factors:
1. Patient age
2. Smoking history
3. Diagnosis of diabetes
4. History of periodontal surgery
5. Pocket depth
6. Bleeding on probing
7. Furcation involvement
8. Subgingival restorations
9. Calculus below the gingival margin
10. Radiographic bone height
11. Vertical bone lesions

The disease score ranges from 0 (no disease) to 100 (severe periodontitis).

| Healthy | Gingivitis | Beginning gum disease | Moderate gum disease | Severe gum disease | Tooth loss |
|---|---|---|---|---|---|
| 1 | 2–3 | 4–10 | 11–36 | 37–100 | |

## Risk Model: Periodontal Risk Assessment Model

In 2003, Lang and Tonetti developed the PRA model. This model evaluates the severity of periodontal disease by probing depth and radiographic evaluation of alveolar bone loss with other systemic factors in consideration. The risk diagram is a functional hexagon diagram consisting of 6 vectors, each of which has a scale from 0 to 10. It allows the assessment of the risk level on individual basis[17] **(Fig. 32.3)**.

*Risk variables*: Six key factors/parameters:
1. BOP
2. Probing pocket depth PPD ≥5 mm
3. Tooth loss
4. Bone loss/age ratio
5. Environmental factors, such as smoking status

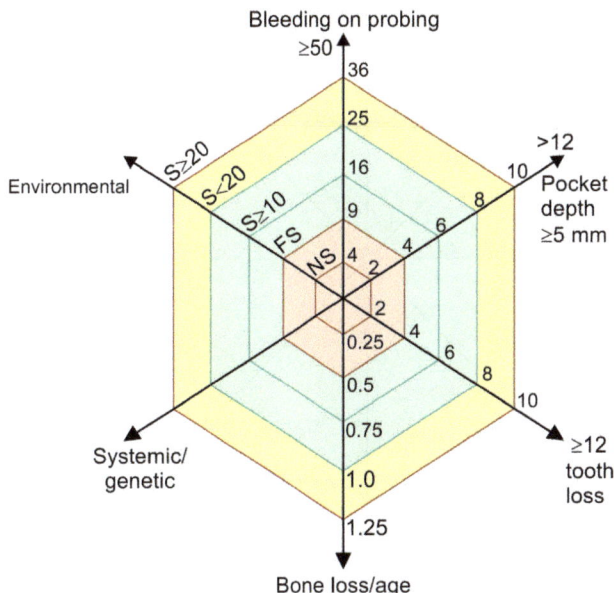

**Fig. 32.3:** Periodontal risk assessment model by Lang and Tonetti.

6. Systemic/genetic status (IL-1, diabetes mellitus, osteoporosis)

A risk score (PRAS) corresponding to diagram surface is calculated with a trigonometric equation and assigned to each patient.
- Score ≤ 20: Low to moderate periodontal risk
- Score ≥ 20: High periodontal risk.

A comprehensive evaluation of the functional diagram will assess patients' risk during supportive periodontal therapy (SPT) visits after active therapy is completed.

## Risk Model: Modified PRA Model

In 2007, Chandra developed this model:[18] The original model had the following limitations:
1. It mainly assessed the cumulative status of periodontitis patients.
2. No proper identification of risk factors and determinants.
3. The presence of the systemic disease is assessed or high-risk factor with no emphasis on current disease status.
4. Smoking is assessed, but diabetics not evaluated separately.
5. Various dental factors which may modify or initiate disease progression not included.

*Risk variables*: It includes eight key factors/parameters. In Modified PRA factors (diabetes and tooth deposits or factors which retain deposits) and other risk determinants such as socioeconomic factors and stress are included. It measures clinical attachment loss (CAL) instead of bone loss (BL) **(Fig. 32.4)**.

## Section 5: Diagnosis

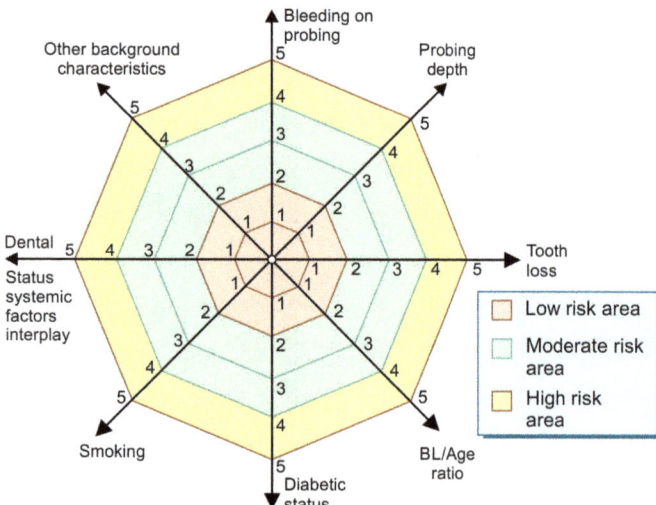

**Fig. 32.4:** Modified PRA model—by Chandra.

|  | **Modified model** | **Original model** |
|---|---|---|
| Low risk | All parameters in low-risk area + two parameters in the modified or high-risk area | All in low-risk area + one parameter in medium risk |
| Moderate risk | 3 parameters in moderate risk + one parameter in high risk | Two parameters in moderate risk + one parameter each in moderate and high risk or one parameter each in moderate and high risk |
| High risk | At least two parameters in high risk | Only two parameters in high risk |

### Points to Ponder

- Various risk factors related to periodontal diseases are tobacco smoking, diabetes, pathogenic bacteria, and microbial tooth deposits.
- Various risk determinants related to periodontal diseases are genetic factors, age, gender, socio-economic status, and stress.
- Various risk indicators related to periodontal diseases are HIV/AIDS, osteoporosis, and infrequent dental visits.
- Various risk predictors/markers related to periodontal diseases are the previous history of periodontal diseases and bleeding on probing.

### REFERENCES

1. Novak KF, Novak MJ. Risk assessment. In: Newman MG, Takei HH, Carranza FA (Eds). Clinical Periodontology, 9th edition. Philadelphia: WB Saunders. 2003;469-74.
2. American Academy of Periodontology statement on risk assessment. J Periodontol. 2008;79:202.
3. Papapanou PN, Lindhe J. Epidemiology of Periodontal Diseases. In, Lindhe J, Karring T, Lang NP (Eds). Clinical Periodontology and Implant dentistry, 4th edition. Blackwell Munksgaard. 2003;50-80.
4. Papapanou PN. Risk assessments in the diagnosis and treatment of periodontal diseases. J Den Edu. 1998;62:822-39.
5. American Academy of Periodontology: Position paper. Epidemiology of periodontal diseases. J Periodontol. 1996; 67:935-45.
6. Consensus report. Periodontal diseases: pathogenesis and microbial factors. Ann Periodontol. 1996;1(1):926-32.
7. Michalowicz BS, Aeppli D, Virag JG, Klump DG, Hinrichs JE, Segal NL, et al. Periodontal findings in adult twins. J Periodontol. 1991;62(5):293-9.
8. Burt BA, Periodontitis and aging: reviewing recent evidence. J Am Dent Assoc. 1994;125:273-9.
9. Shields WD. Acute necrotizing ulcerative gingivitis. A study of some of the contributing factors and their validity in an Army population. J Periodontol. 1977;48:346-9.
10. Kribbs PJ. Comparison of mandibular bone in normal and osteoporotic women. J Prosthet Dent. 1990;63:218-22.
11. Van Wowern J, Klausen B, Kollerup G. Osteoporosis: a risk factor in periodontal disease. J Periodontol. 1994;65:1134-8.
12. Page RC, Beck JD. Risk assessment for periodontal diseases. Int Den J. 1997; 47:61-87.
13. Ronderos M, Ryder MI. Risk assessment in clinical practice. Periodontol 2000. 2004;34:120-35.
14. Grossi SG, Zambon JJ, Ho AW, Koch G, Dunford RG, Machtei EE, et al. Assessment of risk for periodontal disease. I. Risk indicators for attachment loss. J Periodontol. 1994;65:260-7.
15. Grossi SG, Genco RJ, Machtei EE, Ho AW, Koch G, Dunford R, et al. Assessment of risk for periodontal disease. II. Risk indicators for alveolar bone loss. J Periodontol. 1995;66:23-9.
16. Page RC, Krall EA, Martin J, Mancl L, Garcia RI. Validity and accuracy of a risk calculator in predicting periodontal disease. J Am Dent Assoc. 2002;133:569-76.
17. Lang NP, Tonetti MS. Periodontal risk assessment (PRA) for patients in supportive periodontal therapy (SPT). Oral Health Prev Dent. 2003;1:7-16.
18. Chandra RV. Evaluation of a novel periodontal risk assessment model in patients presenting for dental care. Oral Health Prev Dent. 2007;5:39-48.

### VIVA VOCE

**Q1. What is the basic difference between risk and diagnosis?**
**Ans.** Risk predicts the disease status at some future point in time, including the rate at which an existing disease condition is likely to progress. In contrast, diagnosis is an expression of current disease status.

**Q2. What is the association between obesity and periodontal disease?**
**Ans.** Obesity may be considered as a low grade systemic inflammatory disease. Obese patients have elevated serum levels of C-reactive proteins, interleukin-6, tumor necrosis factor-α and leptin which are known markers of inflammation.[22]

**Q3. What are the main measures used to express health risks?**
**Ans.** Absolute risk; relative risk; odds ratio and attributable risk.

**Q4. Who proposed previser risk calculator risk model?**
**Ans.** Page et al., in 2002.

**Q5. Who proposed the periodontal risk assessment diagram surface risk model?**
**Ans.** Leininger in 2010.

**Q6. What is the absolute risk?**
**Ans.** It is the probability that an individual will develop the disease over a specified period of time.

**Q7. What is the relative risk?**
**Ans.** It is the comparison of the health risk between two populations.

**Q8. What are the various risk indicators?**
**Ans.** HIV/AIDS, osteoporosis, and infrequent dental visits.

**Q9. What are the various risk predictors/markers?**
**Ans.** Previous history of periodontal diseases and bleeding on probing.

**Q10. What are the various risk determinants?**
**Ans.** Genetic factors, age, gender, socioeconomic status, and stress.

# Prognosis

*Rajan Gupta*

## Chapter Outline

- Definition
- Prognostication Systems
- Prognostic Factors
- Diagnosis and Prognosis Interrelationship
- Prognosis of Patients

## INTRODUCTION

Prognosis is essentially a clinical prediction of outcomes under various circumstances, such as systemic disease, orthodontic therapy, endodontic therapy, and periodontal therapy. Prognosis is affected by diagnosis and intimately associated with the treatment plan. Thus, determining a prognosis for a patient before any treatment is often difficult.

## DEFINITION

It is a *Greek* word, "pro" means before, and "gignoskein" means to foreknow or to know. Prognosis is a prediction of the probable course, duration, and outcome of a disease based on general knowledge of the disease's pathogenesis and the presence of risk factors for the disease.[1]

## PROGNOSTICATION SYSTEMS

- *McGuire and Nunn*: Based on clinical and radiographic findings:[2,3] Between the extremes of hopeless and good, it is an entire range of gradations: Good, fair, poor, questionable, and hopeless prognosis. Careful analysis of prognostic factors allows the clinician to establish one of the following prognosis **(Table 33.1)**.
- *Hirschfeld and Wasserman 1978*: Based on the extent and configuration of periodontal destruction at the time of examination **(Table 33.2)**: Questionable and favorable prognosis.[4]
- *Becker et al., 1984*: Divided into three types of prognosis:[5]
  1. Good prognosis
  2. *Questionable prognosis*: More than one of the following problems associated:
     - Bone loss close to 50% of the root length.
     - Pocket depths of 6–8 mm.
     - Class II furcation involvement with minimal interradicular space.
     - Presence of a deep vertical groove on the palatal aspect of maxillary incisors.
     - Mesial furcation involvement of maxillary first bicuspids.
     - Teeth with extensive decay, which might not be restorable.
  3. *Hopeless prognosis*: More than one of the following problems associated:
     - Loss of over 75% of the supporting bone.
     - Probing depths greater than 8 mm.
     - Class III furcation involvement.
     - Class III mobility with tooth movement in mesial, distal, and vertical directions.
     - Poor crown-root ratios.
     - Root proximity with minimal interproximal bone and evidence of horizontal bone loss.
     - History of repeated periodontal abscess formation.
- *Kwok et al., 2007*: Based on the probability of disease progression:[6]
  - *Favorable*: When the periodontal condition can be stabilized with extensive periodontal treatment and comprehensive maintenance. Future loss of the periodontal supporting tissues is unlikely if these conditions are met.

**TABLE 33.1:** Types of prognosis.

| Parameters | Good prognosis | Fair prognosis | Poor prognosis | Questionable prognosis | Hopeless prognosis |
|---|---|---|---|---|---|
| One or more of the factors | | | | | |
| Remaining bone support | Adequate | Less than adequate | Moderate-to-advanced bone loss | Advanced bone loss | Advanced bone loss |
| Possibilities to control etiologic factors and maintainable dentition | Adequate | Adequate | Difficult to maintain | Difficult to maintain | Nonmaintainable |
| Tooth mobility | No | Some | Present | Present | Present |
| Furcation involvement | No | Grade I | Grades I and II | Grades II and III | Grades III and IV |
| Patient cooperation | Adequate | Acceptable | Doubtful | Noncooperation | Noncooperation |
| Systemic/environmental factors | No (if present they are well-controlled) | Present (but limited) | Present | Present | Present (uncontrolled) |

**TABLE 33.2:** Classification of questionable and favorable prognosis.

| Parameters | Questionable prognosis | Favorable prognosis |
|---|---|---|
| Furcation involvement | Yes | No |
| Pocket | Deep, noneradicable | Absent |
| Alveolar bone loss | Extensive | No |
| Mobility | Marked mobility in conjunction with probing depth (2° or 2.5° on a scale of three) | No |

- *Questionable*: Periodontal status of tooth influenced by systemic or local factors that may or may not be able to be controlled. The periodontal condition can be stabilized with comprehensive periodontal treatment and periodontal maintenance if these factors are controlled; otherwise, the future periodontal breakdown may occur.
- *Unfavorable*: The tooth's periodontal status is influenced by local and/or systemic factors that cannot be controlled. The periodontal breakdown is likely to occur even with comprehensive periodontal treatment and maintenance.
- *Hopeless*: Tooth must be extracted.

## PROGNOSTIC FACTORS

The prognostic factors are the factors which forecast disease outcome once the disease is present. Prognosis assessment is the process of using prognostic factors to predict the course of a disease.

## Factors Affecting Prognosis

- *Patient's age*: Of two patients with equally advanced bone loss, one of whom is 25 years old, and the other is 70 years old, the younger will have a poorer prognosis. The prognosis is not good for younger patients because the rate of progression was more rapid in a shorter time frame for the younger patient as compared to the older patient.
- *Disease severity and distribution*: The severity of the disease might be slight, moderate, or severe. Severity depends on pocket depth, level of attachment, bone loss, and osseous defect. The distribution of disease may be localized or generalized.
    - *Pocket depth*: Shallow pockets have a better prognosis than do deep pockets. Deep pockets have a favorable prognosis if attachment and bone levels are high.
    - *Level of attachment*: The determination of the level of clinical attachment discloses the approximate extent of root surface lacking periodontal ligament. Pocket depth is not usually related to bone loss, and hence, it is less important than the level of attachment. A tooth with deep pockets; little attachment and bone loss exhibit good prognosis compared to the tooth with shallow pockets; severe attachment and bone loss.
    - *Bone loss and osseous defect*: Greater the bone loss, poorer is the prognosis. Three-walled osseous defect provides a scaffold for repair and thus have good regenerative potential. The two-walled osseous lesion has poorer and one-walled the poorest prognosis for bone regeneration. Therefore, the prognosis is related to the height of the remaining bone.[7]
- *Plaque control*: Cooperation of the patient is necessary for the satisfactory control of plaque, and also for the control of the predisposing and aggravating etiological factors.
- *Patient cooperation*: The prognosis in patients diagnosed with gingival and periodontal disease is significantly affected by several factors, such as:
    - Patient's attitude
    - Motivation to maintain good oral hygiene
    - Dexterity of the patient

If the patient receives information about the nature of the problem and explanation of the rationale behind the treatment plan, it positively affects the patient's cooperation in the treatment plan and its outcome. Thus, it enhances the chances of achieving a good prognosis.[8]

## Systemic Factors

- *Smoking*: Smoking significantly affects—(1) severity of periodontal destruction; (2) healing capacity of periodontal tissues. Smoker with slight-to-moderate periodontitis commonly exhibits fair-to-poor prognosis. However, the prognosis may be poor to hopeless in the case of a smoker with severe periodontitis.
- *Systemic disease*: Patient's health and associated capacity for repair is an important factor to consider in developing the treatment plan and prognosis.
- *Genetic factors*: The nature of the host response is largely determined by the role played by the genetic factors.
- *Stress*: Emotional condition usually interferes with the patient's oral hygiene regime.

## Local Factors

- *Plaque and calculus*: The patient who shows a severe response to minimal amounts of plaque has a poorer prognosis than the patient who exhibits a resistant response in the presence of a considerable plaque. The microbial challenge associated with plaque and calculus is the dominant local factor determining the prognosis of periodontal disease. Thus, a good prognosis is dependent on the ability of the patient and clinician to remove plaque. However, when the teeth are drifted or rotated, oral hygiene may be more difficult; in such cases, the prognosis is poorer.
- *Subgingival restorations*: Tooth with overhangs or subgingival margin discrepancies exhibit poor prognosis compared to a tooth with well-contoured, supragingival margins.
- *Anatomical factors*:
  - *Short, tapered roots*: Teeth with short, tapering roots have a poorer prognosis than those with long and broad roots. The more favorable the crown-root ratio, the better the prognosis. An upper molar with widespread roots and a large root base exhibit a good prognosis compared to a conical-rooted premolar or incisor with an equal amount of bone loss.
  - *Cervical enamel projections (CEPs) and enamel pearls*: These enamel projections on the root surface impart a negative effect on the prognosis.
  - *Root concavities*: Prominent root proximal concavities are present on maxillary 1st premolars, the mesiobuccal root of maxillary 1st molar, both roots of mandibular 1st molars and mandibular incisors. These are the areas that can be difficult for the therapist and patient to clean and, thus, worsen the prognosis.
  - *Developmental grooves*: Grooves on the root are the invaginations are resulting from the incorrect formation of the root. The grooves often begin at the cingulum and extend a variable distance apically on the root-surface between the midpalatal line and the line angle. That is why they are called as "cinguloradicular groove" **(Figs. 33.1A and B)**. These grooves are found on maxillary lateral incisors (5.6%) and maxillary central incisors (3.4%) which act as a plaque-retentive area that is difficult to instrument.[9]
  - *Furcation involvement*: Multirooted teeth having short root trunks with furcation involvement have less favorable prognosis than longer root trunks.[10] Maxillary 1st premolars exhibit more difficulties and hence unfavorable prognosis when the lesion reaches the mesial or distal furcation. Maxillary molars also impose some degree of difficulty and therefore require resection of one of the buccal roots to improve access to the area. This resection procedure helps to improve prognosis. When mandibular 1st molars or buccal furcations of maxillary molars offer good access to the furcation area, their prognosis is usually better.
  - *Tooth mobility*: If the cause of tooth mobility can be eliminated, and if the mobility can be controlled, the prognosis is better. Tooth mobility associated with

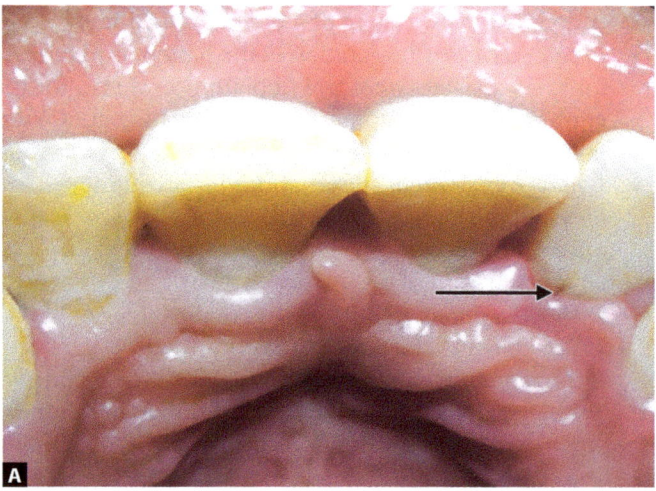 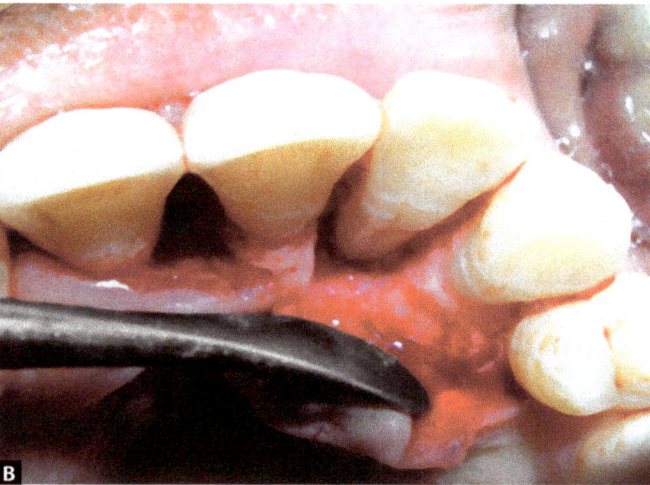

**Figs. 33.1A and B:** Clinical picture showing cinguloradicular/palatogingival groove.

inflammation and trauma from occlusion is usually corrected. However, tooth mobility induced by loss of alveolar bone is unsuitable for correction. Thus, the prognosis is poor in the presence of advanced bone loss. A tooth that can be rotated or depressed has a poorer prognosis than a tooth with horizontal mobility. Mobility must be correlated with other clinical and radiographic findings in determining prognosis.

## DIAGNOSIS AND PROGNOSIS INTERRELATIONSHIP

Many of the criteria used in the diagnosis and classification of the different forms of periodontal disease are also used in developing a prognosis. Significant factors involved in the diagnosis of such a condition are:
- Age of patient
- The severity of the disease
- Genetic susceptibility
- Presence/absence of systemic disease

These are also important in developing a prognosis. These common factors suggest that for any given diagnosis, there should be an expected prognosis under ideal conditions.

## PROGNOSIS OF PATIENTS

### Prognosis of Patients with Gingival Diseases

*Gingivitis associated with dental plaque only*: Prognosis for patients with gingivitis associated with dental plaque is good, provided all local irritants, and other local factors contributing to plaque retention are also eliminated.

*Plaque-induced gingival diseases modified by systemic illness/factors*: Factors that affect the long-term prognosis for patients with systemic illnesses are adequate to control bacterial plaque and the correction of systemic illness/factors.

*Plaque-induced gingival diseases modified by medications*: The severity of drug-induced gingival enlargement can be limited by controlling the plaque. Alterations in gingival contour are commonly corrected by surgical intervention. Continued use of the drug results in recurrence of the enlargement, even following surgical intervention. Long-term prognosis depends on whether the patient's systemic problem can be treated with an alternative medication that does not have gingival enlargement as a side effect.

*Gingival diseases modified by malnutrition*: The prognosis in these patients may depend on the severity and duration of the deficiency and the likelihood of reversing the deficiency through dietary supplementation.

*Nonplaque-induced gingival lesions*: In such cases, the prognosis depends on the removal of the infectious agent's source. In patients with atypical gingivitis seen in dermatologic disorders, the prognosis is linked to the management of the associated dermatologic disorder. Prognosis of patients with allergic, toxic, and foreign body reactions and mechanical and thermal trauma depend on eliminating the causative agent.

### Prognosis of Patients with Periodontitis

*Chronic periodontitis*: In slight-to-moderate periodontitis, where the clinical attachment loss and bone loss are minimal, the prognosis is usually good. However, the inflammation should be controlled with good oral hygiene, and local plaque-retentive factors must be removed adequately. In cases with more severe disease characterized by furcation involvement, increased tooth mobility, or non-compliant patients, the prognosis is usually downgraded from fair to poor.

*Aggressive periodontitis*: In aggressive periodontitis, clinical, microbiologic, and immunologic features usually indicate a poor prognosis. In localized aggressive periodontitis, the patients typically show a strong serum antibody response to the infecting agents, which leads to localization of the lesions. If diagnosed early, conservative therapy with oral hygiene instructions and systemic antibiotic therapy gives an excellent prognosis.

*Periodontitis is a manifestation of systemic diseases*: Systemic diseases alter the host's ability to respond to the microbial challenge presented, which may affect the progression of the disease and, therefore, the prognosis. Unless the systemic disease can be corrected, these patients usually exhibit a fair-to-poor prognosis. In the case of genetic disorders that alter the host response, the prognosis is generally fair to poor.

*Necrotizing periodontal diseases*: The prognosis for a patient with necrotizing ulcerative gingivitis (NUG) is usually good, provided both the bacterial plaque and the secondary factors including acute psychological stress, tobacco smoking, and poor nutrition are adequately controlled. In repeated episodes of NUG, the prognosis may be downgraded to fair. In patients with necrotizing ulcerative periodontitis (NUP), the prognosis depends on the control of local and secondary factors and the management of the systemic problem.

> **Points to Ponder**
> - Prognosis needs to be described at two levels: Overall and individual teeth.
> - Short-term prognosis usually refers to a period of fewer than 5 years.
> - Long-term prognosis usually refers to a period of 5 years or more.
> - The prognosis of three-walled intrabony defects is usually favorable.

## REFERENCES

1. Goodman SF, Novak KF. Determination of prognosis. In: Newman MG, Takei HH, Carranza FA (Eds). Carranza's Clinical Periodontology, 9th edition. Philadelphia, PA, USA: WB Saunders; 2003. pp. 475-86.
2. McGuire MK. Prognosis versus actual outcome: A long-term survey of 100 treated periodontal patients under maintenance care. J Periodontol. 1991;62(1):51-8.
3. McGuire MK, Nunn ME. Prognosis versus actual outcome. II. The effectiveness of clinical parameters in developing an accurate prognosis. J Periodontol. 1996;67(7):658-65.
4. Hirschfeld L, Wasserman B. A long-term survey of tooth loss in 600 treated periodontal patients. J Periodontol. 1978;49(5): 225-37.
5. Becker W, Becker B, Berg L. Periodontal treatment without maintenance. A retrospective study in 44 patients. J Periodontol. 1984;55(9):505-9.
6. Kwok V, Caton JG. Prognosis revisited: A system for assigning periodontal prognosis. J Periodontol. 2007;78(11):2063-71.
7. Grant DA, Stern IB, Listgarten MA. Prognosis. In: Periodontics, 6th edition. St. Louis: CV Mosby; 1988. pp. 573-91.
8. Eley BM, Soory M, Manson JD. Diagnosis, prognosis, and treatment plan. In: Periodontics, 5th edition. Edinburgh, UK: Wright Publishing; 2004. pp. 149-60.
9. Kogon SL. The prevalence, location, and conformation of palato-radicular grooves in maxillary incisors. J Periodontol. 1986;57(4):231-4.
10. Thomas MV, Mealey BL. Formulating a periodontal diagnosis and prognosis. In: Rose LF, Mealey BL, Genco RJ, Cohen DW (Eds). Periodontics: Medicine, Surgery, and Implants, 2nd edition. St. Louis: Elsevier Mosby; 2004. pp. 172-99.

## VIVA VOCE

**Q1. How does the patient's age affect the overall prognosis?**
**Ans.** The prognosis is not good for younger patients because of the shorter time frame in which the periodontal destruction has occurred.

**Q2. Write the factors that are common for both prognosis and diagnosis of the disease.**
**Ans.** Factors common for both prognosis and diagnosis of the disease are:
- Patient's age
- Severity of disease
- Genetic susceptibility
- Presence of systemic disease

**Q3. If there is a question as to which prognosis a tooth should be given?**
**Ans.** The operator should assign better of the two prognosis, e.g., if there is confusion between fair and poor prognosis, the tooth should be given fair one.

**Q4. What is the prognosis of the first maxillary premolar with furcation involvement?**
**Ans.** Poor prognosis.

**Q5. What is the prognosis of a three-walled defect?**
**Ans.** The three-walled osseous defect has a good prognosis.

**Q6. What is the prognosis?**
**Ans.** Prognosis is a prediction of the probable course, duration, and outcome of a disease based on general knowledge of the disease's pathogenesis and the presence of risk factors.

**Q7. What is the range of gradations given by McGuire and Nunn?**
**Ans.** Good, fair, poor, questionable, and hopeless prognosis.

**Q8. What are the types of prognosis given by Hirschfeld and Wasserman?**
**Ans.** Questionable and favorable prognosis.

**Q9. What is the cinguloradicular groove?**
**Ans.** The grooves begin at the cingulum and extend a variable distance apically on the root surface between the midpalatal line and the line angle; that is why they are called "cinguloradicular groove."

**Q10. Where are cinguloradicular grooves usually found?**
**Ans.** Maxillary lateral incisors and maxillary central incisors.

# Section 6: Treatment: Nonsurgical Therapy

- Treatment Plan
- Halitosis
- Dentin Hypersensitivity
- Mechanical Plaque Control
- Chemotherapeutic Agents
- Host Modulation
- Periodontal Instruments
- General Principles of Instrumentation
- Manual Scaling and Root Planing
- Sonic and Ultrasonic Scaling
- Splinting

# Chapter 34

# Treatment Plan

*Shalu Bathla*

## Chapter Outline

- Phases of Periodontal Therapy
- Sequence
- Palliative Treatment
- Explaining the Treatment Plan to the Patient
- Referral

## INTRODUCTION

The treatment plan is the sequential outline of the essential services and procedures that must be carried to eliminate disease and restore the oral cavity to health and normal function. It is as individualistic as are the patient and the disease. Each patient presents an individual problem, and one cannot adhere to a rigid pattern of treatment always. Thus, the treatment plan should be tailored to both the physical and psychological needs of the patient. It is the blueprint for care management.[1] The aim of the treatment plan is total treatment, i.e., the coordination of all treatment procedures to create a well-functioning dentition in a healthy periodontal environment. At all times during treatment, the primary focus is on the patient's welfare.

The treatment plan depends on the following major factors:[2]
- Patient's degree of interest and compliance, as well as the ability to participate in therapy.
- Findings of the examination.
- Nature and extent of the disease diagnosed.
- The prognosis of individual tooth segment and arch.

## PHASES OF PERIODONTAL THERAPY

Phases of periodontal therapy include the following:
- Emergency/preliminary phase.
- *Phase I*: Etiotropic phase.
- *Phase II*: Surgical phase.
- *Phase III*: Restorative phase.
- *Phase IV*: Maintenance phase.

### Emergency/Preliminary Phase

When the patient has pain, swelling, and infection, the emergency condition must be resolved before phase I therapy, just after the history taking and examination of the area involved in the chief complaint. These emergencies take priority over other treatment scheduling.
- *Alleviate pain*: The control of pain comes before any other treatment.[3]
- Swelling, even without pain, requires immediate attention.
- Acute lesions in the periodontium, such as abscesses and necrotizing periodontal diseases, are among the few conditions in periodontics where the patient requires emergency care, mostly because of the associated pain. Endodontics may be necessary as an emergency measure where there is pulpitis, apical abscess, or a combined periapical-periodontal abscess.
- Traumatic lesions.
- *Extraction of hopeless teeth*: Extremely mobile teeth, which seriously interfere with function, should be extracted.
- Repairing of the defective prosthesis.

### Phase I: Etiotropic Phase

It is called the etiotropic treatment phase because its goal is to eliminate periodontal disease's etiologic factor.

The terms phase I, initial phase, and hygienic phase are commonly used to refer to this stage of therapy.

## Objectives

The objectives of phase I therapy are:
- To reduce or eliminate gingival inflammation.
- To eliminate periodontal pocket produced by the edematous enlargement of inflamed gingiva.
- To achieve surgical manageability of the gingiva (i.e., firm consistency and minimal bleeding).
- To improve healing after periodontal surgery.

Thus, the primary goal of phase I is to eliminate inflammation and plaque control which includes the following:
- Patient education and motivation.
- *Mechanical plaque control*: Scaling and root planing.
- *Correction of restorative and prosthetic irritational factors*: Overhanging margins of dental restorations can be removed using a flame-shaped stone or flat-diamond stone mounted on a handpiece.
- *Excavation of caries and temporary restoration*: Caries control or temporary fillings can be performed in the phase I therapy. Amalgam and composite restorations may be performed to close contacts and to correct food impaction.
- *Topical and systemic antimicrobial medication*: Chemical control of plaque can be achieved by mouth rinses, irrigation, or antibiotics.
- *Occlusal therapy*: Occlusal adjustment should follow scaling and root planing. If a tooth is extremely mobile, a gross occlusal adjustment may be done before scaling to reduce mobility.
- *Minor orthodontic tooth movement*: It may precede or follow any surgical interventions. It is performed as part of phase I when there is inflammation or bony deformities due to tooth malalignment. But major orthodontic tooth movement done for purposes of reconstruction or esthetics may follow surgery. Orthodontic therapy is now becoming a more integral part of the treatment of patients undergoing periodontal therapy.
- *Provisional splinting and prosthesis*: Wire ligation and composite acid-etched splinting is generally performed during the phase I therapy. Temporary splinting (short-term stabilization for short periods of up to 6 months) or provisional splinting (long-term stabilization for up to 2 years) may be employed to control secondary occlusal trauma period before decisions about surgery are made.
- Diet changes/modifications.
- Additional preventive measures, such as fluorides, can be advised to the caries-prone patient. Evaluation of response to etiotropic phase—thorough, recorded evaluations of the appearance of tissue, the depth of pocket and level of attachment, mobility, and plaque control should be done. The patient's response should be evaluated to determine whether surgical procedures are indicated and would be beneficial. The frequency of recall visits depends upon the response of the patient.

## Phase II: Surgical Phase

Necessary surgery should be carried out in as few stages as possible over the shortest possible time, and it includes the following:
- Periodontal surgery
- *Implant surgery*: Surgery for first phase insertion of osseointegrated dental implants
- Endodontic therapy

Evaluation of response to surgical procedures should be done before phase III.

## Phase III: Restorative Phase

The restorative phase should follow periodontal surgery, and it includes the following:
- Final restorations
- Fabrication of fixed or removable prosthesis, if needed

Evaluation of response to restorative procedures should be done.

## Phase IV: Maintenance Phase

It is an essential part of a periodontal treatment plan. Patients require recall for inspection, oral hygiene monitoring, and scaling at 3-month, 6-month, 9-month, or 12-month intervals, depending upon the previous disease experience, and susceptibility.[3] Periodic rechecking of plaque and calculus, gingival condition, occlusion, tooth mobility, and other pathological changes should be done. Oral hygiene procedures are also reinforced to the patient during this phase.[4]

## SEQUENCE

It is the scheduled sequence of therapeutic measures used to cure or arrest the patient's periodontal disease. It is divided into four phases mentioned above for each patient according to his needs **(Flowchart 34.1)**.[1]

**Flowchart 34.1:** Sequence of periodontal therapy.

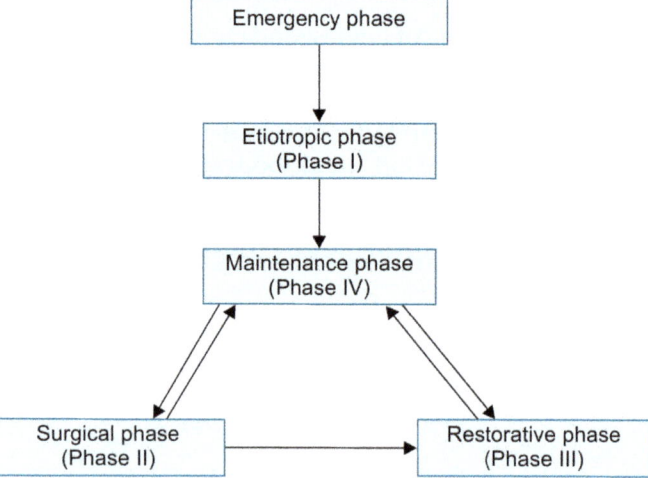

## PALLIATIVE TREATMENT

Following are the candidates for palliative treatment:
- Patients with short-life expectancy either due to advanced age/systemic diseases with poor survival prognosis, such as poorly controlled diabetes or valvular heart defects.
- Patients with severe mental and physical disabilities.
- Patients with severe furcation involvement.
- Patients with limited financial ability.
- Noncooperative patients for existing procedures.

## EXPLAINING THE TREATMENT PLAN TO THE PATIENT

Begin your discussion on a positive note and explain the treatment plan to the patient specifically about the condition, how it is treated, and its prognosis after treatment.

First, talk about the teeth that can be retained and the long-term service they can be expected to render and later inform about the teeth to be extracted. Because telling first the teeth to be extracted will create a negative impression, which adds to the flawed attitude of hopelessness that the patient already may have regarding his or her mouth.

Present the entire treatment plan as a unit. "Plan is not for the site but for the patient." Avoid creating the impression that treatment consists of separate procedures; some may be selected by the patient and get the treatment later on. Make it clear that restorations and prostheses contribute as much to the health of the gingiva as does the elimination of inflammation and periodontal pockets.

Explain to the patient that doing nothing or holding onto hopelessly diseased teeth as long as possible is inadvisable because periodontal disease is a microbial infection, which is an important risk factor for severe life-threatening diseases, such as stroke, cardiovascular disease, pulmonary disease, diabetes and for premature low-birth-weight babies in women of childbearing age.

## REFERRAL

There are three basic reasons for referral:[5]
1. *Professional referrals:* (Maybe medical or dental) Medical referral is indicated when the patient's medical history discloses significant information that may contribute to or influence the course of the treatment. A dental referral is indicated when the general dentist cannot provide the entire periodontal therapy. If clinically observable signs of inflammation and/or ongoing attachment loss are present after treatment, the general dentist should consider other treatment modalities. If advanced periodontal therapy is among those choices, the general dentist has to discuss a possible referral. Other forms of gingivitis and aggressive forms of periodontitis should be referred to the periodontist.
2. *Moral and ethical*: The specialists or consulting dentists will return the patient to the referring dentist upon completion of their therapy.
3. *Legal*: Dentists are obligated by-laws to keep their diagnostic and treatment capabilities up to the standards. Dentists must exercise reasonable judgment in deciding whether to treat or refer their patients.

Other reasons for referral are patient relocation, dentist's preference, and dentist-patient personality conflict.[6]

## Referral Process

Once the general dentist decides to refer, the process should proceed with equal concern for the same communication and quality care expected of the periodontist. During the referral consultation, the patient should be informed about the treatment benefits presented by the specialist. The timing of referral may be fundamental to treatment success. Delay in a referral could change a treatable situation into a hopeless one.

The termination of a referral relationship should always be accompanied by an explanation. Lastly, both the periodontist and the referring dentist should be willing to work together at moderate fees and therapy with those patients who are highly motivated but may not be financially competent.

> **Points to Ponder**
>
> The sequence of periodontal therapy:
> - Emergency/preliminary phase.
> - *Phase I*: Etiotropic phase.
> - *Phase IV*: Maintenance phase.
> - *Phase II*: Surgical phase.
> - *Phase IV*: Maintenance phase.
> - *Phase III*: Restorative phase.
> - *Phase IV*: Maintenance phase.

## REFERENCES

1. Carranza FA, Takei HH. The treatment plan. In: Newman MG, Takei HH, Carranza FA (Eds). Carranza's Clinical Periodontology, 9th edition. Philadelphia, PA, USA: WB Saunders; 2003. pp. 503-6.
2. Genco RJ, Goldman HM, Cohen DW. Periodontal diagnosis, prognosis, and treatment planning. In: Contemporary Periodontics, 1st edition. St. Louis: CV Mosby; 1990. pp. 348-59.
3. Eley BM, Manson JD, Soory M. Diagnosis, prognosis, and treatment plan. In: Periodontics, 5th edition. Edinburgh, UK: Wright Publishing; 2004. pp. 149-60.
4. Philstrom BL. Periodontal risk assessment, diagnosis, and treatment planning. Periodontol 2000. 2001;25:37-58.
5. Grant DA, Stern IB, Listgarten MA. Treatment plan. In: Periodontics, 6th edition. St. Louis: CV Mosby; 1988. pp. 592-10.
6. Wilson RD. Referrals to specialists. In: Wilson TG, Kornman KS (Eds). Fundamentals of Periodontics. Chicago, USA: Quintessence Publishing; 1996. pp. 465-70.

**Section 6:** Treatment: Nonsurgical Therapy

### VIVA VOCE

**Q1.** In which phase, extraction of a hopeless tooth is done?
**Ans.** Emergency/preliminary phase.

**Q2.** In which phase, occlusal therapy is done?
**Ans.** Phase I: Etiotropic phase.

**Q3.** In which phase, an implant is placed surgically?
**Ans.** Phase II: Surgical phase.

**Q4.** In which phase, excavation of caries is done?
**Ans.** Phase I: Etiotropic phase.

**Q5.** What is the primary goal of phase I?
**Ans.** Elimination of inflammation and plaque control.

**Q6.** In which phase, the correction of restorative and prosthetic irritational factors is done?
**Ans.** Phase I: Etiotropic phase.

**Q7.** In which phase, provisional splinting is done?
**Ans.** Phase I: Etiotropic phase.

**Q8.** In which phase, fabrication of fixed or removable prosthesis is done?
**Ans.** Phase III: Restorative phase.

**Q9.** In which phase, root canal therapy is done?
**Ans.** Phase II: Surgical phase.

**Q10.** What are the three basic reasons for a referral?
**Ans.** Professional referrals; moral and ethical; legal.

# Chapter 35: Halitosis

*Shalu Bathla*

## Chapter Outline

- Classifications
- Etiology
- Pathogenesis
- Diagnosis
- Treatment

## INTRODUCTION

Halitosis or more simply "bad breath" is derived from the *Latin* words "Halitus (breath) + Osis (bad)." It is a symptom characterized by unpleasant odor experienced on the exhaled breath. Halitosis is known by various names, including bad breath, fetor ex ore, or fetor oris. The embarrassment associated with bad breath hampers one's self-image and reduces confidence. It is one of the well-known reasons for social, emotional, and psychological anxieties. As most of the causes for halitosis originate from an oral cavity, the patient usually seeks the treatment from a dentist.[1]

## CLASSIFICATIONS

Classification of halitosis has been described in **Table 35.1**.[2]

## ETIOLOGY

There are various physiologic and pathologic causes of halitosis which may be extraoral or intraoral **(Fig. 35.1)**.[3]

### Physiologic Halitosis

It includes food containing lactose (dairy products, such as milk, cheese, yoghurt, ice-cream), food containing sulfur (onion, garlic), lack of salivary flow during sleep, menstruation, smoking, and alcoholic drinks.

### Pathologic Halitosis

#### Intraoral

*Diseases of the oral cavity*: Dental caries, dental plaque, gingivitis, periodontitis, stomatitis, fissured and hairy

**TABLE 35.1:** Classification of halitosis.

| Classification | | Treatment needs | Description |
|---|---|---|---|
| I. Genuine halitosis | | | |
| Physiologic halitosis | | TN-1 | Malodor arises through putrefactive processes within the oral cavity. Neither a specific disease nor a pathologic condition that could cause halitosis is found. Origin is mainly the dorsoposterior region of the tongue |
| Pathologic halitosis | Oral | TN-2 | Halitosis is caused by disease, pathologic condition or malfunction of oral tissues. Halitosis derived from tongue coating, modified by pathologic condition (e.g., periodontal disease, xerostomia) is included in this subdivision |
| | Extraoral | TN-3 | Malodor originates from nasal, paranasal and/or laryngeal region, pulmonary tract or upper digestive tract, diabetes mellitus, hepatic cirrhosis, uremia, internal bleeding |
| II. Pseudohalitosis | | TN-4 | Obvious malodor is not perceived by others, although the patient stubbornly complains of its existence |
| III. Halitophobia | | TN-5 | After treatment for genuine halitosis or pseudohalitosis, the patient persists in believing that he/she has halitosis |

## Section 6: Treatment: Nonsurgical Therapy

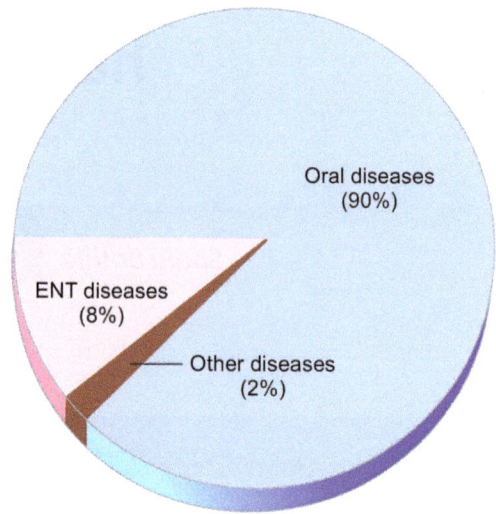

**Fig. 35.1:** Schematic representation showing causes of halitosis.

tongue, acute primary herpetic gingivostomatitis, oral carcinoma, necrotizing ulcerative gingivitis (NUG), open gangrenous pulp and pericoronitis.

### Extraoral

- *Diseases of the upper respiratory tract*: Mouth breathing due to upper respiratory tract blockage, chronic sinusitis, foreign bodies, Wegener's granulomatosis, tuberculosis, adenoiditis, syphilis, nasopharyngeal abscess and carcinoma of the larynx.
- *Diseases of the lower respiratory tract*: Pulmonary abscess, bronchiectasis, chronic fetid bronchitis, pulmonary tuberculosis, carcinoma of the lung, necrotizing pneumonitis, and empyema.
- *Diseases of the upper gastrointestinal tract*: Salivary gland dysfunction, peritonsillar abscess, retropharyngeal abscess, Vincent's angina, pharyngitis sicca, carcinoma of tonsils or pharynx, gangrenous angina, Zenker's diverticulum, and congenital bronchoesophageal fistula.
- *Diseases of the lower gastrointestinal tract*: Gastric carcinoma, hiatus hernia, pyloric stenosis, and enteric infections.
- *Neurological diseases*: Dysgeusia, dysosmia, and zinc deficiency.
- *Oral medications*: Lithium salts, penicillamine, griseofulvin, thiocarbamide, chloral hydrate, amphetamine, antihypertensives, antihistamines, disulfiram, dimethyl sulfoxide (used in interstitial cystitis) and cysteamine (used in nephropathic cystinosis).
- *Systemic causes*: Hepatic failure (mousy odor, sweetish), azotemia/kidney failure (uremic/fishy odor), diabetic ketoacidosis (acetone, fruity odor), chronic glomerulonephritis, lung abscess (foul, putrefactive), and Sjögren's syndrome (fetid).
- *Functional disorders*: Psychosis and depression.

## PATHOGENESIS

### Role of Bacteria

The common microorganisms involved in halitosis are *Peptostreptococcus micros*, *Campylobacter rectus*, *Porphyromonas gingivalis*, *Prevotella intermedia*, *Prevotella nigrescens*, *Aggregatibacter actinomycetemcomitans*, *Fusobacterium nucleatum*, *Tannerella forsythia*, *Eubacterium* species and *spirochetes*.[4,5]

All these causative bacteria use proteins, peptides, or amino acids as a source of nutrition. The degradation of these compounds leads to the formation of volatile sulfur compounds and other odoriferous substances. The tongue is the most common intraoral site for the production of malodor. Others are interdental and subgingival areas, denture, overhanging restorations, leaking crowns, large carious lesions, sites of food impaction, and abscess. In the case of a tongue, the large surface area of it is constantly exposed to the expired air, and tongue flora can degrade available substrates into malodorous molecules.[6] Topographically the dorsal tongue mucosa with an area of 25 cm² exhibits very irregular surface with innumerable depressions, and this acts as an ideal place for bacterial adhesion and growth. Furthermore, it acts as a shelter for bacteria during cleansing processes.[7]

### Role of Volatile Organic Compounds

The existence of odorous gases in the exhaled air from the oral cavity can also lead to halitosis. To term a compound as odoriferous, it must be volatile, just like a phenomenon shown by perfumes. Putrefactive activities of bacteria present on the tongue surfaces, in the saliva, gingival sulcus and other areas mainly release volatile sulfur compounds. Volatile sulfur compounds **(Box 35.1)** increase the permeability of oral mucosa and crevicular epithelium. Proteoglycans and glycoproteins in the extracellular matrix are held together by disulfide bonds, and volatile sulfur compounds break these disulfide bonds. This hampers the process of oxygen utilization by host cells, and induces the reaction with cellular proteins, and interferes with collagen maturation. It also makes collagen more soluble. Additionally, it reduces the deoxyribonucleic acid (DNA)

---

**BOX 35.1:** Volatile organic compounds.

Volatile organic compounds that give rise to malodor:[8]
- *Sulfur compounds*: Methyl mercaptan ($CH_3SH$), hydrogen sulfide ($H_2S$), and dimethyl sulfide
- *Phenyl compounds*: Indole, skatole, and pyridine
- *Short-chain fatty acids*: Butyric acid, propionic acid, and valeric acid
- *Alkanes*: 2-methyl-propane
- *Polyamines*: Cadaverine and putrescine
- *Alcohols*: 1-propoxy-2-propanol
- *Nitrogen-containing compounds*: Urea and ammonia
- Ketones

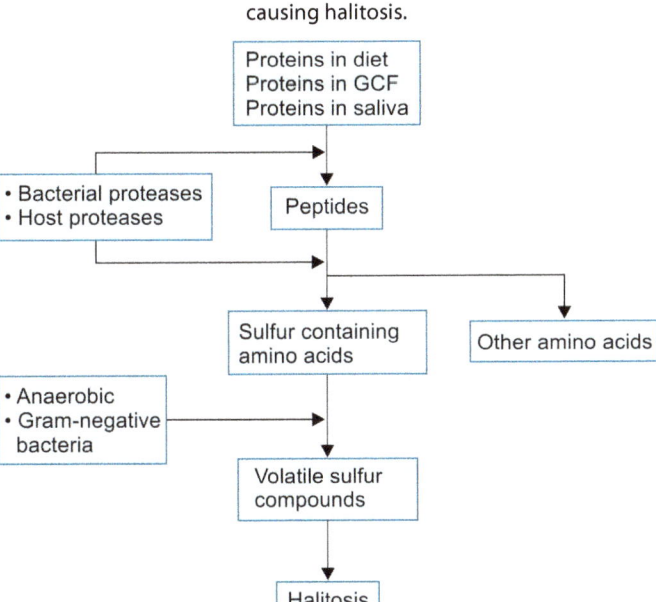

**Flowchart 35.1:** Production of volatile sulfur compounds causing halitosis.

(GCF: gingival crevicular fluid)

synthesis and proline transport reduction of total protein content and collagen synthesis of fibroblasts. It increases the secretion of collagenases, prostaglandins from fibroblasts, ultimately leading to the conversion of mature collagen to a product susceptible to enzymatic degradation. Thus, volatile sulfur compounds reduce the intracellular pH, inhibit cell growth, and periodontal cell migration **(Flowchart 35.1)**.

Extraoral causes, such as hormonal, renal or gastrointestinal factors, produce additional molecules that enter the circulation and get expressed through the exhaled air.[8]

## Role of Saliva

Saliva has a dual action of inhibiting and favoring malodor formation. When the salivary flow rate is slow, and oxygen availability is low, saliva favors the malodor formation. When the flow of saliva is rapid, and there is greater availability of oxygen, the inhibitory property of saliva dominates.

## Role of pH

Acidic pH inhibits whereas neutral and alkaline pH favor malodor production.[9]

## Role of Oxygen

The low partial pressure of oxygen ($pO_2$) helps in the proliferation and growth of Gram-negative anaerobic odoriferous bacteria. In deep periodontal pockets, the low oxygen tension favors the conversion of decarboxylation of amino acids (e.g., lysine) to cadaverine and putrescine. Both of these products act as malodorous diamines and promote bad breath.

## DIAGNOSIS

### Medical History

During history taking, try to get all information regarding the relevant pathologies contributing to bad breath. "Listen to the patient, and the patient will tell you the diagnosis." Thus, proper questioning about medical history will help to achieve an appropriate differential diagnosis.

### Examination

#### Clinical Examination

- *Self-examination*: Self-testing commonly employed for detecting halitosis are as follows:
    - Smelling a metallic spoon after scraping the back of the tongue.[10]
    - Smelling toothpick or dental floss after introducing it in an interdental region.[11]
    - Smelling saliva that is spit in a spoon or cup.[11]
    - Licking the wrist and allowing it to dry (reflects the saliva contribution to malodor).[11]
- *Organoleptic/hedonic measurement*: In this method, based on the examiner's perception of the subject's oral malodor, a sensory test scored is calculated. A plastic tube of 10 cm length and diameter of 2.5 cm is placed into the patient's oral cavity. Upon placing the tube, the patient is asked to exhale slowly. So, the examiner at the other end of the tube can decide the odor. The use of a privacy screen of 50 cm × 70 cm helps to avoid the patient from seeing the examiner sniffing the tube.[12] The examiner smells the patient's breath for the initial 1–2 seconds. The examiner rechecks the patient's breath after taking his/her nose away from the tube for 3–4 seconds. Lung air should be checked after cleaning the tongue and rinsing the mouth with 0.12% chlorhexidine. For examining nasal breath odor, a tube of 3–5 mm in diameter and 10 cm in length is inserted into one of the nostrils, and the other nostril is pushed closed by a finger.
    - *Instructions to patient*: Avoid:
        - Taking antibiotics 3 weeks before the assessment.
        - Consumption of the foods containing onion, garlic, and spices 48 hours before the assessment.
        - Eating, drinking, smoking, oral hygiene practices, and use of breath fresheners for 12 hours before assessment.
    - *Instructions to the examiner*:
        - Should possess a normal sense of smell.
        - Abstain from drinking alcohol and using scented cosmetics before the assessment.
        - Not to wear gloves because its odor may interfere with organoleptic assessment.[13-15]

Normally, breath odor varies dramatically from day-to-day. Hence, assessments must be carried out at several

**Section 6:** Treatment: Nonsurgical Therapy

**TABLE 35.2:** Organoleptic scoring scale.

| Grade | Category of odor | Description |
|---|---|---|
| 0 | Absence of odor | Odor cannot be detected |
| 1 | Questionable odor | The odor is detectable, although the examiners could not recognize it as malodor |
| 2 | Slight odor | The odor is deemed to exceed the threshold of malodor recognition |
| 3 | Moderate odor | Malodor is definitely detected |
| 4 | Strong odor | Strong malodor which can be tolerated |
| 5 | Severe malodor | Overwhelming malodor is detected, which cannot be tolerated |

appointments on different days. The judge has to smell a series of different air samples to reach a proper diagnosis.

Organoleptic scoring scale (0–5 point scale)[2] is explained in **Table 35.2**.

The advantage associated with organoleptic measurement is that there is no dilution of malodor with room air. But the objectivity and reproducibility of organoleptic measurements are poor.

## Laboratory Examination

### Sulfide monitor (halimeter)

This method uses disposable plastic straw, which is placed into the air inlet. During the measurement, the patient is advised to slightly open the mouth and place over the straw allowing the straw to extend approximately 4 cm into the mouth. The procedure requires three measurements to calculate the mean of these values in parts per billion (ppb) sulfide equivalents. The portable sulfide meter uses electrochemical, voltammetric zinc oxide thin film semiconductor sensors, which generate a signal on exposure to sulfide and mercaptan gases. Without discriminating between the two gases, halimeter analyzes the concentration of both methyl mercaptan ($CH_3SH$) and hydrogen sulfide ($H_2S$). It needs regular calibration.

*Advantages*:
- No need for skilled personnel
- Portability
- Noninvasive
- Fewer chances of cross-infection
- Relatively low cost
- Rapid turnaround time of 1–2 minutes between measurements

*Disadvantages*:
- Inability to distinguish between individual sulfides
- With the passage of time instrument exhibits loss of sensitivity and hence needs periodic recalibration
- High levels of ethanol or essential oils interfere with precise measurement

### Gas chromatography

Gas chromatography, coupled with flame photometric detection, was designed by Tonzetich et al. for the analysis of oral malodor. For any volatile component, this device is useful to analyze air and incubated saliva or gingival crevicular fluid.[9]

*Advantages*:
- It can measure extremely low concentrations of gases
- Separation and quantitative measurement of individual gases[11]

*Disadvantages*:
- Relatively high cost
- Skilled personnel required
- Cumbersome and lack of portability
- More time is required for detection and measurement

### Dark-field/phase-contrast microscopy

The higher concentration of motile organisms and spirochetes is usually detected in gingivitis and periodontitis. Dark-field microscopy assesses directly and rapidly, the presence of these motile bacteria in plaque sample. A high proportion of spirochetes in plaque are found to impart specific acidic malodor.

### Saliva incubation test

In this method, a glass tube with a diameter of 1.5 cm is used to collect 0.5 mL of unstimulated saliva, and the tube is flushed with carbon dioxide ($CO_2$) and sealed. The sealing restricts the inflow of outside air, and the glass avoids the smell of the hardware. In an anaerobic chamber at 37°C, this tube is incubated for over 3 hours under an atmosphere of 80% nitrogen ($N_2$), 10% hydrogen ($H_2$), and 10% $CO_2$.

### BANA test

It is an alternative option to detect bacteria or their enzymes producing volatile sulfur compounds in plaque or the tongue coating in a patient presenting with halitosis. Three species, particularly associated with periodontal diseases are *Treponema denticola*, *P. gingivalis* and *T. forsythia*, which produces both volatile sulfur compounds and volatile fatty acids. These organisms can be detected in plaque samples.

### Diamond probe

It is a recently developed instrument carrying integrated sensors into the periodontal probe. The probe has an inbuilt electrical control unit and a disposable sensor tip that combines a standard Michigan 0 style dental probe with a sulfide sensor. It responds to the sulfides when placed into the periodontal pocket or on the tongue. At each site in a digital score, the control unit recorded the sulfide level from 0.0 to 5.0. A score of 0 is considered undetectable, equivalent to $10^{-7}$ M of sulfide while a score of 5 represents more than or equal to $10^{-2}$ M of sulfide.[16]

## TREATMENT

Control of halitosis with folk remedies is a long-run practice and still prevalent across the world. The Bible (Genesis) mentions the use of Labdanum (Mastic) in the Mediterranean countries as a breath freshener for thousands of years. It is a resin and considered as the original chewing gum. Other folk cures tried in various parts of the world are guava peels in Thailand, parsley in Italy, eggshells in China, and cloves in Iraq.

In routine dental practice, TNs for halitosis have been categorized into five classes. These provide absolute guidelines to clinicians in the management of halitosis patients. Treatments of physiologic halitosis (TN-1), oral pathologic halitosis (TN-1 and TN-2), and pseudohalitosis (TN-1 and TN-4) are usually managed by a dentist. However, management of extraoral pathologic halitosis (TN-3) or halitophobia (TN-5) needs the consultation of a physician or medical specialists, such as a psychiatrist or psychologist.[2] Treatment needs (TNs) for breath malodor are described in (**Table 35.3**).[2]

The management of halitosis depends largely on the cause:

- *Mechanical reduction of intraoral nutrients and microorganisms*: Scaling and root planing associated with oral hygiene instructions are effective in controlling halitosis. Tongue cleaning is done either by a brush or a tongue scraper. Small tongue scrapers are used with light pressure designed to reach as far back on the tongue as possible. This will help to dislodge the trapped food debris and microorganisms accumulated in between the filiform papillae and subsequently reduce the amount of volatile sulfur compounds. Rinse and clean the tongue scraper well after each use.
- *Chemical reduction of oral microorganisms*: Chlorhexidine,[17] listerine,[18] cetylpyridinium chloride, hydrogen peroxide, triclosan, and zinc chloride are common mouthwashes used in cases of halitosis. Various mouth rinses contain zinc because of its strong affinity towards thiol groups present in the volatile sulfur compound. This helps to convert volatile $H_2S$, and $CH_3SH$ to nonvolatile sulfides.[19] Penicillins, metronidazole, tetracyclines, ciprofloxacin, and tinidazole are commonly used antimicrobials/antibiotics for halitosis.
- *Baking soda dentifrices and zinc salt solutions*: They render *malodorous* gases nonvolatile.
- *Masking the malodor*: Commercially available oxidizing lozenges provide a considerable antimalodor effect. The peroxide-mediated oxidation of ascorbate *present* in the lozenges produces dehydroascorbic acid, which hides the bad breath. The beneficial effect of chewing gum is due to tea extracts present in it for its deodorizing mechanism. Green tea contains epigallocatechin gallate (EGCG), the main deodorizing agent, which reacts with $CH_3SH$ and results in a nonvolatile product.
- *Dietary recommendations*: Advice to drink plenty of liquids, eat fresh, fibrous vegetables, and rinse their mouth after eating fish, meat, and consuming milk or milk products. Avoid coffee, smoking, and foods such as garlic that might cause halitosis.
- *Consultation to a physician*: Bad breath may indicate the presence of an underlying systemic condition. Therefore, whenever local measures prove ineffective, a physician's consultation is indicated for the systemic cause. Pseudohalitosis almost always requires referral to a clinical psychologist for management.

### Points to Ponder

- Almost 90% of all bad breath has their origin in the oral cavity, and the remaining 10% are due to systemic or extraoral cause.[20]
- The fetid odor is characteristic of NUG, which is easily identified.
- Tea catechin EGCG suppresses the mgl gene, which encodes for L-methionine-α-deamino-γ-mercaptomethane-lyase. This enzyme is responsible for the production of methyl mercaptan by oral anaerobes.
- $CH_3SH$ and $H_2S$ contain free thiols which have the potential to react with DNA and proteins both.[21]
- Morning bad breath experienced on awakening is due to decreased salivary flow and increased putrefaction during the night, which spontaneously disappears after breakfast or oral hygiene. Thus, it is transient in nature.

## REFERENCES

1. Rosenberg M. Clinical assessment of bad breath: current concepts. J Am Dent Assoc. 1996;127(4):475-82.
2. Miyazaki H, Arao M, Okamura K, Kawaguchi Y, Toyofuku A, Hoshi K, et al. Tentative classification of halitosis and its treatment needs. Niigata Dent J. 1999;32:7-11.
3. Grant DA, Stern IB, Listgarten MA. Plaque control, root sensitivity and halitosis. In: Periodontics, 6th edition. St. Louis: CV Mosby; 1988. pp. 611-45.
4. Quirynen M, Zhao H, van Steenberghe D. Review of the treatment strategies for oral malodor. Clin Oral Investig. 2002;6(1):1-10.
5. Persson S, Edlund MB, Claesson R, Carlsson J. The formation of hydrogen sulfide and methyl mercaptan by oral bacteria. Oral Microbiol Immunol. 1990;5(4):195-201.

**TABLE 35.3:** Treatment needs (TNs) for breath malodor.

| Category | Description |
|---|---|
| TN-1 | Explanation of halitosis and instructions for oral hygiene |
| TN-2 | Oral prophylaxis, professional cleaning, and treatment for oral diseases, especially periodontal diseases |
| TN-3 | Referral to a physician or medical specialist |
| TN-4 | Explanation of examination data, further professional instruction, education, and reassurance |
| TN-5 | Referral to a clinical psychologist or psychiatrist |

6. Steenberghe DV, Quirynen M. Breath malodor. In: Lindhe J, Karring T, Lang NP (Eds). Clinical Periodontology and Implant Dentistry, 4th edition. Chicago, USA: Blackwell Munksgaard; 2003. pp. 512-18.
7. De Boever EH, Loesche WJ. Assessing the contribution of anaerobic microflora of the tongue to oral malodor. J Am Dent Assoc. 1995;126(10):1384-93.
8. Krespi YP, Shrime MG, Kacker A. The relationship between oral malodor and volatile sulfur compound-producing bacteria. Otolaryngol Head Neck Surg. 2006;135(5):671-6.
9. Tonzetich J. Production and origin of oral malodor: a review of mechanisms and methods of analysis. J Periodontol. 1977;48(1):13-20.
10. Greenstein RB, Goldberg S, Marku-Cohen S, Sterer N, Rosenberg M. Reduction of oral malodor by oxidizing lozenges. J Periodontol. 1997;68(12):1176-81.
11. Rosenberg M, McCulloch CA. Measurement of oral malodor: current methods and future prospects. J Periodontol. 1992;63(9):776-82.
12. Yaegaki K, Coil JM. Examination, classification, and treatment of halitosis; clinical perspectives. J Can Dent Assoc. 2000;66(5):257-61.
13. Vandekerckhove B, Van den Velde S, De Smit M, Dadamio J, Teughels W, Van Tornout M, et al. Clinical reliability of non-organoleptic oral malodour measurements. J Clin Periodontol. 2009;36(11):964-9.
14. Loesche WJ, Kazor C. Microbiology and treatment of halitosis. Periodontol 2000. 2002;28:256-79.
15. Scully C, Greenman J. Halitosis (breath odour). Periodontol 2000. 2008;48:66-75.
16. Torresyap G, Haffajee AD, Uzel NG, Socransky SS. Relationship between periodontal pocket sulfide levels and subgingival species. J Clin Periodontol. 2003;30(11):1003-10.
17. Rosenberg M, Kulkarni GV, Bosy A, McCulloch CA. Reproducibility and sensitivity of oral malodor measurements with a portable sulphide monitor. J Dent Res. 1991;70(11):1436-40.
18. Pitts G, Brogdon C, Hu L Masurat T, Pianotti R, Schumann P. Mechanism of action of an antiseptic, anti-odour mouthwash. J Dent Res. 1983;62(6):738-42.
19. Wåler SM. The effect of zinc-containing chewing gum on volatile sulfur-containing compounds in the oral cavity. Acta Odontol Scand. 1997;55(3):198-200.
20. Sanz M, Roldan S, Herrera D. Fundamentals of breath malodor. J Contemp Dent Pract. 2001;2(4):1-17.
21. Ratcliff, PA, Johnson PW. The relationship between oral malodor, gingivitis, and periodontitis. A review. J Periodontol. 1999;70(5):485-9.

## VIVA VOCE

**Q1. What is the upper limit of a volatile sulfur compound for social acceptance?**
**Ans.** The upper limit of a volatile sulfur compound for social acceptance is 75 ppb.

**Q2. Which mineral is added in mouthwash to treat halitosis?**
**Ans.** Zinc is added in mouthwash to treat halitosis.

**Q3. Which is the gold standard for the examination of halitosis?**
**Ans.** Organoleptic assessment[13-15] is the gold standard for the examination of halitosis.

**Q4. What is halitophobia?**
**Ans.** Halitophobia is delusion halitosis. After treatment for genuine halitosis or pseudohalitosis, the patient persists in believing that he/she has halitosis.

**Q5. Name various volatile sulfur compound responsible for halitosis.**
**Ans.** Methyl mercaptan ($CH_3SH$), hydrogen sulfide ($H_2S$), and dimethyl sulfide.

**Q6. Which functional disorder causes halitosis?**
**Ans.** Psychosis and depression.

**Q7. Which pH favors malodor production?**
**Ans.** Neutral and alkaline pH.

**Q8. What are the advantages of gas chromatography?**
**Ans.** It can measure extremely low concentrations of gases; separation and quantitative measurement of individual gases can also be done.

**Q9. What are the dietary recommendations for the management of halitosis?**
**Ans.** Advice to drink plenty of liquids, eat fresh, fibrous vegetables and rinse their mouth after eating fish, meat, and consuming milk or milk products. Avoid coffee, smoking, and foods such as garlic that might cause halitosis.

**Q10. In which systemic condition, uremic/fishy odor is present?**
**Ans.** Azotemia/Kidney failure.

# Chapter 36

# Dentin Hypersensitivity

*Shalu Bathla*

## Chapter Outline

- Definition
- Etiology
- Theories
- Diagnosis
- Hypersensitivity Measurement
- Management
- Prevention

## INTRODUCTION

Dentin hypersensitivity is a relatively common problem in periodontal practice, which may occur spontaneously when the root becomes exposed as a result of the gingival recession or after scaling and root planing and surgical periodontal procedures. The diagnosis of which can be made by careful case history and clinical examination. The treatment options for managing dentin hypersensitivity is based on the extent and severity of the problem.

## DEFINITION

Dentin hypersensitivity is an exaggerated response to non-noxious stimuli. It is characterized by short, sharp pain arising from exposed dentin in response to stimuli typically thermal, evaporative, tactile, osmotic/chemical, and, which cannot be ascribed to any other form of dental defect/pathology.

## ETIOLOGY

Dentin hypersensitivity is mainly due to the dentin's exposure that can occur from one of these processes: either removal of the enamel covering the crown or denudation of the root surface due to loss of cementum and overlying periodontal tissues.[1]

### Loss of Enamel

Removal of the enamel may result from tooth wasting diseases, i.e., attrition, abrasion, erosion, or combination. Loss of enamel, which occurs by attrition, is associated with occlusal function and may be exaggerated by habits or parafunctional activity such as bruxism. Loss of enamel may occur by abrasion from dietary components and habits such as toothbrushing; or by erosion associated with environmental and dietary components, particularly acids.

### Loss of Covering Periodontal Structures

Denudation of the root surface is multifactorial. Acute and chronic periodontal diseases, incorrect toothbrushing or chronic trauma from other habits, and some forms of periodontal surgery are important causal factors. Factors such as method and frequency of brushing, the brush type, and the dentifrice used all are related to the effects produced on soft and hard tissues. Erosive agents, primarily acids, environmental, dietary, or endogenous, are known to cause the damage, e.g., workers exposed to fumes of hydrochloric, sulfuric, nitric, and tartaric acids.

The prevalence and distribution of recession and dentin hypersensitivity strongly implicate toothbrushing as an etiologic factor, particularly in the localization of lesions.

The buccal cervical site predilection for dentin exposure and sensitivity is consistent with the toothbrushing practices, with lingual sites receiving little attention during brushing. The left-sided shift to increased recession and sensitivity but decreased plaque scores in preponderantly right-handed toothbrushing groups support the relevance of tooth-cleaning to condition. Interestingly, the finding that females are more commonly affected by dentin hypersensitivity than males, if correct, would also relate in part to oral hygiene practices. Females have increased grooming behavior compared with males, and this is associated with better oral hygiene.

The plaque's role as an etiologic factor in dentin hypersensitivity would appear to be an area of controversy. Thorough, over-enthusiastic toothbrushing has long been associated with gingival recession and sensitivity.

An exaggerated response to stimuli or the continuation of pain even after the removal of stimuli applied to dentin is suggestive of inflammatory changes in the pulp. Such pulpal changes may be due to bacteria or their toxins. Bacteria do penetrate into tubules of dentin left open to the oral environment, and their toxins may diffuse to the pulp. This diffusion would have to occur over relatively large distances and against the outward flow of dentinal fluid.

## THEORIES

The literature described three major theories demonstrating activation of dental nerve fibers in response to the application of stimuli to enamel or dentin (Fig. 36.1):[2,3]
1. Neural theory
2. Odontoblastic transduction theory
3. Hydrodynamic theory

### Neural Theory

The neural theory advocates that thermal or mechanical stimuli directly excite nerve endings, which are within the dentinal tubules. These nerve signals get conducted with the parent primary afferent nerve fibers in the pulp into the dental nerve branches and then transmitted into the brain.

### Odontoblastic Transduction Theory

The theory suggested that the hypersensitivity producing stimuli at first excite the odontoblast's process—the membrane of this odontoblast approximate with nerve endings present in the pulp or in the dentinal tubule.

The odontoblast further transfers the excitation to these associated nerve endings.

### Hydrodynamic Theory

Brannstrom in 1963 proposed that dentin hypersensitivity was the response to the movement of fluids within dentinal tubules. The fluid, when subjected to temperature changes or physical osmotic changes, the resultant movement stimulates the nerve receptor sensitive to pressure. Nerve receptor stimulation leads to the transmission of the stimuli.[4]

## DIAGNOSIS

The diagnosis of dentin hypersensitivity can be made by visual examination of the teeth, detailed dietary history, occlusion assessment, and diagnostic tools. The various diagnostic tools are following:[5]
- Air syringe
- Osmotic method
- Tactile method
- Thermal test

### Air Syringe

A burst of air (temperature between 65 and 70°F and a pressure 60 psi) from a dental syringe when directed at right angles on to the cut dentin causes evaporative fluid movement across the dentin. The evaporation of fluid occurs from the dentin when relatively dry 25°C air is directed at a 32°C tooth, which occurs very quickly (within 1 second). If longer blasts of air are used, one begins to cool the tooth, and the stimulus becomes complex owing to the addition of a thermal stimulus with an evaporative stimulus. Air blasts are useful stimuli during patient screening. They quickly identify individual sensitive teeth, but they are not useful at identifying sensitive tooth surfaces. The exact location of dentin sensitivity is important because it often dictates the type of therapy that might be employed. Air blasts are too diffuse to permit identification and quantitation of specific sites of sensitivity (Table 36.1).

### Osmotic Method

This method is based on the principle of osmosis, i.e., movement of fluid from higher concentration to lower

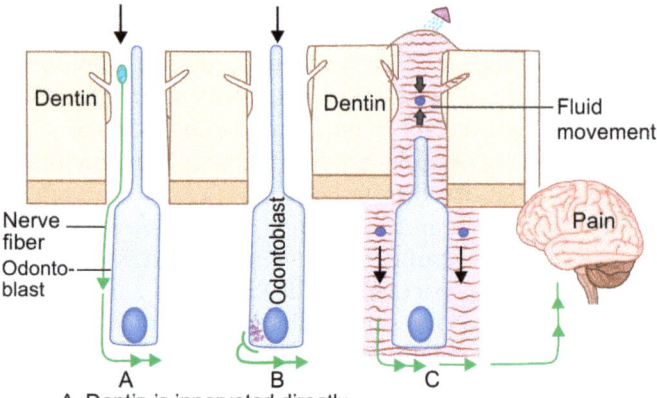

**Fig. 36.1:** Schematic representation showing theories of dentin sensitivity: (Panel A) Neural theory: Dentin is innervated directly; (Panel B) Odontoblastic transduction theory: Odontoblast acts as a receptor and (Panel C) Hydrodynamic theory: receptors are in the pulp and stimulated by fluid movement through the tubules.

| TABLE 36.1: Identification and quantitation of specific sites of sensitivity. | |
|---|---|
| Level of sensitivity | Description |
| 0 | No discomfort |
| 1 | Discomfort but no severe pain |
| 2 | Severe pain during application |
| 3 | Pain persists even after removal of stimuli |

concentration. In 1987, Mcfall and Hamrick introduced an osmotic method that consists of the subjective pain response to a sweet stimulus to measure the impact of several test dentifrices on dentinal sensitivity. After isolation of the test tooth with cotton rolls, a cotton applicator saturated with sucrose solution is applied to the tooth's root surface and allowed to remain in place for 10 seconds or until discomfort was perceived.

## Tactile Method

Dental explorer is used in identifying the regions of sensitive dentin. It is simple yet effective. The explorer's movement across dentin produces hydrodynamic stimulus causing displacement of fluid inwardly at a rapid rate, which activates mechanoreceptors. The amount of displacement is presumably proportional to the depth of the scratch and the compressed volume of the surrounding dentin. There may be recoil and outward movement of fluid when the pressure is taken off.

## Thermal Test

Thermoelectric devices are useful for delivering cold or warm stimuli in a controlled quantitative manner. Patients are generally more sensitive to cold than to hot stimuli. In using cold water, each tooth to be tested is isolated with a rubber dam. Water at a known temperature slowly flows on the exposed dentin surface for a maximum of 3 seconds from a disposable plastic syringe. The patient is asked whether that temperature causes pain or not, and then the next lower temperature is tried until the patient responds unequivocally. Thermal stimuli exhibited differences in thermal conductivity and coefficient of expansion or contraction of pulpal/dentinal fluids, enamel, and dentin and, hence, considered effective hydrodynamic stimuli. Cold application is found to lead to more rapid volumetric contraction of dentinal fluid compared to dentin. Mismatch in volumetric changes leads to the development of negative intrapulpal pressures, which moves mechanoreceptors and stimulates pain. Thermal stimuli to vital dentin cause sharp, well-localized pain (i.e., activation of A-δ fibers), before there is a change in dentin temperature near the pulp where the nerves are located.

## Differential Diagnosis

Dentin hypersensitivity can be differentiated by cracked tooth syndrome, chipped teeth, dental caries, post-restorative sensitivity, and irreversible pulpitis. Incomplete tooth fracture can be associated with several symptoms ranging from mild discomfort to severe pain. The most common complaint is pain on pressure. Tapping the teeth or having the patient bite down on an orangewood stick almost invariably evokes a sharp pain in the affected tooth. Exposure of dentin due to chipped enamel is obvious.

Differentiating dentinal hypersensitivity from caries is relatively easy, particularly in the case of a deep carious lesion. New amalgam or crown that has been placed without proper adjustment of the occlusion can cause post-restorative sensitivity. Pain in irreversible pulpitis frequently occurs without provocation. In the case of thermal test, the intense pain persists after the stimulus has been removed. Thus, it is important to determine chronology, nature, location, radiation, aggravating and alleviating factors that influence the pain.[6,7]

## HYPERSENSITIVITY MEASUREMENT

### Verbal Rating Scale

Verbal rating scale (VRS) records the patient's response after scratching and doing air-cold tests on a severity scale. The investigator should test all sensitive areas on all teeth of all subjects with the same tactile pressure. Immediately after the cold air blast, the subject usually reports the sensitivity level via VRS **(Table 36.2)**.[8]

### Visual Analog Scale

The visual analog scale (VAS) would be a more appropriate device than the VRS for measuring levels of sensitivity pain during the subject assessment, and for measuring tactile and thermal stimuli of hypersensitivity. The VRS is associated with a restrictive choice of words and hence unable to represent pain experience with sufficient precision for all subjects. Scott and Huskisson gave this scale in 1979. It is a scale of 10 cm commonly used to grade sensitivity. The zero-labeled at the one extreme suggests no pain, while 10 cm at the end of the scale suggests severe pain **(Fig. 36.2)**. Subjects are asked to place a mark on the 10 cm line at a location between no pain, and severe pain ends.[8]

**TABLE 36.2:** Level of sensitivity via a verbal rating scale.

| Level of sensitivity | Description |
|---|---|
| 0 | No response |
| 1 | Slight response but no pain |
| 2 | The pain only when a stimulus is applied |
| 3 | Severe, sudden and lasting pain |

*Note:* Score: Levels 0 and 1 are classified as nonsensitive teeth and levels 2 and 3 as hypersensitive teeth.

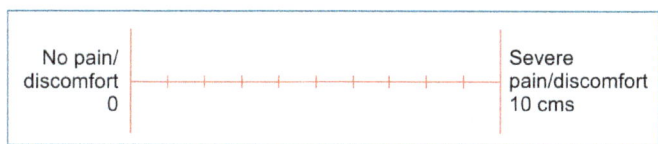

**Fig. 36.2:** Schematic representation showing the visual analog scale.

## MANAGEMENT

### Treatment Approaches for Dentinal Hypersensitivity

*Patient Counseling*
- Oral hygiene practices
- Dietary factors
- Remove risk factors by educating them
  In 1935, Grossman suggested the criteria for the ideal desensitizing agent as follows:[9]
- Non-irritating to the pulp
- Relatively painless on application
- Easily applied
- Rapid in action
- Permanently effective
- Do not discolor tooth structure

*Interventional Treatment*

*At-home treatment options*
At home, desensitizing agents can be **(Fig. 36.3 and Table 36.3)** used to occlude dentinal tubules, which block the hydrodynamic mechanism of dentinal sensitivity. Potassium nitrate ($KNO_3$) occludes the tubules and reduces fluid flow through them. Diffusion of potassium ($K^+$) ions of $KNO_3$ through the dentinal tubules and their entry at the pulp sensory complex leads to the formation of a region of high concentration of $K^+$ ions. This depolarizes the pulpal sensory complex and minimizes the pain transmission.[10]

*In-office treatment options*
- *Noninvasive methods:*[11]
  *Oxalates*: They have been used popularly as a desensitizing agent. They are relatively inexpensive, easy to apply and well-tolerated by the patients. 6% ferric oxalate, 30% potassium oxalate, and 3% monohydrogen monopotassium oxalate solutions are used as desensitizing agents. The oxalate ions usually interact with calcium ions in the dentinal fluid and lead to the formation of insoluble calcium oxalate crystals. These crystals usually get deposited within the apertures of dentinal tubules.
- *Cavity varnishes*: When using desensitizing agents that have a caustic effect on the soft tissue, care must be exercised to prevent them from contacting the alveolar mucosa. The teeth should be isolated and dried with warm air. Dentin often becomes insensitive when open tubules are covered with a thin film of varnish. This may be an effective means of providing temporary relief.
- *Strontium chloride*: Local application of concentrated strontium chloride ($SrCl_2$) on an abraded dentin surface leads to the formation of strontium deposits which usually passes to a depth of approximately 20 µm and spread into the dentinal tubules.
- *Composite resins*: They seal out the dentinal tubules and avoid the entry of pain-producing stimuli at the pulp.
- *GLUMA*: This dentin bonding system composed of 5% glutaraldehyde primer and 35% hydroxyethyl methacrylate (HEMA) provide immediate and strong attachment to dentin.
- *Calcium hydroxide [$Ca(OH)_2$]*: It is a well-known agent for the treatment of dentin hypersensitivity for many years, especially after root planing. The exact mechanism of action is unknown, but evidence suggests that it may block dentinal tubules or promote peritubular dentin formation.
- *LASER*: Argon, carbon dioxide ($CO_2$), Ho: YAG (holmium: yttrium aluminium garnet), Nd: YAG (neodymium-doped yttrium aluminium garnet),

**TABLE 36.3:** Various desensitizing agents.

| Trade name | Agents |
|---|---|
| Sensodyne | 10% strontium chloride ($SrCl_2$) and sodium fluoride |
| Thermodent | 10% $SrCl_2$ |
| Protect | 2% dibasic sodium citrate in a pluronic gel |
| Promise | 5% potassium nitrate ($KNO_3$), dicalcium phosphate and sodium monofluorophosphate |
| Denquel | 5% $KNO_3$ |
| Isodan | $KNO_3$, sodium fluoride, HEMA (hydroxyethyl methacrylate) |
| Sensodyne F | Potassium chloride (KCl) and sodium monofluorophosphate |
| Colgate sensitive care | Potassium citrate and sodium monofluorophosphate |
| Macleans sensitive | Strontium acetate and sodium monofluorophosphate |

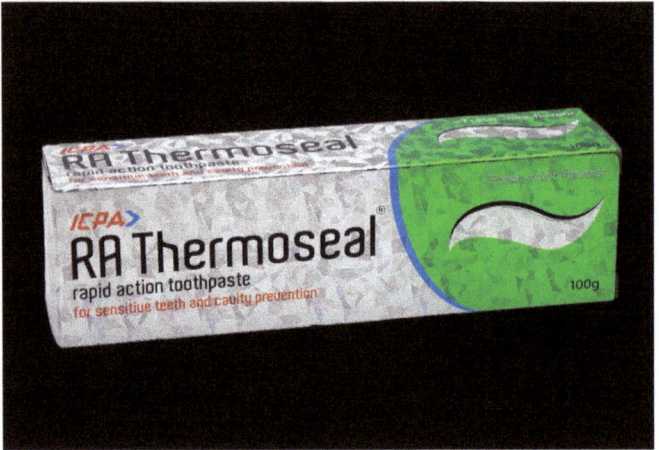

**Fig. 36.3:** Photograph showing desensitizing agent (dentifrice containing potassium nitrate) (Reproduced with permission from ICPA Health Products Ltd.).

erbium YAG is the LASER types used for desensitizing. These systems have become available, which are tailored specifically for dental surgery using fiberoptic delivery to a handpiece, smaller than a conventional rotary dental instrument. The availability of laser would potentially satisfy all the requirements of a desensitizing agent. They block the tubules probably by fusion of crystals (hydroxyapatite), as the low-intensity defocused beam is used.

- *Iontophoresis*: Fluoride iontophoresis is a mean to drive fluoride ions more deeply into dentinal tubules. It involves the placement of a negative electrode to dentin and a positive electrode to the patient's face or arm. Saliva becomes a medium in which ions commence their selective motion. Negative ions flow through the positively charged teeth and positive ions to the negatively charged bristles. Iontophoresis devices are expensive and somewhat difficult to use.[12]

- *Invasive methods*:
  - Pulpectomy
  - Class V restorations
  - Gingival graft surgery

### Block Neural Transmission of the Pulp
- By endodontics
- Tooth extraction

## PREVENTION

### Patient Education and Dietary Counseling

Dietary acids are commonly responsible for the erosive loss of tooth structure resulting in the removal of cementum and opening of dentinal tubules. Hence, dietary counseling should target on controlling the quantity and frequency of acid intake. Counseling should also focus on acid intake in relation to tooth-brushing. Any treatment may fail if these factors are not controlled. Obtain a written diet history from the patients with dentinal hypersensitivity so that it is easy to identify the possible sources of acid in the diet. This knowledge will help to advise the patient on suitable eating habits. Red and white wine, citrus fruit juices, apple juice, and yoghurt, are found to dissolve the smear layer in vitro and hence should be avoided in such patient.[6]

### Toothbrushing Techniques

Toothbrushing, when associated with decalcification of superficial dentin, accelerates the loss of tooth structure. Because the loss of dentin is greatly increased when brushing is performed immediately after exposure of tooth surface to dietary acids. Thus, patients should be cautioned against brushing their teeth soon after the ingestion of citrus food. Improper way of tooth-brushing enhances dentin hypersensitivity, and hence patients should receive instructions on proper brushing techniques to avoid further loss of dentin and hypersensitivity.

#### Clinical Tips

For managing dentin hypersensitivity:
- Avoid hard-bristled tooth-brushes without rounded-end bristles.
- Avoid tooth-brushing immediately after the consumption of acidic food or beverages.
- Avoid over brushing and flossing with excessive pressure for a long duration.
- Avoid over instrumentation of the root surfaces during calculus removal.
- Avoid over-polishing of exposed roots during stain removal.
- Avoid violating the biologic width while positioning crown margins.

#### Points to Ponder

- Robinson's remedy consists of equal parts of carbolic acid and caustic potash.
- Desensitizing agents should be used continuously for at least 2 weeks to show an effective response.
- Localized hypersensitivity can be treated by applying varnishes, dentin bonding agents.
- Generalized hypersensitivity can be treated by prescribing desensitizing dentifrices.

## REFERENCES

1. Addy M. Etiology and clinical implications of dentin hypersensitivity. Dent Clin North Am. 1990;34(3):503-14.
2. Pashley DH. Mechanisms of dentin sensitivity. Dent Clin North Am. 1990;34(3):449-73.
3. Curro FA. Tooth hypersensitivity in the spectrum of pain. Dent Clin North Am. 1990;34(3):429-37.
4. Brannstrom M. Dentin sensitivity and aspiration of odontoblasts. J Am Dent Assoc. 1963;66:366-70.
5. Kleinberg I, Kaufman HW, Confessore F. Methods of measuring tooth hypersensitivity. Dent Clin North Am. 1990;34(3):515-29.
6. Trowbridge HO, Silver DR. A review of current approaches to in-office management of tooth hypersensitivity. Dent Clin North Am. 1990;34(3):561-81.
7. West NX. Dentine hypersensitivity: preventive and therapeutic approaches to treatment. Periodontol 2000. 2008;48:31-41.
8. Clark GE, Troullos ES. Designing hypersensitivity clinical studies. Dent Clin North Am. 1990;34(3):531-44.
9. Grossman LI. A systemic method for the treatment of hypersensitive dentine. J Am Dent Assoc. 1935;22:592-602.
10. Kanapka JA. Over-the-counter dentifrices in the treatment of tooth hypersensitivity. Review of clinical studies. Dent Clin North Am. 1990;34(3):545-60.
11. Klokkevold PR, Carranza FA, Takei HH. General principles of periodontal surgery. In: Newman MG, Takei HH, Carranza FA (Eds). Carranza's Clinical Periodontology, 9th edition. Philadelphia, PA, USA: WB Saunders; 2003. pp. 725-36.
12. Gillam DG, Newman HN. Iontophoresis in the treatment of cervical dentinal sensitivity—a review. J West Soc Periodontol Periodontal Abstr. 1990;38(4):129-33.

## VIVA VOCE

**Q1. Which LASERS are used for desensitizing?**

**Ans.** Argon, carbon dioxide ($CO_2$), Ho: YAG (holmium: yttrium aluminium garnet), Nd: YAG (neodymium-doped yttrium aluminium garnet), and erbium: YAG is the LASER types used for desensitizing.

**Q2. How LASERS cause desensitization?**

**Ans.** LASERS cause desensitization by melting effect with the crystallization of dentin inorganic component and the coagulation of fluids contained into the dentinal tubules.

**Q3. Name ADA approved desensitizing dentifrices.**

**Ans.** Sensodyne and Thermodent ($SrCl_2$)
- Denquel and Promise ($KNO_3$)
- Protect (Sodium Citrate)

**Q4. Which beverages and food should be avoided to prevent dentin hypersensitivity?**

**Ans.** Red and white wine, citrus fruit juices, apple juice, and yoghurt.

**Q5. Which is the most accepted theory related to dentinal hypersensitivity?**

**Ans.** Brannstrom gave the hydrodynamic theory in 1963.

**Q6. What is GLUMA?**

**Ans.** This dentin bonding system composed of 5% glutaraldehyde primer and 35% HEMA (hydroxyethyl methacrylate).

**Q7. Who gave the visual analog scale?**

**Ans.** Scott and Huskisson in 1979.

**Q8. What is iontophoresis?**

**Ans.** Fluoride iontophoresis is a means to drive fluoride ions more deeply into dentinal tubules. It involves the placement of a negative electrode to dentin and a positive electrode to the patient's face or arm.

**Q9. What are the disadvantages associated with iontophoresis?**

**Ans.** Iontophoresis devices are expensive and somewhat difficult to use.

**Q10. How can localized hypersensitivity be treated?**

**Ans.** By applying varnishes or dentin bonding agents.

# Chapter 37

# Mechanical Plaque Control

*Satish C Narula*

## Chapter Outline

- Traditional Oral Hygiene Methods
- Toothbrushes
- Dentifrices
- Interdental Cleaning Aids
- Other Aids
- Oral Hygiene Methods Causing Trauma
- Assessment of Home Care
- Hawthorne Effect

## INTRODUCTION

Plaque control is the removal of dental plaque and prevention of its accumulation on the teeth and adjacent gingival surfaces. Maintaining adequate oral hygiene practices are essential for controlling supragingival plaque. The conventional toothbrush is the cleaning device most frequently used to remove dental plaque. Self-care mechanical plaque control methods prove highly effective when conducted under the supervision and with proper use of oral hygiene aids and manual dexterity. The process requires great motivation and adequate knowledge about maintaining dental hygiene. The prerequisite for achieving a successful outcome in needs-related tooth cleaning habits is a well-motivated, well-informed, and well-instructed patient.

## TRADITIONAL ORAL HYGIENE METHODS

Worldwide traditional oral hygiene methods have been practiced for a long time. Easy availability and low cost make such methods an integral part of religious and/or traditional beliefs. Chewing sticks available from certain plants have been practiced in certain countries of Asia and Africa for decades. They are considered as naturally available good oral hygiene tools. In practice, a chewing stick is cut from the plant's twigs, stems, or roots. This stick is chewed or tapered at one end until it gets to wear out into a brush-like tool. Then this stick is useful to brush the facial aspects of teeth, gingiva, and tongue. When this stick is kept in the mouth for a more extended period after brushing, it can stimulate salivation.

Additionally, extracts leaking out from these sticks into the user's mouth are supposed to impart biological properties, including potential antibacterial effects. It is considered that plants contain antimicrobial substances, which naturally protect against invading microorganisms or other parasites. Furthermore, these substances have innate resistance potential against cariogenic and periodontopathic bacteria.

Earlier, toothbrush bristles were obtained from the hair of the hog or wild boar. Toothbrushes with natural bristles wear rapidly, and their hollowness permits microorganisms and debris to get collect inside. Moreover, they are water absorbent also. Hence, such toothbrushes are not advocated these days. Furthermore, their physical qualifications cannot be standardized. Current toothbrushes have nylon bristles or polyester filaments, which are durable and resistant to bacteria accumulation than natural bristles.

## TOOTHBRUSHES

### Historical Perspective

Historically, the toothbrush was developed and evolved over the years in the following manner:[1,2]

- *1600*: Bristle toothbrush appeared in China.
- *1728*: Pierre Fauchard, in his book "The Surgeon Dentist," advocated wet sponges and specially prepared herb roots.
- *1780*: William Addis of England made the first toothbrush.
- *1840*: England, France, and Germany started producing bristle toothbrush.

- *1857*: HN Wadsworth patented the first American toothbrush.
- *1900*: Celluloid handles were used.
- *1919*: The American Academy of Periodontology (AAP) defined specifications.
- *1938*: Nylon was first applied to toothbrush construction.
- *1939*: Synthetics were substituted for natural materials.

## Designs

### Manual Toothbrushes

Toothbrushes vary in size, design, bristle hardness, length, and arrangement. The choice is a matter of individual preference rather than a demonstrated superiority of any one type. Parts of the toothbrush are shown in **Figure 37.1**.

- *Handle*: Purpose of the handle is to grasp the brush in the hand during toothbrushing. Commonly, handles are composed of plastic, which is sufficiently rigid and durable. The dimension of the handle of an adult is 6-inches; the junior is one-sixth smaller than adult size, and the child is one-third smaller than adult size. The handle should be thick enough to allow a firm grip and good control.
- *Shank*: Shank connects the head with the handle. It varies as per brands, and maybe twisted, curved, or with the angle with or without thumb rests **(Fig. 37.2)**.
- *Head*: Head is the working end of a toothbrush, which consists of tufts of bristles. The head's length is approximately 1–1.25-inch, and the width is 5/16–3/8-inch. Bristle length-to-height is 7/16-inches. The

**BOX 37.1:** American Dental Association (ADA) specifications of toothbrush.[3]
- *Length*: 1–1.25-inches
- *Width*: 5/16–3/8-inches
- *Rows*: 2–4 rows of bristles
- *Tufts*: 5–12 per row

**BOX 37.2:** Bass recommendation for toothbrush.[4]
- *Handle*: Plain straight handle of 6-inch long and width about 7/16-inch
- *Head*: High-quality nylon bristles
- *Rows*: 3 rows of bristles
- *Tufts*: 6 tufts per row, evenly spaced tufts
- *Bristles*: 80–86 bristles per tuft
- *Bristles diameter*: 0.007-inch (0.18 mm)
- *Bristles length*: 0.406-inch (10 mm)
- Round-ended bristles

**BOX 37.3:** Diameter of bristles.[5]
- Bristle diameter ranges from soft to hard
- *Soft*: 0.2 mm/0.007-inches
- *Medium*: 0.3 mm/0.012-inches
- *Hard*: 0.4 mm/0.014-inches
- Filament stiffness $\alpha \dfrac{diameter^2}{length^2}$

brushing plane is the trim that presents the peculiar arrangement of the tips of filaments at the brushing surface.[1] It usually varies from filaments of equal length, i.e., flat planes to those with variable lengths, such as bi-level, dome-shaped. Bristles in adult toothbrushes are usually 10–11 mm long. However, the entire filament should have a rounded end to avoid trauma to the oral tissues **(Boxes 37.1 to 37.3)**.[3-5]

### Care of Toothbrushes

- *Cleaning*: Hold the brush head under a strong stream of warm water to remove dentifrices and bacteria present between filaments and then tap the brush handle on the edge of the sink to remove excess water. Use another toothbrush to clean and remove resistant debris of other toothbrushes.
- *Brush storage*: It should be kept in the open air with head in an upright position, apart from contact with other brushes. Keep the brushes in a portable brush container having sufficient holes after being dried completely.
- *Brush replacement*: Toothbrush should be replaced before filaments frayed, at least every 2–3 months. But patients, who are debilitated, have a known infection or are about to undergo surgery should be advised to disinfect their brush or use a disposable brush.

### Powered Toothbrushes

Electrically powered toothbrushes were invented in 1939. They are also called as mechanical, automatic or electric

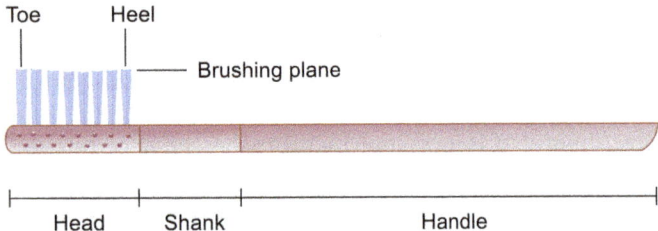

**Fig. 37.1:** Schematic representation showing parts of a toothbrush.

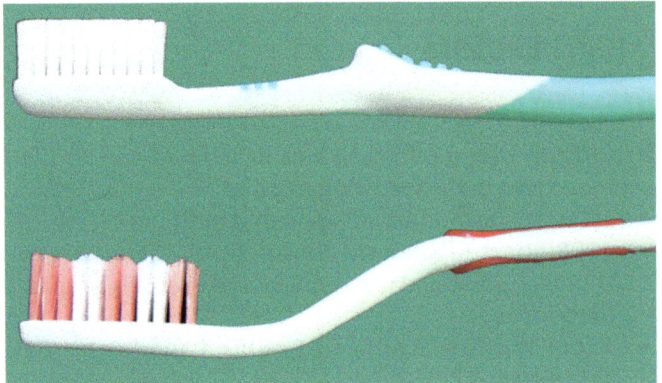

**Fig. 37.2:** Photograph showing straight and angled shank toothbrushes.

brushes. Speed varies from low to high among different models. The thick handles of power-assisted brushes are easily handled and manipulated by patients with disabilities. The action is inbuilt in a powered toothbrush. The only muscle training required is to turn the handle to apply the brush to each surface of each tooth and hold it on each surface for a reasonable time in a correct position **(Figs. 37.3 and 37.4)**.

## Classifications

Classifications of powered toothbrushes based on different forms of movements[6] are as following:
- *Lateral motion powered toothbrush (Philips Sonicare)*: Brush head action that moves from side-to-side laterally.
- *Circular-powered toothbrush*: Whole brush head rotates in one direction.
- *Rotation oscillation-powered toothbrush (Braun Oral-B and Colgate Actibrush)*: Whole brush head rotates in one direction, followed by the other.
- *Counter oscillation powered toothbrush (Interplak brush)*: Adjacent half of the tufts rotate in one direction and then counter-rotate with adjacent tufts moving in opposite directions.
- *Sonic and ultrasonic-powered toothbrush* (Ultrasonex): They transmit high-frequency, low-intensity sound waves through the bristles to soft tissues and plaque deposits. These high-frequency waves disrupt bacterial cell walls due to the phenomenon of acoustic streaming and cavitation.
- *Ionic-powered toothbrush (Hukuba)*: These toothbrushes charge the surface of a tooth by an influx of positively charged ions. The plaque with a similar charge is then repelled from the tooth surface and is attracted by the negatively charged bristles of the toothbrush.

### Indications
- In patients wearing orthodontic appliances.
- Children and adolescents.
- In patients undergoing complex restorative and prosthodontic treatment.
- In patients with dental implants.
- Patients with physical or mental disabilities.
- Hospitalized patients, elder ones who need to have their teeth cleaned by caregivers.
- Poorly compliant patient for periodontal maintenance.[7]

## Orthodontic Toothbrushes

The head of the brush features soft bristles that are shorter down the center with hedges of taller bristles on either side, allowing the brush to pass over the appliance without causing abrasion to the teeth. It is also called as a bi-level toothbrush **(Figs. 37.5 and 37.6)**.

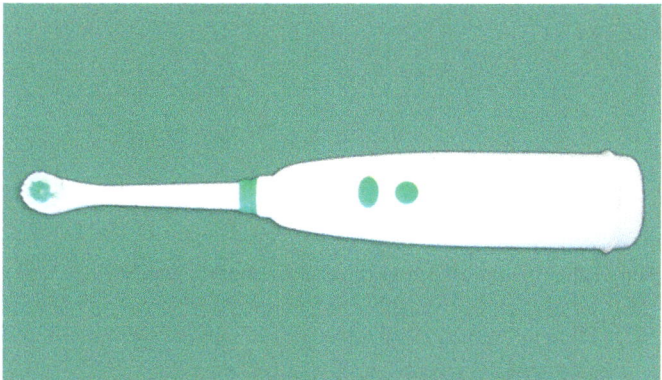

**Fig. 37.3:** Photograph showing powered toothbrush.

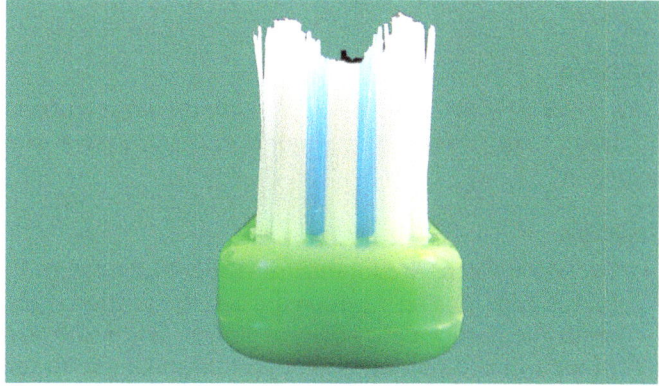

**Fig. 37.5:** Photograph showing an orthodontic brush.

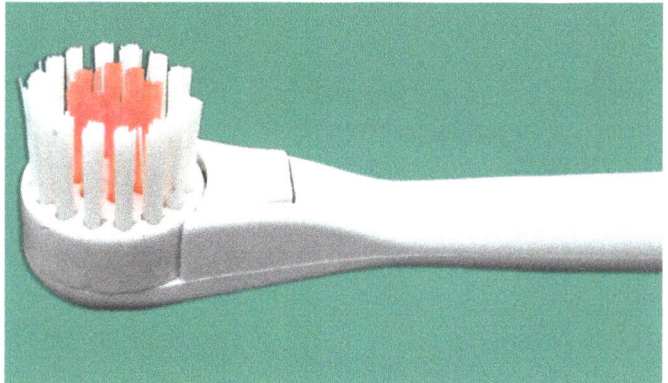

**Fig. 37.4:** Photograph showing head of a powered toothbrush.

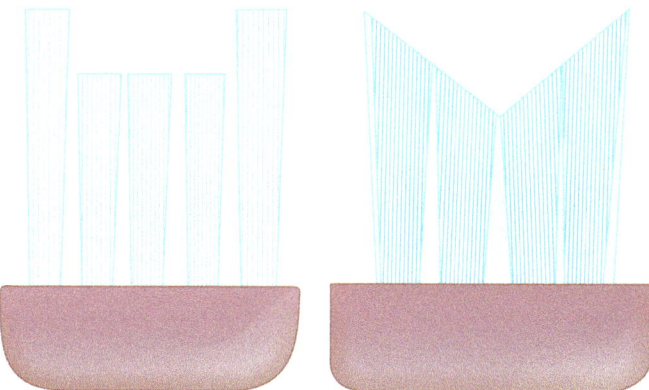

**Fig. 37.6:** Schematic representation showing the bi-level orthodontic brush.

### Novel Toothbrushes

The majority of the individuals use a simple horizontal brushing action and regular flat-headed brush. These toothbrushes are unable to reach the approximal surfaces in the dentition. Hence, novel toothbrushes are introduced to overcome these brushing difficulties. The head of the novel toothbrush has been changed, and multiple tufts of bristles are angled in different directions **(Fig. 37.7)**. Thus, when the head is located horizontal to the tooth surface, there are bristles angled in the direction of the approximal tooth surfaces.

## Methods

Following are the toothbrushing methods which are categorized according to the pattern of motion during the action of brushing:
- *Roll*: Roll and modified Stillman method
- *Vibratory*: Stillman, Charter, and Bass method
- *Sulcular*: Bass method
- *Circular*: Fones method
- *Vertical*: Leonard method
- *Horizontal*: Horizontal and scrub method
- *Physiologic*: Smith method

### Modified Stillman Method

Paul R Stillman described the modified Stillman method in 1932.[8]

#### Indication

This method is advised to reduce abrasive tissue destruction in areas with progressing gingival recession and root exposure.

#### Technique

- *Facial surfaces*: The toothbrush is positioned with its bristle ends, posing partly on the cervical portion of the teeth and partly on the adjacent gingiva. It is positioned in an apical direction and at an oblique angle to the teeth' long axis. Sides of the bristles are placed against the teeth and gingiva while moving the brush with short, back and forth strokes in a coronal direction. This process must be repeated on all tooth surfaces, proceeding systematically around the mouth.
- *Lingual surfaces:* To reach the lingual surfaces of the maxillary and mandibular incisors, the handle of the brush can be held in a vertical position.
- *Occlusal surfaces*: The occlusal surfaces of molars and premolars are cleaned with the bristles placed perpendicular to the occlusal plane and penetrating the grooves and interproximal embrasures **(Figs. 37.8 and 37.9)**.

### Charters Method

Leonard Koecker first described this technique in 1819. However, it was William J Charters in 1932 who endorsed and documented this technique.[9]

#### Indications

- For cleaning purposes in areas of wound healing after periodontal surgery.
- The patients wearing orthodontic appliances.

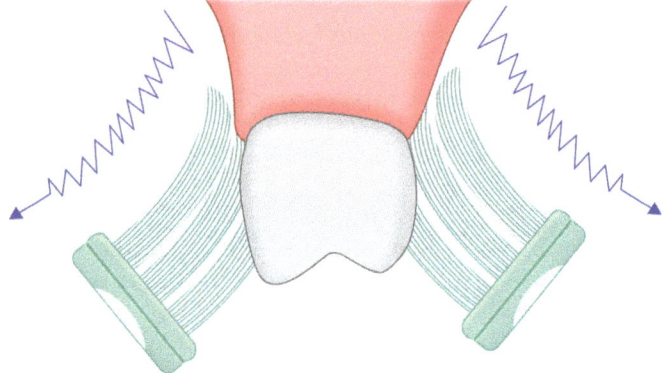

**Fig. 37.8:** Schematic representation showing modified Stillman method: Brush is moved with short back and forth strokes in the coronal direction.

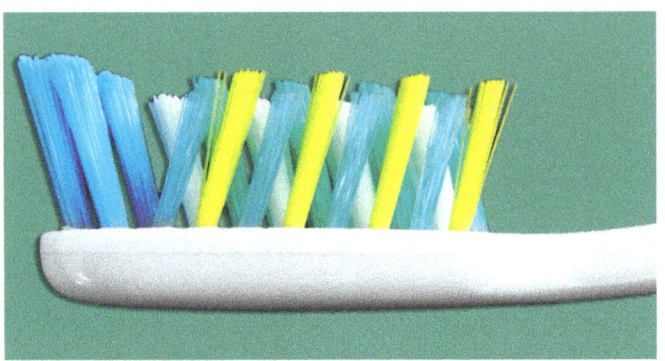

**Fig. 37.7:** Photograph showing novel design toothbrush.

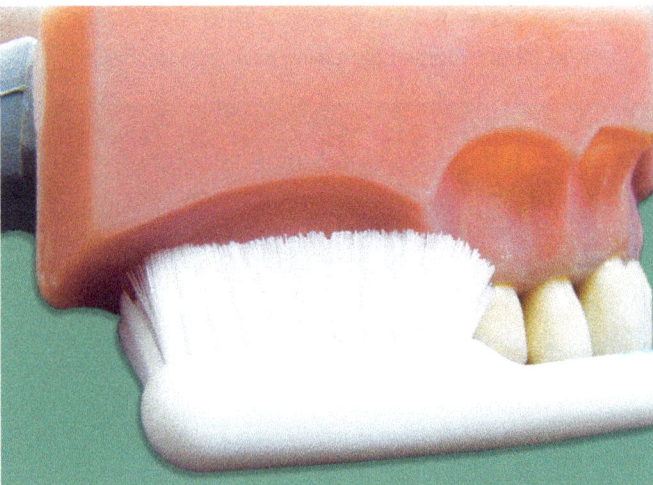

**Fig. 37.9:** Photograph showing Stillman method: Side of the bristles are placed against the teeth and gingiva.

Chapter 37: Mechanical Plaque Control

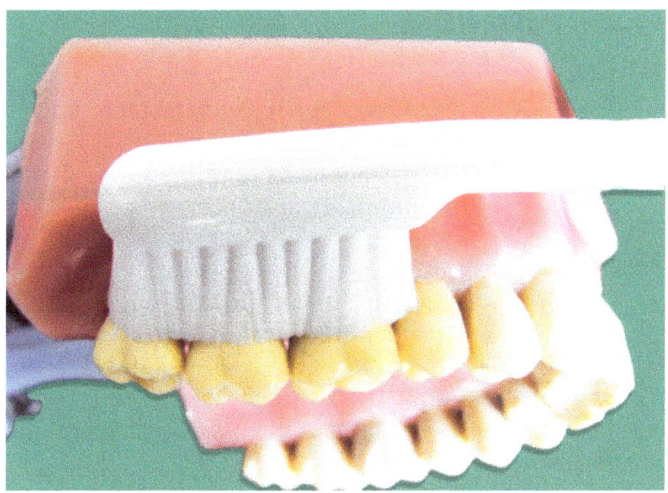

Fig. 37.10: Photograph showing Charters method.

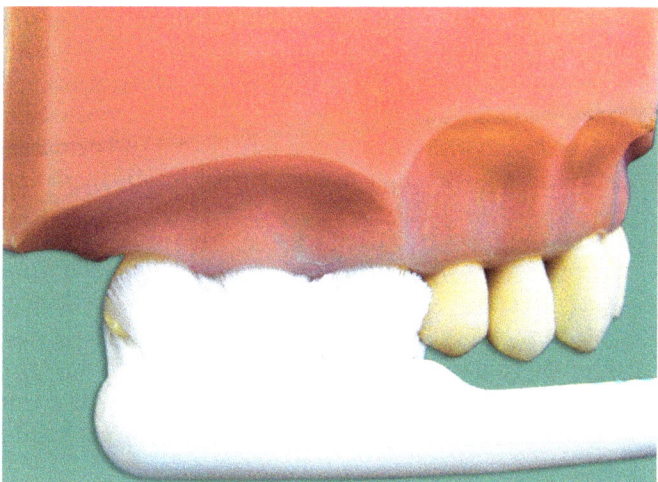

Fig. 37.11: Photograph showing Bass method (facial view).

- Remove bacterial plaque from abutment teeth and under the gingival border of a fixed partial denture (bridge) or from the undersurface of the sanitary bridge.

**Technique**

Hold brush with filaments towards the occlusal or incisal plane of the teeth to be brushed and angle the filaments at 45° to the long-axis of teeth **(Fig. 37.10)**. The sides of the bristles should be bending against the gingiva, and a back and forth vibratory motion is helpful to brush teeth. The technique was designed to massage the gingiva gently, so the bristle tips should not drag across the gingiva.

## *Bass Method*

It is also called the intrasulcular method, which was advocated by Talbot. This toothbrushing technique was then introduced by Charles Cassedy Bass in 1948, utilizing a soft-multi tufted brush with bristles 0.007-inch in diameter.[10]

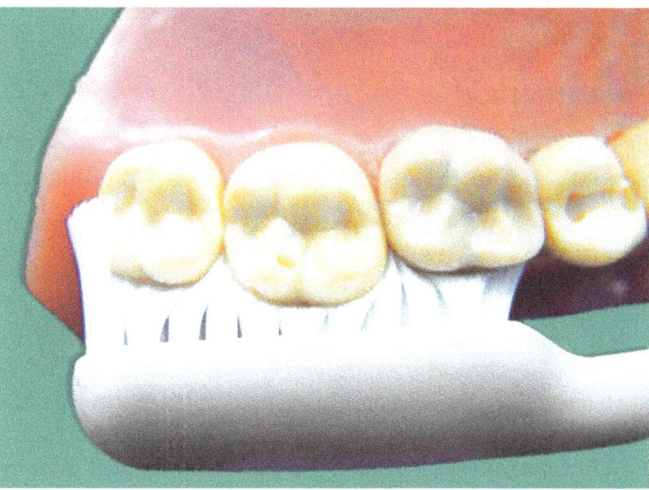

Fig. 37.12: Photograph showing Bass method (occlusal view).

**Indications**

- For open interproximal areas, cervical areas beneath the height of contour of the enamel and exposed root surfaces.
- Recommended for any patient with or without periodontal involvement.

**Technique**

- *Facial surfaces*: Place the head of a soft brush at the start of the most distal tooth in the arch. It should be parallel with the occlusal plane with the brush head covering 3–4 teeth. Filament tips of the brush are directed straight into gingival sulcus and interproximal embrasures at approximately 45° to long-axis of the tooth **(Figs. 37.11 to 37.13)**. Brush vibrates back and forth with very short strokes without removing the filaments' tips from the sulci. Complete approximately 20 strokes in the same

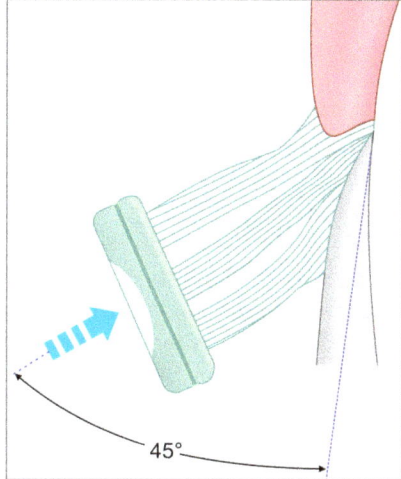

**Fig. 37.13:** Schematic representation showing the Bass method: Bristle tips are in the sulcus, and the position of the brush is at 45° to long-axis of tooth.

position. Continue applying the brush to the next group of 2 or 3 teeth in an overlapping manner.
- *Lingual surfaces*: Place the brush vertically to approach the lingual surface of anterior teeth and press the heel of the brush into the gingival sulcus area and proximal surfaces at a 45° angle to the long axis of the teeth and brush with multiple short vibratory strokes.
- *Occlusal surfaces*: Bristles should be pressed firmly into the pits and fissures and brush with about 20 short back and forth strokes. Repeat the entire stroke at each position around the maxillary and mandibular arches, both facially and lingually.
- In the modified Bass method, bristles are swept towards the occlusal surface after completing the gingival sulcus' vibratory motion.

### Advantages
- It cleans the gingival sulcus.
- It also cleans the interproximal and cervical portion of teeth.

## Fones Method

### Indication
School children or young children because of simplicity.

### Technique
Dr Fones advocated this circular method. The method involves closing the teeth and lightly pressing bristles of the toothbrush against posterior teeth and gingiva. The brush head should be revolved in a fast circular motion with large diameter circles. Continue circular motion. Hold maxillary and mandibular teeth apart and continue same circular motion on maxillary lingual surfaces and then on mandibular lingual surfaces.[11]

### Disadvantages
- It may traumatize soft tissues.
- It does not clean teeth adequately, especially in interproximal areas.

## Vertical Method
Leonard described and advocated the vertical method of toothbrushing.[12]

### Technique
Hold teeth in an edge-to-edge position. Direct the toothbrush bristles at a right angle to the long-axis of teeth. Vigorously move the brush up and down on tooth surfaces. It demands to put sufficient pressure to force the filaments into the embrasures.

### Disadvantages
- It does not clean the teeth adequately.
- It may push debris towards gingival sulci.
- It may cause McCall's festoons.

## Horizontal Method

### Technique
- Place bristle tips at the right angle on facial or lingual surfaces of teeth.
- Draw bristles across adjacent teeth and interdental papillae in a horizontal direction.

### Disadvantages
- This method does not clean the teeth adequately, especially the proximal surfaces.
- It injures free gingiva if performed forcefully can cause gingival recession.
- It can abrade cementum and dentin, leading to tooth abrasion.

## Scrub Method

### Indication
Very young children get the feeling of brushing his/her teeth.

### Technique
This method involves combined horizontal, vertical, and circular strokes performed forcibly with some vibratory motions for specific areas.

## Physiologic Method
In 1940, T Sidney Smith described the physiological method for plaque control, which was recommended later by Bell in 1948. The method was based on the concept that the toothbrush should follow the same physiologic pathway that food follows when it traverses over the tissues in a natural masticating act. With a soft toothbrush, brush the gingival tissues towards apices of teeth in a gentle sweeping motion. Brushing strokes should be directed down over the lower teeth onto the gingiva for the mandibular and upward over the teeth for the maxillary.

### Disadvantages
- It causes injury to soft tissues.
- It does not clean the teeth adequately.

## Sequence of Brushing
The following sequence of toothbrushing should be followed:[1]
- Maxillary teeth first, then mandibular to avoid the deposition of loosened debris from maxillary teeth on brushed mandibular teeth.
- Initiate brushing from the facial aspect of the molar region of one arch around to the opposite side, then back around the lingual aspect. Repeat the same in the opposing arch.
- There should be adequate overlapping between each brush placement with the previous one for thorough coverage.

- Motivate the patient to start brushing at the area that is commonly neglected or difficult to reach for brush placement.
- The sequence is varied at least once each day.

## Toothbrush Contamination

The toothbrush can be a mode of indirect transmission for pathogenic organisms. It can act as a fomite (an inanimate object that houses and transmits potentially infectious agents). Its caps, holders, and plastic coverings encourage microbial growth, so air drying is preferred.

The harmful effects of overzealous horizontal brushing are gingival recession, bacteremia, wedge-shaped abrasion defects in the cervical area of root surfaces, and painful ulceration of the gingiva.

## DENTIFRICES

Dentifrices date back over 2000 years. It was well accepted with the reinvention of the toothbrush by William Addis in 1770. In 1892, Dr Washington Wentworth Sheffield invented a toothpaste tube. In 1942, Bibby conducted the first clinical trial of fluoride toothpaste.

Dentifrice is a substance used with a toothbrush or any other applicator to remove bacterial plaque and debris from the gingiva and teeth. Thus, they aid in cleaning and polishing tooth surfaces. They are used in the form of pastes, powders, and gels.

Different abrasives differ not only with their chemical composition but also in particle size and shape (round, angular). These differences determine the polishing effect of product and abrasiveness of the dentifrices on dentin [which is measured in vitro as radioactive or relative dentin abrasion (RDA) value]. Therapeutic dentifrice has a chemical agent added for a specific preventive or treatment action, e.g., fluoride, desensitizing agent, tartar control agents containing dentifrices **(Table 37.1)**. Colgate® Total™ is the first and only toothpaste approved by the Food and Drug Administration (FDA). To avoid fluorosis in children, a pea-sized amount of toothpaste is sufficient. An adult requires enough toothpaste to cover the whole length of the toothbrush bristles.

## Therapeutic Ingredients

- *Fluoride agents*: Fluorides currently used in dentifrices are sodium fluoride (NaF), sodium monofluorophosphate ($Na_2PFO_3$), and stabilized stannous fluoride ($SnF_2$).
- *Plaque-inhibiting agents*: Sanguinarine, chlorhexidine, lactoperoxidase, triclosan, zinc, and stabilized $SnF_2$ are the plaque-inhibiting agents used in dentifrices.
- *Desensitizing agents*: Fluoride agents have been claimed to have desensitizing properties and are contained in specialized dentifrices (e.g., $SnF_2$); non-fluoride agents commonly used in desensitizing agents include strontium chloride, potassium nitrate, and sodium citrate.

**TABLE 37.1:** Constituents of dentifrices.

| Compositions | Constituents | Purpose | Paste or gel | Powder |
|---|---|---|---|---|
| Abrasives | ◆ Calcium carbonate<br>◆ Calcium phosphate<br>◆ Hydrated alumina<br>◆ Hydrated silica | Cleaning or stain removal | 20–25% | 90–98% |
| Detergent | Sodium lauryl sulfate | Surfactant or foam builder | 1–2% | 1–6% |
| Binder | Carrageenan | Hold ingredients together | 3% | 0 |
| Humectants | ◆ Sorbitol<br>◆ Glycerin | ◆ Provide creamy texture<br>◆ Moisturizing agent | 20–35% | 0 |
| Colorants | ◆ Food colorants<br>◆ Titanium oxide | Make opaque or transparent | 1–2% | 1–2% |
| Water | | Solvent | 15–25% | 0 |
| Flavoring | ◆ Spearmint<br>◆ Wintergreen<br>◆ Cinnamon | Improves taste | 1–2% | 1–2% |
| Tartar control agents | ◆ Triclosan<br>◆ Disodium pyrophosphate<br>◆ Tetrasodium pyrophosphate<br>◆ Tetrapotassium pyrophosphate | Inhibit calculus formation | 0–1% | 0 |
| Fluorides | ◆ Sodium fluoride<br>◆ Stannous fluoride | Anticariogenic reduces caries | 0–1% | 0 |
| Desensitizing agent | ◆ Potassium nitrate<br>◆ Strontium chloride | Reduce hypersensitivity | 0–5% | 0 |

- *Tartar control agents*: They interfere with the calcium phosphate bond in the calculus matrix, thus allowing easier removal of soft calculus during toothbrushing; they are effective only on the formation of supragingival calculus on enamel surfaces.
  - *Pyrophosphate system*: Pyrophosphate has a negative charge, attracts positively charged calcium ions, and interferes with calculus formation.
  - *Zinc system*: Zinc has a positive charge, attracts negatively charged phosphate ions, and interferes with calculus formation.
- *Whitening agents*: Several dentifrices are marketed for their ability to remove stains; several whitening dentifrices have low-abrasive levels; may be effective for maintenance of cosmetic restorations.
- *Baking soda*: Manufacturers claim benefits from the addition of baking soda or baking soda and peroxide to dentifrices; however, therapeutic benefits have not been demonstrated in controlled clinical trials.

## INTERDENTAL CLEANING AIDS

Interdental cleaning aids are dental floss, dental tape, interdental brushes, interdental tips, wooden tips, rubber tips, and plastic tips.

The various factors that should be taken into consideration while recommending an interdental cleaning method are the type and size of the interproximal embrasure (**Figs. 37.14A to C**):[13,14]
- Type 1 embrasures where no gingival recession present,
- there dental floss is used.
- Type 2 embrasures where there is a moderate papillary recession, there interdental brush is used.
- Type 3 embrasures where there is a complete loss of papillae, there unitufted brush is used.

Other factors that affect the interdental cleaning methods are contour and consistency of gingival tissues, tooth position, and alignment, ability and motivation of the patient, presence of orthodontic appliance or fixed prosthesis, and presence of furcation lesion.

## Dental Floss

It is the most widely recommended interdental aid for removing plaque from proximal tooth surfaces.

### Indication

It is indicated where interdental papillae fill the embrasure space.

### Types

- Bonded or nonbonded.
- Twisted or nontwisted.
- *Waxed or unwaxed*: The wax covering waxed dental floss facilitates the movement of floss, prevents excessive absorption of moisture, and shredding.
- *Powered flossing devices*: Now, they have also been introduced.

### Technique

About 12–18-inches of dental floss is wrapped around fingers or ends may be tied together to form a loop (**Fig. 37.15**). The floss is stretched tightly between thumb and forefinger or between both forefingers. It is allowed to pass through each contact area with a firm back-and-forth motion (**Figs. 37.16 to 37.18**). Wrap the floss around the proximal surface of one tooth once it is placed apical to the teeth' contact area. The floss is then moved firmly along the line angle of the tooth up to the contact area and gently down into sulcus. Repeat the same up and downstrokes for several times. Then, move floss across the interdental gingiva and perform the procedure on the adjacent tooth's proximal surface.

Commercially available floss holders are helpful to patients having difficulty in flossing. They are available as plastic handles to hold the floss, which can serve as "substitute fingers" (**Fig. 37.19**). Initially, the patient can find difficulty in using such floss. However, it is very

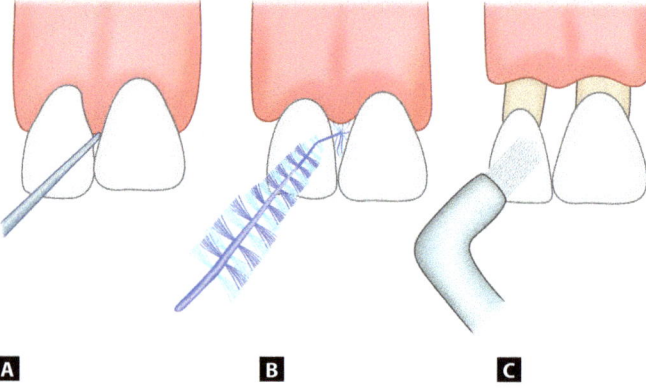

**Figs. 37.14A to C:** Schematic representation showing interproximal embrasure spaces: (A) Type I; (B) Type II; (C) Type III.

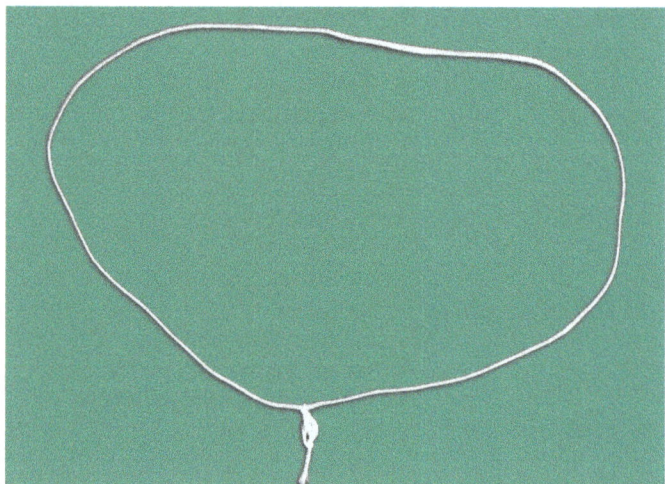

**Fig. 37.15:** Photograph showing dental floss in a loop.

Chapter 37: Mechanical Plaque Control

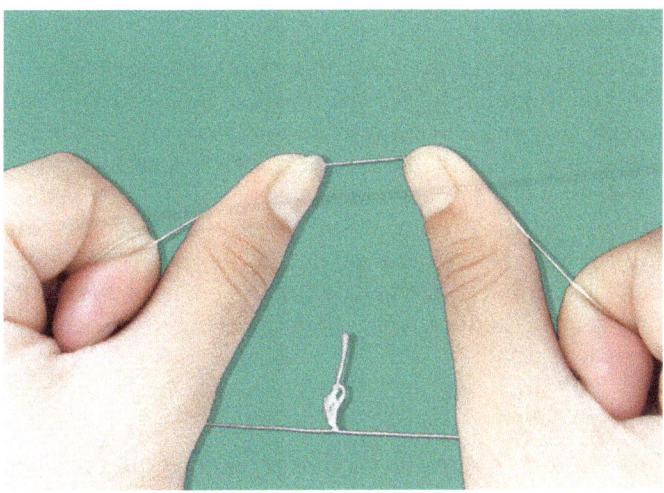

**Fig. 37.16:** Photograph showing holding of floss between thumbs for use in maxillary teeth.

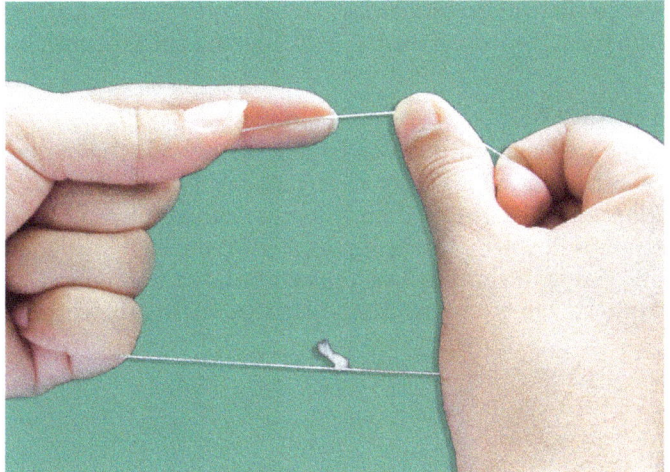

**Fig. 37.17:** Photograph showing holding of floss between the thumb and index finger for use in maxillary teeth.

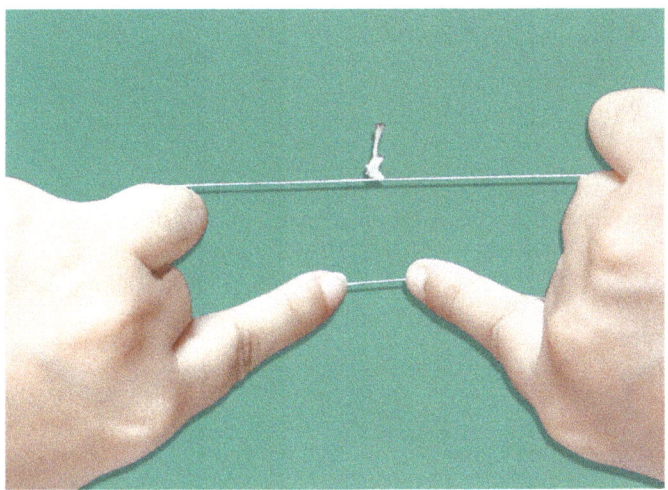

**Fig. 37.18:** Photograph showing holding of floss for use in mandibular teeth.

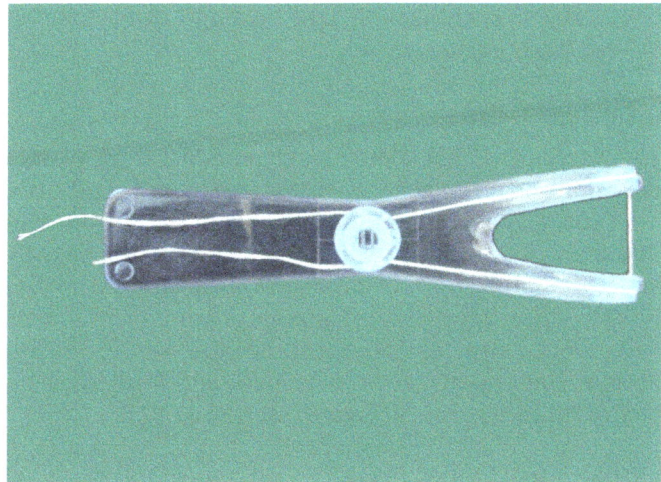

**Fig. 37.19:** Photograph showing reusable floss holder.

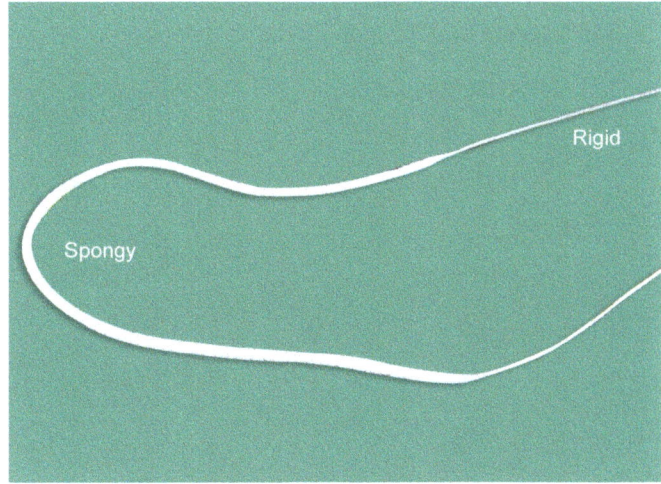

**Fig. 37.20:** Photograph showing super floss.

beneficial in a patient, especially those who have a problem with manual dexterity.

Superfloss, an alternative to the floss threader, is a type of floss with a rigid plastic portion that can be introduced under fixed bridges. The spongy region, which is distal to the rigid plastic portion, is effective for plaque removal **(Fig. 37.20)**. The terminal portion of super floss is similar to standard dental floss. Superfloss is easy to use as compared to floss threaders. The rigid portion is passed into the embrasure space between the retainer and the pontic and pulled through the lingual aspect. Then spongy region is used in an apicocoronal stroke along the intaglio surface of the pontic in a shoeshine approach.[15]

## Dental Tape

It is used with fluoride dentifrice and usually advised for cleaning the approximal surfaces of molars and premolars.

**Section 6:** Treatment: Nonsurgical Therapy

It is used with rubbing motion by holding it by the hand or in a special holder provided.

## Interdental Brush

The interdental area is the most common site for plaque retention and the most inaccessible area to the toothbrush.

Thus, a special method of cleaning is required. The diameter of the interproximal brush should be slightly larger than the gingival embrasures to be cleaned so that bristles can exert pressure on both proximal surfaces as well as root concavities. These brushes are inserted through interproximal spaces and moved back-and-forth between teeth with short strokes **(Figs. 37.21 and 37.22)**.

### Types

The types of interdental brushes are:
- Small insert brushes with reusable handles.
- *Brush with wire handle*: They are recommended in exposed root surfaces having concavities or grooves, and through and through furcation defects.

### Advantages

The advantages of interdental brushes over dental floss are that interdental brushes clean concave root surface and furcations more efficiently than dental floss and are much easier to use than dental floss **(Figs. 37.23A and B)**. When the floss is placed over a concave surface in the furcation region, contact is not possible, and thus supplementary interdental devices are needed to remove plaque and deposits completely. When dentifrices are used, the dental tape may be better than floss in retaining the dentifrices against the tooth.

## Unituft Brush

In a single-tufted brush, there is present a group of small tufts 3–6 mm in diameter, which may be flat or tapered **(Fig. 37.24)**. These are recommended in furcation areas, distal surfaces of the most posterior molars. These brushes are adaptable around and under fixed partial dentures, pontic, and implant abutment easily. The end of the tuft is directed into the interproximal area and along the gingival margin.

## Toothpick

They are usually 2-inch long made of softwood (basswood or birchwood) and are triangular in shape. They are inserted into gingival embrasure with the base of the triangle towards the gingiva. They repeatedly move in and out of the embrasure, thereby removing soft deposits from the teeth and mechanically stimulating the gingiva.

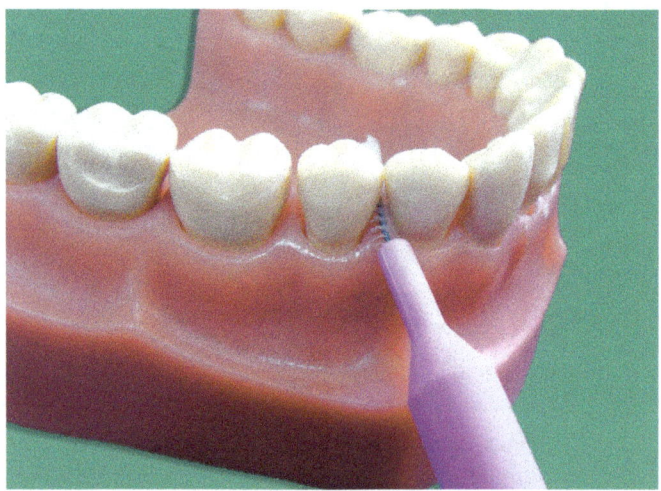

**Fig. 37.21:** Photograph showing an interdental brush.

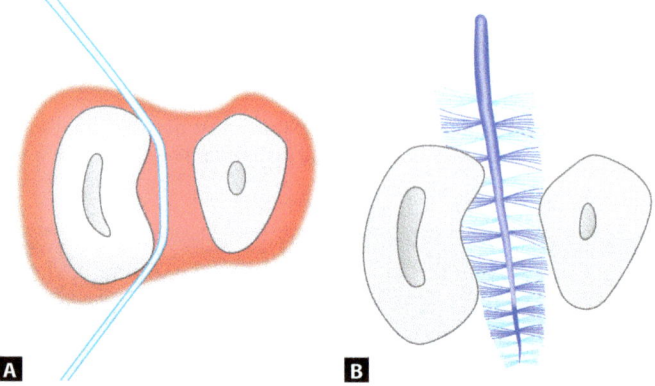

**Figs. 37.23A and B:** Schematic representation showing effective cleaning of the concave proximal tooth surface with an interdental brush (B) compared to dental floss (A).

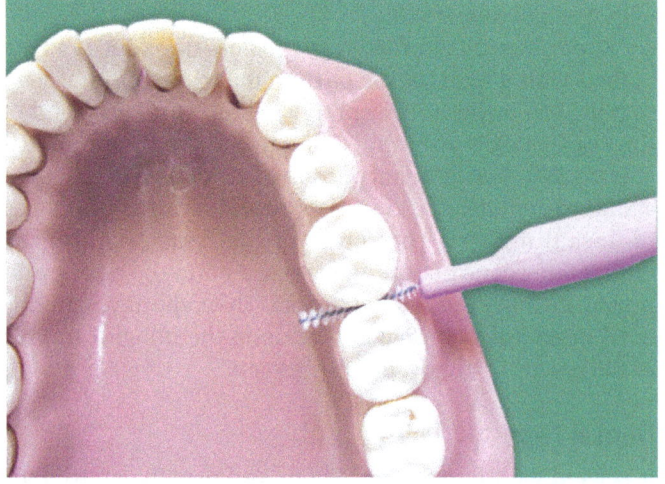

**Fig. 37.22:** Photograph showing an interdental brush (occlusal view).

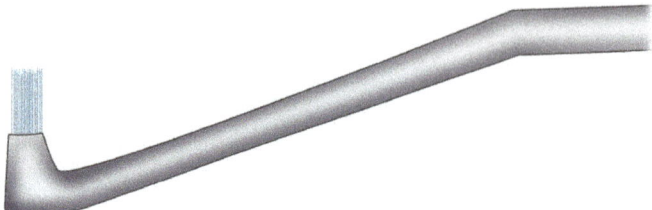

**Fig. 37.24:** Schematic representation showing unituft brush.

They are recommended in patients with open interdental spaces. In fluoridated wooden toothpick, wood can store NaF crystals both on the surface and in porosites. NaF crystal dissolves readily in contact with liquids, such as water or saliva. Toothpicks should be moistened in the saliva for a few seconds just before use to accelerate the release of fluoride. It is contraindicated in children and young adults because interdental space is filled by normal papilla.

## OTHER AIDS

### Tongue Scraper

It may be made of plastic, stainless steel, or other flexible metal. It is indicated in high caries risk, periodontal risk patients, and patients suffering from halitosis. The rationale behind tongue cleaning is that periodontal pathogens produce volatile sulfur compounds (VSC), which are responsible for halitosis and accumulate mostly within the filiform papillae and on the back of the tongue. The tongue brush or scrapers are placed as far back on the tongue as possible **(Fig. 37.25)**. Once the scraper is in position, gently drag it forward and repeat 2 or 3 times or until the tongue is cleaned.[16]

### Gingival Massage

"It is the methodical application of stroking or kneading pressure to the gingival tissue to stimulate blood circulation."[17] Massaging the gingiva improves blood circulation increases keratinization and epithelial thickening. They provide substantial protection against microorganisms and local factors, and thus, are beneficial for gingival health. It is usually done with a toothbrush or interdental cleaning aids.

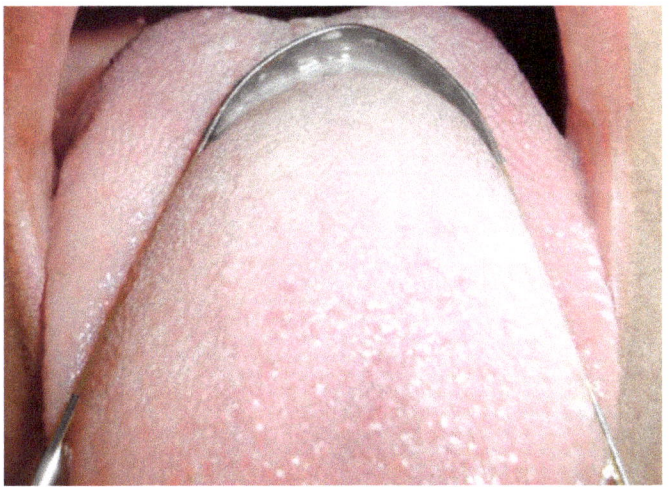

**Fig. 37.25:** Photograph showing tongue scraper which facilitates removal of microorganism accumulations from the dorsum of the tongue, which is the main cause of halitosis.

### Oral Irrigation Devices

Oral irrigators clean nonadherent debris and bacteria around orthodontic appliances or any inaccessible areas.

### Types

There are several types of oral irrigators available depending upon irrigation pressure, water stream characteristics and jet type design.[18,19]

- *Syringe*: A syringe can also be used for delivering a solution to irrigate the pocket. Simple irrigating syringes are usually equipped with blunt or side-port cannulas for subgingival irrigation.
- *Pulsating monojet irrigators*: These are preferred for supragingival irrigation, e.g., Waterpik.
- *Multistreamed irrigators*: These are available for supragingival irrigation.

In most units, the irrigation pressure is produced by an electrical pump, and it is delivered in a continuous or pulsating stream. The alternating compression and decompression phases in pulsating irrigators may facilitate the displacement of plaque bacteria. A continuous flow of water during irrigation causes constant tissue compression and may impair the removal of bacteria.

### Indications

- *Patients undergoing orthodontic therapy*: When other oral hygiene aids fail due to the presence of local factors, such as orthodontic appliances or intermaxillary fixation.
- *Patients with*:
  - Crown and bridgework
  - Implants
  - Surgical indication but unable to undergo surgery because of medical, behavioral, or financial constraints.

### Contraindications

In infective endocarditis, patient irrigation may cause bacteremias. Hence, the method is not suitable for high-risk patients.

### Efficacy

The efficacy of professionally delivered irrigation depends upon penetration, concentration, and duration of irrigation.

- *Penetration*: Initially, the agent must be able to penetrate the base of the pocket to reach the periodontal infection. It is accomplished with a blunt cannula using a hand syringe, or a mechanized device placed 1–3 mm of the pocket. The penetration of the solution through this mechanism ranges from 70 to 95% of the depth of the pocket. Both side-port and end-port cannulas can achieve the same penetration; however, side-port cannulas have the lowest ejection site pressure. The

presence of calculus deposits impairs the subgingival penetration into deep pockets of 7–10 mm.
- *Concentration*: The agent should be of sufficient concentration to be bacteriostatic or bactericidal. The biofilm structure of subgingival plaque may affect antimicrobial agents' activity, potentially limiting the agents' efficacy. Concentrations of agents that kill planktonic cells may not be effective on cells in a biofilm. The biofilm structure of subgingival plaque may affect antimicrobial agents' activity, potentially limiting the efficacy of agents.
- *Duration*: The agent must maintain this concentration for a sufficient duration to be effective against the biofilm. The duration of a solution irrigated into a pocket is affected by the flushing action of gingival crevicular fluid (GCF). The greater outward flow of GCF causes solutions that are put into the periodontal pocket to be rapidly washed out. Because of this phenomenon, antimicrobial agents irrigated subgingivally may not be in contact with the subgingival microflora for a sufficient duration to be effective. To compensate for this, other delivery vehicles that prolong duration have been developed.

## ORAL HYGIENE METHODS CAUSING TRAUMA

Followings are the oral hygiene devices and methods which can cause traumatic lesions:[20]
- *Toothbrush*: Hard toothbrush bristles with horizontal brushing can cause tooth abrasion. Overzealous brushing can cause gingival recession. Pointed unrounded bristles can lead to gingival bleeding. Toothbrushing can also lead to transient bacteremia in the high-risk patient (infective endocarditis). Abrasion of tooth structure is mostly associated with the dentifrice while gingival lesions are associated with toothbrush.[21]
- *Floss*: Flossing can produce gingival clefts if not done properly.[22]
- *Water irrigation devices*: Oral irrigation can cause periodontal abscess and transient bacteremia.
- Dentifrices, mouthwashes, disclosing agents can cause allergic reactions.

## ASSESSMENT OF HOME CARE

In the assessment of adequate dental home care, determining the causes of insufficient dental care is the first and the most important step.

The following three are the possible causes of inadequate home care:
1. The patient does not know what to do (lacks knowledge of oral hygiene).
2. The patient is aware of what to do but is unable to perform (lacks dexterity).
3. The patient is aware of what to do and able to perform it. However, he/she simply does not follow the expected regimen (lacks motivation).

Assessment of the effectiveness of patient plaque control is a continuous process. It starts at the initial evaluation of the oral cavity and continues throughout the therapy, including maintenance. Various methods are available for the assessment of home care. The first method involves a simple visual inspection of the teeth for the presence or absence of plaque. However, this method is not so effective because plaques are usually difficult to see. The second assessment method involves the inspection of plaque by making it visible with the use of a disclosing solution.

Various indices have been developed for this purpose. One widely used index is the O'Leary plaque index. Such indices are helpful in the following two purposes:
1. It is helpful in monitoring patient's progress (e.g., assessing whether home care is sufficient to permit surgical intervention).
2. It acts as a motivational tool for patients.

## Disclosing Agents

Disclosing solution contains a dye or other coloring substance, which gives color to calculus, plaque, and films on the surface of teeth, tongue, and gingiva. Available over-the-counter in liquid or tablet form (**Fig. 37.26**), disclosants contain ingredients that temporarily stain plaque so that it can be observed. Before using disclosing agents, a nonpetroleum based lubricant should be applied to the lips and esthetic dental restorations to prevent staining. Solutions are applied as a concentrate with a cotton swab or diluted with water in a cup to use as an oral rinse. Tablets are chewed and swished around in the mouth. Clean tooth surfaces do not absorb the dye unless roughened. Acquired pellicle, plaque biofilm, debris, and calculus absorb the disclosing agent. After the application of disclosant, the excess is

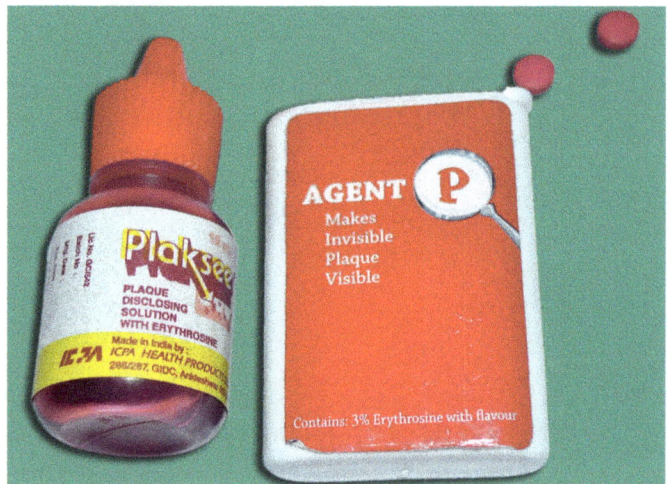

**Fig. 37.26:** Photograph showing disclosing agents: Liquid and tablet form (Reproduced with permission from ICPA Health Products Ltd.).

expectorated or suctioned from the mouth and patient is given a hand mirror to identify the stained deposits.[23]

It is an excellent oral hygiene aid because it can act as an additional motivational tool to improve the efficiency of plaque control procedures carried out by patients. It also conserves operating time by making inconspicuous deposits more evident.

Factors to be considered in the selection of a disclosing solution are:
- The intensity of color
- Taste
- Nonirritating to the mucous membrane
- *Diffusibility*: Neither too thin nor too thick
- Astringent and antiseptic

The various disclosing agents are skinner iodine, iodine disclosing solution, diluted tincture of iodine, Berwick's solution, Buckley's solution, Talbot iodoglycerol, metaphen, basic fuchsin, Bismarck brown, Easlick's solution, Bender's solution, mercurochrome solution, erythrosin [the United States Federal Food, Drug, and Cosmetic Act (FDC) red no. 3], DC yellow no. 8 fluorescein, two-tone dye (FDC red no. 3 and FDC green no. 3). Two-tone dye test uses FDC red No. 3 and FDC green No. 3 solution which stains thick accumulation of plaque as blue and thin deposits as stained red or pink.[24]

## Limitations

- Do not selectively disclose bacteria plaque, but rather stain all soft debris and pellicle.
- Exposed cementum, in particular, can stain vividly, although it is free of bacterial plaque.
- Disclosing solution may stain silicate cement or resin restoration.
- Disclosing solutions containing alcohol should not be kept for more than 2–3 months since the alcohol will evaporate and render the solution highly concentrated.

## Strategies for Improving Home-care

Strategies for improving home-care performance include proper demonstration, instructions, and motivation of the patient.

### Demonstration and Instructions

Toothbrushing techniques can be demonstrated both on a model and in the patient's mouth. Ideally, brushing should be performed before a mirror with good light so that the patient can check the brush and bristles' placement. This allows checking whether the patient has purchased the correct size and type of toothbrush and dentifrice.

Instructions can be given through one-to-one chairside or audio-visual aids. The patient should brush at night before going to bed. Thus, during the hours of sleep, the mouth will be as clean as possible, and plaque will not be left in situ for 12 or more hours.[25]

**Clinical Tips**
- Brushing before going to bed is the most important due to reduced salivary flow when asleep.
- There is no single toothbrushing technique that is ideal for every patient.

### Motivation

To achieve success in attempting to establish needs-related tooth cleaning habits, the first prerequisite is a well-motivated, well-informed, and well-instructed patient. Motivation is defined as readiness to act or the driving force behind a person's actions. It is a powerful force that dictates whether and how a person will act in a given situation and as such must be comprehended so that we can aid the patient in deciding to treat his periodontal disease or understand why many people even when well informed will not act to save their teeth by dental therapy.[26]
- Recognize the patient's needs
- Discover what motives your patient
- Formulate a plan
- Give positive reinforcement

The dentist should accomplish the following during the consultation:
- Determining the patient's needs, motives, and desires
- Making the patient feel important and accepted
- Giving the patient some recognition and attention as an active partner in the treatment plan
- Using visual aids, especially the patient's mouth
- Becoming a good listener, especially in the earlier stages of consultation

## HAWTHORNE EFFECT

A particular psychological phenomenon called the "Hawthorne effect" refers to the tendency of some people to work harder and perform better when they are participants in an experiment. Research subjects behave differently because they realize that they are being observed. This may change their behavior due to the attention they are receiving from researchers rather than the manipulation of independent variables.

Hawthorne was a Western Electric Company plant in Chicago where studies were conducted between 1924 and 1932, examining the influence of different work environment variables on productivity. "Hawthorne effect" has been used frequently to account for gains made by placebo control groups when none were expected. The study or trial participants are always informed about the study objectives and the nature of the research taking place. This enhances the possibility of the patient to spend more time and effort on practicing oral hygiene measures on the day of the visit to the trial unit. In such studies, subjects or patient may improve their tooth-cleaning habits which possibly reduces plaque scores irrespective of the therapy provided.[27]

> **Points to Ponder**
> - Adjunctive aids used for cleansing the oral cavity are irrigators, tongue scrapers, and dentifrices.
> - Tooth powders contain about 95% abrasives and five times more abrasive than pastes. Detergents found in dentifrices denature lectin adhesins.
> - Approximal areas are the visible spaces between teeth not under the contact area, and the interproximal regions refer to the area under and related to the contact point.
> - "Hawthorne effect," which occurs when research subjects behave differently because they realize that they are being observed.

## REFERENCES

1. Wilkins EM. Oral infection control: toothbrushes and toothbrushing. In: Wilkins EM (Ed). Clinical Practice of the Dental Hygienist, 8th edition. Philadelphia, PA, USA: Lippincott Williams & Wilkins; 1999. pp. 350-69.
2. Perry DA. Plaque control for the periodontal patient. In: Newman MG, Takei HH, Carranza FA (Eds). Carranza's Clinical Periodontology, 9th edition. Philadelphia, PA, USA: WB Saunders; 2003. pp. 651-74.
3. The American Dental Association. Accepted Dental Therapeutics, 1969/1970, 33rd edition. Chicago, USA: American Dental Association; 1976.
4. Bass CC. The optimum characteristics of toothbrushes for personal oral hygiene. Dent Items Int. 1948;70(7):697-718.
5. Hine MK. The toothbrush. Int Dent J. 1956;6:15-25.
6. Claydon NC. Current concepts in toothbrushing and interdental cleaning. Periodontol 2000. 2008;48:10-22.
7. Eley BM, Manson JD. Prevention of periodontal disease. In: Periodontics, 5th edition. Edinburgh, Scotland: Wright Publishing; 2004. pp. 133-43.
8. Stillman PR. A philosophy of the treatment of periodontal disease. Dent Digest. 1932;38:314.
9. Charters WJ. Eliminating mouth infections with the toothbrush and other stimulating instruments. Dent Digest. 1932;38:130.
10. Bass CC. An effective method of personal oral hygiene. Part 11. J La State Med Soc. 1954;106(2):57-73.
11. Fones AC. Mouth Hygiene, 4th edition. Philadelphia, PA, USA: Lea & Febiger; 1934.
12. Leonard JF. Conservative treatment of periodontoclasia. J Am Dent Assoc. 1939;26:1308-18.
13. Wilkins EM. Interdental care and chemotherapy. In: Clinical Practice of the Dental Hygienist, 8th edition. Philadelphia, PA, USA: Lippincott Williams & Wilkins; 1999. pp. 370-93.
14. Perry DA, Schmid MO. Plaque control. In: Carranza FA, Newman MG (Eds). Carranza's Clinical Periodontology, 8th edition. Philadelphia, PA, USA: WB Saunders; 2003. pp. 493-511.
15. Thomas MV. Oral physiotherapy. In: Rose LF, Mealey BL, Genco RJ, Cohen DW (Eds). Periodontics: Medicine, Surgery, and Implants. St. Louis: Elsevier-Mosby; 2004. pp. 214-36.
16. Echeverria JJ, Sanz M. Mechanical supragingival plaque control. In: Lindhe J, Karring T, Lang NP (Eds). Clinical Periodontology and Implant Dentistry, 4th edition. Oxford, UK: Blackwell Munksgaard; 2003. pp. 449-63.
17. Dummett CO. Prophylactic periodontics. J Periodontol. 1960;31:40-6.
18. Greenstein G. Position paper: the role of supra- and subgingival irrigation in the treatment of periodontal diseases. J Periodontol. 2005;76(11):2015-27.
19. Hardy JH, Newman HN, Strhan JD. Direct irrigation and subgingival plaque. J Clin Periodontol. 1982;9:57.
20. Oral physiotherapy. Periodontal literature reviews. 1996;1(6):106-11.
21. Sangnes G. Traumatization of teeth and gingiva related to habitual tooth cleaning procedures. J Clin Periodontol. 1976;3(2):94-103.
22. Hallmon WW, Waldrop TC, Houston GD, Hawkins BF. Flossing clefts: clinical and histologic observations. J Periodontol. 1986;57(8):501-4.
23. Tan AE. Disclosing agents in plaque control: a review. J West Soc Periodontol Periodontal Abstr. 1981;29(3):81-6.
24. Gallagher IH, Fussell SJ, Cutress TW. Mechanism of action of a two-tone plaque disclosing agent. J Periodontol. 1977;48(7):395-6.
25. Grant DA, Stern IB, Listgarten MA. Plaque control (oral hygiene, chemical plaque control), root sensitivity and halitosis. In: Periodontics, 6th edition. St. Louis: CV Mosby; 1988. pp. 611-49.
26. Renz AN, Newton JT. Changing the behavior of patients with periodontitis. Periodontol 2000. 2009;51:252-68.
27. McCarney R, Warner J, Iliffe S, van Haselen R, Griffin M, Fisher P. The Hawthorne Effect: a randomized, controlled trial. BMC Med Res Methodol. 2007;7:30.

## VIVA VOCE

**Q1. What is oral prophylaxis?**
**Ans.** Physical resources described by the dentist to prevent oral diseases, especially periodontal diseases.[17]

**Q2. What is a novel toothbrush design?**
**Ans.** The head is located horizontally to the tooth surface; multiple tufts of bristles are angled in the different directions of the approximal tooth surfaces. This design aims to improve plaque removal in approximal areas and based on the fact that the majority of the subjects use a simple horizontal brushing action.

**Q3. What is the difference between bass and modified bass toothbrushing method?**
**Ans.** In the modified bass method, bristles are swept towards the occlusal surface after completing the gingival sulcus' vibratory motion.

**Q4. After how much time toothbrush should be changed?**
**Ans.** The brush should be replaced before filaments fray, at least every 2–3 months. But patients who are debilitated, have a known infection, or are about to undergo surgery should be advised to disinfect their brushes or use disposable brushes.

## Chapter 37: Mechanical Plaque Control

**Q5. Which disclosing agents differentiate between old or thick plaque accumulations and recent or thin plaque accumulations?**
**Ans.** Two-tone dye test that uses FDC red no. 3 and FDC green no. 3. The solution stains thick accumulation of plaque as blue and thin deposits are stained red or pink.

**Q6. Where modified Stillman method is indicated?**
**Ans.** Gingival recession and root exposure.

**Q7. Which toothbrushing technique is advised after periodontal surgery?**
**Ans.** Charters toothbrushing method.

**Q8. What is superfloss?**
**Ans.** It is a type of floss that consists of both a rigid plastic portion and a spongy portion.

**Q9. Which interdental aid is used in Type 1 embrasures where no gingival recession present?**
**Ans.** Dental floss.

**Q10. What are the advantages of interdental brushes over dental floss?**
**Ans.** The advantages of interdental brushes over dental floss are that interdental brushes clean concave root surface and furcations more efficiently than dental floss and are much easier to use than dental floss.

# Chapter 38

# Chemotherapeutic Agents

*MM Dayakar, Shalu Bathla*

## Chapter Outline

- Terminologies
- Chemotherapeutic Agents
- Chemical Antiplaque Agents
- Anticalculus Agents
- Antimicrobials
- Local Drug Delivery System

## INTRODUCTION

Although mechanical plaque removal remains the primary method to prevent gingival and periodontal diseases and maintain oral health, chemical antiplaque and anticalculus agents can be used as adjuncts. To control the disease process of aggressive periodontitis, periodontitis as a manifestation of systemic diseases and chronic periodontitis, and adjunctive chemotherapeutic agents, such as antimicrobials/antibiotics are required. Thorough knowledge of these chemotherapeutic agents is necessary due to their side effects and interactions among them.

## TERMINOLOGIES

*Chemotherapeutic agent*: Chemotherapeutic agent is a general term for a chemical substance that provides a clinical therapeutic benefit. Chemotherapeutic agents can be administered locally, orally, or parenterally.[1]

*Antimicrobial agent*: An antimicrobial agent is a chemotherapeutic agent that works by reducing the number of bacteria present.

*Antibiotics*: These are naturally occurring, semisynthetic or synthetic types of antimicrobial agents that destroy or inhibit the growth of selective microorganisms, generally at low concentrations.

*Antiplaque agents*: Chemicals that inhibit plaque formation to such an extent that they prevent the development of gingivitis.

*Antiseptic*: An antiseptic is a chemical antimicrobial agent applied to living tissues to prevent or arrest the growth or action of microorganisms. In dentistry, antiseptics are widely used as the active ingredient in antiplaque and antigingivitis mouth rinses and dentifrices.

*Disinfectant*: It is an antimicrobial agent that is generally applied to inanimate surfaces to destroy microorganisms.[1]

## CHEMOTHERAPEUTIC AGENTS

- Desensitizing agents
- Corticosteroids
- Analgesics
- Sedatives and hypnotics
- Muscle relaxants
- Anesthetics
- Hemostatics and vasoconstrictors
- Postoperative periodontal dressings
- Dentifrices
- Chemical antiplaque agents
- Anticalculus agents
- Antibiotics
- Anti-edematous substances

In this chapter, only chemical antiplaque agents, anticalculus agents, and antimicrobials or antibiotics are discussed in detail.

## CHEMICAL ANTIPLAQUE AGENTS

Subgingival plaque is derived from supragingival plaque and is intimately associated with the advancing lesions of chronic periodontal diseases. On the basis that plaque-induced gingivitis usually precedes the occurrence and reoccurrence of periodontitis, the mainstay of primary and secondary prevention of periodontal diseases is the control of supragingival plaque. Mechanical tooth cleaning through toothbrushing with dentifrice is arguably the most common and potentially effective form of oral hygiene. The chemical preventive agents should be used as adjuncts and not as replacements for the most conventional and accepted effective mechanical methods. The advantage of an antiplaque agent's chemical approach is that the zone of diffusion achieved with the chemical agent is greater than the limited radius of the effect of a mechanical agent.

The action of the chemical antiplaque agent can be categorized into (**Fig. 38.1**):[2]

- *Antiadhesive*: It prevents bacterial attachment to the tooth, e.g., chlorhexidine (CHX), delmopinol, amine alcohol.
- *Antimicrobial*: It stops or slows bacterial proliferation, e.g., CHX, antibiotics.
- Established plaque removal or chemical toothbrush, e.g., amine alcohol, enzymes.
- *Antipathogenic*: It alters the pathogenicity of plaque.

Various chemical antiplaque agents, as described in **Table 38.1**.

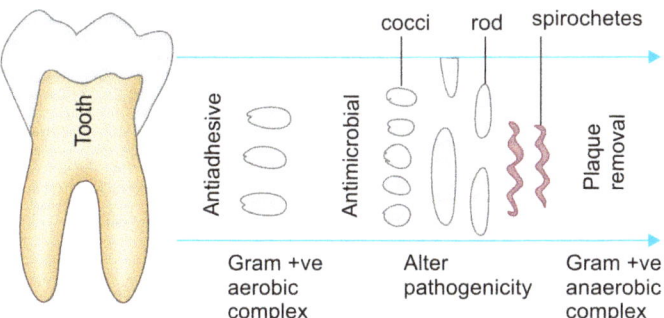

**Fig. 38.1:** Schematic representation showing actions of chemical antiplaque agents.

| TABLE 38.1: Various chemical antiplaque agents. | |
|---|---|
| Antibiotics | Penicillin, vancomycin, kanamycin |
| Bisbiguanide antiseptics | Chlorhexidine, alexidine, octenidine |
| Phenols and essential oils | Thymol, triclosan, hexylresorcinol |
| Natural products | Sanguinarine |
| Quaternary ammonium compounds | Cetylpyridinium chloride |
| Oxygenating agents | Hydrogen peroxide ($H_2O_2$), sodium peroxyborate, sodium peroxycarbonate |
| Detergents | Sodium lauryl sulfate |
| Enzymes | Protease, lipase, nuclease, dextranase, mutanase-glucose oxidase, amyloglucosidase |
| Amine alcohol | Octapinol, delmopinol |
| Metal salts | Tin, zinc, copper |
| Fluorides | Sodium fluoride, stannous fluoride, amine fluoride |

## Generations of Antiplaque Agents

In 1986, Kornman classified these agents into first- and second-generation agents according to their substantivity mainly as:[3]

- *First-generation agents*: They reduce plaque score by 20–50%. Poor substantivity and thus used 4–6 times daily, e.g., sanguinarine, quaternary ammonium compounds, antibiotics.
- *Second-generation agents*: They reduce plaque score by 70–90% and are used twice daily, e.g., CHX and triclosan.
- *Third-generation agents*: They are effective against specific periodontal pathogens, e.g., delmopinol.

The antiplaque agents accepted by the Food and Drug Administration (FDA) for treatment of gingivitis are CHX (prescription drug) and Listerine (over-the-counter or nonprescription drug). In September 1987, Listerine antiseptic mouthwash was the first nonprescription product awarded by the American Dental Association (ADA) Council on the dental therapeutic seal of acceptance as an aid in controlling supragingival dental plaque.

## Chlorhexidine

Chlorhexidine was developed by Imperial Chemical Industries, England, in the 1940s and marketed in 1954 as an antiseptic for a skin wound. Schroeder[4] first investigated plaque inhibition by CHX in 1969, but Loe and Schiott[5] performed the definitive study in 1970.

Chlorhexidine is available in three forms as (1) digluconate, (2) acetate, and (3) hydrochloride (HCl) salts. It is the front-runner and benchmark against which most of the other topical supragingival antiplaque agents have been compared.[6]

### Structure

It is a symmetrical molecule made up of (**Fig. 38.2**):
- Two 4-chlorophenyl rings.
- Two biguanide groups.

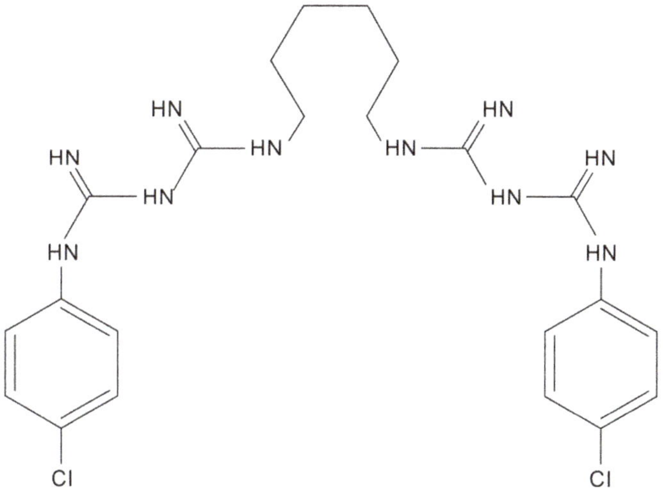

**Fig. 38.2:** Schematic representation showing the structure of chlorhexidine molecule.

**Section 6:** Treatment: Nonsurgical Therapy

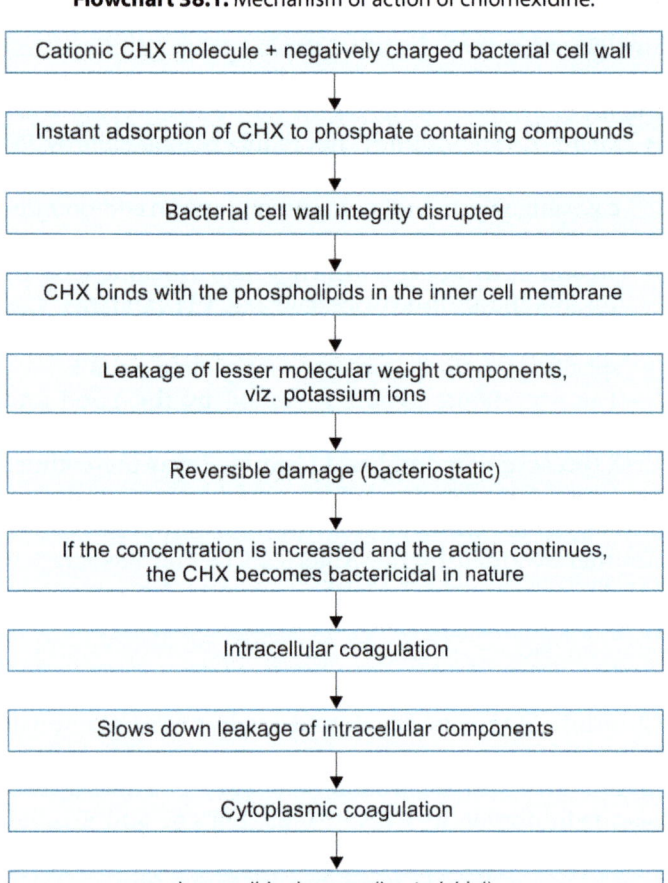

Flowchart 38.1: Mechanism of action of chlorhexidine.

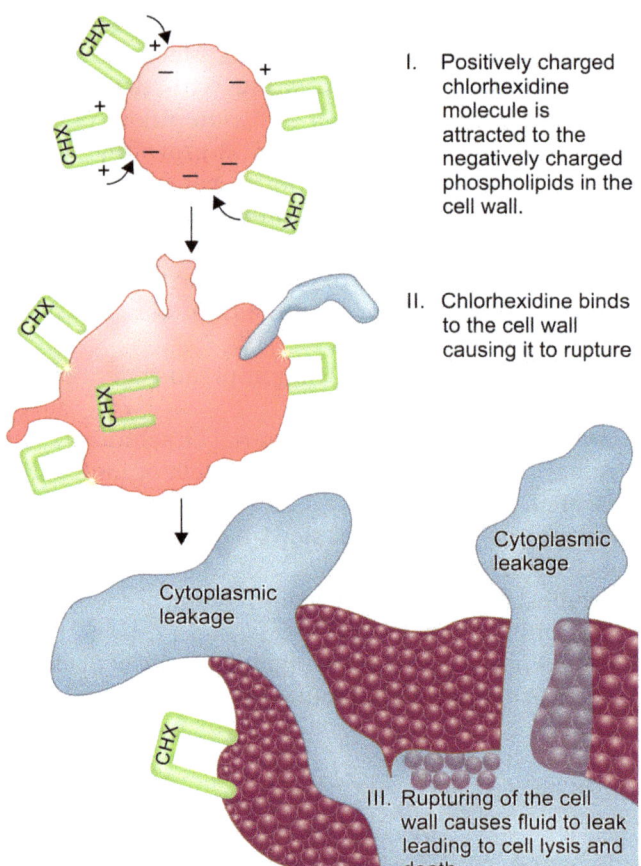

**Fig. 38.3:** Schematic representation showing the mechanism of action of chlorhexidine (CHX): I. Positively charged CHX molecule is attracted to the negatively charged phospholipids in the cell wall; II. CHX binds to the cell wall causing it to rupture and III. Rupturing of the cell wall causes fluid to leak leading to cell lysis and death.

- A central hexamethylene bridge connecting chlorophenyl rings and biguanide groups.

### Mechanism of Action
- *Antibacterial activity*: CHX molecule exhibits a wide range of activity covering gram-positive and gram-negative bacteria, yeasts, and some lipophilic viruses. CHX effects vary with different concentrations **(Flowchart 38.1)**. CHX, at its lower concentration, hampers the cellular transport across the bacterial cell leading to the formation of pores in the cellular membrane and acts as a bacteriostatic agent. However, in higher concentrations, the solution penetrates the bacterial cell and kills the microorganism imparting bactericidal effect[7,8] **(Fig. 38.3)**.
- *Antiplaque activity*:
  - Chlorhexidine molecules occlude the acidic groups on the salivary glycoproteins and retard pellicle formation.
  - In sublethal amounts, CHX molecules directly bind to the bacterial surface and avoid adsorption of bacteria onto the tooth surface.
  - It inhibits acid production in established plaque.[7,8]

### Peculiar Features
- *Substantivity property*: The quality of prolonged contact time between a substance and substrate is known as substantivity. It is influenced by the concentration of medication, its pH and temperature, and length of contact of the solution with oral surfaces. Substantivity property for CHX was first described in the 1970s by Bonesvoll.[9] Its period for CHX is around 12 hours. The substantivity of the plaque-inhibitory substance depends on pharmacokinetics, concentration, and dose, effectiveness over time, and application site.

### Pin-Cushion Effect
One charged end of chlorhexidine molecule binding to the tooth surface and the other remaining available to interact with the bacterial membrane as microorganism approaches the tooth surface as a pin-cushion effect. This explains the lack of effectiveness of other antimicrobials in terms of them lacking a large, rigid molecule with two charged interactive ends.

- Chlorhexidine can be more suitable for repeated use as it does not suffer from the potential drawback of inducing bacterial resistance. Studies have shown that CHX is less effective in changing the bacterial flora than tetracycline and metronidazole.
- No teratogenic potential detected on long-term use.

## Clinical Uses

- Presurgical preparation of periodontal patients.
- Postoral surgery, including periodontal surgery or root planing.
- For patients with jaw fixation.
- Immunocompromised patients are susceptible to oral infections.
- Mentally and physically disabled patients.
- High caries risk patients.
- Frequent susceptibility to oral ulceration.
- Removable and fixed orthodontic appliance wearers.
- In the denture stomatitis patients.
- Preoperative rinsing during ultrasonic scaling and polishing with high-speed instruments.

## Adverse Effects

- *Staining*: Brown discoloration of teeth, restoration, and dorsum of the tongue.[10] The various proposed mechanisms of CHX staining are as follows:[11]
  - Degradation of the CHX molecule liberates para chloroaniline.
  - *Precipitation of anionic dietary chromogens*: CHX reaction with ketones and aldehydes from the dietary breakdown or intermediate products results in the formation of insoluble, colored compounds. Cationic group of CHX molecule gets attached to dietary factors such as gallic acid derivatives present in food and many beverages including tea, coffee and tannins.[12]
  - *Protein denaturation with metal sulfide formation*: CHX splits the sulfide bridges and denatures the proteins in pellicles, leading to free sulfhydryl groups. These sulfhydryl groups react with iron or tin ions to form brown or yellow pigmented products.
  - Catalysis of Maillard reactions.
- *Taste alteration*: An alteration in taste sensation is commonly caused by denaturation of surface proteins present on the taste buds, particularly affecting salt taste.[13]
- *Oral mucosal erosion*: It is due to precipitation of the mucin layer, thus reducing its lubricating effect. It is considered as an idiosyncratic reaction which is usually concentration dependent.[14]
- *Increased calculus formation*: The dead microbes due to the use of CHX may act as an initiator for calculus formation, which is based on the seeding mechanism of calculus formation but involves localized supersaturation, nucleation, crystal growth and the transformation of precursor phases, such as dicalcium phosphate dehydrate, octacalcium phosphate and amorphous calcium phosphate into more stable, crystalline deposits of hydroxyapatite.[15]
- *Unilateral or bilateral parotid swelling*: Stenosis of the parotid duct has also been reported.[14]

*Availability*

Over the years, CHX in the form of gels (chlosite), sprays, varnishes, chewing gums, chips (periochip) and mouthwashes has been developed, and of these, mouthwash is the most commonly used.[16]

The instructions given to the patient after prescribing CHX mouthwash are that the patient is asked to brush with dentifrice at least half an hour and ideally 2 hours before CHX rinsing. Otherwise, the binding of cationic CHX to anionic components of the dentifrice results in the reduction of activity by decreasing the number of active cationic sites. The patients are advised to immediately refrain from consuming tea, coffee, and red wine immediately after CHX use. The corsodyl available in the United Kingdom contains 0.2% CHX (contain 20 mg/volume), and 10 mL volume/rinse is recommended. CHX mouthwash available in the United States of America is "Peridex" and in India "Periogard," which contains 0.12% CHX (contain 18 mg/volume) and 15 mL volume/rinse is recommended. The rationale for lowering the concentration of CHX is to reduce the side effects while maintaining comparable efficacy. Possible ways to reduce staining are using mouthwash only at night, using an oxidizing agent, using the wash with stannous fluoride, and adding a copolymer anti-adhesive agent into the mouthrinse.[17]

## *Quaternary Ammonium Compounds*

Cetylpyridinium chloride has been widely used as mouthrinse at a 0.05% concentration, mainly as an antimicrobial agent. Cetylpyridinium chloride molecule has both hydrophilic and hydrophobic interactions. Interaction with bacteria is assumed to be similar to that achieved by CHX, i.e., via cationic binding. Initial retention of cetylpyridinium chloride is higher than that of CHX, but the clearance of the former is more rapid. The substantivity of cetylpyridinium chloride appears to be only 3–5 hours due to either loss of activity once adsorbed or rapid desorption.

## *Listerine*

It is phenol-related essential oil consisting of thymol (0.064%), eucalyptol (0.092%), methanol (0.042%), methyl salicylate (0.060%) in HCl solution and benzoic acid (0.15%).[18]

The advantages of Listerine are that there is no taste alteration or staining, as seen with CHX usage. It is less expensive and is easier to obtain than CHX, as it is sold over the counter.[19]

Listerine's disadvantage is its high alcohol concentration (ranging from 21.6 to 26.9%), which may exacerbate xerostomia. It is contraindicated in patients under the treatment of alcoholism who take antabuse drugs (disulfiram). The addition of alcohol in mouthrinses helps to solubilize antimicrobial compound that enhances bioavailability and improves the shelf-life of the mouthrinse. The added alcohol also helps to enhance the pleasurable characteristic of mouthrinsing.

### Triclosan

It is an off-white, odorless, tasteless, crystalline powder with a molecular weight of 289.5 and a melting point of 57°C ± 1°C. It is a non-ionic antimicrobial that has been widely used over many years in antiperspirants and soaps. Recently, it has been formulated into toothpaste and mouthrinses. It acts on the microbial cytoplasmic membrane causing leakage of cellular constituents and thereby causing bacteriolysis. Presumably, the hydrophobic portion of the triclosan molecule adsorbs to the lipid portion of the bacterial cell membrane functions. It is bacteriostatic at low concentrations and bactericidal at high concentrations. Wide range of antimicrobial activity is reported against yeasts, gram-positive and gram-negative bacteria. Triclosan has a substantivity period of approximately 5 hours.[20] Activity of triclosan is enhanced by the addition of zinc citrate and polyvinyl methyl ether maleic acid.

*Advantages:*
- It has no staining.
- It can inhibit several important mediators of gingival inflammation.
- It has a dual effect both as an antibacterial and anti-inflammatory.
- It is not significantly impaired by the presence of sodium lauryl sulfate, as CHX does.

### Povidone-Iodine

In the late 1960s, povidone-iodine was introduced in Anglo-American countries. It is iodophor, a compound composed of iodine plus a solubilizing agent, i.e., polyvinylpyrrolidone (PVP) (povidone) from which iodine is continually delivered.

An available iodine equivalent is calculated by dividing the PVP-1 concentration by 10. For example, povidone-iodine (10%) actually contains 1% iodine.[21]

Polyvinylpyrrolidone 1 is microbicidal agent exhibiting wide antimicrobial activity for gram-positive and gram-negative bacteria, mycobacteria, fungi and viruses.[22]

The antibacterial activity of povidone-iodine is mainly because of the oxidation of amino, thiol, and hydroxyl groups. A strong reaction of PVP-1 with double bonds of unsaturated fatty acids in cell walls and organelle membranes results in transient or permanent pore formation. This leads to loss of cytoplasmic material and deactivation of enzymes due to direct contact with iodine. The substantivity of povidone-iodine is around 60 minutes. PVP-1 is contraindicated in pregnant women, nursing mothers, and those who are allergic to iodine. Side effects of povidone-iodine are the staining of teeth and surrounding tissues and interfere with thyroid function due to excessive incorporation of iodine.

### Peroxide

Hydrogen peroxide ($H_2O_2$) is an antiseptic agent that is toxic to many bacteria because of its strong oxidizing properties. The critical factor in peroxide activity is that $H_2O_2$ and other reduction products of $O_2$ (superoxide anions) can generate more toxic hydroxyl radicals. These reactive $O_2$ species damage cell membranes, inactivate bacterial enzymes via oxidation of the sulfhydryl group, and disrupt bacterial chromosome and destroy the bactericidal action of myeloperoxidase enzyme. The disadvantage of peroxide is that it is toxic to the host, causing peroxidation of lipids in the cell membrane and certain chromosomal changes.

### Natural Products

- *Sanguinarine*: It is a benzophenanthridine alkaloid obtained from alcoholic extraction of powdered rhizomes of bloodroot plant *Sanguinaria canadensis*, grown in the USA and Canada. After precipitation and putrefaction of alcohol extract, an orange powder containing 30–35% of sanguinarine is obtained. The trade name of the sanguinarine product is Viadent. It is an antimicrobial agent that is effective against gram-positive and gram-negative bacteria. The exact mode of action is not clear; however, it seems to interfere with the essential steps in the synthesis of the bacterial cell wall. Oxidation of the thiol group from sanguinarine suppresses the activity of several enzymes. Sanguinarine containing mouthrinses have been shown to increase the chances of the oral precancerous lesion.
- *Propolis*: It is a naturally occurring bee product made up of wax and plant extracts. It is commonly used by bees to seal openings in their hives. It is used as plaque-inhibitory mouthwash because of its antiseptic, anti-inflammatory, and bacteriostatic property.
- *Viokase*: It is a dehydrated pancreas preparation containing trypsin, chymotrypsin, carboxypeptidase, amylase, lipase, and nucleases.
- *Dextranase*: Dextran is a polysaccharide synthesized by plaque-forming and cariogenic microbes. The preparation of the dextranase enzyme is effective in preventing the formation of dextran.

## ANTICALCULUS AGENTS

Following are the generations of anticalculus agents:[23]

### First Generation

- *Dissolution via*:
    - *Acid*: The use of acid as an anticalculus agent is one of the older techniques that use a wooden stick moistened with aromatic sulfuric acid. It is inserted into a periodontal pocket to dissolve calculus. 20% trichloroacetic acid and 10% sulfuric acid are some of the other commonly used acids. However, the use

of acid is discontinued because it is caustic to soft tissues and decalcifies tooth structure.
- Sodium ricinoleate is the salt of fatty acids derived from castor oil. It hinders the attachment of microorganisms to teeth and proved as an anticalculus agent. However, it has an unacceptable taste and requires high concentrations for effective action.
- *Plaque attachment via*:
  - Silicone
  - *Ion exchange resins*: The resin is sulfonated polystyrene with negatively charged ions. These negatively charged ions repel the positively charged calcium ions and minimize the degree of calcium mineralization.
- *Plaque inhibition via*:
  - *Antibiotics (niddamycin)*: Effects of penicillin on gram-positive cocci initiated its testing for anticalculus activity.
  - Antiseptics (chloramine T)
- *Matrix disruption via*:
  - *Enzymes*: Normally, enzyme formulations break down the matrix from a plaque or impede the calculus's binding to the tooth. These modes of actions of enzyme preparations make them suitable for anticalculus activity. Mucinase is the first enzyme detected with proteolytic and amylolytic activity. It is theoretically considered that mucinase breaks down the mucin, which is thought to bind the calculus to the tooth.
  - Ascoxal
  - *30% urea*: The urea is found to dissolve the mucoproteinaceous material, especially with the deposition of calcium salts. It is also known to enhance the solubility of calcium salts in saliva. Both of these mechanisms of actions make urea as an anticalculus agent.

## Second Generation

- *Inhibition of crystal growth via*:
  - *Vitamine C (chlomethyl analog)*: It is a surface-active organophosphorus. It reduces crystal growth because of its crystal poisoning mechanism. It has a characteristic taste which is thought to promote saliva flow and reduces calculus levels.
  - *Pyrophosphates*: They breakdown amorphous calcium phosphate to hydroxyapatite and thus prevent the calcification process.
  - *Diphosphonates*: They are a group of synthetic pyrophosphate analogs. They interact strongly with minerals and inhibit crystal growth, thus prevent calculus deposition.
  - *Metal salts (zinc salts)*: They inhibit calculus formation by two mechanisms. In the first mechanism, they considerably inhibit plaque growth. This inhibition is produced due to uptake of the metal salt by bacteria and consequent disruption of intracellular metabolic processes. It may occur due to the extracellular binding of the metal ion with bacteria and the consequent change in the bacterial cell wall. Both of these processes lead to changes in the plaque's adhesive and cohesive nature, resulting in problems with bacterial accretion and binding. Stannous and stannic salts act by this mechanism of action. In the second mechanism of action, metal salts act as strong inhibitors of mineralization. By getting adsorbed to the surface of the growing crystal, metal ion prevents the attachment of lattice ions. This process results in slowing or inhibition of crystal growth. Metal ions can also bind to hydroxyapatite, which is reversible and commonly inhibited due to an increase in the local concentration of calcium. This suggests the competitive nature of calcium for binding sites in the crystal lattice and subsequent displacement of other metal ions from that lattice.
  - *Pyrophosphates, sodium fluoride, Gantrez copolymer*: Gantrez A is found to inhibit the hydrolysis of pyrophosphate by alkaline phosphatase. This copolymer is thought to bind tightly with magnesium ions, which act as a necessary substrate for alkaline phosphatase activity.
  - Citroxain and sodium citrate.
  - Calcium lactate.

## ANTIMICROBIALS

In the general category of systemic chemotherapeutic agents, antimicrobials constitute the majority of agents.[24]

## Rationale

- Mechanical therapy alone is not sufficient to effectively control infection, especially in deep pockets.
- Poor plaque control enhances the rate of reinfection of the pocket.
- Pathogenic bacteria are commonly present in root surface, tongue, tonsils, and other niches in the oral mucosa. This microbiota can recognize the periodontal pocket and initiate reinfection in the oral cavity.
- *Aggregatibacter actinomycetemcomitans* and other tissue invading pathogens are usually difficult to eradicate without concomitant antibiotic therapy.
- Acts as an additional helpful therapy in the management of specific disease profiles (refractory disease) with periodontitis usually needed more aggressive treatment.
- In the prevention of post-surgical complications, including infection.
- In periodontal surgery, especially in the early healing phase, the regeneration of tissues is controlled by controlling the subgingival microflora.

## Indications

- Therapeutic therapy is used to treat established clinical infections such as chronic or aggressive periodontitis.
- Prophylactic therapy means the administration of antimicrobial agents to individuals who may be susceptible to develop clinical disease. Antimicrobial prophylaxis for the prevention of infective endocarditis is an excellent example of prophylactic antibiotic therapy.
- Preemptive therapy is the administration of antimicrobial therapy to individuals before the onset of clinical disease. The therapy is based on clinical, epidemiological, or laboratory findings, which indicate the development of disease in the near future. An example of preemptive therapy is an administration of antimicrobial agents against A. actinomycetemcomitans in younger siblings of adolescents with localized aggressive periodontitis or children of parents with localized aggressive periodontitis.

Parameters used to determine the dosage of an antimicrobial agent are as follows:
- Susceptibility of the infecting pathogen(s)
- The severity of the disease infection
- Body mass (standard dose should be adjusted for under- and overweight patients)
- Other medications

## Combination and Serial Antimicrobial Therapy

A bactericidal antibiotic (e.g., amoxicillin) should not be used simultaneously with a bacteriostatic agent (e.g., tetracycline) because the bactericidal agent exerts activity during cell division that is impaired by the bacteriostatic drugs. When both types of drugs are required, they are administered serially instead of giving in combination.[25]

Combined and serial antimicrobial therapy may help:
- To prevent the emergence of bacterial resistance with the use of agents covering overlapping antimicrobial spectra.
- To reduce the dose of individual antibiotics by exploiting the possible synergy between two drugs against targeted organisms.
- To broaden the antimicrobial range of the therapeutic regimen that is difficult to achieve by any single antibiotic.

For example, metronidazole and ciprofloxacin combination has both therapeutic as well as prophylactic benefit. Metronidazole acts on obligate anaerobes and ciprofloxacin targets against facultative anaerobes, thus providing therapeutic benefits. Ciprofloxacin has minimal effect on *Streptococcus* species which maintain periodontal health and provide prophylactic benefit.[26]

## Various Antibiotics

Various antibiotics used for periodontal diseases are given in **Table 38.2**.

**TABLE 38.2:** Suggested antibiotic dosage for periodontal diseases.

| Antibiotic drugs | Adult dosage | Length of treatment |
|---|---|---|
| Amoxicillin | 500 mg TID | 10 days |
| Tetracycline | 250 mg QID | 21 days |
| Doxycycline | 100 mg BID 1st day followed by 100 mg once daily | 10–14 days |
| Clindamycin | 300 mg TID | 10 days |
| Azithromycin | 500 mg 1st day followed by 250 mg once daily | 5 days |
| Ciprofloxacin | 500 mg BID | 8 days |
| Metronidazole | 500 mg TID (400 mg is available in India) | 10 days |

### Penicillins

The penicillins are a large group of bactericidal compounds with a broad spectrum of antimicrobial activity. They act by inhibiting bacterial cell wall synthesis and directly result in the death of the cell. Penicillins are classified into four groups: (1) natural penicillins (G and V), (2) antistaphylococcal (penicillinase-resistant) penicillins, (3) aminopenicillins (ampicillin and amoxicillin), and (4) antipseudomonal penicillins. All penicillins carry a common structure of a β-lactam ring fused with a thiazolidine nucleus. This β-lactam ring is responsible for the potential antimicrobial activity of penicillin.

However, occasionally penicillin administration is responsible for anaphylactic reactions in susceptible individuals. Anaphylaxis is an adverse effect characterized by severe but rare allergic responses with an occurrence rate between 0.004 and 0.015% of penicillin courses. Allergic reactions to penicillin are immediate immunoglobulin (Ig) E-mediated type I immune responses. Clinical features of such allergic reactions include urticaria, pruritus, bronchospasm, angioedema, laryngeal edema, and hypotension.[27]

### Amoxicillin

It is semisynthetic penicillin covering a wide antimicrobial spectrum that includes both gram-positive and gram-negative bacteria. It demonstrates excellent absorption after oral administration. It is susceptible to penicillinase, a penicillin ring structure, and thereby renders penicillins ineffective.[27]

Amoxicillin is effective in the control of aggressive periodontitis, both in the localized and generalized forms. The recommended dosage for management is 500 mg TID for 8 days.

*Amoxicillin-clavulanic acid (augmentin)*: It is a β-lactamase inhibitor combination. The addition of the β-lactamase inhibitor enhances an antibacterial spectrum against β-lactamase-producing organisms. Hence, augmentin is useful in the treatment of patients with refractory or localized aggressive periodontitis.

Augmentin is the combination drug with broad-spectrum antibacterial activity, good oral bioavailability, and whose elimination takes place by renal excretion.

## *Tetracyclines*

Though all tetracyclines exhibit different chemical structures and are produced by different species of *Streptomyces,* but they have a similar mechanism of action. Tetracycline HCl, doxycycline, and minocycline are all semisynthetic tetracyclines, with tetracycline HCl being derived from oxytetracycline. It consists of four fused cyclic rings. The fourth carbon ring has a dimethyl amino group which is responsible for its antimicrobial action. Tetracyclines are divided into subclasses based on significant differences in serum half-life: short-acting tetracycline (tetracycline, chlortetracycline, and oxytetracycline), intermediate-acting tetracycline (demeclocycline and methacycline) and long-acting tetracycline (minocycline and doxycycline). They are broad-spectrum antibiotics with activity against gram-negative and gram-positive bacteria as well as mycoplasma infections. Tetracyclines bind to the 30S ribosome and thereby prevent the binding of aminoacyl transfer RNA (tRNA) to the A site (acceptor site) on the 50S ribosomal unit.[28] It has antimicrobial, anticollagenase, anti-inflammatory, antiproteolytic, and fibroblast stimulating activity. Tetracyclines are known to exert significant antimatrix metalloproteinase effects and act as potent inhibitors of osteoclast function. Antiresorptive action occurs due to the alteration of intracellular calcium concentration and interaction with a putative calcium receptor. Other actions that occur are: Decrease in the ruffled border area, reduction in acid production, decrease in the secretion of cathepsins, inhibition of osteoclast gelatinase activity and induction of apoptosis or programed cell death of osteoclasts.[29]

*Dosage*: 250 mg QID.

### Interactions

- *Antacid and iron preparation*: Tetracycline HCl is a chelating agent and chelates $Ca^{+2}$, $Mg^{+2}$, and $Al^{+3}$ in the gastrointestinal tract. These ions, especially calcium, are present in a variety of food substances. Thus, it is advisable to take tetracycline either half an hour before or after food.
- *Phenytoin*: It decreases the concentration of doxycycline.
- *Oral contraceptives*: Tetracycline causes the failure of oral contraceptives.
- *Warfarin*: Tetracycline increases the anticoagulant activity of warfarin.
- *Insulin*: Tetracycline with insulin increases hypoglycemia.

### Side Effects

Gastrointestinal tract intolerance, candidiasis, renal diseases, diarrhea, vomiting, nausea, esophageal ulceration, skin rashes, vestibular disturbances, photosensitivity, and increased intracranial pressure are a few side effects of tetracycline.

### Contraindications

Hepatic diseases, renal diseases, insulin-dependent diabetes, pregnancy, lactating mothers, females taking oral contraceptives, children below eight years of age, and systemic lupus erythematosus (SLE) patients are few contraindications of using tetracycline.

## *Doxycycline*

The advantages of doxycycline over other tetracyclines are that calcium, antacids, and milk do not alter absorption and have to be given once daily, thus shows better compliance.

*Dosage*: 100 mg twice daily the 1st day, then 100 mg once daily.[25]

## *Minocycline*

Minocycline is administered twice daily that facilitates compliance as compared to tetracycline. It exhibits less phototoxicity and renal toxicity compared to tetracyclines. However, it is not advised in some light-skinned patients. It is because minocycline causes severe dark bone pigmentation visible through the mucosa of the alveolar ridges in the mouth and other areas where bone directly adheres to the skin (black bone disease).

## *Macrolides*

The macrolide antibiotics consist of a large lactone ring with attached sugars. Antibiotics belonging to this group are erythromycin, clarithromycin, azithromycin, and oleandomycin. All these macrolides exhibit a similar mechanism of action. These antibiotics get to bind to the 50S ribosomal subunit of bacteria but not to the 80S mammalian ribosome by which they produce selective toxicity. Ribosomal binding occurs at a site near peptidyl transferase and results in inhibition of translocation, peptide bond formation, and release of oligopeptidyl tRNA. Erythromycin was the first macrolide, which has been used clinically for some 40 years. Azithromycin and clarithromycin are commercially available newer macrolides. All the macrolide-related compounds are administered orally, while clarithromycin can also be used as an intravenous infusion.

## *Erythromycin*

It is a macrolide antibiotic commonly useful in the management and prevention of *Streptococcus pyogenes* and other streptococcal infections. It is effective against *Staphylococci* and hence can be used as an alternative drug for the penicillin-hypersensitive individual. Side effects are rarely noted with erythromycin. However, mild gastrointestinal upset with nausea, diarrhea, and abdominal pain can occasionally occur with erythromycin therapy.[30]

### Clindamycin

It is a chloroderivative of lincomycin. It is bacteriostatic and inhibits the synthesis of bacterial protein by binding to the 50S ribosomal subunit and interfering with the peptidyl transfer. Antibacterial spectrum of clindamycin consists of gram-positive cocci, including many penicillin-resistant *staphylococci* and anaerobic species such as bacteroides species. It is effective against anaerobic bacteria. The significant side effects of clindamycin are pseudomembranous ulcerative colitis (due to an overgrowth of toxin-producing *clostridium difficile*)[25] and hepatitis.

### Azithromycin

It is a member of the azalide class of macrolides. Broad-spectrum activity of azithromycin covers a number of bacteria, including gram-negative anaerobes. Azithromycin is taken by gingival epithelial cells[31] and penetrates fibroblasts and phagocytes (neutrophils).[32] The drug concentration is usually 100–200 times more than the extracellular compartment and is transported and released directly into the site of inflammation through phagocytes.[33] In gingival crevicular fluid (GCF), its therapeutic levels sustain for at least 2 weeks after the last dose.[34] It is thought to reduce the severity of cyclosporine-induced gingival enlargement.

*Therapeutic dose*: Initial loading dose of 500 mg is followed by 250 mg/day for 5 days. Convenient dosing is a significant advantage.

### Ciprofloxacin

It is the most potent first-generation fluoroquinolone, effective against a broad range of microorganisms. It is a bactericidal drug that is effective against gram-negative rods and anaerobic bacteria. The advantages of ciprofloxacin over other antibiotics for combating aggressive periodontitis are that it has minimal effect on *Streptococcus* species, which is associated with periodontal health. Moreover, all strains of *A. actinomycetemcomitans* are susceptible to ciprofloxacin.

### Metronidazole

It is a nitroimidazole compound with a bactericidal action against anaerobic microorganisms (*Porphyromonas gingivalis* and *Prevotella intermedia*). Hydroxymetabolite of metronidazole disrupts bacterial DNA synthesis. It was initially used in trichomoniasis and amoebiasis.[35] It is used as an alternative drug to penicillin for the management of oral infections or infections associated with β-lactamase-producing anaerobes. It is the first choice of drug for the treatment of acute necrotizing ulcerative gingivitis, pericoronitis, and aggressive periodontitis (along with amoxicillin and ciprofloxacin).[36] It is available in tablets, rectal and intravenous preparations. On oral administration, the drug gets well absorbed, reaching its mean peak plasma concentration within 1–2 hours. The plasma half-life is 8 hours. Metronidazole penetrates into body tissues and fluids and is metabolized in the liver. GCF and serum levels have been shown to reach minimal inhibitory concentration (MIC) levels for most periopathogens. Unchanged drugs and metabolites are excreted in the urine.

The major side effects associated with metronidazole are:
- Gastrointestinal disturbances are the most common adverse reactions associated with metronidazole. Other common side effects are nausea, headache, anorexia, and vomiting. Occasionally drowsiness, depression, skin rashes, and vaginal or urethral burning also occur.

> **Clinical Tip**
> Alcohol and its products should be avoided during metronidazole therapy, and at least 1 day after drug is discontinued.

- *Disulfiram-like reaction or antabuse effect of alcohol*: Disulfiram or metronidazole irreversibly inhibits aldehyde dehydrogenase (ALDH) enzyme **(Flowchart 38.2)**, which leads to accumulation of toxic levels of acetaldehyde in the liver and systemic circulation causing vomiting, visual disturbances, postural fainting, and circulatory collapse.
- Metronidazole crosses the placental barrier and enters the fetal circulation system. It is also secreted in breast milk. The drug is contraindicated in pregnant women and nursing mothers because of its association with tumorigenicity in some animals.

#### Interactions

- *Alcohol*: Metronidazole, when taken with alcohol, shows a disulfiram-like reaction.
- *Anticoagulant*: Simultaneous administration of metronidazole and anticoagulant inhibits warfarin metabolism.
- *Lithium*: Metronidazole, when taken with lithium, elevates serum lithium levels.
- *Phenytoin*: When a patient on phenytoin takes metronidazole, phenytoin accelerates the elimination of metronidazole, resulting in reduced plasma levels.

## LOCAL DRUG DELIVERY SYSTEM

The success of any drug delivery system designed to target periodontal infections depends upon its ability to deliver the antimicrobial agents to the base of the pocket at a bacteriostatic or bactericidal concentration. The rationale behind local drug delivery (LDD) is to disinfect pathogen reservoirs by delivering a high concentration of antibiotics or antimicrobial directly to the site of periodontal infection and facilitating the retention of the medicament long enough to ensure efficacious results **(Table 38.3)**. LDD system was pioneered by Goodson of the Forsyth Dental Research Center.[33,37]

## Chapter 38: Chemotherapeutic Agents

**Flowchart 38.2:** Disulfiram-like reaction or antabuse effect of alcohol.

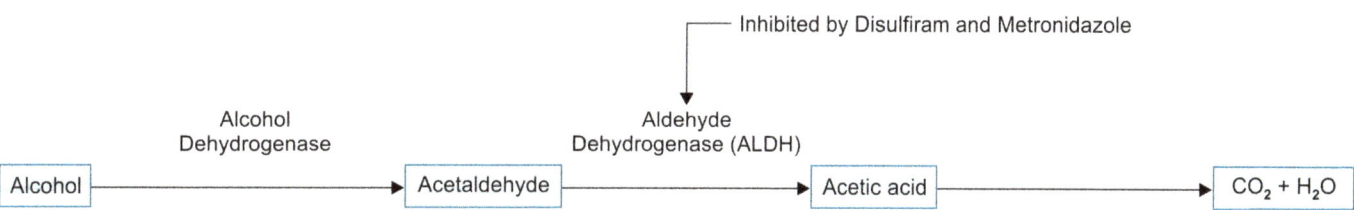

| TABLE 38.3: Comparison of local and systemic antimicrobial therapy. | | |
|---|---|---|
| | **Antimicrobial therapy** | |
| **Parameters** | **Local** | **Systemic** |
| Effective range | Narrow | Wide |
| Drug concentration at the site | High dose | Low |
| Compliance | Less | More |
| Systemic side effects | Less | More |
| Cost | Expensive | Inexpensive |
| Drug dose | Less | More |
| Therapeutic potential | Acts better locally on biofilm-associated microorganisms | Reaches widely distributed microorganisms better |
| Super infections | More chances | Fewer chances |

**Flowchart 38.3:** Classifications of local drug delivery.

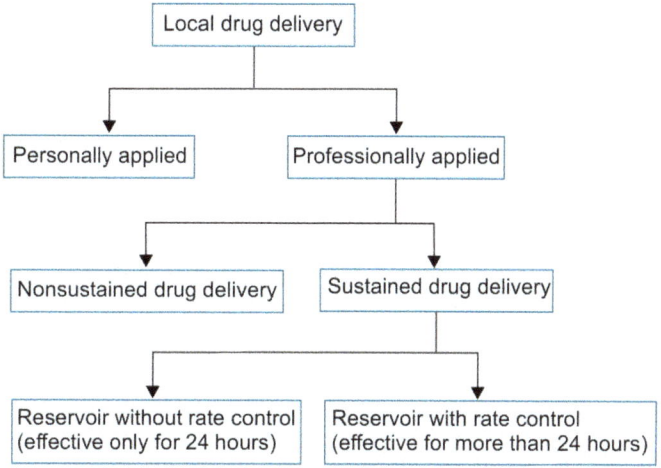

Local drug delivery system should meet the following criteria to be effective in treating the disease:
- It inhibits or kills the putative pathogen.
- It should be able to reach the site.
- It should be in adequate concentration.
- It should be there long enough.
- It should not be toxic.

## Classifications

Various subgingival delivery devices are hollow cellulose fiber, dialysis tubing, gels, acrylic strips, and ethylcellulose strips **(Flowchart 38.3)**.

## Actisite

It is composed of a polymer ethylene vinyl acetate with 25% of saturated tetracycline HCl. It is marketed in the form of flexible yellow fibers of length 23 cm and 0.5 mm diameter containing 2.7 mg of tetracycline HCl.[25]

### Technique

Tetracycline fibers have a slight amount of memory and thus can be bent easily. The optimal site for the use of fibers is the periodontal pocket of 5 mm or more in the depth that bleeds on probing and is resistant to mechanical therapy. Take 2–3-inch of fiber in a forceps and place it in the opening of the pocket. This fiber should be folded on itself and packed into the pocket until it is filled to slightly below the gingival margin because gingival shrinkage is known to occur **(Fig. 38.4)**. Interproximal pockets are packed from both facial and lingual sides. With the completion of fiber placement, isolate the area with an air syringe and applies a drop of tissue adhesive at each interdental as well as facial and lingual area. The patient is advised to avoid using brush and floss in the treated area until fibers are removed, and CHX mouthwash is prescribed twice daily.

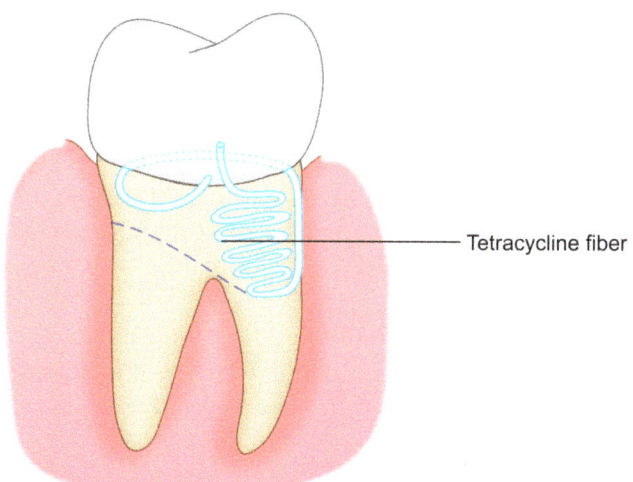

**Fig. 38.4:** Schematic representation showing tetracycline fibers packed till the base of the pocket.

### Disadvantages

- Need for a second appointment for the removal of fibers.
- Sometimes results in oral candidiasis.

## Atridox

It is a gel system containing 10% of doxycycline in a syringe. It comes in two syringes that are coupled together before use and mixed by moving the contents of the syringes back and forth for 100 cycles. The delivery syringe is attached to a 23-gauge blunt cannula, and the material is injected into the periodontal pocket. This product is also available premixed in a single syringe. Overflown material is gently packed in the pocket with a cord packing instrument or the back of a curet. Periodontal dressing or adhesive may aid in retaining the material. The patient is advised to avoid brushing, flossing, or eating from the treated area for a minimum of 7 days. Because the material is biodegradable, no additional appointments for removal are required. The patient is instructed to remove any residual material with his/her toothbrush and dental floss at the end of 1 week.

## Arestin

It is a minocycline microsphere consisting of minocycline HCl microencapsulated in a bioabsorbable polymer of polyglycolide-co-dl lactide. With the help of disposable plastic cartridge (containing 1 mg of minocycline) placed on a stainless steel handle, the microspheres are dispensed in subgingival space. It is achieved by inserting the tip to the base of the periodontal pocket and applying the material while withdrawing the tip. The material is bioadhesive on contact with moisture, and it does not require additional adhesives or periodontal dressings to hold it in place subgingivally. The patient should be instructed to avoid brushing for 12 hours, with no interproximal cleaning for ten days. No additional appointments are needed for the removal of the material because it is bioabsorbable. The minocycline microspheres maintain therapeutic drug concentrations for 14 days.

## Dentomycin or Periocline

Minocycline ointment contains 2% minocycline HCl and is applied using a syringe with a blunt cannula.

## Elyzol

It is a metronidazole gel composed of 25% metronidazole in a glyceryl monooleate and sesame oil base. It is applied into the pocket with the help of a syringe and blunt cannula.

## Periochip

It is a degradable baby's thumbnail size of 4 mm × 5 mm × 0.35 mm orange color chip composed of hydrolyzed gelatin matrix, cross-linked with glutaraldehyde, and also contains glycerin and water with the inclusion of 2.5 mg CHX

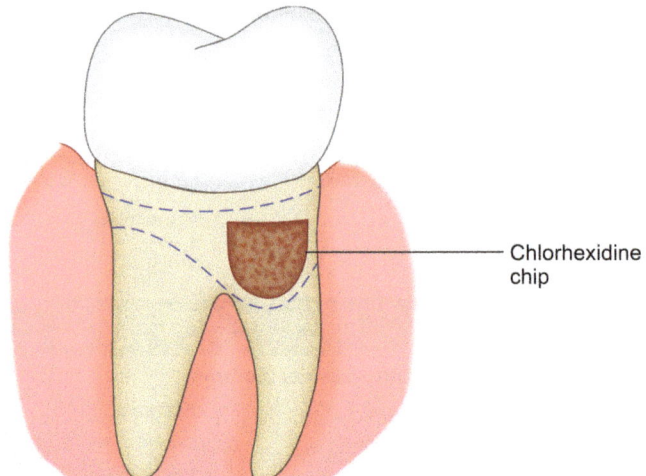

**Fig. 38.5:** Schematic representation showing chlorhexidine chip inserted at the base of the pocket.

gluconate. The chip is introduced into periodontal pockets that are 5 mm or more **(Fig. 38.5)**. The chip's dimensions prevent placement into small, tortuous pockets, so placement into pockets of less than 5 mm may be difficult and not recommended. CHX concentration is 800–1,000 ppm in GCF in the first 48 hours after the placement of periochip. Later on, 100–500 ppm concentration of CHX is present over the next six days.

Since the chip biodegrades, no postoperative appointment for removal is necessary. The patient is advised to avoid brushing or flossing the area for seven days, and twice-daily CHX rinses may be recommended for 2 weeks after placement.

## Atrigel

A biodegradable drug delivery system incorporates 5% sanguinarine. This delivery system consists of poly (DL-lactide) in an N-methyl-2-pyrrolidone carrier in a syringe.

The complicating issues related to LDD are cost-effectiveness (cost includes the price of the local delivery agents), the cost associated with the clinician's time, and the patient's perspective, i.e., number of trips to the clinician.

### Points to Ponder

- *Pin-cushion effect*: One charged end of chlorhexidine (CHX) molecule binding to the tooth surface and the other remaining available to interact with the bacterial membrane as microorganism approaches the tooth surface as the pin-cushion effect.
- The substantivity of CHX is around 12 hours.
- The substantivity of triclosan is around 5 hours.
- The substantivity of cetylpyridinium is around 3–5 hours.

## REFERENCES

1. Ciancio SG. Antiseptics and antibiotics as chemotherapeutic agents for periodontitis management. Compend Contin Educ Dent. 2000;21(1):59-62,64.
2. Addy M. The use of antiseptics in periodontal therapy. In: Lindhe J, Karring T, Lang NP (Eds). Clinical Periodontology and Implant Dentistry, 4th edition. Oxford, UK: Blackwell Munksgaard; 2003. pp. 464-93.
3. Kornman KS. The role of supragingival plaque in the treatment and prevention of periodontal treatment. J Periodontal Res. 1986;21:5-22.
4. Schroeder HE. Formation and Inhibition of Dental Calculus. Berlin, Germany: Hans Huber; 1969. pp. 145-72.
5. Loe H, Schiott CR. The effect of mouthrinses and topical application of chlorhexidine on the development of dental plaque and gingivitis in man. J Periodontal Res. 1970;5(2):79-83.
6. Hammond BF, Genco RJ. Sensitivity of periodontal organisms to antibiotics and other antimicrobial agents. In: Genco RJ, Goldman HM, Cohen DW. Contemporary Periodontics, 1st edition. St. Louis: Elsevier-CV Mosby; 1990. pp. 161-9.
7. Rolla G, Melsen B. On the mechanism of plaque inhibition by chlorhexidine. J Dent Res. 1975;54(Spec No B):B57-62.
8. Denton GW. Chlorhexidine. In: Disinfection, Sterilization and Preservation, 4th edition. Philadelphia, PA, USA: Lea and Febiger; 1991. pp. 274-89.
9. Bonesvoll P, Lökken P, Rölla G, Paus PN. Retention of chlorhexidine in the human oral cavity after mouth rinses. Arch Oral Biol. 1974;19:209-12.
10. Flötra L, Gjermo P, Rölla G, Waerhaug J. Side effects of chlorhexidine mouth washes. Scand J Dent Res. 1971;79(2):119-25.
11. Watts A, Addy M. Tooth discolouration and staining: a review of the literature. Br Dent J. 2001;190(6):309-16.
12. Eley BM, Manson JD. The possible use of antibiotics as adjuncts in the treatment of chronic periodontitis. In: Periodontics, 5th edition. Edinburgh, Scotland: Wright Publishers; 2004. pp. 223-50.
13. Lang NP, Catalanotto FA, Knöpfli RU, Antczak AA. Quality specific taste impairment following the application of chlorhexidine digluconate mouthrinses. J Clin Periodontol. 1988;15(1):43-8.
14. Addy M. Chlorhexidine compared with other locally delivered antimicrobials. A short review. J Clin Periodontol. 1986;13(10):957-64.
15. Leach SA. Mode of action of chlorhexidine in the mouth. In: Lehner T (Ed). The Borderland between Caries and Periodontal Disease. London: Academic Press; 1977. pp. 105-28.
16. Kolahi J, Soolari A. Rinsing with chlorhexidine gluconate solution after brushing and flossing teeth: a systematic review of effectiveness. Quintessence Int. 2006:37(8):605-12.
17. Addy M, Wade W. An approach to efficacy screening of mouthrinses: studies on a group of French products (I). Staining and antimicrobial properties in vitro. J Clin Periodontol. 1995;22(9):718-22.
18. Pihlstrom BL, Ammons WF. Treatment of gingivitis and periodontitis. Research, Science, and Therapy Committee of the American Academy of Periodontology. J Periodontol. 1997;68(12):1246-53.
19. Perry DA. Plaque control for the periodontal patient. In: Newman MG, Takei HH, Carranza FA (Eds). Carranza's Clinical Periodontology, 9th edition. Philadelphia, PA, USA: WB Saunders; 2003. pp. 651-74.
20. Jenkins S, Addy M, Newcombe RJ. A dose-response study of triclosan mouthrinses on plaque re-growth. J Clin Periodontol. 1993;20(8):609-12.
21. Greenstein G. Povidone-iodine's effects and role in the management of periodontal diseases: a Review. J Periodontol. 1999;70(11):1397-405.
22. Schreier H, Erdos G, Reimer K, König B, König W, Fleischer W. Molecular effects of povidone-iodine on relevant microorganisms: an electron-microscopic and biochemical study. Dermatology. 1997;195(Suppl 2):111-6.
23. Fairbrother KJ, Heasman PA. Anticalculus agents. J Clin Periodontol. 2000;27(5):285-301.
24. Drisko CH. Nonsurgical periodontal therapy. Periodontol 2000. 2001;25:77-88.
25. Jolkovsky DL, Ciancio SG. Chemotherapeutic agents in the treatment of periodontal diseases. In: Newman MG, Takei HH, Carranza FA (Eds). Carranza's Clinical Periodontology, 9th edition. Philadelphia, PA, USA: WB Saunders; 2003. pp. 675-87.
26. Rams TE, Feik D, Slots J. Ciprofloxacin/metronidazole treatment of recurrent adult periodontitis. Abstract. J Dent Res. 1992;71:319.
27. Tripathi KD. Beta-lactam antibiotics. In: Essentials of Medical Pharmacology, 4th edition. New Delhi, India: Jaypee Brothers Medical Publishers; 2003. pp. 700-17.
28. Tripathi KD. Tetracyclines and chloramphenicol. In: Essentials of Medical Pharmacology, 4th edition. New Delhi, India: Jaypee Brothers Medical Publishers; 2003. pp. 718-29.
29. Seymour RA, Heasman PA. Tetracyclines in the management of periodontal diseases. A review. J Clin Periodontol. 1995;22(1):22-35.
30. Tripathi KD. Macrolide and other antibacterial drugs, treatment of urinary tract infections. In: Essentials of Medical Pharmacology, 4th edition. New Delhi: Jaypee Brothers Medical Publishers; 2003. pp. 739-50.
31. Lai PC, Walters JD. Azithromycin kills invasive *Aggregatibacter actinomycetemcomitans* in gingival epithelial cells. Antimicrob Agents Chemother. 2013;57(3):1347-51.
32. McDonald PJ, Pruul H. Phagocyte uptake and transport of azithromycin. Eur J Clin Microbiol Infect Dis. 1991;10(10):828-33.
33. Malizia T, Tejada MR, Ghelardi E, Senesi S, Gabriele M, Giuca MR, et al. Periodontal tissue disposition of azithromycin. J Periodontol. 1997;68(12):1206-9.
34. Jain N, Lai PC, Walters JD. Effect of gingivitis on azithromycin concentrations in gingival crevicular fluid. J Periodontol. 2012;83(9):1122-8.
35. Tripathi KD. Antiamoebic and other antiprotozoal drugs. In: Essentials of Medical Pharmacology, 4th edition. New Delhi, India: Jaypee Brothers Medical Publishers; 2003. pp. 804-15.
36. Walker C, Karpinia K. Rationale for use of antibiotics in periodontics. J Periodontol. 2002;73(10):1188-96.
37. Killoy WJ, Polson AM. Controlled local delivery of antimicrobial in the treatment of periodontitis. Dent Clin North Am. 1998;42(2):263-83.

## Section 6: Treatment: Nonsurgical Therapy

### VIVA VOCE

**Q1. What is the advantage of chemical plaque control over mechanical plaque control?**

**Ans.** The advantage of the chemical approach is that the zone of diffusion achieved with the chemical agent is greater than the limited radius of effect of a mechanical therapy.

**Q2. Which mouthwashes produce staining?**

**Ans.** Chlorhexidine, stannous fluoride, and cetylpyridinium chloride produce staining.

**Q3. Classify mouthrinses.**

**Ans.** Mouthrinses have been classified into the following agents:
- *Group A agents*: They are described as antiplaque agents that inhibit plaque formation to such an extent that they prevent the development of gingivitis. This group includes CHX, acidified sodium chlorate, salifluor, and delmopinol. Their efficacy is reflected in the mouthwash form, and they can be used instead of conventional mechanical plaque removal, such as when the individual cannot effectively clean their teeth.
- *Group B agents* are described as plaque inhibitory, which should be used as adjuncts to mechanical cleanings, such as toothbrushing. This group includes cetylpyridinium chloride, essential oil (Listerine), and triclosan rinses.
- *Group C agents* are rinses with little or no effect on plaque accumulation and would be expected to have a largely cosmetic role, such as breath freshening. Rinses in this group include products containing sanguinarine, oxygenating agents and rinses containing hexetidine.

**Q4. All strains of *Actinobacillus* are susceptible to which antibiotic?**

**Ans.** Ciprofloxacin is susceptible to all strains of *Actinobacillus*.

**Q5. What are the advantages of ciprofloxacin over other antibiotics for combating aggressive periodontitis?**

**Ans.** The advantages of ciprofloxacin over other antibiotics for combating aggressive periodontitis are:
- It has minimal effect on *Streptococcus* species, which is associated with periodontal health.
- All strains of *A. actinomycetemcomitans* are susceptible to ciprofloxacin.

**Q6. What are anti-edematous drugs?**

**Ans.** For the prevention of traumatic edema and the treatment of postoperative and traumatic edema, certain enzymes and antihistamines, such as Hyaluronidase, Streptokinase, and Serratiopeptidase are used.

**Q7. What is Serratiopeptidase?**

**Ans.** This proteolytic enzyme hydrolyzes inflammatory mediators responsible for edematous conditions, including bradykinin, histamine, and serotonin. It exerts potential anti-inflammatory, antiedemic, and fibrinolytic activity with a rapid impact on localized inflammation. Dosage: 10–20 mg, 6-hourly.

**Q8. Which drugs concentrate in GCF? Write their concentration in GCF and serum.**

**Ans.**
- *Doxycycline*: Dose 200 mg; Crevicular fluid concentration 2–8 µg/mL; Serum concentration 2–3 µg/mL.
- *Tetracycline*: Dose 500 mg; Crevicular fluid concentration 5–12 µg/mL; Serum concentration 3–4 µg/mL.
- *Metronidazole*: Dose 500 mg; Crevicular fluid concentration 8–10 µg/mL; Serum concentration 6–12 µg/mL.
- *Amoxicillin*: Dose 500 mg; Crevicular fluid concentration 3–4 µg/mL; Serum concentration 8 µg/mL.
- *CHX*: Periochip; Crevicular fluid concentration 100 µg/mL.
- *Actisite*: Crevicular fluid concentration 1,300 µg/mL; Serum concentration 5–12 µg/mL.
- *Clindamycin*: Serum concentration 1–2 µg/mL.

**Q9. What is substantivity?**

**Ans.** The quality of prolonged contact time between a substance and substrate is known as substantivity.

**Q10. What are the adverse effects of CHX?**

**Ans.** Staining, taste alteration, oral mucosal erosion, and increased calculus formation.

# Host Modulation

Shashikant Hegde, Manikandan GR

## Chapter Outline

- Host Modulatory Agents

## INTRODUCTION

Direct damage to the periodontal tissues occurs by bacterial plaque through the release of hydrogen sulfide, butyric acid, and various enzymes and mediators. However, it is concluded from research findings that most of the destruction of periodontal tissues is the result of the activation of the destructive events mediated by the immune-inflammatory response of the host to the plaque bacteria. The host immune response is usually protective. However, the tissue damage and breakdown of connective tissue fibers in the periodontal ligament and resorption of alveolar bone is the result of an inflammatory response.

Host modulatory therapy (HMT), an advanced treatment concept, is unable to "switch off" standard defense mechanisms or inflammation. Paradoxically, HMT downregulates pathologically elevated inflammatory processes, promoting the process of wound healing and developing periodontal stability.[1]

Host modulatory therapy is an emerging treatment concept associated with a reduction in tissue destruction, stabilization, or even regeneration of the periodontium (**Flowchart 39.1**). HMT agents either modify or downregulate the destructive aspects of the host response and upregulate the protective or regenerative responses.[2]

**Flowchart 39.1:** Host modulatory agents.

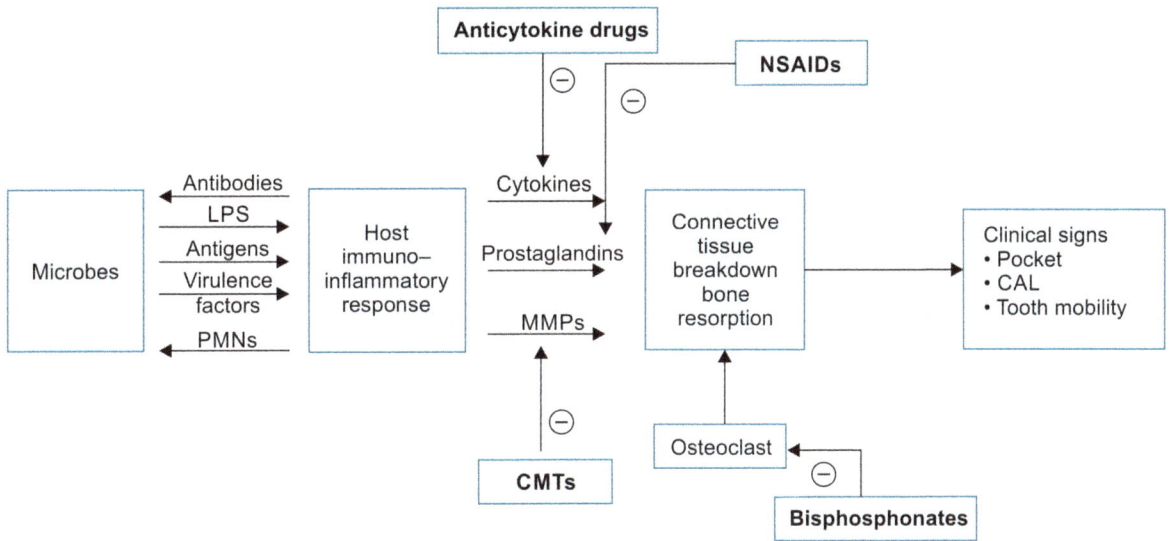

(NSAIDs: nonsteroidal anti-inflammatory drugs; PMNs: polymorphonuclear neutrophil; LPS: lipopolysaccharide; MMPs: matrix metalloproteinases; CAL: clinical attachment loss; CMTs: chemically-modified tetracyclines)

## HOST MODULATORY AGENTS

Various HMTs that have been developed to block the pathways leading to the breakdown of periodontal tissue are as follows **(Flowchart 39.1)**:[3]
- *Inhibition of matrix metalloproteinases (MMPs)*: Through chemically-modified tetracyclines (CMTs).
- *Inhibition of arachidonic acid (AA) metabolites*: Through nonsteroidal anti-inflammatory drugs (NSAIDs) **(Flowchart 39.2)**.
- Modulation of bone metabolism **(Flowchart 39.3)**.
- Regulation of immune and inflammatory responses **(Flowchart 39.4)**.

## Inhibition of Matrix Metalloproteinases

Matrix metalloproteinases are a group of zinc-dependent enzymes. Normally, these enzymes are secreted by the keratinocytes, fibroblasts, neutrophils macrophages, and endothelial cells. Collagenases and gelatinases are some of the common MMPs. These MMPs lead to remodeling of the extracellular matrix, including collagen and proteoglycans. MMP-8 and MMP-9 are the predominant MMPs produced by neutrophils and degrade type I collagen.

### Chemically-modified Tetracyclines

Chemically-modified tetracyclines usually lack dimethylamino group on the 4th carbon atom **(Fig. 39.1)**.[4] Mechanism of action of CMT **(Fig. 39.2)**:[4,5]
- Inhibits or chelates the calcium atoms and subsequently hinders the action of MMPs due to the lack of calcium.
- Inhibits already active MMPs.
- Downregulates MMPs expression.
- Acts as reactive oxygen species (ROS) scavengers.
- Modulates the osteoclast functions.

*Periostat*: It is a subantimicrobial dose of doxycycline hyclate capsule of 20 mg prescribed to patients with chronic periodontitis twice daily.[6]

*Indications*: Periostat is indicated for use in the following patients:
- Not responding to nonsurgical therapy.
- Generalized recurrent sites of pocket depth more than or equal to 5 mm and which also bleed on probing.
- With mild-to-moderate chronic periodontitis.
- Those who are highly susceptible to the rapid progression of periodontal disease.

*Contraindication*: Periostat is contraindicated in patients allergic to tetracycline.

## Inhibition of Arachidonic Acid Metabolism

As a consequence of the periodontal diseases, prostaglandins are synthesized and released within the periodontal tissues and the other AA metabolites. AA is usually metabolized through the cyclooxygenase (COX) or lipoxygenase (LOX) pathways **(Flowchart 39.5)**. In such cases, the host response modulation can be possible with the inhibition of the enzymes responsible for the release of these destructive products.

### Systemically Administered Agents NSAIDs

These drugs are propionic acid derivatives, which act by inhibiting the COX pathway of AA metabolism, thereby reducing prostaglandin formation. Prostaglandins,

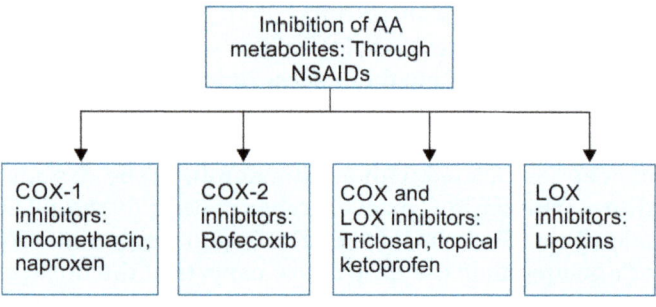

**Flowchart 39.2:** Inhibition of AA metabolites: Through NSAIDs.

(AA: arachidonic acid; COX: cyclooxygenase; LOX: lipoxygenase; NSAIDs: nonsteroidal anti-inflammatory drugs)

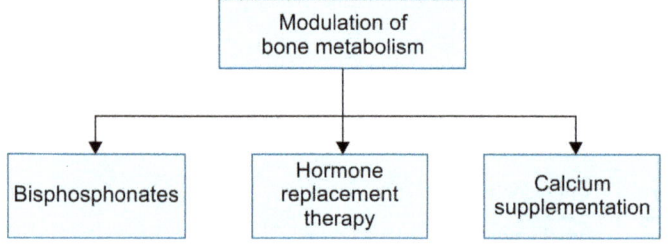

**Flowchart 39.3:** Modulation of bone metabolism.

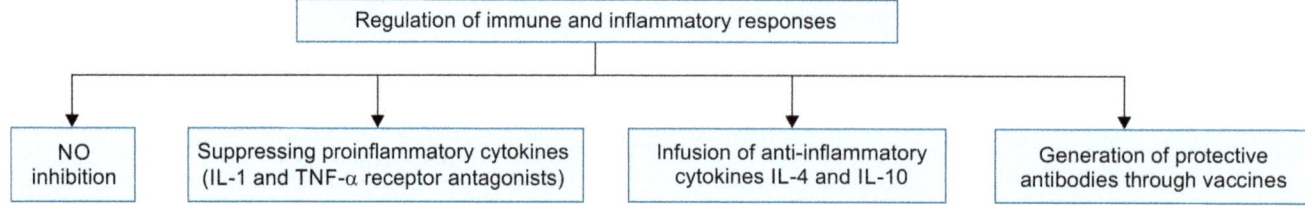

**Flowchart 39.4:** Regulation of immune and inflammatory responses.

(NO: nitric oxide; IL: interleukin; TNF-α: tumor necrosis factor-alpha)

## Chapter 39: Host Modulation

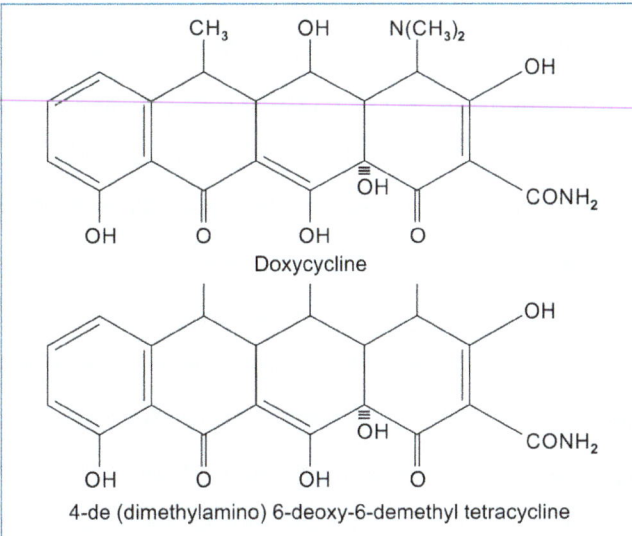

**Fig. 39.1:** Structure of doxycycline and chemically-modified tetracyclines-3.

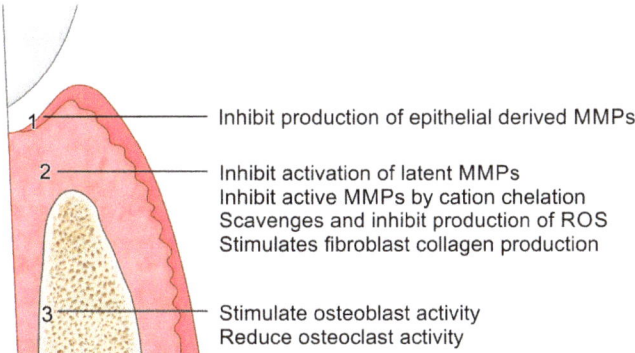

Action of chemically modified tetracyclines on:
1. Epithelium
2. Connective tissue
3. Alveolar bone

**Fig. 39.2:** Schematic representation showing modes of action of CMTs. (MMPs: matrix metalloproteinases; ROS: reactive oxygen species; CMTs: chemically-modified tetracyclines)

including prostaglandin $E_2$ ($PGE_2$), are produced by gingival epithelial cells, neutrophils, macrophages and fibroblast through the COX pathway. Prostaglandins are released in response to the lipopolysaccharide (LPS) present in the Gram-negative bacteria cell wall. $PGE_2$ induces bone loss; thus, NSAIDs control the alveolar bone loss.[7] Mechanism of action of NSAIDs is explained in **Flowchart 39.5**.

### Locally Administered Agents NSAIDs

An alternative to systemic administration, NSAIDs can be applied topically in affected areas. Generally, the topical application of NSAIDs is effective due to its lipophilic nature and absorbance into gingival tissues. Ketorolac tromethamine rinse and S-ketoprofen dentifrice are the NSAIDs that have also been evaluated for the topical administration.

### COX and LOX Inhibitors (Triclosan)

Cyclooxygenase and LOX inhibitors are compounds that have both antibacterial and anti-inflammatory properties. Triclosan (2,4,4'-trichloro-2'-hydroxydiphenyl ether) is a nonionic agent that has an antibacterial property. It also inhibits COX and LOX and, hence can interfere with the production of AA metabolites.[8]

### Omega-3 Fatty Acid

Omega-3 polyunsaturated fatty acids are essential fatty acids that must be derived from dietary sources, i.e., fatty fish such as salmon, sardines, mackerel, herring, and tuna; canola oil, flaxseed oil, soybean oil, walnut oil; pumpkin seeds; soyabean and green leafy vegetables. Omega-3 fatty acids show anti-inflammatory, anti-thrombotic, anti-arithmic, hypolipidemic, and vasodilator effects.[9] It inhibits LOX and COX (AA cascade). It inhibits the production of prostanoids derived from the COX pathway and the leukotrienes, especially leukotriene $B_4$ derived from the LOX pathway.[10]

**Flowchart 39.5:** Mechanism of action of nonsteroidal anti-inflammatory drugs (NSAIDs).

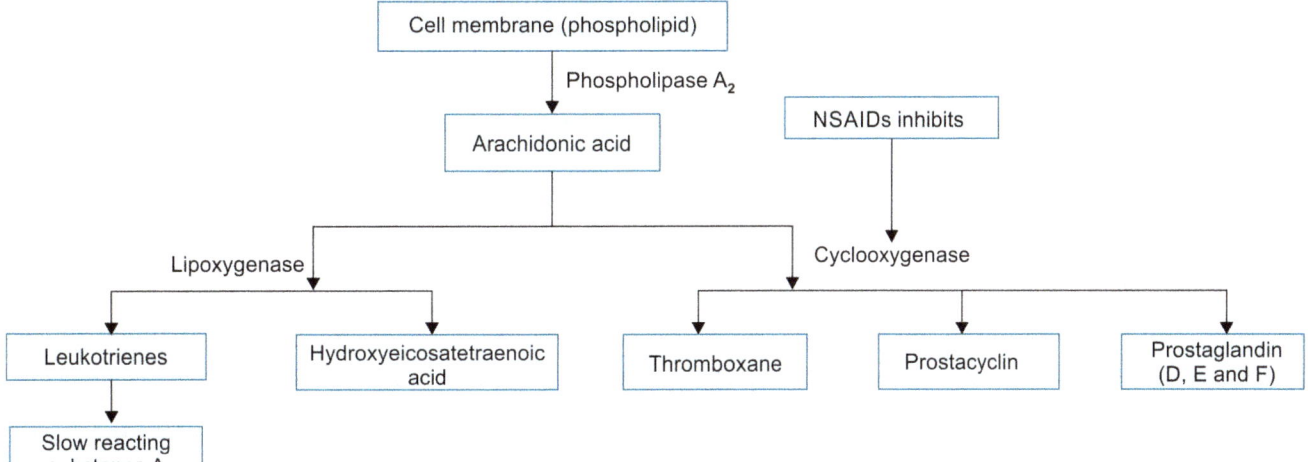

## Lipoxins

These are lipid-derived mediators that are released during the resolution of periodontal inflammation. It blocks interleukin-1β (IL-1β) secretion from neutrophils[11] and also blocks neutrophil migration following exposure to *Porphyromonas gingivalis*.[12]

## Modulation of Bone Metabolism

The following are the two molecules involved in the regulation of osteoclast formation and bone resorption **(Fig. 39.3)**:
- Receptor activator of nuclear factor-kappa B ligand (RANKL).
- Osteoprotegerin (OPG).

Osteoprotegerin blocks osteoclast differentiation and activation induced by RANKL by acting as a decoy receptor for RANKL (See Flowchart 2 in "Chapter 24: Bone Defects.").[13]

### Inhibitor of RANK/RANKL

Inhibitor of RANK/RANKL includes denosumab (a human monoclonal antibody that targets RANKL).

### Osteoprotegerin

Osteoprotegerin is a natural inhibitor of RANKL.

### Bisphosphonates

They are nonbiodegradable analogs of pyrophosphate. They have a high affinity for the calcium phosphate crystals and bring inhibition of osteoclast activity. Bisphosphonates may inhibit MMP activity due to their involvement in the chelation of cations.

Bisphosphonates are divided into three generations depending on the associated side chain:
1. *First-generation bisphosphonates*: It consists of alkyl side chains (e.g., etidronate).
2. *Second-generation bisphosphonates*: They have amino bisphosphonates with an amino-terminal group (e.g., alendronate and pamidronate).
3. *Third-generation bisphosphonates*: It is composed of cyclic side chains (e.g., risedronate).

The antiresorptive properties of bisphosphonates increase approximately 10-fold between drug generations. Suggested modes of action of bisphosphonates are as follows:[14]
- Bisphosphonates inhibit the development of osteoclasts.
- They help in the reduction of the activity of osteoclast.
- They help in the induction of osteoclastic apoptosis.
- They prevent the development of osteoclasts from the hematopoietic precursors.
- They stimulate the production of an osteoclast inhibitory factor.

*Contraindications to the use of bisphosphonates*: Sensitivity to phosphonates and gastrointestinal upset.

The long-term side effect of bisphosphonates is osteonecrosis of the jaw.

### Teriparatide (Bone Forming Drugs)

Teriparatide, a biosynthetic human parathyroid hormone, which consists of the first 34 amino acids of parathyroid hormone, is an anabolic agent. It has been known since 1932 that the parathyroid hormone has anabolic effects on bone.

*Mechanism of action*: Teriparatide and PTH mediate their biological effects via specific, G-protein-dependent, high-affinity membrane cell-surface receptors expressed on osteoblasts and renal tubular cells; both these molecules bind to the receptors with the same affinity and exert the same physiological effects on bone and kidney. Ligand binding induces a cascade that activates protein kinase-1, cyclic adenosine monophosphate, protein kinase C and phospholipase C. The activation of these pathways increases the number of active osteoblasts, a decrease in osteoblast apoptosis and probably, recruitment of bone lining cells as newly formed osteoblasts, thereby increasing bone strength, mass and diameter, and bone structural integrity, as well as increasing serum and urinary levels of markers of bone formation and resorption. Teriparatide upregulates basic fibroblast growth factor 2 (bFGF-2), helping in the proliferation and differentiation of osteoblast progenitors. PTH may transcriptionally suppress Osteocytic Sclerostin (SOST) gene. As a result, reduction in sclerostin, a potent inhibitor of bone formation, could account for part of the anabolic response to PTH.[15]

## Regulation of Immune and Inflammatory Responses

Nitric oxide (NO) is a short-lived molecule having an integral role in biological processes. It is produced by the epithelial and the inflammatory cells in response to the cytokines. It shows cytotoxic effects towards the host cells only when its concentration is elevated as in periodontitis. It is a highly reactive free radical molecule that reacts with metal and also the thiol residues, leading to the lipid peroxidation,

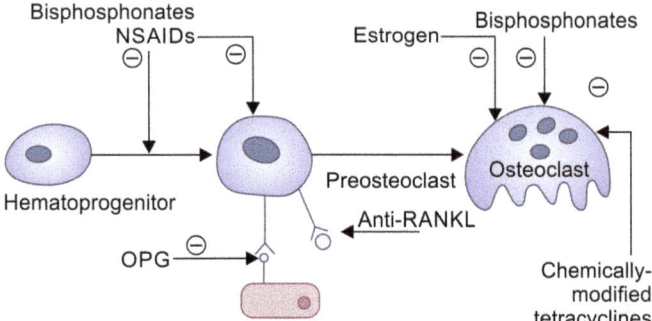

**Fig. 39.3:** Schematic representation showing therapeutic strategies to treat bone resorption.

(NSAIDs: nonsteroidal anti-inflammatory drugs; OPG: osteoprotegerin; RANKL: receptor activator of nuclear factor-kappa B ligand)

destruction of protein and deoxyribonucleic acid (DNA), and the stimulation of cytokine release.[16] Nitric oxide synthase (NOS) is an enzyme that generates NO in tissues.

### Modulation of Nitric Oxide Activity

- *Inhibitors of NOS and NO*: Mercaptoethyl guanidine inhibits inducible NOS and scavenges peroxynitrite, the product of NO and superoxide radical. NOS inhibitor inhibits bone resorption.
- *Inhibitors of downstream mediator*: Nuclear poly (ADP-ribose) polymerase-1 (PARP) enzyme is a mediator of downstream NO toxicity. Inhibition of PARP enzyme reduces alveolar bone resorption.[17]

### Cytokines

- They are the regulatory proteins controlling the survival, growth, differentiation, and functions of cells. The process of bone resorption is stimulated by IL-1 and TNF-α, through $PGE_2$ and MMPs release from fibroblasts and monocytes.[18] TNF-α is an inflammatory cytokine that is released by activated macrophages, T lymphocytes. TNF-α stimulates osteoclast formation thus, blocking it inhibits osteoclast formation.[19]
- *Suppressing proinflammatory cytokines*: Cytokine antagonists, such as IL-1 receptor antagonist (IL-1Ra) and TNF-α receptors antagonist, inhibit the progression of inflammatory cell infiltration and recruitment osteoclasts.[20] IL-4 stimulates the production of IL-1Ra.
- *Anticytokine agents*: Anakinra (recombinant human IL-1Ra); AMG 714 (a human monoclonal antibody against IL-15); recombinant human IL-11 inhibits the production of TNF-α and IL-1.
- *Other locally administered agents*: Various locally acting host modulation agents have been tested to use as an adjunct to surgical procedures. Growth factors and bone morphogenetic proteins are an example of enamel matrix proteins. They improve the wound healing process and stimulate the regeneration of cementum, lost bone, and periodontal ligament. These properties help to restore the complete periodontal attachment apparatus. Currently, the Food and Drug Administration (FDA) approved only one local host modulation agent Emdogain to use as an adjunctive during surgery **(Fig. 39.4)**.[21]

### Probiotics

- The term probiotics were adopted in 2003 by Guarner. The concept of beneficial-for-health microorganisms dates back to the ideas of Nobel Prize laureate Ilya Mechnikov in the early years of the 20th century. By definition, probiotics are live microorganisms that when administered in adequate amounts confer health benefits upon the host. Live microorganisms are administrated in the host, which allows the beneficial bacteria to repopulate and help to kill pathogenic bacteria and fight against infection. The most common probiotic strains belong to the genera *Lactobacillus* and *Bifidobacterium*.[22]

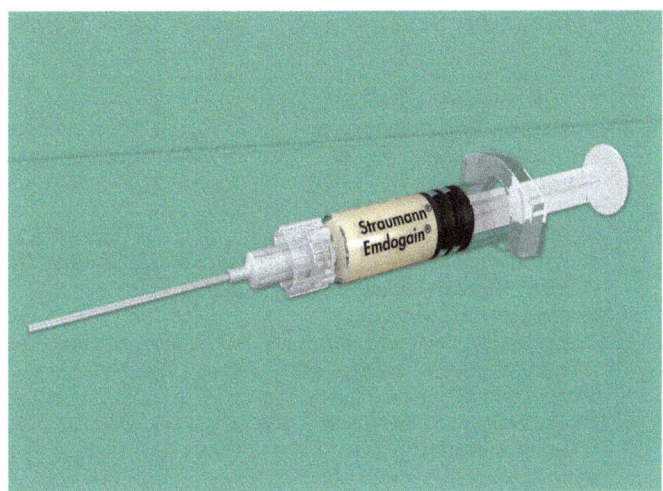

**Fig. 39.4:** Photograph showing emdogain
(© Institut Straumann, Basel, Switzerland; Reproduced with permission from Straumann Holding AG).

- *Mechanism of action*: Probiotics interacts with and strengthen the immune system and helps to prevent periodontal disease in the following manner: Induces the expression of cytoprotective proteins on host cell surfaces; prevents cytokine-induced apoptosis and modulates proinflammatory pathways induced by pathogens.[23]
- Disadvantages associated with probiotics are the transfer of antibiotic-resistance genes in between microorganisms; translocation of living organisms from the intestine to other areas of the body and into the bloodstream and cause systemic infection and; persistence in intestine resulting in fungemia or development of adverse reactions relating to interactions with host's microflora.

> **Points to Ponder**
> 
> ❑ Williams and Golub et al., introduced the concept of host modulation
> ❑ Generations of bisphosphonates are:
>   – First generation: Short-chain molecules that inhibit the Krebs cycle; Etidronate.
>   – Second generation: Long-chain molecules that inhibit fatty chain pathways; Alendronate.
>   – Third generation: Risedronate.
> ❑ Future host modulation agents are Resolvins, Lipoxins, and Probiotics.

## REFERENCES

1. Preshaw PM, Ryan ME, Giannobile WV. Host modulation agents. In: Newman MG, Takei HH, Klokkevold PR, Carranza

## Section 6: Treatment: Nonsurgical Therapy

FA (Eds). Carranza's Clinical Periodontology, 10th edition. St. Louis: Elsevier; 2006. pp. 813-27.
2. Preshaw PM. Host response modulation in periodontics. Periodontol 2000. 2008;48:92-110.
3. Oringer RJ; Research, Science, and Therapy Committee of the American Academy of Periodontology. Modulation of the host response in periodontal therapy. J Periodontol. 2002;73(4):460-70.
4. Golub LM, McNamara TF, Angelo GD, Greenwald RA, Ramamurthy NS. A non-antibacterial chemically-modified tetracycline inhibits mammalian collagenase activity. J Den Res. 1987;66(8):1310-14.
5. Greenstein G, Lamster I. Efficacy of subantimicrobial dosing with doxycycline. Point/counterpoint. J Am Dent Assoc. 2001;132(4):457-66.
6. Preshaw PM, Hefti AF, Jepsen S, Etienne D, Walker C, Bradshaw MH. Subantimicrobial dose doxycycline as an adjunctive treatment for periodontitis: A review. J Clin Periodontol. 2004;31(9):697-707.
7. Offenbacher S, Heasman PA, Collins JG. Modulation of host $PGE_2$ secretion as a determinant of periodontal disease expression. J Periodontol. 1993;64(5 Suppl):432-44.
8. Gaffar A, Scherl D, Affitto J, Coleman EJ. The effect of triclosan on mediators of gingival inflammation. J Clin Periodontol. 1995;22(6):480-4.
9. Vardar S, Buduneli E, Türkoğlu O, Berdeli AH, Baylas H, Başkesen A, et al. Therapeutic versus prophylactic plus therapeutic administration of omega-3 fatty acid on endotoxin-induced periodontitis in rats. J Periodontol. 2004;75:1640-6.
10. Vardar S, Buduneli E, Baylas H, Berdeli AH, Buduneli N, Atilla G. Individual and combined effects of selective cyclooxygenase-2 inhibitor and omega-3 fatty acid on endotoxin-induced periodontitis in rats. J Periodontol. 2005;76(1):99-106.
11. Pouliot M, Serhan CN. Lipoxin A4 and aspirin-triggered 15-epi- LXA4 inhibit tumor necrosis factor-alpha-initiated neutrophil responses and trafficking: novel regulators of a cytokine-chemokine axis relevant to periodontal diseases. J Periodontal Res. 1999;34(7):370-3.
12. Pouliot M, Clish CB, Petasis NA, Van Dyke TE, Serhan CN. Lipoxin A(4) analogues inhibit leukocyte recruitment to Porphyromonas gingivalis: a role for cyclooxygenase-2 and lipoxins in periodontal disease. Biochemistry. 2000;39(16):4761-8.
13. Bartold PM, Cantley MD, Haynes DR. Mechanisms and control of pathologic bone loss in periodontitis. Periodontol 2000. 2010;53:55-69.
14. Tenenbaum HC, Shelemay A, Girard B, Zohar R, Fritz PC. Bisphosphonates and periodontics: potential applications for regulating bone mass in the periodontium and other therapeutic/diagnostic uses. J Periodontol. 2002;73(7):813-22.
15. Brixen KT, Christensen PM, Ejersted C, Langdahl BL, Teriparatide (biosynthetic human parathyroid hormone 1-34): a new paradigm in the treatment of osteoporosis Basic Clin Pharmacol Toxicol. 2004;94:260-70.
16. Salve GE, Lang NP. Host response modulation in the management of periodontal diseases. J Clin Periodontol. 2005;32(Suppl 6):108-29.
17. Lohinai Z, Mabley JG, Feher E, Marton A, Komjati K, Szabo C. Role of the activation of the nuclear enzyme poly(ADP-ribose) polymerase in the pathogenesis of periodontitis. J Dental Res. 2003;82(12):987-92.
18. Birkedal-Hansen H. Role of cytokines and inflammatory mediators in tissue destruction. J Periodontal Res. 1993;28(6 Pt 2):500-10.
19. Cheng X, Kinosaki M, Murali R, Greene MI. The TNF receptor superfamily: role in immune inflammation and bone formation. Immunol Res. 2003;27(2-3):287-94.
20. Delima AJ, Oates T, Assuma R, Schwartz Z, Cochran D, Amar S, et al. Soluble antagonists to interleukin-1 (IL-1) and tumor necrosis factor (TNF) inhibits loss of tissue attachment in experimental periodontitis. J Clin Periodontol. 2001;28(3):233-40.
21. Ryan ME, Kinney J, Kim Amy S, Giannobile WV. The host modulatory approach. Dent Clin North Am. 2005;49:624-35.
22. Deepa D, Mehta DS. Is the role of probiotics friendly in the treatment of periodontal diseases. J Indian Soc Periodontol. 2009;13(1):30-1.
23. Stamatova I, Meurman JH. Probiotics and periodontal disease. Periodontol. 2009;51:141-51.

## VIVA VOCE

**Q1. What are the three categories of host modulating agents?**
**Ans.** Basic three categories of host modulating agents are:
1. Antiproteinases: Tetracyclines, CMTs.
2. Anti-inflammatory drugs: NSAIDs.
3. Bone-sparing drugs: Bisphosphonates.

**Q2. What are CMTs?**
**Ans.** Chemically-modified tetracyclines are those which lack the dimethylamino group on the 4th carbon atom.

**Q3. Name the novel host modulatory therapies.**
**Ans.** The novel host modulatory therapies are proresolving lipid mediators of inflammation lipoxins, protectins, and resolvins.

**Q4. Which is a natural inhibitor of RANKL?**
**Ans.** Osteoprotegerin.

**Q5. Name the local host modulation agent approved by the FDA.**
**Ans.** Emdogain.

**Q6. What is periostat?**
**Ans.** Periostat is a subantimicrobial dose of doxycycline hyclate capsule of 20 mg prescribed to patients with chronic periodontitis twice daily.

**Q7. What are the contraindications to the use of bisphosphonates?**
**Ans.** Sensitivity to phosphonates and gastrointestinal upset.

**Q8. Which molecules are involved in the regulation of osteoclast formation and the process of bone resorption?**
**Ans.** Receptor activator of nuclear factor-kappa B ligand; and OPG.

**Q9. Who introduced the Host modulation concept?**
**Ans.** Williams and Golub et al.

**Q10. What is the long-term side effect of bisphosphonates?**
**Ans.** Osteonecrosis of the jaw.

# Chapter 40: Periodontal Instruments

*Shalu Bathla*

## Chapter Outline

- General Characteristics
- Parts of Instruments
- Classification

## INTRODUCTION

A proper treatment approach, including the removal of local factors and diseased tissue, helps to get clean root surface free of plaque and calculus and achieve periodontal health. In such cases, the use of specially designed periodontal instruments help to remove calculus, plane root surfaces, and also remove diseased tissue. Currently, various instruments are available for the removal of supra- and subgingival calculi. Ultrasonic devices, sickles, hoes, chisels, and curettes are some of them. However, a thorough knowledge of instruments is compulsory for their proper usage and satisfactory outcomes.

## GENERAL CHARACTERISTICS

A large variety of periodontal instruments are available. Each group of instruments has characteristic features; individual therapists often develop variations with which they operate most effectively. Stainless and high carbon steels are used in manufacturing instruments. Commercially available periodontal instruments come in two forms as single- or double-ended instruments. Single-ended instruments are usually safe to use. However, double-ended instruments are more efficient because they reduce instrument exchange. Double-ended instruments are commonly available with paired working ends, that act as exact mirror images of each other. Occasionally, double-ended instruments have unpaired (dissimilar) working ends available as an explorer and a probe combination.

### Balanced Instrument

When the working ends are centered on a line running through the long axis of the handle, it is called as balanced instrument.[1]

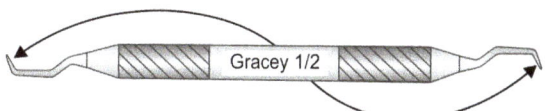

**Fig. 40.1:** Schematic representation showing name and number marked: Along.

### Nomenclature

A double-ended periodontal instrument is recognized with the design name and number provided with it. If the design name and number are imprinted along the length of the handle, each working end is recognized with the number closest to it **(Fig. 40.1)**. When the design name and number are printed across the instrument handle, the first number (on the left side) indicates the working end at the top, and the second number suggests the working end at the bottom of the handle.

The design name suggests the school or individual responsible for the original design or development of an instrument or group of instruments. Usually, instruments are named after the original designer or an academic institution that developed them. The most famous example is the design name "Gracey," which originated in the late 1930s. Dr Clayton H Gracey designed the 14-original single-ended instruments in this series bearing his name. Other commonly known examples are TU-17 in which TU stands for Tufts University School of Dental Medicine; the University of North Carolina developed UNC-15 probe, and 15 indicates the markings that are incremented to 15 mm.[2]

## PARTS OF INSTRUMENTS

The parts of periodontal instruments are the handle, the shank, and the working end **(Fig. 40.2)**. Commercially

## Section 6: Treatment: Nonsurgical Therapy

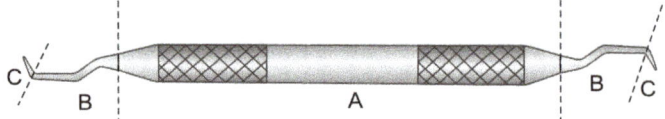

**Fig. 40.2:** Schematic representation showing parts of the periodontal instrument: (A) Handle, (B) Shank and (C) Working end.

available periodontal instruments exist in single- and double-ended forms.

## Handle

Instrument handles are designed in various sizes and shapes, and the design of handle depends upon features like:[3,4]

- *Weight*: Hollow handles increase tactile transfer and minimize fatigue.
- *Diameter*: Small diameter handle (~3/17-inch) decreases control and increases muscle fatigue. Large diameter handle (~3/8-inch) enhances control and decreases muscle cramps. However, they are associated with restricted movement in areas with limited access (e.g., posterior areas).
- *Textures*: Knurled handles increase control and reduces hand fatigue. While smooth handles reduce control and enhance muscle fatigue **(Fig. 40.3)**.

### *Shank*

#### Design Features of Shank

The functional shank length is the distance from the working end to the shank bend near the instrument handle **(Fig. 40.4A)**. Terminal or lower shank is the part of the shank near the working end **(Fig. 40.4B)**. The functional shank length may be short, long, or intermediate. Long functional shanks help to reach the tooth surfaces of posterior teeth or the root surfaces of teeth within periodontal pockets. Short functional shanks are commonly used to get rid of supragingival calculus deposits or to reach the surfaces of anterior teeth. An instrument shank is curved if it has bends that deviate from the long axis of the shank. Instruments with curved shanks can usually be used on both posterior and anterior teeth and are referred to as universal instruments. Instruments with straight shanks are limited to use on anterior sextants and thus are referred to as anterior instruments. Instruments shank maybe flexible, moderately flexible, or rigid in design. Shank flexibility is related to the instrument's use **(Table 40.1)**.

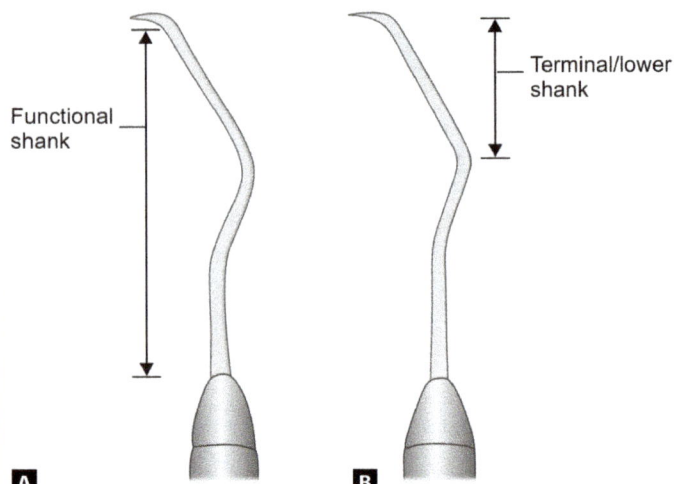

**Figs. 40.4A and B:** Schematic representation showing shank's design: (A) Functional shank; (B) Terminal or lower shank.

## Working End

The design of the working end is an important part of the instrument because it determines the working function of that respective instrument. Working ends may vary from wire-like, rod-shaped with sharp/blunt point (explorers, probes) to others, which have a blade, face, back, toe, lateral surfaces, and cutting edges (scalers, curettes). The face of the instrument is the surface between the two cutting edges. The surface opposite to the face is the back of the instrument. The surface on either side of the face forms the lateral surfaces of the instrument. The cutting edge is a

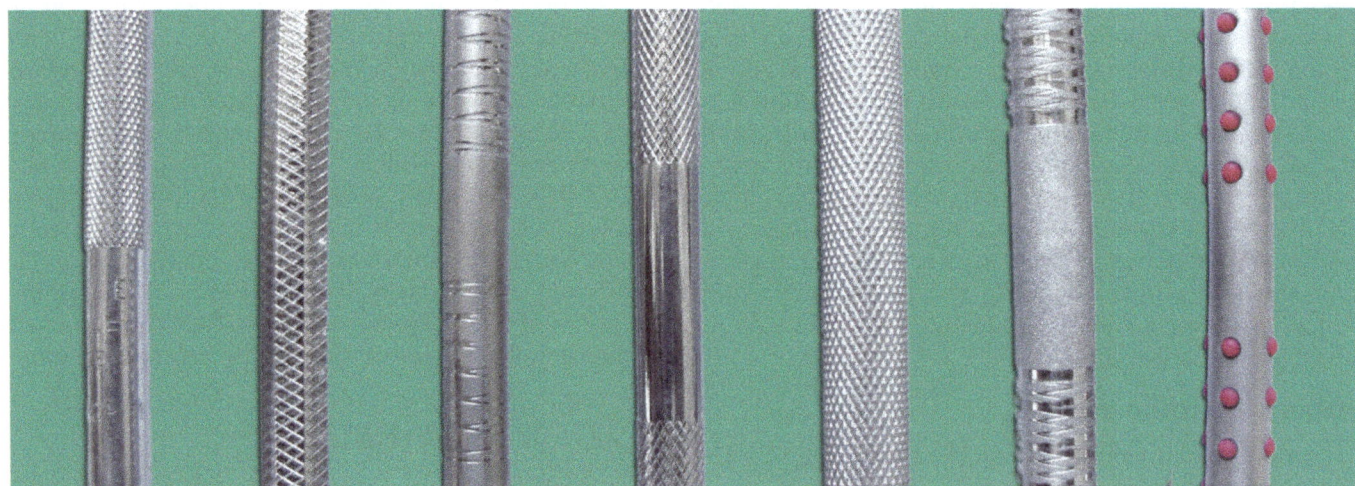

**Fig. 40.3:** Photograph showing handle textures.

| TABLE 40.1: Shank types and its uses.[5] | | |
|---|---|---|
| Shank types | Uses | Examples |
| Rigid shank | • Removal of heavy calculus deposits<br>• Limit tactile conduction so that calculus detection is difficult | Sickle scalers, periodontal files |
| Moderately flexible shank | • Removal of moderate or light calculus<br>• Provide a good level of tactile transfer, by allowing detection and removal of moderate subgingival deposits | Universal curettes |
| Flexible shank | • Detection of subgingival calculus<br>• Removal of fine calculus<br>• Provide the best tactile information to the operator's finger pads through the shank and handle | Explorers, Gracey curettes |

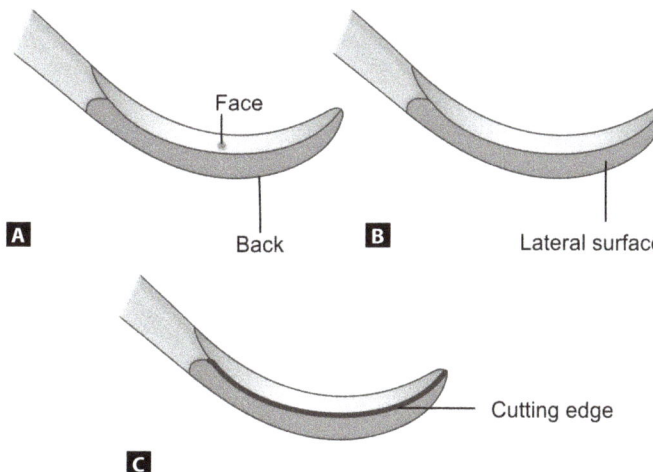

**Figs. 40.5A to C:** Schematic representation showing curette blade: Working end design.

sharp edge formed due to meeting of the face with lateral surfaces **(Figs. 40.5A to C)**.

## CLASSIFICATION

Periodontal instruments have been classified into the following groups:
- Nonsurgical periodontal instruments **(Flowchart 40.1)**.
  - Diagnostic instruments
  - Scaling, root planing, and curettage instruments
  - Periodontal endoscope
  - Cleansing and polishing instruments
- Surgical periodontal instruments **(Flowchart 40.2)**.

## Diagnostic Instruments

### Mouth Mirror

Mouth mirror is composed of the small, cylindrical metal shaft attached to a metal disk at its end. The metal disk holds the mirror.

*Types of the dental mirror*: The various types of dental mirror surfaces are:[6]
- *Plane/flat surface mirror*: The reflecting surface is at the back of the mirror lens and creates a double image.
- *Concave surface mirror*: It produces a magnified image that may be distorted.
- *Front surface mirror*: The reflecting surface is positioned on the front of the lens that eliminates double image, producing the actual image. The front surface mirror is the mirror of choice for dental procedures.
- *Double-sided mirror*: It is helpful to retract the cheek or tongue and subsequently useful to view the indirect image produced on the opposite sides of the mirror.

*Sizes of the dental mirror*:
- Size No. 1: 16 mm
- Size No. 2: 18 mm
- Size No. 3: 20 mm
- Size No. 4: 22 mm
- Size No. 5: 24 mm

Size No. 4 and 5 are regularly used mirrors for a dental examination. Size No. 2 is used to view inaccessible areas of the mouth.

*Uses of the dental mirror*
- *Specific uses*:
  - *Indirect vision*: It is used to see oral structures that cannot be seen directly without compromising the operator's positioning. It is essential for instrumentation in the maxillary right palatal and lingual aspects of anterior teeth.
  - *Indirect illumination*: Mirror is helpful to get good reflection of light from the dental overhead light to any area of the oral cavity.
  - *Retraction*: Before using a mirror for retraction initially, apply water-based lubricant on dry or cracked lips and corners of the mouth. Also, adjust the mirror's position to avoid damage to the angles of the mouth from the undue pressure of the shank of the mirror.
  - *Transillumination (the reflection of light through the teeth)*: Mirror is useful to get a light reflection from the lingual aspect during examining facial surfaces of the teeth for recording translucency of teeth.
- *Nonspecific uses*: Checking mobility, percussion.

### Explorer

*Uses of the explorer*:
- Calculus detection in normal sulci or shallow pockets.

> **Clinical Tip**
> The fogging of mirror is prevented by rubbing the mirror along buccal mucosa to coat mirror with thin transparent film of saliva, using warm mirror with water and requesting patient to breathe through the nose to prevent condensation of moisture on the mirror.

**Section 6:** Treatment: Nonsurgical Therapy

**Flowchart 40.1:** Classification of nonsurgical periodontal instruments.

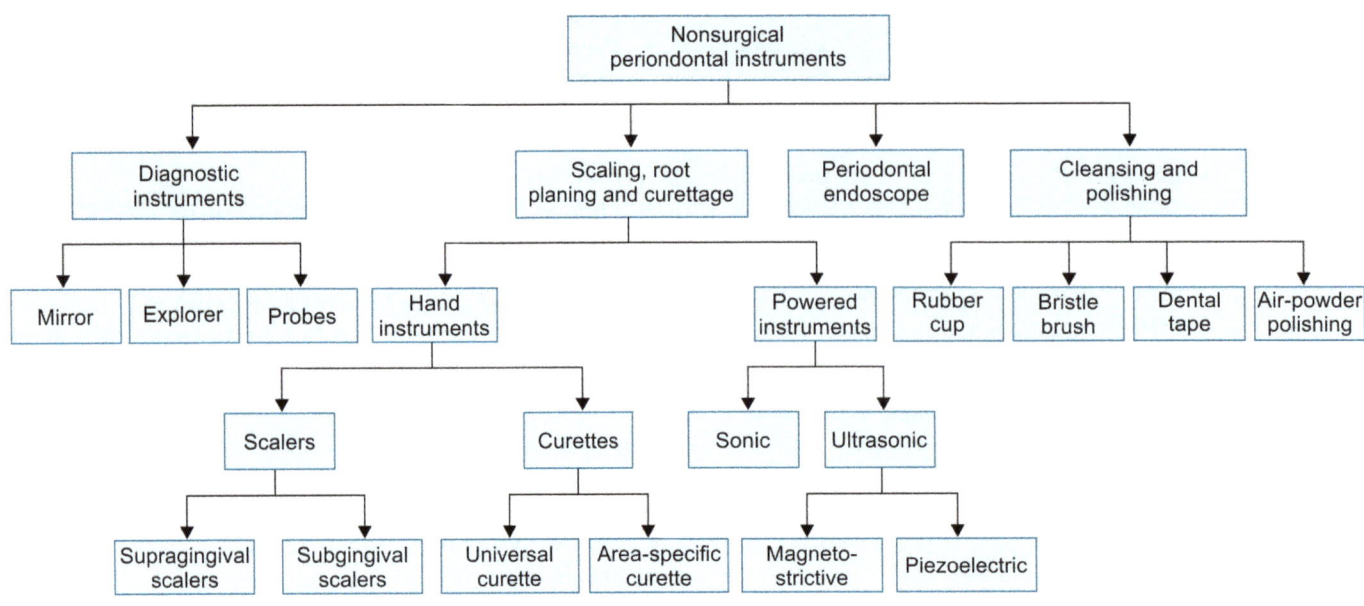

**Flowchart 40.2:** Classification of surgical periodontal instruments.

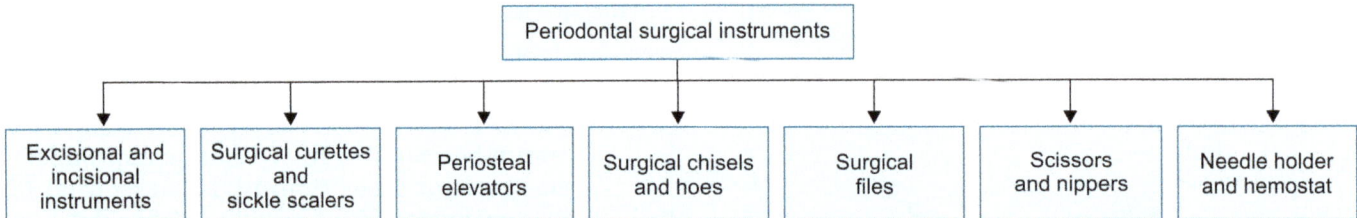

- Assessment of root surfaces of posterior and anterior teeth.
- Supragingival examinations for dental caries and irregular margins of restorations.

*Types of the explorer:*
- *23-Shepherd's hook explorer*: Single-ended/paired with 17. It has a thicker shank and working end than other explorers, which makes it more rigid. Rigidity enhances the role in caries detection but limits its role in subgingival calculus detection **(Fig. 40.6A)**.
- *17-Orbans explorer*: It is an ideal instrument for calculus detection interproximally and in a deep periodontal pocket. Its long, thin shank with a fine tip less than 2 mm that curves at the right angle to the lower shank facing upwards and do not injure soft tissue when placed subgingivally **(Fig. 40.6B)**.
- *Pigtail/Cowhorn/3CH explorer No. 21 and 22*: Double-ended instrument that is easily adapted throughout the

**General Design Features:** Explorer
- Fine, wire-like working end
- Sharp point
- Circular in cross-section

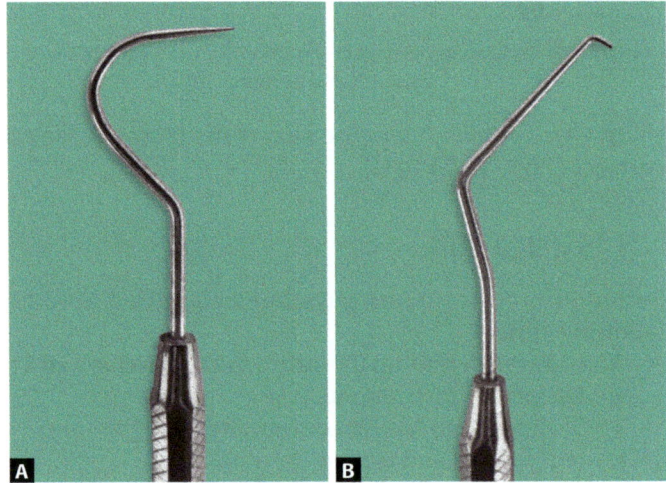

**Figs. 40.6A and B:** Photograph showing 23 and 17 end explorer: (A) 23-Shepherd's hook explorer; (B) 17-Orban explorer.

mouth. The working end is curved, and the shank is thin for calculus detection. Because shank is curved and relatively short, the instrument is best used in children/adults with minimal periodontal pocket depth less than 1 mm, it can also be used for detecting calculus in areas

of furcation involvement (similar instrument design to Nabers probe), detecting proximal and cervical caries. Ineffective in evaluating occlusal caries because the instrument's design limits the force needed to determine occlusal caries.
- *3A explorer*: It has a long, fine, arc-like tip. It adapts well in a deep pocket and furcation areas. Its fine tip allows for good tactile sensitivity, especially for calculus detection.
- *Old Dominion University (ODU) 11/12 Gracey type explorer or EXD 11–12*: Shank design of ODU is similar to that of Gracey 11/12 curette. It was developed by the faculty of ODU, thus named as ODU 11/12. Double-ended, paired instrument used for calculus detection.[7]

## Tweezers

These instruments have a serrated handle for a secure grip. Tweezers have angled beak, which is available in different sizes. They are used to place and remove small items, cotton rolls, and gauze from the mouth.

## Periodontal Probe

The periodontal probe is a tapered rod-like instrument with blunt rounded working end calibrated in millimeter and color-coding. Based on the type of the probe, the markings vary from 1 to 15 mm. This makes it easy in reading and determining the probing pocket depth. The angled shank form an angle of 45° with the working end in relation to the handle. The thin narrow working end is placed slowly up to the depth of the periodontal pocket.

*Uses of the periodontal probe*
- To locate, mark, and measure pocket depth
- To determine pocket course and topography
- To measure the width of the attached gingiva
- To determine and measure clinical attachment loss
- To measure the gingival recession
- To check bleeding on probing
- To evaluate bone support in the furcation areas

> **General Design Features:** Probe
> - Smooth, rounded tip
> - Rod-shaped working ends
> - Rounded or rectangular in cross-section
> - Calibrated with color coding and millimeter graduations

- To determine the amount of bone level that is present.
- To evaluate the completeness of treatment and its success.

*Types of periodontal probes*: Various types of periodontal probes are:
- *William's probe*: This stainless-steel probe is available in a diameter of 1 mm and 13 mm length with markings at 1 mm, 2 mm, 3 mm, 5 mm, 7 mm, 8 mm, 9 mm, and 10 mm **(Fig. 40.7A)**. In this probe, 4 mm and 6 mm readings

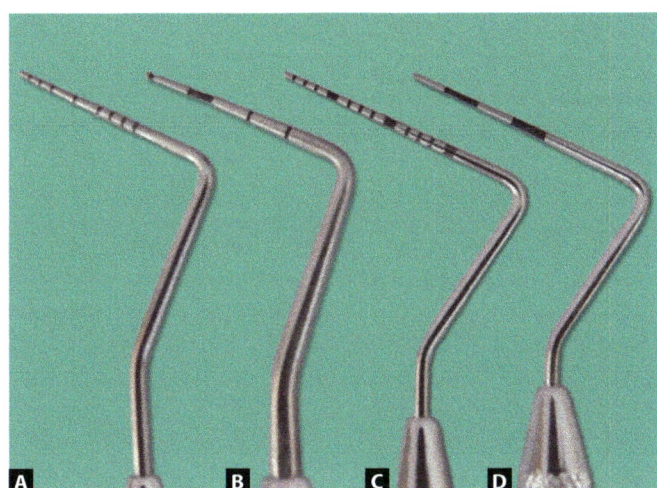

**Figs. 40.7A to D:** Photograph showing various periodontal probes: (A) William's probe; (B) WHO probe; (C) UNC-15; (D) Marquis color-coded probe.
(WHO: World Health Organization; UNC: University of North Carolina)

are absent that enhance the visibility and clear out the confusion in reading the markings.
- *World Health Organization (WHO)/Community Periodontal Index of Treatment Needs (CPITN) probe*: 0.5 mm ball at the tip and millimeter markings at 3.5 mm, 8.5 mm and 11.5 mm and black color-coding from 3.5 to 5.5 mm **(Fig. 40.7B)**.
  Types:
  - *CPITN-E (epidemiological)*: They have 3.5 mm and 5.5 mm markings.
  - *CPITN-C (clinical)*: They have 3.5 mm, 5.5 mm, 8.5 mm and 11.5 mm markings.

> **Clinical Tip**
> Higher grading should be considered as final reading when the gingival margin appears at a level between two markings of the probe.[8]

- *UNC-15 probe*: 15 mm long probe with markings at each mm and color at 5th, 10th, and 15th mm **(Fig. 40.7C)**.
- *Marquis color-coded probe*: Calibrations are in 3 mm sections. The colored band on the periodontal probe is designed to make periodontal examination readings more objective and faster **(Fig. 40.7D)**.
- Michigan "O" probe with markings at 3 mm, 6 mm, and 8 mm.
- *Goldman-Fox probe*: Flat, rectangular probe with William's markings at 1 mm, 2 mm, 3 mm, 5 mm, 7 mm, 8 mm, 9 mm, and 10 mm **(Fig. 40.8)**.
- *Nabers probe*: It is a curved probe designed to get access and determine the extent of the interradicular bone loss at furcation sites **(Fig. 40.9)**.
- *Moffitt/Maryland probe*: WHO design with William's markings.
- *National Institute of Dental Research (NIDR) probe*: Color-coded and graduated in 2 mm increments at

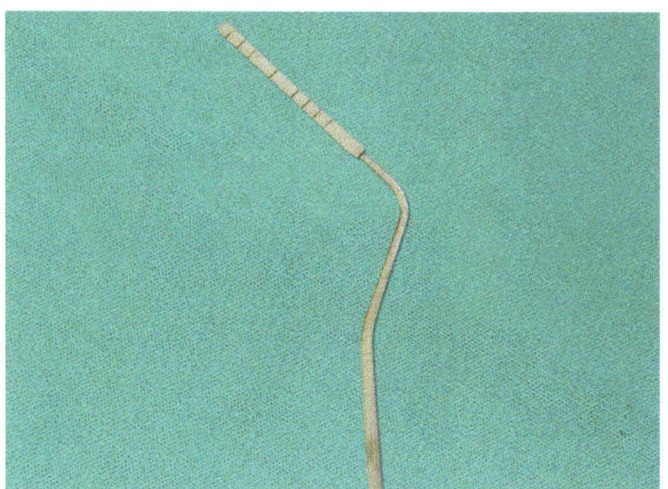

**Fig. 40.8:** Photograph showing Goldman-Fox probe.

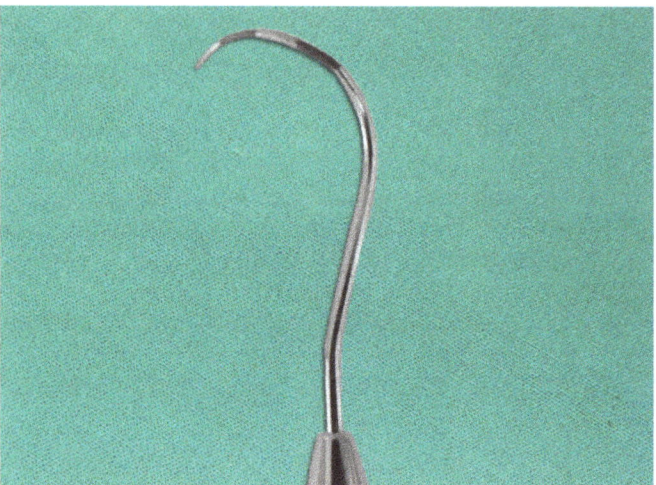

**Fig. 40.9:** Photograph showing Naber's probe for detection of furcation lesion.

2 mm, 4 mm, 6 mm, 8 mm, 10 mm, and 12 mm with alternating increments colored in yellow.
- *Florida probe*: The Florida Research Group met the criteria given by NIDR. Gibbs et al., in the year 1988, developed the Florida probe system.[9] This system incorporates constant probing force, precise electrical measurement, and computer storage of data. The parts are probe handpiece, digital readout, switch, computer interface, and computer. Two models have been developed which differ in their fixed reference point:
  - *Stent model*: The probe has a 1 mm metal collar that rests on a prepared ledge on a prefabricated vacuform stent.
  - *Disk model*: The probe has an 11 mm disk, which rests on the occlusal surface or incisal edge of the tooth.
- *Toronto automated probe*: Researchers at the University of Toronto developed it. Likewise, the Florida probe, the occlusal-incisal surface, is measured with this probe to get clinical attachment levels. The sulcus is probed with 0.5 mm nickel-titanium wire, which extended under air pressure. The probe is useful to control angular discrepancies with the help of a mercury tilt sensor that limits angulation within ±30°. But it requires reproducible positioning of the patient's head and cannot easily measure 2nd and 3rd molars.
- *InterProbe*: Also known as perioprobe, which is a third-generation probe and developed by Goodson and Kondon in 1988. This has an optical encoder transduction element with a flexible probe tip. The tip takes a curve with the tooth when the probe enters the pocket area. The probe optical encoder handpieces uses constant probing pressure to get the repeatable measurement of pocket depth and attachment loss.
- *The Jeffcoat probe (or Foster-Miller probe)*: Jeffcoat developed it in 1986. It is capable of coupling pocket depth measurement with the detection of the cementoenamel junction (CEJ). The probe extends a thin metal fiber along the tooth surface into the sulcus, and detects a slight acceleration rise when encountering the CEJ and then undergoes final extension, under constant force, on reaching the base of the pocket.

The periodontal probes were classified into three generations by BL Pihlstrom in 1992.[10] In 2000, Watts expanded this classification by adding two more generations, namely, fourth and fifth generations **(Table 40.2)**.

## Scaling, Root Planing, and Curettage Instruments

### Hand Instruments

*Sickle scaler*: A sickle scaler is mainly used for the removal of supragingival calculus. Sickles with straight shanks are designed to adapt to anterior teeth while those with contra-angled shanks (called Jacquettes) adapt to posterior teeth. Sickle scalers have a flat surface and two cutting edges that converge in a sharply pointed tip **(Figs. 40.10 and 40.11)**. The shape of the instrument makes the tip durable so that it will not break off during use. Because of the design of this instrument, it is difficult to insert a large sickle-blade under the gingiva without damaging the surrounding gingival tissues.

These are available in either anterior or posterior designs.
- *Anterior sickle scalers*: They are limited to use on anteriors, e.g., OD-1, Jacquette-33, Towner-U15, Goldman-H6, Goldman-H7.
- *Posterior sickle scalers*: They are designed not only for use on posterior sextants but also may be used on anterior teeth. They have two cutting edges: Inner and outer cutting edges. Inner cutting edges are used to instrument distal surfaces. Outer surfaces are used to instrument facial, lingual, and mesial surfaces.[12] For example Jacquette-34/35, Jacquette-14/15, Jacquette-31/32.

## Chapter 40: Periodontal Instruments

**TABLE 40.2:** Generations of the periodontal probe.

| Classification | Periodontal probe | Descriptions |
|---|---|---|
| First-generation | Conventional probes; manual probes | The usual clinical instrument with a thin tapering line marked to be read in millimeter |
| Second-generation | Constant force probes; pressure-sensitive probes | In 1971, Gabathuler and Hassel introduced second-generation probes.[11] Similar to the first-generation probe but with a spring or electronic cut-out when the appropriate force is reached. Force 30 g probe tip remains in cementoenamel junction and force of 50 g are necessary to diagnose osseous defects, e.g., Vine Valley, Vivacare TPS |
| Third-generation | Automated probes | When a probe is in place with a specified force, a device is activated that reads the measurement accurately. Automated and computerized probe, e.g., Florida, Foster-Miller, Toronto automated |
| Fourth-generation | Three-dimensional probes | Presently, these are under the developmental phase. The main objective of developing these probes is to record sequential probe positions along the gingival sulcus |
| Fifth-generation | Noninvasive three-dimensional probes | These will add ultrasound or another device to a fourth-generation probe |

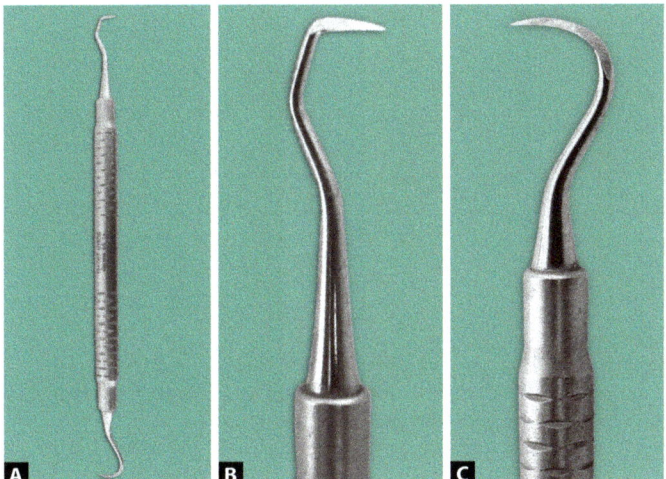

**Figs. 40.10A to C:** Photograph showing sickle scaler.

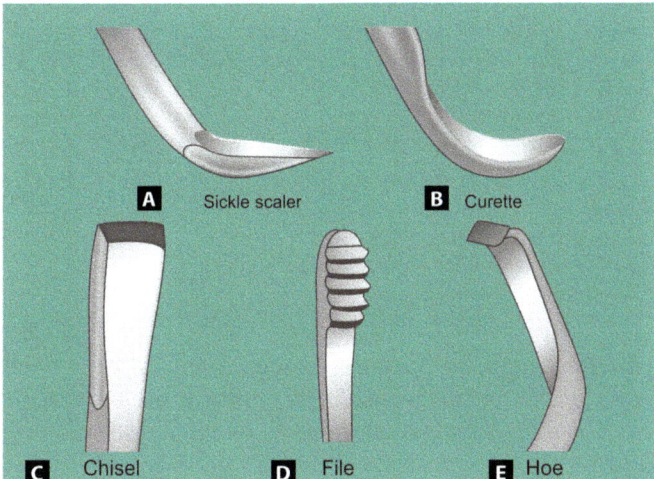

**Figs. 40.11A to E:** Schematic representation showing scaling and root planing instruments: (A) Sickle scaler; (B) Curette; (C) Chisel; (D) File; (E) Hoe.

*Chisel:* Practically, a periodontal chisel scaler has limited usefulness. It is used only to get rid of the heavy supragingival calculus deposits that bridge the open interproximal spaces of the anterior teeth **(Fig. 40.11C)**. The instrument is activated with a push motion while the side of the blade is held firmly against the root.

*Periodontal file:* Each working end of a periodontal file is available with several cutting edges. These edges are useful to crush large calculus deposits and to make smooth the tooth surface.[13] The angulation of the blade in relation to the shank may be from 90° to 105° **(Fig. 40.11D)**.

*Hoe:* Hoe scalers are used for scaling of ledges or rings of calculus. The blade is bent at a 99° angle **(Fig. 40.12A)**. The cutting edge is formed by the junction of the flattened terminal surface with the inner aspects of the blade. The cutting edge is beveled at 45° **(Fig. 40.12B)**. The blade is slightly bowed so that it can maintain contact at two points on a convex surface. This stabilizes the instrument and prevents the nicking of the root. The instrument is activated with a firm pull stroke towards the crown, with every effort being made to preserve the two-point contact with the tooth **(Fig. 40.12C)**.[14] This instrument is heavy and bulky lacking in tactile sensitivity that generally precedes additional scaling by curettes. Hoes can be considered as an adjunctive instrument and may not be routinely included in a standard tray setup for scaling and root planing. Examples are McCall's hoe scalers set of six scalers No. 3–8.

### General Design Features: Sickle Scaler

- Two cutting edges
- Cutting edges meet at pointed tip
- Triangular in cross-section
- Scaler face is at 90° to lower shank **(Fig. 40.18A)**

### General Design Features: Periodontal File

- Many cutting edges
- Cutting edges at 90–105° angle to the shank
- Have strong, rigid shank

## Section 6: Treatment: Nonsurgical Therapy

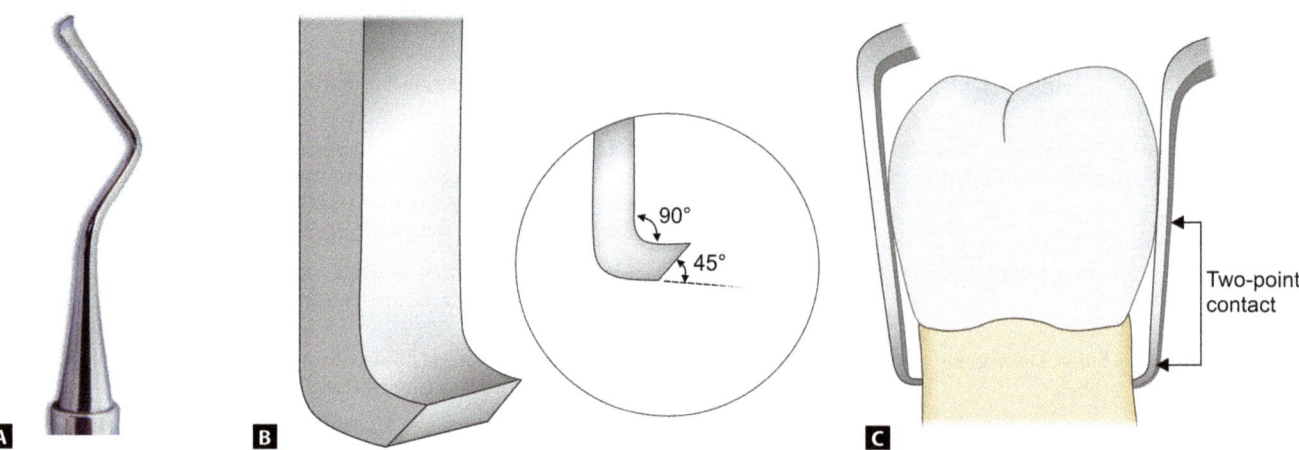

**Figs. 40.12A to C:** Photograph showing Hoe scaler (A) Single-cutting edge; (B) Cutting edge beveled at 45°; (C) Two-point contact.

### General Design Features: Chisel
- One straight cutting edge
- Heavy, straight shank

### General Design Features: Hoe
- One straight cutting edge
- Working end at 99°–100° angle to the shank
- Strong, rigid shank

*Curette*: The term "curette" comes from a *French* word *curer*, meaning "to cleanse." The curette is the instrument of choice for subgingival calculus removal, root planing, and removing soft tissue from the periodontal pocket. The working ends of curettes have a spoon-shaped face and a rounded back. In a cross-section, the curette blade appears in a semicircular fashion instead of a triangular shape (shape of the sickle scaler) **(Fig. 40.13)**.

Two basic types of curettes, namely, the universal and the area-specific, are available for conducting periodontal procedures.
- *Universal curette*: These are paired instruments available in various sizes and shank lengths. They are designed to adapt to most areas of the dentition by altering and adapting the finger rest, fulcrum, and hand position. During procedures, it forms two parallel cutting edges with one on either side of the face **(Fig. 40.14)**. Each cutting edge is useful for conducting procedures.[15] Commonly available universal instruments are the Columbia 2R-2L and 4R-4L **(Figs. 40.15A and B)**.

### General Design Features: Universal Curette
- Two cutting edges
- The spoon-shaped working end
- Cutting edges meet in a rounded toe
- It has a rounded back
- Semicircular in cross-section

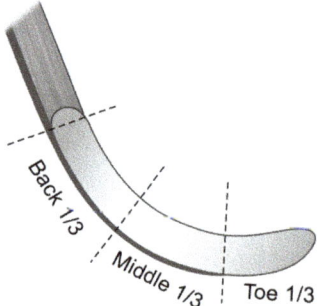

**Fig. 40.13:** Schematic representation showing curette blade: Spoon-shaped blade and rounded tip.

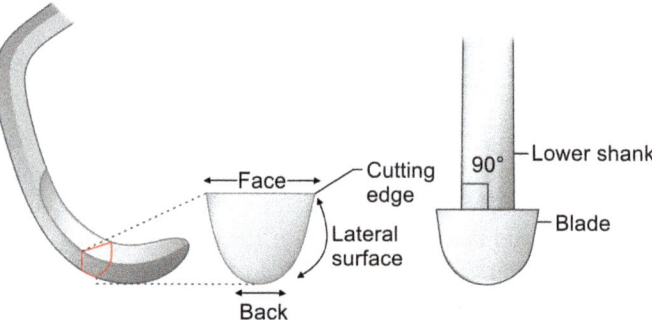

**Fig. 40.14:** Schematic representation showing universal curette blade design.

Columbia 13/14 has a short lower shank and working end, limiting its use within normal sulci/shallow pocket. Barnhart 1/2 has a long lower shank, and the working end thus can be used to instrument root surfaces within deep pockets.
- *Area-specific curettes (Gracey)*: They are different from the universal curettes in various aspects. They come as a set of several instruments, which are designed and angled to adapt as per the specific anatomic area of the dentition; furthermore, these curettes are designed with

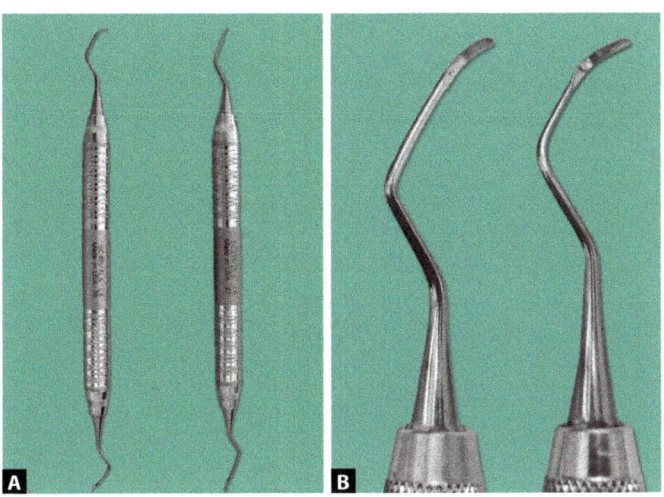

**Figs. 40.15A and B:** Photograph showing universal curettes.

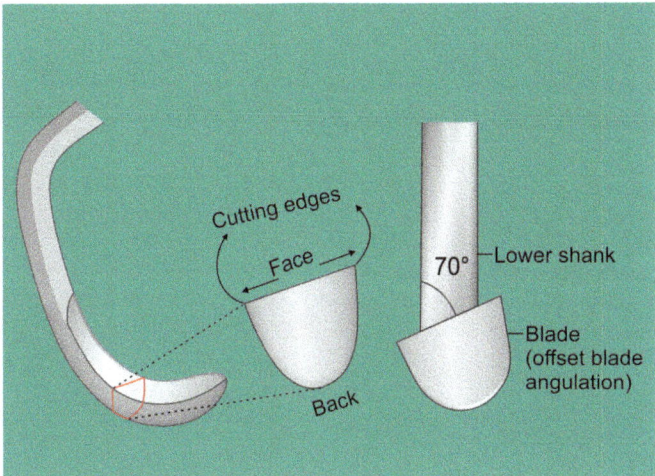

**Fig. 40.16:** Schematic representation showing area-specific curette design.

only one cutting edge. They give the best adaptation to the complex root anatomy and hence are most suitable for subgingival scaling and root planing. Examples of area-specific curettes are Gracey curettes, Kramer-Nevins series, Turgeon series, Hu-Friedy After Five series, Hu-Friedy Mini Five series, Hu-Friedy curvette series, and Furcation curettes.

- *Gracey curettes:* In the 1940s, Dr. Clayton H Gracey, a dentist and educator from the University of Michigan and Hugo Friedman (founder of Hu-Friedy) jointly developed a series of 14 area-specific curettes, namely Gracey curette.

  The Gracey curettes are paired and area-specific instruments consisting of similar blades with different angulations and contra-angulations of the shank **(Figs. 40.16 and 40.17; Tables 40.3 and 40.4)**.[14]

- *Mini-bladed curettes:* The blade is commonly half in length compared to After Five or Standard Gracey curettes **(Fig. 40.19A)**. The short length of blade permits easy insertion and adaptation of curette in deep, narrow pockets; furcations; developmental grooves; line angles; and deep, facial, lingual, or palatal pockets. The Mini Five curettes are available in both the rigid and finishing designs. Rigid Mini Five are recommended for calculus removal. The more flexible shanked, finishing Mini Five are recommended for light subgingival scaling and root planing in periodontal maintenance patients. These curettes come in all standard Gracey numbers except for the no. 9–10.

  *Micro* Mini Five Gracey curettes have blade 20% thinner than Mini Five Gracey curettes to reduce tissue distension further and ease subgingival insertion. These curettes are manufactured by Ever Edge technology, which keeps curettes sharper for a longer duration.

- *After Five curettes:* These are modifications of the standard Gracey curette. The terminal shank is 3 mm longer, which permits insertion into deeper periodontal pockets of 5 mm or more **(Fig. 40.19B)**. The blade of After Five curettes is thin and facilitate smooth entry into the subgingival sulcus and reduced tissue distention. All standard Gracey numbers except for the No. 9-10 (i.e., No. 1-2, 3-4, 5-6, 7-8, 11-12, 13-14) are available in the After Five series. After Five curettes also come in finishing or rigid designs.

  - *Langer curettes:* The design characteristics of Langer curettes **(Table 40.5)** differ from Universal curettes in the following manner:
    - More than one Langer curette is needed to instrument the entire dentition
    - These curettes are designed with the combination of the shank design of standard Gracey 5-6, 11-12, and 13-14 curettes with Universal blade honed at 90° and hence known as the marriage of Gracey and Universal curette design
  - *Curvette area-specific curettes:* The design characteristics of curvette curettes **(Table 40.6)** differ from those of standard Gracey curettes in the following manner:
    - 50% shorter working end
    - Increased curvature of the working end
    - Straighter shank on the anterior instrument
    - Extended lower shank on the posterior instrument
  - *Quentin furcation curettes:* These are specialized instruments used to debride furcation areas and root concavities. The working end of these has a single, straight cutting edge. The corners of cutting edges and back of the working end are rounded to minimize the potential for gouging the tooth surface.

### Powered Instruments

Powered instruments are also used for periodontal debridement **(Table 40.7)**. They can be classified into two

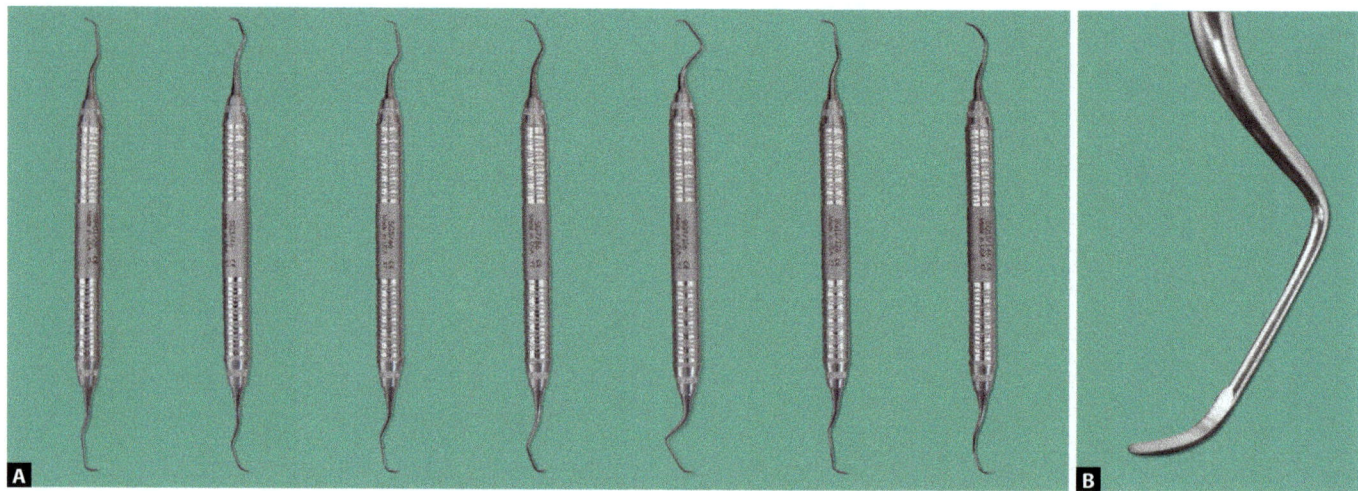

**Figs. 40.17A and B:** Photograph showing Gracey curettes.

**TABLE 40.3:** Area-specific instruments: Gracey curettes.

| Instrument | Area of use |
|---|---|
| Gracey 1–2 and 3–4 | Anterior teeth |
| Gracey 5–6 | Anterior teeth and premolars |
| Gracey 7–8 and 9–10 | Posterior teeth; facial and lingual surfaces |
| Gracey 11–12 | Posterior teeth; mesial surfaces |
| Gracey 13–14 | Posterior teeth; distal surfaces |
| Gracey 15–16 | Posterior teeth; mesial surfaces |
| Gracey 17–18 | Posterior teeth; distal surfaces |

**TABLE 40.4:** Differences between area-specific and universal curettes.

| Parameters | Area-specific curettes | Universal curettes |
|---|---|---|
| Area of use | These are designed for specific areas and surfaces | Designed for all areas and surfaces |
| Cutting edge used | One cutting edge, i.e., the outer edge is used | Both cutting edges are used |
| Curvature | Curved in two planes, blade curves up and to the side | Curved in one plane |
| Blade angle | Offset blade: Face of blade beveled at 60° to 70° to the shank **(Fig. 40.18C)** | Not offset: Face of blade beveled at 90° to the shank **(Fig. 40.18B)** |
| Examples | • Gracey series<br>• Kramer-Nevin series<br>• Turgeon series<br>• After Five series<br>• Mini Five series<br>• Curvette series | • Columbia 2R/2L<br>• Columbia 4R/4L<br>• Columbia 13–14<br>• Barnhart 1/2<br>• Barnhart 5/6 |

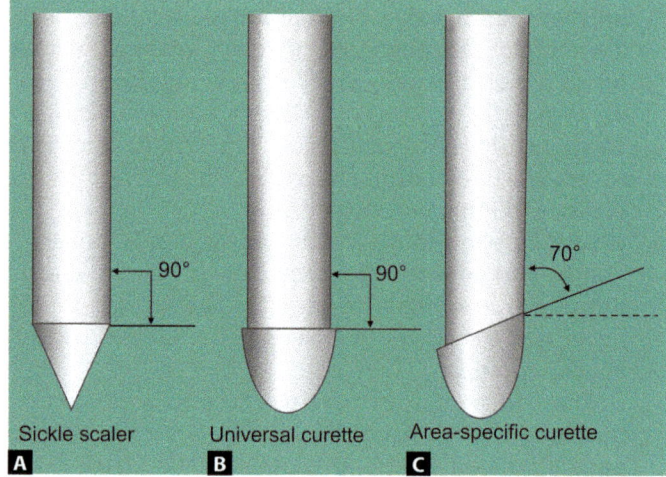

**Figs. 40.18A to C:** Schematic representation showing relation of face to the lower shank: (A) Sickle scaler; (B) Universal curette; (C) Area-specific curette.

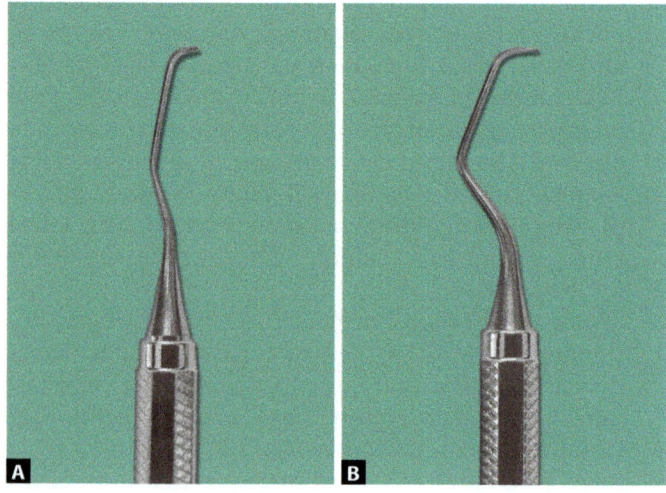

**Figs. 40.19A and B:** Photograph showing (A) Mini-bladed curette; (B) After Five curette.

**TABLE 40.5:** Langer curettes.

| Instrument | Area of use |
|---|---|
| Langer 1/2 | Mandibular posterior teeth |
| Langer 3/4 | Maxillary posterior teeth |
| Langer 5/6 | Mandibular and maxillary anterior teeth |
| Langer 17/18 | Mandibular and maxillary 2nd and 3rd molars |

**TABLE 40.6:** Curvette area-specific curettes.

| Instrument | Area of use |
|---|---|
| Curvette sub-zero | Anterior teeth and premolars (facial and lingual surfaces) |
| Curvette 1/2 | Anterior teeth and premolars (interproximal surfaces) |
| Curvette 11/12 | Mesial surfaces of molars |
| Curvette 13/14 | Distal surfaces of molars |

**TABLE 40.7:** Comparison between ultrasonic and manual instrumentation.[16]

| Ultrasonic instrument | Hand instrument |
|---|---|
| *Mechanism of action*: Vibration, acoustic streaming, and cavitation | Mechanical removal of deposit |
| Used on heavy tenacious deposits and stains | Used on all amounts of deposits |
| Instrument tip is dull and bulky | Sharp and thin |
| Less tactile sensitivity | Good tactile sensitivity |
| Digital motion activation is used with light pressure | Hand motion activation is used with firm pressure |
| Inaccessible to some areas because of tip design | Greater accessibility |
| Less time required | More time required |
| Less clinician fatigue | More clinician fatigue |
| Water spray causes discomfort to the patient | No water spray, no discomfort |
| Possibility of damage to the tooth from heat build-up | No heat build-up |
| Aerosols are produced | No aerosols are produced |
| Contraindicated in patients with a pacemaker and having contagious diseases | No such contraindications |
| Sharpening not needed frequently | Sharpening frequently required |
| Smaller tip size 0.3–0.55 mm | Larger tip size 0.76–1.00 mm |

groups based on their operating frequencies: Sonic and ultrasonic.

### Sonic and Ultrasonic Instruments

- *Sonic scalers*: They operate at a relatively low frequency of 3,000–8,000 cycles per second and are driven by compressed air from the dental unit. The stroke pattern of sonic scalers is elliptical to orbital, and all the surfaces of the tip can be adapted to root surfaces.

- *Ultrasonic scalers*: They can be further categorized into magnetostrictive and piezoelectric, based on the mechanism used to convert the electrical current used for energy to activate the tips.
    - *Magnetostrictive ultrasonics*: They operate inaudibly and transfer electrical energy to metal stacks made of nickel-iron alloy or to a ferrous rod. Electrical energy applied to the magnetostrictive insert changes its shape resulting in vibrations. The tip vibrates in an elliptical to orbital motion at 18–45 kHz (cycles per second). The instrument is comprised of an electronic generator, a handpiece assembly containing a coil to energize the insert, and a variety of interchangeable inserts. The generator produces an alternating low voltage electric current in the handpiece. This current produces a magnetic field in the handpiece that causes the insert to expand and contract along its length and, in turn, causes the insert tip to vibrate.
    - *Piezoelectric scalers* (**Figs. 40.20A and B**) also are inaudible, operating within a range of 25–50 kHz. This type of powered scaler uses electrical energy to activate crystals within the handpiece to vibrate the tip. In contrast to the magnetostrictive scalers, the motion of the tip is linear in nature resulting in activation of mainly the lateral surfaces of the tip. This system is comprised of an electronic generator, a handpiece assembly containing piezo (ceramic) crystals to energize a scaling tip, and a variety of interchangeable screw-on tips. The generator produces an alternating, high voltage in the handpiece. This voltage produces an electric field in the handpiece that causes the piezo crystals to expand and contract along their diameter and, in turn, causes the scaling tip to vibrate.

*Acoustic streaming*: The pressure produced by the continuous stream of fluid flowing into the confined space of the periodontal pocket is known as acoustic streaming or turbulence. Bacteria and Gram-negative motile rods, in particular, are sensitive to acoustic energy.

*Cavitation*: The vibratory motion of the tip and the continuous stream of water cause tremendous pressure, creating powerful bursts of the collapsing bubbles. This is referred to as cavitation. It is a combination of the vibrating instrument's tip against the deposit, high-frequency sound waves, and exploding bubbles that allow for calculus removal.

Preprocedural antiseptic mouth rinse and use of high-volume evacuators can reduce hazards of aerosols production by ultrasonic instrumentation.

*Contraindications*:
- Patients with contagious diseases
- Patients with a pacemaker, especially magnetostrictive
- Composite resin restorations
- Porcelain inlays or crowns

**Section 6:** Treatment: Nonsurgical Therapy

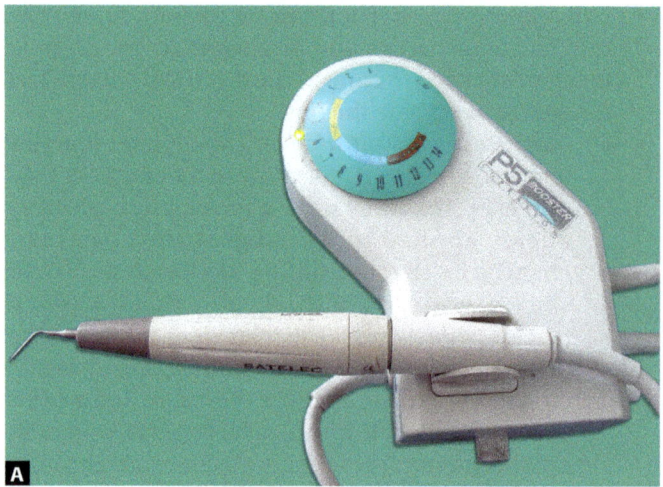
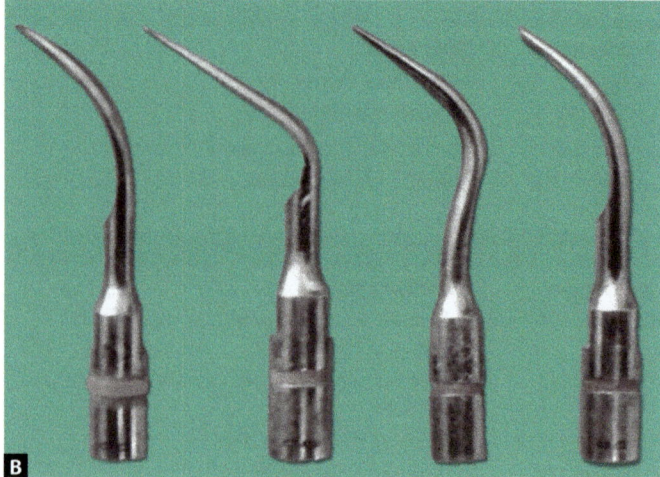

**Figs. 40.20A and B:** Photograph showing (A) Piezoelectric ultrasonic unit; (B) Ultrasonic tips.

## Periodontal Endoscope

It consists of a 0.99 mm-diameter reusable fiberoptic endoscope over which is fitted a disposable, sterile sheath. The fiberoptic endoscope fits onto periodontal probes and ultrasonic instruments that have been designed to accept it. The sheath delivers water irrigation that flushes the pocket while the endoscope is in use and keeps the field clear. The fiberoptic endoscope attaches to a medical-grade charged coupled device (CCD) video camera and a light source that produces an image on a flat panel video monitor for viewing during the subgingival exploration and the instrumentation. This device allows clear visualization of deep subgingival pockets and furcations. It enables the operator to detect the presence and location of subgingival deposits and guides the operator in their thorough removal.

## Cleansing and Polishing Instruments

The primary objective of polishing is the removal of extrinsic stain and supragingival plaque. The rationale for this procedure includes improving the appearance of the dentition, demonstrating a standard of oral cleanliness for the patient to attain on a daily basis, and motivating the patient to improve plaque control, as well as the belief that the outcome of quality periodontal service should be a plaque-free mouth.

### Various Cleansing and Polishing Instruments

- *Bristle brushes:* They are available in the wheel and cup shapes. The brush is used in the handpiece along with a polishing paste. Brush bristles are usually stiff, and hence its use should be restricted to the crown to prevent injury to the cementum and the gingiva.
- *Rubber cups:* They consist of a rubber shell with or without webbed configurations in the hollow interior **(Fig. 40.21)**. They are used in the handpiece with a special prophylaxis angle. A good cleaning and polishing paste that contains fluoride should be used and kept

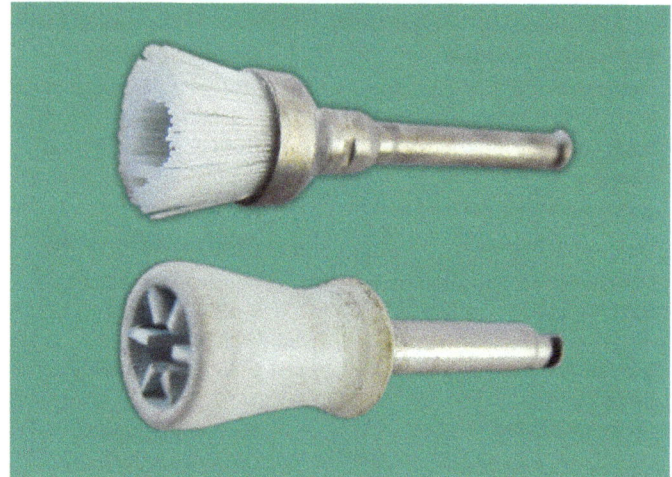

**Fig. 40.21:** Photograph showing bristle brush and rubber cup.

moist to minimize frictional heat as the cup revolves **(Fig. 40.22)**. Polishing pastes come as a fine, medium, or coarse grits and are packaged in small, convenient containers.
- *Dental tape with the polishing paste*: It is used for polishing the proximal surface that is inaccessible to other polishing instruments.
- *Air-powered polishing*: Prophy-jet is composed of air-powered slurry of warm water and sodium bicarbonate. This system is beneficial in the removal of extrinsic stains and soft deposits. The slurry removes stains rapidly and efficiently by mechanical abrasion and provides warm water for rinsing and lavage.

### Contraindications of Polishing

- Patients who have a communicable disease that could be spread by aerosols.
- Patients who are susceptible to bacteremia.
- Areas of thin or deficient enamel, cementum or dentin surfaces, areas of hypersensitivity.

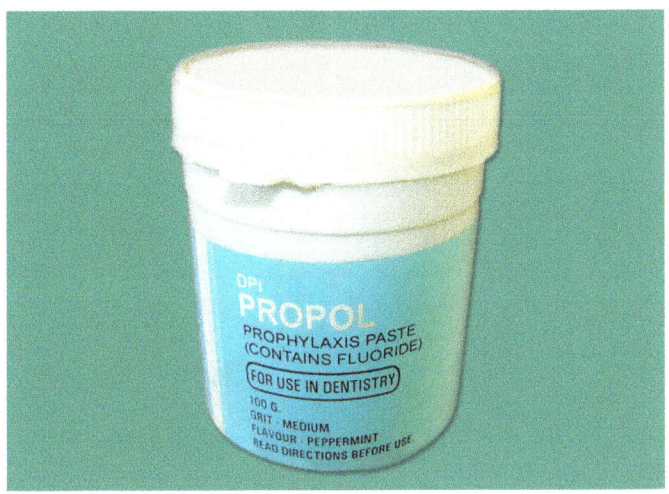

**Fig. 40.22:** Photograph showing cleansing and polishing paste (Reproduced with permission from Dental Products of India a division of The Bombay Burmah Trading Corpn. Ltd.)

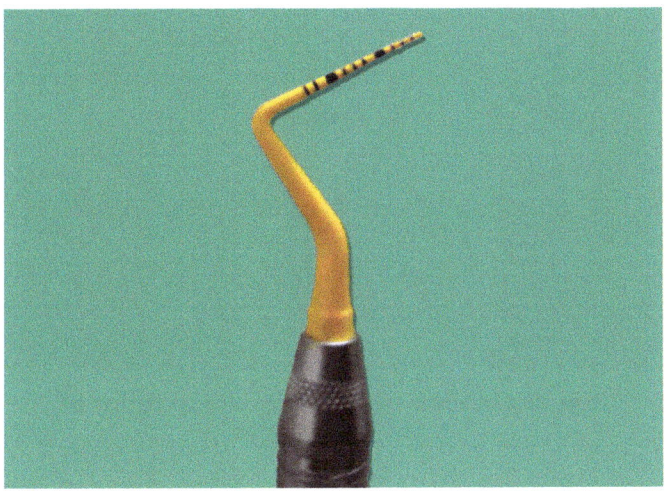

**Fig. 40.23:** Photograph showing a polymeric color-coded plastic probe.

- Caries susceptible teeth; areas of white spot demineralized mottled teeth.
- Gold restorations.
- A restricted sodium diet, including patients with controlled hypertension.
- Composite restorations.[17]

*Dental implant instruments*: Plastic probes are available for probing around the implant **(Fig. 40.23)**. Special scalers composed of plastic or nonmetallic materials are developed for cleaning the abutment of dental implants. The special material gives an effective cleaning solution without damaging the abutment surface. Implacare implant instruments have autoclavable stainless steel handles with different plastic tip designs **(Figs. 40.24A and B)**. Metal scaler curettes and ultrasonic tips should be avoided to prevent damage to the surface topography of the implant.[18]

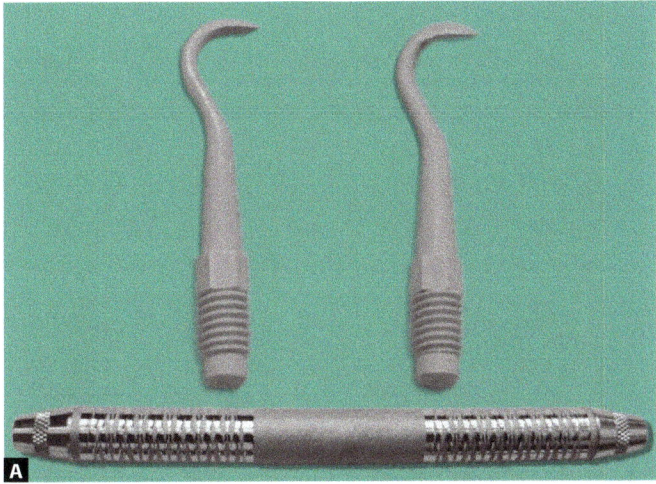
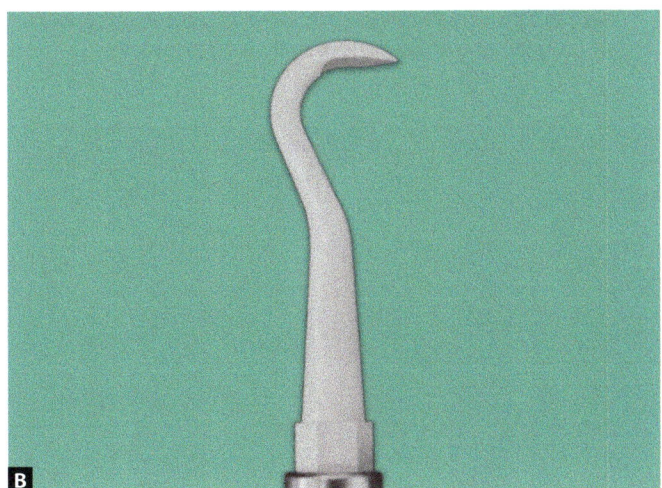

**Figs. 40.24A and B:** Photograph showing (A) Implacare implant maintenance instrument; (B) Plastic tip.

## Surgical Instruments

Surgical periodontal instruments have been classified into the following categories:
- Excisional and incisional instruments
- Surgical curettes and sickle scalers
- Periosteal elevators
- Surgical chisels and hoes
- Surgical files
- Scissors and nippers
- Needle holders and hemostats

### Excisional and Incisional Instruments

*Flat-bladed gingivectomy knives (kidney-shaped knife)*: These knives have broad, flat blades that are nearly perpendicular to the lower shank of the instrument. The curved cutting edge extends around the entire outer edge of the blade and is formed by bevels on both the front and back surfaces of the blade, e.g., Kirkland knife **(Fig. 40.25A)**.

*Interdental knives/interproximal knives (spear-shaped knife)*: The blades of interproximal knives have two long,

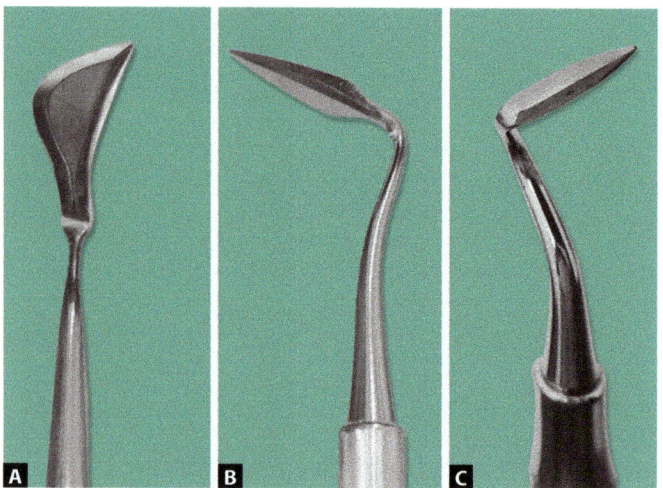

**Figs. 40.25A to C:** Photograph showing gingivectomy knives: (A) Kirkland knife; (B) Buck knife; (C) Orban's knife.

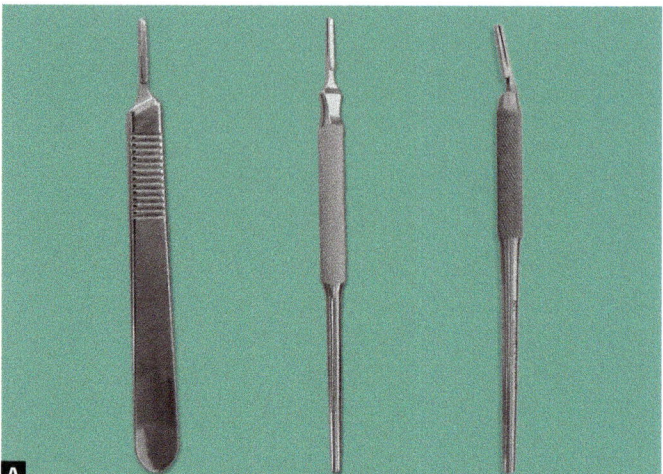

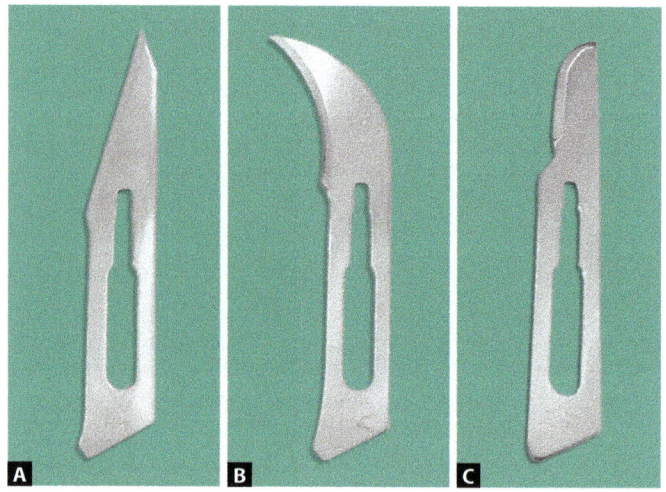

**Figs. 40.26A to C:** Photograph showing surgical blades: (A) No. 11; No. 12; (C) No. 15.

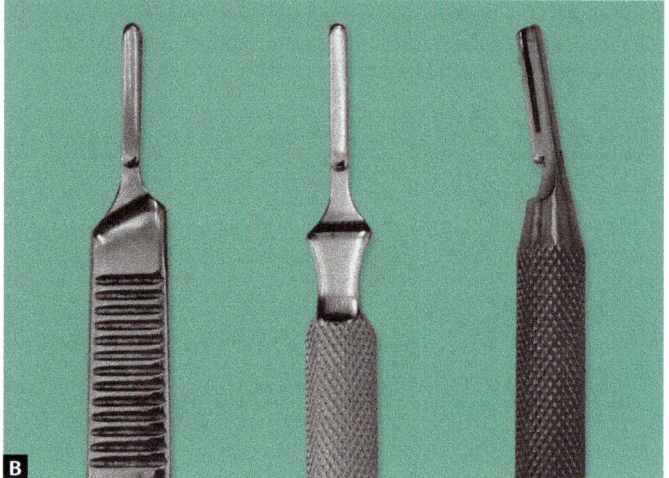

**Figs. 40.27A and B:** Photograph showing scalpel handle: Bard-Parker handles.

straight cutting edges that come together at the sharply pointed tip of the instrument. Bevels form the cutting edges on the front and back surfaces of the blade. The entire blade is roughly perpendicular to the lower shank of the instrument. Examples are the Buck knife **(Fig. 40.25B)**, Orban's knife **(Fig. 40.25C)** and Merrifield Waerhaug knife.

*Surgical blades*: The most commonly used scalpel blades in periodontal surgery are No. 11, No. 12, No. 15, and No. 15C **(Figs. 40.26A to C)**. The 12 No. blade is available as a beak-shaped blade with cutting edges on both sides. The 15 No. blade is used for thinning flaps and for all-around use. The 15C No. blade is commonly used for making the initial, scalloping type incision. When mounted in ordinary handles, such as Bard-Parker (BP), they are used for releasing incisions and reverse bevel incisions in flap procedures and periodontal plastic surgeries. The No. 3 handle is the most frequently used handle for periodontal surgery. The tip of a scalpel handle is designed to receive various differently shaped scalpel blades to the inserted onto the slotted portion of the handle.

Bard-Parker scalpel handle has the real advantage of using a disposable blade so that sharpening is unnecessary. All of these blades and disposable BP handles are discarded after a single-use. The perfectly balanced round handle allows easy rotation in difficult-to-reach areas **(Figs. 40.27A and B)**. Special handles, such as Blakes handle, make it possible to mount blades in angulated positions, which facilitates the use of such knives for both gingivectomy excisions and reverse bevel incisions.[19]

The scalpel blade must be carefully positioned onto the handle holding the blade with a needle holder. This minimizes the possibility of injury to the fingers. The blade is placed in such a way to get support from a small rib, and the handle is held in a position with the male portion of the fitting is pointing upward. With this, the scalpel blade is allowed to slide onto the handle along the grooves in the male portion until it fits into the position. The unloading of the scalpel is carried out in a similar manner. The needle holder is used to grasps the end away from the blade and lifts it to loosen it from the male fitting. The scalpel is then slid off the handle. The used blade must be discarded immediately into a specifically designed, rigid-sided sharp container.

*Electrosurgery techniques and instrumentation*: Following are the four types of electrosurgical techniques:[20,21]
1. *Electrosection*: It is one of the electrosurgical techniques used for incisions, excisions and tissue planing with single-wire active electrodes. The bending of the wire helps to adapt and conduct various types of cutting procedures.
2. *Electrocoagulation*: The use of fine tungsten wire for electrosection is much easier compared to the active electrodes used for coagulation. Electrocoagulation prevents bleeding primarily when it enters into soft tissue. However, it unable to stop bleeding when blood is already present. In all forms of hemorrhage, the bleeding should be controlled initially by direct pressure, such as compression or hemostat. It is useful in the final sealing of the capillaries or large vessels with a short application of the electrocoagulation current.
3. *Electrofulguration*: It is used to destroy and remove tissue (malignant tumor).
4. *Electrodesiccation*: It is used for the treatment of basal cell cancers of the skin.

Electrofulguration and electrodesiccation are not generally used in dentistry.

The electrosurgical unit consists of a passive/conductive plate, an active electrode handle with tip, and a footswitch. Various active electrodes are as follows **(Fig. 40.28)**:
- Loop electrodes are used for planing tissue;
- Single-wire electrodes are used for incising/excising
- Heavy bulkier electrodes are used for coagulation procedures.

## Surgical Curettes and Sickle Scalers

Surgical curettes and sickles are larger and heavier. Both are commonly used during surgical debridement of granulation tissue, fibrous interdental tissue, and tenacious subgingival deposits, e.g., Prichard curettes, Kramer curettes 1, 2, and 3; Kirkland curettes and Ball scalers B2–B3. Lucas bone curettes are available with mirror image ends. The terminal shank is angled at 50° with a maximum of 20 mm reach. The spoon-shaped blades come with an elongated radius. Miller bone curettes also have mirror image ends. The terminal shank is angled at 40° and has a 22 mm reach. The spoon-shaped blades are available with a scooped radius.

### Clinical Tips for Electrosurgery
- Keep the tip moving.
- Interrupted application at intervals adequate of 5–10 seconds.
- It is contraindicated in noncompatible or poorly shielded cardiac pacemaker patients.

## Periosteal Elevators

Most of the periosteal elevators have a pointed or triangular end on one side, to release the interdental papillae and the broad end on the other side to elevate the mucoperiosteal flap from the bone or to retract soft tissue. These instruments are used to reflect full-thickness flap and to move or to displace the flap after the incision has been made during flap surgery, e.g., Goldman-Fox 14; Glickman 24G **(Figs. 40.29A and B)**; Molt No. 9 and Allen No. 9A.
- *Molt No. 9*: It is a combination of a large curved blade with a 7.5 mm width and a rounded tip with a curved blade of 3.5 mm width and pointed tip **(Figs. 40.30A to C)**.
- *Allen No. 9A*: This periosteal elevator combines the same tips as the traditional Molt No. 9 periosteal elevator but comes with a rounded end with a 3 mm suture hole **(Fig. 40.31)**.

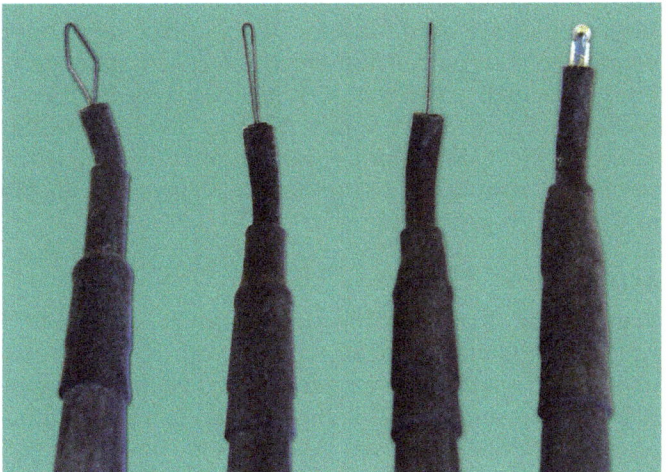

**Fig. 40.28:** Photograph showing active electrosurgery electrodes.

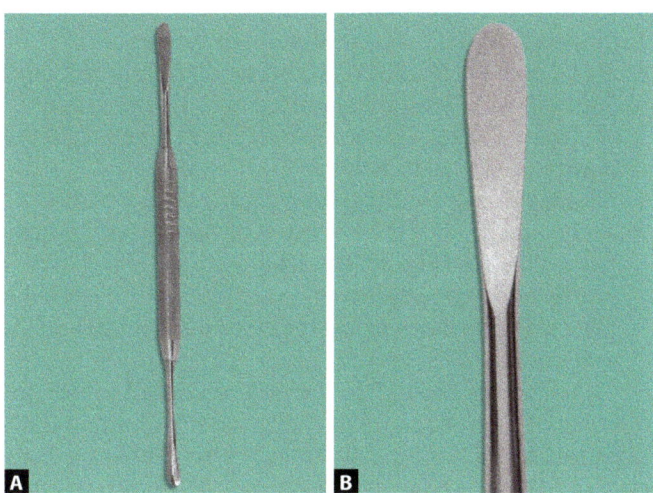

**Figs. 40.29A and B:** Photograph showing a periosteal elevator (Glickman 24G).

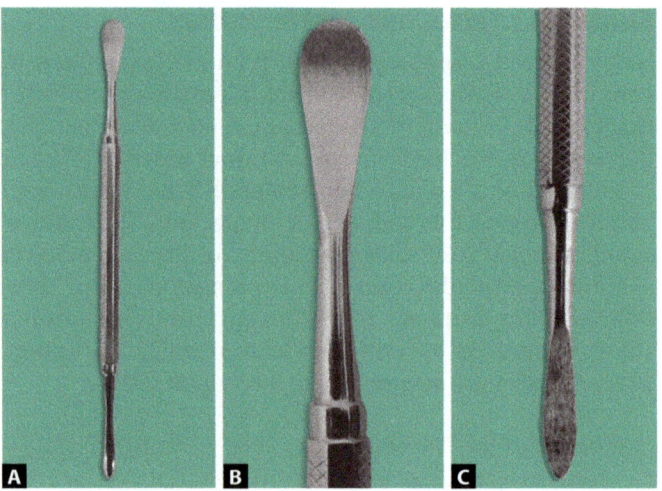

**Figs. 40.30A to C:** Photograph showing molt No. 9 periosteal elevator.

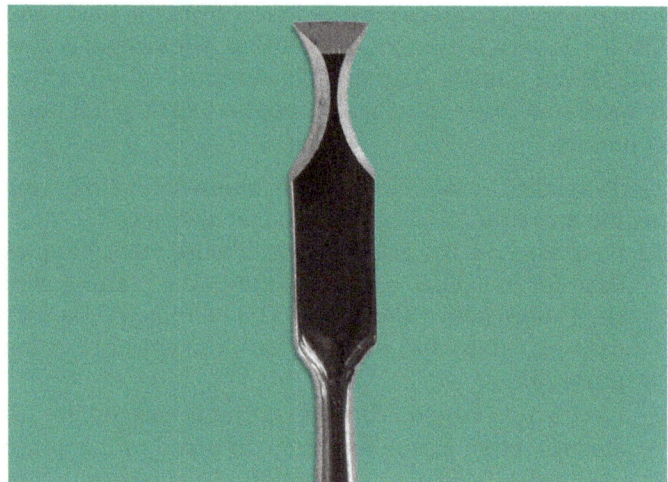

**Fig. 40.32:** Photograph showing Ochsenbein chisels.

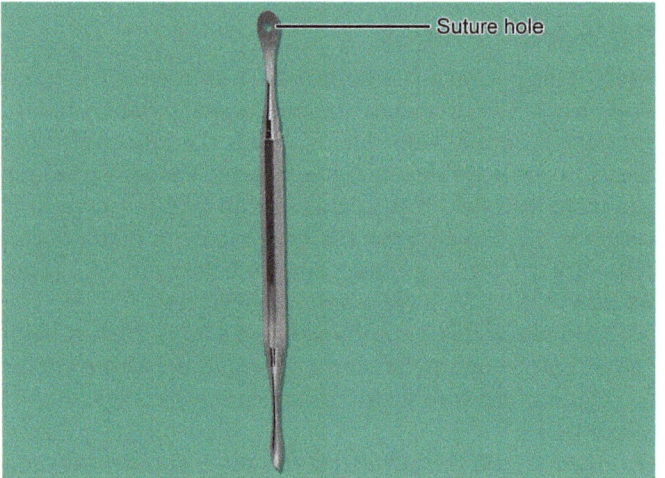

**Fig. 40.31:** Photograph showing Allen No. 9A periosteal elevator.

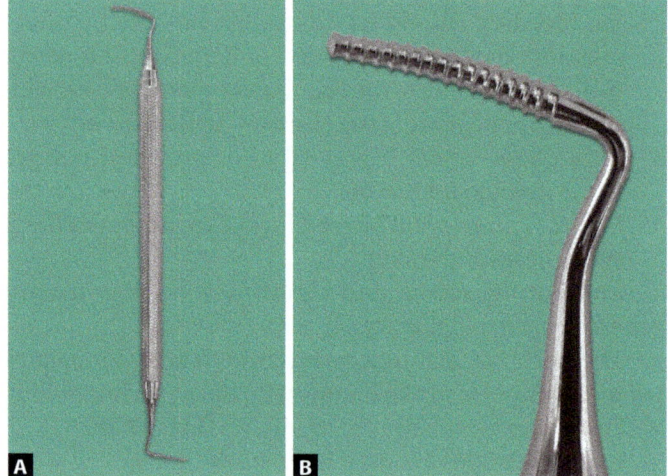

**Figs. 40.33A and B:** Photograph showing Schluger surgical file.

## Surgical Chisels and Hoes

Chisels and hoes are used for removing and reshaping bone during periodontal osseous surgery. Examples are:
- Rhodes chisel No. 36/37 is used for distal interproximal and radicular bony margin correction. The instrument is designed so that the correct parabolic curve to osseous morphology can be achieved.
- Thodes chisel No. 38/39 is used on mesial surfaces.
- Ochsenbein chisels have three beveled cutting edges on each blade **(Fig. 40.32)**. They feature a chisel edge at the tip and two semicircular indentations that will allow the cutting surfaces to engage around the tooth into the interdental area.

Ochsenbein chisel No. 1 and 2 are excellent for the removal of bone because of their shape and angulation. Ochsenbein No. 1 is a single-ended chisel that has a 6 mm width and cutting edges on the front of the blade curvature, whereas Ochsenbein No. 2 has cutting edges on the back of the blade curvature.

## Surgical Files

These are usually double-ended instruments. Periodontal surgical files are used for removing and reshaping bone primarily to smooth rough bony ledges in all areas of bone. The teeth of many bone files are arranged in such a fashion that they remove bone only on a pull stroke. Pushing the bone file against bone results in the burnishing and smoothing of the bone. Examples are Schluger **(Figs. 40.33A and B)** and Sugarman files.

## Scissors and Nippers

Scissors **(Fig. 40.34)** and nippers **(Fig. 40.35)** are regularly used in periodontal surgical procedures during the removal of tissue tabs in the gingivectomy procedure, trimming the flap margins and widening the incision in a periodontal abscess. They are also used in periodontal plastic surgery for removing tissue or muscle attachment.

Various types of scissors are used, and they belong to the following categories soft-tissue scissors and suture scissors.

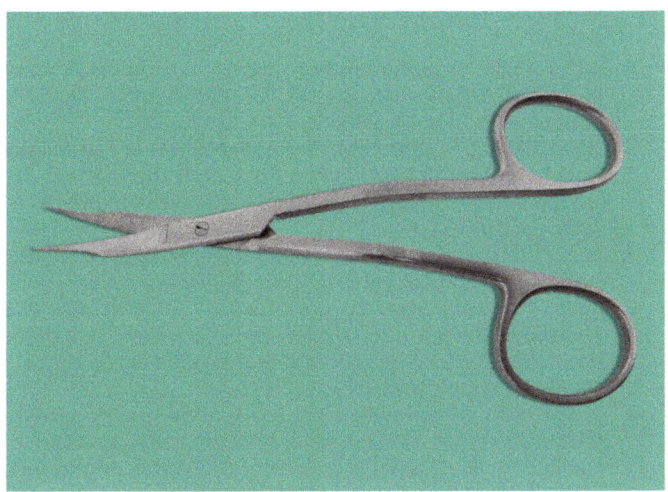

**Fig. 40.34:** Photograph showing scissors.

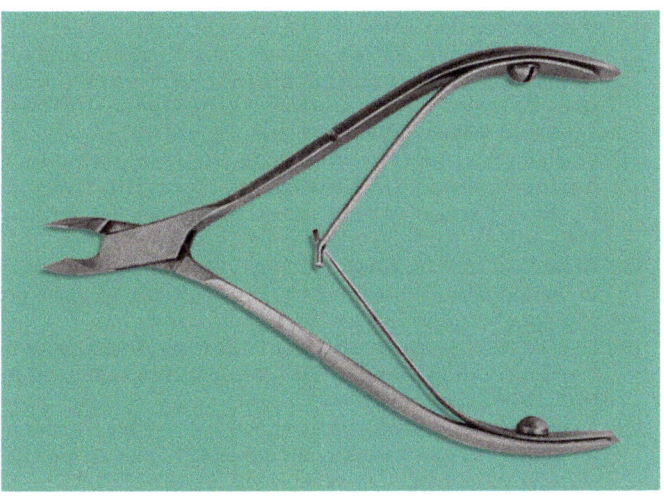

**Fig. 40.35:** Photograph showing tissue nipper.

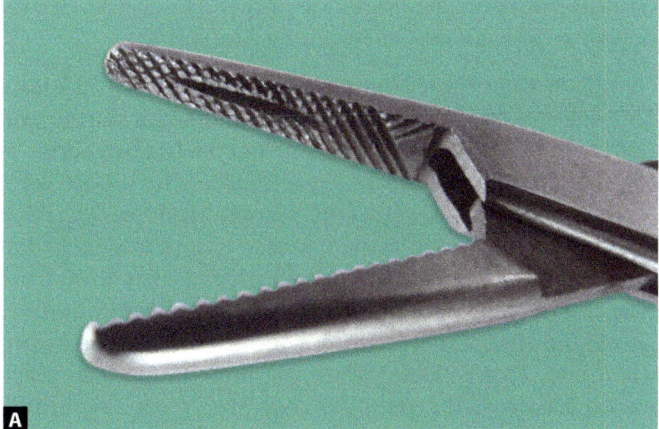

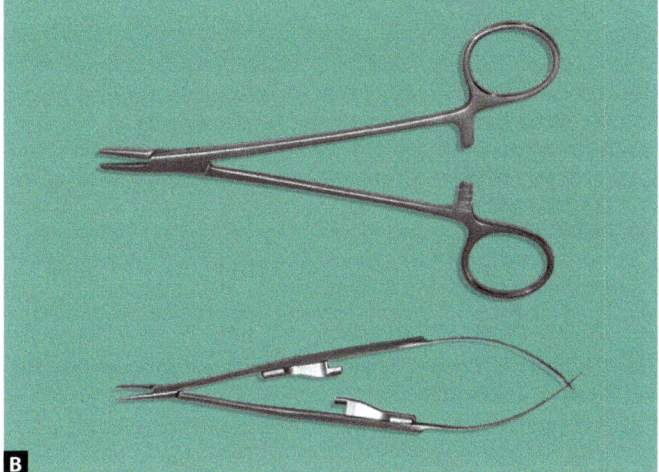

**Figs. 40.36A and B:** Photograph showing (A) Conventional needle holder and (B) Mayo-Hegar and Castroviejo needle holders.

### Soft-tissue Scissors

When tissue scissors are used for cutting sutures, the suture material damages the edges of the blades and reduces their effectiveness or makes them more traumatic while cutting tissue.
- Goldman-Fox scissors.
- Iris scissors are small, sharp-pointed scissors.
- Metzenbaum scissors are longer and delicate scissors. They come in two forms as a sharp-tipped or blunt-tipped.
- Lagrange scissors are narrow scissors with sharp blades and are mainly used for removing excess gingival tissue, while Metzenbaum blunt-nosed scissors are suitable for dissecting and undermining mucosa from underlying soft tissues.

### Suture Scissors

They are purely indicated for cutting sutures and hence available with short cutting edges. Dean scissors are the commonly used suture scissors. These scissors have slightly curved handles and serrated blades to facilitate sutures cutting. Suture scissors usually have long handles and thumb and finger rings. The scissors are held in the same way as the needle holder.

### *Needle Holders and Hemostat*

These instruments come with a locking handle and a short, blunt beak. The inner surface of the beak is serrated criss-crossly with a groove, which gives a better grip for holding a suture needle **(Fig. 40.36A)**. The edges of the hinge are tapered and rounded off to avoid snagging of the suture material. This instrument is held between the ring finger and the thumb; the index and the middle finger support the needle holder.

There are stainless steel and carbide needle holders. The carbide needle holders are recognized with their gold handles and useful for practices having a high volume of surgical procedures, e.g., Mayo-Hegar and Castroviejo needle holder **(Fig. 40.36B)**.

Castroviejo needle holders have beaks with very fine serrations on narrow profile jaws. The locking mechanism of a needle holder is achieved by squeezing the spring-action handle. These needle holders are proved to be effective for periodontal applications requiring fine suture.

*Hemostat (hemostat clamp, arterial forceps)*: It has long and delicate beaks with a locking handle with thumb and finger rings. The locking mechanism consists of a series of interlocking teeth, a few on each handle. The interlocking teeth help the user to adjust the clamping force of the pliers. When locked on, the force between the tips is recorded approximately 40 N. The locking mechanism allows the surgeon to clamp the hemostat onto a vessel and then let go off the instrument, which will remain clamped onto the tissue. This is useful when the surgeon plans to place a suture around the vessel or cauterize it, e.g., Mosquito, Kelly.

### Points to Ponder

- A general rule for working end selection is that the lower shank should be parallel to the surface to be instrumented.
- Instruments with straight shank are used in anteriors and premolars whereas instruments with contra-angle are used on posterior teeth.
- Merritt and Gilmore periodontal probes are not calibrated probe.
- The aerosols, which are produced by ultrasonic scaling, remain in the air for minimum of 30 minutes.
- Chisel is the only instrument which is activated with a push motion.
- The beaks of a needle holder are shorter and stronger than the beaks of a hemostat.

## REFERENCES

1. Nield-Gehrig JS. Instrument design and classification. In: Fundamentals of Periodontal Instrumentation & Advanced Root Instrumentation, 6th edition. Philadelphia, PA, USA: Lippincott Williams & Wilkins; 2008. pp. 149-66.
2. Scaramucci MK. Instrument design and principles of instrumentation. In: Daniel SJ, Harfst SA, Wilder RS (Eds). Mosby's Dental Hygiene: Concepts, Cases and Competencies, 2nd edition. St. Louis: Mosby; 2008. pp. 169-87.
3. Plemons J, Eden BD. Nonsurgical therapy. In: Rose LF, Mealey BL, Genco RJ, Cohen DW (Eds). Periodontics: Medicine, Surgery and Implants, 2nd edition. St. Louis: Elsevier-Mosby; 2004. pp. 237-62.
4. Wilkins EM. Instruments and principles for instrumentation. In: Clinical Practice of the Dental Hygienist, 8th edition. Philadelphia, PA, USA: Lippincott Williams & Wilkins; 1994. pp. 525-39.
5. Nield JS, Houseman GA. Instrument design and classification. In: Fundamentals of Dental Hygiene Instrumentation, 2nd edition. Philadelphia, PA, USA: Lea & Febiger; 1988. pp. 179-200.
6. Wilkins EM. Examination procedures. In: Clinical Practice of the Dental Hygienist, 8th edition. Philadelphia, PA, USA: Lippincott Williams & Wilkins; 1994. pp. 201-23.
7. Nield-Gehrig JS. Explorers. In: Fundamentals of Periodontal Instrumentation & Advanced Root Instrumentation, 6th edition. Philadelphia, PA, USA: Lippincott Williams & Wilkins; 2008. pp. 243-73.
8. Parr PW, Gree E, Ratcliff PA, et al. Recognizing periodontal disease, San Francisco, USA: Praxis Publishing; 1978.
9. Gibbs CH, Hirschfeld JW, Lee LG, Low SB, Magnusson I, Thousand RR, et al. Description and clinical evaluation of a new computerized periodontal probe--the Florida probe. J Clin Periodontol. 1988;15(2):137-44.
10. Philstrom BL. Measurement of attachment level in clinical trials: probing methods. J Periodontol. 1992;63(12 Suppl):1072-7.
11. Gabathuler H, Hassell T. A pressure-sensitive periodontal probe. Helv Odontol Acta. 1971;15(2):114-7.
12. Nield-Gehrig JS. Sickle scalers. In: Fundamentals of Periodontal Instrumentation & Advanced Root Instrumentation, 6th edition. Philadelphia, PA, USA: Lippincott Williams & Wilkins; 2008. pp. 285-306.
13. Nield-Gehrig JS. Periodontal file. In: Fundamentals of Periodontal Instrumentation & Advanced Root Instrumentation, 6th edition. Philadelphia, PA, USA: Lippincott Williams & Wilkins; 2008. pp. 361-74.
14. Pattison AM, Pattison GL, Takei HH. The periodontal instrumentarium. In: Newman MG, Takei HH, Carranza FA (Eds). Carranza's Clinical Periodontology, 9th edition. Philadelphia, PA, USA: WB Saunders; 2003. pp. 567-93.
15. Grant DA, Stern IB, Listgarten MA. Scaling and root planing. In: Periodontics, 6th edition. St. Louis: CV Mosby; 1988. pp. 650-718.
16. Drisko CL. Scaling and root planing without over instrumentation: hand versus power-driven scalers. Curr Opin Periodontol. 1993;78-88.
17. Eliades GC, Tzoutzas JG, Vougiouklakis GJ. Surface alterations on dental restorative materials subjected to an air-powder abrasive instrument. J Prosthet Dent. 1991;65(1):27-33.
18. Fox SC, Moriarty JD, Kusy RP. The effects of scaling a titanium implant surface with metal and plastic instruments: an in vitro study. J Periodontol. 1990;61(8):485-90.
19. Wennstrom JL, Heijl L, Lindhe J. Periodontal surgery: access therapy. In: Lindhe J, Karring T, Lang NP (Eds). Clinical Periodontology and Implant Dentistry, 4th edition. Chicago, USA: Blackwell Munksgaard; 2003. pp. 519-60.
20. Gnanasekhar JD, al-Duwairi YS. Electrosurgery in dentistry. Quintessence Int. 1998;29(10):649-54.
21. McKechnie LB. Instrumentation selection and care. In: Genco RJ, Goldman HM, Cohen DW (Eds). Contemporary Periodontics, 2nd edition. St. Louis: CV Mosby; 1990. pp. 525-39.

### VIVA VOCE

**Q1. What is Expros?**
**Ans.** Expros is the double-ended instrument with an explorer on one end and probe on others, e.g., 17/Williams, 23/0 Michigan, 23/Williams.

**Q2. What are Novatech probes?**
**Ans.** These are the probes with a unique right-angle design for improved adaptability in posterior teeth.

**Chapter 40:** Periodontal Instruments

**Q3. What is a balanced instrument?**
**Ans.** When the working ends are centered on a line running through the long-axis of the handle, then the instrument is said balanced instrument.

**Q4. Which mark should be taken as final reading, when the gingival margin appears at a level between two probe marks?**
**Ans.** A higher mark should be taken as final reading when the gingival margin appears at a level between two probe marks.

**Q5. What is the advantage of the color band on some periodontal probes?**
**Ans.** The colored band on the periodontal probe is designed to make periodontal examination readings more objective and faster.

**Q6. What are contra-angled shanks?**
**Ans.** Instruments with longer blades/more complex orientations may require 2 or 3 angles in the shank to bring the cutting edge close to the long axis of the handle. Such shanks are termed as contra-angled shanks.

**Q7. Which instrument shows two-point contact?**
**Ans.** Hoe scalers show two-point contact.

**Q8. Which probe is flat and not round in nature?**
**Ans.** Goldman-Fox probe

**Q9. What is the basic difference between After Five or Standard Gracey Curettes?**
**Ans.** The blade of Mini-bladed curettes is half in length compared to After Five or Standard Gracey curettes.

**Q10. Which instrument is activated with a push motion?**
**Ans.** Chisel is the only instrument that is activated with a push motion.

# Chapter 41: General Principles of Instrumentation

*Shalu Bathla*

## Chapter Outline

- Accessibility
- Visibility, Illumination, and Retraction
- Condition of the Instruments
- Maintaining a Clean Field
- Instrument Stabilization
- Instrument Activation
- Instrumentation Strokes
- Principles of Scaling and Root Planing

## INTRODUCTION

Various general principles apply to all periodontal instruments in order to achieve effective instrumentation. Maintaining a suitable position of both the patient and the operator, illumination, and retraction for optimal visibility and sharp instruments are fundamental prerequisites to get good results. There may be variations in instrumentation based on previous clinical experience to provide accurate judgment and confidence to modify them for personal preferences or special circumstances.

## ACCESSIBILITY

### Position of the Operator

The patient and operator position should be adjusted to achieve maximal accessibility to the operating site, and accessibility facilitates thoroughness of instrumentation. The clinician should be seated on a comfortable operating stool that has been positioned so that:

- The head is relatively erect. It should be erect in the least strained position vertically and horizontally.
- Eyes are directed downward in order to avoid neck and eye strain.
- Maintain adequate distance between the patient's mouth and the clinician's eyes at least about 14–16 inches.
- Shoulders are relaxed.
- The forearm and wrist are kept in a straight line; the wrist is neither flexed nor extended.
- Body-weight is completely supported by the chair.
- The back is straight and erect.
- Thighs parallel with the floor.
- The feet are flat on the floor.

Patient or operator positioning is commonly identified by the position of the small hand on a clock in relation to the face of the clock. The face of the clock represents the patient. The operator is represented by the small hand of the clock.[1] The patient's chin is at 6 O'clock **(Fig. 41.1)**. The right-handed operator sits between 9 O'clock and 12 O'clock.[2]

- *Right-handed operator*:
  - Right front: 7 O'clock
  - Right: 9 O'clock

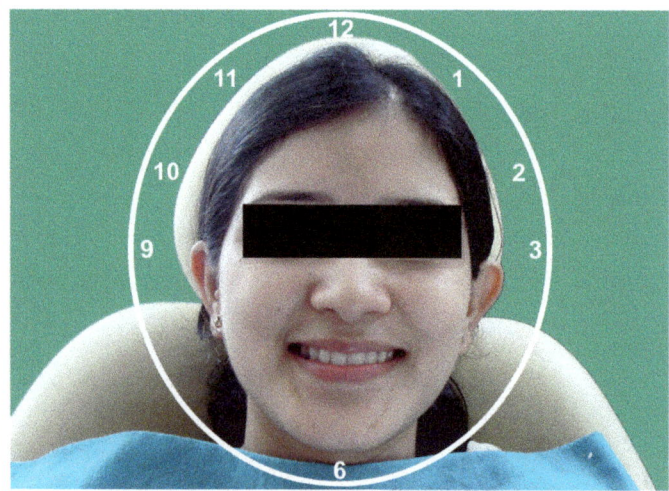

**Fig. 41.1:** Photograph showing operator positioning relative to the patient.

- Right rear: 11 O'clock
- Direct rear: 12 O'clock

The left-handed operator sits on the opposite side between 12 O'clock and 3 O'clock.[2]
- *Left-handed operator*:
  - Left front: 5 O'clock
  - Left: 3 O'clock
  - Left rear: 1 O'clock
  - Direct rear: 12 O'clock

## Position of the Patient

For instrumentation of the maxillary arch, the patient should be asked to raise his or her chin slightly to provide optimal visibility and accessibility. For instrumentation on the mandibular arch, it may be necessary to slightly raise the back of the chair and request that the patient lower his or her chin until the mandible is parallel to the floor. This will especially facilitate work on the lingual aspects of the mandibular anterior teeth. The patient's mouth's distance to the clinician's eyes should be approximately 14–16 inches. The assistant is seated with eye level 4–6 inches above the clinician's eye level and facing towards the head of the dental chair. Following are the various positions of the patient on the dental chair:

- *Upright position*: Initial position from which chair adjustments are made.
- *Semi-upright position*: Respiratory and cardiovascular patients should be in a semi-upright position during treatment.
- *Supine position*: Flat position with head and feet maintained on the same level.
- *Trendelenburg position*: Modified supine position when the head is lower than the heart. The brain is lower than the heart and feet slightly elevated.

## VISIBILITY, ILLUMINATION, AND RETRACTION

Direct vision with direct illumination achieved from the dental light is the most desirable for conducting operating procedures. If this is not possible, indirect vision may be obtained by using the mouth mirror. Indirect illumination may also be obtained by using the mirror to reflect light to where it is needed. Indirect vision and indirect illumination are often used simultaneously. Retraction provides visibility, accessibility, and illumination. Depending on the location of the operation area, the fingers and/or the mirrors are used for retraction. The mirror may be used for retraction of the cheeks (**Fig. 41.2**) or the tongue (**Fig. 41.3**), and the index finger may also be used for retraction of the lips or cheeks. While retracting the lips and cheeks, avoid pulling the cheeks away from the dentition and imposing pressure on the labial commissures. Fogging of the mirror is usually prevented by warming it to body temperature by placing it against the buccal mucosa. Apply petroleum jelly on the angle of mouth and lips before instrumentation is begun, which is a helpful precaution against cracking and bleeding. Careful retraction is especially important for patients with a history of recurrent herpes labialis, because these patients may easily develop herpetic lesions after instrumentation.[3]

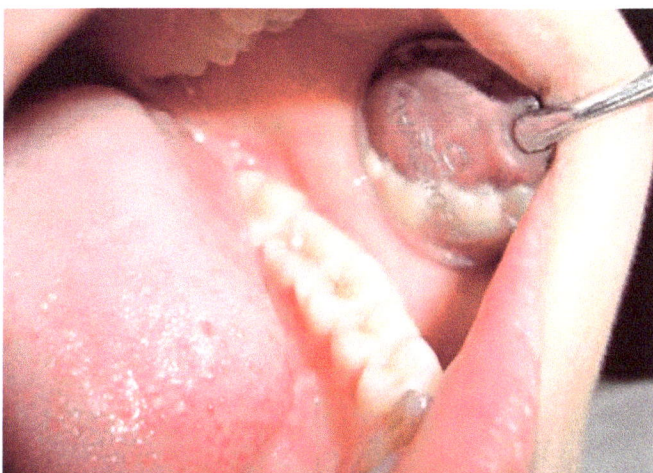

**Fig. 41.2:** Clinical picture showing retraction of the cheek by a mirror.

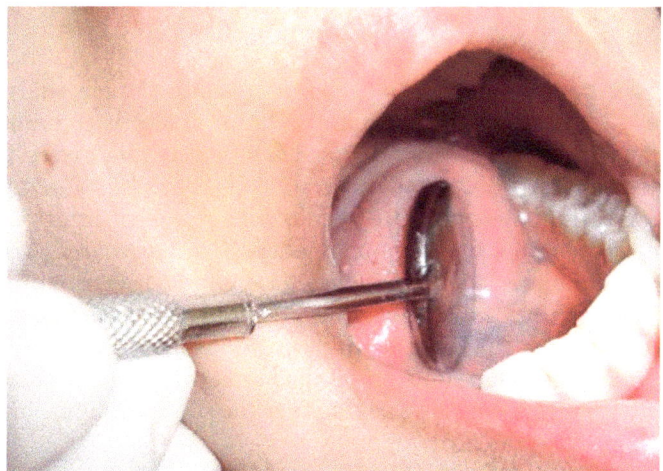

**Fig. 41.3:** Clinical picture showing retraction of the tongue by the mirror.

### Clinical Tip

- *Instrument exchange*: All instrument exchanges between the operator and the assistant should occur in the exchange zone between the patient's chin and a few inches above the patient's chest.
- The assistant should take the instrument from the operator, rather than the operator dropping it into the assistant's hand.

## CONDITION OF THE INSTRUMENTS

Steps in the effective care of instruments:
- Instruments are cleaned after each use by removing blood and debris under running water.
- The instruments are sharpened regularly, and sharpness is checked thereafter.
- Instruments are sterilized thoroughly.

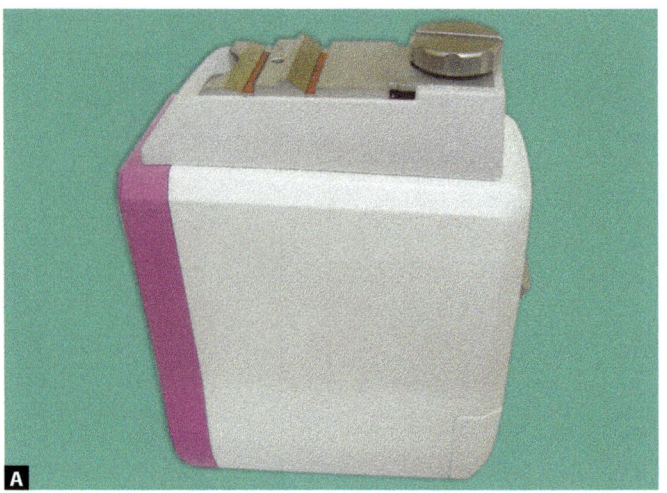
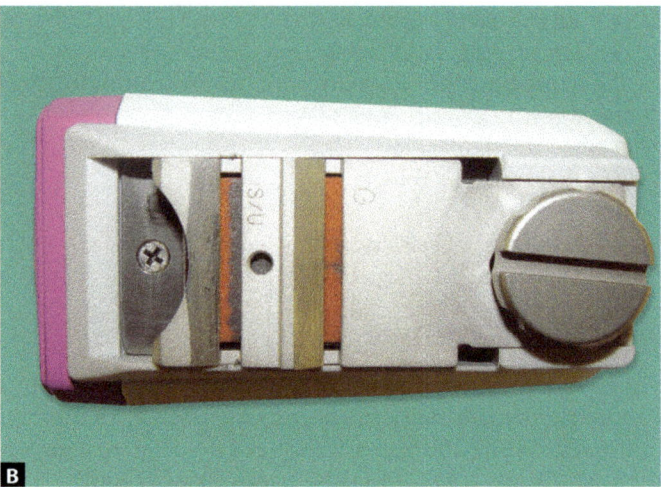

**Figs. 41.4A and B:** Photograph showing automated sharpener.

## Sharpness

Instruments are sharpened to produce a functionally sharp edge to preserve the shape and contour of the instrument. Sharp instruments improve tactile sensations, thus increase the efficiency of deposit removal. Using sharp instruments also requires less pressure for calculus and deposit removal.

The various types of equipment used during sharpening are automated sharpener (**Figs. 41.4A and B**), sharpening stones mounted and unmounted Arkansas stone (**Fig. 41.5**), India stone, carborundum stone, light mineral oil, diamond-coated stone, lubricating fluids, water, acrylic test stick, and gauge. Arkansas stone is the stone of choice for sharpening instruments.[4]

### Principles of Sharpening

- Instruments must be sharpened at the first sign of dullness.
- Choose a suitable sterilized sharpening stone of appropriate shape and abrasiveness for the instrument sharpening.
- Set the proper angle between the sharpening stone and the surface of the instrument.
- A stable firm grasp should be maintained on both instruments and sharpening stone.
- Avoid excessive pressure.
- Make the sharpening stroke by moving the instrument towards and not away from you; this will minimize the formation of a wire edge.
- Do not overheat the instrument during sharpening. Lubricate the stone well during sharpening.

### Sharpening of Individual Instruments

Different instruments are sharpened in different ways:[5-9]

### Chisel and Hoe

To sharpen a chisel, grasp the instrument with a modified pen grasp and stabilize a flat sharpening stone on a flat

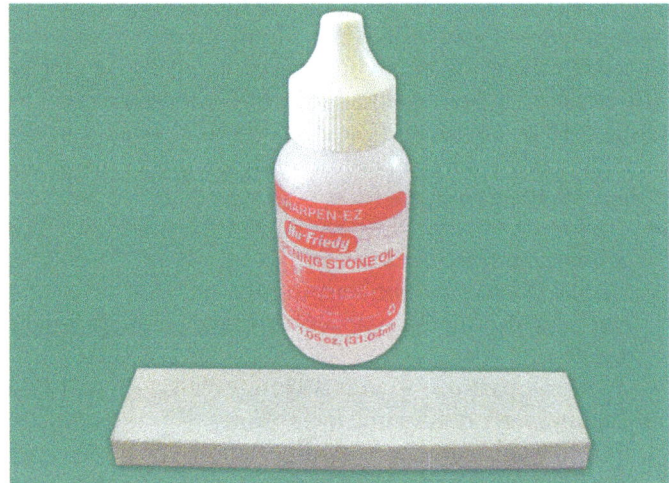

**Fig. 41.5:** Photograph showing flat Arkansas stone and stone oil.

surface. Establish a finger rest with the pads of the 3rd and 4th fingers against the sharpening stone's straight edge. Apply the flat-beveled surface of the chisel to the surface of the stone. If the entire surface of the bevel is contacting the stone, then the 45° angle between the beveled surface and the face of the blade will be maintained, and the design of the instrument will not be altered (**Fig. 41.6A**).

Using moderate, steady pressure, with the hand and arm acting as a unit and the finger resting on the edge of the stone as a guide, push the instrument across the sharpening stone's surface. Release pressure slightly and draw the instrument back to its starting point. Repeat the sharpening stroke until a sharp edge has been obtained.

*Precaution*: Remember to finish with a push stroke to prevent the formation of a wire edge.

Back-action surgical chisels and hoe scalers are sharpened with exactly the same technique described for chisels except that a pull stroke is used rather than a push stroke.

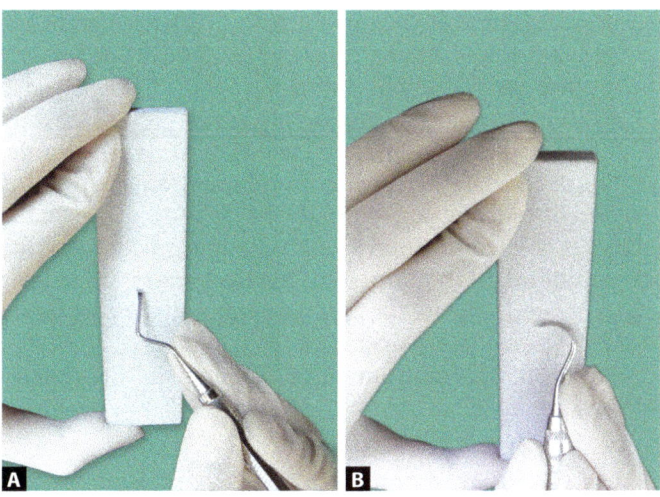

**Figs. 41.6A and B:** Photograph showing recommended hand positions during sharpening of: (A) hoe; (B) sickle scaler.

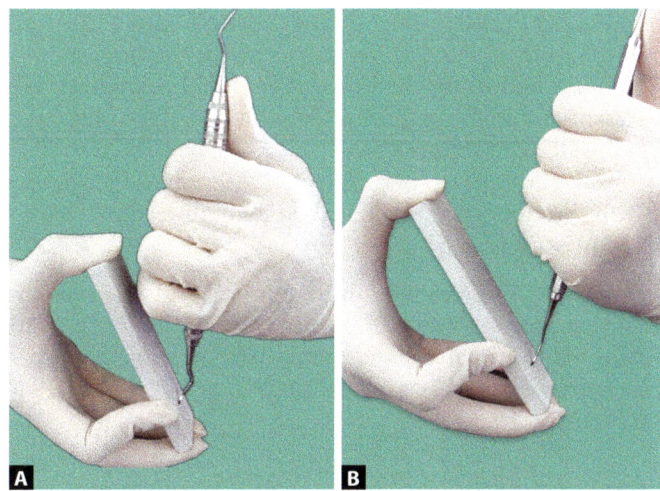

**Figs. 41.7A and B:** Photograph showing recommended hand positions during sharpening of: (A) universal curette; (B) Gracey curette.

## Sickle Scaler

A large, flat stone is used to sharpen sickles **(Fig. 41.6B)**. The stone is stabilized on a table or cabinet with the left hand. The sickle is held in the right hand with a modified pen grasp and applied to the stone in order to maintain the angle between the face of the blade and the stone at 100–110°. The 4th finger is placed on the right-hand edge of the stone to stabilize and guide the sharpening movement. The right hand then pushes and pulls the sickle across the surface of the stone. To avoid a wire edge, finish with a pull stroke, being sure that the proper angulation is always maintained.

The sickle scaler can also be sharpened in a manner much like that described for the curette except that the sickle has a sharp, pointed toe that must not be rounded.

## Universal Curette

Sharpening the lateral surface:
- When a flat, handheld stone is correctly applied to the lateral surface of a curette to maintain the 70–80° angle, the angle formed in between the face of the blade and the surface of the stone will be 100–110°. This can best be visualized by holding the curette so that the face of the blade is parallel to the floor. A palm grasp should be used, and the upper arm braced against the body for support **(Fig. 41.7A)**.
- Beginning at the shank end of the cutting edge and working toward the toe, activate the stone with short up-and-down strokes. Use light and consistent pressure by keeping the stone continuously in contact with the blade. Make sure that the 100–110° angle is constantly maintained.
- Check for sharpness as previously described, and continue sharpening as necessary. In order to avoid the toe of the curette from becoming pointed, the entire blade must be sharpened from shank end to toe. While approaching the toe, care should be taken to sharpen around it to preserve its rounded form.
- As the stone is moved along the cutting edge, finish each section with a downstroke into or towards the cutting edge. This will minimize the formation of a wire edge. Check the cutting edge under a light.
- Sharpening the curette in this manner tends to flatten the lateral surface. This can be corrected by lightly grinding the lateral surface and the back of the instrument, away from the cutting edge, each time the instrument is sharpened.
- When one edge has been properly sharpened, the opposite cutting edge can be sharpened in the same manner.

Sharpening the face of the blade: This may be done by moving a handheld cylindrical or cone-shaped stone back and forth across the face of the blade. A similar stone mounted in a handpiece may also be used by applying it to the blade's face with the stone rotating towards the toe. These methods are not recommended for routine use for the following reasons:
- The angulation between the instrument and the stone is difficult to maintain, and therefore the blade may be improperly beveled.
- Sharpening the face of the blade narrows the working end from face to back. This weakens the blade and makes it likely to bend or break while in use.
- Sharpening the face of the blade with a handheld stone using a back-and-forth motion produces a wire edge that interferes with the blade's sharpness.

## Area-specific (Gracey) Curette

- Hold the curette so that the face of the blade is parallel to the floor. Because the blade is offset, the instrument's shank will not be perpendicular to the floor, as it is with universal curettes **(Fig. 41.7B)**.

- Identify the edge to be sharpened. Remember that only one cutting edge is used, so only that edge must be sharpened. Apply the stone to the lateral surface in order to maintain the angle between the face of the blade and the stone at 100–110°.
- Activate short up-and-down strokes, working from the shank end of the blade to the curved toe. Finish with a downstroke.

*Precaution*: The cutting edge is curved and reserves the curve by turning the stone while sharpening from shank to toe. If the stone is maintained in one place for too many strokes, the chances for flattening of the blade will increase.

### Extended Shank Gracey Curettes

Extended shank Gracey curettes, such as the After Fives, are sharpened in exactly the same manner as the standard Gracey curettes. Although the terminal shank is 3 mm longer, the blade size and shape are very similar, and therefore, there is no difference in the sharpening technique.

*Precaution*: Sharpening too heavily or too often around the toe of a mini-bladed curette should be avoided to prevent excessive shortening of the blade.

### Gingivectomy Knives

- *Kirkland knife*: When sharpening the Kirkland knife, only the bevel on the instrument's back surface needs to be ground. This can be done by drawing the blade across a stationary flat sharpening stone or by holding the instrument stationary and drawing the stone across its blade.
- *Interproximal knife*: As with the flat-bladed gingivectomy knife, only the bevels on the back surface of the interproximal knife need to be sharpened. This can be accomplished by drawing the instrument across a stationary stone or by holding the instrument stationary and moving the stone across it.

## Methods of Testing Sharpness

Different methods of testing sharpness are as follows:[3,10]
- *Effectiveness during use*: A blunt instrument will not bite on the root surface, and the operator will need to apply increased pressure for it to be effective.
- *Visual or glaze test*: If a dull instrument is grasped under a light, the rounded surface of its cutting edge reflects light back to the observer, and it appears as a bright line running the length of the cutting edge. If a sharp instrument is grasped under light, no such bright line is observed. The cutting edge when examined under magnifying viewer (x5 magnification) should not show any reflection.
- *Acrylic stick test*: Tactile evaluation of sharpness is performed by drawing the instrument lightly across an acrylic rod and evaluating the bite. A dull instrument will slide smoothly, but a sharp instrument will bite into the surface, raising a light shaving.

Undesirable edges formed during sharpening are wire edges and beveled edges. Wire edges are undesirable, sawtooth-like projections of metal fragments extending beyond the cutting edge from the lateral side or face of the blade. It is formed when a coarse stone is used, and the instrument is over sharpened. Beveled edges are cutting edges created beneath the original cutting edge by improper stone to instrument placement.

Sterilization of instruments is explained in "Chapter 69: Miscellaneous."

## MAINTAINING A CLEAN FIELD

The operative field is obscured by saliva, blood, and debris. The pooling of saliva interferes with visibility during instrumentation and impedes control because a firm finger rest cannot be established on wet, slippery tooth surfaces. Adequate suction is essential and can be achieved with a saliva ejector, or, if working with an assistant, an aspirator. Blood and debris can be removed from the operative field with suction and by wiping or blotting with gauze squares. Compressed air and gauze squares can be used to facilitate visual inspection of tooth surfaces just below the gingival margin during instrumentation. A jet of air directed into the pocket deflects a retractable gingival margin. Retractable tissue can also be deflected away from the tooth by gently packing the edge of a gauze square into the pocket with the back of a curette. After the gauze is removed immediately, the subgingival area could be clean, dry, and clearly visible for a brief interval.

## INSTRUMENT STABILIZATION

Controlled instrumentation demands the stability of the instrument and the operating hand. The two important factors that determine the instrument's stability are the instrument grasps and the finger rest.

### Instrument Grasps

The various instrument grasps are:[3,10]
- Standard pen grasp
- Modified pen grasp
- Palm and thumb grasp

#### Standard Pen Grasp

Here the thumb, index finger, and middle finger hold the instrument in a manner of holding a pen, and the side of the middle finger rests on the shank **(Fig. 41.8)**.

#### Modified Pen Grasp

A modified pen grasp is considered as the most effective and stable grasp for periodontal instruments. Thumb, index

Chapter 41: General Principles of Instrumentation

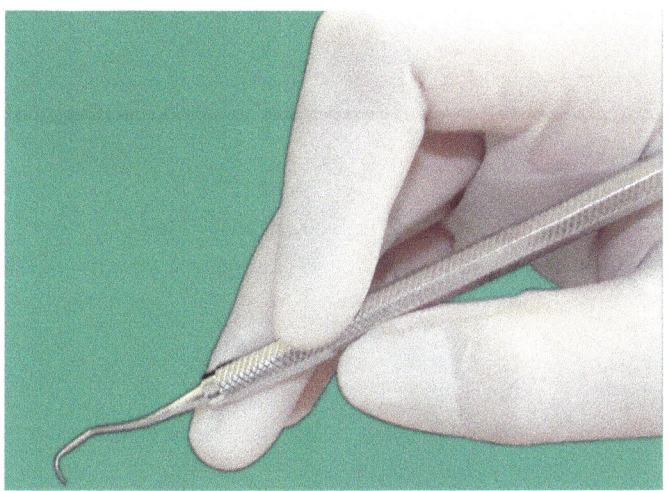

Fig. 41.8: Photograph showing standard pen grasp (the side of middle finger rests on the shank).

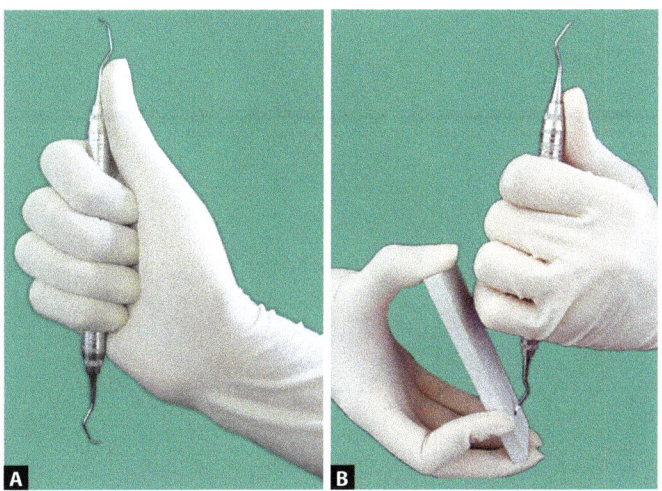

Figs. 41.10A and B: Photograph showing palm and thumb grasp.

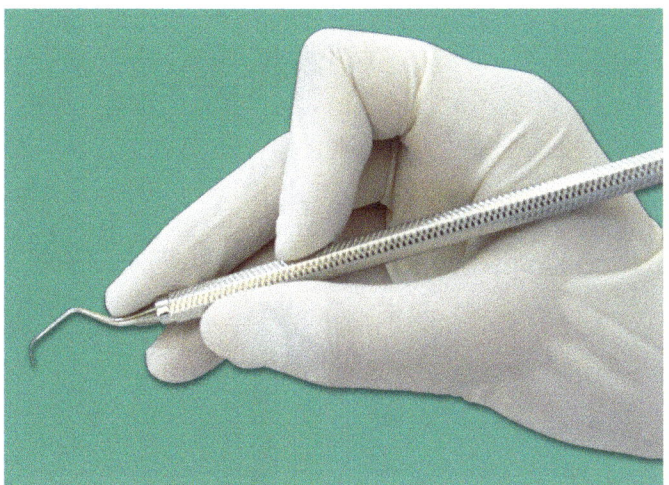

Fig. 41.9: Photograph showing modified pen grasp (the pad of middle finger rests on the shank).

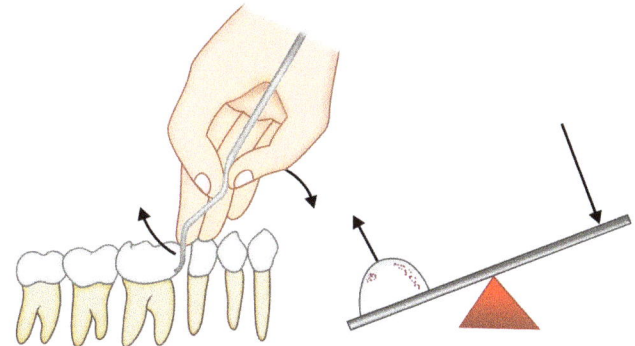

Fig. 41.11: Schematic representation showing fulcrum (for stabilizing and pivotal point from which scaling and root planing is done).

finger, and middle finger are used to hold the instrument while the pad of the middle finger resting on the shank. The pad of the fingers has the maximum nerve receptors. The index finger should be bent at the second joint from the finger's tip and is maintained well above the middle finger on the same side of the handle. The pad of the thumb should be positioned midway between the middle and index fingers on the opposite side of the handle (**Fig. 41.9**).

## Palm and Thumb Grasp

The instrument's handle is grasped in the palm by cupped index, middle, ring, and little fingers. The thumb is free to serve as the fulcrum. The palm grasp limits operation in that there is less tactile sensitivity and less flexibility of movement. Palm and thumb grasp is helpful in instrument stabilization during sharpening, for manipulating air and water syringes and for manipulating porte polisher (**Fig. 41.10A and B**).

## Finger Rests

A scaling instrument operates as a lever, and the ring finger acts as a fulcrum and as a stabilizing point for the hand. A fulcrum is a point on which the lever pivots. The fulcrum permits the instrument to function properly. Also, it provides stability and control over the instrument in order to avoid injury to the surrounding tissues (**Fig. 41.11**). A proper finger rest provides stable fulcrum, optimal angulation of the blade, and enables the use of wrist-forearm motion.

## Various Types of Finger Rests

The various types of finger rests are:[3,10]
- *Intraoral finger rests*: Intraoral fulcrum places the pad of the ring finger on a tooth closer to the tooth to be instrumented in the oral cavity and thus provides stabilization to the clinician's dominant hand.
  - *Conventional finger rest*: Finger rest is established on the immediately adjacent tooth (**Fig. 41.12**).
  - *Cross-arch finger rest*: Finger rest is established on the tooth surface on the other side of the same arch (**Fig. 41.13**).

## Section 6: Treatment: Nonsurgical Therapy

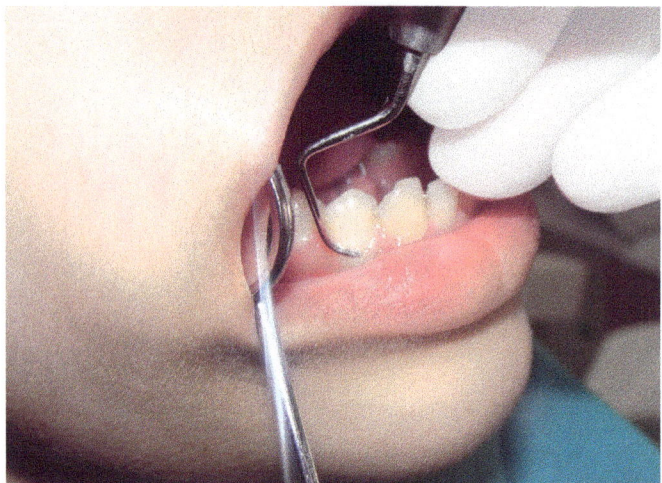

**Fig. 41.12:** Photograph showing intraoral conventional finger rest: 4th finger rests on occlusal surfaces of adjacent teeth.

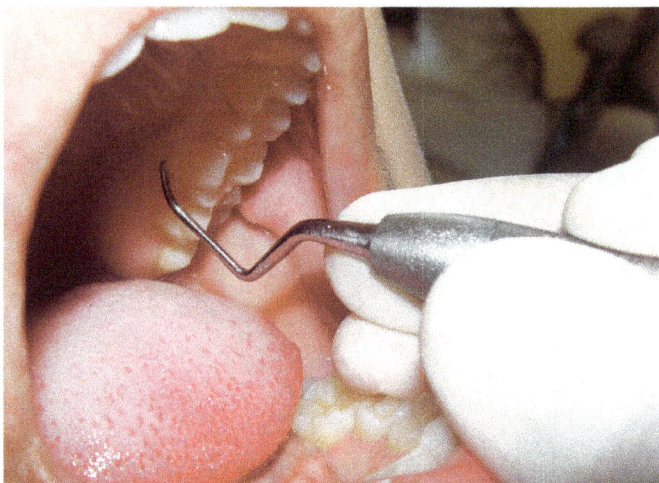

**Fig. 41.14:** Clinical picture showing opposite arch finger rest: 4th finger rests on the mandibular teeth while the maxillary posterior teeth are instrumented.

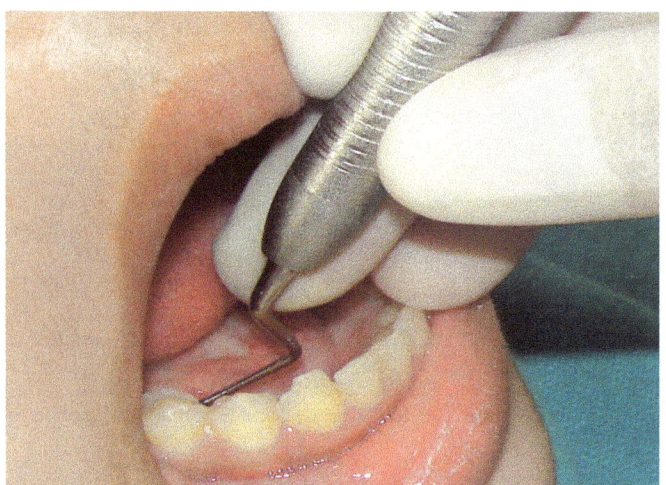

**Fig. 41.13:** Clinical picture showing cross-arch finger rest: 4th finger rests on the incisal surface of teeth on the opposite side of the same arch.

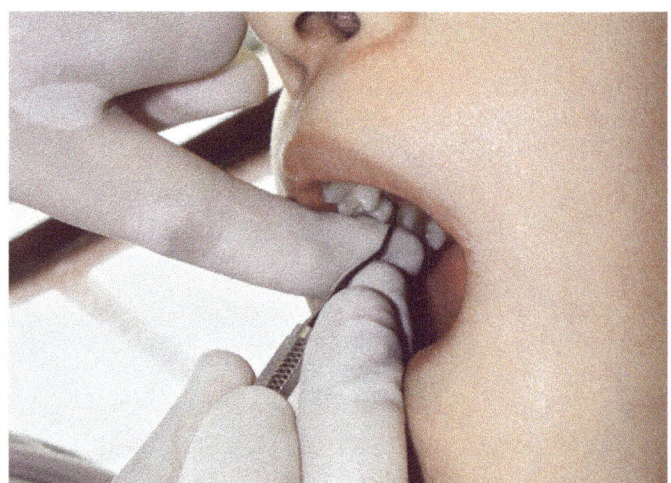

**Fig. 41.15:** Clinical picture showing finger on finger: 4th finger rests on the index finger of the nonoperating hand.

- *Opposite arch finger rest*: Finger rest is a grasp established on the tooth surface on the opposite arch **(Fig. 41.14)**.
- *Finger on finger*: Finger rest is established on the thumb or index finger of the nonoperating hand **(Fig. 41.15)**.
- Extraoral fulcrums: These provide stabilization to the clinician's hand outside the patient's mouth commonly on the chin or cheek. They are essential for effective instrumentation in deep periodontally involved maxillary posterior teeth.
  - *Knuckle rest technique or palm up*: The clinician rests his or her knuckles against the patient's chin or cheek. The back surfaces of the middle and 4th finger are positioned on the skin, covering the mandible lateral aspects on the right side of the face **(Fig. 41.16A)**.
  - *Chin-cup technique or palm down*: Clinician cups the patient's chin in the palm of his or her hand. The front surfaces of the middle and 4th finger are placed on the skin, overlying the mandible lateral aspects on the left side of the face **(Fig. 41.16B)**.

## INSTRUMENT ACTIVATION

### Adaptation

Adaptation is the manner of positioning the working end of a periodontal instrument against the tooth's surface. The primary goal of adaptation is to maintain the instrument tip's continuous contact with the tooth surface during each successive instrument stroke. This can be achieved by adapting the tip of instruments with the varying contours of each surface and periodontal structures just by rolling the

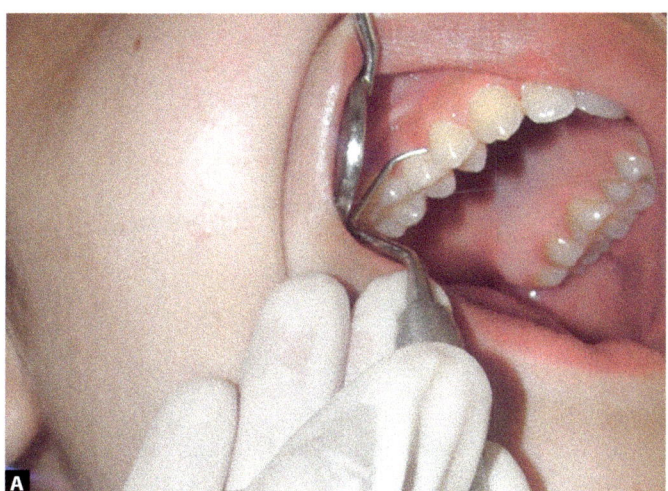 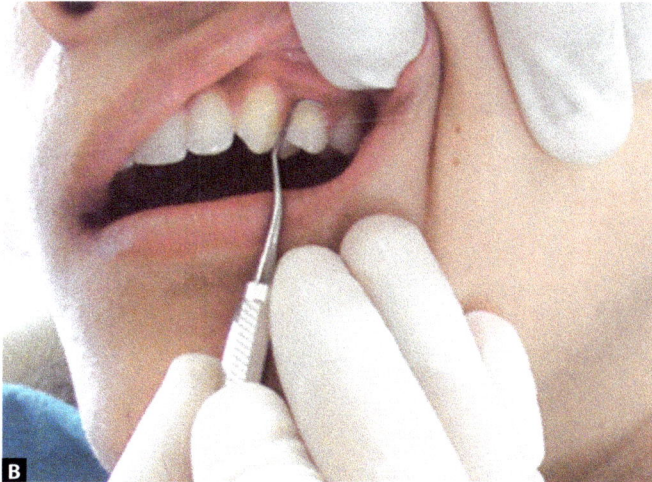

**Figs. 41.16A and B:** Clinical picture showing extraoral (A) palm up fulcrum; (B) palm down fulcrum.

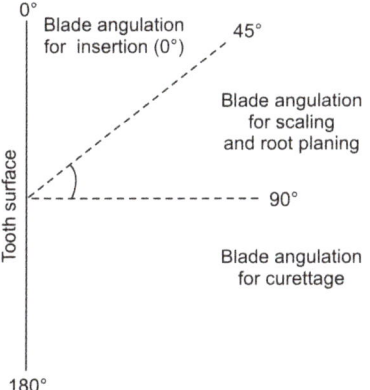

**Fig. 41.17:** Schematic representation showing a geometric representation of blade angulation.

handle between the index finger and thumb. The instrument tip should be in continuous contact with the tooth surface around the circumference of the tooth. Adaptation favors complete coverage of the surface by each stroke overlapping the previous one.

## Angulation

It refers to the angle between the face of a bladed instrument and the tooth surface. It is also called a tooth-blade relationship **(Figs. 41.17 and 41.18)**.

Face to tooth surface angulation for:
- *Insertion beneath the gingival margin*: 0°.
- *Scaling and root planing*: 45–90°.
- *Gingival curettage*: >90°

For successful instrumentation, correct angulation of the working end must be maintained throughout the instrumentation stroke. Lateral pressure refers to the pressure created when force is applied against the surface of a tooth with a bladed instrument's cutting edge. It may be firm, moderate, or light. It is the act of applying equal pressure with the index finger and thumb inward against the instrument handle to press the working end against the calculus deposit or tooth surface before and throughout an instrumentation stroke.

## INSTRUMENTATION STROKES

### Stroke Directions

There are three basic stroke directions **(Figs. 41.19A to C)**:[3,10]

1. *Vertical strokes*: These are commonly performed on the facial, lingual and proximal surfaces of anterior teeth. On posterior teeth, they are particularly used for the mesial and distal surfaces.
2. *Horizontal strokes*: These are made in a perpendicular direction to the long axis of the tooth. This stroke is used at the line angle of posterior teeth, facial and lingual surfaces of anterior teeth, furcation areas, and extremely narrow area where vertical or oblique stokes are difficult to conduct.
3. *Oblique strokes*: These are commonly performed on the facial and lingual surfaces of anterior and posterior teeth.

Following three basic strokes may be activated by pull or push motion in a vertical, oblique or horizontal directions:[3,10]

1. *Exploratory stroke or assessment stroke*: These are light feeling stroke, which is used to assess tooth anatomy, level of attachment, detect calculus, and other plaque retentive factors. They are used with explorers to locate calculus deposits and with periodontal probes to determine periodontal pocket depths and clinical attachment level.

**Section 6:** Treatment: Nonsurgical Therapy

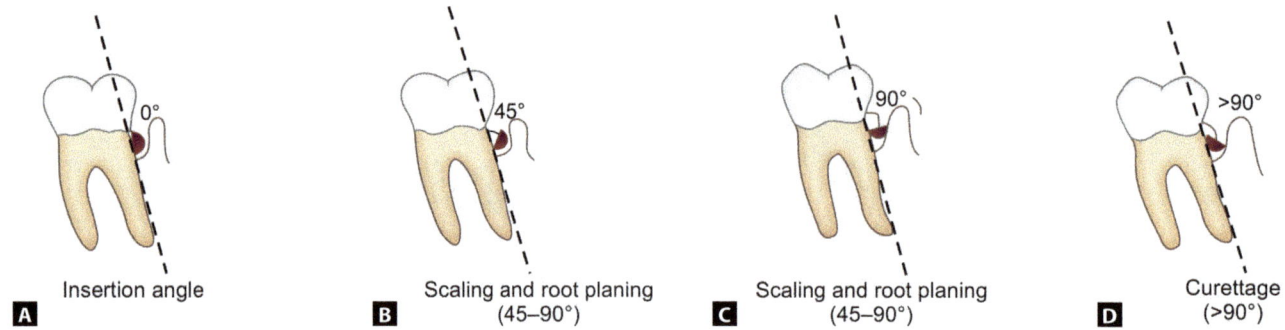

**Figs. 41.18A to D:** Schematic representation showing tooth-blade relationship: (A) Insertion angle (0°); (B) Scaling and root planing at 45°; (C) Scaling and root planing at 90°; and (D) Curettage >90°.

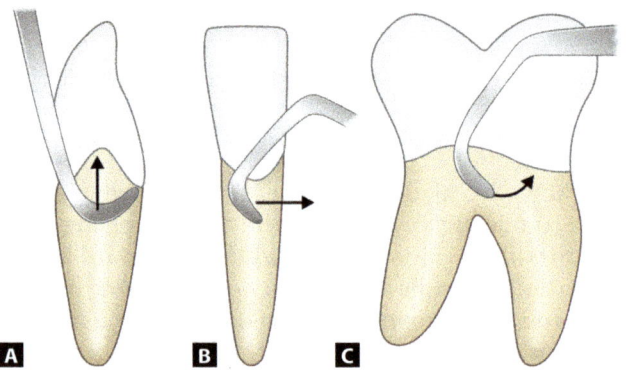

**Figs. 41.19A to C:** Schematic representation showing stroke directions: (A) Vertical stroke; (B) Horizontal stroke; and (C) Oblique stroke.

2. *Scaling stroke*: These are short, powerful pull stroke used to remove supragingival and subgingival calculus with the help of bladed instruments.
3. *Root planing stroke*: These are long, moderate-to-light pull stroke used for final smoothing and planing of the root surfaces with the help of curettes, hoes, files, and ultrasonic instruments.

The walking stroke is the movement of a calibrated probe around the perimeter of the base of a sulcus or pocket. Walking strokes are used to cover the entire circumference of the sulcus or pocket base.

Production of the walking stroke:
- Walking strokes are a series of bobbing strokes commonly performed within the sulcus or pocket. The stroke begins with the insertion of a probe into the sulcus and maintaining the probe tip against the tooth surface.
- The probe should be inserted until the tip experiences the junctional epithelium's resistance that forms the base of the sulcus. When the probe touches the junctional epithelium, it feels as soft and resilient.
- Walking stroke is usually created by moving the probe up and down in short bobbing strokes and forward in 1 mm increments (↔). With each downstroke, the probe returns to touch the junctional epithelium.
- The probe should not be removed from the sulcus with each upward stroke. Frequent removal and reinsertion of the probe can traumatize the tissue at the gingival margin.
- The ideal pressure between 10 g and 20 g should be exerted with the probe tip against the junctional epithelium.

## PRINCIPLES OF SCALING AND ROOT PLANING

Scaling and root planing strokes are confined to the tooth portion where calculus or altered cementum is found; this zone is called an instrumentation zone.

General principles for the use of the curettes for scaling and root planing are as follows:[3]
- The correct cutting edge should be determined by visually inspecting the blade. With the toe pointed in the direction to be scaled, only the back of the blade can be seen if the correct cutting edge has been selected **(Fig. 41.20A)**. If the wrong cutting edge has been adapted, the blade's flat, shiny face will be seen instead **(Fig. 41.20B)**.
- The lower shank should be parallel to the surface to be instrumented.
- When intraoral finger rests are used, the 4th and middle fingers together built-up fulcrum for maximum control and wrist-arm action.
- For working on the maxillary posterior teeth, extraoral fulcrums or mandibular finger rests are used.
- Concentrate on using the lower third of the instrument's cutting edge for calculus removal, especially on line angles or when attempting to remove a calculus ledge by breaking it away in sections, beginning at the lateral edge.
- The wrist and forearm should carry the burden of the stroke, rather than flexing the fingers. The clinician should activate an instrument with wrist-arm motions rolling from the fulcrum finger. Wrist flexion is hand movement at the wrist as performed during waving hand or painting with a brush. Fingers alone are not sufficient to activate the instrument stroke. This is because finger movements are usually smaller and involved less powerful muscles. Moreover, finger's movements have restricted range of motion and lack the involvement of the fulcrum.

## Chapter 41: General Principles of Instrumentation

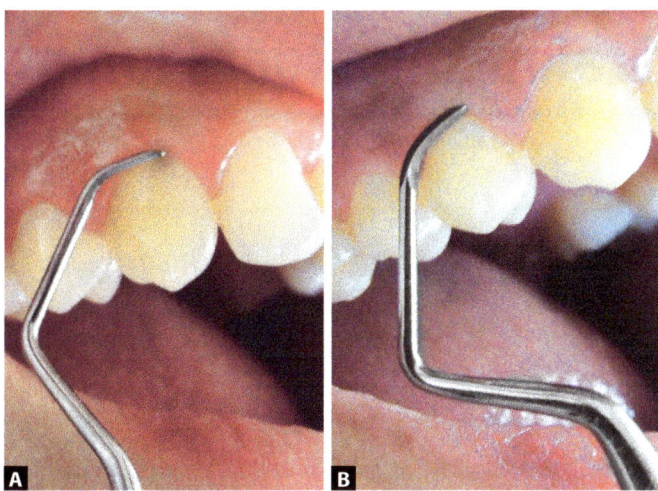

**Figs. 41.20A and B:** Clinical picture showing (A) correct; (B) incorrect cutting edge of Gracey curette adapted to the tooth.

### Points to Ponder
- The major difference between standard pen grasp and modified pen grasp: In standard pen grasp, the side of the pad of middle finger rests on the shank while in a modified pen grasp, the pad of middle finger rests on the shank.
- Exploratory stroke is a light feeling stroke.
- Scaling stroke is a short, powerful pull stroke.
- Root planing stroke is a long moderate-to-light pull stroke.

### REFERENCES
1. Grant DA, Stern IB, Listgarten MA. Scaling, and root planing. In: Periodontics, 6th edition. St. Louis: CV Mosby; 1988. pp. 650-718.
2. Plemons J, Eden BD. Nonsurgical therapy. In: Rose LF, Mealey BL, Genco RJ, Cohen DW (Eds). Periodontics: Medicine, Surgery, and Implants, 2nd illustrated edition. Philadelphia, PA, USA: Elsevier- Mosby; 2004. pp. 236-62.
3. Pattison GL, Pattison AM. Manual instrumentation. In: Newman MG, Takei HH, Carranza FA (Eds). Carranza's Clinical Periodontology, 9th edition. Philadelphia, PA, USA: WB Saunders; 2003. pp. 594-606.
4. McKenzie LB. Instrumentation selection and care. In: Genco RJ, Goldman HM, Cohen DW (Eds). Contemporary Periodontics, 1st edition. St. Louis: CV Mosby; 1990. pp. 525-39.
5. Scaramucci MK. Instrument sharpening. In: Daniel SJ, Harfst SA, Wilder RS (Eds). Mosby's Dental Hygiene: Concepts, Cases, and Competencies, 2nd edition. St. Louis: Mosby; 2008. pp. 188-201.
6. Pattison AM, Pattison GL, Takei HH. The periodontal instrumentation. In: Carranza FA, Newman MG, Takei HH (Eds). Carranza's Clinical Periodontology, 8th edition. Philadelphia, PA, USA: WB Saunders; 1996. pp. 427-50.
7. Paquette OE, Levin M P. The sharpening of scaling instruments: I. An examination of principles. J Periodontol. 1977;48(3):163-8.
8. Paquette OF, Levin MP. The sharpening of scaling instruments: II. A preferred technique. J Periodontol. 1977;48(3):169-72.
9. Wilkins EM. Instruments and principles of instrumentation. In: Clinical Practice of the Dental Hygienist, 8th edition. Philadelphia, PA, USA: Lippincott Williams & Wilkins; 1999. pp. 512-43.
10. Nield-Gehrig JS. Fundamentals of Periodontal Instrumentation & Advanced Root Instrumentation, 6th edition. Philadelphia, PA, USA: Lippincott Williams & Wilkins. 2008.

### VIVA VOCE

**Q1. What should be the patient's mouth's distance to the clinician's eyes during dental treatment?**
**Ans.** The distance from the patient's mouth to the eyes of the clinician during dental treatment is 14–16 inches.

**Q2. What is the major difference between standard pen grasp and modified pen grasp?**
**Ans.** In standard pen grasp, the middle finger's side rests on the shank while in modified pen grasps, the pad of the middle finger rests on the shank.

**Q3. Where is palm and thumb grasp used?**
**Ans.** Palm and thumb grasp is used for:
- Stabilizing instruments during sharpening.
- Manipulating air and water syringes.
- Manipulating porte polisher.

**Q4. What is the instrumentation zone?**
**Ans.** Scaling and root planing strokes are confined to the portion of the tooth where calculus or altered cementum is found, this zone is called as instrumentation zone.

**Q5. What is the optimal blade angulation for subgingival insertion of the instrument, scaling, and root planing and gingival curettage?**
**Ans.** The optimal blade angulation for:
- Subgingival insertion of the instrument: 0°.
- Scaling and root planing: 45–90°.
- Gingival curettage: >90°

**Q6. In which position of the chair, patients with cardiac and respiratory disease should be treated.**
**Ans.** Semi-upright position.

**Q7. What is Trendelenburg position?**
**Ans.** It is a modified supine position when the head is lower than the heart. The brain is lower than the heart and feet slightly elevated.

**Q8. When should the periodontal instruments be sharpened?**
**Ans.** At the first sign of dullness.

**Q9. What is the acrylic stick test?**
**Ans.** Tactile evaluation of sharpness is performed by drawing the instrument lightly across an acrylic rod and evaluating the bite. A dull instrument will slide smoothly, but a sharp instrument will bite into the surface, raising a light shaving.

**Q10. What is a walking stroke?**
**Ans.** Walking stroke is the movement of a calibrated probe around the perimeter of the base of a sulcus or pocket. Walking strokes are used to cover the entire circumference of the sulcus or pocket base.

# Chapter 42: Manual Scaling and Root Planing

*Shalu Bathla*

## Chapter Outline

- Definition
- Objectives
- Scaling and Root Planing
- Instrumentation Approaches
- Full-Mouth Disinfection
- Evaluation of Scaling and Root Planing

## INTRODUCTION

Scaling and root planing remove bacterial plaque and calculus, which are responsible for causing gingival inflammation. Thus, these procedures are carried out during phase I to remove the primary etiological factors and to restore gingival health.

## DEFINITION

Scaling is the process by which plaque and calculus are removed from both supragingival and subgingival tooth surfaces.[1]

Root planing is the process by which residual embedded calculus and portions of cementum are removed from the roots to produce a smooth, hard, and clean surface.

## OBJECTIVES

The primary objectives of scaling and root planing are:[2,3]
- Restoration of gingival health is achieved by complete removal of the dental plaque and calculus and converting inflamed bleeding or suppurating pathologic pockets to healthy gingival tissue.
- To suppress or eliminate the pathogenic periodontal microflora and replacing with healthy microflora.
- To facilitate shrinkage of the deepened pathologic pocket to a shallow and healthy gingival sulcus.
- To provide a root surface compatible with the re-establishment of healthy connective tissue and epithelial attachment.

## SCALING AND ROOT PLANING

### Supragingival Scaling

Supragingival scaling is performed coronal to the gingival margin, which allows direct visibility and freedom of movement. This makes adaptation and angulation of the instruments much more comfortable as compared with subgingival scaling and root planing.

### Instruments

Sickle scalers, curettes, and ultrasonic and sonic instruments are most commonly used during supragingival scaling.

### Technique

Following are the steps to be followed during supragingival scaling:[2-5]
- *Grasp:* Supragingival scaling is performed with sickle scaler or curette by holding them with a modified pen grasp.
- *Finger rest:* A firm finger rest is achieved on the teeth adjacent to the working area.
- *Adaptation and angulation:* The blade is adapted with an angulation of slightly <90° to the surface being scaled. The sharply pointed tip of the sickle can easily lacerate marginal tissue or gouge exposed root surfaces, so careful adaptation is especially important when this instrument is being used.
- *Strokes:* The cutting edge of the blade should engage the apical margin of the supragingival calculus. Short,

powerful, and overlapping scaling strokes should be activated coronally in a vertical or oblique direction.
- *Endpoint:* Final scaling should always follow with the finishing curette. The tooth surface is needed to be instrumented until it appears visually and tactilely free of all supragingival deposits.

## Subgingival Scaling and Root Planing

Subgingival scaling is performed apical to the gingival margin, which impairs the visibility and freedom of movement. Visibility is also obscured by the bleeding that is inevitable during subgingival instrumentation. Adaptation and angulation of the instruments are more difficult during subgingival scaling and root planing. Moreover, subgingival calculus is harder than supragingival calculus and is fixed into root irregularities, making it more tenacious and hard to remove.

## Instruments

Subgingival scaling and root planing are commonly performed with either universal or area-specific (Gracey) curettes. Sickles, hoes, Hirschfeld files, and thin ultrasonic tips can also be useful for the removal of subgingival calculus.

## Technique

Following are the steps to be followed during subgingival scaling:[1,4,6,7]
- *Grasp:* A modified pen grasp is used to hold a curette.
- *Finger rest:* A stable finger rest is established on the teeth adjacent to the working area. The location of the finger rest or fulcrum is important to keep the lower shank of the instrument parallel or nearly parallel to the tooth surface being treated and enable the operator to use wrist-arm motion. The finger rest must be close enough to the working area to fulfill these two requirements, except in some aspects of the maxillary posterior teeth. These requirements can be met only with the use of extraoral or opposite-arch fulcrums.
- *Insertion:* The blade is inserted under the gingiva at 0°.
- *Adaptation and angulation:* The correct cutting edge needs to be adapted to the tooth, and the lower shank is kept parallel to the tooth surface with the face of the blade nearly flush with the tooth surface. With the entry of cutting edge at the base of the pocket, a working angulation is maintained between 45° and 90°, and pressure is applied laterally against the tooth surface.

> **Clinical Tip**
> Engaging a large, tenacious ledge or piece of calculus with the entire cutting edge's length is not recommended because the force is distributed through a longer section of the cutting edge rather than concentrated. Moreover, more lateral pressure is required to dislodge the entire deposit in one stroke, diminishing tactile sensitivity and contributing to loss of control and resulting in tissue trauma.

- *Strokes:* Calculus is removed by a series of controlled, overlapping, short and powerful strokes primarily using wrist-arm motion. Longer, lighter root planing strokes are then activated with less lateral pressure until the root surface is completely smooth and hard. The instrument handle must be rolled carefully between the thumb and the fingers to keep the blade adapted closely to the tooth surface as line angles, and developmental depressions in tooth contour are followed.

  During scaling strokes, force should be maximized by concentrating lateral pressure onto the lower third of the blade. This small section, the terminal few millimeters of the blade, is positioned slightly apical to the lateral edge of the deposit. A short vertical or oblique stroke is used to split the calculus from the tooth surface. Without withdrawing the instrument from the pocket, the lower third of the blade is advanced laterally and repositioned to engage the next portion of the remaining deposit. Another vertical or oblique stroke is made, slightly overlapping the previous stroke. This process is repeated in a series of powerful scaling strokes until the entire deposit has been removed. The overlapping of these pathways or "channels" of instrumentation ensures that the entire instrumentation zone is covered.
- *Endpoint:* Final subgingival scaling and root planing should always follow with the finishing curette. The tooth surface is instrumented until all subgingival deposits are removed.

## INSTRUMENTATION APPROACHES

Different instrumentation approaches for maxillary teeth are discussed below:

*Maxillary anterior sextant: Facial aspect, surface towards the operator* **(Fig. 42.1)**
- *Position:* Front
- *Illumination:* Direct

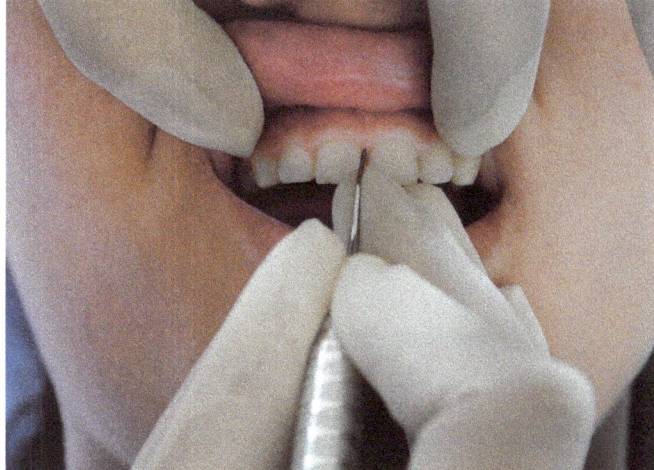

**Fig. 42.1:** Clinical picture showing scaling in maxillary anterior sextant: facial aspect, surface towards the operator.

- *Visibility:* Direct
- *Retraction:* Index finger of the nonoperating hand
- *Finger rest:* Intraoral, palm down. Fourth finger on the incisal edges or the occlusal or facial surfaces of adjacent maxillary teeth.

*Maxillary anterior sextant: Facial aspect, surface away from the operator* (**Fig. 42.2**)
- *Position:* Front
- *Illumination:* Direct
- *Visibility:* Direct
- *Retraction:* Index finger of the nonoperating hand.
- *Finger rest:* Intraoral, palm up. Fourth finger on the incisal edges or the occlusal or facial surfaces of adjacent maxillary teeth.

*Maxillary anterior sextant: Lingual aspect, surface away from the operator* (**Fig. 42.3**)
- *Position:* Back position
- *Illumination:* Indirect

- *Visibility:* Indirect
- *Retraction:* None
- *Finger rest:* Intraoral, palm up. Fourth finger on the incisal edges or the occlusal or facial surfaces of adjacent maxillary teeth.

*Maxillary right posterior sextant: Premolar region only: facial aspect* (**Fig. 42.4**)
- *Position:* Side or back position
- *Illumination:* Direct
- *Visibility:* Direct
- *Retraction:* Mirror or index finger of the nonoperating hand.
- *Finger rest:* Intraoral, palm up. Fourth finger on the occlusal surfaces of the adjacent maxillary posterior teeth.

*Maxillary right posterior sextant: Facial aspect* (**Fig. 42.5**)
- *Position:* Side position
- *Illumination:* Direct

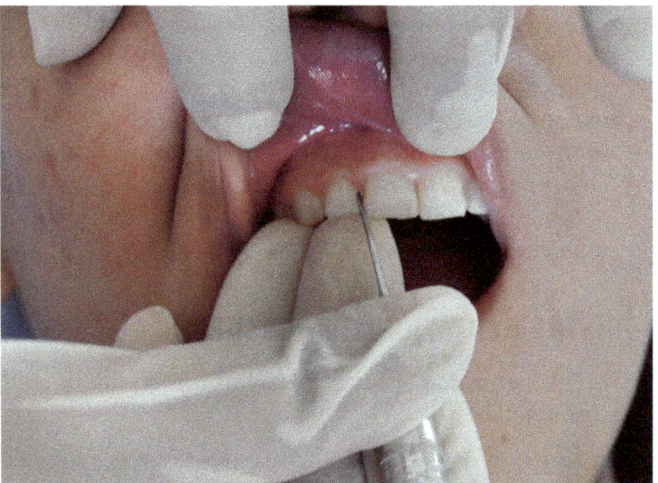

**Fig. 42.2:** Clinical picture showing scaling in maxillary anterior sextant: facial aspect, surface away from the operator.

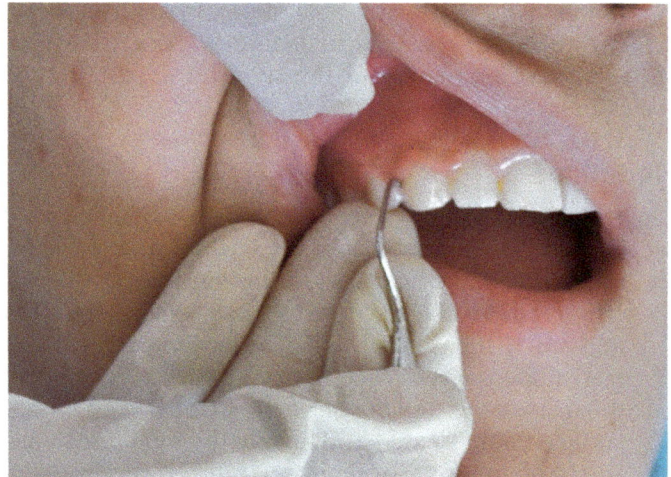

**Fig. 42.4:** Clinical picture showing scaling in maxillary right posterior sextant: premolar region only: facial aspect.

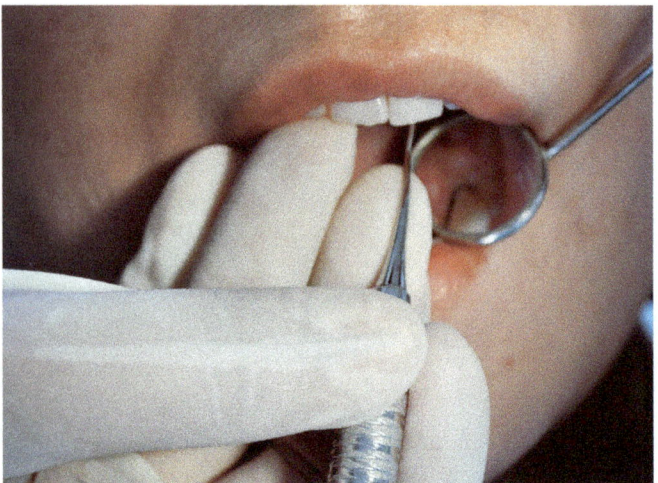

**Fig. 42.3:** Clinical picture showing scaling in maxillary anterior sextant: lingual aspect, surface away from the operator.

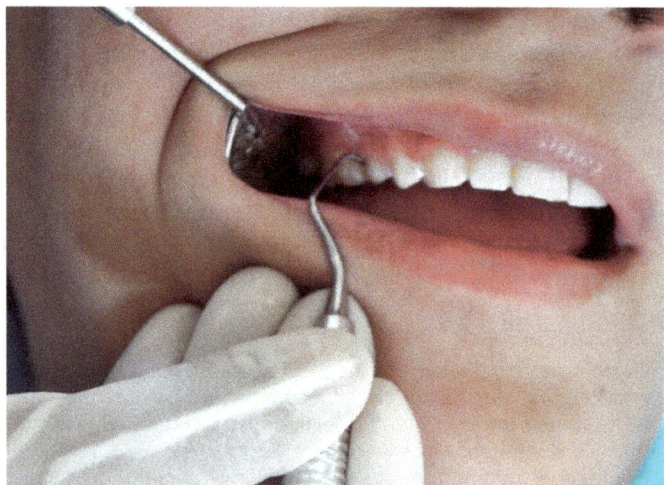

**Fig. 42.5:** Clinical picture showing scaling in maxillary right posterior sextant: facial aspect.

- *Visibility:* Direct (indirect for distal surfaces of molars)
- *Retraction:* Mirror or index finger of the nonoperating hand
- *Finger rest:* Extraoral, palm up. Back of the middle and fourth fingers on the lateral aspect of the mandible on the right side of the face.

*Maxillary right posterior sextant: Lingual aspect* (**Fig. 42.6**)
- *Position:* Side or front position
- *Illumination:* Direct or indirect
- *Visibility:* Direct or indirect
- *Retraction:* None
- *Finger rest:* Extraoral, palm up. Back of the middle and fourth fingers on the lateral aspect of the mandible on the right side of the face.

*Maxillary right posterior sextant: Lingual aspect* (**Fig. 42.7**)
- *Position:* Front position
- *Illumination:* Direct
- *Visibility:* Direct
- *Retraction:* None
- *Finger rest:* Intraoral, palm up, finger on finger

*Maxillary left posterior sextant: Facial aspect* (**Fig. 42.8**)
- *Position:* Side or back position
- *Illumination:* Direct or indirect
- *Visibility:* Direct or indirect
- *Retraction:* Mirror
- *Finger rest:* Extraoral, palm down. Front surfaces of the middle and fourth fingers on the lateral aspect of the mandible on the left side of the face.

*Maxillary left posterior sextant: Facial aspect* (**Fig. 42.9**)
- *Position:* Back or side position
- *Illumination:* Direct or indirect
- *Visibility:* Direct or indirect
- *Retraction:* Mirror
- *Finger rest:* Intraoral, palm up. Fourth finger on the incisal edges or the occlusal surfaces of the adjacent maxillary teeth.

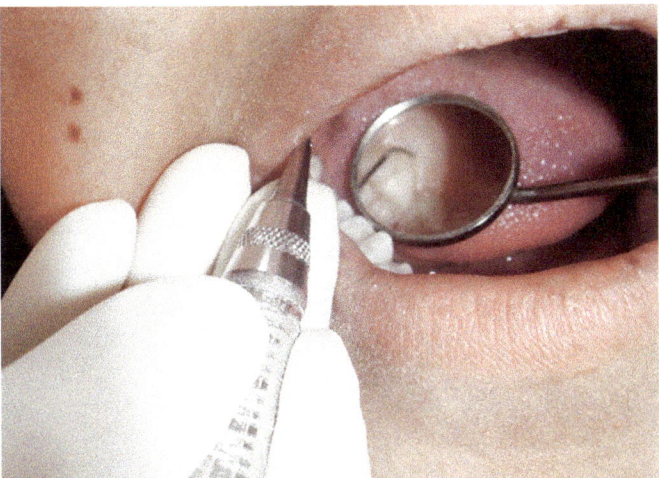

**Fig. 42.6:** Clinical picture showing scaling in maxillary right posterior sextant: lingual aspect.

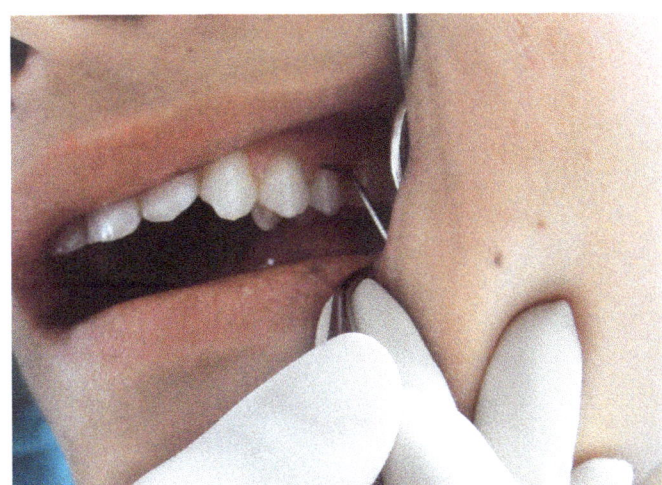

**Fig. 42.8:** Clinical picture showing scaling in the maxillary left posterior sextant: facial aspect.

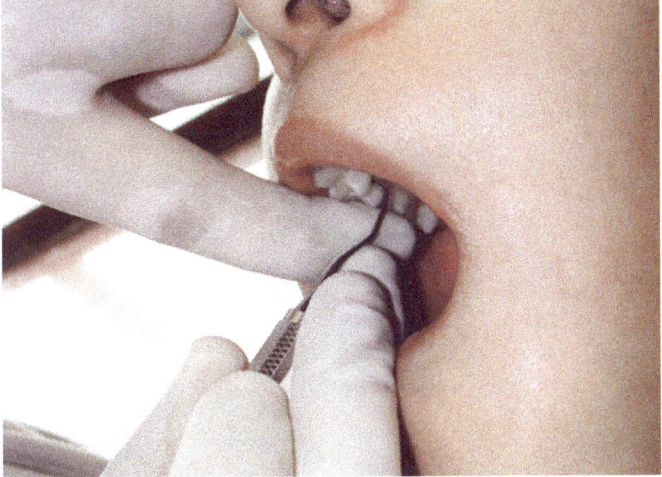

**Fig. 42.7:** Clinical picture showing scaling in maxillary right posterior sextant: lingual aspect.

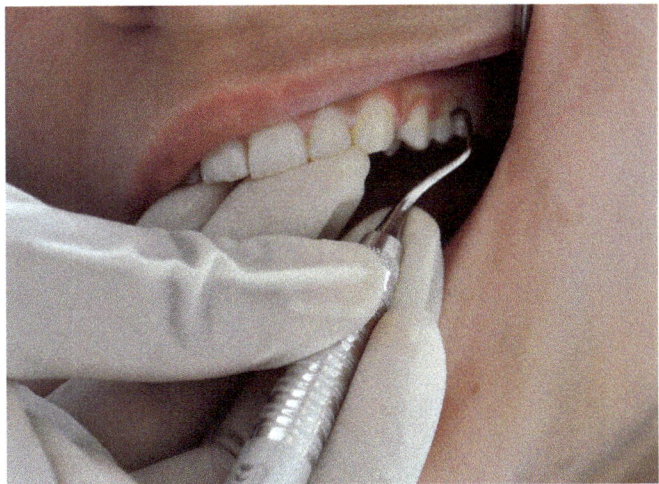

**Fig. 42.9:** Clinical picture showing scaling in the maxillary left posterior sextant: facial aspect.

*Maxillary left posterior sextant: Lingual aspect* (**Fig. 42.10**)
- *Position:* Front position
- *Illumination:* Direct
- *Visibility:* Direct
- *Retraction:* None
- *Finger rest:* Intraoral, palm down, opposite arch, reinforced. Fourth finger on the incisal or facial surfaces of the mandibular teeth.

*Maxillary left posterior sextant: Lingual aspect* (**Fig. 42.11**)
- *Position:* Front position
- *Illumination:* Direct or indirect
- *Visibility:* Direct or indirect
- *Retraction:* None
- *Finger rest:* Extraoral, palm down. The front surface of the middle and fourth fingers on the lateral aspect of the mandible on the left side of the face.

*Maxillary left posterior sextant: Lingual aspect* (**Fig. 42.12**)
- *Position:* Side or front position
- *Illumination:* Direct
- *Visibility:* Direct
- *Retraction:* None
- *Finger rest:* Intraoral, palm up. Fourth finger on the occlusal surfaces of the adjacent maxillary teeth.

The different instrumentation approaches for mandibular teeth are as follows:

*Mandibular anterior sextant: Facial aspect, surfaces towards the operator* (**Fig. 42.13**)
- *Position:* Front position
- *Illumination:* Direct
- *Visibility:* Direct
- *Retraction:* Index finger of the nonoperating hand
- *Finger rest:* Intraoral, palm down. Fourth finger on the incisal edge or the occlusal surfaces of the adjacent mandibular teeth.

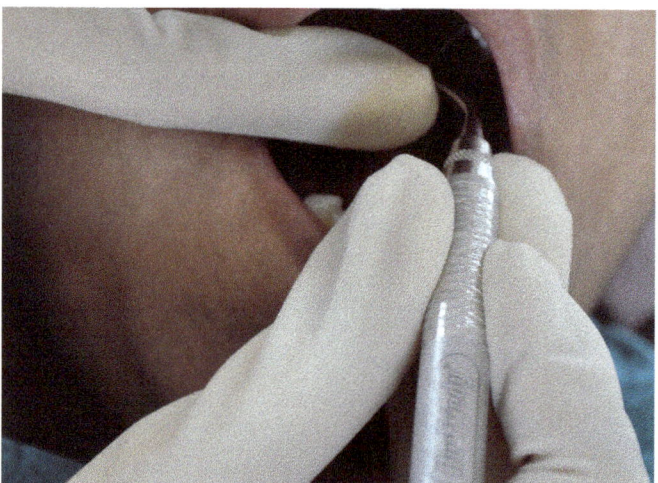

**Fig. 42.10:** Clinical picture showing scaling in the maxillary left posterior sextant: lingual aspect.

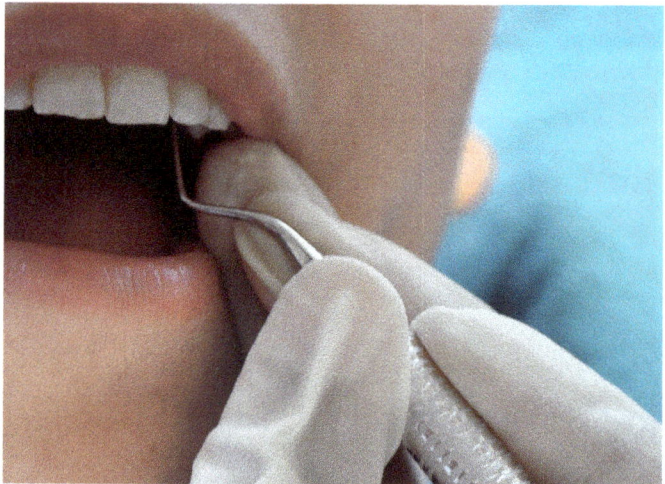

**Fig. 42.12:** Clinical picture showing scaling in the maxillary left posterior sextant: lingual aspect.

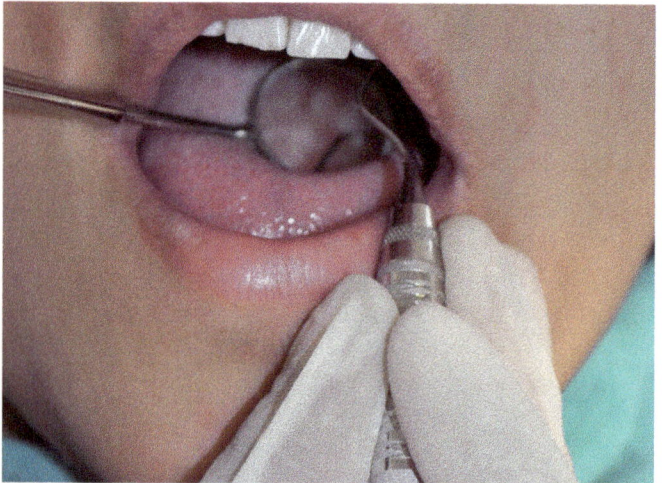

**Fig. 42.11:** Clinical picture showing scaling in the maxillary left posterior sextant: lingual aspect.

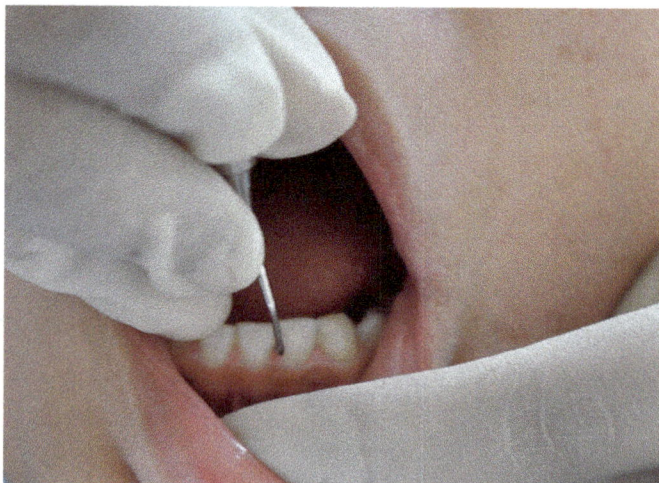

**Fig. 42.13:** Clinical picture showing scaling in mandibular anterior sextant: facial aspect, surface towards the operator.

*Mandibular anterior sextant: Facial aspect, surface away from the operator* (**Fig. 42.14**)
- *Position:* Back position
- *Illumination:* Direct
- *Visibility:* Direct
- *Retraction:* Index finger or thumb of the nonoperating hand
- *Finger rest:* Intraoral, palm down. Fourth finger on the incisal edge or the occlusal surfaces of the adjacent mandibular teeth.

*Mandibular anterior sextant: Lingual aspect, surface away from the operator* (**Fig. 42.15**)
- *Position:* Back position
- *Illumination:* Direct or indirect
- *Visibility:* Direct or indirect
- *Retraction:* Mirror retracts the tongue
- *Finger rest:* Intraoral, palm down. Fourth finger on the incisal edge or the occlusal surfaces of the adjacent mandibular teeth.

*Mandibular anterior sextant: Lingual aspect, surface towards the operator* (**Fig. 42.16**)
- *Position:* Front position
- *Illumination:* Direct or indirect
- *Visibility:* Direct or indirect
- *Retraction:* Mirror retracts the tongue
- *Finger rest:* Intraoral, palm down. Fourth finger on the incisal edge or the occlusal surfaces of the adjacent mandibular teeth.

*Mandibular right posterior sextant: Facial aspect* (**Fig. 42.17**)
- *Position:* Side or front position
- *Illumination:* Direct
- *Visibility:* Direct
- *Retraction:* Mirror or index finger of the nonoperating hand
- *Finger rest:* Intraoral, palm down. Fourth finger on the incisal edge or the occlusal surfaces of the adjacent mandibular teeth.

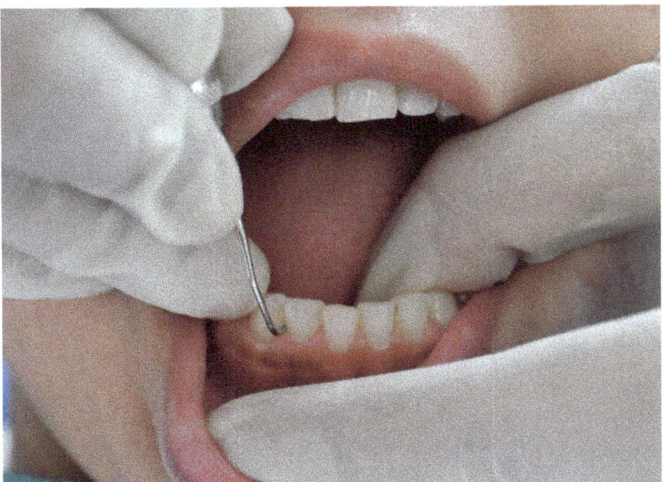

**Fig. 42.14:** Clinical picture showing scaling in mandibular anterior sextant: facial aspect, surface away from the operator.

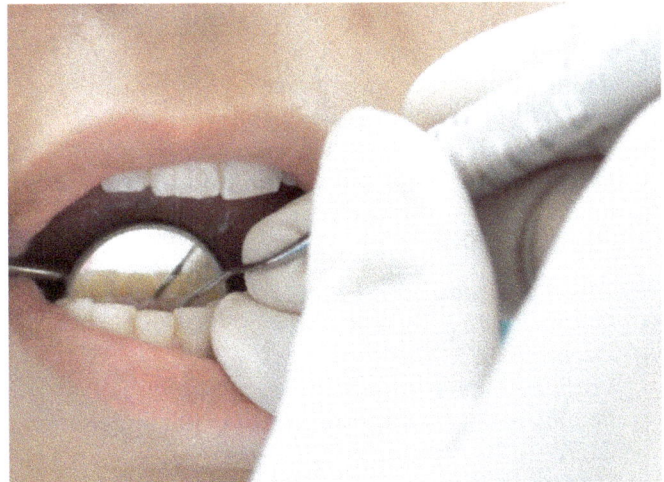

**Fig. 42.16:** Clinical picture showing scaling in mandibular anterior sextant: lingual aspect, surface towards the operator.

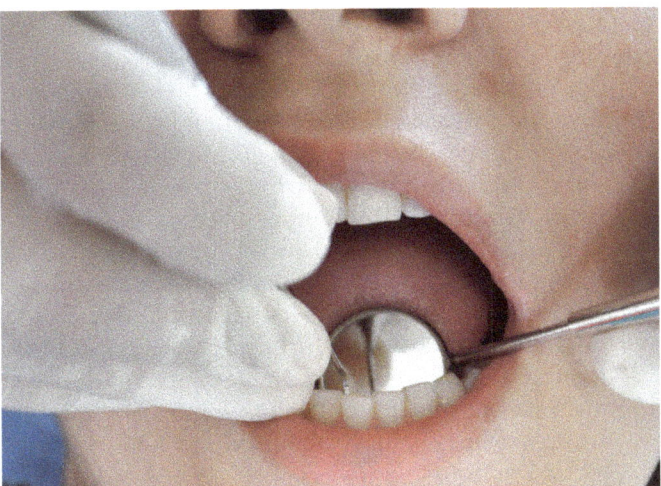

**Fig. 42.15:** Clinical picture showing scaling in mandibular anterior sextant: lingual aspect, surface away from the operator.

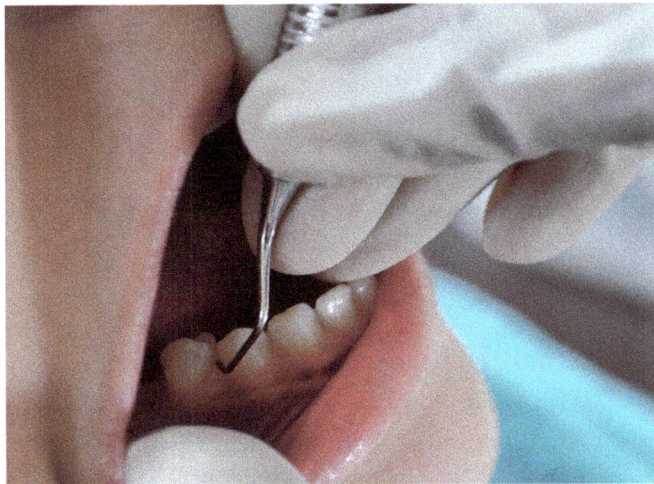

**Fig. 42.17:** Clinical picture showing scaling in mandibular right posterior sextant: facial aspect.

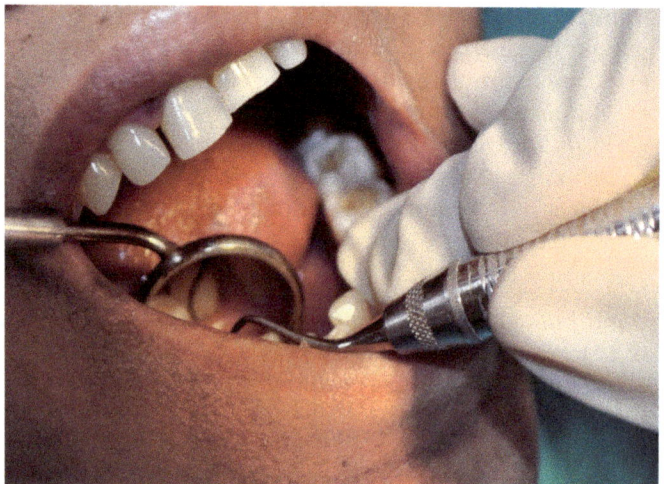

**Fig. 42.18:** Clinical picture showing scaling in mandibular right posterior sextant: lingual aspect.

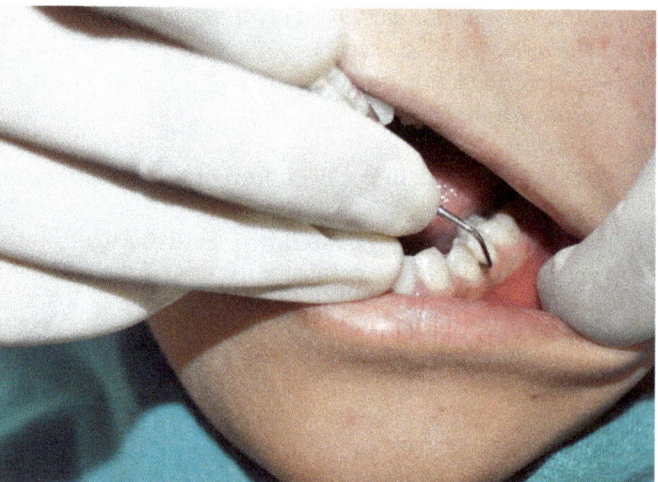

**Fig. 42.19:** Clinical picture showing scaling in mandibular left posterior sextant: facial aspect.

*Mandibular right posterior sextant: Lingual aspect* (**Fig. 42.18**)
- *Position:* Front position
- *Illumination:* Direct or indirect
- *Visibility:* Direct or indirect
- *Retraction:* Mirror retracts the tongue
- *Finger rest:* Intraoral, palm down. Fourth finger on the incisal edge or the occlusal surfaces of the adjacent mandibular teeth.

*Mandibular left posterior sextant: Facial aspect* (**Fig. 42.19**)
- *Position:* Side or back position
- *Illumination:* Direct
- *Visibility:* Direct or indirect
- *Retraction:* Index finger or mirror of the nonoperating hand
- *Finger rest:* Intraoral, palm down. Fourth finger on the incisal edge or the occlusal surfaces of the adjacent mandibular teeth.

*Mandibular left posterior sextant: Lingual aspect* (**Fig. 42.20**)
- *Position:* Front or side position
- *Illumination:* Direct or indirect
- *Visibility:* Direct
- *Retraction:* Mirror retracts the tongue
- *Finger rest:* Intraoral, palm down. Fourth finger on the incisal edge or the occlusal surfaces of the adjacent mandibular teeth.

## FULL-MOUTH DISINFECTION

Conventional periodontal therapy involving scaling and root planing is always conducted in a quadrant- or sextant-wise manner and is usually completed in 4–6 weeks. In 1995, Quirynen et al., introduced a full-mouth disinfection approach for management of periodontal infections, which

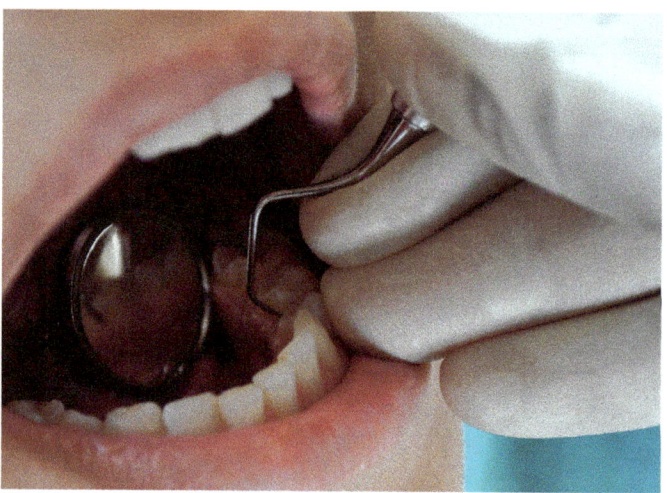

**Fig. 42.20:** Clinical picture showing scaling in mandibular left posterior sextant: lingual aspect.

involves conducting the entire scaling and root planing in one stage within 24 hours.[8]

The rationale behind full-mouth disinfection is to suppress the risk of cross-contamination between treated and untreated sites as well as other ecologic habitats.

Following is the original protocol of full-mouth disinfection introduced by Quirynen et al.:
- Full-mouth scaling and root planing involve the procedure performed on entire dentition in two visits within 24 hours, i.e., two consecutive days under local anesthesia—this minimizes the total number of subgingival pathogenic bacteria and induces an environment suitable for healing.
- Brushing of the dorsum of tongue with 1% chlorhexidine gel for 1 minute.
- Rinsing mouth twice with 0.2% chlorhexidine mouthrinse for 1 minute. During the last 10 seconds,

the patient should gargle in order to reach the tonsils—this helps to eradicate the remaining bacteria.
- Followed by both sessions of scaling and root planing, subgingival irrigation of all pockets, three times within 10 minutes, with chlorhexidine 1% gel and repetition on day 8, using a syringe with marks at 6 mm and 8 mm—this inhibits the bacteria colonizing this habitat.
- Rinsing the mouth with 10 mL of 0.2% chlorhexidine mouthrinse twice daily for 1 minute for the following two weeks at home—this reduces the risk of reinfection of the treated pockets within a short time span and creates a new and less pathogenic subgingival environment composed of beneficial bacteria.
- Oral hygiene instructions on proper toothbrushing, interdental cleansing with interdental brushes or other aids, and tongue brushing also.

Thus, the full-mouth approach helps to minimize the number of visits for patients and time spent on treatment. It also avoids the transmission of pathogens from other intraoral niches and subgingival sites. However, the approach is failed to rule out reinfection by transmission from an extraoral source or person.

## EVALUATION OF SCALING AND ROOT PLANING

*Immediately after scaling and root planing:* Tooth surfaces should be carefully inspected visually with optimal lighting and with the aid of a mouth mirror and compressed air. They should also be examined with a fine explorer or probe. Subgingival surfaces should be hard and smooth. Thus, smoothness is the criterion by which scaling and root planing are immediately evaluated.[9-12]

*After two weeks of scaling and root planing:* The ultimate evaluation of instrumentation is based on tissue response. Probing should not be conducted before two weeks postoperatively because re-epithelialization takes approximately 1–2 weeks.[13] If the treated site still elicits bleeding on probing, assessment of bleeding site should be done. If the bleeding occurs from the margin of the gingiva, that means newly-formed plaque may be the reason, and just reinforcement of oral hygiene may resolve the inflammation. If the bleeding occurs from the base of the pocket, then it is due to persistent inflammation produced by residual plaque or calculus deposits, which were not removed during scaling and root planing.

### Points to Ponder
- Scaling strokes are short and powerful pull strokes.
- Root planing strokes are longer and lighter pull strokes.
- Scaling and root planing strokes should be confined to the instrumentation zone, i.e., the zone where calculus or altered cementum is found. Sweeping the instrument over the crown where it is not needed wastes operating time, dulls the instrument, and causes loss of control.

## REFERENCES

1. Pattison GL, Pattison AM. Scaling and root planing. In: Newman MG, Takei HH, Carranza FA (Eds). Carranza's Clinical Periodontology, 9th edition. Philadelphia, PA, USA: WB Saunders; 2003. pp. 631-45.
2. Cohen DW, Sherwood LA. Scaling and root planing: removal of calculus and subgingival organisms. In: Genco RJ, Goldman HM, Cohen DW (Eds). Contemporary Periodontics, 6th edition. St. Louis: CV Mosby; 1990. pp. 400-18.
3. Grant DA, Stern IB, Listgarten MA. Scaling and root planing. In: Periodontics in the Tradition of Gottlieb and Orban, 6th edition. St. Louis: CV Mosby; 1988. pp. 650-718.
4. Fleischer HC, Mellonig JT, Brayer WK, Gray JL, Barnett JD. Scaling and root planing efficacy in multirooted teeth. J Periodontol. 1989;60(7):402-9.
5. Wilkins EM. Clinical Practice of the Dental Hygienist, 7th edition. Philadelphia, PA, USA: Lippincott Williams & Wilkins; 1994.
6. Barnes JE, Schaffer EM. Subgingival root planing: a comparison using files, hoes, and curettes. J Periodontol. 1960;31:300.
7. Brayer WK, Mellonig JT, Dunlop RM, Marinak KW, Carson RE. Scaling and root planing effectiveness: the effect of root surface access and operator experience. J Periodontol. 1989;60(1):67-72.
8. Quirynen M, Bollen CM, Vandekerckhove BN, Dekeyser C, Papaioannou W, Eyssen H. Full-versus partial-mouth disinfection in the treatment of periodontal infections: short-term clinical and microbiological observations. J Dent Res. 1995;74(8):1459-67.
9. Badersten A, Nilvéus R, Egelberg J. Effect of nonsurgical periodontal therapy. I. Moderately advanced periodontitis. J Clin Periodontol. 1981;8(1):57-72.
10. Garrett JS. Effects of nonsurgical periodontal therapy on periodontitis in humans. A review. J Clin Periodontol. 1983;10(5):515-23.
11. Lowenguth RA, Greenstein G. Clinical and microbiological response to nonsurgical mechanical periodontal therapy. Periodontol 2000. 1995;9:14-22.
12. Sbordone L, Ramaglia L, Gulletta E, Iacono V. Recolonization of the subgingival microflora after scaling and root planing in human periodontitis. J Periodontol. 1990;61(9):579-84.
13. Stahl SS, Weiner JM, Benjamin S, Yamada L. Soft tissue healing following curettage and root planing. J Periodontol. 1971;42:678-84.

### VIVA VOCE

**Q1.** Why is single heavy stroke not used to remove subgingival calculus?
**Ans.** With a single heavy stroke, the blade skips over or skims the surface of the calculus. Subsequent strokes made with the entire cutting edge tend to shave the deposit down layer by layer. When a series of these repeated whittling strokes are applied, the calculus may be reduced to a thin, smooth, burnished sheet that is difficult to distinguish from the surrounding root surface.

**Section 6:** Treatment: Nonsurgical Therapy

**Q2.** **What is the fundamental requirement for optimal working angulation?**
**Ans.** Parallelism is the fundamental requirement for optimal working angulation. The lower shank of the instrument should be parallel or nearly parallel to the tooth surface being treated.

**Q3.** **Why finger rest must be close enough to the working area?**
**Ans.** When finger rest is placed too far from the working area, the clinician in an effort to obtain parallelism and proper angulation separates the middle finger from the fourth finger, i.e., finger rest. Effective wrist-arm motion is possible only when these two fingers are kept together in a built-up fulcrum. Separation of the fingers commits the clinician to the exclusive use of finger flexing for the activation of strokes.

**Q4.** **What is the primary objective of scaling and root planing?**
**Ans.** Restoration of gingival health by complete removal of the dental plaque and calculus.

**Q5.** **Why is subgingival scaling difficult to perform as compared to supragingival scaling?**
**Ans.** Subgingival scaling is performed apical to the gingival margin, which impairs the visibility and freedom of movement. Visibility is also obscured by the bleeding.

**Q6.** **Which instruments are used for subgingival scaling and root planing?**
**Ans.** Universal or area-specific (Gracey) curettes, hoes, Hirschfeld files, and thin ultrasonic tips can also be useful.

**Q7.** **Which instruments are used for supragingival scaling?**
**Ans.** Sickle scalers, curettes, and ultrasonic and sonic instruments are most commonly used during supragingival scaling.

**Q8.** **Who introduced full-mouth disinfection approach for management of periodontal infections?**
**Ans.** Marc Quirynen et al., in 1995.

**Q9.** **What is the instrumentation approach for the maxillary anterior sextant, facial aspect, surface away from the operator?**
**Ans.** Position: Front; Illumination: Direct; Visibility: Direct; Retraction: Index finger of nonoperating hand; Finger rest: Intraoral, palm up. Fourth finger on the incisal edges or the occlusal or facial surfaces of adjacent maxillary teeth.

**Q10.** **For how much time after scaling and root planing probing should not be done?**
**Ans.** Probing should not be conducted before two weeks postoperatively because re-epithelialization takes approximately 1–2 weeks.

# Chapter 43: Sonic and Ultrasonic Scaling

*Shalu Bathla*

## Chapter Outline

- Sonic Scalers
- Ultrasonic Scalers
- Tip Designs
- Mechanism of Action
- Ultrasonic Scaling Technique
- Potential Hazards
- Contraindications

## INTRODUCTION

Since hand scalers were technically demanding, time-consuming, and tiring for both the operator and the patient, and as a result, power-driven scalers have been developed during the last decades **(Table 43.1)**. Ultrasound was first introduced in the periodontal procedure as ultrasonic scalers in 1955 by Zinner. Power-driven instruments are slender with probe-like tips, which allow efficient instrumentation of deep, periodontal pockets with less operator fatigue, these instruments have become an accepted treatment modality for removing subgingival biofilm and calculus. Powered instruments used for periodontal debridement can be classified into two groups on the basis of their operating frequencies: sonic and ultrasonic scalers[1] **(Table 43.2)**.

**TABLE 43.1:** Comparison between ultrasonic and manual scalers.

| Parameters | Ultrasonic scalers | Hand scalers |
|---|---|---|
| Mechanism of action | Vibration, acoustic streaming, and cavitation | Mechanical removal of deposits |
| Uses | Used on heavy tenacious deposits and stains | Used on all amounts of deposits |
| Nature of instrument tip | Dull and bulky | Sharp and thin |
| Tip size | Smaller tip size 0.3–0.55 mm | Larger tip size 0.76–1 mm |
| Tactile sensitivity | Less | Good |
| Activation | Digital-motion activation is used with light pressure | Hand-motion activation is used with firm pressure |
| Accessibility | Inaccessible to some areas because of tip design | Greater accessibility |
| Time requirement | Less time required | More time required |
| Clinician's comfort | Less clinician fatigue | More clinician fatigue |
| Patient's comfort | Water spray causes patient discomfort | No water spray, no discomfort |
| Heat production | Possibility of damage to the tooth from heat build-up | No heat build-up |
| Aerosol production | Aerosols are produced | No aerosols are produced |
| Contraindications | Contraindicated in patients with a pacemaker and having contagious diseases | No such contraindications |
| Sharpening | Not needed frequently | Frequently required |

**TABLE 43.2:** Comparison between sonic and ultrasonic scalers.

| Parameters | Sonic scalers | Ultrasonic scalers |
|---|---|---|
| Separate installation | Not needed as they are used with air pressure | Required |
| Heat production | Less | More |
| Noise production | More | Less |
| Range of vibration | Low | High |
| Tip amplitude | High | Low |

**TABLE 43.3:** Comparison between magnetostrictive and piezoelectric scalers.

| Parameters | Magnetostrictive scalers | Piezoelectric scalers |
|---|---|---|
| Principle of working | Vibrations are produced due to expansion or contraction of ferromagnetic material in an alternating electromagnetic field | Vibrations are produced due to dimensional changes in crystals housed within handpiece as electricity passes over the surface of crystals |
| Tip motion | Elliptical | Linear |
| Vibration | 18–42 kHz | 24–50 kHz |

## SONIC SCALERS

Sonic scaler handpieces were invented during the 1960s. Sonic scalers operate at a relatively low frequency of 3,000–8,000 cycles per second (3–8 kHz) and are driven by compressed air from the dental unit. The stroke pattern of sonic scalers is elliptical to orbital, and all the surfaces of the tip can be adapted to root surfaces. Some sonic scalers are equipped with fiberoptics also. The major disadvantage associated with sonic scalers is high noise level because of the release of air pressure needed for the movement of the tip of the sonic handpiece.[2-4]

## ULTRASONIC SCALERS

Ultrasonic scalers can be further categorized into magnetostrictive and piezoelectric **(Table 43.3)** based on the mechanism used to convert the electrical current used for energy to activate the tips.[2-5]

### Magnetostrictive Ultrasonics

Magnetostrictive ultrasonics operate inaudibly, and the instrument is comprised of an electronic generator, a handpiece assembly containing a coil to energize the insert, and a variety of interchangeable inserts. The insert comprises either a nickel-iron alloy or a ferrous rod. The generator produces an alternating low-voltage electric current in the handpiece. This current produces a magnetic field in the handpiece that causes the insert to expand and contract along its length and, in turn, causes the insert tip to vibrate. The tip vibrates in an elliptical to orbital motion at 18,000–42,000 kHz (cycles per second).

### Piezoelectric Scalers

Piezoelectric scalers **(Fig. 43.1)** are also inaudible, operating within a range of 24,000–45,000 kHz. This type of powered scaler uses electrical energy to activate crystals within the handpiece to vibrate the tip. In contrast to the magnetostrictive scalers, the tip's motion is linear in nature, resulting in the activation of mainly the lateral surfaces of the tip. This system is comprised of an electronic generator, a handpiece assembly containing piezo (ceramic) crystals to energize a scaling tip, and a variety of interchangeable screw-on tips. The generator produces an alternating,

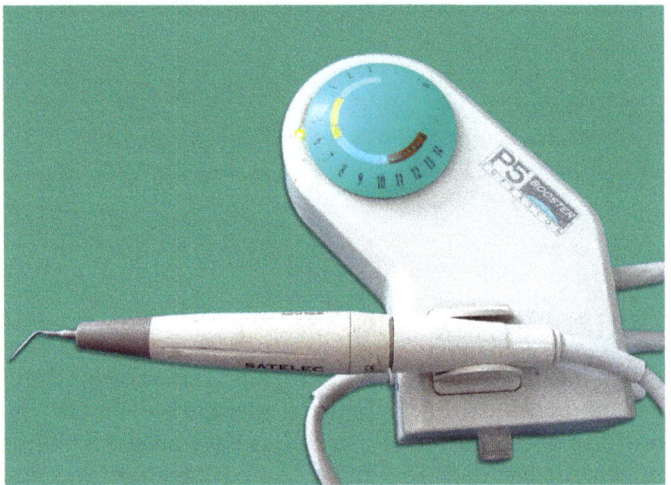

**Fig. 43.1:** Photograph showing piezoelectric scaler.

high voltage in the handpiece. This voltage produces an electric field in the handpiece that causes the piezo crystals to expand and contract along their diameter and, in turn, causes the scaling tip to vibrate.

## TIP DESIGNS

### Sonic Scaler Tips

Sonic scaler tips are large in diameter and universal in design.

### Ultrasonic Tips

Earlier ultrasonic tips were bulky, difficult to adapt, and most efficient for heavy supragingival calculus. Now, a variety of insert tip designs and shapes are available to use, and current tips are smaller and designed to be both site-specific and job-specific **(Fig. 43.2)**. Large diameter tips are created in universal design and are indicated for the removal of large, tenacious deposits; a high-power setting is generally recommended. Thinner diameter tips may have a site-specific design. The straight tip design is ideal for treating patients with gingivitis and for deplaquing

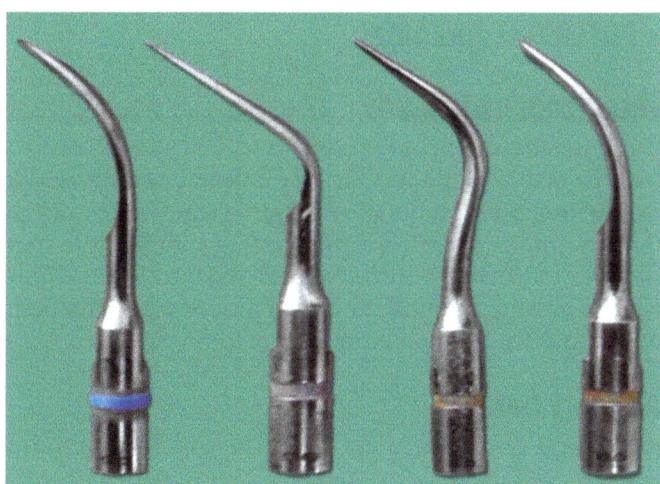

**Fig. 43.2:** Photograph showing ultrasonic tips.

in maintenance patients. The right and left contra-angled instruments to allow for greater access and adaptation to root morphology. These inserts are designed to work at a low-power setting and may even be used for exploration.

## Modified Tips

Tips are designed for furcation to enhance debridement in class II and III furcation defects. Diamond-coated tips have been shown to remove more calculus in moderate- to-deep pockets.

## MECHANISM OF ACTION

### Frequency

It is defined as the number of times per second an insert tip moves back and forth during one cycle in an orbital, elliptic, or linear-stroke path. It is important because it determines the area of the insert tip that is considered active. Only the active portion of the insert can remove hard and soft debris.

### Stroke

It is the maximum distance the insert tip travels during one cycle or stroke path. Amplitude is equal to one-half of the distance of the stroke. The power knob on an ultrasonic unit controls the stroke length of the insert during one cycle. Increasing the power knob increases the distance the tip travels while the frequency remains constant. High-power settings produce a longer stroke pattern, and lower power settings provide a shorter stroke pattern.

### Water Flow

Water knob controls the volume of water being delivered to the insert tip. Manual-tuned units have three control knobs on the front panel labeled: (1) water, (2) tuning, and (3) power. Manual technology allows the clinician to control the frequency of the unit by adjusting the tuning knob. Auto-tuned units have two control knobs, water, and power, and maintain a stable frequency. These units work through feedback that constantly adjusts the insert tip to ensure that it is vibrating at the predetermined frequency level.

Water contributes to the following physiologic effects that enhance the efficacy of power scalers: acoustic streaming, acoustic turbulence, and cavitation.

- *Acoustic streaming*: It is the unidirectional fluid flow caused by ultrasound waves.
- *Acoustic turbulence*: It is created when the movement of the tip causes the coolant to accelerate, producing an intensified swirling effect. This turbulence continues until cavitation occurs.[6]
- *Cavitation*: The vibratory motion of the tip and the continuous stream of water cause tremendous pressure, creating powerful bursts of collapsing bubbles. This is referred to as cavitation. It is a combination of the vibrating instrument's tip against the deposit, high-frequency sound waves, and exploding bubbles that allow calculus removal.

The combination of acoustic streaming, acoustic turbulence and cavitation has been shown to disrupt microflora, since bacteria and gram-negative motile rods, in particular, are sensitive to acoustic energy.

## ULTRASONIC SCALING TECHNIQUE

Ultrasonic scaling is done in the following manner:[7-9]
- *Patient preparation*: Direct the patient to rinse for one minute with an antimicrobial mouthrinse, such as 0.12% chlorhexidine to reduce the contaminated aerosol.
- *Preparation of ultrasonic unit*: Thoroughly wipe the ultrasonic unit with a disinfectant and cover the ultrasonic unit or control knobs with plastic or latex barriers. Use a sterile, autoclavable ultrasonic handpiece. Flush the waterlines and handpiece for approximately 2 minutes to decrease the number of microorganisms in the lines. Whenever possible, use waterline filters or sterile water.
- *Operator preparation*: The operator and the assistant should wear protective eyewear and masks and use high-speed evacuation to minimize the inhalation of the contaminated aerosol produced during instrumentation.
- *Patient and operator positioning*: Slightly raise the back of the patient's chair as it allows easy pooling of water and provides better and direct visibility of certain areas.
- *Power setting*: Depending on the unit used, power setting and water need to be adjusted with each tip application. The sturdier tips can accommodate a higher power setting, whereas finer tips require less power. Medium-to-high power settings are recommended for heavy debris removal, and low-to-

medium settings are recommended for removing light debris. But, the power setting should begin on low and be adjusted not higher than necessary to remove calculus. Medium-to-high power settings have been shown to cause damage to roots when the tip is not parallel to the root surface.

- *Turn on the unit, select tip and place it into the handpiece*: Magnetostrictive device is inserted by pushing downward with a slight twist until the O-ring is within the handpiece and the tip securely in place. For the piezoelectric system, a wrench is used to screw the tip into the handpiece. Adjust the water control knob to produce a light mist of water at the working tip.
- *Pen grasp and finger rest*: The instrument is grasped with a light pen or modified pen grasp. Light grasp increases tactile sensitivity and a patient's comfort and reduces clinician's fatigue.

The bulk of the powered instrument's handpiece and attached cord sometimes requires the use of an extraoral fulcrum to maintain control of the instruments. An extraoral fulcrum provides balance rather than strength. A finger rest or extraoral fulcrum should be established to allow a very light, feather-like touch. For maxillary teeth, extraoral hand rests should be used, and for mandibular teeth, either intraoral or extraoral fulcrums may be used.

> **Clinical Tip**
> Tip to tooth adaptation should be 0–15°. More than 15° causes gouging on the root surfaces and injury to soft tissue.

Powered handpieces are heavier than manual instruments, and moreover, weight from the cord drags, which require adjustments in the cord placement. To reduce tension from the cord and correct the instrument's adaptation, the cord is wrapped around the forearm.

- *Adaptation and angulation*: Like manual instrumentation, an adaptation of the anterior 2–3 mm of the tip is appropriate. Keep the working tip adapted to the tooth surface as it is passed over the deposit. Heavy lateral pressure is unnecessary because the vibrational energy of the instrument dislodges the calculus. However, the working end must touch the deposit for this to occur. The working end should be kept in constant motion, and the tip should be kept parallel to the tooth surface or at not more than a 15° angle to avoid grooving of the tooth surface.
- *Strokes*: Use short, light, vertical, horizontal, or oblique overlapping strokes.
- The instrument should be switched off periodically to allow for aspiration of water, and the tooth surface should be examined frequently with an explorer.
- Any remaining irregularities of the root surface should be removed thereafter with sharp curettes.

## POTENTIAL HAZARDS

### Thrombogenic Hazards

If the oscillating tip of the ultrasonic scaler contacts a tooth, it may be possible that the tooth acts as a waveguide conducting the vibrational energy from the scaler towards the apex of the root. If sufficient energy reaches the root, then it could pose a thrombogenic hazard to the blood vessels passing through the apical foramen into the pulp, which may lead to a potential loss of tooth vitality.

### Auditory Hazards

Ultrasonic scalers may act as a potential hazard to the auditory system of both clinicians and patients. Chronic acoustic trauma is caused by prolonged exposure to lower intensity sound irritant. The damage is irreversible because cochlear hair cells cannot regenerate. Damage to operator hearing is possible through airborne subharmonics of the ultrasonic scaler. For the patient, damage can occur through the transmission of ultrasound through tooth contact to the inner ear via the skull's bones.

### Vibrational Hazards

The vibration amplitude associated with dental scalers is small but has the potential to produce a "white finger." There is a disruption in the blood flow to the fingers, caused by the vibration that is passed from the scaler through to the hand.

### Aerosol Production Hazards

Micik and colleagues defined dental aerosols as being particles smaller than 50 μm, with any particles larger than 50 μm being described as splatter. These particles behaved in a ballistic manner means that these particles are ejected forcibly from the operating site, and they arch in a trajectory similar to that of a bullet until they contact a surface or fall to the floor.

The aerosol produced by sonic and ultrasonic instrumentation may contain potentially infectious blood- and airborne pathogens. *Pneumococci*, *Staphylococci*, alpha-hemolytic streptococci, and *Mycobacterium tuberculosis* are among the bacteria that have been found in dental aerosols.

Both large and small aerosol particles may contain blood elements with attached viral particles, such as herpes simplex virus, influenza virus, common cold viruses, Epstein-Barr virus, cytomegalovirus, human immunodeficiency virus and hepatitis B virus. Of additional concern are pathogens that do not originate from patients but are from the contaminated waterlines of the dental unit or the ultrasonic device. Putative pathogens, such as *Pseudomonas sp.* and *Legionella pneumophila*, have been isolated from dental unit water and can become aerosolized by an ultrasonic scaler. Aerosol from ultrasonic instrumentation always contains blood and lingers in the air for 30 minutes or longer in the entire operatory and in areas of the dental office outside the operatory.[10-13]

Following are the ways that can reduce hazards of aerosols production:[14,15]

- *Protective barriers*: Unprotected patients may be more susceptible to infection from the aerosol than dental personnel who are wearing protective barriers, such as masks, gloves, eyewear, and clinical clothing. A well-fitting surgical facemask, i.e., theater or dome-type facemask is preferable to the paper type, which rapidly becomes permeable and inefficient. Masks should have at least 95% filtration efficiency for particles 3.0–5.0 μm in diameter. Ideally, the mask should be changed for each patient. It should be changed after 20 minutes in aerosol or 60 minutes in nonaerosol environments. Protective glasses with top and side shields must be worn while treating patients.

### Clinical Tip
Preprocedural antiseptic mouthrinse and the use of HVEs are the main ways to reduce the hazards of aerosol's production during ultrasonic instrumentation.

- *Position of the patient*: The position of a patient during dental treatment is also significant. A patient should be treated in the supine position, which, apart from other advantages, makes it possible for a doctor to avoid work in the breath way of a patient.
- *High-volume evacuator (HVE)*: HVE removes a large volume of air within a short period. It usually has an opening of 8 mm or more and evacuates up to 100 cubic feet of air per minute. It can reduce the contamination arising from the operative site by more than 90%.
- *Preprocedural rinsing*: Rinse the oral cavity of a patient with an antiseptic, e.g., chlorhexidine, before the procedure.
- *Flushing of the handpiece and waterlines or a self-contained sterile water source, thorough disinfection of environmental surfaces*: The first flushing assures elimination of microflora whose presence is due to the night stagnation. The second rinsing for 20–30 seconds is recommended, to help reduce the risk of retraction of the oral cavity fluids, and aims at the elimination of potential cross-infection.
- Adequate ventilation and air filtration units with high-efficiency particulate air (HEPA) filters effectively reduce the bacterial load in the operatory environment. A dental unit should be rinsed at the beginning of a working day, and between patients.

## CONTRAINDICATIONS

- *Pacemakers*: Patients with a pacemaker poses electromagnetic interference, especially to magnetostrictive, but newer models of pacemakers are insulated and bipolar, so electromagnetic interference is unlikely.
- *Patients with contagious and communicable diseases*: Hepatitis, tuberculosis, throat, and respiratory infections wherein transmission via aerosols is possible.
- *Composite resin and porcelain inlays or crown*: For demineralized tooth structure, hypersensitive areas, veneers, cast crowns, and implants, ultrasonic instrumentation may harm the surfaces.
- *Children*: Primary and newly erupted teeth have larger pulp areas and are more susceptible to heat.
- *Immunocompromised patient*: The creation of aerosols may increase the patient's risk of infection.

### Points to Ponder
- The magnetostrictive tip moves in an elliptical pattern.
- The piezoelectric tip moves in a linear pattern.

## REFERENCES

1. Zinner DD. Recent ultrasonic dental studies, including periodontia, without the use of an abrasive. J Dent Res. 1955;34:748-9.
2. Menne A, Griesinger H, Jepsen S, Albers H, Jepsen K. Vibration characteristics of oscillating scalers. J Dent Res. 1994;73:434-9.
3. Loos B, Kiger R, Egelberg J. An evaluation of basic periodontal therapy using sonic and ultrasonic scalers. J Clin Periodontol. 1987;14(1):29-33.
4. Drisko CL, Cochran DL, Blieden T, Bouwsma OJ, Cohen RE, Damoulis P, et al. Position paper: sonic and ultrasonic scalers in periodontics. Research, Science and Therapy Committee of the American Academy of Periodontology. J Periodontol. 2000;71(11):1792-801.
5. Flemmig TF, Petersilka GJ, Mehl A, Hickel R, Klaiber B. Working parameters of a magnetostrictive ultrasonic scaler influencing root substance removal in vitro. J Periodontol. 1998;69(5):547-53.
6. Khambay BS, Walmsley AD. Acoustic microstreaming: detection and measurement around ultrasonic scalers. J Periodontol. 1999;70(6):626-31.
7. Nield-Gehrig JS. Basic concepts of ultrasonic instrumentation. In: Fundamentals of Periodontal Instrumentation, 4th edition. Philadelphia, PA, USA: Lippincott Williams & Wilkins; 2000. pp. 538-78.
8. Petersilka GJ, Flemmig TF. Sonic and ultrasonic instrumentation. In: Newman MG, Takei HH, Carranza FA (Eds). Carranza's Clinical Periodontology, 9th edition. Philadelphia, PA, USA: WB Saunders; 2002. pp. 828-35.
9. Pattison AM, Pattison GL. Scaling and root planing. In: Newman MG, Takei HH, Klokevold PR, Carranza FA (Eds). Carranza's Clinical Periodontology, 10th edition. Philadelphia, PA, USA: WB Saunders; 2006. pp. 749-97.
10. Rivera-Hidalgo F, Barnes JB, Harrel SK. Aerosol and splatter production by focused spray and standard ultrasonic inserts. J Periodontol. 1999;70(5):473-7.
11. Timmerman MF, Menso L, Steinfort J, van Winkelhoff AJ, van der Weijden GA. Atmospheric contamination during ultrasonic scaling. J Clin Periodontol. 2004;31:458-62.
12. Trenter SC, Walmsley AD. Ultrasonic dental scaler: associated hazards. J Clin Periodontol. 2003;30(2):95-101.

13. Harrel SK. Airborne spread of disease—the implication for dentistry. J Calif Dent Assoc. 2004;32(11):901-6.
14. Harrel SK, Barnes JB, Rivera-Hidalgo F. Reduction of aerosols produced by ultrasonic scalers. J Periodontol. 1996;67(1):28-32.
15. King TB, Muzzin KB, Berry CW, Anders LM. The effectiveness of an aerosol reduction device for ultrasonic scalers. J Periodontol. 1997;68(1):45-9.

## VIVA VOCE

**Q1.** What is the difference between splatter and aerosol?
**Ans.** The particle of the true aerosol is less than 50 μm in diameter, while the splatter particle is greater than 50 μm.

**Q2.** What are the methods to reduce the hazards of aerosols produced by ultrasonic instrumentation?
**Ans.** The hazards of aerosols produced by ultrasonic instrumentation can be reduced with the help of the following methods:
- Preprocedural antiseptic mouthrinse
- Use of HVEs
- High-risk infective patients should be treated with hand instruments.

**Q3.** For how much minimum time period the aerosols which are produced by ultrasonic scaling remain in the air?
**Ans.** The aerosols produced by ultrasonic scaling remain in the air for at least 30 minutes.

**Q4.** What is cavitation?
**Ans.** The vibratory motion of the tip and the continuous stream of water cause tremendous pressure, creating powerful bursts of collapsing bubbles. This is referred to as cavitation.

**Q5.** What is the major contraindication for ultrasonic scaler?
**Ans.** Patients with a pacemaker.

**Q6.** What is the mechanism of action of ultrasonic scalers?
**Ans.** Vibration, acoustic streaming, and cavitation.

**Q7.** Which scaler produces more noise?
**Ans.** Sonic scalers.

**Q8.** What are the potential hazards of ultrasonic scaling?
**Ans.** Thrombogenic, auditory, vibrational, and aerosol production hazards.

**Q9.** What is the principle of working of Piezoelectric scalers?
**Ans.** Vibrations are produced due to dimensional changes in crystals housed within handpiece as electricity passes over the surface of crystals.

**Q10.** How is acoustic turbulence created?
**Ans.** It is created when the tip's movement causes the coolant to accelerate, producing an intensified swirling effect. This turbulence continues until cavitation occurs.

# Chapter 44: Splinting

Harpreet S Grover

## Chapter Outline

- Historical Perspective
- Definition
- Objectives
- Indications
- Contraindications
- Advantages
- Disadvantages
- Classifications

## INTRODUCTION

Splinting is the stabilization of teeth by splints to provide rest and redistribute functional and parafunctional forces. Splinting can be temporary or long term, which does not prevent or treat periodontal disease.

## HISTORICAL PERSPECTIVE

Early evidence of splinting weakened teeth can be seen in archeological findings. From the period of 8th century BC to the 1st century AD, Etruscans civilization reported the use of wire ligation and small gold rings and bands to stabilize loose teeth. In 1723, Fauchard ligated and banded teeth to stabilize them.[1] In the 1900s, several authors described splinting techniques. Hirschfeld (1950) was one of the first modern periodontal authors to advocate ligation of periodontally diseased teeth using either stainless steel wire or silk. His technique was extracoronal and involved only the anterior teeth. In 1951, Obin and Arvins advocated the use of a self-curing internal splint to achieve temporary stabilization. Harrington (1957) modified the splint by incorporating a cemented stainless-steel wire. Cross, in 1954, suggested the use of an amalgam splint for fixation of mobile posterior teeth.

## DEFINITION

A splint is any appliance that joins two or more teeth to provide support.[2] Splintee is the tooth that needs support. Splinters are the adjacent teeth that provide support.

## OBJECTIVES

Objectives of splinting are as follows:[3,4]
- *To provide rest*: Occlusal rest provided by splint therapy in one form or another helps to eliminate or neutralize some adverse occlusal factors.
- *To redirect forces*: Splint helps to redirect the forces of occlusion in a more axial direction over all the teeth covered by it.
- *To redistribute forces*: Splinting provides stabilization and enhances resistance to the applied force. Such redistribution of forces acts as a safeguard and confirms that forces do not exceed the adaptive capacity.
- *To preserve arch integrity*: By restoring proximal contacts splinting helps to reduce food impaction.
- *Restoration of functional stability*: Splinting restores functional occlusion and brings stabilization of mobile abutment teeth. Splinting also enhances masticatory comfort.
- *Psychological well-being*: Splinting gives the patient comfort from mobile teeth and improves a sense of well-being.
- To stabilize mobile teeth during a surgical procedure, especially regenerative therapy.
- To protect the tooth-supporting tissues during the healing period following surgery or after an accident.
- To prevent the extrusion of unopposed teeth.
- To bring into function the teeth that cannot be used to eat efficiently.

*Ideal requirements of splints*:
- Simple design

- Economical, stable, and efficient
- Hygienic and nonirritating to the soft tissues
- Esthetically acceptable
- Not provoke iatrogenic disease

## INDICATIONS

- To stabilize moderate-to-advanced tooth mobility, which is unable to decrease by occlusal adjustment or periodontal therapy.
- Stabilize teeth in secondary occlusal trauma.
- Stabilize teeth with increased tooth mobility, which interferes with normal masticatory function.
- Make scaling and surgical procedures easy to conduct.
- Stabilize teeth after orthodontic movement.
- Stabilize teeth after an acute dental trauma, i.e., subluxation, avulsion, etc.

## CONTRAINDICATIONS

- Moderate-to-severe tooth mobility associated with periodontal inflammation and/or primary occlusal trauma.
- The inadequate number of firm teeth in order to stabilize mobile teeth.
- Unable to perform a prior occlusal adjustment on teeth with occlusal trauma or occlusal interferences.
- Patient with poor oral hygiene.
- When the sole objective of splinting is to decrease tooth mobility following the removal of the splint.

## ADVANTAGES

- Helps to achieve final stability and comfort for the patient with the history of occlusal trauma.
- Useful to reduce tooth mobility and enhance healing following acute trauma to the teeth.
- Orthodontically splinted teeth permit remodeling of alveolar bone and periodontal ligament.
- Useful in reducing mobility and favoring regenerative therapy.
- Distributes occlusal forces over a wide area.

## DISADVANTAGES

- *Hygienic*: Poor oral hygiene favors the accumulation of plaque at the splinted margins which can further damage periodontal apparatus in a patient with poor periodontal support.
- *Mechanical*: Rigid nature of the splint makes it act as a lever with uneven distribution of forces. This can injure the periodontium of all teeth within the splint when one tooth of the splint gets traumatic occlusion.
- *Biological*: Development of caries is an unavoidable risk and, thus, requires excellent maintenance by the patient.

## CLASSIFICATIONS

- *According to the type of material*:
    - A-splints
    - Braided wire splint
    - Bonded, composite resin splint
- *According to the location on the tooth*:
    - *Intracoronal*:
        - Composite resin with wire
        - Inlays
        - Nylon wire
    - *Extracoronal*:
        - Night guard
        - Welded band
        - Tooth-bonded plastic
- *According to the period of stabilization*:
    - *Temporary stabilization*: Worn for less than six months.
        - Removable: Occlusal splint with wire and Hawley with splinting arch wire.
        - Fixed: Intracoronal and extracoronal
    - *Provisional stabilization*: To be used for 6–12 months, e.g., acrylic splints and metal bands.
    - *Permanent splints*: Used indefinitely
        - Removable/fixed
        - Extra/intracoronal
        - Full/partial veneer crowns soldered together
        - Inlay/onlay soldered together
- *Ross, Weisgold and Wright classification*:[5]
    - *Temporary stabilization*:
        - Extracoronal splints:
            - Removable
            - Fixed
        - Intracoronal splints.
    - *Provisional stabilization*:
        - Acrylic splints
        - Metal-band and acrylic splints
    - *Permanent/long-term stabilization*:
        - Removable splints
        - Fixed splints
        - Combination of removable and fixed splints.
- *Permanent splint classification*:
    - *Removable*: External
        - Continuous clasp devices
        - Swing-lock devices
        - Overdenture (full or partial)
    - *Fixed*: Internal.
        - Full coverage, three-fourths coverage crowns, and inlays
        - Posts in root canals
    - Horizontal pin splints
    - Cast-metal, resin-bonded fixed partial dentures (Maryland splints).

- *Combined*:
  - Partial dentures and splinted abutments
  - Removable and fixed splints
  - Full or partial dentures on splinted roots
  - Fixed bridges incorporated in partial dentures, seated on posts or copings.
- Endodontic posts

## Extracoronal Type of Splints

Extracoronal splints are very simple and reversible, i.e., they do not necessitate any tooth structure loss. These splints require less chairside time and are economical. The disadvantages of extracoronal splint are that they may interfere with plaque removal and maintenance measures. They are cosmetically poor due to bulky contours.

### Welded-band Splints

These are useful for temporary stabilization of posterior teeth. Separate the teeth by placing brass wire ligatures interdentally for 24 hours before splinting. Adapt a strip of stainless steel 0.003–0.005-inch thick to the tooth and weld it to form a band. Weld the next strip to the mesial surface of the first band. Seat the two pieces while adapting the second strip to the tooth, then weld the second strip to form a band. Several strips can be added and formed into bands for successive teeth. Bands should not impinge on the gingiva. Alternatively, the splint can be fabricated on a model and cemented onto teeth.[2]

### Continuous Clasps

These are made of acrylic, gold, or cast stainless steel.[6] These splints are seated and removed in the fashion of a partial denture. Sharp edges should be rounded off. Adequate oral hygiene is possible with the continuous clasps.

### Acrylic Bite Guards

They are made of heat-cured acrylic and completely cover the occlusal surfaces of the teeth. These splints can be made thin enough to be quite comfortable while worn. The splint should cover the teeth' occlusal surface and extend 1–2 mm over the teeth' facial surfaces. The occlusal surface must be designed to allow free excursion of the mandible with no greater than 1 mm increase in vertical dimension in the molar regions. Bite guards are usually worn only at night because they impede normal functions and are unesthetic. But in cases of severe hypermobility caused by parafunction, guards could be worn during the day as well. It is an important adjunct in the treatment of bruxism, temporomandibular joint dysfunction, muscular spasm, and joint pain.[3]

### Rochette Splint

An impression of the teeth to be splinted is taken, and a chrome–cobalt splint, fitting the lingual surface of these teeth, is constructed. The lingual tooth surfaces are dried and etched, and the splint is glued into position with the composite material.[7]

### Wire Ligation

These are satisfactory means of stabilizing anterior teeth. Dead-soft stainless-steel wire of 0.007–0.010-inch thickness is used. Double a 12-inch length to use as an arch wire and bend it about the six anterior teeth. It should be positioned apical to contact points and incisal to the cingula and then loosely twist buccal and lingual strands at one end. Place single, hairpin bent wires interdentally around the arch wire and below the contact points **(Figs. 44.1A to C)**. Tighten them by twisting clockwise with a needle holder. Tighten the last interdental ligature after all the other interdental ligatures, and the arch wires have been tightened. Clip the ends of the wires short 2–3 mm and bend them into the interdental space **(Fig. 44.2)**. Self-cure acrylic or composite acid-etch resin may be placed over the wires.

## Intracoronal Type of Splints

They usually require tooth structure removal and are inconspicuous splints.

### Acrylic Splints (A-splint)

The channel or slot is prepared midway between cingulum and the incisal edge of approximately 3 mm wide and 2 mm deep on the tooth's lingual aspect **(Fig. 44.3)**. Platinized knurled wire (22 to 16 gauge) or stainless-steel wire is placed in the slot. Self-cure acrylic is then placed over the wire to seal the slots. It is an effective method of stabilizing teeth for prolonged periods of time if proper plaque control is achieved. The main disadvantage associated with this type of splint is the leakage and the breakage of acrylic.[2]

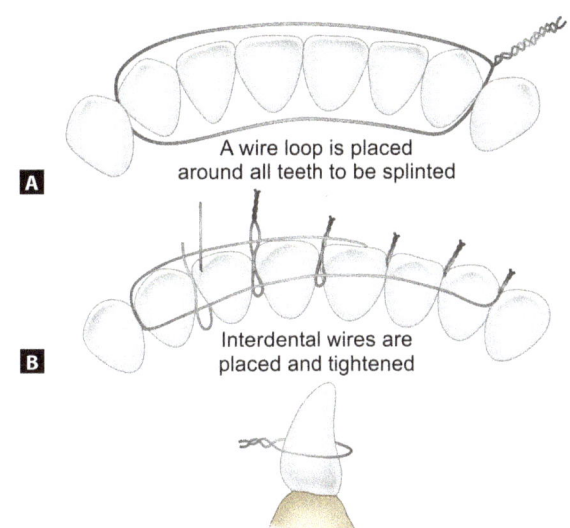

**A** A wire loop is placed around all teeth to be splinted

**B** Interdental wires are placed and tightened

**C** Splint must be placed just apical to contact point

**Figs. 44.1A to C:** Schematic representation showing wire ligation.

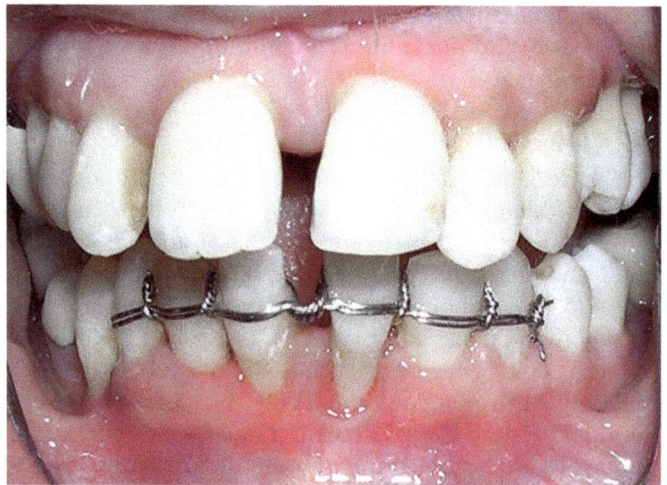

**Fig. 44.2:** Clinical picture showing wire splinting (interdental ligatures are bent in upward direction instead in interdental spaces, as use of interdental aid was being interfered).

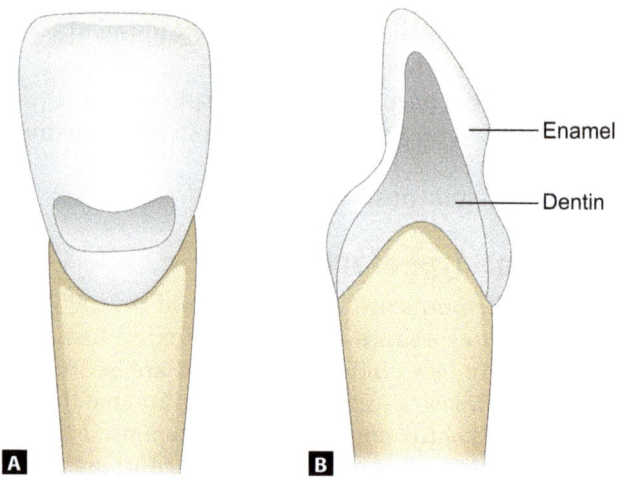

**Figs. 44.4A and B:** Schematic representation showing composite and wire splint: (A) Groove in anterior view; (B) Groove in longitudinal labiolingual section (not extending to dentin).

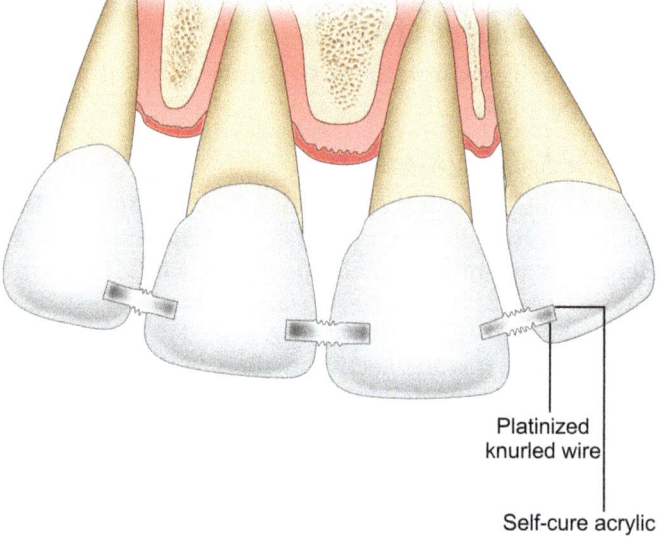

**Fig. 44.3:** Schematic representation showing acrylic A-splint.

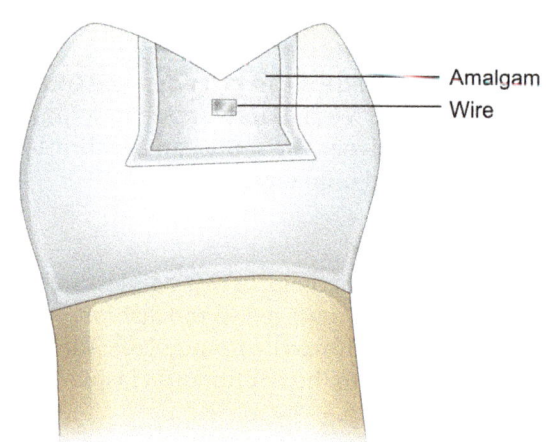

**Fig. 44.5:** Schematic representation showing amalgam and stainless-steel wire splint.

## Composite Splints

The use of composite splints demands consideration of factors, such as the position of the opposing teeth, crowding, spacing, rotations, and size of embrasures.

After proper shade selection, a rubber dam is placed. A large round carbide bur at its high speed with water coolant is used to prepare grooves. A shallow groove is prepared in the enamel layer at a level slightly apical to the contact points without reaching the dentin **(Figs. 44.4A and B)**. Prepared surfaces are completely polished with a slurry of pumice and water, and then it is rinsed and dried with air. The thin layer of hard-setting calcium hydroxide [$Ca(OH)_2$] base is coated over the exposed dentin surfaces to protect the pulp. A 0.010-inch dead, soft single or double wire is placed in the grooves, ligating the teeth continuously with figure-of-eight loops. In order to avoid packing of embrasures with composite material, wood wedges are inserted into all embrasure spaces. 37% phosphoric acid solution is applied to buccal, lingual, and interproximal surfaces of the ligated teeth, and resin is applied. Finishing of the composite is done thereafter.[8]

## Amalgam and Stainless-steel Splint

It is similar to the A-splint but used in posterior teeth. A series of mesio-occluso-distal preparations are made and then restored with an amalgam that has stainless-steel wire of diameter of 0.050-inch embedded in it at the time of condensation.[9] More amalgam is condensed over the wire in one unit **(Fig. 44.5)**. Two or five teeth are splinted together with amalgam splints. The disadvantage associated with it is the frequent fracture of amalgam.

## Chapter 44: Splinting

### Points to Ponder

- The choice of the splint should reflect patients' needs rather than the artistic aspirations of the operator. When the prognosis is doubtful, a simple form of the splint is indicated.
- Splinting should be undertaken only by patients who prove their willingness and ability to perform plaque control.

## REFERENCES

1. Rosenberg S. A new method for stabilization of periodontally involved teeth. J Periodontol. 1980;51(8):469-73.
2. Grant DA, Stern IB, Listgarten MA. Splinting and stabilization. In: Periodontics in the Tradition of Gottlieb and Orban, 6th edition. St. Louis: CV Mosby; 1988. pp. 1056-74.
3. Schluger S, Yuodelis RA, Page RC. Temporary stabilization: Removable and fixed splints. In: Periodontal Diseases. Philadelphia, PA, USA: Lea & Febiger; 1977. pp. 408-22.
4. Lemmerman K. Rationale for stabilization. J Periodontol. 1976;47(7):405-11.
5. Ross SE, Weisgold A, Wright WH. Temporary stabilization. In: Goldman HM, Cohen DW (Eds). Periodontal Therapy, 4th edition. St. Louis: CV Mosby; 1968.
6. Friedman N. Temporary splinting: An adjunct in periodontal therapy. J Periodontol. 1953;24:229.
7. Eley BM, Manson JD. Splinting. In: Periodontics, 5th edition. Edinburgh, UK: Elsevier Science-John Wright; 2004. pp. 366-74.
8. Greenfield DS, Nathanson D. Periodontal splinting with wire and composite resin. A revised approach. J Periodontol. 1980;51(8):465-8.
9. Liatukas EL. The amalgam splints. J Periodontol. 1967;38(5):392-4.

### VIVA VOCE

**Q1. What is a splint?**
Ans. A splint is an appliance that joins two or more teeth to provide support.

**Q2. How are splints classified?**
Ans. According to the location on the tooth: Intracoronal and extracoronal.
According to the period of stabilization: Temporary; provisional and permanent splints.

**Q3. What are the objectives of splinting?**
Ans. Objectives of splinting are to provide rest, redirect, and redistribute the forces.

**Q4. What are the disadvantages associated with A-splint?**
Ans. Leakage and the breakage of acrylic material.

**Q5. What is the disadvantage associated with amalgam and stainless-steel splint?**
Ans. Frequent fracture of amalgam.

**Q6. What are continuous clasps made up of?**
Ans. Acrylic, gold, or cast stainless steel.

**Q7. Who suggested the use of an amalgam splint for the fixation of mobile posterior teeth?**
Ans. Cross, in 1954.

**Q8. What are the ideal requirements of splints?**
Ans. Simple design; economical, stable and efficient; hygienic and nonirritating to the soft tissues; esthetically acceptable; not provoke iatrogenic disease.

**Q9. What is the thickness of stainless steel wire used for wire ligation?**
Ans. 0.007–0.010-inch thickness.

**Q10. What concentration of the phosphoric acid solution is applied in composite splints?**
Ans. 37% phosphoric acid solution.

# Section 7

# Treatment: Surgical Therapy

- ❖ Surgical Anatomy
- ❖ General Principles of Periodontal Surgery
- ❖ Gingival Curettage
- ❖ Gingivectomy
- ❖ Periodontal Flap
- ❖ Resective Osseous Surgery
- ❖ Regenerative Osseous Surgery
- ❖ Furcation
- ❖ Periodontal Plastic Surgery
- ❖ Periodontal Microsurgery
- ❖ Periodontal Treatment of Medically Compromised Patients

# Chapter 45

# Surgical Anatomy

*Nageshwar Iyer, Shalu Bathla*

## Chapter Outline

- Anatomic Structures
- Vital Structures

## INTRODUCTION

Surgical anatomy can be defined as the knowledge of anatomical facts that have local significance in relation to surgical therapy. Knowing the local anatomy is a prerequisite for understanding the principles involved in making proper surgical incisions and designing and managing the surgical flap and graft.

## ANATOMIC STRUCTURES

### Mandible

It is a horseshoe-shaped bone connected to the skull by the temporomandibular joints, which presents several landmarks of great surgical importance.

### Coronoid Process

*Location*: It is located in infratemporal fossa lateral to the pterygoid plate and medial to the zygomatic process of the maxilla **(Fig. 45.1)**.

#### Surgical Implication

Prominent coronoid process approximates maxillary tuberosity, 2nd or 3rd molar during the jaw opening, which hinders surgical access and flap retraction.

### Anterior Border of Ramus

*Location*: It lies laterally to the alveolar process as it extends anteriorly and inferiorly **(Fig. 45.1)**.

#### Surgical Implications

- A prominent or high external oblique ridge may create a shallow vestibular fornix along with the broad flat alveolar process, which can form a shelf of bone.

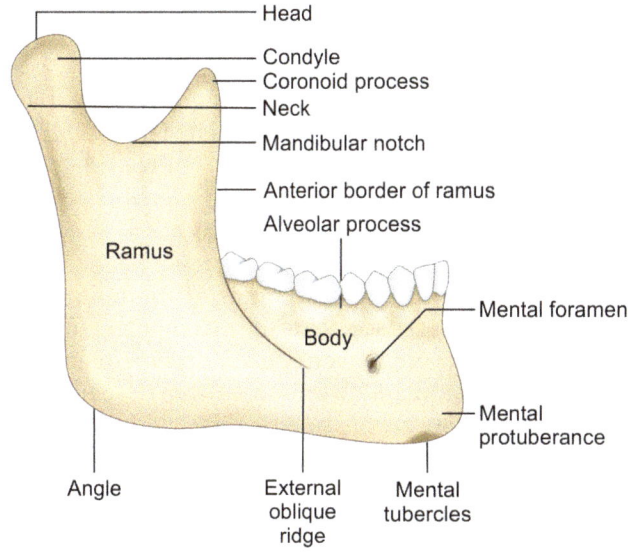

**Fig. 45.1:** Schematic representation showing outer surface of the mandible (showing coronoid process, anterior border of ramus, external oblique ridge).

- Osseous resection to achieve physiologic architecture depends on the depth of the periodontal defect, thickness of the bony shelf, and ability to apically position surgical flap.
- Soft-tissue grafting procedures may be compromised by a shallow vestibule buccinator and muscle attachment.

### External Oblique Ridge

*Location*: Formed as a continuation of the anterior border of ramus, which runs downward and forwards to the margin of 1st or 2nd molar, creating a shelf-like bony area **(Fig. 45.1)**.

## Surgical Implications
- The location and degree of prominence of the external oblique ridge determine the depth of the vestibular fornix in the area of the posterior molars.
- Distal to the 3rd molar, the external oblique ridge circumscribes the retromolar triangle. This region is occupied by glandular and adipose tissue covered by unattached nonkeratinized mucosa. If sufficient space exists distal to the last molar, a band of attached gingiva may be present; only in such case, distal wedge operation can be performed.
- Resective osseous surgery may be difficult or impossible in this area because of the amount of bone that would have to be removed.

### Internal Oblique Ridge
*Location*: It is located medial and posterior to the anterior border of the ramus; as it approaches distal of the last molar, it widens and forms retromolar triangle; together with the laterally located anterior border of ramus it forms the retromolar fossa **(Fig. 45.2)**.

### Surgical Implication
The prominent internal oblique ridge, along with the alveolar process, may form a broad shelf of bone distal and lingual to the last molar.

### Mandibular Canal
*Location*: The mandibular canal, occupied by the inferior alveolar nerve and vessels, begins at the mandibular foramen on the medial surface of the mandibular ramus and curves downward and forward, becoming horizontal below the apices of the molars. The distance from the canal to the molars' apices is shorter in the 3rd molar area and increases as it goes forward. In the premolar area, the canal divides into two parts: (1) The incisive canal, which continues horizontally to the midline, and (2) the mental canal, which turns upward and opens in the mental foramen.

### Surgical Implication
In partially or totally edentulous jaws, there is the disappearance of the mandible's alveolar portion, which brings the mandibular canal closer to the superior border. When these patients are evaluated for placement of implants, the distance between the canal and the superior surface of the bone must be carefully determined to avoid surgical injury to the nerve.

### Mental Foramen
*Location*: It is located on the mandible's buccal surface below the apices of the premolars, sometimes closer to the 2nd premolar and usually halfway between the lower border of the mandible and the alveolar margin. The opening of the mental foramen faces upward and distally, with its posterosuperior borders slanting gradually to the bone surface **(Fig. 45.1)**. The mental nerve and vessels emerge from mental foramen and divide into three branches: one branch of the nerve turns forward and downward to supply the skin of the chin, and the other two branches course anteriorly and upward to supply the skin and mucous membrane of the lower lip and the mucosa of the labial alveolar surface.

### Surgical Implications
- Neurovascular content of mental foramen, i.e., mental artery and nerves, becomes important when mucogingival surgery or apically positioned flap in the premolar region is considered. Long releasing incisions should be avoided in the premolar area to reduce the potential trauma to these structures.
- Surgical trauma to the mental nerve can produce paresthesia of the lip, which recovers slowly. Familiarity with the mental nerve's location and appearance reduces the likelihood of injury; thus, it is important to identify its location by radiographs and palpation.

> **Clinical Tip**
> Careful mucoperiosteal reflection with perhaps a limitation of 3 mm of bone exposed may prevent trauma to the mental nerve.

### Mylohyoid Ridge
*Location*: The inner side of the body of the mandible is traversed obliquely by the mylohyoid ridge, which starts close to the alveolar margin in the 3rd molar area and continues anteriorly, increasing its distance from the osseous margin as it goes forward **(Fig. 45.2)**. The mylohyoid muscle, inserted at this ridge, separates the sublingual space, located more anteriorly and superiorly, from the submandibular space, located more posteriorly and inferiorly.

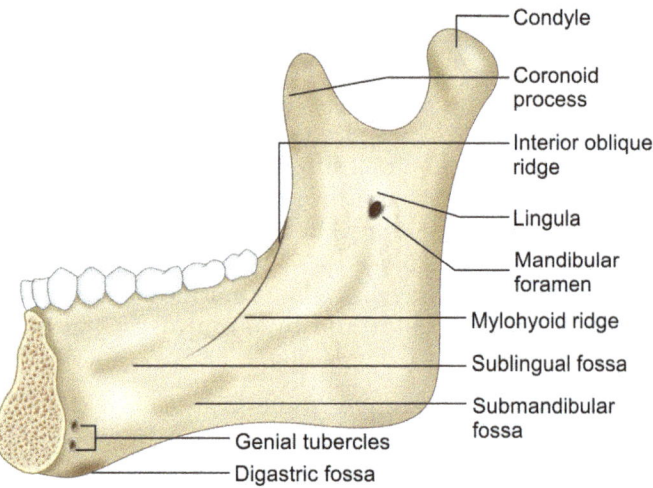

**Fig. 45.2:** Schematic representation showing the inner surface of the mandible.

### Surgical Implications
- The prominent mylohyoid ridge, along with the alveolar process, may create a broad bony ledge opposite to the molars. Horizontal bone loss around the molar teeth may accentuate the ledging effect.
- Prominent mylohyoid ridge can be a source of autogenous bone graft.

## Genial Tubercles
*Location*: It is located at midline near the mandible's inferior border **(Fig. 45.2)**. It provides attachment superiorly for genioglossus and inferiorly for geniohyoid muscles.

### Surgical Implication
It poses a problem during flap reflection and implant placement in case of severe horizontal bone loss or mandibular atrophy.

## Mental Protuberance and Tubercles
*Location*: It is a median triangular prominence present at the mandible lower outer surface, which provides attachment for mentalis muscle **(Fig. 45.1)**.

### Surgical Implications
- A short alveolar process with prominent protuberance and high attachment of the mentalis muscles creates a shallow vestibular fornix, which usually compromises certain soft-tissue grafting procedures to cover roots or deepen vestibule.
- Resective osseous surgery may be limited by the depth of periodontal defects and the ability to apically position the surgical flap.

## Mandibular Torus
*Location*: The most common location of a mandibular torus is the lingual area of canine and premolars, above the mylohyoid muscle **(Fig. 45.3)**.

### Surgical Implications
- They may hinder the removal of plaque by the patient and may have to be removed to improve the prognosis of neighboring teeth.
- Mucosal tissue over tori is usually thin and subject to tearing, so care should be taken in reflecting flaps.
- Exostosis can be a source of autogenous bone graft for intrabony defects.

## Maxilla
The maxilla is a paired pyramidal-shaped bone. Each one consists of a body and four processes, namely:
1. *Zygomatic process*: It extends laterally from the area of the 1st molar and determines the depth of the vestibular fornix **(Fig. 45.4A)**.

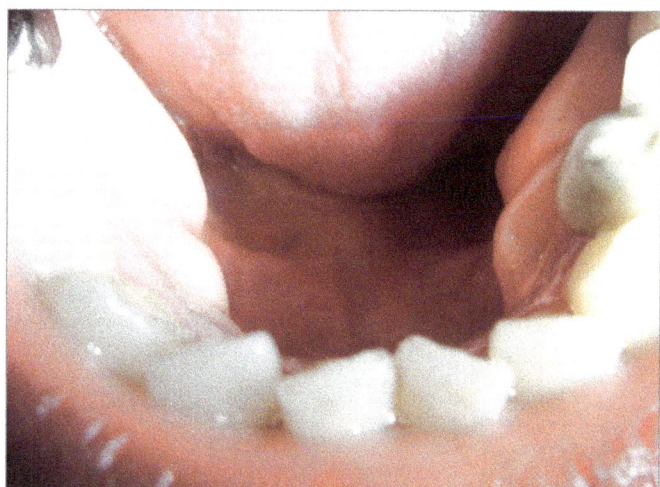

**Fig. 45.3:** Clinical picture showing bilateral mandibular lingual exostosis.

2. *Frontal process*: It extends in an ascending direction and articulates with the frontal bone at the frontomaxillary suture **(Fig. 45.4A)**.
3. *Alveolar process*: It contains the sockets for the upper teeth **(Fig. 45.4A)**.
4. *Palatine process*: It extends horizontally to meet its counterpart from the other maxilla at the midline intermaxillary suture and posteriorly with the palatine bone's horizontal plate to form the hard palate **(Fig. 45.4B)**.

## Incisive Canal and Foramen
*Location*: It is located posterior to the central incisors and deep to the incisive papilla **(Fig. 45.5)**. The terminal branches of the nasopalatine nerves and vessels pass through the incisive canal, and emerge from incisive foramen to supply the anterior palate from canine to canine.

### Surgical Implication
Vessels emerging through the incisive canal are of small caliber, and their surgical interference is of little consequence.

## Greater Palatine Foramen
*Location*: The greater palatine foramen opens 3–4 mm anterior to the hard palate's posterior border and 15 mm from the midline **(Fig. 45.5)**. The greater palatine nerves and vessels emerge through this foramen and run anteriorly in the palate's submucosa, between the palatal and alveolar processes.

### Surgical Implications
- Palatal flaps and donor sites for gingival grafts should be carefully performed and selected to avoid invading these areas, as profuse hemorrhages may occur if vessels are damaged at the palatine foramen.

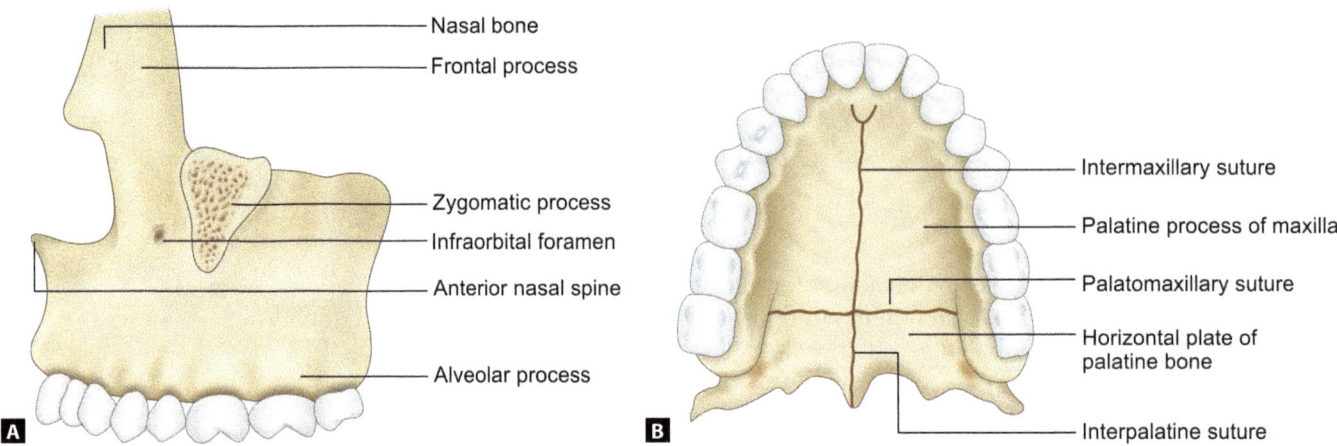

**Figs. 45.4A and B:** Schematic representation showing maxilla as viewed from: (A) Lateral; (B) Palatal aspect.

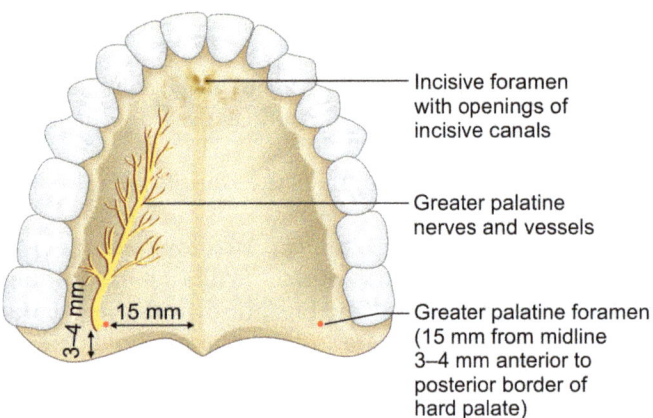

**Fig. 45.5:** Schematic representation showing maxilla as viewed from the palatal aspect (showing incisive foramen, greater palatine foramen, and greater palatine nerves and vessels).

- Avoid vertical releasing incisions, thinning or harvesting connective tissue grafts to or beyond 7 mm from the alveolar crest in a shallow palate, 12 mm in an average palate, and 17 mm in a high palate.

## Palatal Vault

*Location*: The mucous membrane covering the hard palate is firmly attached to the underlying bone. The submucous layer of the palate posterior to the 1st molars contains the palatal glands, which are more compact in the soft palate and extend anteriorly, filling the gap between the mucosal connective tissue and the periosteum and protecting the underlying vessels and nerve.

### Surgical Implications

- The shape of the palatal vault may range from wide and shallow to narrow and high. A wide and shallow palatal vault is usually associated with a broad bony ledge at the alveolar crest, as well as a wide ledge of palatal mucosa. This anatomy is unfavorable for pocket elimination during resective osseous technique. In contrast, high and steep vaults are favorable for treating periodontal defects and achieving a physiologic architecture in both bone and palatal mucosa with resective osseous surgery.
- The amount of soft-tissue grafts that can be harvested from the palate is generally less in a shallow palatal vault than a high vault.

## Palatal Exostosis

*Location*: Maxillary tori are usually located in the midline of the hard palate; smaller tori may be seen over the palatal roots of the molars.

### Surgical Implication

Prominent palatal exostosis makes osseous interproximal ramping difficult.

## Maxillary Tuberosity

*Location*: The area distal to the last molar is called the maxillary tuberosity and consists of the posteroinferior angle of the infratemporal surface of the maxilla; medially, it articulates with the pyramidal process of the palatine bone. It is covered by fibrous connective tissue and contains the terminal branches of the middle and posterior palatine nerves.

### Surgical Implications

- Excision of the area for distal wedge surgery may reach the tensor palati muscle medially, which comes from the greater wing of the sphenoid bone and ends in a tendon that forms the palatine aponeurosis and attaches to the posterior border of the hard palate.
- A flap design for distal wedge procedure is determined by the size of maxillary tuberosity:
  - For long and large tuberosity, a square incision is given.
  - For long and large tuberosity and when the osseous defect is close to the maxillary sinus, pedicle incision is given.

- When the size of the wedge is small, a triangular incision is given.

### *Maxillary Sinus*

*Location*: The maxilla body is occupied by the maxillary sinus or antrum, which is a hollow pyramidal area with its base toward the nose and lined by respiratory epithelium.

#### Surgical Implications

The inferior wall of the maxillary sinus is frequently separated from the apices and roots of the maxillary posterior teeth by a thin, bony plate. In edentulous posterior areas, the maxillary sinus bony wall may be only a thin plate in intimate contact with the alveolar mucosa. Adequate determination of the maxillary sinus's extension into the surgical site is important to avoid creating an oroantral communication, particularly in relation to:

> **Clinical Tip**
> An inferior extension of the sinus into the base of the alveolar process is of special clinical significance because it establishes more intimate relations of the sinus with the maxillary teeth. In extreme cases, the sinus even extends into the alveolar process between the roots of the teeth so that their sockets protrude into the cavity.

- *Placement of implants*: The minimum distance between the implant and maxillary sinus should be approximately 5 mm.
- *Ostectomy to eliminate craters*: Craters, if present between two maxillary molars, which are in close proximity to the floor of the maxillary sinus, elimination of the crater by ostectomy may expose antrum.
- *Curettage to eliminate infrabony pockets*: Infrabony pockets have the base in close proximity to the floor of the sinus. Careless curettage of such pockets at the base may cause entry into the antrum.
- *Osteoplasty to eliminate furcation defects*: Careless osteoplasty near the sinus or buccal trifurcation involvements may cause invasion of the antrum.

In edentulous jaws, determining the amount of available bone in the anterior area, below the floor of the nasal cavity, is also critical.

## MUSCLES

Several muscles may be encountered while performing periodontal flaps, particularly in mucogingival surgery. Tension from high muscle attachments interferes with mucogingival surgery by causing a postoperative reduction in vestibular depth and width of the attached gingiva. These muscles are mentalis, mylohyoid, buccinator, and muscles of mastication.

### Mentalis Muscle

*Location*: These are paired, small, conical muscles arising from the mandible, beginning at the midroot level of the lower incisor teeth and continuing inferiorly to a point below the apices **(Fig. 45.6)**. They are separated from one another by a firm septum and adipose tissue. At the inferior portion of its origin, the mentalis muscle attaches laterally to the *pogonial trigone*. The fibers of this muscle pass from their origin inferiorly, inserting into the skin of the chin at the soft-tissue chin prominence. The most superior fibers are the shortest and pass almost horizontally into the skin of the upper chin. The lower fibers are the longest and pass obliquely or vertically to the skin at the lower part of the chin.

The mentalis muscle is innervated by the marginal mandibular branch of the facial nerve.

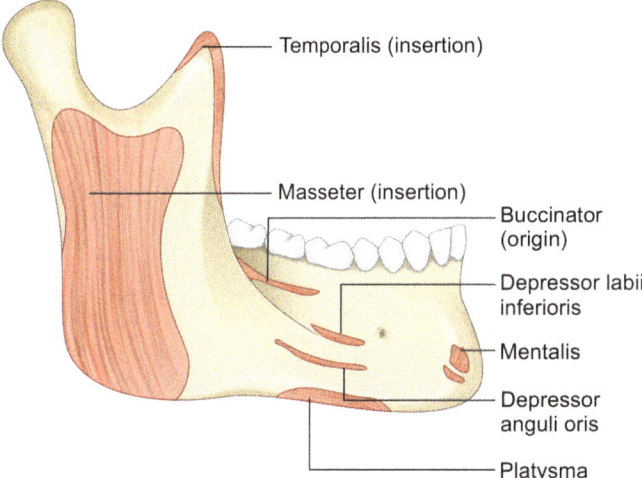

**Fig. 45.6:** Schematic representation showing muscle attachments on the outer surface of the mandible.

#### Surgical Implications
- The mentalis muscle's origin determines the depth of the labial sulcus in the anterior portion of the mouth—a high mentalis muscle attachment results in a very shallow vestibule.
- Elevation of the muscle attachment to gain adequate access during flap surgery exposes the submental space, which may lead to infection originating in this space with the potential to spread posteriorly into the lateral pharyngeal space.

### Mylohyoid Muscle

*Location*: Mylohyoid muscle forms the floor of the mouth and inserts posteriorly along the mylohyoid ridge as far as the 2nd and 3rd molar regions **(Fig. 45.7)**.

### *Surgical Implication*

In the case of mandibular alveolar atrophy, where pre-prosthetic reconstruction requires floor of the mouth vestibuloplasty, the mylohyoid fibers can be completely detached without the change in speech. This also reduces the mylohyoid displacement of the denture.

Section 7: Treatment: Surgical Therapy

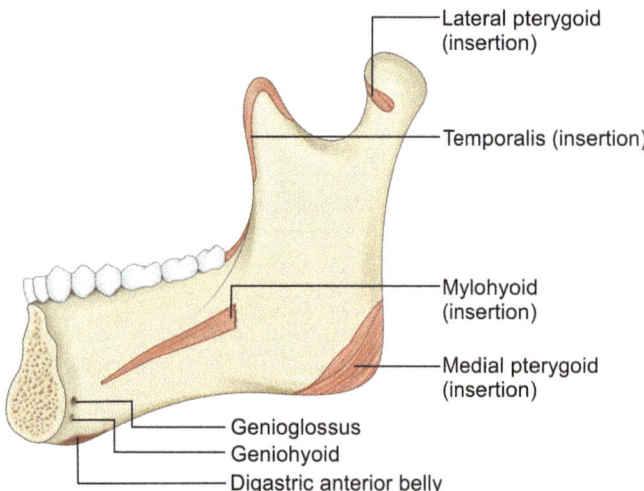

Fig. 45.7: Schematic representation showing muscle attachments on the inner surface of the mandible.

## Buccinator Muscle

*Location*: It is the muscle of the cheek that prevents the accumulation of food in the vestibule.

### Origin

- *Upper fibers*: From maxilla, opposite molar teeth.
- *Lower fibers*: From mandible, opposite molar teeth.
- *Middle fibers*: From pterygomandibular raphe (**Fig. 45.6**).

### Insertion

Upper fibers straight into the upper lip and lower fibers into the lower lip and middle fibers decussate.

### Surgical Implications

- The pterygomandibular raphe is formed by the attachment of buccinators' muscle to the superior pharyngeal constrictor muscle, which lies immediately in front of the anterior border of medial pterygoid muscle.
- The thin attachment of the buccinator muscle to the mandible along the molar teeth may limit the necessary extension of the vestibule.
- Buccinator muscle forms a medial wall of buccal space. If this muscle gets perforated while elevating buccal flap, the buccal space would be entered, producing the buccal space infection.

## MUSCLES OF MASTICATION

Muscles of mastication are namely: lateral pterygoid, medial pterygoid, temporalis, and masseter.

## Lateral Pterygoid Muscle

Short conical muscle having two heads: (1) upper and (2) lower. It depresses mandible to open mouth.

### Origin

- *Upper head*: From infratemporal surface and crest of the greater wing of the sphenoid bone.
- *Lower head*: From the lateral surface of the lateral pterygoid plate.

### Insertion

Pterygoid fovea on the anterior surface of the neck of the mandible (**Fig. 45.7**).

## Medial Pterygoid Muscle

Quadrilateral muscle having a superficial and deep head. It elevates and helps to protrude the mandible.

### Origin

- *Superficial head*: From tuberosity of maxilla.
- *Deep head*: From the medial surface of the lateral pterygoid plate.

### Insertion

The roughened area on the medial surface of the angle and adjoining ramus of the mandible (**Fig. 45.7**).

## Temporalis Muscle

Fan-shaped muscle that fills the temporal fossa. It elevates the mandible and helps in the side-to-side grinding movements.

### Origin

- Temporal fossa
- Temporal fascia

### Insertion

Margins and deep surface of the coronoid process and anterior border of the ramus of mandible (**Figs. 45.6 and 45.7**).

## Masseter Muscle

Quadrilateral muscle, which covers the lateral surface of the ramus of mandible (**Fig. 45.6**). It elevates and helps to protrude the mandible.

### Origin

- *Superficial layer*: From anterior two-thirds of the lower border of the zygomatic arch.
- *Deep layer*: From the deep surface of the zygomatic arch.
- *Middle layer*: From the lower border of the posterior one-third of the zygomatic arch.

### Insertion

- *Superficial layer*—into the lower part of the lateral surface of the ramus of the mandible.
- *Deep layer*—into the rest of the ramus of the mandible.

> **Trismus**
> Trismus during pericoronitis of mandibular molars is due to the irritation of muscles of mastication, namely: Deep belly of masseter muscles, medial pterygoid, and superficial fibers of temporalis muscle which are responsible for closing the mouth.

- *Middle layer*—into the central part of the ramus of the mandible.

## VITAL STRUCTURES

### Neurovascular Bundle

#### Blood Supply

The major arterial supply to the oral cavity comes primarily from the lingual, facial and maxillary arteries, which are branches of the external carotid artery.

#### Lingual Artery

*Location*: It arises between the superior laryngeal artery and the facial artery and runs forward beneath the hyoglossus muscle. The sublingual artery arises from the lingual artery at the anterior border of the hyoglossus muscle. It is found coronal to the mylohyoid muscle supplying the sublingual gland, neighboring muscles, mucosa of the floor of the mouth and the lingual mandibular gingival tissue.

#### Surgical Implication

The arterial blood supply of the floor of the mouth is formed by anastomosis of the sublingual and submental arteries (branch of the facial artery). In the canine area, the vessels are closer to the lingual plate and alveolar crest than in more posterior areas.

Intraosseous hemorrhage is not a serious event, and control of the hemorrhage can be ensured by compressing the area. However, severe bleeding and the formation of massive hematomas on the floor of the mouth are the results of arterial trauma.

#### Facial Artery

*Location and its branches*: Superior to the lingual artery is the facial, which runs forward close to the inferior border of the mandible, lodged in a groove on the posterior surface of the submandibular gland. At the anterior border of the masseter muscle, it curves superiorly over the body of the mandible to travel forward and upward within the cheek to the angle of the mouth.

The main branches of the facial artery are submental, inferior labial, and superior labial. The submental artery arises as the facial artery emerges from the submandibular gland. It then travels on the mylohyoid muscle below the mandible's body toward the symphysis where it turns over the chin to divide into deep and superficial branches. Both of these branches supply the muscles and mucosa of the lower lip. The deep branch anastomoses with the mental artery, as does another branch of the facial artery, the inferior labial, which also supplies the muscles and mucosa of the lower lip.

#### Surgical Implication

Interruption of the facial artery flow by injury or during surgery is usually not significant since its zone of supply is rapidly taken over by transverse facial artery branches, buccal, infraorbital, and sphenopalatine branches of the maxillary artery.

#### Maxillary Artery

It is the larger terminal branch of the external carotid artery, given off behind the neck of the mandible.

- *Inferior alveolar artery:* It runs downward, forward medial to the ramus of the mandible to reach mandibular foramen. Passing through this foramen, the artery enters the mandibular canal in which it runs downward and forwards, giving branches to the mandible and roots of each tooth attached to the bone.
- *Posterior superior alveolar artery:* It arises just before the maxillary artery enters the pterygomaxillary fissures. It descends on the posterior surface of the maxilla and gives branches that enter canals in the bone to supply premolars and molars and maxillary sinus.

#### Surgical Implication

While giving posterior superior nerve block, rapid hematoma may develop due to laceration of the posterior superior alveolar artery (earlier believed due to laceration of pterygoid venous plexus), which is manifested as sudden swelling of the buccal area of the face.

- *Greater palatine artery*: Greater palatine artery (GPA) runs downwards in the greater palatine canal to emerge on the posterolateral part of the hard palate through the greater palatine foramen **(Fig. 45.5)**. It then runs forward near the palate's lateral margin to reach the incisive canal near the midline.

> **Clinical Tip**
> While giving local anesthesia with a vasoconstrictor to the greater palatine nerve, tissue ischemia and necrosis may be seen due to tightly attached mucosa.

#### Surgical Implications

To avoid accidental injury to the GPA in the palatine abscess, following things should be remembered:

- The incision of a palatine abscess, arising for instance from the lingual root of 1st molar, must never be made in a transverse direction but in an anteroposterior line.
- The incision should also be made near the free margin of the gingiva as possible without missing the abscess. Also, the edge of the knife should be directed outward and upward and not straight upward.

## Nerve Supply

The nerves of the oral cavity are primarily branches of the V cranial nerve, i.e., trigeminal nerve, which is made up of large sensory and smaller motor branches. Three major branches of this nerve are ophthalmic, maxillary, and mandibular nerve.

## Nasopalatine Nerve

*Location*: The terminal branches of the nasopalatine nerves and vessels pass through the incisive canal, which opens in the midline anterior area of the palate. The mucosa overlying the incisive canal presents a slight protuberance called the incisive papilla.

### Surgical Implication

Vessels emerging through the incisive canal are of small caliber, and their surgical interference is of little consequence.

## Mandibular Branch of Trigeminal Nerve

Mandibular nerve is the largest mixed branch of the trigeminal nerve, which begins in the middle cranial fossa through a large sensory root and a small motor root. Sensory root arises from the lateral part of trigeminal ganglion and leaves the cranial cavity through foramen ovale. The motor root lies deep in the trigeminal ganglion and to sensory root. The main trunk lies in the infratemporal fossa on the *tensor veli palatani* giving two branches, i.e., meningeal branch and nerve to medial pterygoid. After a short course, the main trunk is divided into small anterior trunks giving various branches, namely: buccal, masseteric, deep temporal and lateral pterygoid nerve; and a large posterior trunk gives three branches, i.e., auriculotemporal, lingual and inferior alveolar nerves.

> **Clinical Tip**
> Postinjection trismus is due to the tearing of masticatory muscle by penetration of needle or by injecting an anesthetic solution directly into the muscle. The most common muscle involved is medial pterygoid muscle during an inferior alveolar nerve block. This can be avoided by keeping needle lateral to pterygomandibular raphe.

## Lingual Nerve

*Location*: The lingual nerve, along with the inferior alveolar nerve, is a branch of the posterior division of the mandibular nerve and descends along the mandibular ramus medial to and in front of the inferior alveolar nerve. It lies close to the surface of the oral mucosa in the 3rd molar area and goes deeper as it goes forward.

### Surgical Implications

- It can be damaged during anesthetic injections and during oral surgery procedures, such as 3rd molar extractions.
- It may be injured when a periodontal partial-thickness flap is raised in the 3rd molar region or releasing incisions are made.
- Due to this, vertical incisions are avoided in these areas.

## Inferior Alveolar Nerve

*Location*: It runs vertically downward lateral to the medial pterygoid and to the sphenomandibular ligament. It enters the mandibular foramen and runs in the mandibular canal. Mylohyoid branch arises before the inferior alveolar nerve enters into the mandibular foramen. While running in the mandibular canal, it gives branches that supply the mandibular teeth and gingiva. The mental nerve emerges at the mental foramen and supplies the lower lip's skin and mucous membrane. Its incisive branch supplies the labial aspect of the gingiva of canine and incisors.

### Surgical Implication

The point of nerve entry into the mandibular foramen is important as the site of inferior alveolar block anesthesia.

> **Points to Ponder**
> - The mental foramen is located below the apices of the mandibular premolars (closer to the second premolar) on the buccal surface and halfway between the lower border of the mandible and the alveolar margin.
> - Incisive foramen is located posterior to the maxillary central incisors and deep to the incisive papilla.
> - The greater palatine foramen is located 3–4 mm anterior to the posterior border of the hard palate and 15 mm from the midline.
> - High mentalis muscle attachment results in a very shallow mandibular vestibule.

## BIBLIOGRAPHY

1. Annibali S, Ripari M, La Monaca G, Tonoli F, Cristalli MP. Local accidents in dental implant surgery: prevention and treatment. Int J Periodontics Restorative Dent. 2009;29(3):325-31.
2. Carranza FA. Surgical anatomy of the periodontium and related structures. In: Newman MG, Takei HH, Carranza FA (Eds). Carranza's Clinical Periodontology, 9th edition. Philadelphia, PA, USA: WB Saunders; 2003. pp. 737-43.
3. Clarke MA, Bueltmann KW. Anatomical considerations in periodontal surgery. J Periodontol. 1971;42(10):610-25.
4. Gregg JM. Surgical anatomy. In: Laskin DM (Ed). Oral and Maxillofacial Surgery, 1st edition. New Delhi, India: AITBS Publishers; 2013. pp. 3-49.
5. Greenstein G, Tarnow D. The mental foramen and nerve: clinical and anatomical factors related to dental implant placement: a literature review. J Periodontol. 2006;77(12):1933-43.
6. Lindhe J, Karring T, Araujo M. Anatomy of the periodontium. In: Lindhe J, Karring T, Lang NP (Eds). Clinical Periodontology and Implant Dentistry, 4th edition. Oxford, UK: Blackwell Munksgaard; 2003. pp. 3-49.
7. McDonnell HT, Mills MP. Principles and practice of periodontal surgery. In: Rose LF, Mealey BL, Genco RJ, Cohen DW (Eds). Periodontics: Medicine, Surgery, and Implants, 1st edition. St. Louis: Elsevier-Mosby; 2004. pp. 693-769.

8. Misch K, Wang HL. Implant surgery complications: etiology and treatment. Implant Dent. 2008;17(2):159-68.
9. Reiser GM, Bruno JF, Mahan PE, Larkin LH. The subepithelial connective tissue graft palatal donor site: anatomic considerations for surgeons. Int J Periodontics Restorative Dent. 1996;16(2):130-7.
10. Stern IB. Oral mucous membrane. In: Bhaskar SN (Ed). Orban's Oral Histology and Embryology, 11th edition. St. Louis: Mosby; 1991. pp. 260-336.
11. Squier CA, Finkelstein MW. Oral mucosa. In: Nanci A, Ten Cate AR, Richard A (Eds). Ten Cate's Oral Histology: Development, Structure, and Function, 8th edition. St. Louis: Elsvier-Mosby; 2013. pp. 278-310.
12. Yu SK, Lee MH, Park BS, Jeon YH, Chung YY, Kim HJ. Topographical relationship of the greater palatine artery and the palatal spine. Significance for periodontal surgery. J Clin Periodontol. 2014;41(9):908-13.

## VIVA VOCE

**Q1. Which muscle separates submandibular space from sublingual space?**
Ans. Mylohyoid muscle separates submandibular space from sublingual space.

**Q2. Which process of the maxilla determines the depth of vestibular fornix?**
Ans. The zygomatic process of the maxilla determines the depth of the vestibular fornix.

**Q3. Which is the most common location of a mandibular torus?**
Ans. Lingual area of canine and premolars is the most common location of a mandibular torus.

**Q4. What is the cause of postinjection trismus?**
Ans. Postinjection trismus is due to the tearing of masticatory muscle by penetration of needle or by injecting an anesthetic solution directly into the muscle. The most common muscle involved is medial pterygoid muscle during an inferior alveolar nerve block. This can be avoided by keeping needle lateral to pterygomandibular raphe.

**Q5. What is the minimum distance between the implant and other vital structures?**
Ans.

| Vital structures | Minimum distance (mm) |
| --- | --- |
| Maxillary sinus | 5 |
| Mental nerve | 2 |
| Inferior alveolar nerve | 2 |
| Adjacent tooth | 1.5 |

**Q6. What is the surgical implication of genial tubercles?**
Ans. It poses a problem during flap reflection and implant placement in case of severe horizontal bone loss or mandibular atrophy.

**Q7. What is the location of palatal exostosis?**
Ans. Maxillary tori are usually located in the midline of the hard palate; smaller tori may be seen over the palatal roots of the molars.

**Q8. What is the origin of the buccinator muscle?**
Ans. Upper fibers from the maxilla, opposite molar teeth; Lower fibers from the mandible, opposite molar teeth; Middle fibers from pterygomandibular raphe.

**Q9. What is the major arterial supply of the oral cavity?**
Ans. Primarily the lingual, facial, and maxillary arteries, which are branches of the external carotid artery.

**Q10. What is the nerve supply of the oral cavity?**
Ans. Primarily branches of the Vth cranial nerve, i.e., trigeminal nerve, are made up of large sensory and smaller motor branches. Three major branches of this nerve are ophthalmic, maxillary, and mandibular nerve.

# Chapter 46

# General Principles of Periodontal Surgery

*Shalu Bathla*

## Chapter Outline

- Objectives
- Preoperative Considerations
- Intraoperative Considerations
- Postoperative Instructions and Care
- Postsurgical Complications
- Wound Healing

## INTRODUCTION

Since a wide range of periodontal surgical therapies is available for the treatment of soft tissue and bony periodontal defects, consideration must be given to the most appropriate surgery for each involved site in each case criteria.

Broad classification of periodontal surgery is given in **Table 46.1**.

**TABLE 46.1:** Classification of periodontal surgery.[1]

| | | |
|---|---|---|
| Pocket reduction surgery | Resective | Gingivectomy, apically displaced flap and undisplaced flap with or without osseous resection |
| | Regenerative | Flaps with grafts and membranes |
| Correction of anatomic or morphologic defects | Plastic surgery techniques to widen attached gingiva | Epithelial grafts |
| | | Connective tissue grafts |
| | Esthetic surgery | Root coverage |
| | | Recreation of gingival papillae |
| | Preprosthetic surgery techniques | Crown lengthening |
| | | Ridge augmentation |
| | | Vestibular deepening |
| | Placement of dental implants | With guided bone regeneration (GBR) |
| | | Sinus grafts |

## OBJECTIVES

Objectives of the surgical phase of periodontal surgery are as follows:
- Regeneration of lost periodontal attachment.
- Improvement of the prognosis of teeth and their replacements.
- Improvement of esthetics.

## PREOPERATIVE CONSIDERATIONS

### Case History

#### Medical History

The operator should determine if specific preoperative modifications are indicated because of the patient's medical history, well before scheduling any surgical procedure. Drug allergy, patient's medication, or systemic disease dictate alterations in the type of anesthetic agent, analgesics, prophylactic antibiotic, and even surgical procedure.

### Indications for Periodontal Surgery

- Correction of gross gingival aberrations.
- Persistent inflammation in areas with moderate-to-deep pockets.
- Areas with irregular bony contours, deep craters.
- When removal of root irritant is not possible due to deep pockets, especially in molars and premolars.
- Furcation lesions.
- Infrabony pockets on the distal areas of last molars, complicated by mucogingival problems.

## Contraindications for Periodontal Surgery

Following are the contraindications for periodontal surgery:[2]
- Uncooperative patient
- *Uncontrolled systemic diseases/hormonal disorders*:
  - Uncontrolled diabetes mellitus
  - Adrenal dysfunction
- Blood disorders
- Smoking
- *Cardiovascular diseases*:
  - Hypertension
  - Myocardial infarction
  - Angina pectoris
  - Anticoagulant therapy
  - Rheumatic fever
- Organ transplantation
- *Neurological disorders*:
  - Multiple sclerosis
  - Parkinson's disease

## Consent

The patient should be fully informed verbally and in writing about the procedure's details and possible complications. The patient should be given agreement for the procedure both with an oral statement and by signing a consent form.[3]

## Premedications

Premedication should be given when indicated. The chemotherapeutic agents used for premedications are as follows:
- *Anxiolytics*: Apprehensive and neurotic patients are given antianxiety, sedative, hypnotic agents, tranquilizers, or barbiturates intramuscularly (IM) or intravenously (IV) prior to surgical therapy.
- *Antibiotics*: It is given to only medically compromised patients, such as infective endocarditis, or patients who require prophylactic antibiotics regimen (valvular heart disease). It should be given 1 hour before surgery to attain adequate levels to prevent bacteremia.
- *Antiseptics*: Oral rinse with 0.12% chlorhexidine (CHX) gluconate mouthwash.
- *Nonsteroidal anti-inflammatory drugs (NSAIDs)*: Ibuprofen can be given as premedication before surgery.

### Clinical Tip
Patients on anticoagulant therapy or aspirin should stop these medicines 7–14 days before surgery and 3–4 days afterward with physician's approval.[4]

## INTRAOPERATIVE CONSIDERATIONS

### Monitoring Presurgical Data

The data necessary to select the surgical procedure includes periapical radiographs, study casts, and probing charts.

## Anesthesia

Periodontal surgery should be performed painlessly; the entire area of the dentition scheduled for surgery, the teeth, and periodontal tissues should be anesthetized by proper anesthesia. Local infiltration and block anesthesia are the methods of choice. After the initial administration of local anesthesia, inject a drop of the anesthetic solution directly into interdental papilla. It makes the gingiva firmer and easier to incise and has a hemostatic effect because of the vasoconstrictor present in the solution. In general, most periodontal surgical procedures are done under local anesthesia. However, in apprehensive patients or patients suffering from neurological disorders, surgery is done under general anesthesia.

## Tissue Management

### Incision

The incision should be made by a sharp blade of proper size. The incision should be clean, firm, and continuous without unnecessarily repeated strokes. Blades should be changed when it does not seem to be incising easily. Repeated strokes increase both the amount of damaged tissue and the amount of bleeding. Thus, long and continuous strokes are preferred over short and interrupted. Surgeon's focus must remain on the blade to avoid accidently cutting lips or tongue while introducing and removing the blade to and from the mouth.[5] The various incisions used in periodontal surgery are explained in "Chapter 49: Periodontal Flap."

### Flap Preparation

The surgical flap is defined as the separation of a section of tissue from the surrounding tissues except at its base. The flap can be full or partial thickness.

### Flap Design

Flap design should be based on the principle of maintaining optimal blood supply to the tissue. The recommended flap length (height-to-base) ratio should not be greater than 2:1 (**Fig. 46.1**). The greater the flap length ratio to flap base, the greater the vascular compromise at the flap margins.[6]

### Flap Reflection

A full-thickness flap is elevated using a sharp periosteal elevator directed beneath the periosteum keeping against the bone. Papillae are reflected first, followed by the marginal gingiva, working across the anterior or posterior extent of the incisions until the flap margin has been freed from the teeth or alveolar crest or both. Once the flap margin has been completely released, the periosteal elevator is directed in both horizontal and vertical planes until adequate access is achieved.

## Section 7: Treatment: Surgical Therapy

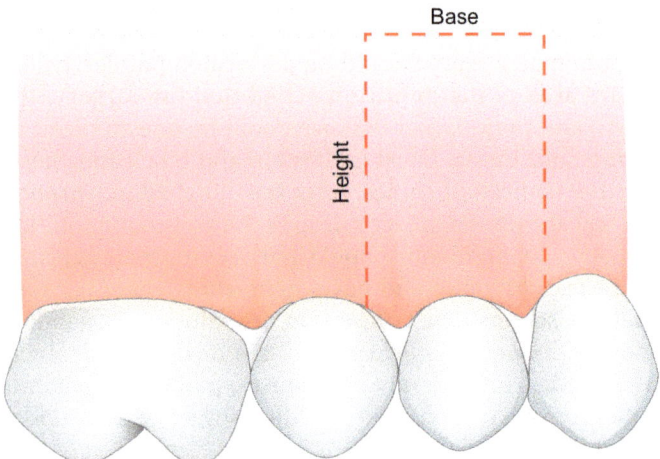

**Fig. 46.1:** Schematic representation showing flap height-to-base ratio (ratio should not exceed 2: 1).

### Flap Retraction

Surgical retractors are used to hold the flap back from the teeth and bone. Retraction should be passive without any tension. Continuous flap retraction for a long period is not advised. When the flap is retracted, the surgical field should be irrigated with sterile saline to keep the tissues moist, reduce contamination, and improve visibility. The periosteal elevator can be used as a retractor. Once the periosteum has been elevated, the periosteal elevator's broad base is held firmly against the bone with the mucoperiosteal flap elevated into reflected position.

### Flap Repositioning

Surgical flaps may be repositioned, apically positioned, coronally positioned, or laterally positioned. The final flap location is determined by the goal of therapy and the specific periodontal surgical technique performed. Thus, in general, tissue should be handled carefully with minimum surgical trauma.
- Use suction during surgery to avoid compression of tissues with a dry sponge. Cotton fibers of dry sponge or gauze could be left behind and maybe a source of future irritation and infection.
- A sterile saline solution should be used.
- Do not blow air into the surgical site as it may induce cervicofacial emphysema, which can be fatal.
- Slow-speed sharp surgical bur and adequate cooling should be used for bone removal. Avoid undue drying of the bone and do not heat the bone above 47°C; otherwise, it will cause necrosis of bone surface.[7]
- Avoid heavy pressure against soft tissues or bone.

### Scaling and Root Planing

Scaling and root planing, in conjunction with periodontal surgery, is done on exposed root surfaces with the help of curettes.

### Hemostasis

Before the approximation of flaps, all areas should be rinsed free of clots, and the surgical site should be checked again for bleeding. Pressure should be applied to the flap to encourage minimal clot thickness. Good closure with suturing discourages postsurgical hemorrhage. Distal wedge and edentulous ridge sites should be well approximated carefully with attention because these areas are a good source of postoperative bleeding. Excessive bleeding from interproximal and infrabony lesions results from inadequate degranulation. Residual granulomatous tissue is a common source of hemorrhage since it is composed largely of capillaries.

### Steps to Control Postsurgical Bleeding

- *Step I—Pressure*: Identify the source of bleeding and do suction carefully. To remove the extravasated blood, just dab the wound with the sponge and do not wipe, as wiping reopen vessels that one plugged with clotted blood. The first step to control bleeding is to apply local pressure with gauze sponges. Small vessels usually take only 20–30 seconds, whereas large vessels take 5–10 minutes of continuous pressure.[5]
- *Step II—Vasoconstrictor*: Judicious injection of vasoconstrictor combined with continuous application of pressure, encourages clot formation.
- *Step III—Hemostatic agents*: Artificial clot may be induced by the use of an oxidized cellulose microfibrillar collagen product. Various topical hemostatic agents are given below in **Table 46.2**.
- *Step IV—Thermal coagulation*: Electrocoagulation can be effective for capillary bleeding sites and small arterioles.
- *Step V—Suturing*: Large arteriole bleeding sites can be controlled by placing sutures in the soft tissue. A knot is drawn tight to occlude vessel by compression from the surrounding tissue[6,7] (**Figs. 46.2A and B**).

| TABLE 46.2: Various topical hemostatic agents. | |
|---|---|
| **Agents** | **Main constituent** |
| Avitene | Collagen |
| CollaCote | Collagen |
| CollaTape | Collagen |
| CollaPlug | Collagen |
| Thrombinar | Thrombin |
| Thrombogen | Thrombin |
| Thrombostat | Thrombin |
| Gelfoam | Gelatin |
| Beriplast | Fibrin |
| Surgicel | Cellulose |

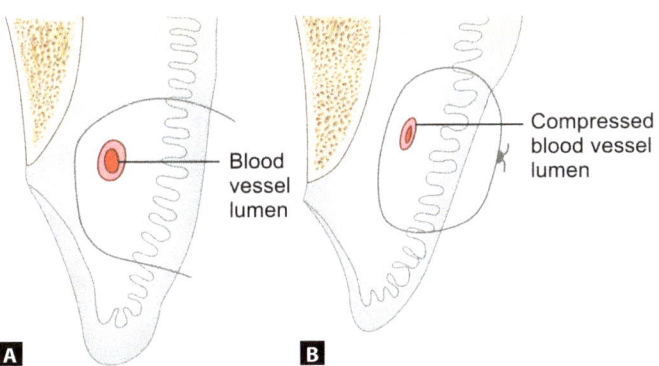

**Figs. 46.2A and B:** Schematic representation showing compression suture to control bleeding.

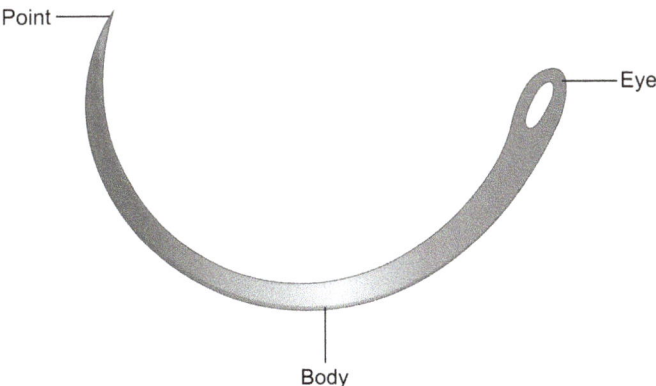

**Fig. 46.3:** Schematic representation showing parts of suture needle: Point, body, and eye.

- *Step VI—Wax*: If bleeding is from an intraosseous site, then it can be controlled by bone wax (beeswax and salicylic acid), which occlude bony canals.
- *Step VII—Suture ligation*: If a large vessel is severed, each end of the vessel is grasped with hemostats, and then nonabsorbable sutures are tied around each end of the vessels and hemostats are removed.

## Wound Closure

The various materials for wound closure are sutures, skin clips or staples, skin tapes, and wound adhesive[8,9] [autologous fibrin glue, fibrin fibronectin sealing system (tissucol), cyanoacrylate, Mussel adhesive protein].

The various intraoral anchoring structures useful in securing movable tissues are:
- *Teeth*: These teeth are the easiest and most secure of all intraoral anchors.
- *Bound down tissue*: Gingiva affixed to the bone via periosteum is the second most reliable anchor.
- Periosteum
- *Loose connective tissue*: It is the least secure anchoring structure in the mouth. Connective tissue in the vestibule and fatty tissue in the retromolar area are the examples of loose connective tissue anchor source.

### Suture and Suturing Techniques

The selection of the type of suture material and needle is dependent on tissue type and thickness, location in the mouth, ease of handling, cost, and the planned time of suture removal.

> **Clinical Tip**
> The length of the needles used generally ranges from 13 mm to 21 mm, and in fact, rarely exceeds 18 mm.

### Suture Needle

Needles are made of either stainless steel or carbon steel and are manufactured in two basic shapes, straight and curved.

*Suture needle anatomy*: Regardless of its intended use, every surgical needle has three basic parts (**Fig. 46.3**):
1. *Eye/point of attachment*: It is the working end of the needle.
2. *Body*: It refers to the grasping area, which forms most of the needle length. It starts where the point of needle ends and ends where the contour change, marking the beginning of the swage of the needle. The needle's body should be as close as possible to the diameter of the suture material to minimize bleeding and leakage.
3. *Eye/swage*: It is the segment at which needle and suture materials are joined.

*Needle size*: It may be measured in inches or in metric units. The following measurements determine the size of a needle:
- *Chord*: The linear distance between eye and tip.
- *Length of the needle*: The distance between eye and tip following the curvature.
- *Radius*: The distance of the needle's body from the center of the circle if the radius of the curve continued to produce a complete circle.

> **Fishermen's Needle**
> - Needles with compound curvature also exist, i.e., with two segments of different radius.
> - These are used where there is little room for maneuver, and the suture thread is very fine.
> - Includes an elliptic portion.
> - It cannot be superimposed on a circle.

- *Diameter*: Gauge or thickness of the metal wire out of which the needle is made. Very small needles of the fine gauge are needed for microsurgery.

### Types of Needles
- *Based on shape*:
  - *Straight*: Straight needles with no curvature, find their principal use in continuous intradermal sutures.
  - *Curved*: Curved needles[10] are designated as 1/4, 3/8, 1/2, 5/8 (**Fig. 46.4**).

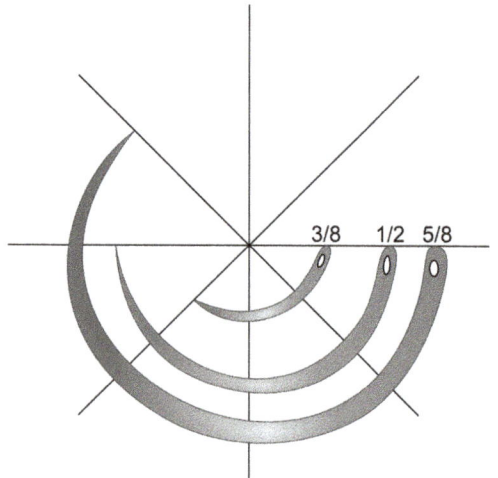

**Fig. 46.4:** Schematic representation showing suture needles: The arc describes as 3/8, 1/2 or 5/8th of a circle.

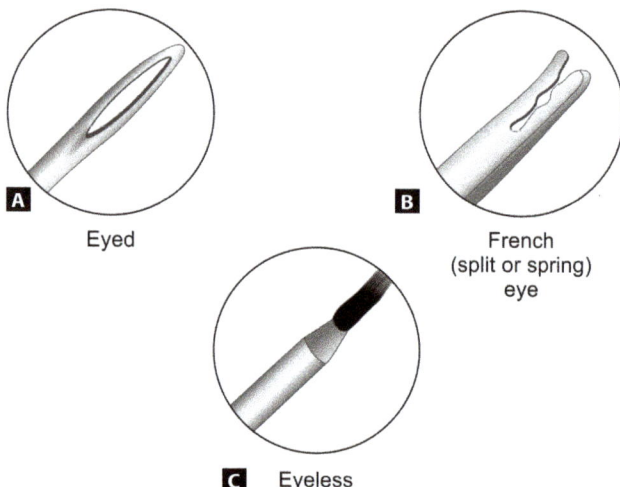

**Figs. 46.5A to C:** Schematic representation showing (A) Eyed needle; (B) French (split or spring) eye needle; (C) Eyeless needle.

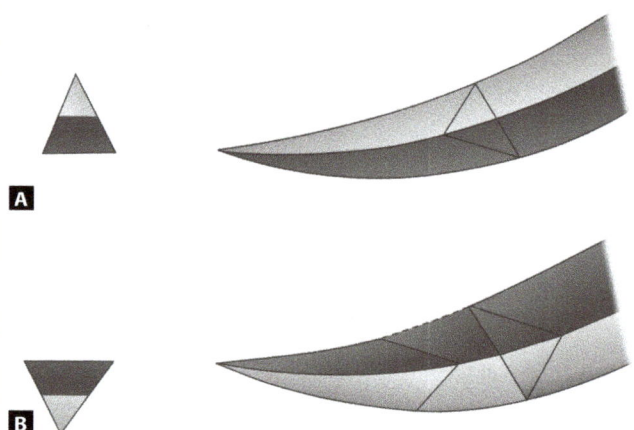

**Figs. 46.6A and B:** Schematic representation showing: (A) Conventional cutting needle; (B) Reverse cutting needle.

- *Based on the eye (Figs. 46.5A to C):*
  - *Eyed*: Suture material is tied to the needle and is designed to reuse. It may be a closed eye or French (split or spring) eye. The closed eye is similar to a household sewing needle. The shape of the eye may be round, oblong, or square. French eye needles have a slit from inside the eye to the end of the needle with ridges that catch and hold the suture in place.
  - *Eyeless or swaged*: The suture material is inserted into a hollow end during manufacturing, and metal is compressed around it. The needle is not reusable.
- *Based on the shape of the tip*, needles may be subdivided into two categories: Cutting and blunt needles.[11]
  1. *Cutting needles*: These are sub-grouped into five categories:
     i. Classical cutting needle (**Fig. 46.6A**): It has a triangular section with the base of the triangle towards the external/convex part of the arc of the circle and has three cutting edges: Two laterally and one superficially on its concave side. Disadvantage: The risk of accidentally cutting tissues from a depth upwards is at a maximum with this type of needle.
     ii. Reverse cutting needle (**Fig. 46.6B**): It has an identical triangular section but with the base of the triangle towards the concave side and with the cutting edge towards the external convex side of the needle.
     Advantages associated with the reverse cutting needle are as follows:
     - The tissue is protected in the case of accidental traction being applied to the needle, since it is the needle's concave side, with no cutting edge that meets the overlying tissues.
     - Due to the engineering and construction of needle, reverse cutting needle is much stronger than a classic cutting needle.
     iii. Lateral cutting needle: Tips with only two lateral cutting edges are also known as spatula tips, from their shape. The section is a trapezoid, with the smaller base on the convex side of the needle and larger base on the concave side. These types of needles are used in ophthalmic surgery.

**Clinical Tips**
- A 5/8th circle needle is used for suturing the palatal mucosa.
- J curvature needle is more useful in placing sutures in the depth.

     iv. Taper cut needle: Combines the characteristics described for reverse cutting needles and those of beveled needles. Immediately distal to the apex of the tapered tip, three sharp cutting edges depart that gradually meet the cylindrical

portion. The characteristics of an aggressive cutting tip are combined with a cylindrical and beveled body. These are used to fix bilaminar grafts in the needle holder.
  v. Beveled needle.
2. *Blunt needles*: Needles without cutting tips are of relative importance when used in high-risk patients [human immunodeficiency virus (HIV), hepatitis C virus (HCV)]. The use of these needles greatly reduces the risks of surgical staff becoming accidentally contaminated, where the precision of suturing is only of moderate importance, like after extraction of inflamed teeth.

### Types of Suture Materials
- *Based on the number of filaments*:
  - Monofilament, e.g., steel and nylon
  - Multifilament, e.g., silk and cotton
- *Based on suture diameter* by US Pharmacopeia in descending order from 5, 4, 3, 2, 1-0 till 11-0 size. 1-0 is the largest diameter and 11-0, the smallest one.
- *Based on the resorbability of suture material*:
  - Nonabsorbable: These are the sutures that are removed manually.
  - Absorbable: These are the sutures which break down harmlessly in the body over time without intervention. Resorbable sutures are preferred to nonresorbable sutures in high-risk infected patients (HIV, HCV), to avoid exposing medical and paramedical staff to additional risks.
    - Application of absorbable sutures:
      - In the case of bilaminar grafts, subepithelial connective tissue grafting procedure. These can only be fixed with resorbable sutures since suture removal would be impossible.

> **Clinical Tips**
> - PERMA-HAND surgical silk is available as an eyeless needled sterile suture in sizes 7–0 to 1–0.
> - Reels as nonsterile sutures are available in sizes 5–0 to 3–0.

      - In bed-ridden patients, hospitalized for the long-term, psychiatric or phobic patients.
      - Young children, to avoid a second trauma.
      - In the case of suturing on more than one plane.
- *Based on the source*:
  - Natural:
    - Absorbable: Plain gut, chromic gut, fast-absorbing gut, plain collagen, chromic collagen.
    - Nonabsorbable: Silk, cotton, linen.
  - Synthetic:
    - Absorbable: Polyglactin, polyglyconate, polyglcolic, polydioxanone.
    - Nonabsorbable: Nylon, polybutester, polyester, decron, polypropylene, nurolon.

### Nonabsorbable Sutures
- *Silk*: It is an organic substance that undergoes slow proteolysis when implanted. It is derived from the cocoon of the silkworm larvae. It is a protein, like keratin of a hair and skin, and is covered initially by an albuminous layer. This layer is removed by the process of degumming prior to the making of sutures. The suture is braided around a core and coated with wax to reduce capillary action. The black color of the silk suture is for better visibility against the red surgical field **(Fig. 46.7)**. It is the most popular suture material for intraoral use. It is braided, which gives it excellent handling characteristics; it produces a moderate tissue response and does not irritate the adjacent mucous membrane. It is an inexpensive suture. There are two disadvantages associated with silk suture—It must be removed postoperatively, as it does not resorb and it is made of many strands of material that permits passage of bacteria and fluid into the surgical wound.[12]
- *Nylon*: It can be obtained in braided or monofilament forms. In its monofilament form, it is the most popular skin suture material. The antibacterial activity (against *Staphylococcus aureus*) accounts in parts for the good tissue response. Nylon, like other synthetic polymeric materials, possesses the property of memory. This memory is actually the built-in orientation of the polymer produced by extruding and stretching during filament manufacture. When tied, the suture tends to "remember" that it was originally a straight fiber and knot slip and untie. A large knot is required due to its stiffness. It is not frequently used intraorally because of the tendency to tear through nonkeratinized tissue.
- *Linen*: It is made from flax and is cellulose material. It is a natural cellulose polymer. It is twisted to form a fiber to make a suture. It gains 10% in tensile strength when wet, and is used for tying pedicles and as ligatures.
- *Cotton*: It is derived from the hair of the seed of the cotton plant. It is twisted to form a suture. It is weaker as compared to linen. Handling is not as good as silk.

### Absorbable Sutures
- *Gut*: It is the oldest known absorbable suture material. The origin of the word "Catgut" is the *Arabic* "kitstring

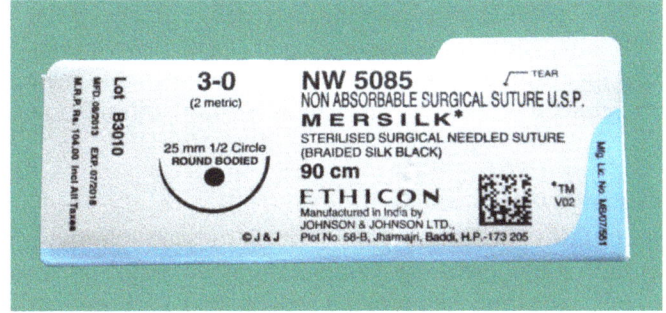

**Fig. 46.7:** Photograph showing silk suture (Black color).

or kitgut," the string of a dancing master's fiddle, which was also made of animal intestine. Catgut is derived from sheep intestinal submucosa or bovine intestinal serosa. The gut has the least tensile strength of any of the commonly used suture materials. Because it is an organic material and highly susceptible to enzymatic degradation, it is packaged in isopropyl alcohol as a preservative, which also serves to condition or softens it. The suture absorbs the alcohol, causing it to swell and increase in diameter. The alcohol is combustible and is also irritating to tissue; it should be removed by a quick rinse in saline prior to use. The gut suture is absorbed by proteolytic degradation and phagocytosis. This is accompanied by considerable inflammation and tissue reaction.

The plain gut is somewhat more difficult to use than other suture materials, as it is stiff and has insecure knot holding characteristics when wet.

Chromic gut, which is plain gut, has been tanned with chromium salts' solution before being spun, ground, and polished. The chromium salts act as a cross-linking agent and increase the tensile strength of the material and its resistance to absorption by the body[13] **(Fig. 46.8)**.

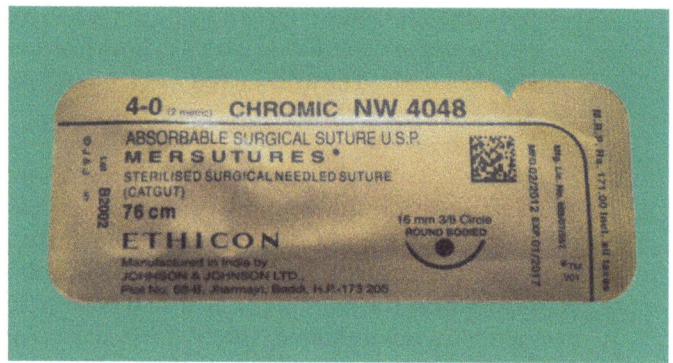

**Fig. 46.8:** Photograph showing the chromic gut suture.

- *Collagen*: Reconstituted collagen sutures are obtained by grinding the native collagen of deep flexor tendons of cattle, which is then acidified to form a gel and extruded into a neutralizing dehydration bath.
- *Polyglycolic acid* is hydroxyacetic acid, which, in the presence of heat and a catalyst, is converted to a high molecular weight linear chain polymer. The suture material is manufactured by orienting these filaments by means of stretching and braiding.
- *Polyglactin 910* is a copolymer of glycolide and lactide, which are derived from hydroxyacetic and lactic acid, respectively **(Fig. 46.9)**. Both polyglycolic acid and polyglactin 910 suture materials, when braided, are the strongest of the absorbable materials.

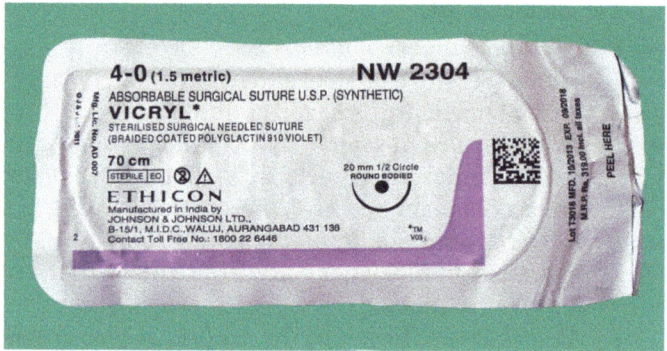

**Fig. 46.9:** Photograph showing polyglactin 910 suture (violet color).

The problem associated with polyglycolic acid and polyglactin 910 is the difficulty in tying the suture material. The material slides easily on itself, making tying difficult. The manufacturer has recommended wetting the material with a saline solution to facilitate tying.

- *Vicryl plus*: This is a polyglactin 910 coated, braided synthetic absorbable antibacterial suture. This suture is the world's first and only antibacterial suture, which offers protection against the suture's bacterial colonization. It contains triclosan, which is a broad-spectrum antibacterial agent. It provides defenses against unwanted bacteria by a zone of inhibition that stops bacterial growth **(Fig. 46.10)**.

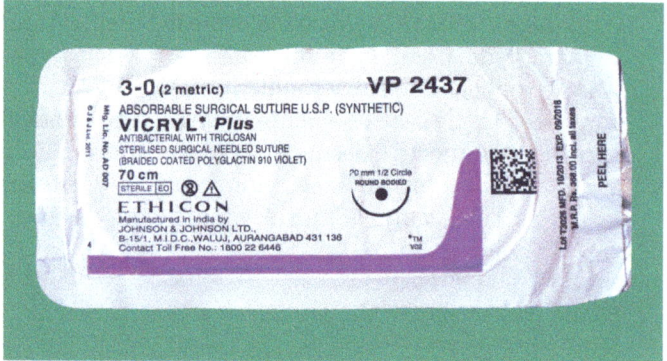

**Fig. 46.10:** Photograph showing vicryl plus suture (violet color).

### Description Over the Suture

It contains the name of the suture, its size, length and atraumatic, the type and size of the needle and number of foils required, e.g., prolene 5-0, 90 cm with atraumatic reverse cutting needle (12 mm 3/8 circle), 1 foil **(Fig. 46.11)**.

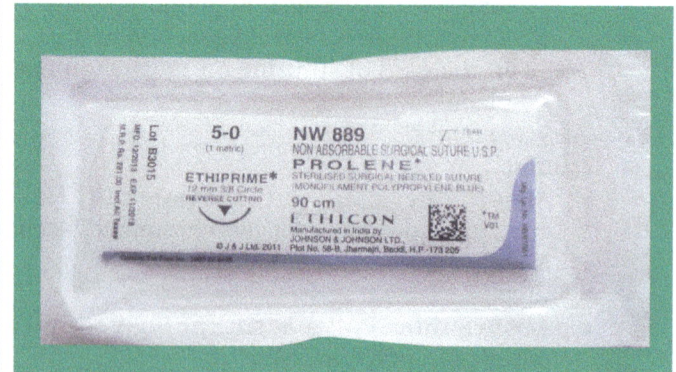

**Fig. 46.11:** Photograph showing description over the suture.

Chapter 46: General Principles of Periodontal Surgery

| TABLE 46.3: Material of choice. | | | | |
|---|---|---|---|---|
| Parameters | Periosteal suturing | Apically positioned flaps suturing | Periodontal regenerative surgery suturing | Periodontal plastic surgery suturing |
| Suture number | 4-0 or 5-0 | 4-0 | 3-0 to 5-0 | 4-0 to 6-0 |
| Needle size | J-1, P-3 | J-1, FS2, P-3 | P-3, RT-16 | P-3 |
| Suture material | Silk | Silk | Gore-Tex, Vicryl | Chromic gut, silk, monofilament |

## Material of Choice

The choice of material depends on the following (**Table 46.3**):[14]
- J-1: 17 mm, 1/2 circle
- FS-2: 19 mm, 3/8 circle
- P-3: 3/8 circle, reverse cutting needle
- RT-16: A CV-5 suture with a 16 mm and 3/8 circle, reverse cutting needle.

## *Objectives of Suturing*

- To stabilize the tissue.
- To secure tissues in the desired locations.
- To maintain hemostasis.
- To permit healing by primary intention.
- As a tool to retract flap for photography or to retrieve free gingiva/connective tissue autografts.

## *Principles of Suturing*

Following are the principles of suturing:[13]
1. Needle holder should grasp the needle approximately three-fourths of the distance from the point.
2. The needle should enter the tissue perpendicular to the surface.
3. The needle should be passed through the tissue following the curvature of the needle.
4. The suture should be placed at an equal distance (2–3 mm) from the incision on both sides and at an equal depth.
5. The needle should be passed from free to the fixed side.
6. The needle should be passed from thinner to thicker side.
7. If one tissue plane is deeper than the other, the needle should be passed from deeper to the superficial side.
8. The distance that the needle is passed into tissue should be greater than the distance from the tissue edge.
9. The tissue should not be closed under tension; it will either tear or necrose.
10. The suture should be tied so that tissue is merely approximated, not blanched.
11. The suture should not be placed over the incision line.
12. The suture should be placed approximately 3–4 mm apart.
13. In the interdental papilla, sutures should enter and exit the tissue at a point located below the imaginary line that forms the base of the triangle of the interdental papilla[15] (**Fig. 46.12**).

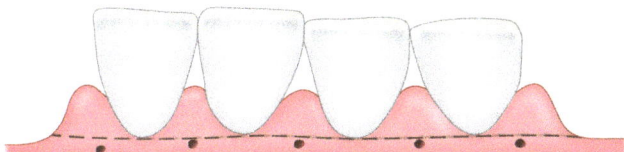

**Fig. 46.12:** Schematic representation showing sutures in the interdental papilla placed below the base of an imaginary triangle of the papilla.

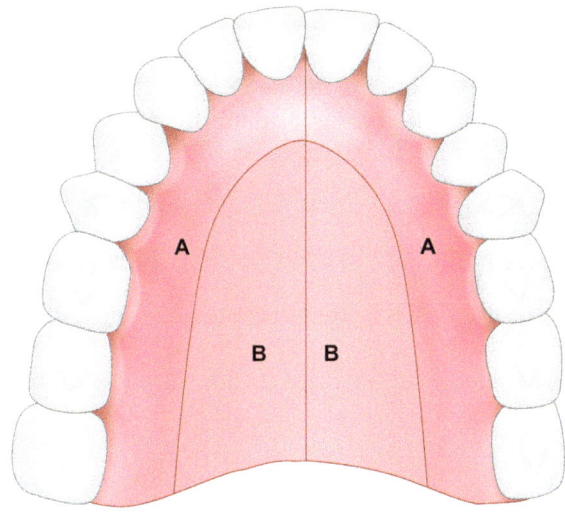

**Fig. 46.13:** Schematic representation showing sutures at the palatal area: For slightly/moderately elevated palatal flap—sutures are placed in "A" area (marginal area) and for more substantial elevated palatal flap—sutures are placed in "B" area (central area).

14. For the palatal flap, the location of sutures depends on the extent of flap elevation. The flap is divided into four quadrants. The sutures should be placed in the quadrant closest to the teeth when the flap's elevation is slight/moderate, but when the flap's elevation is substantial, the sutures are placed in the central portion[15] (**Fig. 46.13**).

## *Suturing Techniques*

Following are the suturing techniques:[14,16,17]
- *Interrupted suturing*:
  - Direct/loop
  - Figure of eight
  - Mattress: Vertical and horizontal
- *Continuous suturing*:
  - Continuous locking
  - Mattress: Vertical and horizontal
- Simple sling suture
- Periosteal sutures

### Interrupted Suturing

- *Direct/loop suture*:
  - Indication: These sutures are used where bone grafts are placed and when a closed apposition of scalloped incision is required.
  - Technique: The needle penetrates the outer surface of the first flap. The undersurface of the opposite flap is engaged, and the suture is brought back to the initial side where the knot is tied **(Figs. 46.14A to D)**.
- *Figure-of-eight suture*:
  - Indication: These sutures are placed when flaps are not in close apposition because of apical flap position or nonscalloped incisions.
  - Technique: The needle penetrates the outer surface of the first flap and the outer surface of the opposite flap. The suture is brought back to the first flap, and the knot is tied **(Figs. 46.15A to D)**. The main advantage of this suturing is easier access between the teeth, but the disadvantage is that there will be interposed suture between the flaps that prevent their approximation.
- *Mattress sutures*: Mattress means that the suture passes through the flap twice. The material does not pass under the incision line, thus minimizing wicking.
  Vertical mattress:
  - Indication: It is used in areas with long and narrow papillae.
  - Technique: The needle penetrates the outer/the epithelized surface of the flap 8–10 mm apical to the tip of the papilla. It is passed through the under the surface of the flap, emerging again from the outer surface of the same flap 2–3 mm from the tip of papilla. Thus, a vertical bite of 6–7 mm is taken with the needle. The needle is passed through the embrasure, where the technique is again repeated with the opposite/second flap. The suture is tied on the first flap **(Figs. 46.16A to D)**. It is of two types: everting and inverting.
  Horizontal mattress:
  - Indication: Interproximal areas of diastema with short and wide papillae.
  - Technique: The needle penetrates the outer surfaces of flap 7–8 mm apical and to one side of the midline of papilla emerging again 4–5 mm through the outer surface on the opposite side of the midline papilla. Thus, the horizontal bite of 4–5 mm is taken with the needle. The needle is passed through the embrasure, where the technique is again repeated with the opposite/second flap. The suture is tied on the first flap **(Figs. 46.17A to C)**.
- *Criss-cross suture*: Criss-cross single horizontal mattress is good for holding osseous grafts in papilla preservation flap **(Fig. 46.18)**.
  - Indication: The use of a criss-cross as the suture passes through the interproximal areas provides

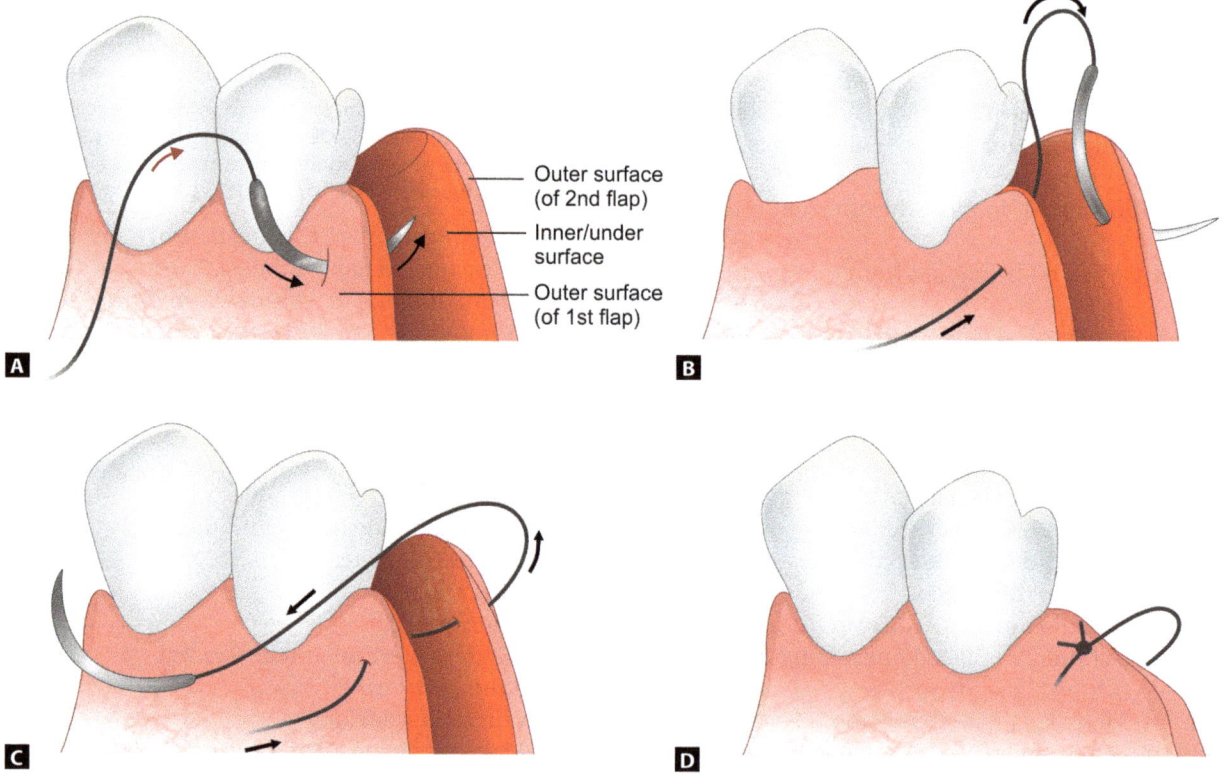

**Figs. 46.14A to D:** Schematic representation showing direct loop suturing.

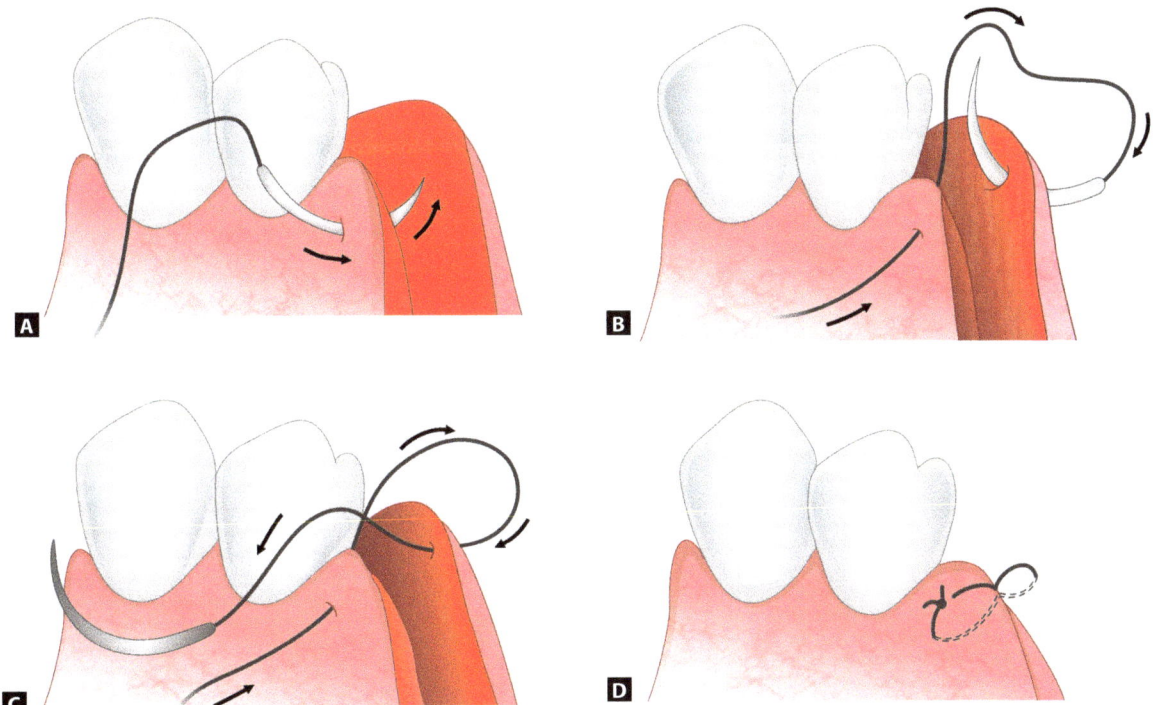

**Figs. 46.15A to D:** Schematic representation showing figure-of-eight suturing.

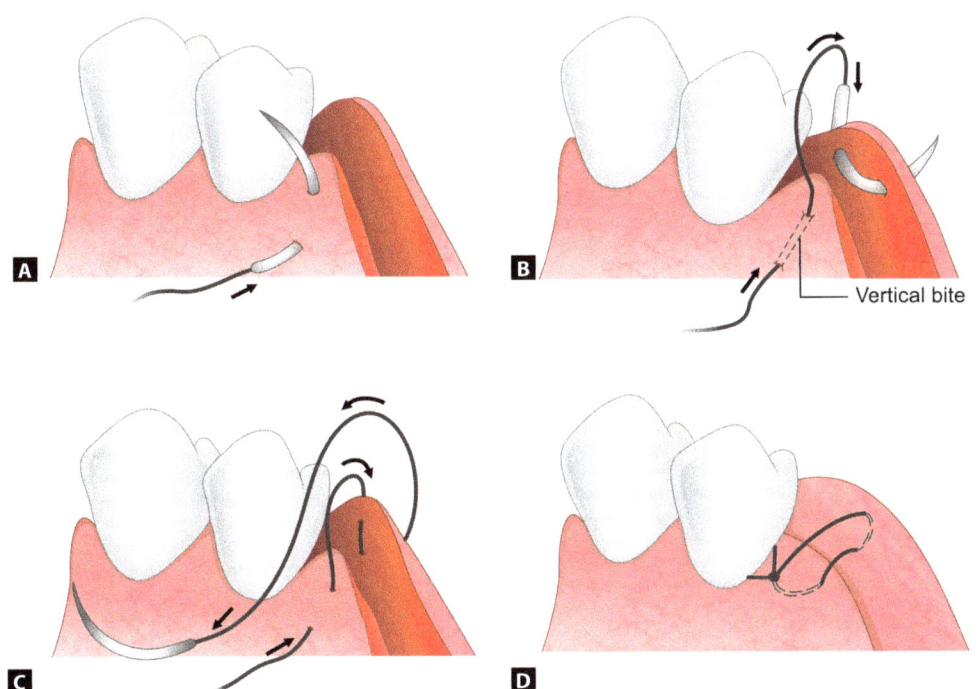

**Figs. 46.16A to D:** Schematic representation showing vertical mattress suturing.

good control of the flap papilla and keeps the suture out of the healing interproximal sulcus area.
- Technique: The needle is passed by entering the outer surface of the mesial lingual aspect (position 1) and the existing distal lingual aspect (position 2); the suture is then crossed over, enters the outer surface of the mesial buccal aspect (position 3), and exits the distal buccal aspect (position 4). The suture at the distal buccal (position 4) is tied to the free end of the mesial lingual (position 1); the knot is positioned towards the lingual aspect **(Fig. 46.18)**.

**Section 7:** Treatment: Surgical Therapy

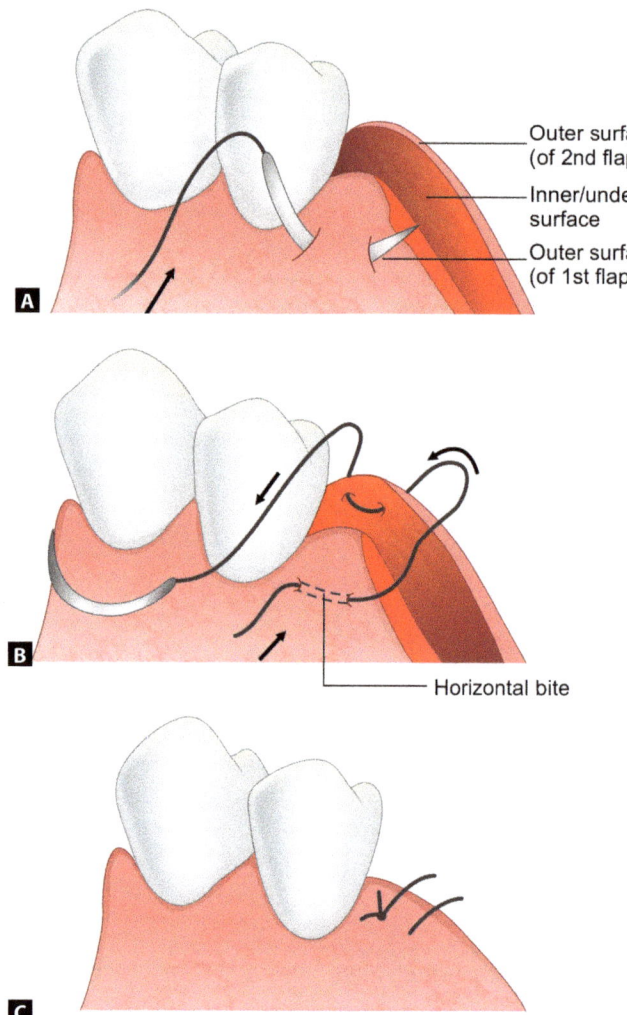

**Figs. 46.17A to C:** Schematic representation showing horizontal mattress suturing.

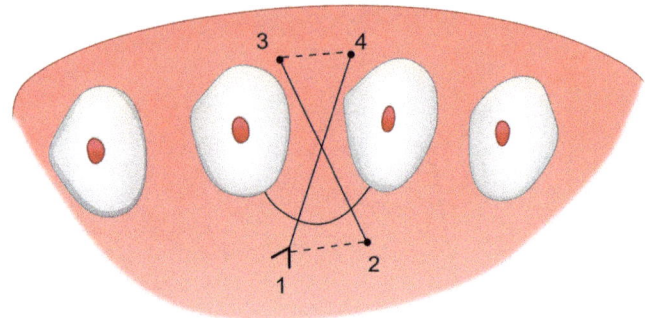

**Fig. 46.18:** Schematic representation showing criss-cross horizontal mattress suture.

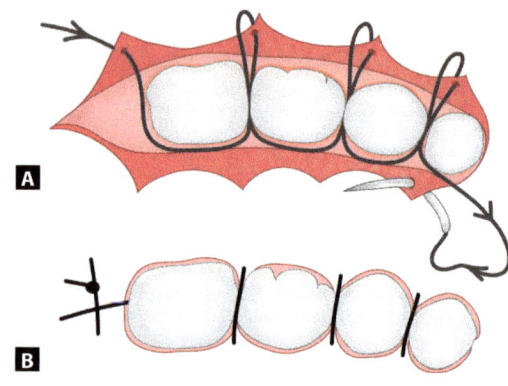

**Figs. 46.19A and B:** Schematic representation showing continuous suturing: The positions of flaps are adjusted and secured in their proper positions by closing the suture.

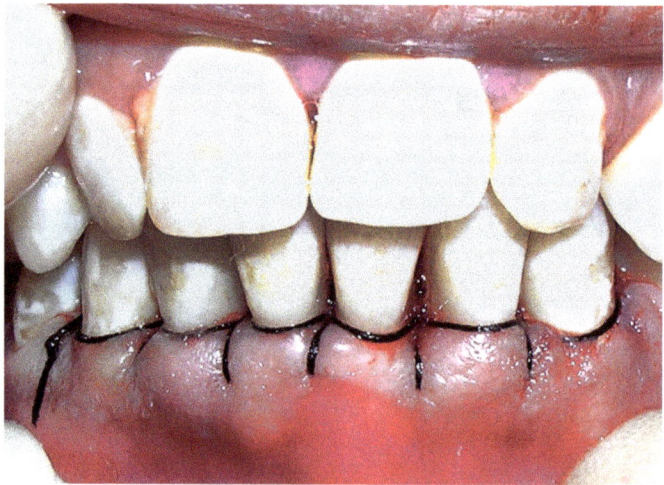

**Fig. 46.20:** Clinical picture showing continuous sutures: Only one knot is needed.

### Continuous Suturing
- *Indication*: The continuous suture is commonly used when flaps involving several teeth are to be apically repositioned. When the flaps have been elevated on both sides of the teeth, one flap at a time is secured in its correct position.
- *Technique*: The suturing procedure is started at the mesial/distal aspect of the buccal flap by passing the needle through the flap and across the interdental area. The suture is laid around the tooth's lingual surface and returned to the buccal side through the next interdental space. The procedure is repeated tooth by tooth until the distal/mesial end of the flap is reached. Thereafter, the needle is passed through the lingual flap, with the suture laid around each tooth's buccal aspect and through each interproximal space. When the suturing of the lingual flap is completed, and the needle has been brought back to the first interdental area, the positions of the flaps are adjusted and secured in their proper positions by closing the suture (**Figs. 46.19A and B**). Thus, only one knot is needed (**Fig. 46.20**).

*Advantages*:
- Minimal use of knots.
- The lesser time required for both placement and removal.
- Teeth are used to anchor the flap.

## Chapter 46: General Principles of Periodontal Surgery

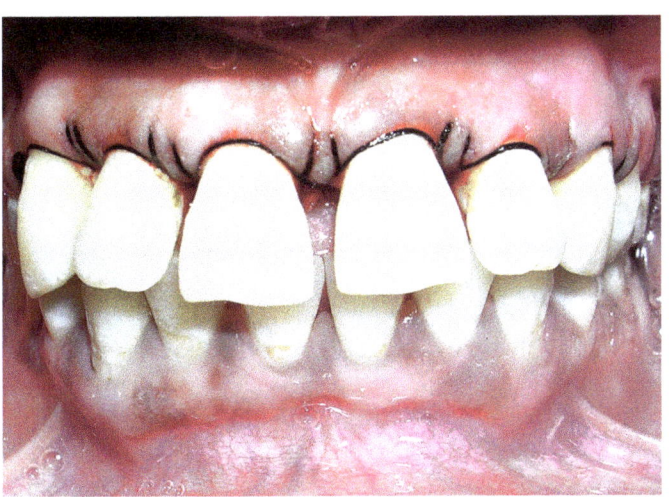

**Fig. 46.21:** Clinical picture showing continuous horizontal mattress sutures.

*Disadvantage*: A disadvantage of the continuous suture is that if one suture pulls through, the entire suture line becomes loose **(Fig. 46.21)**.

### Simple Sling Suturing
- *Indication*: It is used primarily with apically positioned flap and in repositioning the flap.
- *Technique*: The needle engages the outer surface of the flap and encircles the tooth. The outer surface of the same flap of the adjacent interdental area is engaged. The suture is returned to the initial site, and the knot tied **(Figs. 46.22A to D)**.

The sling/suspensory suture is used primarily when the surgical procedure is of a limited extent and involves only the tissue of the buccal or lingual aspect of the teeth. It is also the suture of choice when the buccal and lingual flaps are repositioned at different levels and to place the barrier membrane onto the tooth surface.

### Periosteal Suturing
This is the technique of immobilizing flap or graft to a new position by utilizing the adjacent periosteum to anchor the flap.
- *Indication*: It is used primarily with apically positioned partial-thickness flap and free gingival grafts.
- *Technique*: The flap is pierced perpendicular to the outer surface of the flap by inserting the needle perpendicular to the periosteum-connective tissue. While rotating the needle, periosteal fibers are engaged. The needle is moved coronally along the bone surface and is removed from the periosteum-connective tissue from the inner surface of the flap[18] **(Figs. 46.23A to C)**.

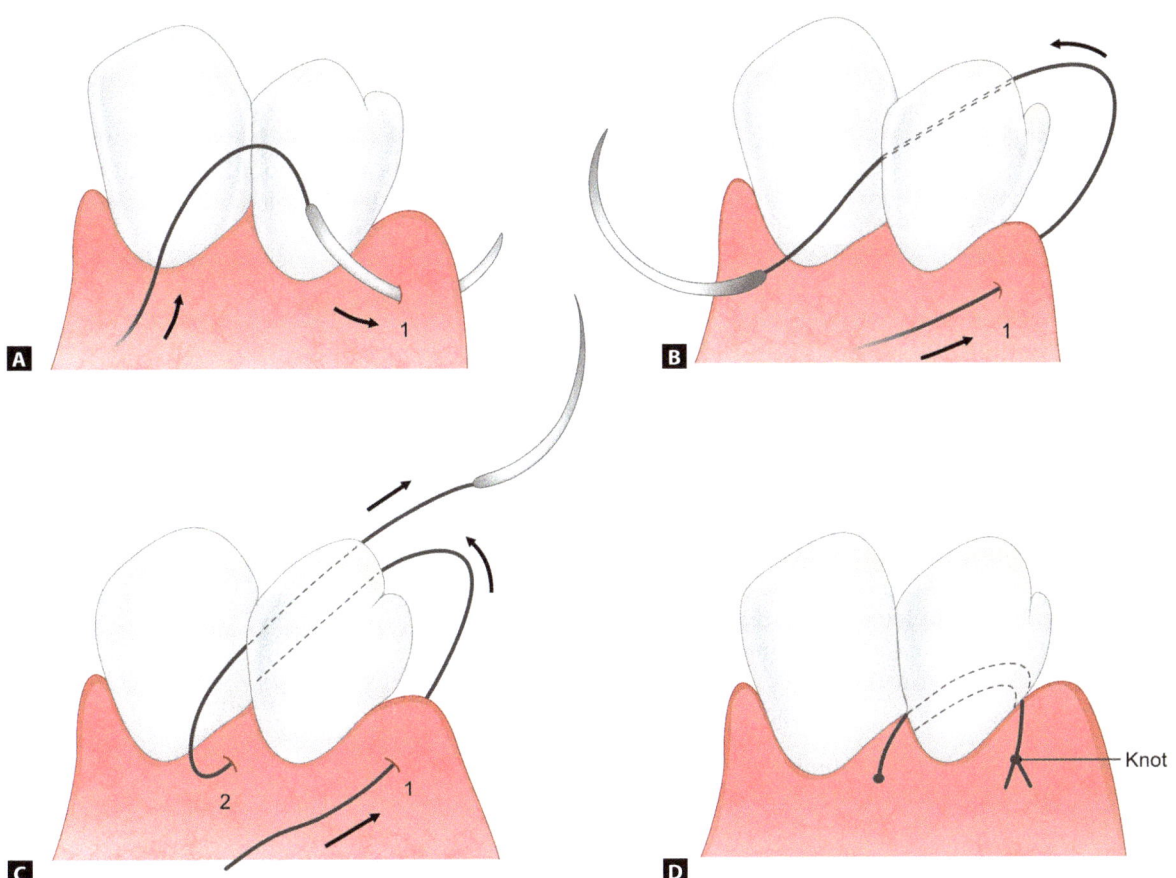

**Figs. 46.22A to D:** Schematic representation showing sling suturing.

**Section 7:** Treatment: Surgical Therapy

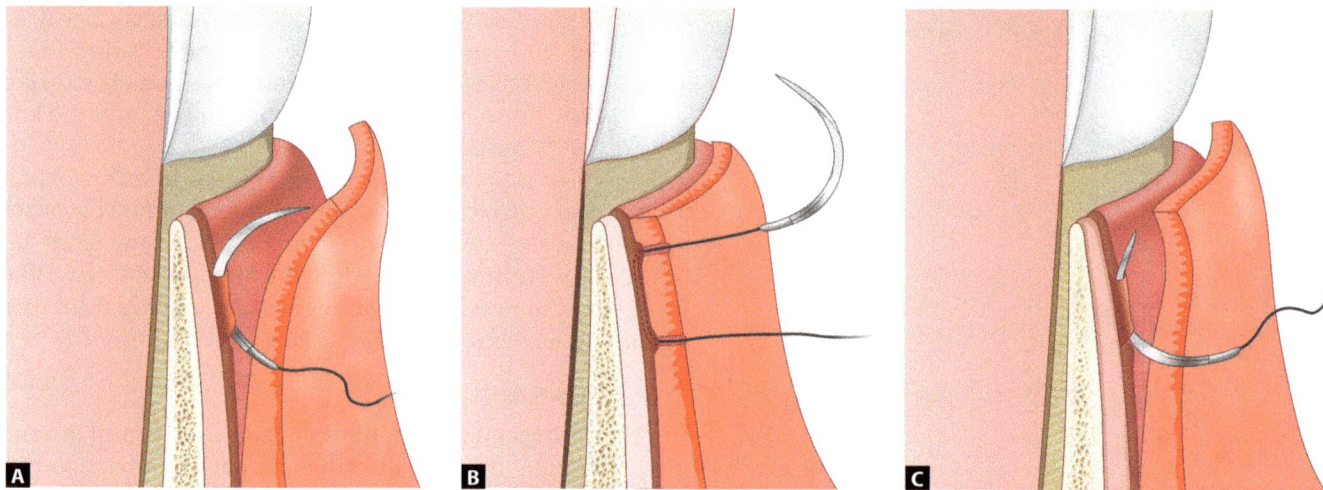

**Figs. 46.23A to C:** Schematic representation showing periosteal suturing.

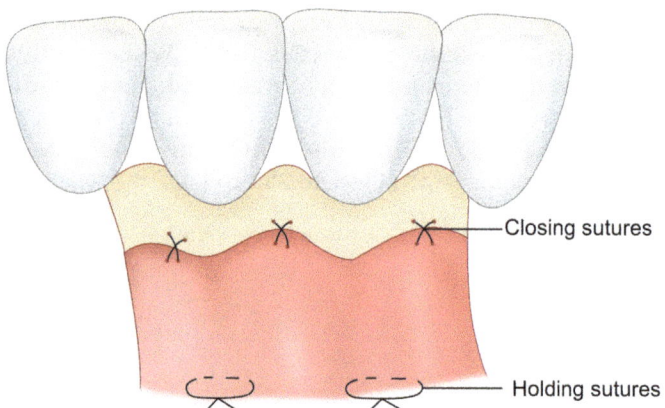

**Fig. 46.24:** Schematic representation showing periosteal sutures: Holding and closing sutures.

### Types of periosteal suture

It is of two types: holding and closing sutures. Holding sutures are done first which are given at the bottom, followed by the closing sutures, which are given at the coronal edge of the flap[15] **(Fig. 46.24)**.

*Sutured knots*: The components of sutured knots are loop, knot, and ears. The knot is composed of a number of tight throws; each throw represents a weave of the two strands and ears that are the suture's cut ends. Knots should be tied as small as possible. Completed knots should be firm to reduce slippage. Tie knots on the facial aspect for access in removal, leaving 2–3 mm suture tail.

Types of knots:
- *Square knot*: Two single ties in the opposite direction.
- *Granny knot*: Two or three ties in the same direction.
- *Surgeon's knot 2-1*: The first tie is a double, and the second tie is single in the opposite direction.
- *Surgeon's knot 2-2*: Both first and second ties are double in the opposite direction.

### Principles of Suture Removal

1. Areas should be swabbed with hydrogen peroxide for removal of encrusted necrotic debris, blood, and serum from the suture.
2. A sharp suture scissor should be used to cut the suture loops, close to the epithelial surface as possible. In this way, a minimal amount of portion of sutures that were exposed to the outside environment and has become laden with debris and bacteria will be dragged through the tissue.
3. A cotton plier is then used to remove the sutures. The knots' location should be noted so that they can be removed first, which will prevent unnecessary entrapment of the flap.

## Periodontal Dressings

Periodontal dressings were first introduced in 1923 when Dr AW Ward advocated the rules and use of packing material around the teeth following gingival surgery.[19] This material was called WondrPak, which consisted of zinc oxide (ZnO) eugenol mixed with alcohol, pine oil, and asbestos fibers.

### Purpose

Following are the purposes of periodontal dressing:[20]
- Protect the wound area from irritants, such as hot or spicy food.
- Enhance the patient's comfort.
- Help to maintain the position of repositioned soft tissues.
- Help to act as a template to prevent the formation of excessive granulation tissue.
- Protect newly exposed root surfaces from temperature changes.
- Stabilize mobile teeth and protect sutures.

## Properties

Dressing should:
- Be soft, but with enough plasticity and flexibility.
- Set within a reasonable time.
- Have sufficient rigidity to prevent fracture and dislocation.
- Have a smooth surface after setting to prevent irritation to the cheeks and lips.
- Be dimensionally stable to prevent salivary leakage and accumulation of plaque debris.
- Preferably have bactericidal properties to prevent excessive plaque formation.
- Not induce allergic reactions.
- Have an acceptable taste.
- Not interfere with healing.

## Classifications

Periodontal dressings have been classified into the following categories:
- *Zinc oxide eugenol dressings*: Kirkland pack, Wonder pack.
- *Zinc oxide non-eugenol dressings*: Coe-Pak, Periocare, Periopac, Perioputty, and Vocopac.
- *Others*: Photocuring periodontal dressing (Barricaid), collagen dressings, methacrylic gel, and cyanoacrylate.

### Zinc Oxide Eugenol Dressings

- *Powder and liquid form (Kirkland pack)*: Powder is composed of ZnO, tannic acid, rosin, kaolin, zinc-stearate, asbestos. The liquid contains eugenol, peanut oil, rosin. When the components of ZnO eugenol dressings are mixed, setting occurs as a result of chemical interaction between ZnO and eugenol forming zinc eugenolate.
- *Paste form*:
  - Tube 1: Base ZnO 87%, fixed vegetable/mineral oil 13%.
  - Tube 2: Accelerator oil of clove 12%, gum/polymerized rosin.

### Zinc Oxide Non-eugenol Dressings

- *Coe-pak*: It is the most common and widely used non-eugenol dressing **(Fig. 46.25)**.
  - Zinc oxide: Main ingredient
  - Vegetable oil: For plasticity
  - Gum: For cohesiveness
  - Lorothidol: Fungicide
  - Liquid coconut: Fatty acids
  - Chlorothymol: Bacteriostatic agent
  - Colophony: Resin
- *Periocare*: Paste contains ZnO, magnesium oxide (MgO), calcium hydroxide [$Ca(OH)_2$], vegetable oils. The gel contains resins, fatty acids, ethylcellulose, lanolin, $Ca(OH)_2$. The setting of Periocare occurs by chemical reaction.

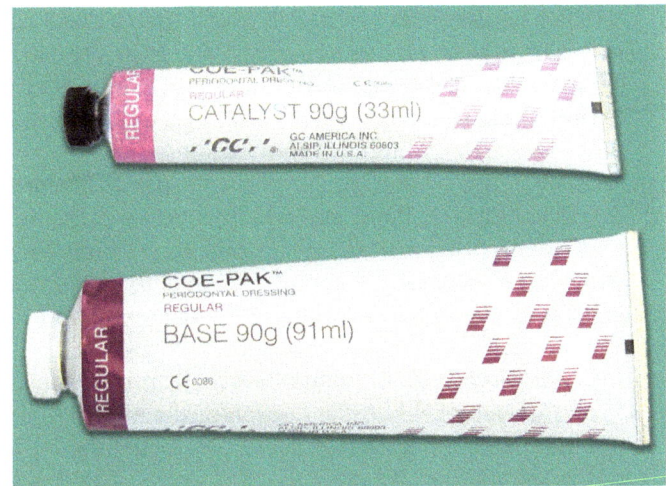

**Fig. 46.25:** Photograph showing Coe-pak: Non-eugenol periodontal dressing.

- *Periopac*: It is premixed ZnO non-eugenol dressing containing tricalcium phosphate [$Ca_3(PO_4)_2$], ZnO, acrylate, organic solvents, flavoring and coloring agents. When this material is exposed to air or moisture, it sets by the loss of organic solvents. After it is set, this dressing becomes quite brittle.
- *Vocopac*: It is a newly formulated product for use as a periodontal dressing. It contains 90 g base and 90 g catalyst. It contains neither eugenol nor coumarin and causes no gingival irritation; it retains its tough elastic qualities throughout its life in the patient's mouth and does not become brittle. It adheres excellently to the teeth and promotes healing. Mixing time is about 20–30 seconds, and its working time is approximately 10–15 minutes.
- *Perioputty*: It is a non-eugenol dressing which contains methyl and propyl-parabens for their effective bactericidal and fungicide properties and benzocaine as a topical anesthetic.
- *Barricaid visible light cure periodontal dressing*: This single component of periodontal dressing eliminates messy, time-consuming mixing of paste. It is available in a syringe for the direct application or dispensing on a mixing pad and placement intraorally. Curing of the material is then accomplished with a visible light curing unit to form a non-brittle, but firm, protective elastic covering. Thus, it provides a more esthetic dressing for the anterior region. The principle ingredients of this material are polyether urethane dimethacrylate resin, silica, visible light cure photoinitiator, accelerator, and stabilizer. It contains polymerizable monomers, which may cause skin sensitization (allergic contact dermatitis) in susceptible persons. Eye protection should be worn while curing with a visible light unit.
- *Collagen dressings*: An example of collagen dressing is CollaCote. Collagen dressing is in the form of collagen sponge, which is a type I collagen derived from bovine

Achilles tendon. It is a completely resorbable dressing that is used to cover and protect palatal graft sites; the sponge is approximately 3 mm thick and can be cut to fit the graft site. It stops bleeding and can absorb 30–40 times its weight in fluid, without swelling.
- *Methacrylate gel dressings*: They have elastic consistency that is soft and resilient and will flow under pressure. They adapt closely to the tissues and are very comfortable with wound site. The major advantage of this material is its ability to carry and release medicaments to the soft tissues.
- *Cyanoacrylate*: In 1964, tissue adhesives were introduced to dentistry. Dr SN Bhaskar conceived the idea of their potential use in periodontics and conducted the bulk of the laboratory and clinical researches.[21] The basic formula of cyanoacrylate is $CH_2=C(CN)COOR$, where R represents methyl, propyl, and butyl radicals. The butyl and isobutyl forms are ideal as periodontal dressings. The use of cyanoacrylate is an alternative to suturing and as a surface adhesive and periodontal dressing. This material has the unique ability to cement together moist, living tissue surfaces. Cyanoacrylate is either applied in drops or sprayed on the tissues. The material is much less bulky than other dressings. Other advantages include lack of apparent side effects, easy adherence to living tissues, immediate hemostasis, lack of evidence of systemic toxicity/sensitivity, precise placement of flaps, decreased suturing time, ease of application, and patient preference over bulky dressings.[22] It is most useful in flap control in concave zones, such as furcal area fluting. Cyanoacrylate has been used for surface application only; adhesives that become trapped under soft tissue flap will delay in wound healing.

Antibacterial properties of packs: Bacitracins, Oxytetracycline (Terramycin), Neomycin and Nitrofurazone, have been tried but may produce hypersensitivity reactions. Incorporation of tetracycline powder in Coe-Pak is generally recommended, particularly when long and traumatic surgeries are performed.

### Preparation and Application

Zinc oxide packs are mixed with eugenol or non-eugenol liquids on a wax paper pad with a wooden tongue depressor. The powder is gradually incorporated with the liquid until a thick paste is formed.

Coe-pak is prepared by mixing equal lengths of paste from tubes containing the accelerator and the base until the resulting paste is of uniform color. The pack is then placed in a cup of water at room temperature for 2–3 minutes so that the paste loses its tackiness and can be molded. It remains workable for 15–20 minutes. The pack is then rolled into two strips of approximately the length of the treated area **(Figs. 46.26A to D)**. The end of one strip is bent into a hook shape and fitted around the distal surface of the last tooth, approaching it from the distal surface. The remainder of the strip is brought forward along the facial surface to the midline. The second strip is applied from the lingual surface. It is joined to the pack at the distal surface of the last tooth and then brought forward along the gingival margin to the midline. The strips are joined interproximally by applying gentle pressure on the pack's facial and lingual surfaces **(Fig. 46.27)**.

### Do Not's

The periodontal dressing should not:
- Extend onto uninvolved mucosa
- Extend over occlusal surfaces of teeth
- Interfere with occlusion

### Placement of Periodontal Dressings

Periodontal dressings are retained mechanically by interlocking in interdental spaces of teeth and joining the lingual and facial portions of the pack. In the case of edentulous areas, the periodontal dressing is retained with the help of splints, Hawley appliance, and stents. In case of isolated teeth, tie dental floss or gauze loosely around the teeth and over which pack is applied.

A periodontal dressing may entrap sutures beneath the dressing and may displace flap.

## POSTOPERATIVE INSTRUCTIONS AND CARE

Appropriate postoperative instructions should be given both verbally and in writing to the patient, including an explanation concerning:
- Discomfort and potential complications.
- All medications, especially analgesics and antibiotics.
- Diet modification.

### Instructions to the Patient after Surgery

#### Dos

- Take two tablets of acetaminophen every 6 hours on 1st day.
- Chew on the nonoperated side.
- Take semisolid food.
- Apply ice, intermittently for alternating 20 minutes on and 20 minutes off, on the face over the operated side on the 1st day.
- Use CHX mouthwash.
- If the bleeding does not stop, take a piece of gauge and form it into U-shape and hold it on thumb and index finger, apply it on both sides of the pack, and hold it there under pressure for 20 minutes.
- Swelling is usual in the extensive surgical procedures. It subsides in 3 or 4 days. Apply moist heat if it persists.
- If any other problem arises, do call the doctor.

### Do Not's

- Avoid hot food.
- Do not smoke or take alcohol.

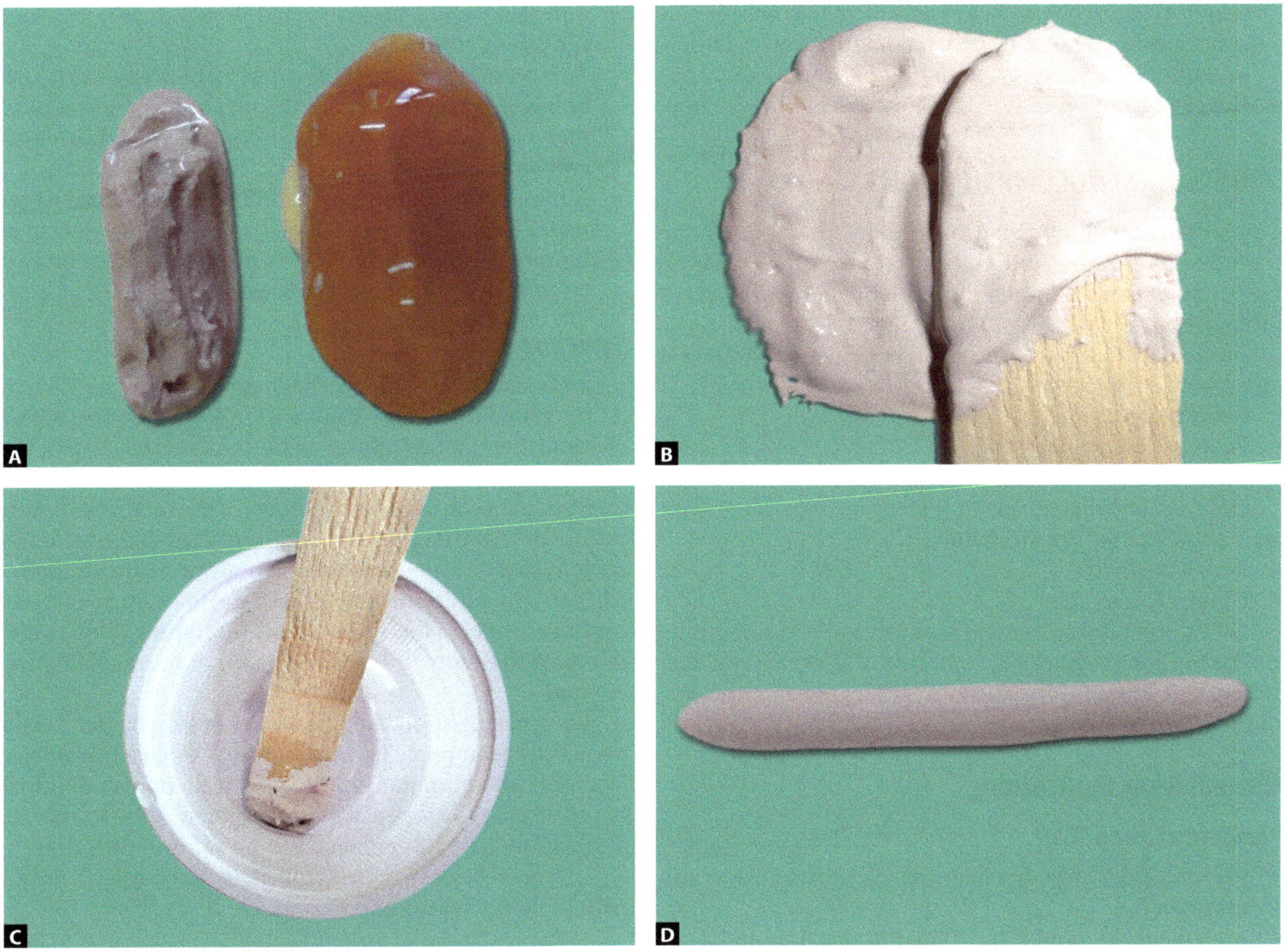

**Chapter 46:** General Principles of Periodontal Surgery

**Figs. 46.26A to D:** Photograph showing (A) Equal lengths of two pastes placed on the paper pad; (B) Pastes are uniformly mixed with wooden tongue depressor; (C) Paste is placed in a cup of water at room temperature to lose its tackiness, and (D) Paste is rolled into a cylinder with lubricated fingers.

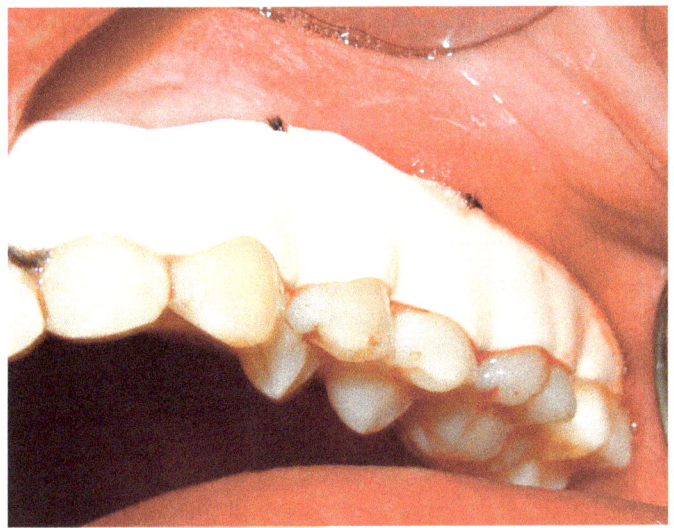

**Fig. 46.27:** Clinical picture showing periodontal pack placement.

- Avoid citrus, highly spicy food.
- Do not brush over the pack/operated site.
- Avoid exertion.
- Do not try to stop bleeding by rinsing.

## Postsurgical Care

- *Day 1*: Analgesics, cold packs, moist gauze locally as needed, total avoidance of wound disturbance.
- *After day 1*: Pain, swelling, bleeding should diminish or disappear. Begin light activity, warm packs as needed, and chemical plaque controls are recommended.
- *After 5–10 days*: Remove dressing and sutures after seven days. Professionally deplaque supragingivally. Begin light oral hygiene.
- *After 4–6 weeks*: Bi-weekly visits for professional deplaqing and oral hygiene instructions. The dentogingival junction should not be probed or

## Section 7: Treatment: Surgical Therapy

instrumented for 6-8 weeks following surgery. A soft toothbrush should be used gently for the 1st few postoperative weeks. The patient should follow the Charter's method of avoiding vigorous toothbrushing.

## POSTSURGICAL COMPLICATIONS

If postoperative complications occur, they should be managed by prompt and appropriate treatment, which may include control of bleeding, adequate analgesics, or antibiotics.

Immediate complications associated with periodontal surgery are as follows:
- Persistent bleeding
- Postoperative pain
- Swelling

Delayed or long-term complications associated with periodontal surgery are as follows:
- Root sensitivity
- Gingival recession

Other potential risks include infection, flap sloughing, root resorption or ankylosis, some loss of alveolar crest, flap perforation, abscess formation, irregular gingival contours, and reaction to medications.

## Immediate Complications

### Persistent Bleeding

- *Primary* postoperative hemorrhage starts at the time of surgery.
- *Intermediate* hemorrhage during the first 48 hours of the surgery, after having stopped temporarily following surgery. It is usually due to the breakdown of an incomplete clot, such as associated with loss of the vasoconstrictor effect of anesthesia.
- *Secondary* hemorrhage occurs after 7-14 days postoperatively. It occurs when the wound becomes infected.
- Persistent bleeding can be stopped with pressure or electrosurgery.

### Postoperative Pain

The severity of postoperative pain varies depending on the patient's threshold level, location, duration, the extent of surgery, and skill with which the soft and osseous tissues are handled during surgery.
- Postoperative pain and discomfort for the patient can be minimized by the surgical handling of the soft and osseous tissues atraumatically.
- The bone should be kept moist as dryness of bone induces severe pain. There should be complete soft tissue coverage of the bone during suturing. Thus, bone exposure should not be extensive.
- The periodontal dressing should not overextend beyond the mucogingival junction, or onto frenum and palate.
- Patients should be instructed to avoid chewing from the operated site.
- Two acetaminophen tablets every 6 hours for the first 24 hours are prescribed for little pain or discomfort. But if pain persists, then acetaminophen plus codeine tablets can be prescribed.
- If the postoperative pain is related to infection, which usually starts after four days following surgery (localized lymphadenopathy and fever), it should be treated with systemic antibiotics and analgesics.

### Swelling

It can be caused by hemorrhage and/or edema. After an injury, bleeding usually stops within 5 minutes because of clotting; therefore, swelling usually is caused by edema. The application of icepack decreases temperature also reduces tissue metabolism and permeability. Depressed metabolism results in less tissue debris, a diminished amount of free protein, and subsequently less osmotic pressure for fluid to exit cells. In addition, reduced cell death because of tissue hypoxia results in fewer mediators (e.g., bradykinin) being released; therefore, there is less vascular permeability and edema.

Reasons for applying icepacks after surgery are to cool tissues to accomplish the following physiological objectives: Decrease inflammation, inhibit swelling (edema), diminish blood supply (vasoconstriction), decrease the metabolic alterations (cold decreases the metabolic rate thereby lessening secondary injuries due to lack of oxygen), relieve pain (cold decreases nerve conduction speed).[23]

> **Clinical Tip**
> Swelling after surgery is best prevented by the use of icepacks. Once swelling develops, hot moist packs and frequent lavage with warm saline solution are preferred.

Generally, swelling subsides by the 4th postoperative day. If swelling persists and becomes worse, then amoxicillin (500 mg) should be taken every 8 hours for one week. Not all postoperative swelling is caused by inflammation; some may be caused by bleeding into tissues which may be accompanied by discoloration under the cheek, chin or eye.[3]

## Delayed or Long-term Complications

### Gingival Recession

The apical movement of gingival margin is common after periodontal surgery. Gingival recession is associated with postoperative problems, like root sensitivity, esthetics, and interproximal food retention. The extent of recession is influenced by the pocket depth and the type of therapy.

### Root Sensitivity

Root sensitivity is manifested as pain induced by hot or cold temperature, more commonly cold. Scaling and root planing during surgical procedures remove the thin cementum present over the cervical area of the root, causing hypersensitivity. The various desensitizing agents are explained in "Chapter 36: Dentin Hypersensitivity."

## WOUND HEALING

To ensure proper healing, atraumatic surgical principles should be followed, including:
- Adequate anesthesia
- Surface disinfection
- Sharp instrumentation
- Minimal, atraumatic tissue handling
- Short operating time
- Preventing unnecessary contamination
- Proper suturing and dressing, if indicated

Healing is a phase of the inflammatory response that leads to a new physiological and anatomical relationship among the disrupted body elements.

Healing of periodontal tissue can be in the form of repair, new attachment, and regeneration (Rest is explained in "Chapter 51: Regenerative Osseous Surgery").

Gingival wounds heal much more rapidly with much less scar formation when compared to skin. The reasons for this reduced scar formation are as follows:
- Gingival fibroblasts, unlike the fibroblasts of other connective tissue, produce more matrix metallopeptidase 13 (MMP13) than MMP1. MMP13 has a broad substantivity and is capable of breakdown or turnover of a number of extracellular matrix proteins. MMP1, on the other hand, has a biological activity that is restricted to collagen I. The greater presence of MMP13 in the wound area is thought to produce a greater turnover and thereby prevent scar formation.
- There is a greater presence of myofibroblasts in the gingiva when compared to skin. Fibroblasts can differentiate to form the more synthetic myofibroblasts under the influence of transforming growth factor-beta (TGF-β). The presence of TGF-β in the wound area enhances the already greater presence of myofibroblasts, thereby leading to lesser wound contraction and scarring.

### Points to Ponder

- Causes of excessive bleeding during surgery include laceration of large blood vessels, incomplete removal of granulation tissue, hypertensive patient, bleeding disorder patient, and patient on anticoagulant therapy.
- However, if the surrounding tissue blanches, the suture is too tight, which may cause necrosis because of poor vascularization.
- Hemostasis should be achieved before and not by the application of a dressing. The only clear indication for dressing is to achieve tissue stasis, such as with a free mucosal graft, or to protect a clot over the bone in the interdental denudation technique. The application of dressing is a matter of individual preference.
- The possible outcomes of surgical periodontal therapy are: Regeneration, new attachment, long junctional epithelium, root resorption or ankylosis and recurrence of pocket.[24]

## REFERENCES

1. Takei HH, Carranza FM. The surgical phase of therapy. In: Newman MG, Takei HH, Carranza FA (Eds). Carranza's Clinical Periodontology, 9th edition. Philadelphia, PA, USA: WB Saunders; 2003. pp. 719-24.
2. Wennstrom JL, Heijl L, Lindhe J. Periodontal surgery: access therapy. In: Lindhe J, Karring T, Lang NP (Eds). Clinical Periodontology and Implant Dentistry, 4th edition. Oxford, UK: Blackwell Munksgaard; 2003. pp. 519-60.
3. Klokkevold PR, Carranza FM, Takei HH. General principles of periodontal surgery. In: Newman MG, Takei HH, Carranza FA (Eds). Carranza's Clinical Periodontology, 9th edition. Philadelphia, PA, USA: WB Saunders; 2003. pp. 725-36.
4. Grant DA, Stern IB, Listgarten MA. Preparations for periodontal surgery. In: Periodontics, 6th edition. St. Louis: CV Mosby; 1988. pp. 719-39.
5. Hupp JR. Principles of surgery. In: Hupp JR, Tucker MR, Ellis E (Eds). Contemporary Oral and Maxillofacial Surgery, 6th edition. St. Louis: Mosby; 2013. pp. 42-8.
6. McDonnell HT, Mills MP. Principle, and practice of periodontal surgery. In: Rose LF, Mealey BL, Genco RJ, Cohen DW (Eds). Periodontics: Medicine, Surgery, and Implants, 1st edition. St. Louis: Elsevier-Mosby; 2004. pp. 358-404.
7. Genco RJ, Rosenberg ES, Evian C. Periodontal surgery. In: Genco RJ, Goldman HM, Cohen DW (Eds). Contemporary Periodontics. St. Louis: CV Mosby; 1990. pp. 554-84.
8. Robinson PJ, Goodman CH. General principles of surgical therapy. In: Genco RJ, Goldman HM, Cohen DW (Eds). Contemporary Periodontics. St. Louis: CV Mosby; 1990. pp. 543-53.
9. Moore RL, Hill M. Suturing techniques for periodontal plastic surgery. Periodontol 2000. 1996;11:103-11.
10. Grant DA, Stern IB, Listgarten MA. Periodontal flap. In: Periodontics, 6th edition. St. Louis: CV Mosby; 1988. pp. 786-822.
11. Siervo S. Technological aspects. In: Suturing Techniques in Oral surgery. Milano, Italy: Quintessenza Edizioni Srl; 2008. pp. 34-71.
12. Levin MP. Periodontal suture materials and surgical dressings. Dent Clin North Am. 1980;24(4):767-81.
13. Evaskus DS. General principles and techniques of surgery. In: Laskin DM (Eds). Clinician's Handbook of Oral and Maxillofacial Surgery, 1st edition. Illinois, USA: Quintessence Publishing; 2013. pp. 255-91.
14. Cohen ES. Sutures and suturing. In: Atlas of Cosmetic Reconstructive Periodontal Surgery, 2nd edition. Philadelphia, PA, USA: Lea & Febiger; 1994. pp. 9-30.
15. Takei HH, Carranza FA. The periodontal flap. In: Newman MG, Takei HH, Carranza FA (Eds). Carranza's Clinical Periodontology, 8th edition. Philadelphia, PA, USA: WB Saunders; 1996. pp. 592-604.
16. Galgut PN. Suturing techniques in periodontal surgery. Br Dent J. 1989;167(1):29-31.
17. Takei H, Carranza FA. The periodontal flap. In: Newman MG, Takei HH, Carranza FA (Eds). Carranza's Clinical Periodontology, 9th edition. Philadelphia, PA, USA: WB Saunders; 2003. pp. 762-73.
18. Sato N. Increasing the attached gingiva. In: Periodontal Surgery: A Clinical Atlas, 1st edition. Illinois, USA: Quintessence Publishing; 2000. pp. 81-140.
19. Ward AW. Inharmonious cusp relation as a factor in periodontoclasia. J Am Dent Assoc. 1923;10:471.
20. Sachs HA, Farnoush A, Checchi L, Joseph CE. Current status of periodontal dressings. J Periodontol. 1984;55(12):689-96.

## Section 7: Treatment: Surgical Therapy

21. Bhaskar SN, Frisch J, Margetis PM, Leonard F. Oral surgery--oral pathology conference No. 18, Walter Reed Army Medical Center. Application of a new chemical adhesive in periodontic and oral surgery. Oral Surg Oral Med Oral Pathol. 1966;22(4):526-35.
22. Forrest JO. The use of cyanoacrylates in periodontal surgery. J Periodontol. 1974;45(4):225-9.
23. Greenstein G. Therapeutic efficacy of cold therapy after intraoral surgical procedure: a literature Review. J Periodontol. 2007;78(5):790-800.
24. Baab DA, Ammons WF, Selipsky H. Blood loss during periodontal flap surgery. J Periodontol. 1977;48(11):693-8.

### VIVA VOCE

**Q1. What are the critical zones in pocket surgery?**
**Ans.** The critical zones in pocket surgery are as follows:
- Zone 1: Soft-tissue wall
- Zone 2: Tooth surface
- Zone 3: Bone
- Zone 4: Attached gingiva

**Q2. What are the causes of excessive bleeding during surgery?**
**Ans.** The causes of excessive bleeding during surgery are as follows:
- Laceration of large blood vessels
- Incomplete removal of granulation tissue
- Hypertensive patient
- Patient with a bleeding disorder
- Patient on anticoagulant therapy

**Q3. Why is increased mobility seen immediately after surgical procedures in periodontally involved teeth?**
**Ans.** These procedures often significantly disrupt/remove the gingival fiber groups, enabling the gingiva to form a rigid cuff around the tooth that adds stability, especially when the periodontal ligament and alveolar support are lost.

**Q4. Who had put forward "No Pack Philosophy"?**
**Ans.** Stahl had put forward "No Pack Philosophy" in 1969.

**Q5. What are the complications that arise in the 1st postoperative week?**
**Ans.** Complications that arise in the 1st postoperative week are as follows:
- Persistent bleeding after surgery
- Sensitivity to percussion
- Swelling
- Feeling of weakness

**Q6. What are the complications that usually arise after 1st postoperative week?**
**Ans.** Root sensitivity, tooth mobility, and gingival recession are complications that usually arise after 1st postoperative week.

**Q7. What is the average blood loss during periodontal surgical procedures?**
**Ans.** According to Baab, an average of 134 mL blood loss occurs during one sextant of periodontal surgery with a wide variability of 16–592 mL.[24]

**Q8. How much time various periodontal tissues take to heal?**
**Ans.** The junctional epithelium takes approximately five days to heal.
Sulcular epithelium takes approximately 7–10 days to heal.
Gingival surface epithelium takes approximately 10–14 days to heal.
Connective tissue takes approximately 21–28 days to heal.
Alveolar bone takes approximately 4–6 weeks to heal.

**Q9. How many days before surgery, the anticoagulant therapy or aspirin should be stopped?**
**Ans.** 7–14 days before surgery, anticoagulant therapy or aspirin should be stopped and can be restarted after 3–4 days of surgery, with the physician's approval.

**Q10. Which type of consent should be taken before surgery?**
**Ans.** Both verbal and written consent.

# Chapter 47

# Gingival Curettage

*Shalu Bathla*

## Chapter Outline

- Terminology
- Indications
- Contraindications
- Procedure
- Present Concept
- Healing after Curettage

## INTRODUCTION

Gingival curettage is a surgical procedure involving the removal of the inflamed soft tissue lateral to the pocket wall. The objective behind the design of gingival curettage was the stimulation of new connective tissue attachment to the tooth by the removal of pocket lining, junctional epithelium, and the subjacent granulation tissue. Gingival curettage results in the promotion of a long junctional epithelium, and the result is similar to the outcomes obtained by scaling and root planing alone. Gingival curettage is a closed procedure though it is a surgical type procedure. The major limitation of the procedure is the lack of accessibility to the root surface and poor visibility to achieve complete mechanical removal of plaque, calculus, and biofilm. This makes gingival curettage inferior compared to flap surgery.

## TERMINOLOGY

- Gingival curettage is a surgical procedure designed to remove the periodontal pocket's soft tissue lining with a curette, leaving only gingival connective tissue lining.
- Inadvertent curettage is the curettage which is done unintentionally when scaling and root planing procedure is performed.[1]
- Subgingival curettage refers to the procedure that is performed apical to the epithelial attachment, severing the connective tissue attachment down to the osseous crest.[1]

## INDICATIONS

- In patients in whom extensive surgery is contraindicated owing to systemic diseases or psychological problems.
- Shallow pocket depths with adequate width and thickness of gingival tissue.
- It is usually recommended as a part of new attachment attempts in moderately deep infrabony pockets located in the accessible areas.
- Can be performed as a part of maintenance treatment for areas of recurrent inflammation during recall visits.[2]
- In suprabony pockets, which are restricted below the mucogingival junction.

## CONTRAINDICATIONS

- Presence of acute infections, such as necrotizing ulcerative gingivitis (NUG).[3]
- Fibrosis of soft tissue wall is the contraindication as little shrinkage can be expected. Fibrous enlargement of the gingiva, such as phenytoin hyperplasia.[4]
- Extension of the base of pocket apical to the mucogingival junction.
- If the patient is medically compromised, the benefits versus the surgical procedure's risks should be carefully weighed before committing the patient to the procedure.

## PROCEDURE

Curettage can be accomplished as a closed procedure with a sharp curette or as an open procedure with a gingival incision followed by root planing, i.e., excisional new attachment procedure.

### Basic Technique (with Curette)

#### Instruments

Instruments include Gracey curettes and Columbia universal curettes.

### Technique

- *Isolate and anesthetize*: Local infiltration is given to anesthetize the isolated selected site.
- *Insertion of curette*: Sharp Gracey or Columbia Universal curette is inserted with cutting edge against the tissue in order to involve the inner lining of the pocket wall and junctional epithelium.
- *Curette the soft tissue wall*: Curette is penetrated along the soft tissue, in a horizontal stroke manner **(Figs. 47.1A and B)**. A gentle finger pressure applied on the external surface helps to support the pocket wall. Several overlapping strokes are used to completely remove the epithelium and underlying granulation tissue. In subgingival curettage, the tissues attached between the bottom of the pocket and alveolar crest are removed with a scooping motion of curette to the tooth surface.[1]
- *Irrigation*: Irrigate the area with sterile normal saline solution to remove debris and press the tissue to the tooth surface gently, which enables the arrest of bleeding and the adaption of soft tissue to the root surface.
- *Suturing*: Suture the tissue, if necessary.
- Postoperative instructions are given thereafter.

## Excisional New Attachment Procedure

Excisional new attachment procedure (ENAP) is a subgingival curettage performed with a knife. This technique was developed by the United States Naval Dental Corps.[5] The aim of the procedure is to properly prepare soft tissue to gain better access to the root surface. This helps the soft tissue to adapt intimately to the root surface.[6]

### Instruments

Instruments include a surgical handle (Bard-Parker No. 3), surgical blades No. 11, No. 12, No. 15, and curettes.

### Technique

- *Anesthesia*: Adequate local anesthesia is given to the selected site.
- *Incision*: Internal bevel incision is given with surgical blade No. 15 or No. 11, from the gingival margin to a point below the bottom of the pocket **(Figs. 47.2A and B)**. The intent is to cut the inner portion of the pocket's soft tissue wall, all around the tooth.
- *Removal of the tissue*: The excised and granulation tissues are removed with a curette. Root planing is done after that.
- *Irrigation*: Irrigate the area with saline.
- *Suturing*: Approximate the wound edges and place suitable sutures.
- Postoperative instructions are given thereafter.

## Chemical Curettage

Sodium sulfide, phenol, camphor, antiformin,[7] citric acid, and sodium hypochlorite[8] are commonly used for chemical curettage.

Anesthesia is given to the selected site. After isolating the site with cotton rolls, the solution of sodium hypochlorite is placed into the pocket for 1 minute. Then 5% citric acid solution is introduced into the pocket for 1 minute to neutralize the sodium hypochlorite. With the help of a curette, the coagulated tissues are removed, and the pocket is flushed with saline to get rid of the connective tissue remnants.

The extent of chemical penetration to the tissue cannot be controlled, and thus, chemical curettage procedure is discarded.

## Ultrasonic Curettage

Ultrasonic curettage involves curettage with ultrasonic devices.[9] Sound energy absorbed at tissue junctions that

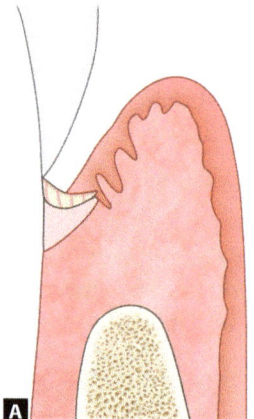 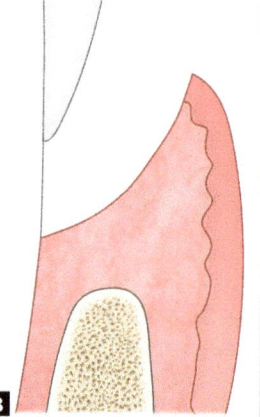

**Figs. 47.1A and B:** Schematic representation showing curettage with a curette.

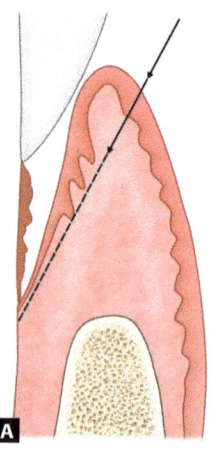 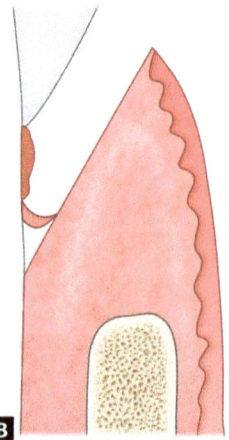

**Figs. 47.2A and B:** Schematic representation showing excisional new attachment procedure (ENAP).

take the form of heat, results in coagulation. The coagulated epithelium is then removed by the mechanical action of the vibrations of the ultrasonic instrument. Ultrasonic curettage is found to be as effective as manual curettage.[10] Moreover, it is associated with less inflammation and less removal of underlying connective tissue as compared to hand instrumentation.

## Laser

Curettage with a dental laser is a new method introduced for epithelial removal. The objectives of laser curettage are to remove epithelial cells as performed in previous methods and to reduce bacteria. However, a short-term study conducted with neodymium-doped: yttrium aluminium garnet (Nd: YAG) laser treatment failed to produce a statistically significant bacterial reduction.

## PRESENT CONCEPT

Recently conducted short- and long-term clinical trials have demonstrated that gingival curettage was insufficient to offer additional benefit in comparison to scaling and root planing alone considering probing depth reduction, attachment gain, or inflammation reduction. When benefits of curettage were compared with scaling and root planing alone and along with scaling and root planing, it was reported that curettage "did not serve any additional useful purpose." In the year of 1989, an extensive discussion happened on the topic of curettage in World Workshop in Clinical Periodontics. The discussion concluded that curettage had "no justifiable application during active therapy for chronic adult periodontitis."[11] In consideration of a lack of evidence of the therapeutic benefit of gingival curettage in the treatment of chronic periodontitis, the American Dental Association has removed the code from the Fourth Edition of Current Dental Terminology (CDT- 4). Additionally, the American Academy of Periodontology did not include gingival curettage as a method of treatment in its guidelines for periodontal therapy. This suggests that gingival curettage has no clinical value in periodontal therapeutic areas.[12]

## HEALING AFTER CURETTAGE

- Clinically, chronically inflamed gingival lesion heals after curettage in the manner described in **Flowchart 47.1**.
- Histologically, chronically inflamed gingival lesion heals after curettage in the manner described in **Flowchart 47.2**.[13]

Gingival wall shrinkage is markedly enhanced by the increased drainage of tissue fluid exudate. The gingival sulcus is totally or partially devoid of the epithelial lining and is filled by blood clot immediately after curettage.

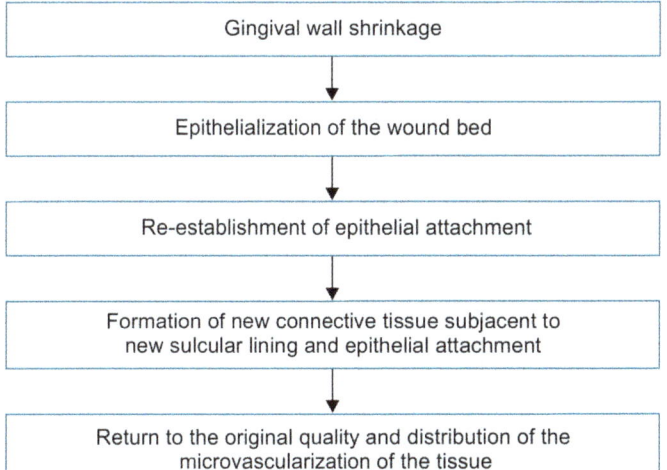

Flowchart 47.1: Clinical healing of chronically inflamed gingival lesion after curettage.

- At 1st day, marginal gingiva is bluish red/purplish red in color with marginal blood clot, oozing of blood and exudate
- After 1st day, marginal gingiva and portion of attached gingiva is edematous and swollen with lighter bluish red hue
- By 4–6 days, reduced edema, greater rigidity and adaptation of gingival wall and concurrent shrinkage
- By 7–10 days, gingival margin acquire pale pink coloration and loses its smooth topography
- By 10–14 days, gingival margin become firm pink that resists bleeding on palpation indicating improved collagen formation and organization in the underlying corium

Flowchart 47.2: Histological healing of chronically inflamed gingival lesion after curettage.

- Gingival wall shrinkage
- Epithelialization of the wound bed
- Re-establishment of epithelial attachment
- Formation of new connective tissue subjacent to new sulcular lining and epithelial attachment
- Return to the original quality and distribution of the microvascularization of the tissue

This is followed by the rapid proliferation of granulation tissue. Granulation tissue, which consists of newly formed blood vessels, connective tissue fibroblasts, and some inflammatory cells, forms subjacent to the clot and may replace it in part as it resorbs and sequesters. The granulation tissue forms between the epithelium and the primary wound bed. Removal of the blood clot postsurgically occurs by both enzymatic and phagocytic activity. In the early phases of the clot's presence, neutrophilic enzymes begin a dissolution process that is completed when the accumulating macrophages phagocytize the clot's residual elements.

## Epithelialization

After an initial lag of 12–24 hours, the epithelium's migration begins from the existing epithelium of the attached gingiva. The rate of cell migration approximates 0.5–1 mm/day over the wound surface. New epithelium begins to cover the exposed gingival connective tissue within 2–3 days and is completed in 7–10 days. The prickle cells of the keratinized epithelium at the periphery of the wound initiate the migration of cells that give rise to the new nonkeratinized epithelium of the dentogingival junction.

## Connective Tissue

At about 4th day as inflammation becomes more chronic and epithelization progresses, collagenation begins in the subepithelial area to eventually form a new and thin lamina propria. The formation and reorganization of the connective tissue fibers are the product of vascular proliferative and fibroblastic elements of the inflammatory response's reparative phase. The connective tissue phase of repair is a comparatively slower process, which takes approximately 21 days to form immature and poorly arranged collagen fibers below the new epithelium.

> **Points to Ponder**
> - The major disadvantage of gingival curettage procedure is limited access, especially in deep, tortuous, and infrabony pockets.
> - While performing curettage, Gracey curette No. 11–12 is used for distal surfaces of posteriors. Gracey curette No. 13–14 is used for mesial surfaces of posteriors (which is opposite for scaling and root planing).
> - For the gingival curettage blade, face to tooth surface angulation is more than 90°.

## REFERENCES

1. Carranza FM, Takei HH. Gingival curettage. In: Newman MG, Takei HH, Carranza FA (Eds). Carranza's Clinical Periodontology, 9th edition. Philadelphia, PA, USA: WB Saunders; 2003. pp. 744-8.
2. Ramfjord SP, Ash MM. Curettage. In: Periodontology and Periodontics: Modern Theory and Practice, 1st edition. USA: Ishiyaku Euroamerica; 1996. pp. 269-74.
3. Genco RJ, Goldman HM, Cohen DW. Periodontal surgery. In: Contemporary Periodontics. St. Louis, United States: CV Mosby; 1990. pp. 553-84.
4. Chace R. Subgingival curettage in periodontal therapy. J Periodontol. 1974;45(2):107-9.
5. US Naval Dental Corps. Periodontics Syllabus. NAVED P5110. United States: US Naval Dental Corps; 1975. pp. 113-5.
6. Grant DA, Stern IB, Listgarten MA. Gingival and subgingival curettage: Curettage of the pocket wall. In: Periodontics, 6th edition. Boca Raton, Florida, USA: CRC Press; 1988. pp. 740-60.
7. Forgas LB, Gound S. The effects of antiformin-citric acid chemical curettage on the microbial flora of the periodontal pocket. J Periodontol. 1987;58(3):153-8.
8. Vieira EM, O'Leary TJ, Kafrawy AH. The effect of sodium hypochlorite and citric acid solution on healing of periodontal pockets. J Periodontol. 1982;53(2):71-80.
9. Goldman HM. Curettage by ultrasonic instruments. Preliminary report. Oral Surg Oral Med Oral Pathol. 1960;13:43-53.
10. Sanderson AD. Gingival curettage by hand and ultrasonic instruments: A histologic comparison. J Periodontol. 1966;37(4):279-90.
11. Kalkwarf K. Tissue attachments. In: Proceedings of World Workshop in Clinical Periodontics. Chicago, USA: American Academy of Periodontology; 1989. pp. V1-19.
12. American Academy of Periodontology. The American Academy of Periodontology statement regarding gingival curettage. J Periodontol. 2002;73(10):1229-30.
13. Ruben MP, Smukler H, Schulman SM, Kon S, Bloom AA. Healing of periodontal surgical wounds. In: Goldman HM, Cohen DW (Eds). Periodontal Therapy, 5th edition. St. Louis: CV Mosby; 1980. pp. 640-754.

## VIVA VOCE

**Q1.** What is the motion of curette in subgingival curettage?
**Ans.** In subgingival curettage, the tissues attached between the bottom of the pocket and alveolar crests are removed with scooping motion of the curette.

**Q2.** Which incision is given in ENAP?
**Ans.** Internal bevel incision is given in ENAP.

**Q3.** Why is extended digital pressure important during curettage?
**Ans.** Extended digital pressure is important during curettage, as it leads to the formation of a very thin blood clot in the sulcular area, which resorbs rapidly and improves the potential for more rapid healing and re-epithelialization.

**Q4.** Why root preparation is a *sine qua non* to successful curettage?
**Ans.** The presence of plaque, calculus, and adsorbed endotoxins delays healing and promote further inflammation. Thus, root preparation is a *sine qua non* to successful curettage.

**Q5.** Which Gracey curette is used for curettage on mesial surfaces of molars?
**Ans.** Gracey curette No. 13–14.

**Q6.** What is inadvertent curettage?
**Ans.** The curettage, which is done unintentionally when scaling and root planing procedure is performed.

**Q7.** Which instruments are used for ENAP?
**Ans.** Surgical handle (Bard-Parker No. 3), surgical blades No. 11, No. 12, No. 15, and curettes.

**Q8.** What is the rate of cell migration over the wound surface?
**Ans.** Approximately 0.5–1 mm/day.

**Q9.** What is the major limitation of gingival curettage?
**Ans.** Lack of accessibility to the root surface and poor visibility to achieve complete mechanical removal of plaque, calculus, and biofilm.

**Q10.** Which chemicals are used in chemical curettage?
**Ans.** Sodium sulfide, phenol, camphor, antiformin, citric acid, and sodium hypochlorite.

# Gingivectomy

*Dhoom S Mehta, Shalu Bathla*

## Chapter Outline

- Historical Perspective
- Definition
- Objectives
- Indications
- Contraindications
- Limiting Circumstances
- Drawbacks
- Gingivoplasty
- Types
- Postoperative Healing

## INTRODUCTION

Gingivectomy is the excision of the gingival pocket wall, which provides visibility and accessibility for complete calculus removal and thorough root planing. It helps to create a favorable environment for the restoration of physiologic gingival contour.

## HISTORICAL PERSPECTIVE

History of gingivectomy can be dated back to 1742 when Fauchard described the procedure to remove excessive tissue. Robicsek, in 1884, later on, described the so-called gingivectomy procedure as a straight incision technique in which the tissues were excised and the granulation tissue eliminated.[1] Pickerill's book "Stomatology in General Practice," published in 1912, described the procedure and very reasonably named the operation gingivectomy. Zentler, in 1918, gave a scalloped incision technique for gingivectomy.[2] Gingivectomy is thought to be introduced as an official periodontal therapy when the idea of periodontal etiology shifts from bone to soft tissue. This is mainly due to Kronfeld, in 1935, who emphasized that periodontal disease is not the disease of the bone only. Gingivectomy was later defined by Grant et al., in 1979 as being the excision of the soft tissue wall of a pathologic periodontal pocket.[3]

## DEFINITION

According to the World Workshop in Periodontics (1989), gingivectomy is defined as the "excision of the soft tissue wall of the periodontal pocket."

## OBJECTIVES

- Pocket elimination by gingival resection.
- Development of physiologic tissue form for disease prevention.

## INDICATIONS

Following are the indications of gingivectomy:[4]
- Elimination of suprabony pocket.
- Elimination of gingival enlargement.
- Elimination of suprabony periodontal abscess.
- To expose additional clinical crown to gain added retention for restorative purposes and to provide access to subgingival caries.
- The presence of furcation involvement (without associated bone defects) where there is a wide zone of attached gingiva.
- Pericoronal flap.

## CONTRAINDICATIONS

- The need for bone surgery or examination of the bone shape and morphology.
- Situations in which the bottom of the pocket is apical to the mucogingival junction, gingivectomy will excise most of the gingiva and leave an inadequate zone of the gingiva.
- Esthetic considerations, particularly in the anterior maxilla.
- If the patient complains of tooth sensitivity before surgery. Although it is a relative contraindication, as

the cause of any complaint should be treated before the surgery and if the sensitivity cannot be controlled, surgery should be contraindicated.

## LIMITING CIRCUMSTANCES

- *Palatal aspects of maxillary posterior teeth*: When the palatal vault is shallow, and the depth of periodontal involvement is near or enters the vault area, gingivectomy on the palatal aspects of maxillary posterior teeth may result in the elimination of most if not all of the palatal gingiva, placing the gingival margin at or near a level of coincident with that of the roof of the mouth.
- *Mandibular retromolar lesions*: When an incision is made on movable and delicate mucosa, this tissue often cuts poorly, bleeds profusely, and may be difficult to resect and shape. Thus, the use of the distal wedge procedure often simplifies the management of retromolar tissue.
- *Maxillary tuberosity areas*: When soft tissue is so great, relative to the depth of periodontal involvement on the distal aspects of the last molar that its level of resection would bring about surgical entry into the mucosa of the hamular notch. It may be more appropriate to perform a distal wedge procedure to immediately eliminate diseased tissue adjacent to the distal portion of the molar.
- *Cases of emotional stress*: With age, diminished patient's cooperation and motivation, retarded healing, etc., have a direct bearing upon the desirability of surgical therapy. Such a patient is a poor surgical risk and requires therapeutic modification.

## DRAWBACKS

- Tissue wound heals by secondary intention.
- Alveolar bone defects are not revealed and, therefore, cannot be treated adequately.
- Gingivectomy is a radical procedure in which the zone of attached gingiva is compromised or may be eliminated. Thus, the attached gingiva is wasted.
- Clinical crowns are lengthened considerably and need to be explained to the patient before surgery.
- It may lead to dentin hypersensitivity due to root exposure.

## GINGIVOPLASTY

Gingivoplasty was first described by Goldman in 1950 as a plastic procedure by which the gingival tissue was removed.[5] Sugarman in 1951 described electrosurgical gingivoplasty in his case report. Gingivoplasty can be defined as the recontouring of the gingiva that has lost its physiologic form. It was introduced to facilitate dealing with the abnormal form of gingiva and was essentially a surgical procedure designed to reshape gingiva without necessarily reducing sulcular depth. Gingivectomy and gingivoplasty are usually performed together with different objectives.[6]

The purpose of gingivoplasty is different from gingivectomy, as gingivoplasty is just reshaping of the gingiva to create physiologic gingival contours, with the sole purpose of recontouring the gingiva in the absence of pockets, while the objective of the gingivectomy is to eliminate pocket.[7]

### Indications

- Need for correction of the grossly thickened gingival margin.
- Gingival clefts and craters caused by necrotizing ulcerative gingivitis interfere with normal food excursion and collect plaque and food debris.
- Sharply varying levels of the gingival margin in adjacent areas.
- Saucer-shaped deformities, buccolingual in the interproximal regions.

### Instruments

Gingivoplasty may be done with a periodontal knife, scalpel, rotary coarse diamond stones or electrodes.[8]

### Gingivoplasty Procedure

Steps in the gingivoplasty procedure are similar and resemble those performed in festooning artificial dentures namely:[7]

- Tapering the gingival margin.
- Creating a scalloped marginal outline.
- Thinning the attached gingiva.
- Creating vertical interdental grooves and shaping the interdental papillae to provide embrasures for the passage of food.

### Scrapping

Use a scalpel as a hoe and pass the instrument tightly but firmly over a firm, tough tissue surface, which results in the shaving of the surface. The use of rotary abrasive consists essentially of abrading tissue until it has assumed the desired form. The rules governing the application of the rotary abrasive to soft tissue are exactly those that apply to hard tissue. A stream of water on the instrument expedites the procedure immeasurably just as it does on bone, enamel or dentin. Accelerated speed ensures smooth, rapid operation while the stream of water provides temperature control and prevents clogging of instruments.

## TYPES

### Surgical Gingivectomy

#### Surgical Instruments

- *Pocket markers*: Goldman-fox; Crane Kaplan (**Figs. 48.1A and B**).

Chapter 48: Gingivectomy

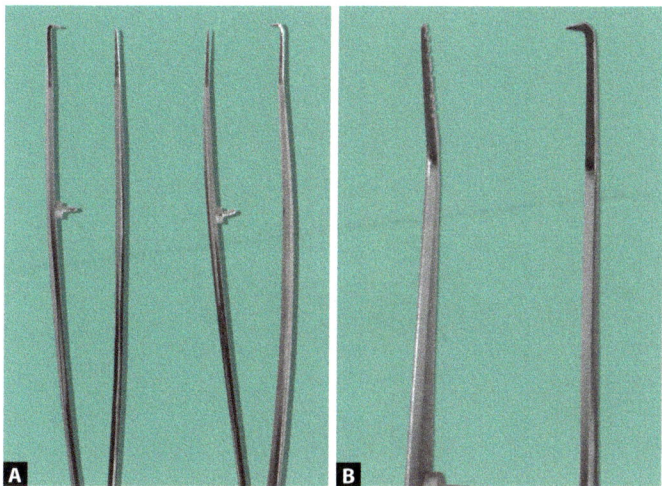

**Figs. 48.1A and B:** Photograph showing pocket markers.

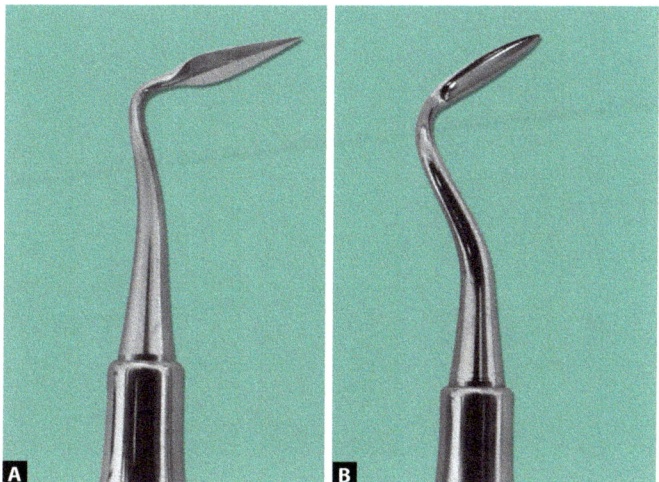

**Figs. 48.3A and B:** Photograph showing interproximal knives: (A) Buck knife; (B) Orban's knife.

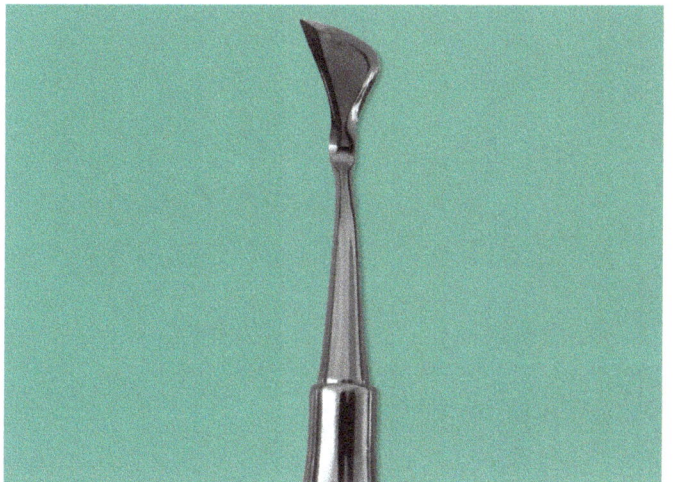

**Fig. 48.2:** Photograph showing a Kirkland knife (kidney-shaped blade).

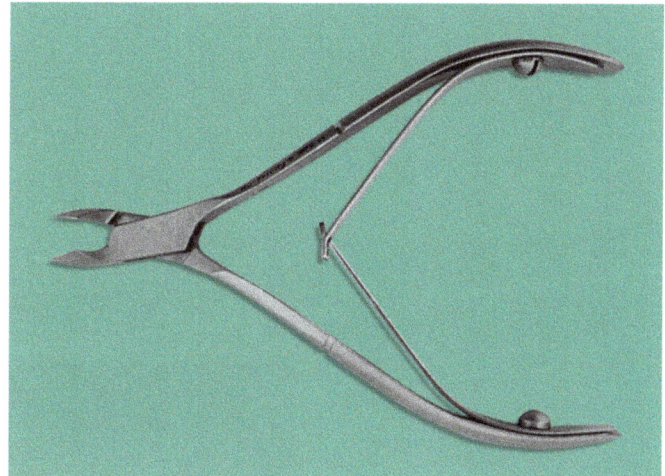

**Fig. 48.4:** Photograph showing tissue nipper.

- *Broad bladed knife*: Goldman-fox No. 7; Kirkland knife **(Fig. 48.2)**.
- *Interproximal knife*: Goldman-fox Nos. 8, 9 and 10; Bucks knife **(Fig. 48.3A)**; Orban's knife **(Fig. 48.3B)**.
- *Surgical handle*: Bard-Parker™ (BP) No. 3 or angulated handle (Blake's handle) with blade Nos. 11, 12, 15, and curettes.
- Tissue nipper **(Fig. 48.4)**; scissors.

## Procedure

The following are the steps of gingivectomy procedure[4,7,9] **(Figs. 48.5A to E)**.

- *Mark bleeding points*: After local anesthesia (LA) is given in the selected site, mark bleeding points with the help of pocket marker systematically, beginning on the distal surface of the tooth, then on the facial and mesial surface. The procedure is repeated on the lingual or palatal surface. The beak of the pocket marker must be parallel to the root surface. Pinpoint perforations individuate pocket depth, which is used as a guideline for the incision.
- *Incisions*: Discontinuous or continuous incision is given apical to the bottom of the bleeding point, beginning at the most terminal tooth **(Figs. 48.6A and B)**. External bevel incision is given at an angle of 45° apical to the base of the pocket with the help of Kirkland knife, or blade No. 11 or 15 with BP handle No. 3 or angulated Blake's handle. The blade must pass fully through the tissue to the tooth in coronal direction[10] **(Fig. 48.7)**. The incision should be as close as possible to the bone without exposing it so as to remove the soft tissue coronal to the bone **(Figs. 48.8A and B)**. The main principle here is to eliminate pocket all the way to the base without exposing the bone. Once the primary incision is completed on the buccal and lingual aspects, Orban's knife or Waerhaug knife is placed at an angle of 45° to free the tissue interproximally.

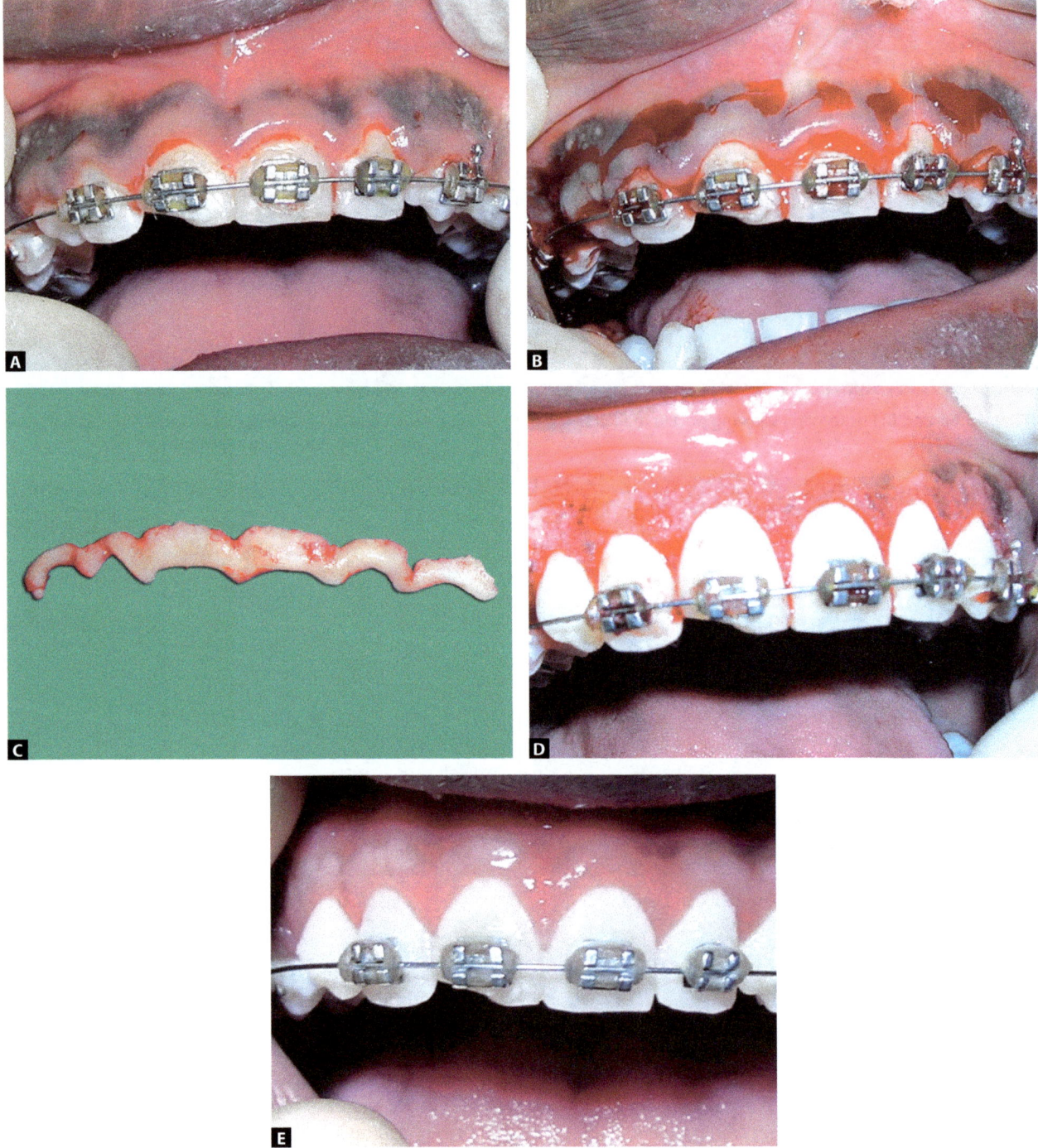

**Figs. 48.5A to E:** Clinical picture showing: (A) Preoperative gingival bleeding points; (B) External bevel incision; (C) Tissue excised; (D) Tissue tabs removed; (E) Postoperative after 1 month.

- *Tissue removed*: The incised tissues are carefully removed with the help of curettes or scalers. The remaining tissue tabs are removed with scissors and tissue nippers. The gingival margins should be thin and beveled and, if necessary, corrected by means of knives or rotating diamond burs.
- *Scaling and root planing*: The calculus and necrotic cementum on the tooth are removed with the help of scalers and curettes.
- *Periodontal dressing*: Bleeding is controlled, and after that, periodontal dressing is applied over the treated site primarily for patient comfort. Thereafter, the patient is given postoperative instructions.

## LASER Gingivectomy

The light amplification by stimulated emission of radiations (LASER) most commonly used for gingivectomy are the carbon dioxide ($CO_2$) having wavelength of 10,600 nm[11] and

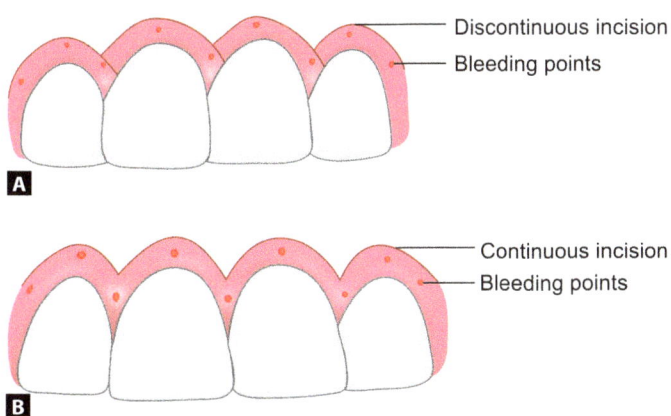

**Figs. 48.6A and B:** Schematic representation showing incisions: (A) Discontinuous incision; (B) Continuous incision.

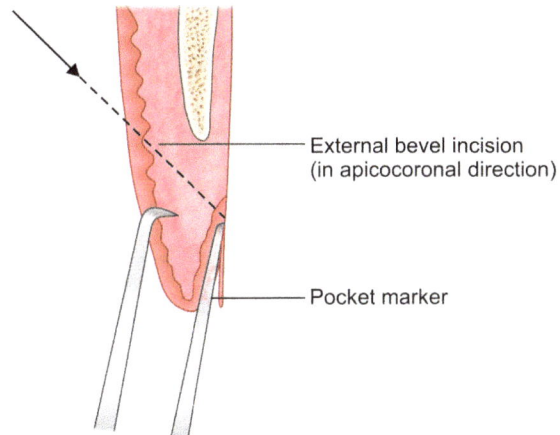

**Fig. 48.7:** Schematic representation showing marking of the depth of pocket with the pocket marker. External bevel incision is given apical to the bleeding point making 45° angle to the long axis of the tooth.

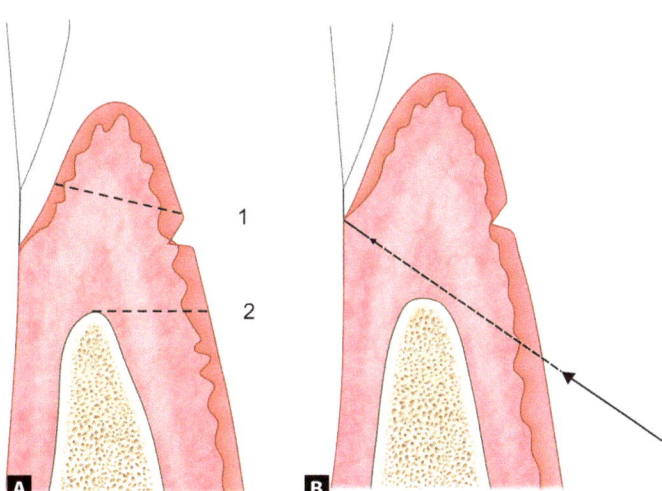

**Figs. 48.8A and B:** Schematic representation showing: (A) Incorrect incisions: 1. Shallow incision (fails to remove pocket) and 2. No bevel incision (results in bone exposure); (B) Correct incision.

neodymium-doped: yttrium-aluminium-garnet (Nd: YAG) having wavelength of 1,064 nm both in the infrared range.

### Advantages

- LASER offers an almost completely dry, bloodless surgery.
- Because of the dried field, surgical time may be reduced.
- There is instant sterilization of the area, decreasing the chances of bacteremia.
- This is noncontact surgery, thus no mechanical trauma to the surgical site.
- There is prompt healing with minimal postoperative swelling and scarring.
- Postoperative pain appears to be greatly reduced.

### Disadvantages

- There is a loss of tactile feedback in using these instruments.
- It is imperative that all operating room personnel wear safety glasses for protection of their eyes.
- There is a high cost of the equipment.

## Electrosurgical Gingivectomy

### Instruments

Instruments include needle electrode (thickness varying from 0.0075-inch to 0.015-inch), small ovoid loop, or diamond-shaped electrodes.

### Procedure

The site must not be too dry; otherwise, excessive sparking will result. Conversely, if excessive moisture is present, considerable surface coagulation will occur instantly. For the best results, the site should be very slightly moist. The removal of gingival enlargements and gingivoplasty is performed with the needle electrode, supplemented by the small ovoid loop or diamond-shaped electrode for festooning. A blended cutting and coagulating (fully rectified) current is used. In all reshaping procedures, the electrode is activated and moved in a concise shaving motion.[7] Electrode should be kept in constant motion in order to prevent a build-up of heat with an appropriate current setting, and the patient should be properly grounded. Clean all debris from electrodes with gauze sponges after each movement through soft tissue (**Figs. 48.9A to D**).

### Advantages

- It provides a clear operating area with little or no bleeding.
- Lack of pressure to incise tissue, thus allowing a more precise incision than is obtained by a scalpel.
- Minor tissue loss after healing.

Section 7: Treatment: Surgical Therapy

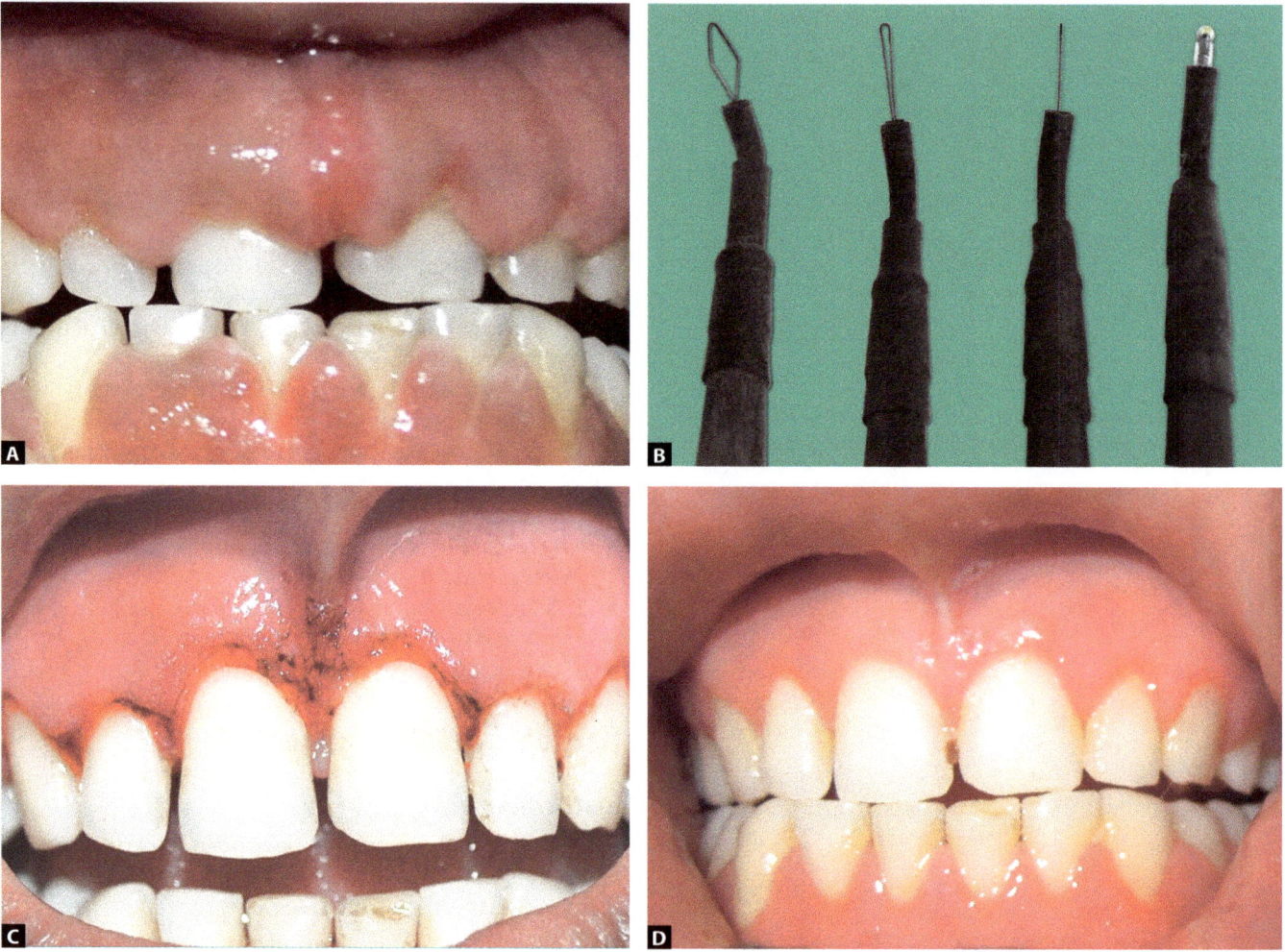

**Figs. 48.9A to D:** Clinical picture showing: (A) Gingival enlargement at maxillary and mandibular anterior regions; (B) Electrosurgical electrodes; (C) Gingivectomy done by electrosurgery, and (D) Postoperative maxillary and mandibular anterior regions.

- Self-sterilization of the tip of the active electrode.
- Greater ease for the patient as well as for the operator.

### Disadvantages

- It causes an unpleasant odor.
- If the electrosurgery point touches the bone, irreparable damage can occur.
- When the electrode touches the root, areas of cementum burns are produced.

### Contraindication

One major contraindication to electrosurgery is a cardiac pacemaker. Since an electrosurgical unit generates radiofrequency energy, it should never be used within 15 feet of an individual with a cardiac pacemaker.[12]

### Chemosurgical Gingivectomy

Five percent paraformaldehyde or potassium hydroxide was the chemicals used to perform gingivectomy which is no longer in use because of the following disadvantages associated with it:

- The depth of chemical action cannot be controlled.
- Gingival remodeling cannot be accomplished effectively.
- Epithelialization and reformation of the junctional epithelium, the reestablishment of the alveolar crest fiber system are slower in chemically treated gingival wounds than in those produced by the scalpel.

## POSTOPERATIVE HEALING

Healing after gingivectomy is done by secondary intention. Bernier and Kaplan reported the following time sequence for healing following gingivectomy in humans: The initial response after gingivectomy is the formation of a protective surface clot; the underlying tissue becomes acutely inflamed with some necrosis.[13]

The outer epithelium heals by approximately 14 days, but sulcular epithelium requires 3–5 weeks to heal. Twelve hours after gingivectomy, there is a slight reduction

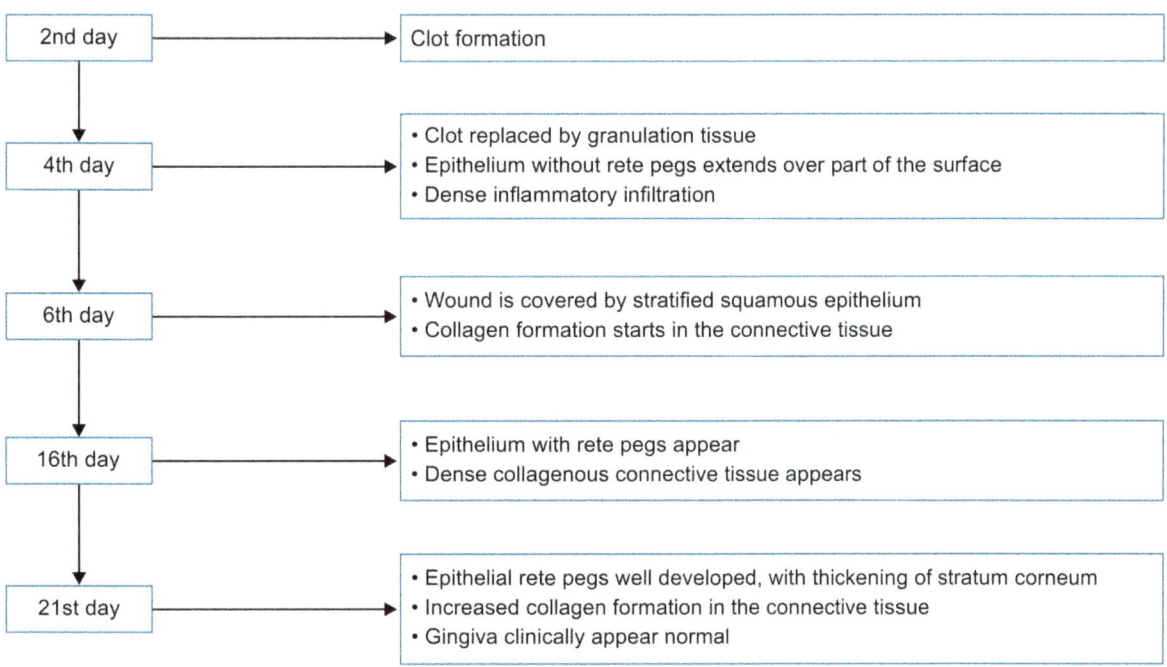

**Flowchart 48.1:** Healing after gingivectomy.

in cementoblasts and some loss of continuity of the osteoblastic layer on the outer aspects of the alveolar crest. New bone formation occurs at the alveolar crest as early as the 4th day after gingivectomy, and new cementoid appears after about 10–15 days **(Flowchart 48.1)**.

Thus, total gingivectomy healing takes place in about 4–5 weeks, and remodeling of the alveolar bone crest has been shown to occur during this phase. Gingivoplasty wounds often heal faster than gingivectomy wound.

The tissue changes that occur in postgingivectomy healing are the same in all individuals. Still, the time required for complete healing varies depending on the local and systemic factors that influence wound healing (interference from local irritation, infection, and age).

### Clinical Tip
In gingivectomy, external bevel incision is given at 45° to the tooth surface in apicocoronal direction.

### Points to Ponder
- Failure to produce beveled incision leaves a broad plateau that takes more time than ordinarily required to develop the gingiva's physiologic contour; thus, the incision should be beveled at approximately 45° to the tooth surface.
- The granulomatous tissue is removed first; then thorough scaling is attempted on the tooth so that hemorrhage from the granulomatous tissue should not obscure the scaling during the surgical procedure.
- Gingivectomy wound heals by secondary intention.

## REFERENCES

1. Robicsek S. Ueber das Wesen und Entstehen der Alveolar-Pyorrhoe und deren Behandlung. 1884. The 3rd Annual Report of the Australian Dental Association. Rev J Periodontol. 1965;36:265.
2. Zentler A. Suppurative gingivitis with alveolar involvement. A new surgical procedure. J Am Med Assoc. 1918;71(19):1530-4.
3. Grant DA, Stern IB, Everett FG. Periodontics in the Tradition of Orban and Gottlieb, 5th edition. St. Louis: CV Mosby; 1979.
4. Eley BM, Manson JD, Soory M. The surgical periodontal treatment. In: Periodontics, 5th edition. Edinburgh, Scotland: Wright Publishing; 2004. pp. 262-75.
5. Goldman HM. The development of physiologic gingival contours by gingivoplasty. Oral Surg Oral Med Oral Pathol. 1950;3(7):879- 88.
6. Grant DA, Stern IB, Listgarten MA. Gingivectomy and Gingivoplasty. In: Periodontics, 6th edition. St. Louis: CV Mosby; 1988. pp. 761-85.
7. Carranza FA. The gingivectomy technique. In: Newman MG, Takei HH, Carranza FA (Eds). Carranza's Clinical Periodontology, 9th edition. Philadelphia, PA, USA: WB Saunders; 2003. pp. 749-53.
8. Genco RJ, Rosenberg ES, Evian C. Periodontal surgery. In: Genco RJ, Goldman HM, Cohen DW (Eds). Contemporary Periodontics, 2nd edition. St. Louis: CV Mosby; 1999. pp. 554-84.
9. Wennstrom JL, Heijl L, Lindhe J. Periodontal surgery: access therapy. In: Lindhe J, Karring T, Lang NP (Eds). Clinical Periodontology and Implant Dentistry, 4th edition. Oxford, UK: Blackwell Munksgaard; 2003. pp. 519-60.
10. Tibbetts LS, Ammons WF. Resective periodontal surgery. In: Rose LF, Mealey BL, Genco RJ, Cohen DW (Eds). Periodontics: Medicine, Surgery, and Implants, 1st edition. United States: Elsevier-Mosby; 2005. pp. 502-52.

## Section 7: Treatment: Surgical Therapy

11. Pick RM, Pecaro BC, Silberman CJ. The laser gingivectomy. The use of the $CO_2$ laser for the removal of phenytoin hyperplasia. J Periodontol. 1985;56(8):492-6.
12. Flocken JE. Electrosurgical management of soft tissues and restorative dentistry. Dent Clin North Am. 1980;24(2):247-69.
13. Bernier JL, Kaplan H. The repair of gingival tissues after surgical intervention. J Am Dent Assoc. 1947;35(10):697-705.

### VIVA VOCE

**Q1. How is gingivoplasty different from gingivectomy?**
**Ans.** The purpose of gingivoplasty is different from gingivectomy, as gingivoplasty is just reshaping of the gingiva to create physiologic gingival contours, with the sole purpose of recontouring the gingiva in the absence of pockets, while the objective of the gingivectomy is to eliminate the pocket.

**Q2. What are the advantages of light amplification by stimulated emission of radiation (LASER) gingivectomy?**
**Ans.** The advantages of LASER gingivectomy are as follows:
- LASER offers an almost completely dry, bloodless surgery.
- Because of dry field, surgical time may be reduced.
- There is an instant sterilization of the area, decreasing the chances of bacteremia.
- This is a noncontact surgery, thus no mechanical trauma to the surgical site.
- There is prompt healing with minimal postoperative swelling and scarring.
- Postoperative pain appears to be greatly reduced.

**Q3. What is the angulation given for the incision in gingivectomy?**
**Ans.** The incision should be beveled at approximately 45° to the tooth surface.

**Q4. How is gingivectomy different from flap procedures?**
**Ans.**

| Parameters | Gingivectomy | Flap procedure |
| --- | --- | --- |
| Reattachment | No | Possible |
| Bleeding postoperatively | High | Low |
| Healing | Secondary intention | Primary intention |
| Preservation of keratinized gingiva | No | Yes |
| Visibility and ability to treat osseous irregularities and defects | Inadequate | Good |
| Time required | Fast | Slow |
| Degree of difficulty | Low | High |

**Q5. What is the major contraindication for the gingivectomy procedure?**
**Ans.** The need for bone surgery or examination of the bone shape and morphology.

**Q6. What is the objective of the gingivectomy procedure?**
**Ans.** Pocket elimination by gingival resection and development of physiologic tissue form for disease prevention.

**Q7. Who described gingivoplasty for the first time?**
**Ans.** Goldman in 1950

**Q8. Which instruments are used in a gingivoplasty procedure?**
**Ans.** Periodontal knife, scalpel, rotary coarse diamond stones, or electrodes.

**Q9. Which laser is used for the gingivectomy procedure?**
**Ans.** Carbon dioxide ($CO_2$) laser has a wavelength of 10,600 nm and neodymium-doped: yttrium-aluminum-garnet (Nd: YAG) having wavelength of 1,064 nm both in infrared range.

**Q10. How much time it takes for the sulcular epithelium to heal after gingivectomy?**
**Ans.** 3–5 weeks

# Periodontal Flap

Shalu Bathla

## Chapter Outline

- Definition
- Objectives
- Principles
- Classifications
- Incisions
- Flap Procedures

## INTRODUCTION

The periodontal flap provides visibility and accessibility to the bone and root surface. The flap also allows the gingiva to be displaced to a different location in various periodontal surgeries. Thus, proper surgical incisions, designing, and managing the surgical flap required are discussed in detail in this chapter.

## DEFINITION

It is the portion of gingiva and/or alveolar mucosa surgically separated from the underlying tissues to provide visibility and access to the bone and root surface.

## OBJECTIVES

- Provide access for root surface detoxification.
- Reducing probing depth, including those that extend to or beyond the mucogingival junction.
- Preserve or create an adequate zone of attached gingiva.
- Permit access to underlying bone for the treatment of osseous defects.
- Facilitate regenerative procedures.

## PRINCIPLES

According to Hupp (1993), the following principles should be followed for flap design:[1]
- *Prevention of flap necrosis*:
  - The apex of the flap should never be wider than the base.
  - The flap sides should either run parallel to each other or preferably converge moving from the base of the flap to the apex of the flap.
  - Length of the flap should be no more than twice the width of the base.
  - The base of the flaps should not be excessively twisted or stretched.
  - Whenever possible, an axial blood supply should be included in the base of the flap.
- *Prevention of flap tearing*:
  - Vertical releasing incisions should be placed one full tooth anterior to the sites of any anticipated bone removal.
  - The vertical incision should be started at the line angle of the tooth or in the adjacent interdental papilla and carried obliquely, apically into the unattached gingiva.

## CLASSIFICATIONS

Classification of periodontal flaps:[2]
- *According to flap reflection or tissue content (Table 49.1)*:
  - Full-thickness flap
  - Split-thickness flap
- *According to the management of papilla*:
  - Conventional flap
  - Papilla preservation flap
- *According to flap placement after surgery*:
  - Nondisplaced flap
  - Displaced flap:
    - Apical displaced flap
    - Coronal displaced flap
    - Lateral displaced flap

# Section 7: Treatment: Surgical Therapy

**TABLE 49.1:** Comparison between the full-thickness flap and partial-thickness flap.

| Parameters | Full-thickness flap | Partial-thickness flap |
|---|---|---|
| Tissue content | Consists of the epithelium, connective tissue, and periosteum | Consists of only epithelium and connective tissue |
| Periosteal retention | No | Yes |
| Raised or reflected by | Reflected with the help of a periosteal elevator | Produced by sharp dissection with the help of a surgical blade |
| Osseous surgery | Possible | Not possible |
| Bleeding | Lesser | Greater |
| Tissue trauma | Limited | More |
| Widen zone of keratinized gingiva | No | Yes |
| Degree of technical difficulty | Moderate | High |
| Healing | Primary intention | Secondary intention |

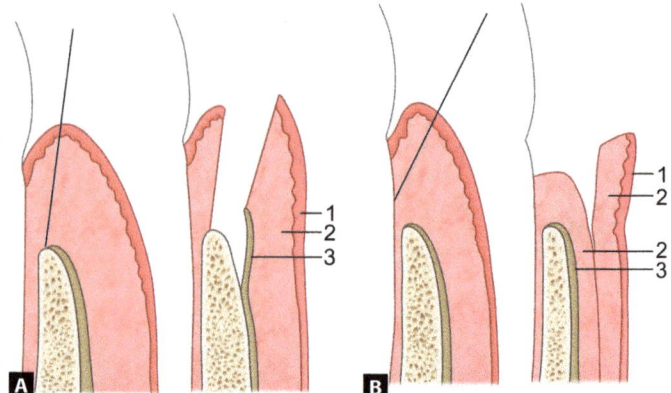

**Figs. 49.1A and B:** Schematic representation showing (A) Full-thickness flap consisting of: 1. Epithelium, 2. connective tissue, and 3. periosteum. Incision ends on the bone; (B) Partial-thickness flap consisting of: 1. Epithelium, 2. connective tissue and 3. periosteum Incision ends on the root surface.

## Full-thickness Flap

It consists of the complete mucoperiosteum, i.e., surface epithelium, connective tissue, and periosteum, which is raised by a periosteal elevator, also known as a mucoperiosteal flap **(Fig. 49.1A)**.

### Indication

A full-thickness flap is used to expose the bone surface in osseous surgery.

### Contraindications

- The area where treatment for an osseous defect with a mucogingival problem is not required.
- Thin periodontal tissue with probable osseous dehiscence and osseous fenestration.
- The area where the alveolar bone is thin.

## Split-thickness Flap

It is also known as the mucosal flap. Gingiva is dissected from the underlying periosteum, which is left on the bone and consists of epithelium and a thin layer of connective tissue **(Fig. 49.1B)**. Sharp dissection is used to produce a partial-thickness flap. The partial-thickness flap is prepared while holding and pulling the flap edge with tissue pliers, turning the blade towards the gingival margin. The flap is dissected slowly from an apico-occlusal direction. To prevent flap penetration, use the side of the blade and hold it parallel to the periosteum to make the incision.

### Indications

Partial-thickness flaps are especially useful for augmentation of the attached gingiva. This is done by positioning the flap apically or laterally. This is employed when the exposure of bone is to be avoided, as in the case of fenestration or dehiscence.

### Advantages

The flap can be attached firmly to the desired position with a periosteal suture if the reflected flap is displaced apically and the thin marginal bone can be protected by the periosteum-connective tissue bed.

### Disadvantages

The biggest problem of a partial-thickness flap is with the thickness of the remaining periosteum-connective tissue bed on the bone. If it is less than 0.5 mm, the remaining periosteum-connective tissue may become necrotic, with decreased protective effect for the alveolar bone. However, the partial-thickness flap is a difficult technique and causes much discomfort because of postoperative swelling.

## INCISIONS

The incision defines the boundary between tissue to be moved or removed and tissue to remain in place **(Box 49.1)**.

## Horizontal Incisions

### Internal Bevel Incision: First or Basic Incision

It starts from a designated area on the gingiva and is directed to an area at or near the crest of the alveolar bone

**BOX 49.1:** Incisions used in periodontal surgery.

- Horizontal incisions:
  - Internal bevel incision
  - Crevicular or sulcular incision
  - Interdental incision
- Vertical incision
- Thinning incision
- Cut-back incision
- Periosteal incision

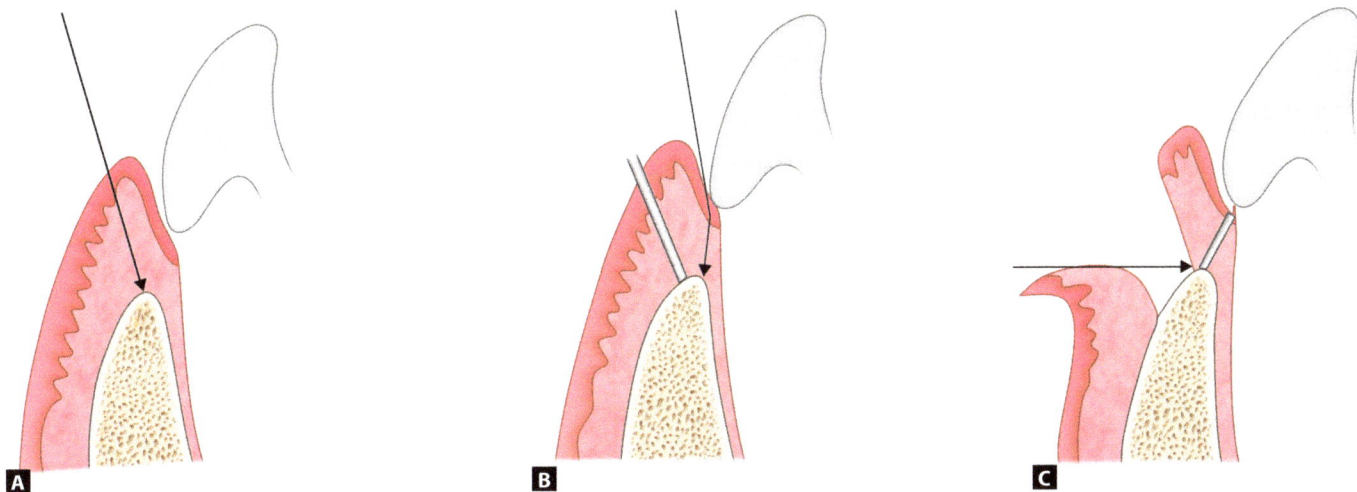

**Figs. 49.2A to C:** Schematic representation showing horizontal incisions: (A) Internal bevel incision; (B) Crevicular incision; (C) Interdental incision.

**(Figs. 49.2A and 49.4A)**, given with the help of 11 No. or 15 No. surgical blade. Morris, in 1965 introduced internal bevel incision, which separated the pocket wall from the rest of the mucoperiosteal flap and produced a healthy thin and flexible margin. It is also called as reverse bevel incision because its bevel is in the reverse direction from that of gingivectomy incision.

### Objectives

It accomplishes three important objectives:
1. It removes the pocket lining.
2. It produces a sharp, thin flap margin for adaptation to the bone-tooth junction.
3. It conserves the relatively uninvolved outer surface of the gingiva.

### Indications

Primary incision of flap surgery is given if:
- There is a sufficient band of attached gingiva.
- Thick gingiva (such as palatal gingiva).
- Deep periodontal pockets and bone defect.
- Desire to lengthen the clinical crown.

There are important variations in the way internal bevel incision is performed for the different types of flaps:
- *Modified Widman flap*: It does not intend to remove the pocket wall, but it does eliminate the pocket lining. Therefore, the internal bevel incision starts close, not more than 1–2 mm apically, to the gingival margin, and follows the gingival margin's normal scalloping margin **(Fig. 49.3)**.
- *Apically displaced flap*: For the apically displaced flap, the internal bevel incision should be made as close to the tooth as possible, 0.5–1.0 mm **(Fig. 49.3)**. The pocket wall must be preserved to be positioned apically while its lining is removed. The purpose of this surgical technique is to preserve the maximum amount of keratinized gingiva of the pocket wall to displace it apically and transform it into the attached gingiva.
- *Undisplaced flap*: For an undisplaced flap, however, the internal bevel incision is initiated at or near a point just coronal to the projection of the bottom of the pocket on the outer surface of the gingiva **(Fig. 49.3)**. This incision can be accomplished only if sufficient attached gingival remains apical to the incision.

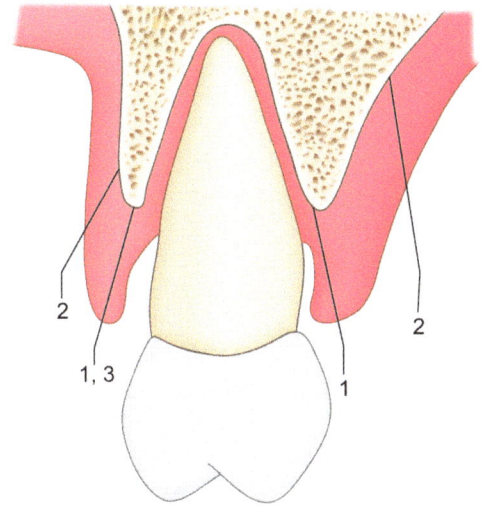

**Fig. 49.3:** Schematic representation showing varying locations of internal bevel incision for different flaps: 1. Modified Widman flap, 2. Undisplaced flap, and 3. Apically displaced flap.
(*Courtesy*: Dr SK Salaria)

### Crevicular or Sulcular Incision: Second Incision

It is made from the base of the pocket to the crest of the alveolar bone[3] **(Figs. 49.2B and 49.4B)**. This incision is

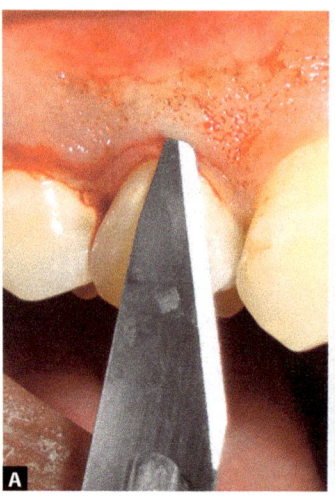
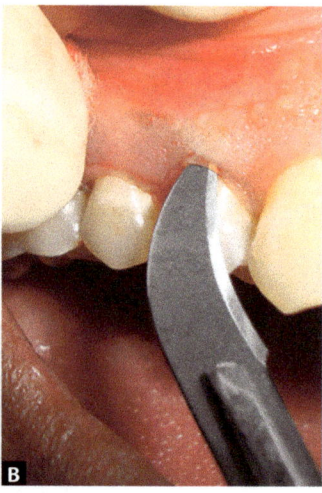

**Figs. 49.4A and B:** Clinical picture showing: (A) Internal bevel incision; (B) Crevicular incision.

carried around the entire tooth with the help of 12 No. surgical blade. Its purpose is to facilitate the removal of the inflammatory granulation tissue surrounding the cervical area (cervical wedge) left after reflecting the primary flap.

### Indications
- A narrow band of attached gingiva.
- Thin gingiva and alveolar process.
- Shallow periodontal pocket.
- Desire to lessen postoperative gingival recession for esthetic reasons in the maxillary anterior region.
- As a secondary incision of usual flap surgery.
- Bone graft or guided tissue regeneration (GTR) procedure: Desire to preserve as much periodontal tissue (especially interdental papilla) as possible to completely cover grafted bone and membrane by the flap.

### *Interdental Incision: Third Incision*
This incision is made in a horizontal direction and close to the bone crest's surface, thereby separating the soft tissue collar from the root surfaces and alveolar bone **(Fig. 49.2C)**. Given by Orban's knife, the third incision facilitates secondary flap removal as a single piece.

## Vertical Incision or Oblique Releasing Incision
A vertical incision can relieve the mechanical tension that often disrupts circulation and tears the tissue. It must extend beyond the mucogingival line. It should be made at the tooth's line angles, either to include the papilla in the flap or to avoid it completely. Thus, it should be placed on the tooth surface rather than on interdental gingiva **(Figs. 49.5A and B)**, given with the help of an 11 or 15 No. surgical blade. Vertical incisions in lingual and palatal areas are avoided. These should be designed so as to avoid short flap mesiodistally with long apically directed horizontal incision because this could jeopardize the blood supply to the flap.

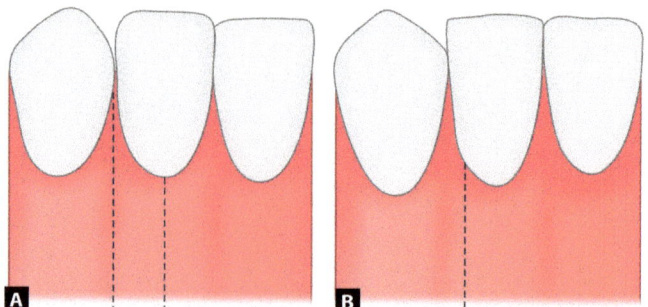

**Figs. 49.5A and B:** Schematic representation showing vertical incision: (A) Incorrect: Not in the center of interdental papilla and not at radicular surface; (B) Correct: At line angle.

As a rule, no vertical incision should be made on the lingual surface because of the following reasons:
- When one equates the tissue area covering the alveolar process to a circle, it is obvious that the tissue must be stretched to a greater circumference to gain access to the facial surfaces. In contrast, the lingual tissue tends to drape itself toward the center of the circle, negating the need for a releasing incision to obtain access. Adequate access in the 2nd and 3rd molar areas can be obtained by extending the flap mesially.
- As on the gingival aspect of the mandible, there is thin and fragile tissue.
- A vertical incision usually opens into the subgingival space and, if beyond the mylohyoid muscle, into the submandibular space. A vertical incision with full-thickness mucogingival flap potentially opens a number of potential tissue spaces other than the subperiosteal space.
- Vertical incision frequently in the 2nd molar area or distally involves unnecessary hemorrhage due to the vascularity of the area.
- Vertical incision gapes widely and heals slowly over the dense bone on the lingual surface due to the elastic fibers in the mucosa and the frequently lengthened mesial-distal distance following interdental osseous grooving.
- But if it has to be made, then vertical incision should extend only to the mucogingival junction so that no tissue spaces are endangered.

## Thinning Incision
The thinning incision extends from gingiva toward the base of the flap in the palatal flap and distal wedge procedures, given with the help of 11 No. or 15 No. surgical blade.

## Cut-back Incision
Cut-back incision is made at the apical aspect of releasing incision and directed toward the base of the flap in laterally positioned flap **(Fig. 49.6)**. This is given with the help of 11 No. or 15 No surgical blade.

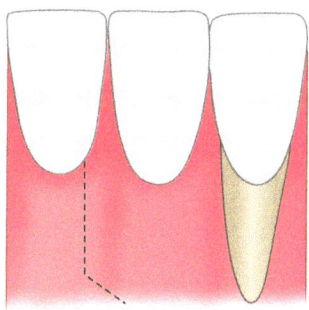

**Fig. 49.6:** Schematic representation showing cut-back incision.

## Periosteal Releasing Incision

The periosteal releasing incision is made at the base of flap severing the underlying periosteum, given with the help of a 15 No. or 15C No. surgical blade.

## FLAP PROCEDURES

Several flap techniques can be used for the treatment of periodontal pockets, namely: modified Widman flap, undisplaced flap, apically displaced flap, papilla preservation flap, palatal flap, and distal molar surgery. The decision of which flap technique to perform depends on two important landmarks, i.e., pocket depth and location of the mucogingival junction. These landmarks establish the attached gingiva's presence and width, which is the basis for the decision. These flap techniques have different objectives **(Table 49.2)**.

## Modified Widman Flap

### Historical Perspective

In 1918, Widman introduced Widman flap surgery. In 1965, Morris revived this technique and called it an unrepositioned mucoperiosteal flap.[4] The same procedure was presented in 1974 by Ramfjord SP and Nissle RR who called it the modified Widman flap.[5]

The advantages of "Modified Widman flap" over "Original Widman flap" procedure **(Table 49.3)** are as follows:
- Close adaptation of soft tissue to root surface
- Minimum trauma to the alveolar bone
- Access to adequate instrumentation of the root surface

### Objectives
- To facilitate instrumentation on root surfaces by exposing them. Residual deposits of subgingival calculus left in deep pockets are thus removed.
- To remove the pocket lining.[5]

### Indications

Shallow-to-moderate pocket depth with the base of the pockets located coronal to the mucogingival junction.[6]

**TABLE 49.2:** Objectives of flap procedures.

| Flap procedures | Objectives |
| --- | --- |
| Modified Widman flap | To facilitate root instrumentation |
| | To remove the pocket lining |
| | Does not eliminate pocket |
| Undisplaced flap | To remove the pocket wall, thereby reducing or eliminating the pocket |
| Apically displaced flap | To eliminate the pocket |
| | To increase the width of the attached gingiva |

**TABLE 49.3:** Differences between original and modified Widman flap.

| Parameters | Original Widman flap | Modified Widman flap |
| --- | --- | --- |
| Given by | Leonard Widman, 1918 | Ramfjord and Nissle, 1974 |
| Purpose | For pocket elimination | Provide access for adequate instrumentation |
| The collar of tissue attached to the teeth torn | With curettes | With Orban's knife |
| Releasing incision | Given | Not given |
| Flap reflection | High-flap reflection | Minimal-flap reflection |
| Bone contouring | Done | No bone contouring |
| After suturing | Flaps do not cover interproximal bone, remains exposed | Flaps cover interproximal bone |

### Contraindications
- Gingival enlargement
- Large bony thickening or exostoses

### Surgical Instruments

Surgical instruments include:
- Blade Nos. 11, 12, and 15
- Bard-Parker handle No. 3
- Periosteal elevator
- Curettes

### Procedure

Following are the steps of Modified Widman flap procedure:[5]
- *Step I—First incision:* The internal bevel incision is the first incision starting 0.5–1.0 mm from the gingival margin to the alveolar crest **(Fig. 49.7A)**. Scalloping follows the gingival margin. Care should be taken to insert the blade in such a way that the papilla is left with a thickness similar to that of the remaining facial flap.
- *Step II—Flap reflection:* The gingiva is reflected with a periosteal elevator.
- *Step III—Crevicular incision:* A crevicular incision is made from the bottom of the pocket to the alveolar bone,

**Section 7:** Treatment: Surgical Therapy

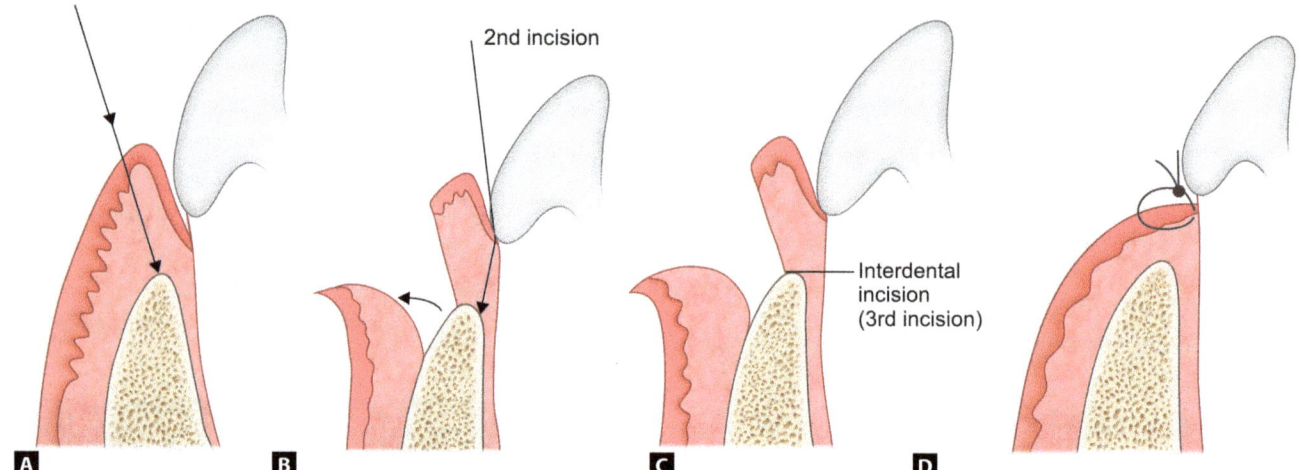

**Figs. 49.7A to D:** Schematic representation showing: (A) Internal bevel; (B) Crevicular; (C) Interdental incisions of modified Widman flap; and (D) Modified Widman flap sutured.

circumscribing the triangular wedge of tissue containing the pocket lining **(Fig. 49.7B)**.
- *Step IV—Interdental incision*: A third incision, i.e., an interdental incision is made in the interdental space, coronal to the bone, with an interproximal knife **(Fig. 49.7C)**.
- *Step V—Removal of the cervical wedge*: The gingival collar is removed with the help of a curette.
- *Step VI—Curettage, scaling, and root planing*: Tissue tags and granulation tissue are removed with a curette. The root surfaces are checked and are scaled and planed, if necessary. Residual periodontal fibers attached to the tooth surface should not be disturbed. Bone architecture is not corrected unless it prevents good tissue adaptation to the neck of the teeth. Every effort is made to adapt the facial and lingual interproximal tissue adjacent to each other in such a way that no interproximal bone remains exposed at the time of suturing. The flaps may be thinned to allow for close adaptation of the gingiva around the tooth's entire circumference and to each other interproximally.
- *Step VII—Suturing*: The flaps are replaced in their original position and secured by interdental suturing **(Fig. 49.7D)**.
- *Step VIII—Postoperative management*: The operated site is covered with the periodontal surgical pack and postoperative instructions are given thereafter.

## Undisplaced Flap

It is also called as internal bevel gingivectomy because the soft-tissue pocket wall is removed with the initial incision.[7]

### Objectives
- To reduce or eliminate pocket by removing the pocket wall.
- To improve accessibility for instrumentation.

### Indications
Gingival enlargement

### Surgical Instruments
Surgical instruments include:
- Pocket marker
- Blade Nos. 11, 12, and 15
- Bard-Parker handle No. 3
- Periosteal elevator
- Curettes

### Procedure
Following are the steps of undisplaced flap procedure **(Figs. 49.8A and B)**:
- *Step I—Mark bleeding points*: The pockets are measured with a periodontal probe, and bleeding points are produced on the gingiva's outer surface to mark the pocket bottom with the help of a pocket marker.
- *Step II—Incisions*: The initial, internal bevel incision is made following the scalloping of the bleeding marks on the gingiva. The incision is usually carried to a point apical to the alveolar crest, depending on the thickness of the tissue. The thicker the tissue is, the more apical will be the ending point of the incision. Then, a crevicular incision is made from the bottom of the pocket to the bone to detach the connective tissue from the tooth.
- *Step III—Flap reflection*: Full-thickness flap is reflected with a periosteal elevator.
- *Step IV—Interdental incision*: The third incision, i.e., an interdental incision, is made with an interdental knife.
- *Step V—Removal of the cervical wedge*: The triangular wedge of tissue created by the three incisions is removed with a curette.
- *Step VI—Removal of granulation tissue*: The area is debrided, removing all tissue tags and granulation tissue with sharp curettes.

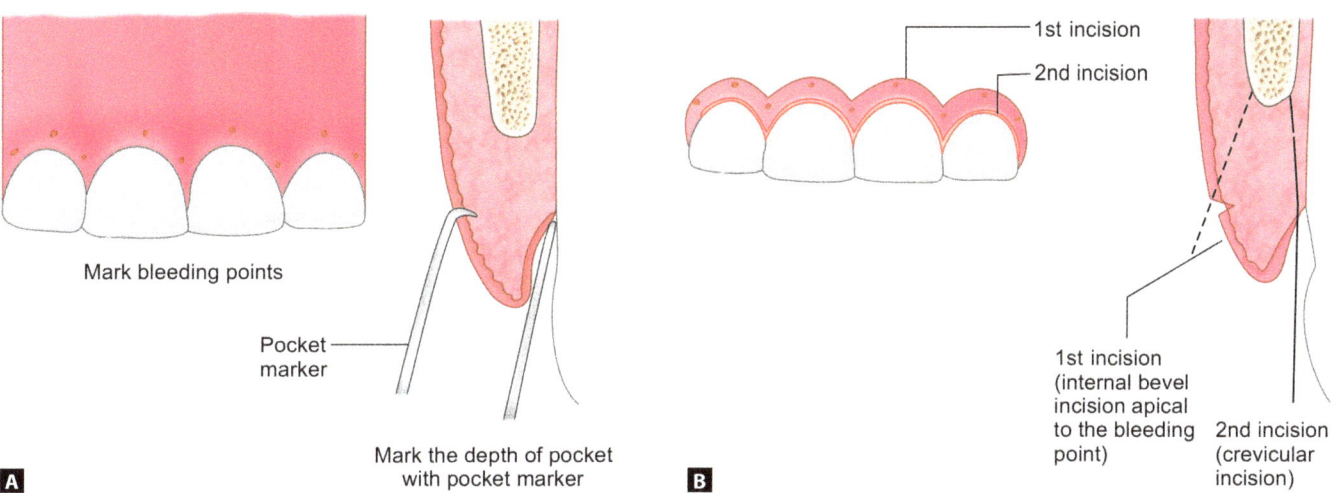

**Figs. 49.8A and B:** Schematic representation showing an undisplaced flap.

- *Step VII—Curettage, scaling, and root planing*: After the necessary scaling and root planing, the flap edge should rest on the root–bone junction.
- *Step VIII—Suturing*: A continuous sling suture is utilized to hold the flap edges at the root–bone junction. This type of suture, which uses the tooth as an anchor, is advantageous to position and hold the flap edges at the root-bone junction. The area is covered with a periodontal pack.
- *Step IX—Instructions*: Postoperative instructions are given thereafter.

## Apically Displaced Flap

### Historical Perspective

In 1954, Naber's described the repositioning of the attached gingiva. For the first time, a mucoperiosteal flap was apically positioned after treatment.[8] He utilized one vertical releasing incision, which is placed mesially to the area of the deepest pocket. Later in 1957, he introduced the inverse bevel incision of which he called the "repositioning incision," which includes the internal incision from the gingival margin to the alveolar crest. This incision, he stated, would permit an easier flap reflection and result in a thinner gingival margin. In that same year, Ariaudo and Tyrrell modified Nabers' technique and recommended two vertical releasing incisions instead of just one to facilitate the mobilization of the flap.[9] At this point, the only difference from the flap design of Widman is the apical positioning. Finally, in 1962, Friedman published the technique in his paper and coined the term "apically repositioned flap".[10] In his paper, he described the use of inverse beveled incision to thin the marginal tissue and the papillae. This thinning incision eliminates thick gingival margin and papillae with large triangular pieces of interdental tissue. A thick tissue would be difficult to eliminate from the already raised flap and created a problem in the approximation of tissue for primary intention healing, resulting in bulbous or ledging tissue upon healing. This flap design could be referred to as the partial-full-thickness flap since the marginal papillae was partially dissected with the inverse bevel incision, then this incision continues to include the mucoperiosteum of the full-thickness flap. In 1982, Goldman introduced another variation of which he followed the full-thickness flap with a partial dissection, allowing the use of periosteal suture to position the flap. This flap design, he called the tertiary flap or the partial-full partial-thickness flap. Today, the word "reposition" is replaced by the term "position" since reposition means to place the flap back to where it was before. The flap can be positioned apically or reposition, depending on each individualized case. The sling suture is recommended for better flap placement. Pocket elimination is achieved only by the apical positioning of the flap.

### Objectives

- To eliminate pocket by apically positioning the soft tissue wall of the pocket.
- To preserve or increase the width of the attached gingiva.
- To improve accessibility.

### Indications

- Moderate or deep pockets with the base of the pocket apical to the mucogingival junction.
- Crown lengthening.[7]

### Contraindications

- Anterior regions because of esthetics.
- Exposed roots.
- Patients who are at risk for root caries.

The position of the flap displacement varies depending on the:

- The thickness of the alveolar margin in the operating area.
- Width of attached gingiva.
- Clinical crown length necessary for an abutment.

### Surgical Instruments

Surgical instruments include:
- Blade Nos. 11, 12, and 15
- Bard-Parker handle No. 3
- Periosteal elevator
- Curettes

### Procedures

Following are the steps of apically displaced flap procedure (Figs. 49.9A to D):
- *Step I—Incisions*:
  - The first incision, internal bevel incision, is made 1 mm from the gingiva's crest and directed towards the crest of the alveolar bone. The beveling incision should be given a scalloped outline to ensure maximal interproximal coverage of the alveolar bone when the flap is subsequently repositioned.
  - The second incision, a crevicular incision, is made, followed by the elevation of the full-thickness mucoperiosteal flap.
  - The third incision, an interdental incision is given and the wedge of the tissue that contains a pocket wall is removed.
  - Vertical incisions extending out into alveolar mucosa (i.e., past the mucogingival junction) are made at each endpoint of the internal bevel incision, making the apical repositioning of the flap.
- *Step II—Flap reflection*: For the full-thickness flap, the periosteal elevator is used to reflect the flap.
- *Step III—Removal of granulation tissue*: Marginal collar tissue and granulation tissue are removed with curettes.
- *Step IV—Scaling and root planing*: Scaling and root planing is done carefully with scalers and curettes.
- *Step V—Osseous recontouring*: Alveolar bone crest is recontoured with the help of bur and bone chisels.

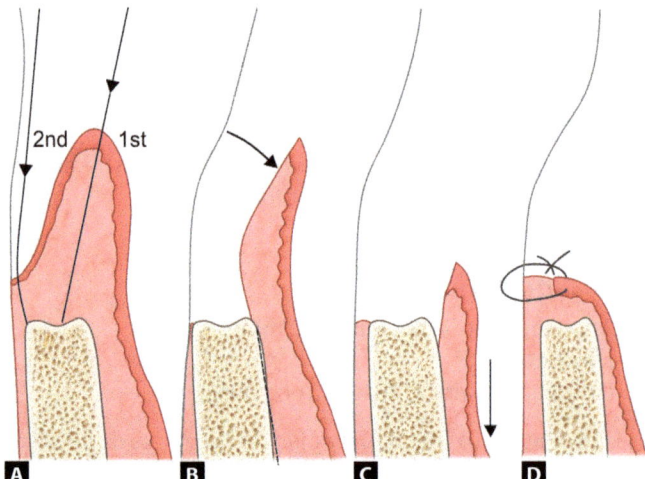

**Figs. 49.9A to D:** Schematic representation showing apically positioned flap: (A) First inverse bevel incision, second crevicular incision; (B) Flap reflected and dissected from the alveolar process; (C) Flap moved in an apical direction; (D) Flap sutured in an apical position.

- *Step VI—Apical positioning and suturing*: The flap is reflected to the base of the vestibule. Once released, the flap tends to contract and fold up so that apical positioning takes place. The flap is displaced apically, so that edge just covers the newly recontoured alveolar crest. Interrupted sutures should be placed first at the mesial and distal vertical incisions. The full-thickness flap is sutured using sling suture while the partial-thickness flap is secured with a direct loop suture or a combination of loop and anchor suture. A periodontal dressing is applied on the operated site over the dry foil.
- *Step VII—Instructions*: Postoperative instructions are given thereafter.

### Advantages

- *Eliminates periodontal pocket*: Apically repositioned flap results in pocket elimination and the formation of a normal or physiological length of junctional epithelium, whereas the replaced flap results in the formation of a long junctional epithelium which may adhere to the root surface. The long junctional epithelium is inherently less stable than the physiological junctional epithelium and demands much higher frequencies of recall for maintenance than pocket elimination procedures.
- It preserves the attached gingiva and increases its width.
- It establishes gingival morphology by facilitating good hygiene.
- It ensures a healthy root surface necessary for the biologic width on the alveolar margin and lengthens clinical crown.

### Disadvantages

- It may cause:
  - Esthetic problems due to root exposure
  - Attachment loss due to surgery
  - Hypersensitivity
- It may increase the risk of root caries
- Possibility of exposure of furcations and roots, which complicates postoperative supragingival plaque control.

## Papilla Preservation Flap

In 1985, Takei et al., proposed a surgical approach called "papilla preservation technique."[11] Later, Cortellini et al., described modifications of this flap design. It is the procedure that incorporates the entire papilla in one of the flaps by means of crevicular and interdental incisions to sever the connective tissue attachment and a horizontal incision at the base of the papilla, leaving it connected to one of the flaps.

### Indications

- Diastema region
- Bone grafting areas

### Contraindication
Narrow embrasures

### Procedure
Following are the steps of papilla preservation flap procedure **(Figs. 49.10 and 49.11)**:
- *Step I—Incisions*:
  - Crevicular incisions are made at the facial, palatal, and proximal aspects of the teeth without making incisions through the interdental papillae **(Fig. 49.10A)**.
  - Semilunar incisions are made across each interdental area with the blade perpendicular to the outer surface of gingiva and extending through the periosteum to the alveolar process **(Fig. 49.10B)**. The semilunar incision should dip apically at least 5 mm from the line angles of teeth, which will allow the interdental tissue to be dissected from the lingual or palatal aspect so that it can be elevated intact with the facial flap.
- *Step II—Reflection of flap*: A curette or interproximal knife is used to carefully free the interdental papilla from the underlying hard tissue. The detached interdental tissue is pushed through the embrasure with a blunt instrument **(Fig. 49.10C)**. A full-thickness flap is reflected with a periosteal elevator on both facial and palatal surfaces.
- *Step III—Scaling and root planing*: The exposed root surfaces are thoroughly scaled and root planed and bone defects carefully curetted.
- *Step IV—Removal of granulomatous tissue*: While, holding the reflected flap, the margins of the flap and the interdental tissue are scrapped to remove pocket epithelium and excessive granulation tissue. In anterior areas, the trimming of granulation tissue should be limited so as to maintain the thickness of tissue. After the reflection of the flap, access to the interdental bony defect will be obtained. The bony defect is cleaned out using a curette.
- *Step V—Placing graft material*: The bone graft material is placed if required.
- *Step VI—Suturing*: The flaps are repositioned and sutured using the criss-cross mattress. The cross-mattress suture results in optimal flap closure without having suture material in direct contact with the graft material. Alternatively, a direct suture of the semilunar incisions can be done as the only means of flap closure **(Fig. 49.10D)**. A periodontal dressing may be placed to protect the surgical area.
- *Step VII—Instruction*: Postoperative instructions are given thereafter.

### Advantages
- Esthetically pleasing
- Primary coverage of the implant
- Prevent postoperative tissue craters

### Disadvantages
- Technically difficult
- Time-consuming

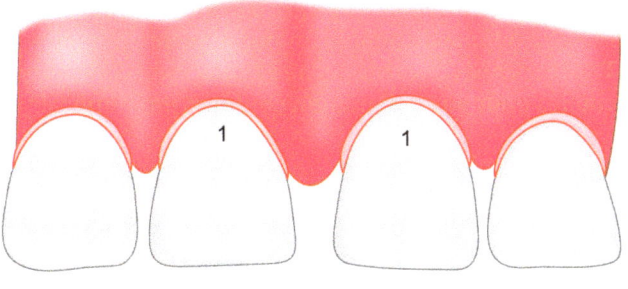

A

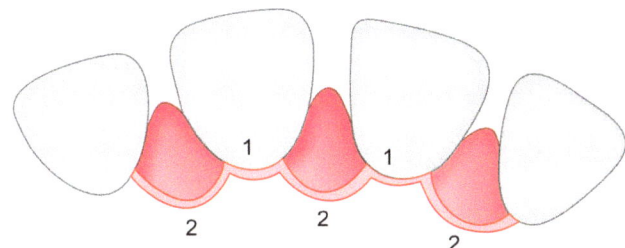

B

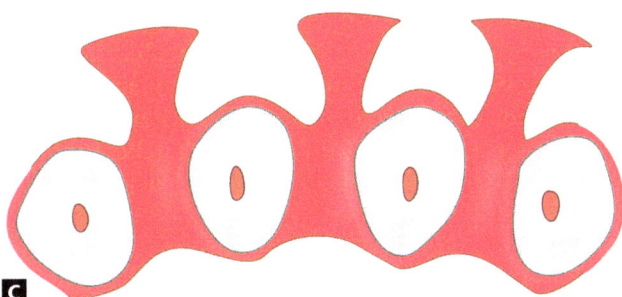

C

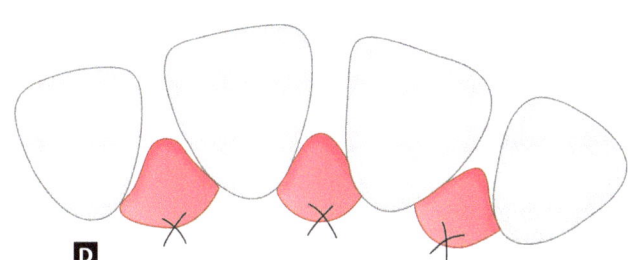

D

**Figs. 49.10A to D:** Schematic representation showing papilla preservation flap incisions: (A) Facial view, 1. Intrasulcular incision; (B) Palatal view, 1. Intrasulcular incision, 2. semilunar incision; (C) Incisal view reflected papilla preservation flap; (D) Palatal view papilla preservation flap sutured.

## Section 7: Treatment: Surgical Therapy

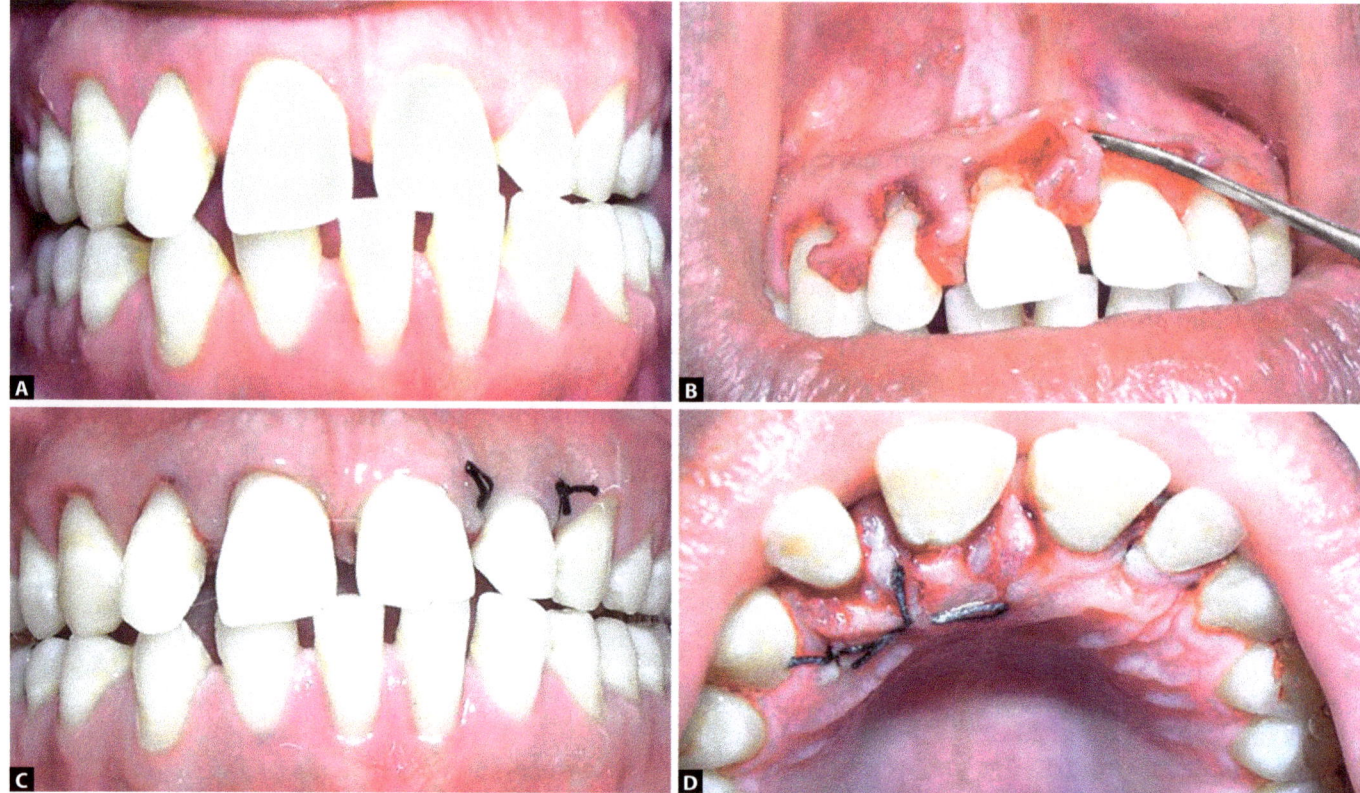

**Figs. 49.11A to D:** Clinical picture showing: (A) Preoperative; (B) Both papilla in a facial flap; (C) Facial view after suturing; (D) Palatal view after suturing.

## Palatal Flap

The surgical approach for the palatal flap is different from other flaps because of the nature of palatal tissue, which is attached and keratinized with no elastic properties. The apical portion of the scalloping should be narrower than the line angle area because of the taper of palatal root apically. The palatal flap cannot be displaced apically, nor can a split-thickness palatal flap be accomplished.[12]

### Indications

- Areas that require osseous surgery
- Pocket elimination
- Reduction of enlarged and bulbous tissue

### Contraindication

A palatal flap is contraindicated when the palate is broad and shallow.

### Precautions

Special care must be taken performing a palatal flap due to several anatomic structures:
- Greater palatine artery and nerve may be damaged if flap reflection is extensive in the molar region.
- Palatal exostoses present in the molar region in one-third of the patient. It creates thin tissue in the region and makes proper flap margin placement difficult.
- Incisive papilla present in anterior palate.
- The presence of palatal rugae at or near the flap margin creates poor gingival margin contours postsurgically.

### Procedure

The outline of initial incision for palatal flap varies and is determined with consideration for the:
- The thickness of palatal soft tissue
- Depth of periodontal pocket
- Necessity for osteoplasty
- The clinical crown length required for restorative treatment. If the purpose of surgery is debridement, then internal bevel incision is given such that palatal flap is adapted at the root–bone junction, when sutured. If osseous resection is to be done, then the palatal incision is planned to compensate for a lowered level of the bone when the flap is closed.
  - *Step I—Incisions:* The initial incision, i.e., internal bevel incision, followed by crevicular and interdental incisions, are given. If the tissue is thick, a horizontal

gingivectomy incision may be made, followed by an internal bevel incision that starts at the edge of this incision and ends on the lateral surface of the underlying bone. The placement of the internal bevel incision must be done in such a way that the flap fits around the tooth without exposing the bone. The blade should be parallel to the palatal soft tissue to prepare a thin and uniform primary flap (1.5-2.0 mm thickness). Caution must be taken to avoid perforating the flap or making the flap too thin, which will cut-off the necessary blood supply.

- *Step II—Flap reflection*: Before the flap is reflected in the final position for scaling and managing the osseous lesions, its thickness must be checked. Flaps should be thin to adapt to the underlying osseous tissue and provide a thin, knife-like gingival margin. The full-thickness flap is reflected.
- *Step III—Scaling and root planing*: With the help of scalers and curettes, scaling and root planing is performed. Osteoplasty is done only if required.
- *Step IV—Suturing*: Suture the flap's edge at the level of the bone margin or slightly over the alveolar crest (approximately 1-2 mm above the bone margin).
- *Step V—Instruction*: Postoperative instructions are given thereafter.

## Distal Molar Surgery

The treatment of periodontal pockets on the terminal molar's distal surface is often complicated by the presence of bulbous fibrous tissue over the maxillary tuberosity or prominent retromolar pad in the mandible. Deep vertical defects are also commonly present in conjunction with the redundant fibrous tissue. This procedure enables the removal of thick gingival tissue on the adjacent edentulous site. If there is an osseous defect, it corrects the bone morphology by flattening it, and the intrabony defect may be eliminated. The periodontal pocket is eliminated, and a shallow gingival sulcus favorable for postoperative maintenance is created.

### *Objectives*

- To maintain and preserve the attached gingiva.
- To eliminate periodontal pocket.
- To lengthen clinical crown.
- To create easily cleansable gingiva-alveolar form.

### *Incisions*

The various incisions for distal molar surgery[13] (**Figs. 49.12A to D**):
- Linear incision
- Triangular incision
- Pedicle incision
- Square, parallel incision

### *Indications*

- Long and large edentulous ridge, maxillary tuberosity, and retromolar triangle.
- Much tissue to be removed in the wedge area.
- Sufficient existing band of attached gingiva.
- Deep periodontal pockets and osseous defects on the mesial and distal aspects of the abutment.

### *Maxillary Molars*

Two parallel incisions, beginning at the distal portion of the tooth and extending to the mucogingival junction distal to the tuberosity, are made. These incisions are usually interconnected with the incisions for the remainder of the surgery in the quadrant involved. The amount of wedge tissue to be removed (the distance between the two internal bevel incisions) is determined by a number of factors, such as:

- Depth of periodontal pocket.
- The thickness of the soft-tissue wedge.
- Whether osteoplasty or osseous resection is necessary.
- The clinical crown length required for the abutment.

A transversal incision is made at the distal end of the two parallel incisions so that a long, rectangular piece of tissue can be removed. The parallel distal incisions should be confined to the attached gingiva because bleeding and flap management becomes a problem when the incision is extended into the alveolar mucosa. When the tissue between the two incisions is removed, and the flaps are thinned, the two flap edges must approximate each other at a new apical position without overlapping.

### *Mandibular Molars*

The mandibular arch's incisions differ from those used for the tuberosity, owing to differences in the anatomy and histologic features of the areas. The retromolar pad area does not usually present as much fibrous attached gingiva. The two incisions distal to the molar should follow the area with the greatest amount of attached gingiva. Therefore, the incisions could be directed distolingually or distofacially, depending on which area has more attached gingiva. Before the flap is completely reflected, it is thinned with a 15 No. blade. It is easier to thin the flap before it is completely free and mobile. After the reflection of the flap and the removal of the redundant fibrous tissue, any necessary osseous surgery is performed. The flaps are approximated similarly to those in the maxillary tuberosity area.

### *Advantages*

- Maintenance of attached tissue.
- Accessibility for treatment of both distal furcation and underlying osseous irregularities.

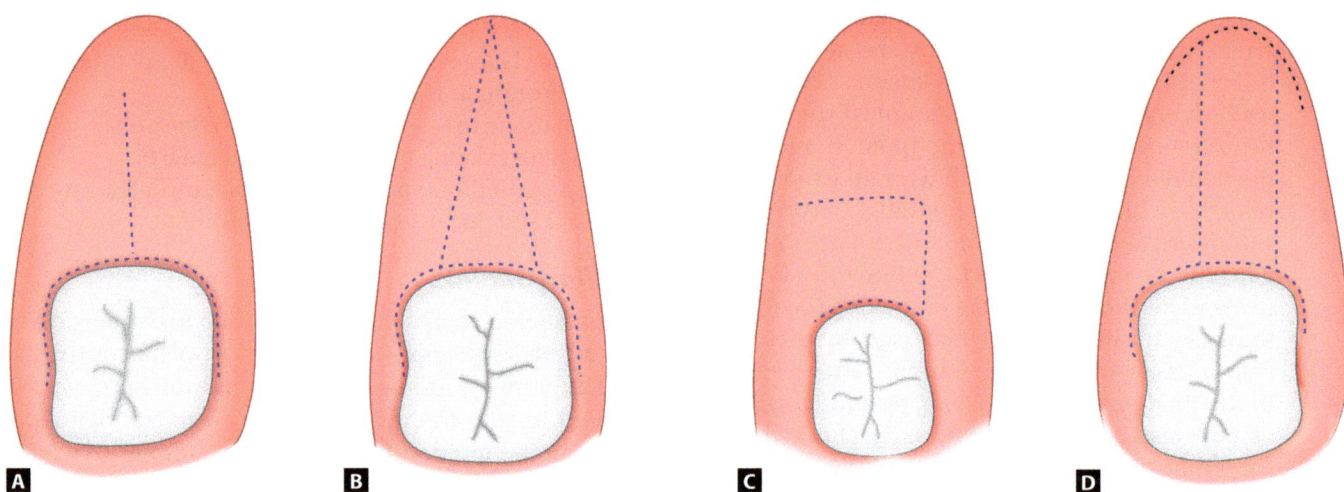

**Figs. 49.12A to D:** Schematic representation showing various incisions for distal molar surgery: (A) Linear incision; (B) Triangular incision; (C) Pedicle incision; (D) Square, parallel incision.

## Coronally Displaced Flap

Coronally displaced flap is explained in "Chapter 53: Periodontal Plastic Surgery".

## Laterally Positioned Pedicle Flap

It was originally developed by Grupe and Warren in 1956. In this procedure, a pedicle graft is taken from a donor site and is placed on the adjoining site by moving the flap towards the recipient site, and sutures are placed[14] (Rest is described in "Chapter 53: Periodontal Plastic Surgery").

## Double Papilla Pedicle Flap

Double papilla pedicle flap is explained in "Chapter 53: Periodontal Plastic Surgery".

### Points to Ponder

- Incisions are either coronally directed incisions (external bevel incision) or apically directed incisions (internal bevel, sulcular incision).
- The undisplaced flap is considered as internal bevel gingivectomy. Undisplaced flap and gingivectomy procedures surgically remove the pocket wall.
- Apically positioned flap surgery is one of the most reliable techniques for the elimination of periodontal pockets.
- The flap without vertical incision is called envelope flap.
- The tissue, which is left on the surface of the tooth when the flap is raised, is called a cervical wedge.
- Neumann flap: Neumann, in 1911, introduced the flap in which the intrasulcular incision was made along with two vertical releasing incisions, a full-thickness flap raised, and the area was curetted thoroughly to eliminate all the granulation tissue to prevent reinfection. Root was planed smooth, and bone was superficially removed.
- The conventional flap is the flap in which the papilla is split into facial half and lingual or palatal half.

## REFERENCES

1. Hupp JR, Ellis E, Tucker MR. Contemporary Oral and Maxillofacial Surgery, 2nd edition. Singapore: Harcourt Brace and Company, Asia Private Limited; 2014.
2. Takei HH, Carranza FA. The periodontal flap. In: Newman MG, Takei HH, Carranza FA (Eds). Carranza's Clinical Periodontology, 9th edition. Philadelphia, PA, USA: WB Saunders; 2003. pp. 762-73.
3. Friedman N. Mucogingival surgery. The apically repositioned flap. J Periodontol. 1962;33:328-40.
4. Morris ML. The unrepositioned muco-periosteal flap. Periodontics. 1965;3:147-51.
5. Ramfjord SP, Nissle R. The modified Widman flap. J Periodontol. 1974;45(8):601-7.
6. enco RJ, Rosenberg ES, Evian C. Periodontal surgery. In: Genco RJ, Goldman HM, Cohen DW (Eds). Contemporary Periodontics, 2nd edition. St. Louis: CV Mosby; 1999. pp. 554-84.
7. Carranza FM, Takei HH. The flap technique for pocket therapy. In: Newman MG, Takei HH, Carranza FA (Eds). Carranza's Clinical Periodontology, 9th edition. Philadelphia, PA, USA: WB Saunders; 2003. pp. 774-85.
8. Nabers CL. Repositioning the attached gingiva. J Periodontol. 1954;25:38-9.
9. Ariaudo AA, Tyrell HA. Repositioning and increasing the zone of attached gingiva. J Periodontol. 1957;28:106-10.
10. Friedman N. Mucogingival surgery: The apically repositioned flap. J Periodontol. 1962;33:328-40.
11. Takei HH, Han TJ, Carranza FA, Kenney EB, Lekovic V. Flap technique for periodontal bone implants. Papilla preservation technique. J Periodontol. 1985;56(4):204-10.
12. Wennstrom JL, Heijl L, Lindhe J. Periodontal surgery: access therapy. In: Lindhe J, Karring T, Lang NP (Eds). Clinical Periodontology and Implant Dentistry, 4th edition. Chicago, USA: Blackwell Munksgaard; 2003. pp. 519-60.
13. McDonnell HT, Mills MP. Principles and practice of periodontal surgery. In: Rose LF, Mealey BL, Genco RJ, Cohen DW (Eds). Periodontics: Medicine, Surgery, and Implants, 1st edition. St. Louis: Elsevier-Mosby; 2004. pp. 358-404.
14. Grupe HE, Warren RF. Repair of gingival defects by a sliding flap operation. J Periodontol. 1956;27:92.

## Chapter 49: Periodontal Flap

### VIVA VOCE

**Q1. Which incision is called as reverse bevel incision?**
**Ans.** Internal bevel incision is called as reverse bevel incision because its bevel is in the reverse direction from that of the gingivectomy incision.

**Q2. Why is the surgical approach for the palatal flap different from other flaps?**
**Ans.** The surgical approach for the palatal flap is different from other flaps because of the nature of palatal tissue, which is attached and keratinized with no elastic properties.

**Q3. Which flap procedure is considered as internal bevel gingivectomy?**
**Ans.** The undisplaced flap is considered as internal bevel gingivectomy.

**Q4. Which surgical procedures remove the pocket wall?**
**Ans.** Surgical procedures which remove the pocket wall are: undisplaced flap and gingivectomy.

**Q5. What are the differences in incision and flap for regenerative surgery from other surgical procedures?**
**Ans.** The differences in incision and flap for regenerative surgery from other surgical procedures are as follows:
- Papilla preservation or conventional flap are raised during a regenerative surgical procedure.
- Sulcular incision is given so as to preserve the maximum amount of gingival tissue for regenerative surgical procedures.
- Do not make the flap thin in regenerative surgery as for other surgical procedures.

**Q6. What is the thickness of the primary flap?**
**Ans.** The thickness of the primary flap is about 1.5 mm. If the flap is too thin, there will be insufficient connective tissue support, and because of which, there will be insufficient blood supply, and the flap will get necrosed.

**Q7. Comparison between modified Widman flap, undisplaced flap, and apically displaced flap procedure.**
**Ans.**

| Parameters | Modified Widman flap | Undisplaced flap | Apically displaced flap |
|---|---|---|---|
| Nature of procedure | The incisional procedure of the gingiva | The excisional procedure of the gingiva | The incisional procedure of the gingiva |
| Objectives | To facilitate root instrumentation | To reduce pocket wall | To eliminate the pocket |
|  | To remove the pocket lining |  | To increase the width of the attached gingiva |
| Indications | Shallow to moderate pocket depth with the base of the pockets located coronal to the mucogingival junction | Gingival enlargements | Moderate or deep pockets with the base of the pocket apical to the mucogingival junction |
|  |  |  | To lengthen crown |
| Vertical incisions | Not given | Not given | Given |
| Bleeding points | Not marked | Marked | Not marked |
| Ability to treat osseous irregularities and defects | No | No | Yes |
| Degree of difficulty | Low | Low | High |

**Q8. What are the basic flap requirements?**
**Ans.**
- Base of the flap must be wide enough to maintain an adequate blood supply.
- The flap must be big enough to expose any underlying bone defects.
- No important vessels or nerves should be damaged in raising the flap.
- Incisions must allow movement of flap without tension.

**Q9. What is the indication for full-thickness flap?**
**Ans.** To expose the bone surface in osseous surgery.

**Q10. What are the objectives of an apically displaced flap?**
**Ans.** To eliminate the pocket and to increase the width of the attached gingiva.

# Resective Osseous Surgery

*Shaili Pradhan, Shalu Bathla*

## Chapter Outline

- Definitions
- Objectives
- Rationale
- Osteoplasty Indications
- Ostectomy Indications
- Examination
- Instruments
- Procedure
- Disadvantages
- Postoperative Healing

## INTRODUCTION

Schluger, considered the "Father of Resective Osseous Surgery," advocated osseous resective treatment of periodontitis, rather than scaling and root planing or the gingivectomy. In resective osseous surgery, there is the combined use of both osteoplasty and ostectomy to re-establish the marginal bone morphology around the teeth to resemble normal bone with a positive architecture.

## DEFINITIONS

- *Resective osseous surgery*: The procedure designed to restore the form of pre-existing alveolar bone to the level existing at the time of surgery or slightly more apical to this level is called as resective osseous surgery.
- *Osteoplasty*: It is a procedure to create a physiologic form of alveolar bone without removing any supporting bone.
- *Ostectomy*: It is a procedure in which supporting bone, i.e., bone involved in the attachment of tooth is removed to reshape deformities.
- *Ideal architecture*: The bone level is more coronal in the interproximal areas, with a gradual slope around and away from the tooth.
- *Positive architecture*: The level of radicular bone is apical to the interdental bone (**Fig. 50.1A**).
- *Negative architecture*: The level of interdental bone is more apical to the radicular bone. It is also called as reversed architecture (**Fig. 50.1B**).
- *Flat architecture*: The interdental bone is at the same level as that of radicular bone (**Fig. 50.1C**).

## OBJECTIVES

The objectives of osseous resection are to:[1,2]
- Remove osseous defects.
- Correct bone morphology.
- Create a harmonious relationship between the gingiva and the alveolar bone by eliminating periodontal pockets.
- Create a favorable postoperative gingival morphology.

## RATIONALE

To achieve a physiologic architecture of marginal alveolar bone conducive to gingival flap adaption with minimal probing depth. The endpoints of osseous resective surgery are minimal probing depths and a gingival tissue morphology that enhances good self-performed oral hygiene and periodontal health.[1,2]

## OSTEOPLASTY INDICATIONS

Following are the indications of osteoplasty:[3,4]
- Removing exostoses (**Figs. 50.2A and B**).
- Tori that interferes with plaque control and persistent pocket.
- Early grade I furcation lesion.
- To contour alveolar ridge to make room for pontics.
- Open furcation in tunneling procedure.

# Chapter 50: Resective Osseous Surgery

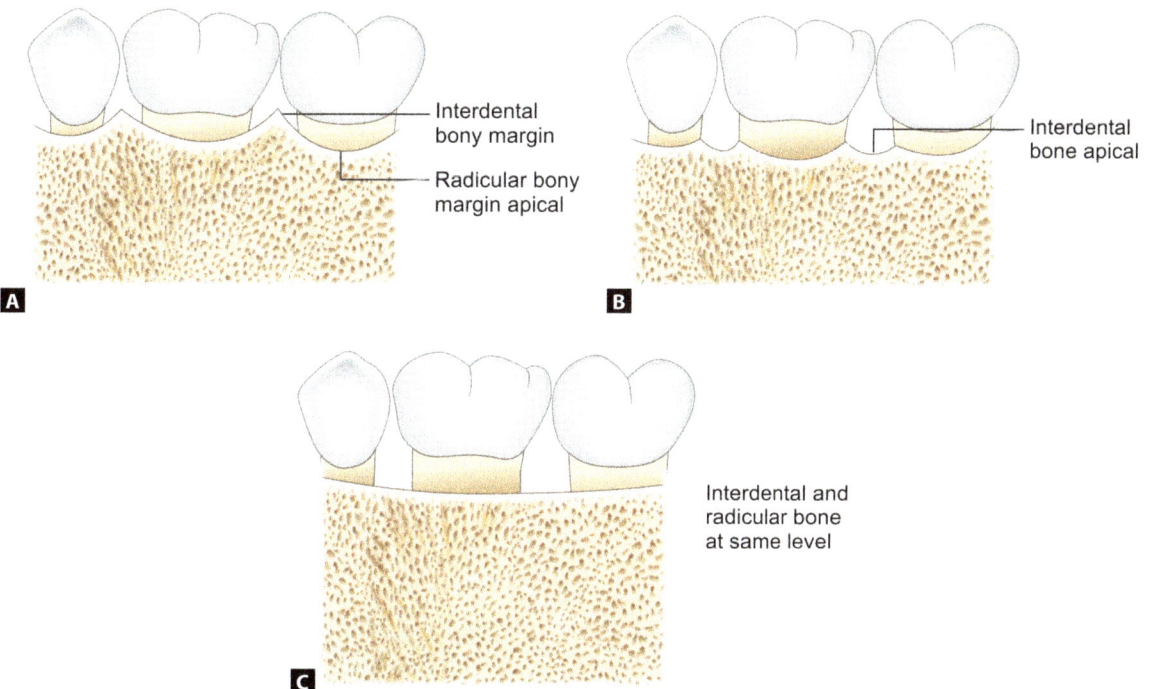

**Figs. 50.1A to C:** Schematic representation showing bone architecture: (A) Positive; (B) Reversed or negative; (C) Flat.

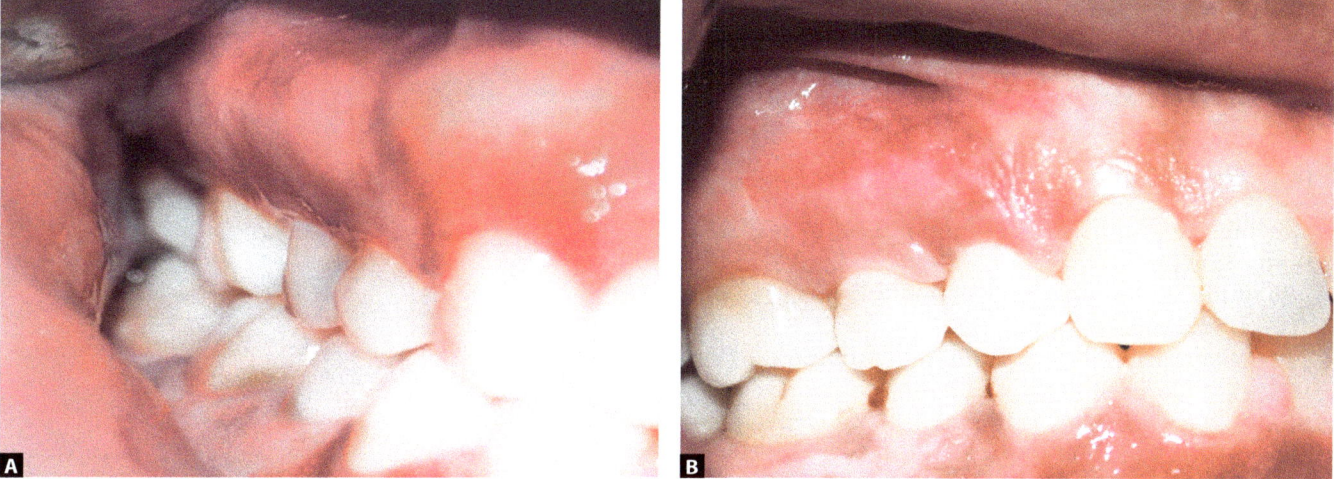

**Figs. 50.2A and B:** Clinical picture showing exostoses at right buccal maxillary region: (A) Preoperative; and (B) Postoperative.

## OSTECTOMY INDICATIONS

Following are the indications of ostectomy:[3]
- Crown lengthening.
- Exposure of sound dentin apical to caries or fractures.
- Opening of interradicular spaces for the treatment of furcation involvement.

## EXAMINATION

The potential need for a resective osseous surgery is usually recognized during the following comprehensive periodontal examination:[5-10]
- Soft-tissue palpation
- *Radiographic examination*: It provides information about:
  - The interproximal bone loss and/or the presence of angular or irregular bone loss.
  - The extent of bony defect or the number of bony walls remaining.
- *Probing*: It reveals the presence of:
  - Pocket depth greater than that of the normal gingival sulcus.
  - Location of the base of pocket relative to mucogingival junction and attachment level on adjacent teeth.
  - The number of bony walls.
  - Furcation defects.

**Section 7:** Treatment: Surgical Therapy

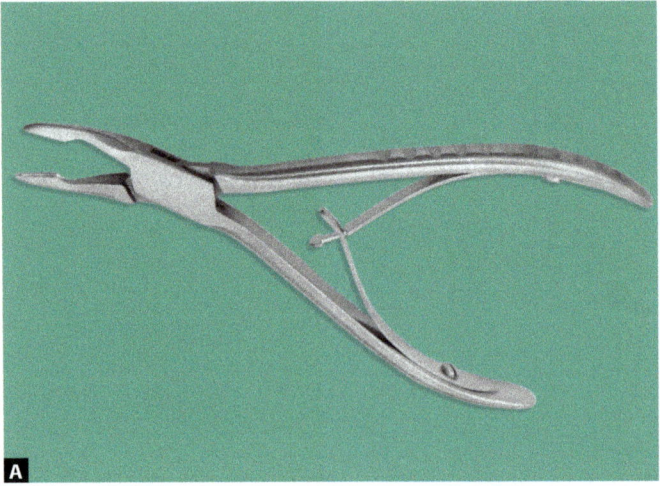

**Figs. 50.3A and B:** Photograph showing bone rongeurs.

- *Transgingival probing (sounding)*:[2]
  - Under local anesthesia, it confirms the extent and configuration of the intrabony component of the pocket or furcation defects.
  - The probe walks along the tissue-tooth interface to feel the bony topography.
  - The probe may pass horizontally through the tissue to provide three-dimensional information regarding bony contours.

## INSTRUMENTS

Following are the instruments often used in resective osseous surgery:[2,4]
- *Rongeurs*: Blumenthal rongeur and Friedman rongeur **(Figs. 50.3A and B)**.
- *Files*: Sugarman file **(Fig. 50.4A)** and Schluger file **(Fig. 50.4B)**.
- *Chisels*: Rhodes back action chisel and Ochsenbein chisel **(Fig. 50.5)**.
- *Burs*: Carbide and diamond burs.

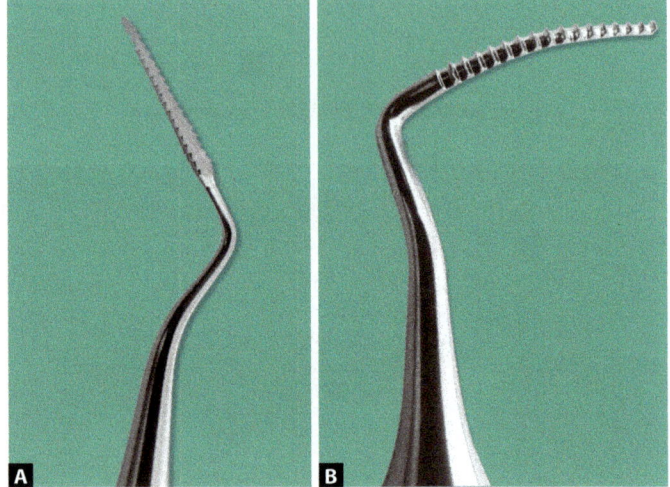

**Figs. 50.4A and B:** Photograph showing files: (A) Sugarman file; (B) Schluger file.

## PROCEDURE

- *Anesthesia*: Appropriate local anesthesia is given in the selected area.
- *Incision and flap reflection*: Mucoperiosteal flap is reflected by giving horizontal and vertical incisions in the surgical area **(Fig. 50.6)** (for the apically displaced flap, a vertical incision should be given).
- *Resective osseous technique*: It is carried out in four steps **(Figs. 50.7A to D)**:
  1. Step I: Vertical grooving or festooning.
  2. Step II: Radicular blending.
  3. Step III: Flattening of interproximal bone.
  4. Step IV: Gradualizing marginal bone.

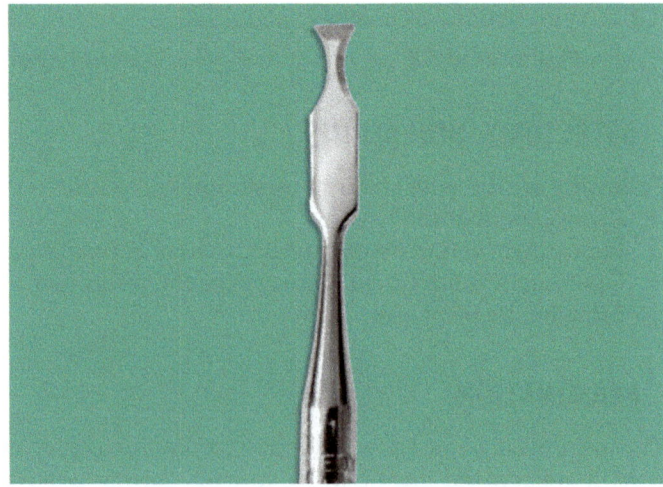

**Fig. 50.5:** Photograph showing Ochsenbein chisel.

## Chapter 50: Resective Osseous Surgery

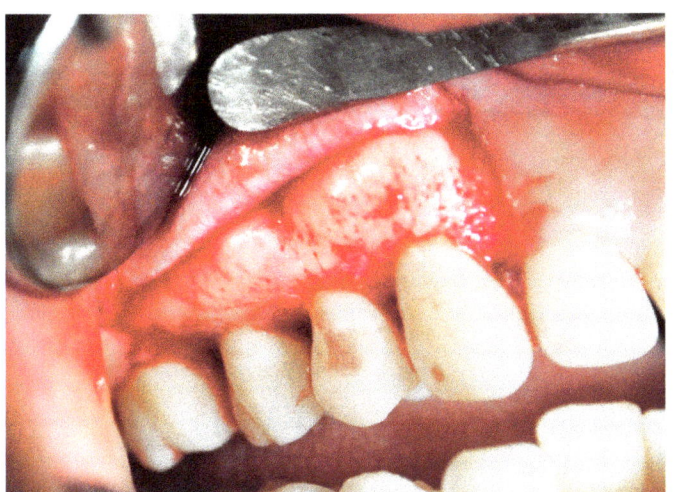

**Fig. 50.6:** Clinical picture showing exostoses after the reflection of mucoperiosteal flap.

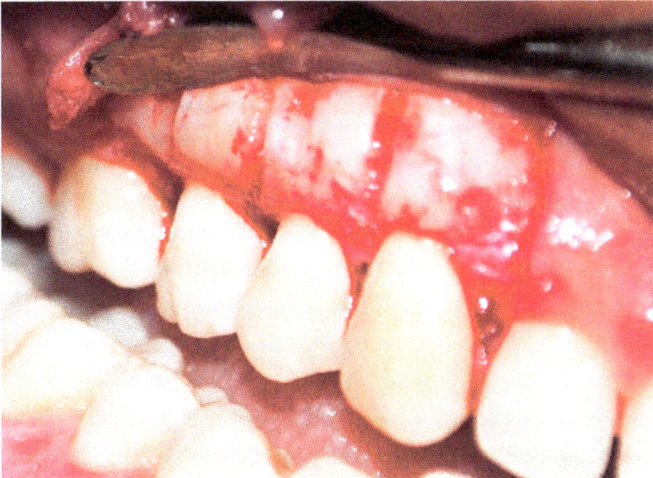

**Fig. 50.8:** Clinical picture showing vertical grooving at the surgical site.

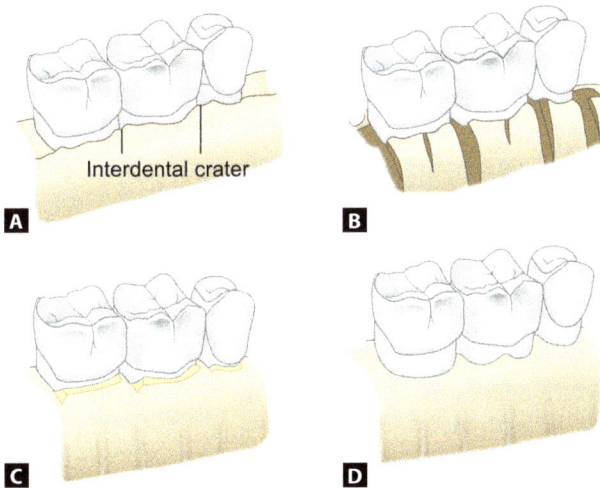

**Figs. 50.7A to D:** Schematic representation showing resective osseous technique: (A) Bony topography showing interdental craters; (B) Vertical grooving; (C) Radicular blending and flattening of interproximal bone; (D) Gradualizing the marginal bone.
(*Courtesy*: Dr SK Salaria)

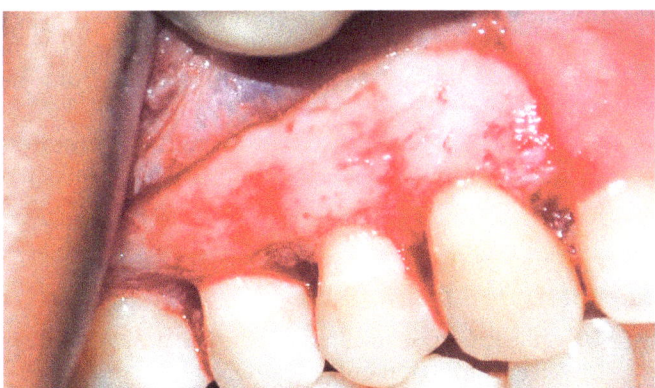

**Fig. 50.9:** Clinical picture showing radicular blending at the surgical site.

*Step I—Vertical grooving or festooning*: It is the first step of the resective osseous surgery designed to reduce the thickness of the alveolar housing and to provide prominence to the radicular aspects of the teeth **(Fig. 50.8)**. Slow speed (2,000 rpm) handpiece with a sharp carbide surgical bur is used to perform the vertical grooving. Cooling with a copious spray of sterile saline is necessary so that the bone's temperature is not raised beyond 47°C. It is contraindicated in close root proximity or thin alveolar housing areas.[3]

It is designed:
- To reduce the thickness of the alveolar housing.
- To provide relative prominence to the radicular aspect of the teeth.
- To provide continuity from the interproximal surface onto the radicular surface.

*Step II—Radicular blending*: It is the extension of vertical grooving, which gradualize the bone over the entire radicular surface to produce a smooth and blended surface for good flap adaptation **(Fig. 50.9)**. It is indicated where thick ledges of bone is present on the radicular surface, whereas it is contraindicated where thin, fenestrated radicular bone is present.

Both vertical grooving and radicular blending may be used for the treatment of:
- Thick osseous ledges of bone on the radicular surface.
- Class I and early class II furcation involvement.

*Step III—Flattening of interproximal bone*: This is done where interproximal bone levels vary horizontally. There is a small amount of supporting bone that is removed with the help of chisel.

*Step IV—Gradualizing marginal bone*: It is the minimal bone removal to provide a sound, regular base for gingival tissue to follow. The bone is removed with a chisel. Saline

irrigation should also be carried out during chiseling since this generates heat.
- *Suturing*: After removal of the osseous tissue, the flap is adapted closely to cover the bone with the flap apically displaced, which is then sutured in place.
- *Postoperative instructions*: The patient is followed postoperatively as with other flap procedures.

## Specific Osseous Reshaping Situations

### Correction of One-walled Hemiseptal Defect

- The bone should be reduced to the level of the most apical portion of the defect. It requires the removal of some bones on the side with the greatest coronal bony height. This results in a significant reduction in attachment on relatively unaffected adjacent teeth to eliminate the defect.
- If the tooth has a one-wall defect on both of its mesial and distal surfaces, the severely affected tooth may be extruded by orthodontics during disease control to minimize the need for resection of bone from the adjacent teeth.
- If a one-walled defect occurs next to the edentulous area, the edentulous ridge is reduced to the level of the osseous defect **(Fig. 50.10)**.

### Correction of Exostoses, Malpositioned or Supraerupted Tooth

- Osteoplasty is done to eliminate the exostoses or reduce the buccal or lingual bulk of bone.
- It is common to incorporate a degree of vertical grooving during the reduction of the bony ledges since it facilitates the process of blending the radicular bone into interproximal areas.[10]
- Follow all the four steps explained above.

## DISADVANTAGES

- It causes recession and hypersensitivity.
- Reduces tooth bone support.

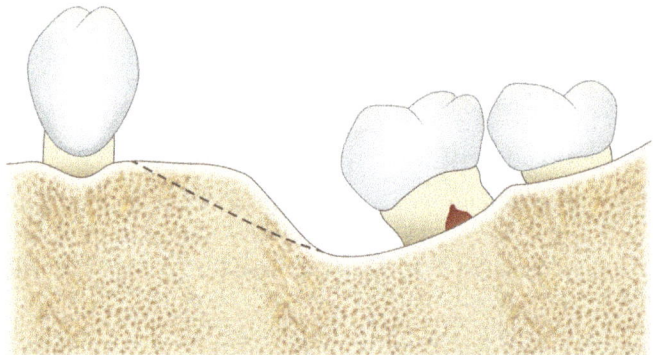

**Fig. 50.10:** Schematic representation showing reduction of one- wall angular defect by ramping.

**Flowchart 50.1:** Healing after resective osseous surgery.

Soon after surgery, blood clot is formed bordered by viable and nonviable granulocytes (blood clot over bone is a complex of exudate and cellular and tissue debris, loosely complexed with fibrin)
↓
Hydrolytic enzymes from neutrophils leads to
↓
Within 2 days: Necrosis and resorption of osseous surface demineralization
↓
At 10–14 days: Osteoclast-mediated resorption continues
↓
Loss of axial periodicity of collagen molecules
↓
Granulation tissue is formed over the previously denuded bone and is of periosteal and endosteal origin (centripetal lateral ingrowth from peripherally located periosteum and outgrowth from exposed marrow cavities and vascular channels)
↓
By 2–3 weeks: Osteoid and woven bone is formed
↓
By 4 weeks: Periodontal ligament is restored
↓
By 3 months: Parital compact bone is formed

- Removes bone that may be needed if implants are desired.
- Exposed roots could be at higher risk for caries in patients with poor oral hygiene.
- More access for a brush but more challenges for the patients to maintain.

## POSTOPERATIVE HEALING

Clinically, healing after resective osseous surgery occurs in the following manner: both in radicular and interdental bone areas, loss of bone occurs during the initial healing stages. In interdental areas, which have cancellous bone, the subsequent repair stage results in total restitution without any loss of bone; whereas in radicular bone, particularly if thin and unsupported by cancellous bone, bone repair results in loss of marginal bone.[11]

Histologically, healing after resective osseous surgery occurs in the following manner **(Flowchart 50.1)**:[12]

### Points to Ponder

- Resective osseous surgery is the most predictable pocket reduction technique.
- *Spheroiding or parabolizing*: It is the removal of supporting bone to produce a positive gingival and osseous architecture.
- *Scribing*: It is the technique by which high-speed rotary instruments are used to outline the radicular bone, which is to be removed by hand instrumentation.

## REFERENCES

1. Carnevale G, Kaldahl WB. Osseous resective surgery. Periodontol 2000. 2000;22:59-87.
2. Sims TN, Ammons WF. Resective osseous surgery. In: Newman MG, Takei HH, Carranza FA (Eds). Clinical Periodontology, 9th edition. Philadelphia: WB Saunders; 2003. pp. 786-803.
3. Genco RJ, Rosenberg ES, Evian C. Periodontal Surgery. In: Genco RJ, Goldman HM, Cohen DW (Eds). Contemporary Periodontics. St. Louis: CV Mosby; 1990. pp. 554-84.
4. Grant DA, Stern IB, Listgarten MA. Periodontal osseous resection. In: Periodontics, 6th edition. St. Louis: CV Mosby; 1988. pp. 838-59.
5. Tibbetts LS, Ammons WF. Resective periodontal surgery. In: Rose LF, Mealey BL, Genco RJ, Cohen DW (Eds). Periodontics: Medicine, Surgery, and Implants, 2nd edition. St. Louis: Elsevier-Mosby; 2004. pp. 502-52.
6. Ochsenbein C. Current status of osseous surgery. J Periodontol. 1977;48(9):577-86.
7. Ochsenbein C. A primer for osseous surgery. Int J Periodontics Restorative Dent. 1986;6(1):8-47.
8. Ochsenbein C, Ross S. A reevaluation of osseous surgery. Dent Clin North Am. 1969;13(1):87-102.
9. Prichard J. Reflections on osseous therapy. Int J Periodontics Restorative Dent. 1986;6:5-6.
10. Selipsky H. Osseous surgery--how much need we compromise? Dent Clin North Am. 1976;20(1):79-106.
11. Wilderman MN, Pennel BM, King K, Barron JM. Histogenesis of repair following osseous surgery. J Periodontol. 1970;41(10):551-65.
12. Ruben MP, Smukler H, Schulman SM, Kon S, Bloom AA. Healing of periodontal surgical wounds. In: Goldman HM, Cohen DW (Eds). Periodontal Therapy, 5th edition. St. Louis: CV Mosby; 1980. pp. 640-754.

## VIVA VOCE

**Q1. What are the endpoints of osseous resective surgery?**
**Ans.** The endpoints of osseous resective surgery are minimal probing depths and a gingival tissue morphology that enhances good self-performed oral hygiene and periodontal health.

**Q2. What are the widow's peaks?**
**Ans.** Schluger, in 1949, described widow's peaks as the residual pieces of cortical bone leftover facial or lingual line angle from the horizontal grooving that forms a crater in a mesiodistal direction.
They will not be absorbed and will result in immediate postoperative tissue pocketing. Hand instrumentation with Ochsenbein chisel is used to eliminate the widow's peak.

**Q3. Which is the most predictable pocket reduction technique?**
**Ans.** Resective osseous surgery is the most predictable pocket reduction technique.

**Q4. What is ramping?**
**Ans.** If one-walled defects occur next to an edentulous space, the edentulous ridge is reduced to osseous defect, which is called ramping.

**Q5. What are the major contraindications for vertical grooving?**
**Ans.** Close root proximity or thin alveolar housing.

**Q6. Who is considered to be the "Father of Resective Osseous Surgery"?**
**Ans.** Schluger

**Q7. What is an ideal architecture?**
**Ans.** The bone level is more coronal in the interproximal areas, with a gradual slope around and away from the tooth.

**Q8. How much time does it take for the periodontal ligament to be restored after resective osseous surgery?**
**Ans.** Four weeks.

**Q9. What are the indications of ostectomy?**
**Ans.** Crown lengthening; exposure of sound dentin apical to caries or fractures and opening of interradicular spaces for the treatment of furcation involvement.

**Q10. Which instruments are used in resective osseous surgery?**
**Ans.** *Rongeurs*: Blumenthal rongeur and Friedman rongeur; *Files*: Sugarman file and Schluger file; *Chisels*: Rhodes back action chisel and Ochsenbein chisel and *Burs*: Carbide and diamond burs.

# Chapter 51: Regenerative Osseous Surgery

*Shalu Bathla*

## Chapter Outline

- Terminologies
- Regenerative Surgical Management
- Recent Advancements
- Postoperative Tissue Changes
- Factors Influencing Regenerative Procedures
- Postoperative Healing

## INTRODUCTION

New attachment with periodontal regeneration is the best result of periodontal therapy. It not only results in obliteration of the pocket but also leads to the marginal periodontium reconstruction. On the cellular level, periodontal regeneration is a complex process requiring coordinated proliferation, differentiation, and development of various cell types to form the periodontal attachment apparatus.

## TERMINOLOGIES

Following are the terminologies related to regenerative osseous surgery:[1]

- *Repair*: Healing of a wound by a tissue that does not fully restore the architecture or function of the part.
- *Regeneration*: It refers to the reproduction or reconstruction of a lost or injured tissue.
  *New attachment*: It is defined as the union of connective tissue or epithelium with a root surface that has been deprived of its original attachment apparatus. It can also be defined as the embedding of new periodontal ligament (PDL) fibers into new cementum and the gingival epithelium's attachment to a tooth surface previously denuded by the disease.
- *Reattachment*: It describes the reunion of epithelial and connective tissue with a root surface.
- *Periodontal regeneration*: It is defined as the restoration of lost periodontium or supporting tissues and includes the formation of new alveolar bone, new cementum, and new PDL.

## REGENERATIVE SURGICAL MANAGEMENT

*Incision*: Usually, sulcular incision is given in regenerative surgical procedures. The incision for regenerative surgery is given, such as to preserve the maximum amount of gingival tissue.

*Flap design*: The flap design of choice in regenerative surgery is the papilla preservation flap, which retains the entire papilla covering the defect. However, to use this flap, there must be adequate interdental space to allow the intact papilla to be reflected with the facial or lingual or palatal flap. When the interdental space is very narrow, making it impossible to perform a papilla preservation flap, a conventional flap with only sulcular incisions is made. Surgical flap design should be such that after sulcular incision, buccal and lingual full-thickness flaps are reflected, extending to at least 1 to 3 teeth mesially and distally to the treated tooth. Interdental tissues should be preserved in their entirety, so that flap margins cover the graft or membrane completely preventing their exposure during healing. The flap in regenerative surgery is not thinned out as for other surgical procedures.

Regenerative surgical techniques can be subdivided into two major areas:
1. Nongraft-associated new attachment.
2. Graft-associated new attachment.

### Nongraft-associated New Attachment

Meticulously treated three-wall defects (intrabony defects) and periodontal abscess do not require the use of grafts in periodontal reconstruction.

*Removal of junctional and pocket epithelium*: The presence of junctional and pocket epithelium interferes with the direct apposition of connective tissue and cementum. This restricts the height to which periodontal fibers can be inserted into the cementum and thus, creates limitations in successful therapy. Methods usually performed to remove junctional, and pocket epithelium are curettage, chemical agents, ultrasonic methods, and surgical techniques, such as excisional new attachment procedure (ENAP).

*Prevention of epithelial migration*: Mostly, the epithelium from the excised margin gets rapidly proliferated and interposed between the healing connective tissue and the cementum. Thus, the prevention of epithelial migration is required.

## Root Biomodification

*Biological concept*: It is reported that the acid treatment leads to demineralization of the root planed dentin and exposes the dentin matrix's collagen fibrils. This exposure of collagen fibrils probably facilitates the blood clot's adhesion to the root surface; it facilitates the migration of fibroblasts and that the exposed collagen fibrils of the dentin matrix may interdigitate with newly formed collagen fibrils in the adjacent healing tissues. This forms the biological concept behind root biomodification. Root surface conditioning was initially introduced due to the ability of acid to modify the root surface by "detoxifying." Thus, the rationale of root biomodification is to make contaminated root surfaces biologically acceptable.[2]

Various physical and chemical methods that have been tried to enhance new attachment by root conditioning are as follows:[3,4]

- *Physical methods*: They include root conditioning by lasers.
- *Chemical methods*: They include the use of various chemicals like citric acid, tetracycline, ethylenediamine tetra acetic acid (EDTA), fibronectin (tissucol), laminin, sodium deoxycholate, human plasma fraction Cohn IV and growth factors including platelet-derived growth factor (PDGF), basic fibroblast growth factor (bFGF), insulin-like growth factor (IGF) and transforming growth factor (TGF).

*Lasers*: They are capable of sterilizing the diseased root surface and thus, ultimately promoting cell reattachment. The laser's ability to sterilize, vaporize, and ablate appears to offer an effective means of removing or altering adsorbed endotoxin, calculus, plaque, and other root surface contaminants. Carbon dioxide, neodymium: yttrium-aluminium-garnet (Nd: YAG) and erbium: yttrium-aluminium-garnet (Er: YAG) are commercially available laser systems.

*Citric acid*: The potential of acid demineralization of root surface as an adjunct to new attachment procedures gained new popularity following Urist (1965) studies. He suggested that dentin following acid demineralization possessed inductive properties. Register and Burdick (1975) showed that citric acid (pH = 1) was the acid of choice with an optimal application time of 2–3 minutes. 61 g of citric acid per 100 mL of distilled water is added to achieve a pH of 1. It has been shown that citric acid demineralization enhances new attachment or reattachment and regeneration by one or more of the following mechanisms:

- Antibacterial effect
- Root detoxification
- Exposure of root collagen and opening of dentinal tubules
- Removal of smear laser
- Initial clot stabilization
- Demineralization prior to cementogenesis
- Enhanced fibroblasts growth and stability
- Attachment by direct linkage with or without cementogenesis
- Prevention of epithelial migration along with the denuded roots
- Accelerated healing and new cementum formation after detachment of the gingival tissues and demineralization of the root surface by means of citric acid

The use of citric acid has also been recommended in conjunction with coverage of denuded roots using free gingival grafts.

*Fibronectin*: This is a high-molecular-weight glycoprotein (molecular weight = 440,000) that is found in the extracellular tissue and is the main component that holds the clot together. It promotes cell adhesion to both collagen and scaled root surfaces and has a chemotactic effect on fibroblasts and mesenchymal cells.

The use of fibronectin as a supplement to demineralization is, therefore, strongly supported by the following:

- The initial stage after demineralization and prior to new attachment is fibrin formation and linkage.
- The coronal growth of cells from the PDL is usually responsible for new attachment, and fibronectin stimulates this growth.
- Fibronectin favors the growth and attachment of fibroblasts over epithelial cells to the root surface.
- It speeds the linkage process by being chemoattractive for fibroblasts and stabilizing the clot between the exposed root surface collagen and new fibers within the tissue.

*Laminin*: It is a glycoprotein of high-molecular-weight. It is capable of adhering to various substrates. It promotes gingival epithelial and fibroblast chemotaxis. It also promotes epithelial cell adhesion and growth to tetracycline and glycoprotein conditioned surfaces.

*Sodium-deoxycholate and human plasma fraction Cohn IV*: These agents can dissociate endotoxin into subunits and might thereby detoxify the diseased root surface. The human plasma fraction possibly contains fibronectin.

*Technique*: The recommended technique of root biomodification is as follows:
- *Step I*: Raise the mucoperiosteal flap.
- *Step II*: Thoroughly instrument the root surface removing calculus and underlying cementum.
- *Step III*: Apply cotton pellets soaked in a saturated solution of citric acid (pH 1) or EDTA or any other root biomodifier and leave on for 2–4 minutes.
- *Step IV*: Remove pellets and irrigate root surface profusely with water.
- *Step V*: Replace the flap and suture.

## Guided Tissue Regeneration

*Historical perspective*: A technique pioneered by Nyman et al.,[5] in 1982, was introduced in periodontal therapy, which was later named by Gottlow as "guided tissue regeneration (GTR)" in 1986 and slowly became acceptable for regenerative therapy.[6] Nyman et al., in 1982, carried out the first human study to test the hypothesis that new attachment may form on a previously periodontitis involved root surface, provided the cells originating from the transforming were enabled to repopulate the root surface first during healing.[5]

*Definition*: The 1996 World Workshop in periodontics defined GTR as procedures attempting to regenerate lost periodontal structures through differential tissue responses. Barriers are employed in the hope of excluding epithelium and gingival corium from the root surface in the belief that they interfere with regeneration.[7]

The rationale behind using GTR barrier membranes (**Fig. 51.1**) include the following:
- Exclusion of epithelium and gingival connective tissue.
- The barrier membrane maintains space between the defect and tooth.
- Stabilize the clot.

*Biological requirements*: Scantlebury introduced the historical development of barrier membranes. He proposed five general criteria required in the design of membranes intended for use in regenerative applications in the oral cavity. Membranes intended to be used for dentoalveolar regeneration should exhibit the following characteristics:[8]
- *Tissue integration*: Tissue can build up into the material without penetrating all the way through. Hence, tissue integration aims to avoid rapid epithelial down growth on the outer surface of the material or encapsulation of the material and provide stability to the overlying flap.
- *Cell occlusivity*: George Winter, an English researcher, had proposed the phenomenon of contact inhibition describing the ingrowth of specific porosities with connective tissue, which stopped or slowed the migration and pocketing of epithelial tissues. The material should act as a barrier to exclude undesirable cell types from entering the secluded space adjacent to the root surface. It is also considered as an advantage that the material should facilitate the transfer of nutrients and gases.
- *Clinical manageability*: Barrier should be provided in configurations that are easy to trim and place.
- *Space making*: Barrier material should be capable of creating and maintaining the space adjacent to the root surface, allowing the ingrowth of tissue from the PDL. Some materials may be so soft and flexible that they collapse into the defect, and others are too stiff that they may perforate the overlying tissues.
- *Biocompatibility*: The material should not elicit an immune response, sensitization, or chronic inflammation, which may interfere with healing and present a hazard to the patient.

*Indications for GTR procedures*:[9,10]
- Narrow 2- or 3-wall infrabony defects.
- Circumferential defects
- Class II furcation defects
- Recession defects

*Contraindications for GTR procedures*:[9,10]
- Any medical condition contraindicating surgery
- Infection at the defect site
- Poor oral hygiene
- Smoking (heavy)
- Tooth mobility more than 1 mm
- Defect less than 4 mm deep
- Width of attached gingiva at the defect site less than or equal to 1 mm
- The thickness of the attached gingiva at the defect site less than or equal to 0.5 mm
- Furcation with short root trunks
- Generalized horizontal bone loss
- Advanced lesions with little remaining support
- Multiple defects

*Materials used for GTR*:[10,11]
- *First-generation material*: Nonresorbable membranes include: Expanded polytetrafluoroethylene (ePTFE),

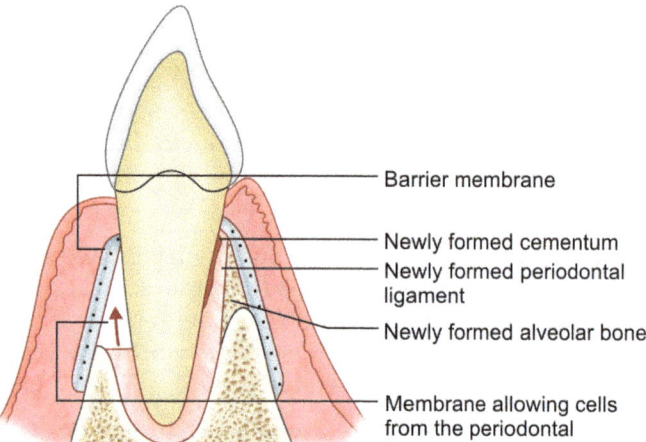

**Fig. 51.1:** Schematic representation of the barrier membrane, which prevents epithelium and gingival connective tissue.

GORE-TEX® membrane, dense polytetrafluoroethylene (dPTFE), nucleopore, millipore filters, ethyl cellulose, and semipermeable silicone barrier. ePTFE is one of the most inert materials known which has an extremely long carbon chain protected by a dense sheath of fluorine atoms. As the body cannot react with it chemically, tissue "accepts" it, while exhibiting a healthy tissue reaction.
- *Second-generation material*: Resorbable membranes:
  - Collagen: BioMend, BioMend-extend, periogen, paroguide, biostite, biogide, tissue guide and biobar.
  - Polylactide and polyglycolide-guidor, vicryl **(Fig. 51.2)**, atrisorb, resolute, epiguide, and biofix.
  - Others: Periosteum, connective tissue graft, alloderm, emdogain, surgicel, gelform, gengiflex, capset, hapset, and cargile membrane.
- *Third-generation material*: Resorbable bioactive barrier membranes with added growth factors: Chorion, amnion membrane **(Fig. 51.3)**.

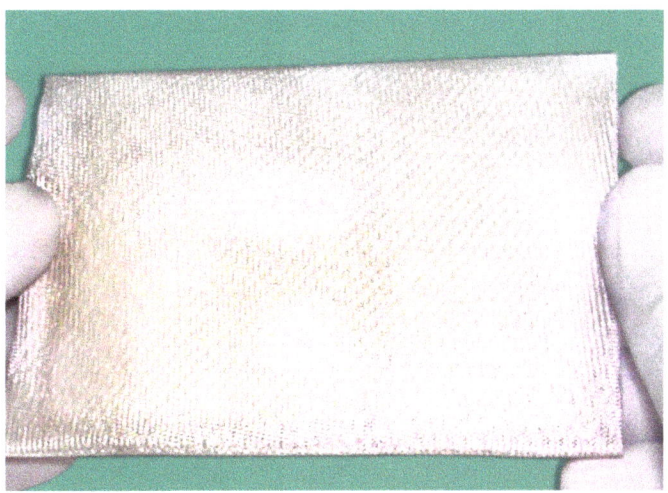

**Fig. 51.2:** Photograph showing vicryl knitted mesh: Resorbable membrane.

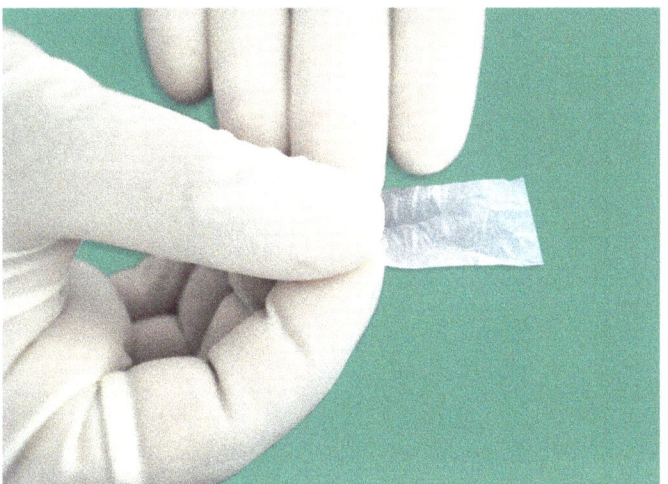

**Fig. 51.3:** Photograph showing amnion membrane.

*Bioresorbable GTR barrier materials*:
- *Guidor*: It is a hydrophobic barrier material made from polylactic acid (PLA) combined with a citric acid ester softening agent. It is a bilayer consisting of an external layer having large rectangular perforations (400–500/$cm^2$) and an internal layer having smaller circular perforations (4,000–5,000/$cm^2$).
- *Vicryl*: It is made from a copolymer of glycolide and lactide. It is available in two forms:
  1. *Knitted mesh*: These have large pore size with better handling property.
  2. *Woven mesh*: These have smaller pore sizes but tend to fray.

  These membranes degrade to produce polylactide and polyglycolide, that are converted to lactic acid and pyruvate, respectively, and metabolized by the enzymes of the Krebs cycle and are eliminated as carbon dioxide and water.
- *Atrisorb*: It is a polymer of lactic acid and poly (D, L-lactic acid), dissolved in N-methyl-2-pyrrolidone. It is prepared as a solution that coagulates or sets to a firm consistency on contact with water or other aqueous solution; this principle is used in forming a barrier that is partially coagulated to a semirigid state in a chairside mixing kit, which can be trimmed to the dimensions of the defect. Kit contains sufficient material for the fabrication of up to 10 membranes. However, excess material cannot be stored for future use and may result in wastage of material.
- *Resolute*: It is a copolymer of polyglycolic acid and PLA, which is supplied with a bioresorbable suture.
- *Epiguide*: It is a hydrophilic membrane formed from PLA (D, L-form). It contains a flexible open cell structure and internal void spaces.
- *Collagen membrane*: Its antigenicity and rate of degradation can be controlled by varying its cross-linkage. They are degraded by collagenases and subsequently by gelatinases and peptidases. The various advantages associated with collagen membranes are: Hemostasis, chemotaxis for PDL fibroblasts and gingival fibroblasts, weak immunogenicity, easy manipulation and ability to augment tissue thickness.[12]

*Bio-Gide*: The collagen membrane is prepared from a pig, which involves several technological processing steps. An alkaline treatment is carried out for several hours to eliminate any viral or bacterial contamination of the material. The structural quality of the membrane is controlled by segment analysis. Collagen fibers are obtained without any other organic residues. The collagen membrane should be devoid of antigenicity. For this, terminal peptides or telopeptides are split off, and fat and protein residues are also removed by specific purification process for the same reason of reducing antigenicity. The collagen membranes are cross-linked to extend absorption time and to reduce antigenicity. Cross-linking agents used in the collagen barrier membrane are physical agents (gamma and ultraviolet radiation) and chemical agents (formaldehyde and diphenylphosphoryl azide). The resorption of collagen membranes starts with the action of collagenase, which splits the molecule at specific sites. The resultant fragments are denatured at 37°C to gelatin, and then gelatinases and other proteinases degrade gelatin to oligopeptides and amino acids.

*Advantages of resorbable GTR barrier materials*:
- Elimination of second surgery for barrier removal
- Reduce operatory time
- Increase patient acceptance
- Reduce the risk of loss of regenerated attachment owing to reentry surgery
- More tissue friendly

*Disadvantages of resorbable GTR barrier materials*:
- Instability of barrier against the root, as they lack rigidity
- High cost
- The biodegradation rate cannot be controlled
- In case of infection or strong tissue response, if there is a need to remove the membrane, the disintegration of the material in its various stages, makes it impossible

*Surgical technique*
Following are the steps[13-15] **(Figs. 51.4A to D)**:
- *Step I—incision*: Intrasulcular incision is made to preserve as much as attached gingiva as possible, including the adjacent interdental papilla. Mucoperiosteal or full-thickness flap is raised by making vertical incisions involving a minimum of two teeth anteriorly and one tooth distally to the tooth being treated.
- *Step II—defect preparation and membrane placement*: It consists of debridement of the osseous defect and thorough planing of the roots. An appropriate membrane is selected among the several membranes available. With the help of sharp scissors, the membrane should be trimmed to the approximate size of the area being treated. The extension of the apical border of the material should be 3–4 mm apical to the margin of the defect and laterally 2–3 mm beyond the defect. The occlusal border of the membrane should be at 2 mm apical to the cementoenamel junction **(Fig. 51.5)**.

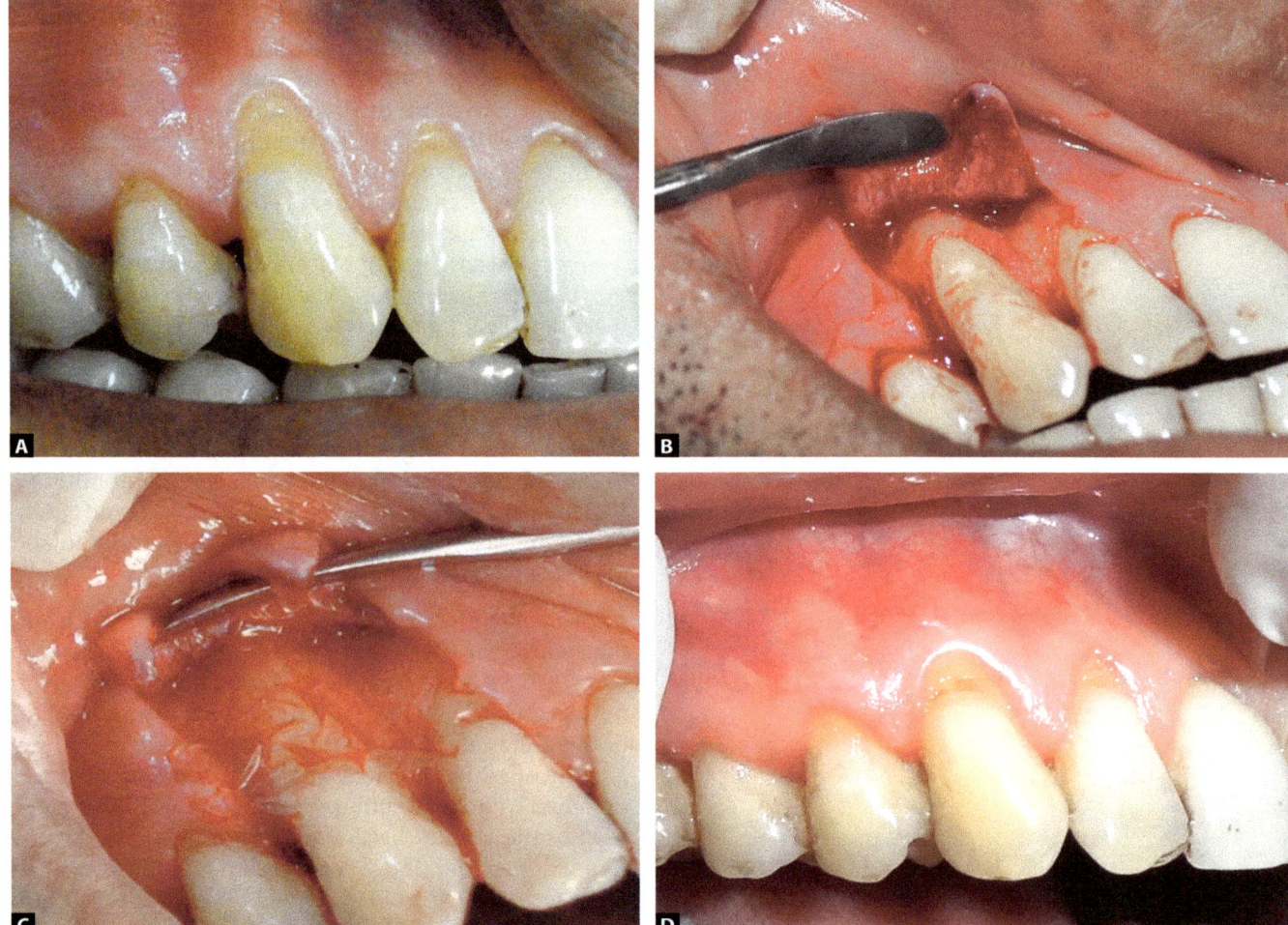

**Figs. 51.4A to D:** Clinical picture showing (A) Preoperative site where the membrane is to be placed; (B) Flap reflected; (C) Amnion membrane placed; (D) Postoperative site.

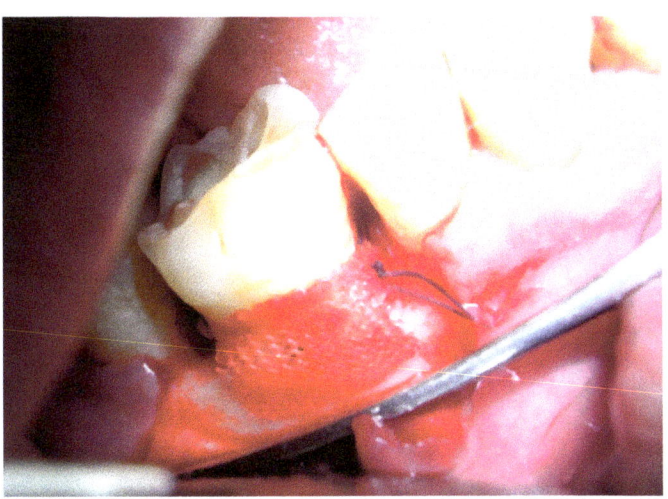

**Fig. 51.5:** Clinical picture showing the placement of resorbable guided-tissue regeneration membrane (vicryl membrane).

- *Step III—suturing*: With the help of sling suture, the membrane should be tightly sutured around the tooth if necessary. The flap should be sutured back in its original position or slightly coronal to it with the help of independent sutures interdentally and in the vertical incisions. The flap should cover the membrane entirely. The use of periodontal dressing is optional, and antibiotic therapy is administered for 1 week.
- *Step IV—removal of the membrane*: If the nonresorbable membrane is used, then remove it after 4–6 weeks of placement. The material is removed by making a sharp access incision for dissection of the material from the flap. The flap is then dissected from the membrane.
  Sutures holding the membrane are cut, and the membrane is removed.

## Graft-associated New Attachment

### Bone Graft Materials

There are numerous therapeutic grafting modalities for reconstructing periodontal osseous defects.[16-18]

Classification of bone graft materials are as follows:
- *According to the type of graft (Flowchart 51.1)*:
  - Autografts or autogenous bone grafts
  - Isografts
  - Allografts or allogenic grafts
  - Xenografts or xenogenic grafts
  - Alloplasts or inert biologic fillers
  - Composite grafts
- *According to their mode of action*:
  - Osteogenetic or osteoproliferative means that new bone is formed by bone-forming cells contained in the graft.
  - Osteoinductive means that bone formation is induced in the surrounding soft tissues immediately adjacent to the graft.
  - Osteoconductive means that the grafted material does not contribute to new bone formation but serves as a scaffold for bone formation originating from adjacent host bone.

### Autografts or Autogenous Bone Grafts

Grafts are transferred from one position to another within the same individual. Autogenous bone is certainly the best since it has both osteogenetic and osteoinductive potencies. Its availability is nevertheless limited, and its use generally results in additional inconvenience for the patient. They are resorbed and replaced by few viable bones. Autogenous bone grafts can be harvested from intraoral or extraoral sites and can be cortical bone or cancellous bone.

**Flowchart 51.1:** Classification of bone grafts.

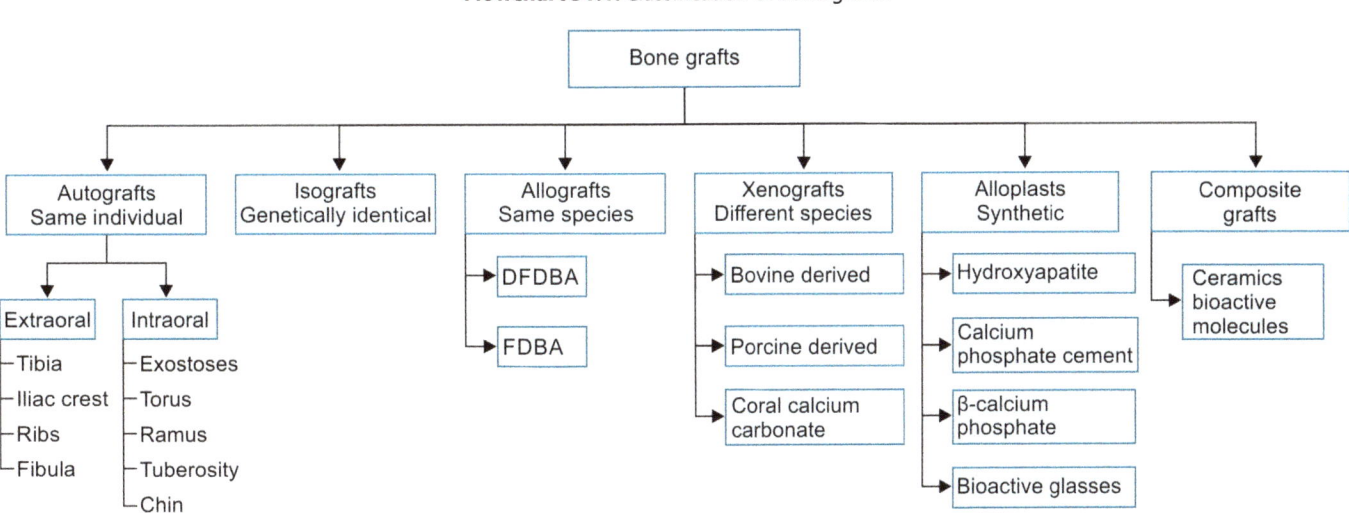

(DFDBA: demineralized freeze-dried bone allograft; FDBA: freeze-dried bone allograft)

**Section 7:** Treatment: Surgical Therapy

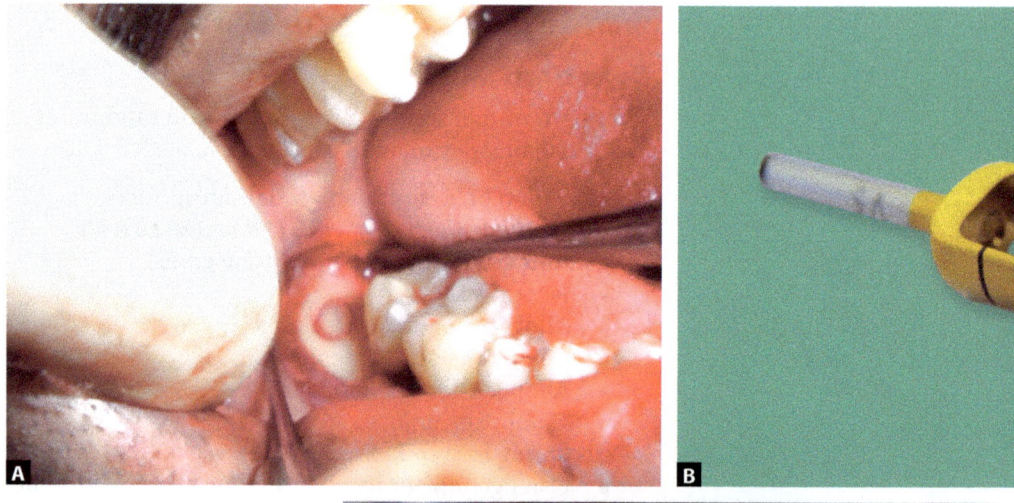

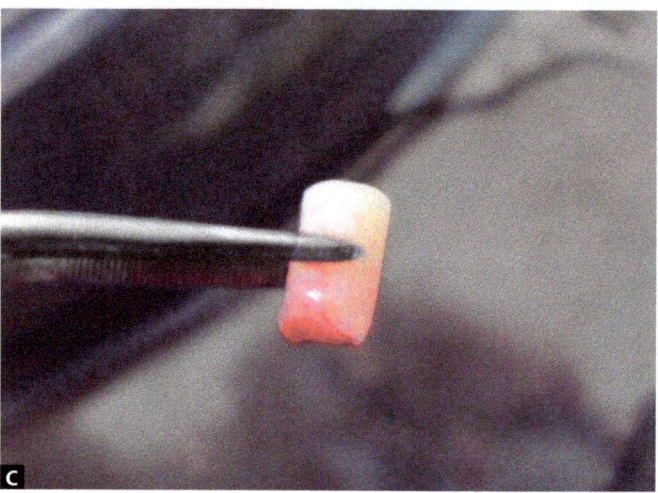

**Figs. 51.6A to C:** Clinical picture and photographs showing autogenous bone graft from the mandibular retromolar area by trephine.
(*Courtesy:* Dr Vikrender Yadav)

The various sites for procuring autogenous bone grafts are as follows:
- *Intraoral sites*: Healing extraction wounds, edentulous ridges, exostosis, the lingual ridge on the mandible, bone distal to the terminal tooth, the lingual surface of the mandible at least 5 mm from the roots, maxillary tuberosity and mandibular retromolar area **(Figs. 51.6A to C)**.
- *Extraoral sites*: Iliac autografts-posterior iliac crest. Problems associated with iliac autografts are postoperative infection, exfoliation, sequestration, varying rates of healing, root resorption, and rapid recurrence of the defect. Root resorption is very common with fresh iliac. According to Dragoo and Sullivan, fresh iliac material was so highly inductive that both clasts, as well as blast activity, were stimulated more than in other graft materials or in the same material used after storage. It has been observed clinically that frequent curettage of the resorbed area, particularly in the crestal areas of newly forming bone, often reverses the process. Due to the morbidity associated with donor site and root resorption, the iliac crest marrow grafts are not used now in regenerative periodontal therapy.

### Osseous Coagulum

It is a mixture of bone dust obtained by grounding cortical bone and blood. Round carbide bur revolving at 25,000–30,000 rpm is used within the surgical site to reduce donor bone to small particles, which is then coated with the patient's blood to make coagulum.

*Advantages:*
- Relatively rapid technique.
- Complements osseous resective procedures that may be required at the surgical site.
- Particle size provides additional surface area for the interaction between cellular and vascular elements.

*Disadvantages:*
- It cannot be used in larger defects because of the inability to procure adequate material.
- Poor surgical visibility.
- Relatively low predictability.

- Inability to use aspiration during accumulation of the coagulum.
- The fluidity of the material makes it difficult to transfer the coagulum to the defect.

### Bone Swaging

The piece of bone is incompletely detached from its base by a chisel and swung into a neighboring bone defect with some of its blood supply maintained. It is the technique that requires the existence of an edentulous area adjacent to the defect. It represents a contiguous or pedicle bony autograft utilizing the principle of greenstick fracture of long bones.

### Bone Blend

It involves removing bone (cortical, cancellous, or both) from an accessible intraoral donor site by chisel or rongeur forceps, placing it in a sterile plastic amalgam capsule with a pestle and then triturating.

## Isografts

It is an autograft taken from monozygous twins or related persons. It is also called as "syngenous grafts."

## Allografts or Allogenic Grafts

Allografts are the grafts transferred between genetically dissimilar members of the same species. They can be demineralized freeze-dried bone allograft (DFDBA) or freeze-dried bone allograft (FDBA) **(Table 51.1)**.

Commercial bone allografts are available from tissue banks. They are usually obtained from cortical bone within 12 hours of the death of the donor. They are defatted, cut in pieces, washed in absolute alcohol, and deep-frozen for further use. The material may then be demineralized and subsequently ground and sieved to a particle size 250–750 µm, freeze-dried, and vacuum-sealed in glass vials. The various methods to suppress the antigenic potential of allograft and xenograft are as follows:
- *Radiation treatment*: 6 mega rads of high intensity of gamma radiation is adequate.
- *Freezing*: Deep frozen –197°C liquid nitrogen freezer for a period of at least 4 weeks.
- *Chemical treatment*: Through keeping in merthiolate solution.

Demineralization in cold, diluted hydrochloric acid exposes the bone matrix components, closely associated with collagen fibrils that have been termed "bone morphogenetic protein" (BMP).

Bone allografts do not require an additional surgical site for the removal of donor material from the same patient, but can provoke an immune response in the recipient patient.[16]

## Xenografts or Xenogenic Grafts

They are commonly obtained from a donor of another species. They are usually referred to as "anorganic bone." Proprietary processes remove all cells and proteinaceous material and result in the formation of inert and absorbable bone scaffolding. It is considered that on this scaffolding revascularization, osteoblast migration and woven bone formation occur. Resorption of xenografts has been reported to occur very slowly.

Sclera as nonbone graft material. There are some structural similarities of the sclera to the PDL. It is derived from mesoderm and consists of obliquely arranged collagen fibers of 640–700 Å axial periodicity. It is easily sterilized and show low levels of antigenicity due to minimal cellularity and poor vascularity. But, it has tissue memory and tends to return to its original curvature; this limits its application to wide and shallow defects.

## Alloplasts or Inert Biologic Fillers

Synthetic or inorganic implant materials, which are used as substitutes for a bone graft, function primarily as defect fillers.

Alloplasts bone substitutes should possess the following properties:[19]
- Biocompatibility
- Minimal fibrotic reaction
- The tendency to undergo remodeling and support the formation of new bone
- Similar strength is comparable to cortical or cancellous bone
- Similar modulus of elasticity compared to the bone in order to avoid fatigue fracture under cyclic loading.[19]

These are namely polymers, tricalcium phosphate (TCP), hydroxyapatite (HA), and bioactive glasses

Biocompatible composite polymer (Bioplant HTR) consists of polymethyl methacrylate and poly hydroxyethyl methacrylate beads coated by calcium hydroxide. This calcium hydroxide surface forms a calcium carbonate apatite when introduced into the body.

*Tricalcium phosphate*: It has a calcium-to-phosphate ratio of 1.5 and are β-whitlockite crystals. It is partially bioresorbable.

*Hydroxyapatite*: It has a calcium-to-phosphate ratio of 1.67, similar to that found in bone material. It is generally non-bioresorbable.

**TABLE 51.1:** Comparison between freeze-dried bone allograft (FDBA) and demineralized freeze-dried bone allograft (DFDBA).

| FDBA | DFDBA |
|---|---|
| Not demineralized | Demineralized |
| More radiopaque | More radiolucent |
| Breakdown by way of foreign body reaction | Rapid resorption |
| Primary indication: Bone augmentation associated with implant treatment | Primary indication: Periodontal disease associated with natural tooth |
| Osteoconductive | Osteoinductive |
| No bone morphogenetic protein (BMP) expression | More BMP |

*Bioactive glass-ceramics*: They are made of calcium oxide (CaO), sodium oxide ($Na_2O$), silicon dioxide ($SiO_2$) and phosphorus pentoxide ($P_2O_5$) in the same proportions as in bone and teeth and are referred to as 45S5 bioactive glass. This material was initially introduced as an amorphous material (BioGlass). The material was subsequently produced in a particulate form with a 90-710 μm diameter (PerioGlas) and a 300-350 μm diameter (BioGran). Bioactive glass facilitates the process of bone formation. It brings ionic dissolution of the ceramic particles in such a way that a silica gel layer forms over the particles on contact with body fluid. On this silica gel layer, a calcium phosphate layer forms, which rapidly get transformed into a hydroxycarbonate apatite layer. This apatite layer is found to be similar to bone mineral and provides the surface for osteoblast cell attachment and bone deposition. The continuous ionic exchange results in the dissolution of the ceramic particles such that after 1-3 years, the particles have been shown to be replaced by bone.

*Calcium carbonates*: They are processed natural coral skeletons from porites coral, which can serve as resorbable bone graft substitutes.

### Bone Grafting Technique[20,21]

- *Step I—incision*: Sulcular incision is made on facial and lingual aspects with the conservation of interproximal space and preservation of papilla.
- *Step II—flap design*: In regenerative techniques, tissue flap preservation is important to ensure coverage and containment of the graft postsurgically. While flap preservation, care should be taken to prevent flap perforation or the papilla's loss from the granulomatous tissue of the lesion that usually attaches to the inner aspect of the flap. Moreover, excessive thinning of the flap can hamper blood supply and flap survival.
- *Step III—root debridement*: Meticulously remove all hard and soft accretions on the root surface. Root biomodification is done by using a saturated solution of citric acid (pH 1).

> **Clinical Tip**
> The osseous defects should not be overfilled. Any donor bone and attendant cellular elements can become necrotic above the area where they are unprotected by the fibrin seal of the clot, especially when get exposed to the environment of the oral cavity. The osteoclastic response marshaled to resorb the exposed necrotic bone may well endanger cemental and dentinal surfaces to unwanted resorption and also delays repair.

- *Step IV—defect debridement*: Debride the defect of all soft tissue using hand, ultrasonic and rotating instruments.
- *Step V—preparation of graft material*: Bone grafts should be wetted with the patient's own blood from the surgical site, rather than sterile water or saline.

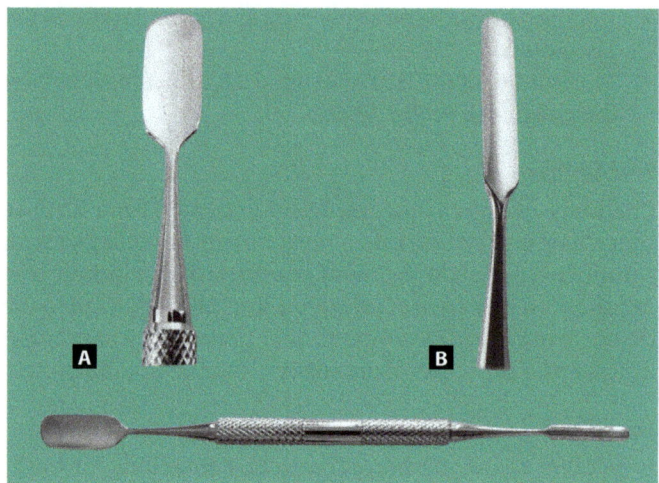

**Figs. 51.7A and B:** Photograph showing bone scoop which is used to place a bone graft into the osseous defect.

- *Step VI—promotion of bleeding surface*: In the case of a more chronic bone lesion, i.e., lined with an intact cortical plate, a one-quarter or one-half round bur is used to perforate the bone. This helps to form a bleeding environment. The concept behind cortical or intramarrow penetration is that bone marrow, like the PDL, functions as a repository for the pluripotent progenitor cells essential for regeneration. Intramarrow penetration is required to facilitate rapid revascularization and incorporation of the graft.
- *Step VII—presuturing*: Loose sutures are placed prior to filling the defect to reduce the displacement of bone graft during the suturing process.
- *Step VIII—placement of the graft into the osseous defect*: A bone graft is transferred with the help of bone graft scoop (**Figs. 51.7A and B**). The graft is contoured, and the graft material is packed firmly but not too tight, as some space is necessary for the development of granulation tissue. Defects should be filled with grafts only to the level of defect wall and not overfilled.
- *Step IX—final suturing*: The flaps are closed using a monofilament suture with an interrupted or vertical mattress suture technique.
- *Step X—postoperative instructions*: They are given thereafter.

## RECENT ADVANCEMENTS

### Growth Factors

Growth factors are polypeptide molecules released by cells in the inflamed area, which regulate events in wound healing. These factors primarily secreted by macrophages, endothelial cells, fibroblasts, and platelets include PDGF, IGF, bFGF, and transforming growth factor-alpha (TGF-α). These factors could be used to control events during periodontal wound healing (e.g., promoting the proliferation of fibroblasts from the PDL and favoring bone formation). A combination of PDGF and IGF-1 would be effective in promoting the growth of all the components of the periodontium.[22]

### Bone Morphogenetic Protein

The history of the identification and purification of BMPs began in 1965 when Marshall Urist demonstrated that the cellular events associated with embryonic bone development could be reproduced in heterotrophic sites by implants of demineralized bone segments. In the late 1960s and early 1970s, it was recognized that dentin also contained bone morphogenetic activity. BMPs form a subgroup of a larger family of structurally related proteins known as the TGF-β superfamily.[23]

*Types*: At least 15 BMPs have been identified up-to-date. Most of them are identified by their capacity to induce bone in vivo or extra-skeletal sites in mammals.
- *BMP-1*: Protease; not osteoinductive.
- *BMP-2*: Osteoinductive; located in bone, spleen, liver, brain, and kidney.
- *BMP-3*: Osteogenin osteoinductive; located in the lung, kidney, and brain.
- *BMP-4*: Osteoinductive; located in the apical ectodermal ridge, meninges, lung, kidney, and liver.
- *BMP-5*: Osteoinductive; located in the lung, kidney, and liver.
- *BMP-6*: Not osteoinductive; found in lung, brain, kidney, uterus, muscle, and skin.
- *BMP-7*: Osteoinductive; located in adrenal glands, placental, spleen, and skeletal muscle.
- *BMP-8*: Osteoinductive.
- *BMP-9*: Osteoinductive; stimulates hepatocyte proliferation; hepatocyte growth and function.
- *BMP-12 and BMP-13*: Inhibition of terminal differentiation of myeloblasts.

### Tissucol

A fibrin-fibronectin sealing system (FFSS) has been commercially available (Tissucol-Tisseel) in Europe since 1975. It is a human plasma cryoprecipitate, which consists of highly concentrated fibrinogen, fibronectin, factor XIII, PDGF, antiplasmins, and plasminogen. Aprotinin (bovine antiplasmin), thrombin and calcium chloride ($CaCl_2$) are added at the moment of use.[24]

Highly concentrated fibrinogen, fibronectin, PDGF plays a significant role in the coagulation process and wound healing. Activated thrombin induces the clotting of cryoprecipitate. Aprotinin in different concentrations can modulate the stability of artificial clot. Fibrinogen is a high-molecular-weight 340 kDa protein, which is transformed into fibrin by thrombin to form the bulk of the blood clot, thereby providing hemostasis. It is arranged to form a network, lining collagen and glycosaminoglycans in such a way that tissue adhesion occurs. Fibronectin is found in plasma on the cell surface, in the extracellular matrix, and in the epithelium's basement membrane. It promotes cell-to-cell adhesion and cell mobility. Thus, it promotes migration, adhesion, attachment, and synthetic activity of fibroblasts. Factor XIII is a transglutaminase, an enzyme that mediates the clot's links and the collagen and glycosaminoglycans of the connective tissue. Plasminogen is a glycoprotein (90 kDa) that is transformed into plasmin under the effect of active thrombin. The protease activity of plasmin causes the lysis of fibrin. The plasminogen-to-fibrinogen ratio in tissucol is reduced up to 30 times less than in human plasma. This reduced proportion is more favorable to clot stability. Antiplasmin is macroglobulin that modulates the rate of coagulum lysis inhibiting plasmin activity. Thrombin is a serino protease (40 kDa) that activates fibrinogen and factor XIII in the presence of $Ca^{+2}$, which is provided by $CaCl_2$ in Tissucol. It stimulates the growth of fibroblasts and the synthesis of fibronectin and collagen. Aprotinin is a polypeptide extracted from bovine lungs, and it inhibits plasmin activity. PDGF is a major human serum polypeptide growth factor. It is stored in granules of circulating platelets and is released into serum during blood clotting. It is a potent mitogen and chemoattractant for fibroblasts. Thus, there are several promising research areas for the use of biologic mediators, such as in GTR procedures, coronally positioned flaps for furcations, ridge augmentation, and implant surgery.

### Emdogain

It is a resorbable, implantable material that consists of enamel matrix proteins extracted from developing embryonic enamel of porcine origin supplied in sterile, lyophilized form.

Emdogain contains a protein preparation that mimics the matrix proteins that induce cementogenesis. During root development, the Hertwig's epithelial sheath deposits enamel matrix proteins on the newly formed root dentin surface. These proteins stimulate the differentiation of surrounding mesenchymal cells into cementoblasts, which form acellular cementum. Once a new cementum layer is formed, collagen fibers form in the adjacent PDL, attaching into the new cementum.

The major constituents are amelogenins, which are highly hydrophobic proteins that aggregate and serve as a nidus for crystallization. Other proteins identified include: Ameloblastin and enamelin. This protein preparation uses PGA as a carrier. The enamel matrix derivative (EMD)-containing PGA remains highly viscous when stored in the cold or at room temperature. Once it is applied to the tissue at a neutral pH and at body temperature, the PGA carrier decreases in viscosity, and the EMD preparation precipitates. EMD gets absorbed into the HA and collagen fibers of the root surface. Here, EMD stimulates cementum formation followed by periodontal regeneration.[25,26]

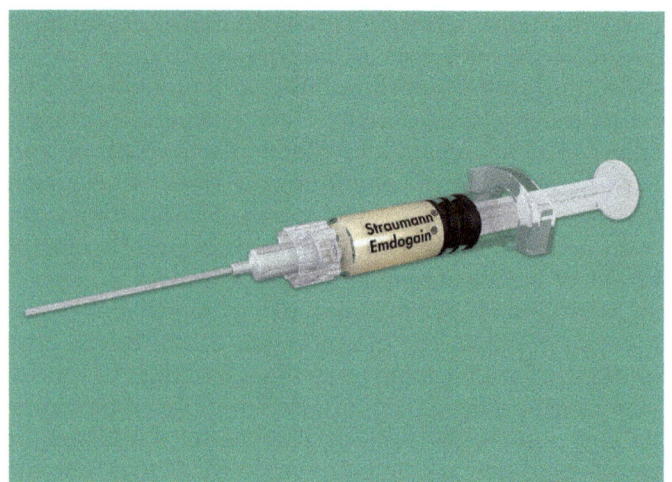

**Fig. 51.8:** Photograph showing emdogain gel: (© Institut Straumann, Basel, Switzerland; Reproduced with permission from Straumann Holding AG).

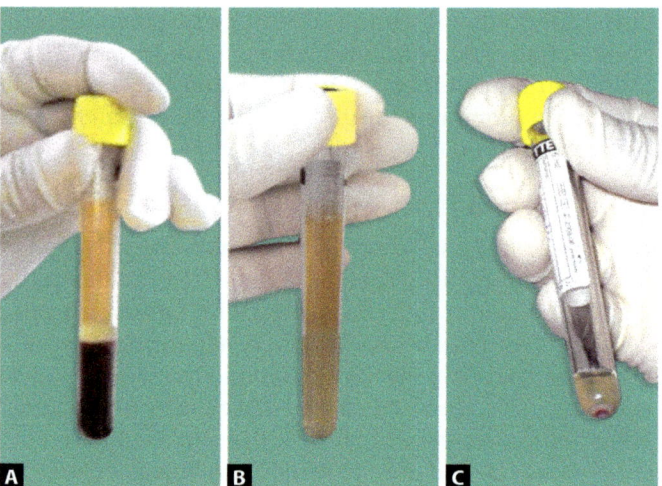

**Figs. 51.9A to C:** Photograph showing (A) After the first spin, platelet-poor plasma (PPP), platelet-rich plasma (PRP) and RBC base; (B) PPP and PRP were separated from RBC base and transferred into another empty vacutainer tube; (C) After the second spin, PRP settled at the bottom.

(*Courtesy*: Dr Deepak Kochar)

*Emdogain has two presentation forms*: One is in liquid and powder form, in two separate bottles containing the vehicle and the protein powder, and the other is in the form of a gel in a syringe **(Fig. 51.8)**. The material is stored at 2–8°C in the refrigerator. It should be used within 2 hours from opening because it usually gelifies and hardens. Emdogain is used in various osseous and recession defects.

## Platelet Concentrate

Generations of platelet concentrate:[27]
- *First-generation platelet concentrate*: Platelet-rich plasma (PRP).
- *Second-generation platelet concentrate*: Platelet-rich fibrin (PRF).
- *Third-generation platelet concentrate*: Titanium-prepared PRF (T-PRF).

### Platelet-rich Plasma

It is an autologous thrombocyte concentrate. It is composed of different components with hemostatic effects and factors stimulating the healing process. It stimulates the neoformation of blood vessels, which accelerate the process of regeneration. It has an osteostimulant effect and is not osteoinductive. Hence, while using synthetic materials, it is better to add a small amount of autologous bone to accelerate bone maturation and bone quality. PRP is derived from direct centrifugation from the patient's blood and required to be applied as early as possible.

*Preparation* **(Figs. 51.9A to C)**: Procedure requires one-unit of whole blood, i.e., approximately 450 mL collected into a standard collection bag containing a citrate-phosphate-dextrose anticoagulant. At first, the blood is centrifuged at 5,600 rpm in order to separate the platelet-poor plasma (PPP) from the erythrocytes, platelets, and leukocytes. The centrifuge speed then reduced to 2,400 rpm for further separation of the platelets and leukocytes from the red blood cell (RBC) pack. Separation of RBC pack yields 30 mL of plasma containing the concentrated platelets in the range of 500,000 to 1 million. A mixture of 10,000 units of bovine thrombin in powder form and 10 mL of 10% $CaCl_2$ is prepared. Next, 7 mL of PRP and 2 mL of air are drawn into a 10 mL syringe. 1 mL of the thrombin/$CaCl_2$ mixture is aspirated into the syringe and gently rocked to allow the air bubble to mix the components. Within 5–30 seconds, gel formation occurs once the citrate gets neutralized, and the thrombin activates polymerization of the fibrin and degranulation of the platelets.

*Components*: Platelet count in PRP often ranges from 500,000 to 1 million. Hence, PRP acts as a factor that accelerates and enhances the body's natural wound healing mechanisms.
- Growth factors (PDGFs)
- White blood cell, phagocytic cells
- Native fibrinogen concentration
- Vasoactive and chemotactic agents
- A high concentration of platelets

*Disadvantages*:
- Long preparation time
- Risk of immunogenicity

### Platelet-rich Fibrin

It was first described by Choukroun et al.,[28] in France in 2001. It is the second generation of platelet concentrate. The PRF clot forms a strong natural fibrin matrix, which

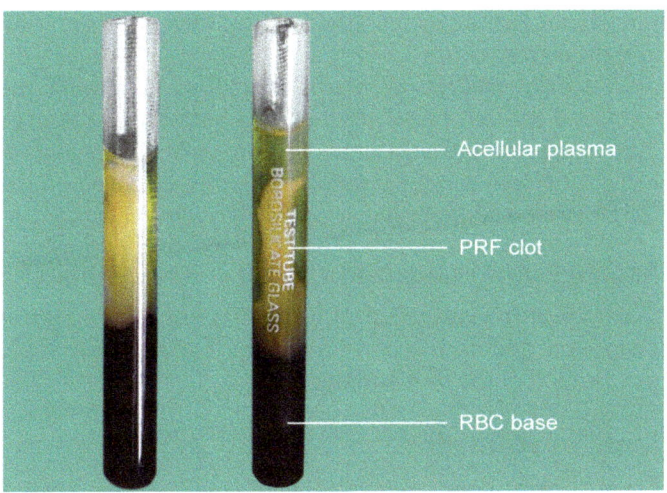

**Fig. 51.10:** Photograph showing platelet-rich fibrin (PRF) clot in between acellular plasma and red blood cells (RBCs).

concentrates almost all the platelets and growth factors of the blood harvest. PRF releases high amounts of growth factors [such as TGF-β1, PDGF-AB, vascular endothelial growth factor (VEGF), and matrix glycoproteins (such as thrombospondin-1)] during at least seven days in vitro. It upregulates phosphorylated extracellular signal-regulated protein kinase expression and suppresses osteoclastogenesis by promoting the secretion of osteoprotegerin.[29,30]

*Preparation*: There is a simple, natural, and inexpensive technique for its production. Blood is collected without anticoagulant and immediately centrifuged (3,000 rpm for 10 minutes). Coagulation starts during the centrifugation with the quick formation of three parts in the tube: (1) RBC base at the bottom of the tube, (2) acellular plasma forms as a supernatant PPP, and (3) PRF clot formation in between them **(Fig. 51.10)**.

Platelet-rich fibrin was easily separated from the red corpuscles base using sterile tweezers and scissors just after the removal of poor platelet plasma.

The PRF clot can be transformed into a membrane by compression between two sterile gauzes.

Platelet-rich fibrin is a consistent fibrin biomaterial, which failed to improve fibrin glue from the PRP family.

Each PRF membrane concentrates most platelets and more than half of the leukocytes from a 9-mL blood harvest.

*Advantages:*
Platelet-rich fibrin is the most preferred among platelet concentrates in fibrin technology because of the following reasons:
- *The slow release of growth factors*: There is functional, intact platelet in the fibrin matrix and a slow release of growth factors.
- *Quickly prepared*: It is quickly prepared as no second spin is required.
- *Simplified and cost-effective processing*: No chemical additives like anticoagulant, bovine thrombin, $CaCl_2$ required during its preparation. Conversion of fibrinogen to fibrin occurs slowly due to small quantities of physiologically available thrombin available in the blood sample itself.
- *Easily prepared*: It is easily prepared, and approximately 10 mL of the blood is required.
- Platelet-rich fibrin has a supportive effect on the immune system.
- Platelet-rich fibrin helps in hemostasis.

*Disadvantages*:
- *Quick handling of blood is needed, immediately after collection*: For better outcome, the technique demands speedy blood collection and immediate transfer to the centrifuge. The blood sample starts to coagulate quickly once it comes in contact with the tube glass due to lack of anticoagulant.
It will take just a few minutes of centrifugation to concentrate fibrinogen in the middle and upper part of the tube. Hence, quick handling is the best way to derive a clinically usable PRF.
- *Storage*: Another disadvantage of PRF is its storage after preparation. After preparation, PRF should be used immediately as it will get shrink, and resulting dehydration may alter the structural integrity of PRF. Dehydration reduces growth factor content in PRF and adversely affect the leukocyte viability by altering its biologic properties.
- *The amount available is low*: The quantity of PRF obtained is low, and only a limited volume can be used because it is obtained from an autologous blood sample.

*Clinical application*: PRF can be used to promote wound healing and hemostasis; thus, can be used for the following:
- Treatment of periodontal intrabony defects
- Treatment of furcation defects
- Sinus-lift procedures

### Titanium-prepared, Platelet-rich Fibrin (T-PRF)

The hypothesis behind the T-PRF method is that titanium may be more effective in activating platelets than the silica activators used with glass tubes in Choukroun's leukocyte-platelet-rich fibrin (L-PRF) method.

Health hazards probably occur while preparing L-PRF due to the use of glass-evacuated blood collection tubes with silica activators. During treatment, the chances of reaching silica particles in the patient are high. Noncorrosive properties of titanium provide it excellent biocompatibility. The material passivates itself in vivo by forming an adhesive oxide layer. T-PRF is prepared like the L-PRF method but with tubes made up of biocompatible material, titanium.

## POSTOPERATIVE TISSUE CHANGES

Various methods used to quantify tissue changes after regenerative periodontal surgery are as follows:[31-33]

## Histological Evaluation of Biopsy Material

Human histology is the most reliable outcome variable useful for evaluating periodontal regeneration. However, it is suitable only in isolated case studies due to associated morbidity. This technique is used in studies designed to prove the efficacy of a drug, device, or technique capable of regenerating the lost periodontium, including bone, cementum, and PDL. If this variable is unavailable, other "surrogate" variables must be used.

## Clinical Evaluation of Hard Tissue Changes (Bone Formation)

New bone formation is considered the primary alternative of all the surrogate variables available in regenerative clinical trials. It is suitable to directly measure the formation of one of the three components required for successful regeneration. Sometimes new bone formation turned out as a "stand-alone" phenomenon without accompanying cementum and functional PDL. Various alternative methods are available for measuring new bone formation:

### Direct Bone Measurements

*Linear measurements*: A series of linear measurements are conducted with the use of a fixed reference point, such as the CEJ, restorative margins, or tooth notch at baseline and at the final evaluation. The net changes are calculated from these two observations.

Three sets of measurements performed in linear measurements are as follows:
1. Distance from a landmark to the bone crest.
2. Distance from a landmark to the base of the defect.
3. Distance from the bone crest to the base of the defect.

*Volumetric measurements*: The alveolar defect is filled with elastomeric impression material, either in vivo or on a plaster model of the teeth and surrounding bone is reproduced from an impression of the surgical site. After setting, the material in the defect is removed carefully and weighed. Weight values are translated into volumetric units based on the material's specific gravity. However, a significant drawback of this method is the distortion of the impression material, which might affect the measurements. The method fails to discriminate between defect resolutions that arise from the bone fill and crestal resorption. Hence, it is likely to overestimate positive changes.

### Indirect Bone Measurements

Indirect bone measurements include sounding bone measurement and radiographic bone measurement.

## Clinical Evaluation of Attachment Levels and Other Soft Tissue Parameters

They include clinical attachment level measurements, probing depth measurements, gingival recession, measurements of gingival infection, and inflammation and tissue formation.

A scanning electron microscopy helps investigate the nature of the cell population on the barrier membrane's inner surface. Fibroblast-like cells, along with inflammatory cells, RBC, and some bacterial cells, were reported on the inner surface of the middle portion of the membrane.

## Radiographic Evaluation of Hard Tissue Changes

Radiographic evaluation of bone regeneration requires careful standardized techniques for reproducible positioning of the film and the tube.

## Ancillary Methods

Gingival bone count index (GCBI): Dunning JM and Leach DB (1960).

## Surgical Re-entry

The surgical reentry of the operated site after a healing period gives a good view of the state of the bone crest that can be compared with the view taken during the initial surgical intervention and can also be subject to measurements. But the disadvantages associated with surgical reentry are that it requires an unnecessary second operation and does not show the type of attachment. Moreover, it is an unethical issue.

# FACTORS INFLUENCING REGENERATIVE PROCEDURES

Factors that can adversely affect clinical outcome after regenerative therapy are as follows:
- *Barrier-dependent factors*:
  - *Inadequate root barrier adaptation*: Absence of barrier effect
  - *Nonsterile technique*: Plaque or saliva contamination of barrier
  - Instability (movement) of barrier against the root
  - Premature exposure of barrier to oral environment and microbes
  - Premature loss or degradation of the barrier
- *Barrier-independent factors*:
  - Poor plaque control
  - Smoking
  - *Occlusal trauma*: Hyperocclusion
  - *Suboptimal tissue health*: Inflammation persists
  - *Mechanical habits*: Aggressive toothbrushing techniques
  - *Overlying gingival tissue*:
    - Inadequate zone of keratinized tissue.
    - Inadequate tissue thickness.
  - *Surgical technique*:
    - *Improper incision placement*: Excessive loss of marginal tissue.

- Traumatic flap elevation and management
- *Excessive surgical tissue*: Tissue or flap desiccation
- *Inadequate closure or suturing*: Failure to achieve and maintain primary closure.
  - *Postsurgical factor*:
    - Premature tissue challenge
    - Plaque recolonization
    - Mechanical insult
    - Loss of wound stability: Loose sutures, loss of early fibrin clot

The above-mentioned factors usually limit regenerative healing after GTR surgery. The presence of smoking habits, poor plaque control, and premature exposure of barrier material are the most important of them.

## POSTOPERATIVE HEALING

Transfer of a free bone graft from donor to the recipient site results in an interruption of microcirculation and cell death in the grafted tissue. Thus, the grafted bone itself is initially not capable of new bone formation. Therefore, the incorporation process is entirely dependent on nutrition, cellular migration, and revascularization from the adjacent tissues at the recipient site.

Grafted tissue (autograft, allograft) contains chemotactic inflammatory mediators and growth factors facilitating the healing process, which is in contrast to bone substitute materials (alloplast, xenograft).

When autograft (compact bone) is placed in a freshly prepared recipient site, most of the osteocytes die except osteocytes present at the surface. Once the blood supply has been severed, surface osteocytes obtain all their nourishment via tissue fluids through canaliculi and, thus, survive. Surface osteocytes and osteogenic cells have the best opportunity for continued existence in newly transplanted bone. During cytolysis, dead osteocytes release and inductive organic substance capable of promoting osteogenesis in the underlying connective tissues. Bone formation occurs by the proliferation of the cells from the osteogenic layer of periosteum, endosteum, and marrow of the host bone that are brought outwardly in the granulation tissue towards the graft forming new trabeculae that eventually unite with the graft. After the union of the graft and recipient site, the general process of resorption and replacement occur simultaneously. Resorption occurs along the outer surfaces of the transplant between areas where the new bone's trabeculae have joined and on the inner surfaces of the Haversian canal.

Cancellous bone graft has greater endurance and growth of covering and lining cells (osteoblasts) of the cancellous fragment as compared to the compact bone graft. The endosteum of autogenous hematopoietic bone marrow may act as a possible source of osteogenic cells. The undifferentiated mesenchymal cell that is stem cells of donor marrow may differentiate into osteoblasts by the inductive effect of damaged recipient bone tissues. Donor marrow cells may undergo disruption and liberate inductive factors that act as a stimulus for the undifferentiated mesenchymal cells of the receptor site to differentiate into osteoblasts.[34]

### Points to Ponder

- Various stars of healing are as follows:
  - *One-star healing*: Control of inflammation
  - *Two-star healing*: Long junctional epithelium
  - *Three-star healing*: New attachment
  - *Four-star healing*: Partial regeneration
  - *Five-star healing*: Complete regeneration
- Root conditioning, now also called as chemically GTR.
- The advantage of autogenous grafts over allografts is that there is no problem of disease transmission or histocompatibility.
- Radiographically, FDBA appears radiopaque because it is not demineralized.

## REFERENCES

1. American Academy of Periodontology. Glossary of Periodontal Terms, 4th edition. Chicago, IL, USA: American Academy of Periodontology; 2001.
2. Polson AM, Hanes PJ. Root surface and periodontal regeneration. In: Polson AM (Ed). Periodontal Regeneration: Current Status and Directions. Chicago, United States: Quintessence Publishing; 1994. pp. 21-40.
3. Aravind B, Koshy C, Bhat GS, Bhat KM. Root conditioning: A review. JISP. 2003;6:88-93.
4. Lowenguth RA, Blieden TM. Periodontal regeneration: root surface demineralization. Periodontol 2000. 1993;1:54-68.
5. Nyman S, Lindhe J, Karring T, Rylander H. New attachment following surgical treatment of human periodontal disease. J Clin Periodontol. 1982;9(4):290-6.
6. Gottlow J, Nyman S, Lindhe J, Karring T, Wennström J. New attachment formation in the human periodontium by guided tissue regeneration. Case reports. J Clin Periodontol. 1986;13(6):604-16.
7. Proceedings of the 1996 World Workshop in Periodontics. Lansdowne, Virginia, July 13-17, 1996. Ann Periodontol. 1996;1(1):1-947.
8. Scantlebury TV. 1982-1992: a decade of technology development for guided tissue regeneration. J Periodontol. 1993;64(11 Suppl):1129-37.
9. Wang HL, Cooke J. Periodontal regeneration techniques for treatment of periodontal diseases. Dent Clin North Am. 2005;49(3):637-59.
10. Greenstein G, Caton JG. Biodegradable barriers and guided tissue regeneration. Periodontol 2000. 1993;1:36-45.
11. Greenstein G, Caton JG. Resorbable barriers and periodontal regeneration. In: Polson AM (Ed). Periodontal Regeneration: Current Status and Directions. Chicago, United States: Quintessence Publishing; 1994. pp. 151-66.
12. Bunyaratavej P, Wang HL. Collagen membranes: a review. J Periodontol. 2001;72(2):215-29.
13. Becker W. Guided tissue regeneration for periodontal defects. In: Polson AM (Ed). Periodontal Regeneration: Current

Status and Directions. Chicago, United States: Quintessence Publishing; 1994. pp. 137-50.
14. Carranza FM, Mclain PK, Schallhorn RG. Regenerative osseous surgery. In: Newman MG, Takei HH, Carranza FA (Eds). Carranza's Clinical Periodontology, 9th edition. Philadelphia, PA, USA: WB Saunders; 2003. pp. 804-24.
15. Karring T, Lindhe J, Cortellini P. Regenerative periodontal therapy. In: Clinical Periodontology and Implant Dentistry, 4th edition. Oxford, United Kingdom: Blackwell Munksgaard; 2003. pp. 650-704.
16. Rosenberg E, Rose LF. Biologic and clinical considerations for autografts and allografts in periodontal regeneration. Dent Clin North Am. 1998;42(3):467-90.
17. Grant DA, Stern IB, Listgarten MA. Bone grafts and transplants. In: Periodontics, 6th edition. St. Louis: CV Mosby; 1988. pp. 860-82.
18. Mellonig JT, Brunsvold MA. Osseous grafts and periodontal regeneration. In: Polson AM (Ed). Periodontal Regeneration: Current Status and Directions. Chicago, United States: Quintessence Publishing; 1994. pp. 71-102.
19. Yukna RA. Synthetic grafts and regeneration. In: Polson AM (Ed). Periodontal Regeneration: Current Status and Directions. Chicago, United States: Quintessence Publishing; 1994. pp. 103-12.
20. AlGhamdi AS, Shibly O, Ciancio SG. Osseous grafting part I: autografts and allografts for periodontal regeneration--a literature review. J Int Acad Periodontol. 2010;12(2):34-8.
21. Hiatt WH, Genco RJ. Regenerative therapy in periodontics. In: Genco RJ, Goldman HM, Cohen DW (Eds). Contemporary Periodontics. St. Louis: CV Mosby; 1990. pp. 585-604.
22. Lynch SE. The role of growth factors in periodontal repair. In: Polson AM (Ed). Periodontal Regeneration: Current Status and Directions. Chicago, United States: Quintessence Publishing; 1994. pp. 179-98.
23. Polson AM, Prove MP. Fibrin linkage: a precursor for new attachment. J Periodontol. 1983;54(3):141-7.
24. Cochran DL, Wozney JM. Biological mediators for periodontal regeneration. Periodontol 2000. 1999;19:40-58.
25. Hammarström L, Heijl L, Gestrelius S. Periodontal regeneration in a buccal dehiscence model in monkeys after application of enamel matrix proteins. J Clin Periodontol. 1997;24(9 Pt 2):669-77.
26. Miron RJ, Wei L, Yang S, Caluseru OM, Sculean A, Zhang Y. Effect of enamel matrix derivative on periodontal wound healing and regeneration in an osteoporotic model. J Periodontol. 2014;85(11):1603-11.
27. Tunali M, Özdemir H, Küçükodacı Z, Akman S, Yaprak, E, Toker H, et al. A novel platelet concentrate: titanium-prepared platelet-rich fibrin. Biomed Res Int. 2014;2014:209548.
28. Choukroun JI, Adda F, Schoeffler C, Vervelle A. An opportunity in perio-implantology: The PRF (in French). Implantodontie. 2001;42:55-62.
29. Dohan DM, Choukroun J, Diss A, Dohan SL, Dohan AJ, Mouhyi J, et al. Platelet-rich fibrin (PRF): a second-generation platelet concentrate. Part I: Technological concepts and evolution. Oral Surg Oral Med Oral Pathol Oral Radiol Endod. 2006;101(3):e37-44.
30. Dohan Ehrenfest DM, de Peppo GM, Doglioli P, Sammartino G. Slow release of growth factors and thrombospondin-1 in Choukroun's platelet-rich fibrin (PRF): a gold standard to achieve for all surgical platelet concentrates technologies. Growth Factors. 2009;27(1):63-9.
31. Caffesse RG, Nasjleti CE. Clinical and histologic results of regenerative procedures. In: Polson AM (Ed). Periodontal Regeneration: Current Status and Directions. Chicago, United States: Quintessence Publishing; 1994. pp. 113-36.
32. Kao RT. Periodontal regeneration and reconstructive surgery. In: Rose LF, Mealey BL, Genco RJ, Cohen DW (Eds). Periodontics: Medicine, Surgery, and Implants. United States: Elsevier-Mosby; 2004. pp. 572-609.
33. Lynch SE. Methods for evaluation of regenerative procedures. J Periodontal. 1992;63(12 Suppl):1085-92.
34. Ruben MP, Smukler H, Schulman SM, Kon S, Bloom AA. Healing of periodontal surgical wounds. In: Goldman HM, Cohen DW (Eds). Periodontal Therapy, 5th edition. St. Louis: CV Mosby; 1980. pp. 640-754.

## VIVA VOCE

**Q1. What are the various methods to suppress the antigenic potential of allograft and xenograft?**
**Ans.** The various methods to suppress the antigenic potential of allograft and xenograft are as follows:
- *Radiation treatment*: 6 mega rads of high intensity of gamma radiation is adequate.
- *Freezing*: Deep frozen −197°C liquid nitrogen freezer for a period of at least 4 weeks.
- *Chemical treatment*: Through keeping in merthiolate solution.

**Q2. What are the disadvantages of surgical reentry?**
**Ans.** The disadvantages of surgical reentry are as follows:
- It requires an unnecessary second operation.
- It does not show the type of attachment.
- It is an unethical issue.

**Q3. Why is root resorption very common with fresh iliac autograft?**
**Ans.** According to Dragoo and Sullivan, fresh iliac material is so highly inductive that both clast and blast activity is stimulated more than in other graft materials or in the same material used after storage. It has been observed clinically that frequent curettage of the resorbed area, particularly in the crestal areas of newly forming bone, often reverses the process.

**Q4. What is isograft?**
**Ans.** Isograft is an autograft taken from monozygous twins or related persons. It is also called as syngenous grafts.

## Chapter 51: Regenerative Osseous Surgery

**Q5. What is the basic difference between biodegradable, bioresorbable and bioabsorbable?**

**Ans.** The basic difference between biodegradable, bioresorbable, and bioabsorbable is as follows:
- *Biodegradable*: Macromolecular degradation takes place, and degradation by-products move from their site of action but not necessarily from the body.
- *Bioresorbable*: Macromolecular degradation by-products are eliminated through natural pathways by simple filtration.
- *Bioabsorbable*: Polymer molecules undergo dissolution in body fluids, which may or may not be excreted.

**Q6. What should be the minimum gingival thickness for the GTR procedure?**

**Ans.** A 1.5 mm should be the minimum gingival thickness, to maintain blood supply and to prevent flap necrosis from achieving favorable results.

**Q7. What are the differences in the preparation of PRP and PRF?**

**Ans.** None of the additives, such as anticoagulant, calcium chloride, and thrombin are required during PRF preparation as required in PRP preparation. In PRF preparation, only one spin is required.

**Q8. Who coined the term GTR?**

**Ans.** Gottlow, in 1986.

**Q9. What is Osteoconduction?**

**Ans.** Grafted material does not contribute to new bone formation but serves as the scaffold for bone formation originating from adjacent host bone.

**Q10. Which BMP is not osteoinductive in nature?**

**Ans.** BMP-1 and BMP-6.

# Chapter 52

# Furcation

*Shalu Bathla*

## Chapter Outline

- Terminologies
- Classifications
- Etiology
- Factors Influencing Furcation Management
- Diagnosis
- Prognosis
- Management

## INTRODUCTION

The furcation lesion defect represents a serious complication in periodontal therapy due to inaccessibility to adequate instrumentation, presence of root concavities, and furrows making proper cleaning of the area difficult. Thus, loss of periodontal attachment in the furcation area is a condition that requires careful evaluation and management in order to achieve stability of dentition.

## TERMINOLOGIES

Following are the terminologies related to furcation:[1]
- Furcation is the area located between individual root cones.
- Furcation involvement is the extension of pocket formation into the interradicular area of the bone of a multirooted tooth.
- Furcation entrance is the transitional area between the undivided and divided parts of the root.
- Furcation fornix is the roof of the furcation.
- The degree of separation is the angle of separation between two roots (cones) **(Fig. 52.1A)**.
- The coefficient of separation is the length of root cones in relation to the length of the root complex **(Fig. 52.1B)**.
- Root amputation is the removal of one or more roots from a multirooted tooth, leaving the majority of crown intact.
- Sectioning is the surgical sectioning of a tooth into segments consisting of the root and overlying crown.

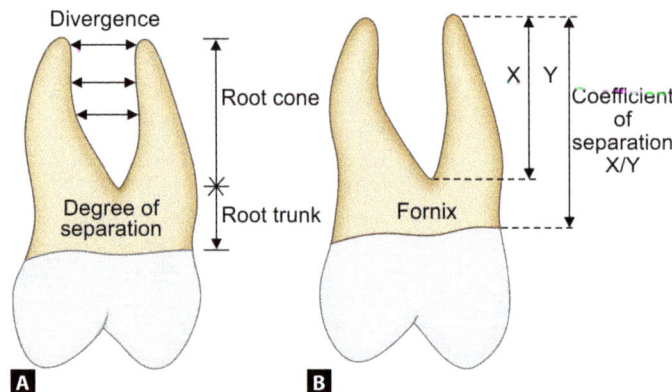

**Figs. 52.1A and B:** Schematic representation showing terminology in relation to furcation: (A) Degree of separation; (B) Coefficient of separation.

## CLASSIFICATIONS

Various classifications have been proposed to categorize furcation defects:
- *According to Glickman (1953):*[2]
    - *Grade I*: It is the incipient stage of furcation involvement, but radiographically changes are not usually found.
    - *Grade II*: The furcation lesion is a cul-de-sac with a definite horizontal component. Radiographs may or may not depict the furcation involvement **(Fig. 52.2)**.
    - *Grade III*: The bone is not attached to the dome of the furcation. This grade of furcation displays the defect as a radiolucent area in the crotch of the tooth **(Fig. 52.3)**.

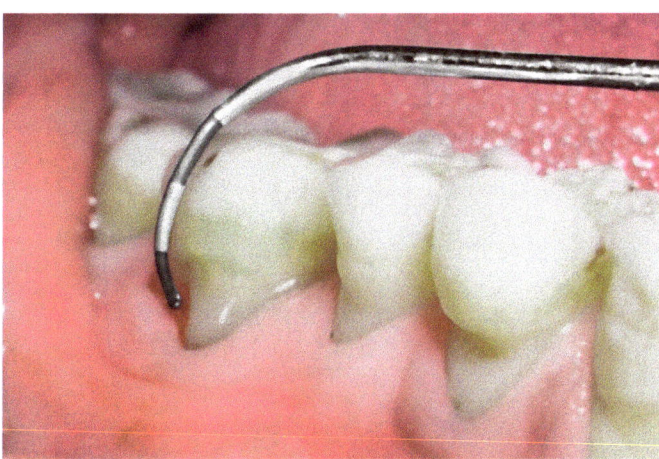

**Fig. 52.2:** Clinical picture showing grade II furcation defect.

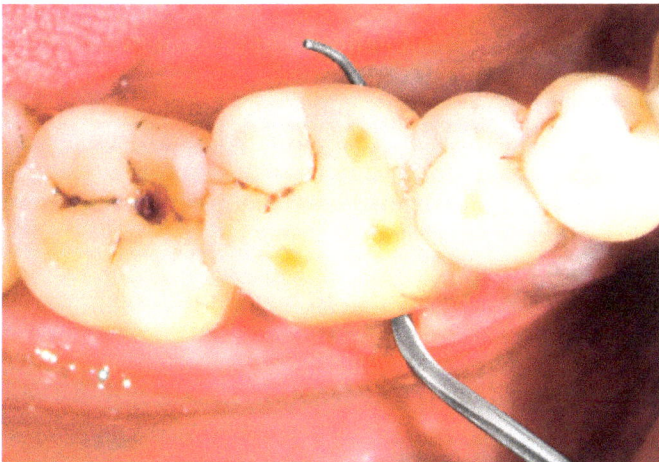

**Fig. 52.3:** Clinical picture showing grade III furcation defect (occlusal view). Naber's probe passes through and through the furcation lesion.

- *Grade IV*: The interdental bone is destroyed, and soft tissues have receded apically so that the furcation opening is clinically visible.
- *According to Goldman and Cohen (1958):*[3]
  - *Grade I*: Incipient lesion
  - *Grade II*: Cul-de-sac lesion
  - *Grade III*: Through and through the lesion

- *According to Staffileno (1969):*[4]
  - *Grade I*: Soft tissue lesion extending to the entrance of the furcation with a minor degree of bone loss.
  - *Grade II*: Loss of furcal bone but not through and through.
  - *Grade III*: Through and through.
- *According to Easley and Drennan*[5] **(Figs. 52.4A to D):**
  - *Class I*: Incipient involvement in which the fluting coronal to the furcation entrance is affected, but there is no definite horizontal component to the furcation involvement. In this classification system, class II and III furcations are separated into subtypes 1 and 2 on the basis of the configuration of the alveolar bone at the entrance to the furcation. Horizontal resorption into the furca is subtype 1, whereas subtype 2 indicates a significant vertical component to the defect.
  - *Class II*: Type 1—a definite horizontal loss of attachment into the furcation, but the pattern of bone loss is essentially horizontal. There is no definite buccal or lingual ledge of bone. Type 2—there is a buccal or lingual bony ledge and a definite vertical component to the attachment loss.
  - *Class III*: A through-and-through loss of attachment in the furcation. As with class II furcation defects, the pattern of attachment loss may be horizontal type 1, or there may be a vertical component type 2 of varying depth.
- *According to Hamp et al. (1975)*[6] **(Figs. 52.5A to C):**
  - *Degree I*: Horizontal loss of periodontal support not exceeding one-third of the width of the tooth (<3 mm).
  - *Degree II*: Horizontal loss of periodontal support exceeding one-third of the width of the tooth (≥3 mm).
  - *Degree III*: Horizontal through-and-through destruction of periodontal tissue in the furcation area.
- *According to Ramfjord and Ash (1979):*[7]
  - *Class I*: Beginning involvement. Tissue destruction of less than 2 mm (one-third of tooth width) into the furcation.

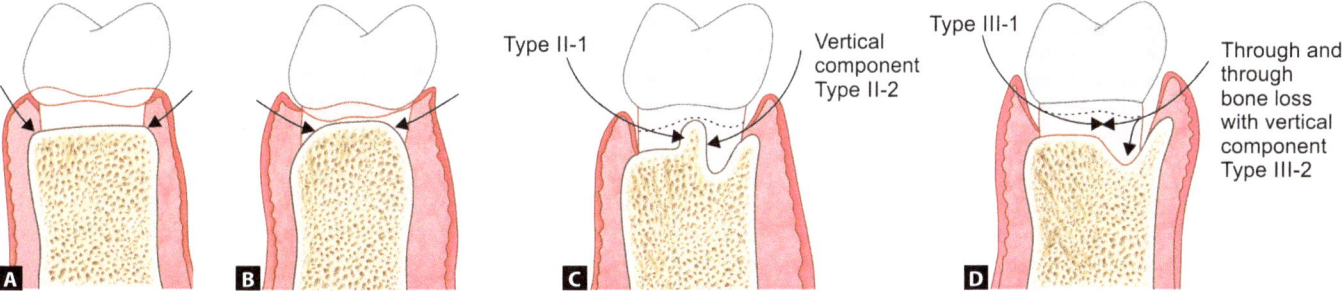

**Figs. 52.4A to D:** Schematic representation showing Easley and Drennan defect classification. (A) No furcation involvement; (B) Class I: incipient involvement; (C) Class II: Type-1 and Type-2; (D) Class III: Type-1 and Type-2.

**Section 7:** Treatment: Surgical Therapy

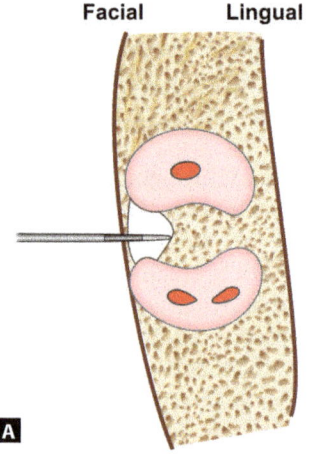
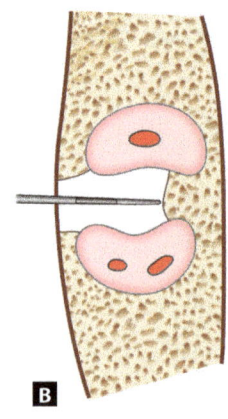
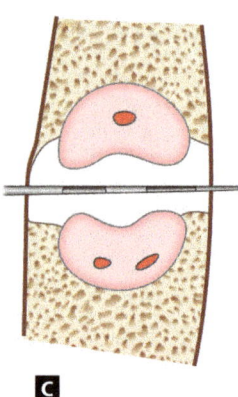

**Figs. 52.5A to C:** Schematic representation showing (A) Furcation probed up to the depth of 3 mm; (B) Furcation probed more than 3 mm but not through and through; (C) Furcation probed through and through.

- *Class II*: Cul-de-sac, tissue destruction more than 2 mm (more than one-third of tooth width), but not through-and-through.
- *Class III*: Through-and-through involvement.
- *According to Tarnow and Fletcher (1984)*:[8] Based on the vertical component of furcation involvement depending on the distance from the base of the defect to the roof of the furcation, they are classified into:
    - *Subgroup A*: Vertical destruction of bone up to one-third of the interradicular height (1–3 mm).
    - *Subgroup B*: Vertical destruction of bone up to two-thirds of the interradicular height (4–6 mm).
    - *Subgroup C*: Vertical destruction beyond the apical-third (7 mm or more).
- *According to Eskow and Kapin (1984)*:[9] Based on the vertical component of furcation involvement:
    - *Subgroup A*: Vertical osseous defect up to one-third of the root.
    - *Subgroup B*: Vertical osseous defect up to two-thirds of the root.
    - *Subgroup C*: Vertical osseous defect greater than two-thirds of the root.
- *According to Fedi (1985)*:[10]
    - Combined Glickman and Hamp classifications.
    - Grades are the same as Glickman's grades I through IV, but grade II is subdivided into degrees I and II.
    - *Degree I*: The furcation bone loss possesses a vertical component of greater than 1 but less than 3 mm.
    - *Degree II*: The furcation bone loss possesses a vertical component of greater than 3 mm, but still does not Communicate through-and-through.
- *According to Hou (1998)*:[11] Classification based on root trunk length and horizontal and vertical bone loss. Types of root trunk:
    - *Type A*: Furcation involving a cervical third of the root length.
    - *Type B*: Furcation involving cervical third and cervical two-thirds of root length.
    - *Type C*: Furcation involving cervical two-thirds of root length.

The different classes of furcation are as follows:
- *Class I*: Horizontal loss of periodontal tissue support less than 3 mm.
- *Class II*: Horizontal loss of support greater than 3 mm, but does not encompass the total width of the furcation area.
- *Class III*: Horizontal "through-and-through" loss of periodontal tissue in the furcation.

Subclasses of furcation involvement relate to alveolar bone loss from the furcation roof apically to the root apex by radiographic assessment of the periapical view.
- *Subclass "A"*: Suprabony defect.
- *Subclass "B"*: Infrabony defect.

Classifications of furcation:
- *AI, AII, and AIII*: Type A root trunks with class I, class II and class III furcations.
- *BI, BII, and BIII*: Type B root trunks with class I, class II and class III furcations.
- *CI, CII, and CIII*: Type C root trunks with class I, class II and class III furcations.

## ETIOLOGY

There is no difference in basic etiology and pathology between furcation involvements and other periodontal pockets. However, the anatomical and morphological features of the furcations and their relationship to the adjacent structures pose specific problems in the treatment of involved teeth.[12]

- The primary cause of furcation involvement is the progressive loss of attachment that results from inflammatory periodontal disease. Bacterial plaque is the most common cause of marginal periodontitis, which progressively invades one or more furcation areas to varying degrees, resulting in irreversible bone loss in the interradicular area. In most patients, the response to bacterial plaque, in the absence of therapy, is a progressive and site-specific attachment loss. Although the rate of response may vary from individual to individual, local anatomic factors that affect the deposition of plaque or hamper its removal can significantly impact the development of attachment loss.[13]

- *Predisposing factors*:[14,15]
  - *Cervical enamel projections (CEPs)*: CEPs present on the root surface in the furcation region have been considered a predisposing etiologic factor for periodontal attachment loss.
  - *Trauma from occlusion*: Trauma from occlusion acting as a predisposing cofactor for the rapid formation of furcation involvement is controversial. Glickman (1961) assigned a key role to trauma since furcation areas are most sensitive to injury from excessive occlusal forces. Waerhaug (1979) denied the initiating effect of trauma and considered that inflammation and edema caused by plaque in the furcation area tend to extrude the tooth, which becomes traumatized and sensitive.
  - *Pulpal periodontal disease*: The high percentage of molar teeth with patent accessory canal opening into the furcation suggest that pulpal disease could be an initiating cofactor in the development of furcation involvement.
  - *Iatrogenic cofactors*: Iatrogenic predisposing cofactors, i.e., pin and endodontic perforations and overhanging restorations, can lead to the formation of isolated furcation lesion by therapists themselves. Overhanging restorations harbor dental plaque, which causes periodontal inflammation and attachment loss.
  - *Root fractures involving furcations*: If these root fractures involve the trunk of a multirooted molar and extend into the furcation, this can result in a rapidly forming isolated furcation defect. The prognosis for these situations is poor and usually results in loss of the tooth.[13]

## FACTORS INFLUENCING FURCATION MANAGEMENT

- *Root trunk length*: Root trunk length is a key factor that affects both the development of furcation involvement and the mode of treatment. If root trunk is short, less attachment has to be lost before furcation is involved. When the root trunk is long, furcation will be invaded later but will be difficult to instrument.[15] Short-root trunk facilitates surgical procedure. It is more accessible to maintenance therapy than the long-root trunk.
  - Maxillary molars—mesial furcation entrance is located about 3 mm from the cementoenamel junction (CEJ), while the buccal furcation entrance is approximately about 4 mm and distal furcation entrance is located about 5 mm from CEJ.
  - Maxillary premolars—length of root trunk is approximately 8 mm.
  - Mandibular molars—the length of root trunk at the lingual entrance is 4 mm, and at the buccal entrance, it is approximately 3 mm.
- *Root length*: Root length is directly related to the quantity of attachment supporting the tooth.
- *Root form*: The roots of molars may be fused, partially fused, closely approximated, or widely divergent **(Figs. 52.6A to D)**. Curvature and fluting increase the potential for root perforation during endodontics and vertical root fracture. Marked concavities appear in the mesiobuccal root of the maxillary first molar and both roots of the mandibular first molar.
- *Interradicular dimensions*: Narrow and interradicular zone complicate the surgical procedure, whereas widely separated roots have more treatment options as this can be easily hemisected and readily treated. In divergent rooted teeth, adequate instrumentation can be done during scaling, root planing, and surgery. The dimensions of the furcation entrance should be taken into consideration during the selection of instruments.
  - *Maxillary premolars*: The width of the furcation entrance of maxillary premolars is approximately 0.7 mm.

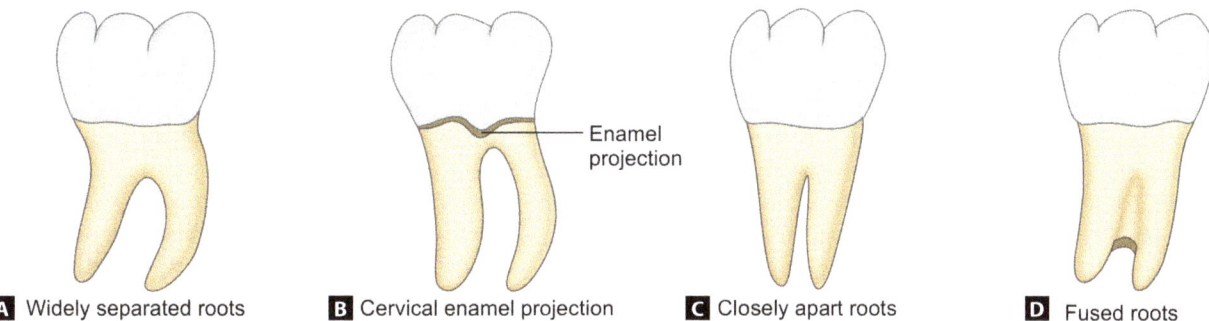

**A** Widely separated roots  **B** Cervical enamel projection  **C** Closely apart roots  **D** Fused roots

**Figs. 52.6A to D:** Schematic representation showing the anatomic variation of furcation areas.

(*Courtesy:* Dr SK Salaria)

- *Maxillary molars*: The width of the buccal entrance is 0.5 mm, mesial entrance is 0.75 mm, and the distal entrance is approximately 0.5–0.75 mm.
- *Mandibular molars*: The buccal entrance is often less than 0.75 mm, while the lingual entrance is more than 0.75 mm.
- *Anatomy of furcation*: An intermediate bifurcation ridge has been described in 73% of mandibular first molars, crossing from the mesial to the distal root at the mid-root of the bifurcation. Furcation ridges have a core of dentine but are composed predominantly of cellular cementum, which increases in thickness with age. Ridges are natural obstructions to both plaque control procedures and professional debridement of furcation lesions.
- *Cervical enamel projections*: They favor plaque accumulation and complicate scaling and root planing. Enamel projections act as a local factor in the development of gingivitis and periodontitis.

Masters and Hoskins in 1964 classified CEPs into three grades:[16]
- *Grade I*: The enamel projection extends from CEJ towards the furcation entrance.
- *Grade II*: Enamel projection approaches the entrance of the furcation without entering the furcation with no horizontal component.
- *Grade III*: Enamel projection extends horizontally into the furcation. The prevalence of CEPs is highest in mandibular and maxillary second molar teeth.

## DIAGNOSIS

The furcation region's position and morphology complicate the clinician's ability to identify the location and extent of the furcation defect. Furcation must be diagnosed at the earliest possible time.[17,18]

- *Radiographically*: Radiographs are useful in assessing root morphology and apicocoronal position of the furcation but do not allow the clinician to determine attachment loss in the furcation.[19] Thus, two-dimensional radiographic pictures provide meager information about furcation involvement, especially in the maxilla. High-resolution spiral computed tomography (CT), computer-assisted densitometric image analysis (CADIA), and digital radiography will allow cross-section views of interior furcation lesions (**Fig. 52.7**). It appears that radiographs alone do not detect the furcation lesion with any predictable accuracy and that probing the furcation areas is necessary to confirm the presence and severity of the furcation defect.
- *Clinically*: Periodontal probes are useful for determining the probing depth in a vertical direction but less useful for determining the degree of horizontal involvement. For this purpose, either curved Cowhorn explorer or Naber's probe are very useful. Furcation probes have

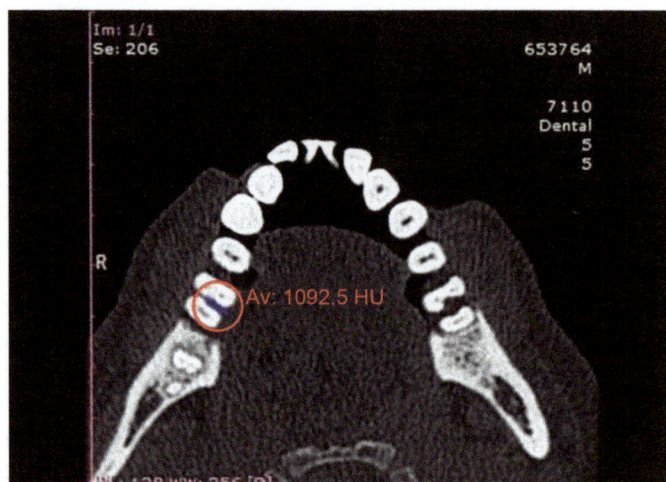

**Fig. 52.7:** Computed tomography scan image showing a bone loss at the furcation area.

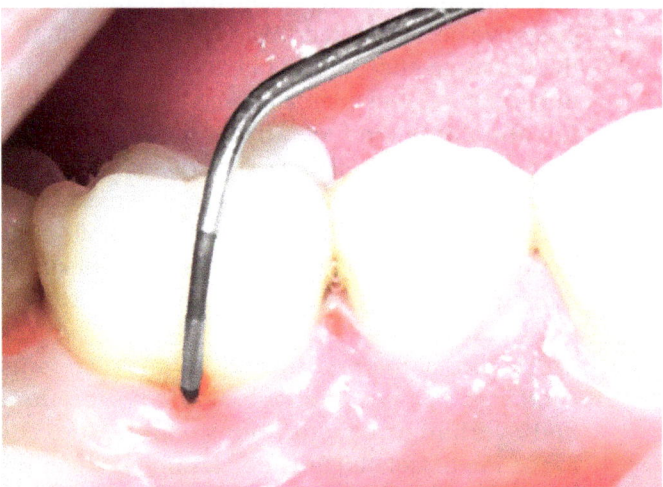

**Fig. 52.8:** Clinical picture showing probing of molar furcation with Naber's probe.

a curved, blunt tip that allows easy access to furcation areas. An example of furcation probes is Naber's 1N and Naber's 2N. The probe is directed beneath the gingival margin. At the base of the pocket, rotate the probe tip toward the tooth to fit the tip into the furcation entrance. The terminal shank of Naber's probe is positioned parallel to the long axis of the tooth surface being examined (**Fig. 52.8**).
- Probing of mandibular molar furcations is relatively easy because there are only buccal and lingual entrances, each of which is located midway mesiodistally.
- *Probing of maxillary molar furcations*: Buccal entrance is accessible midway mesiodistally. Distal furcation is present midway buccolingually, thus can be probed from either buccal or palatal aspect. Mesial furcation of maxillary molar is easily probed from the palatal aspect because mesial furcation

opens about two-thirds of the way towards the palate, rather than midway buccolingually.[1]
- *Transgingival probing/bone sounding*: To determine the bone contours associated with furcation lesions more accurately, transgingival probing can be accomplished through anesthetized soft tissues (Rest is explained in "Chapter 29: Clinical Diagnosis").

## PROGNOSIS

In general, teeth with furcation involvements have a poor prognosis.[18]
- Prognosis of furcation involvement in maxillary first premolar has a poor prognosis.
- Prognosis of maxillary molars is not good, whereas the prognosis of mandibular first molar is considered good. The following factors should be considered in projecting a prognosis of the tooth with furcation involvement:
- The extent of involvement
- Status of bone support
- Root separation
- Health of neighboring teeth

Other factors involved in establishing a treatment prognosis are related to personal, psychological, sociological, and financial considerations.

## MANAGEMENT

### Objectives

- To facilitate maintenance of existing furcation defect through scaling and root planing.
- To increase access to the furcation through gingivectomy, apically positioned flap, odontoplasty, ostectomy/osteoplasty, and tunnel preparation.
- To prevent further attachment loss or eliminate the furcation through root amputation, tooth resection, and hemisection.
- To obliterate the furcation defect by filling furcation defects with a biocompatible material, such as polymeric reinforced zinc oxide eugenol ionomer restorative material (IRM) and glass ionomer cement (GIC).
- To regenerate the lost attachment through guided tissue regeneration (GTR) procedures and bone grafting.

Following are the factors to be considered during treatment of furcation lesion:[14]
- *Tooth-related factors*:
  - Degree of furcation involved
  - Amount of remaining periodontal support
  - Probing depth
  - Tooth mobility
  - Root trunk length
  - Root length
  - Root form
  - Interradicular dimensions
  - Anatomy of furcation
  - Cervical enamel projections
  - Tooth position and occlusal antagonisms
  - Endodontic conditions and root canal anatomy
- *Patient-related factors*:
  - The strategic value of the tooth in relation to the overall plan
  - Patient's age and health condition
  - Oral hygiene capacity

### Treatment Modalities

The keys to successful treatment of molar furcation involvement are the same as for any other periodontal problem, i.e., early diagnosis, thorough treatment planning, good oral hygiene by the patient, careful technical execution of the therapeutic modality, and a well-designed and implemented program of periodontal maintenance. Various therapeutic methods are attempted depending upon the severity of furcation involvement and tooth position in either maxilla or mandible.

### Class I Furcation Defects

- *Furcation plasty*: In 1975, Hamp, Nyman, and Lindhe described furcation plasty as raising a mucoperiosteal flap to provide access to the furcation area and combining scaling and root planing, osteoplasty and odontoplasty to remove local irritants and to open the furcation to allow the patient access to clean the area. It is done in grade I and early grade II furcation lesions.
- *Scaling and root planing*: In grade I, furcation lesions have not lost bone within the furcation, so closed, or open scaling and root planing procedures can resolve inflammation. If inflammation is not resolved, then gingivectomy or apically positioned flap can be done depending upon the width of the attached gingiva.
- *Odontoplasty*: Odontoplasty is defined as the reshaping of a tooth coronal to the furcation. It widens and shallows the furcation by raising the roof of furcation. The rationale behind this technique is to create improved access for plaque control and maintenance. If CEP is found, then it is removed, and the area is recontoured. Odontoplasty must be approached with caution due to the potential complications of hypersensitivity, pulpal exposure, and increased risk of root caries.
- *Osteoplasty*: It is done to provide better gingival form by grooving the bone between the roots and then, festooning and beveling the bone over the roots.
- *Gingivectomy/apical positioned flap*: It can be used to reduce or eliminate the soft tissue pockets over the furcation region to increase access for plaque control and allow the resolution of periodontal inflammation.

### Class II Furcation Defects

- *Open flap debridement*: If sufficient subgingival access is not possible with a closed approach, for furcated

molars with deep lesions, then open flap debridement or modified Widman flap yields more effective plaque and calculus removal.
- *Guided tissue regeneration:* Organic or synthetic barrier membranes are used based on the principles of guided tissue regeneration.[20]
- *Bone grafting:* The strong focus on bone formation as a prerequisite for new attachment formation has led to bone graft implantation or different types of bone substitutes into furcation defects. Among these are bone autografts, allografts, xenografts and alloplastic materials designed as either bone substitutes or biologic barriers.[21]

## Class III and Class IV Furcation Defects

- *Tunnel preparation:* Tunneling is the process of deliberately removing bone from the furcation to produce an open tunnel through the furcation. It is a resective technique and used to treat advanced class II and class III furcation defects. This technique aims to make the furcal area accessible to home care instruments by the patient.

  The factors to be considered while selecting the case of tunnel preparation are as follows:
  - The tooth should be mandibular molar for clear two ways access.
  - Patients should have a low caries index.
  - Good patient compliance towards plaque control.
  - Root trunk should be short with high furcation entrance and long roots.
  - Root should have a wide furcal entrance with the degree of divergence of more than 30°.
  - The floor of the pulp chamber should not be close to the roof of the furcation to allow for possible odontoplasty of the entrance.

### Procedure

Buccal and lingual flaps are reflected, and the involved area is widened by the removal of some of the interradicular bone. Some of the interfurcal bone is sacrificed vertically and is recontoured to obtain a flat outline of the bone. Following bone resection, enough space is established in the furcation area to allow access for cleaning devices to be used by the patient itself. The main advantage associated with tunneling is the avoidance of prosthetic reconstruction and endodontic therapy.

The drawbacks associated with tunnel preparation are the threat of root caries, subsequent pulpal pathology, reverse architecture, and retained plaque in furcation cavities leading to progressive periodontal breakdown.

- *Root resection:* It is often the treatment of choice for deep grade II and III furcation lesions when regeneration is unpredictable. Root with the greatest bone loss should be considered for amputation.

Indications for root resection include:
- Severe and disproportionate attachment loss around the affected root
- Furcation defects that can be eliminated by root amputation
- Elimination of cracked or deeply fissured roots
- Elimination of an endodontically untreatable root
- Inoperable root caries
- Recession exposing most or all of the roots in a multirooted tooth

Factors determining the root resection are as follows:
- Bone levels in the furcation
- Accessibility for plaque removal
- Root proximity
- Position of the root in the arch
- Root morphology
- Endodontic complications

### Procedure

- *Root selection of mandibular molar:* The mesial root concavities are less accessible for plaque removal, and two narrow pulp canals of the mesial root are more difficult to treat endodontically than distal root. Post and core restoration are easily constructed on the distal root. Thus, mesial root of the mandibular molar is preferred over distal root for root resection.[22,23]
- *Root selection of maxillary molar:* The most commonly performed root resection is the distobuccal root of the maxillary first molar **(Figs. 52.9A to D)**. When both the mesial and distal furcation is involved, palatal root amputation should be considered if buccal furcation is intact. Palatal root has an unfavorable axial inclination and unfavorable prosthetic relationship with the first bicuspid.[22,23]
- *Endodontic phase:* In a nonvital root resection, endodontic therapy (root canal therapy) is done prior to root resection, and in vital root resection, the root resection is accomplished first and then endodontic therapy.
- *Resective phase:*
  - *Flap reflection:* After local anesthesia (LA) is given to the selected site, through the crevicular incision,

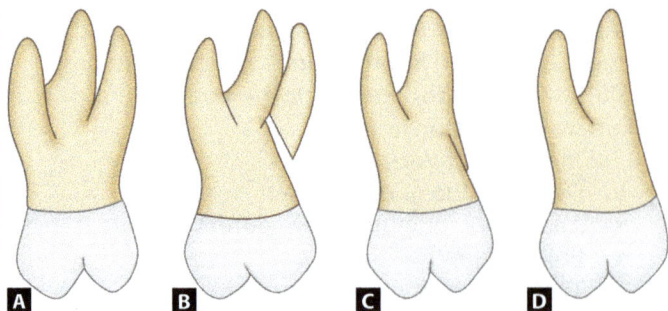

**Figs. 52.9A to D:** Schematic representation showing root resection of maxillary molar. (A) Maxillary molar; (B) Root resection cut to separate the root from root trunk; (C) Extraction of the separated root; (D) Final recontouring of the root trunk.

full-thickness mucoperiosteal buccal and lingual flaps are reflected.
- *Cut*: Small amount of bone covering the root (which is to be resected) is removed to provide access for elevation and root removal. The cut is made with high-speed surgical length fissure or cross-cut fissure carbide bur. The cut is then directed from just apical to the contact point of the tooth, through the tooth, to the other orifices of furcation. In a vital root resection, the cut is made more horizontally, so as to expose less surface area of the pulp chamber.
- *Root removal*: After sectioning, the root is elevated from its socket. Before flap closure, it is important to check for any residual root spurs and ledges that can act as subgingival overhangs to retain plaque and cause future periodontal destruction.
- *Suturing*: Sutures are placed over the approximated flap.

- *Restorative phase*: The removal of a root alters the direction of occlusal forces on the remaining roots. The occlusion of that tooth is evaluated and adjusted. Crowns should be placed. But before giving permanent restoration the quality of the endodontic filling, residual ledges should be examined radiographically and clinically.
- *Hemisection:* Hemisection is the splitting of a two-rooted tooth into two separate teeth. This process is also called as bicuspidization.

### Indications
- Strategic teeth with grade III furcation involvement.
- Teeth with divergent well-supported roots.

### Contraindications
- When the remaining periodontal support is inadequate.
- A tooth that cannot be treated endodontically.
- Where adequate restorations of the remaining tooth, including splinting, cannot be performed.

### Procedure
- *Cut*: The vertically oriented cut is made faciolingually through the buccal and lingual developmental grooves of the tooth, through the pulp chamber and through the furcation. The metallic portion of the cut should be made before flap elevation, which will prevent the contamination of the surgical field with metallic particles **(Figs. 52.10A to C)**.
- *Flap raised*: Buccal and lingual flaps are raised, and the area is curetted. Osseous surgery is completed by removing the residual internal osseous crater on the mesial or distal aspect of the remaining root.
- *Tooth reshaping*: Roof of furcation is carefully perforated with a dull, rounded bur in a slow handpiece. Each half of the tooth is reshaped into a single-rooted tooth and will be prepared to receive a crown.
- Orthodontic separation of the roots is required to allow restoration with adequate embrasure form.

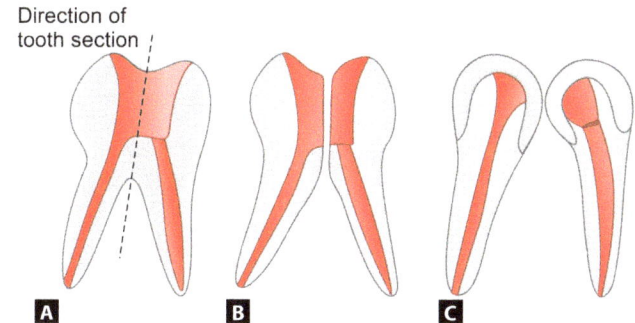

**Figs. 52.10A to C:** Schematic representation showing hemisection of mandibular molar.

- *Tooth resection*: Tooth resection involves the removal of one or more roots of the tooth as well as the corresponding portion of the crown.

### Advanced Class IV Furcation Defects

*Tooth extraction:* Indications for removal of a tooth with a grade III and IV furcal defects are as follows:[24]
- Individuals who do not maintain oral hygiene.
- Patients with a high level of caries activity.
- The existence of an unopposed molar which is the terminal tooth in the arch.
- Financial consideration precludes acceptance of treatment.
- If an otherwise heroic effort for a tooth with a questionable prognosis would be better handled by an implant.

### Failures in Surgical Furcation Therapy

Failures in surgical furcation therapy are due to the following reasons:[24]
- Inadequate plaque control and maintenance
- Poor root resection
- Improper restoration
- Endodontic failures
- Cracked roots
- Root caries
- Patients who respond poorly despite the best treatment

### Points to Ponder
- The dimensions of the furcation entrance should be taken into consideration during the selection of instruments.
- Furcation defects of maxillary molars are more difficult to interpret on radiographs because of the large palatal root's superimposition.
- In hemisection, a two-rooted molar tooth is converted into two single-rooted teeth.

## REFERENCES

1. Carnevale G, Pontoriero R, Lindhe J. Treatment of furcation involved teeth. In: Lindhe J, Karring T, Lang NP (Eds). Clinical Periodontology and Implant dentistry, 4th edition. Oxford, UK: Blackwell Munksgaard; 2003. pp. 705-30.

2. Glickman I. The treatment of bifurcation and trifurcation involvement. In: Clinical Periodontology, 2nd edition. Philadelphia, USA: WB Saunders; 1958. pp. 693-704.
3. Goldman HM. Therapy of the incipient bifurcation involvement. J Periodontol. 1958;29:112.
4. Staffileno HJ. Surgical management of the furca invasion. Dent Clin North Am. 1969;13(1):103-19.
5. Easley JR, Drennan GA. Morphological classification of the furca. J Can Dent Assoc (Tor). 1969;35(2):104-7.
6. Hamp SE, Nyman S, Lindhe J. Periodontal treatment of multirooted teeth. Result after 5 years. J Clin Periodontol. 1975;2(3):126-35.
7. Ramjford SP, Ash MM. Periodontology and periodontics. In: Modern Theory and Practice, 1st edition. Philadelphia USA: WB Saunders; 1979. p. 666.
8. Tarnow D, Fletcher P. Classification of the vertical component of furcation involvement. J Periodontol. 1984;55(5):283-4.
9. Eskow RN, Kapin SH. Furcation invasions: correlating a classification system with therapeutic considerations. Part II. Periodontal and restorative considerations in furcation management. Compend Contin Educ Dent. 1984;5(7): 527-32.
10. Fedi PF. The Periodontal syllabus, 2nd edition. Philadelphia, USA: Lea and Febiger; 1985. pp. 169-70.
11. Hou GL, Chen YM, Tsai CC, Weisgold AS. A new classification of molar furcation involvement based on the root trunk and horizontal and vertical bone loss. Int J Periodontics Restorative Dent. 1998;18(3):257-65.
12. Ammons WF, Harrington GW. Furcation: the problem and its management. In: Newman HN, Takei HH, Carranza FA (Eds). Clinical Periodontology, 9th edition. Philadelphia, USA: WB Saunders; 2003. pp. 825-39.
13. Newell DH. The diagnosis and treatment of molar furcation invasions. Dent Clin North Am. 1998;42(2):301-37.
14. Kalkwarf KL, Reinhardt RA. The furcation problem. Current controversies and future directions. Dent Clin North Am. 1988;32(2):243-66.
15. Mcclain PK, Schallhorn RG. Focus on furcation defects—guided tissue regeneration in combination with bone grafting. Periodontol 2000. 2000;22:190-212.
16. Masters DH, Hoskins SW. Projection of cervical enamel into molar furcations. J Periodontol. 1964;35:49.
17. Zappa U, Grosso L, Simona C, Graf H, Case D. Clinical furcation diagnosis and interradicular bone defects. J Periodontol. 1993;64(3):219-27.
18. Waerhaug J. The furcation problem, etiology, pathogenesis, diagnosis, therapy and prognosis. J Clin Periodontol. 1980;7(2):73-95.
19. Graetz C, Plaumann A, Wiebe JF, Springer C, Sälzer S, Dörfer CE. Periodontal probing versus radiographs for the diagnosis of furcation involvement. J Periodontol. 2014;85(10):1371-9.
20. Sanz M, Giovannoli JL. Focus on furcation defects: guided tissue regeneration. Periodontol 2000. 2000;22:169-89.
21. Garette S, Bogle G. Periodontal regeneration with bone grafts. Curr Opin Periodontol. 1994;168-77.
22. Genco RJ, Rosenberg ES, Evian C. Periodontal surgery. In: Genco RJ, Goldman HM, Cohen DW (Eds). Contemporary Periodontics. St. Louis, USA: CV Mosby; 1999. pp. 554-84.
23. de Sanctis M, Prato GP. Root resection and root amputation. Curr Opin Periodontol. 1993;105-10.
24. Grant DA, Stern IB, Listgarten MA. In: Periodontics. The Periodontally Diseased furcation, 6th edition. St. Louis, USA: CV Mosby; 1988. pp. 921-49.
25. Hardekopf JD, Dunlap RM, Ahl DR, Pelleu GB. The "furcation arrow." A reliable radiographic image? J Periodontol. 1987;58(4):258-61.

## VIVA VOCE

**Q1. Why should the dimensions of the furcation entrance be taken into consideration during the selection of instruments?**
Ans. According to Bower, 81% of furcations of maxillary and mandibular permanent first molar has orifices that are 1 mm or less wide, while in 58% molars, furcation entrance is narrower (0.75 mm or less) than the width of the blade of standard curettes (>0.75 mm).

**Q2. From which aspect mesial furcation of maxillary molar is easily probed?**
Ans. Mesial furcation of maxillary molar is easily probed from the palatal aspect because mesial furcation opens about two-thirds of the way towards the palate, rather than midway buccolingually.

**Q3. What is nonvital and vital root resection?**
Ans. Nonvital root resection—the endodontic therapy is done prior to root resection.
Vital root resection—the root resection is accomplished first and then endodontic therapy.

**Q4. What is furcation arrow?**
Ans. Furcation arrow is a small triangular radiographic shadow noted in the radiographs of maxillary molars over an either mesial or distal root in the proximal class II or III, furcation defects.[25]

**Q5. Why prognosis of the furcation defect of a maxillary first premolar is the worst?**
Ans. The maxillary first premolar has a long root trunk of approximately 8 mm, which makes instrumentation at the furcation defect much difficult.

**Q6. What is furcation entrance?**
Ans. It is the transitional area between the undivided and divided parts of the root.

**Q7. What are the predisposing factors for furcation involvement?**
Ans. Cervical enamel projections; trauma from occlusion; pulpal periodontal disease; iatrogenic cofactors and root fractures involving furcations.

**Q8. Which factors should be considered in projecting the prognosis of the tooth with furcation involvement?**
Ans. The extent of involvement, the status of bone support, root separation, and health of neighboring teeth.

**Q9. Who described furcation plasty?**
Ans. Hamp, Nyman, and Lindhe in 1975.

**Q10. How is furcation classified according to Goldman and Cohen?**
Ans. Grade I: Incipient lesion; Grade II: Cul-de-sac lesion; Grade III: Through and through the lesion.

# Periodontal Plastic Surgery

*Ajay Mahajan, Neeraj Deshpande*

## Chapter Outline

- Objectives
- Selection Criteria
- Techniques for Increasing Attached Gingiva
- Root Coverage Gingival Recession
- Techniques for Frenectomy
- Techniques for Vestibular Extension
- Techniques for Papilla Reconstruction
- Techniques for Alveolar Ridge Augmentation

## INTRODUCTION

Mucogingival therapy was defined as the correction of defects in morphology, position, or amount of soft tissue and underlying bone. This is the most comprehensive definition because it includes both nonsurgical and surgical mucogingival therapy of the gingiva, alveolar mucosa, and bone, such as papilla reconstruction by means of orthodontics or restorative dentistry. The term "mucogingival surgery" was initially used in the literature by Friedman in 1957; he referred to corrective surgery of the alveolar mucosa and the gingiva which included problems with attached gingiva, aberrant frenum and shallow vestibule.[1]

The 1996 World Workshop renamed mucogingival surgery as periodontal plastic surgery,[2] a term proposed initially by Miller in 1993, because the term "mucogingival surgery" did not adequately describe all the periodontal procedures that were being performed under this section.[3] The goal is the creation of form and appearance that is acceptable and pleasing to both patient and therapist. The word "plastic" means "to mold or shape," therefore periodontal plastic surgery, literally means "to mold or shape the tissues around the teeth or implants to create optimal esthetics."

Periodontal plastic surgery is defined as the surgical procedures performed to correct or eliminate anatomic, developmental or traumatic deformities of the gingiva or alveolar mucosa.[2] It includes the following:
- Periodontal prosthetic corrections
- Crown lengthening
- Ridge augmentation
- Esthetic surgical corrections
- Coverage of the denuded root surface
- Reconstruction of papillae
- Esthetic surgical correction around implants
- Surgical exposure of unerupted teeth for orthodontics

## OBJECTIVES

The objectives of the periodontal plastic surgery are to deal with the problems associated with:[4]
- *Attached gingiva*: Widening the attached gingiva enhances plaque removal around the gingival margin, improves esthetics, and reduces inflammation around restored teeth.
- *Shallow vestibule*: The sulcular brushing technique requires toothbrush placement at the gingival margin, which may not be possible with reduced vestibular depth. Adequate vestibular depth may also be necessary for proper placement of the removable prosthesis.
- *Aberrant frenum*: A frenum that encroaches on the margin of the gingiva may interfere with plaque removal, and tension on this frenum may tend to open the sulcus.
- Papilla
- *Resorbed alveolar ridge*.

## SELECTION CRITERIA

- *Surgical site free of plaque, calculus, and inflammation*: Periodontal plastic surgery procedures should be undertaken in a plaque and inflammation free environment to enable precise incisions on the firm gingival tissue.

- *Adequate blood supply to the donor tissue*: Root coverage procedures present a portion of the recipient site (denuded root surface) without blood supply. A pedicle displaced flap has a better blood supply than a free graft, with the base of the flap intact. If the anatomy is favorable, the pedicle flap is the best procedure for localized root coverage. The subepithelial connective tissue graft and the pouch and tunnel techniques use a split-flap with the connective tissue sandwiched between the flaps. This flap design maximizes the blood supply to the donor tissue. If large areas require root coverage, these sandwich-type recipient sites provide the best flap design.
- *Anatomy of the recipient site*: The presence or absence of vestibular depth is an important anatomic criterion at the recipient site for gingival augmentation. If gingival augmentation is indicated apical to the area of recession, there must be adequate vestibular depth apical to the recessed gingival margin to provide space for either a free or pedicle graft. When split-thickness, sandwich-type flap, e.g., the subepithelial connective graft is indicated, then an adequate amount of gingival thickness is required at the recipient site.
- *Anatomy of the donor site*: Pedicle displacement of tissue necessitates the presence of an adjacent donor site that presents gingival thickness and width. Palatal tissue thickness is also necessary for the connective tissue donor autograft.
- Stability of the grafted tissue to the recipient site.
- *Minimal trauma to the surgical site*: Poor incisions, flap perforations, tears, traumatic and excessive placement of sutures can lead to tissue necrosis. The selection of proper instruments, needles, and sutures are mandatory to minimize tissue trauma. Sharp contoured blades, smaller diameter needles, and resorbable monofilament sutures should be used for atraumatic surgery.

## TECHNIQUES FOR INCREASING ATTACHED GINGIVA

### Techniques

Following are the techniques for increasing attached gingiva:
- *Gingival augmentation apical to recession*:
  - Free epithelial autograft
  - Free connective tissue autograft
  - Apically positioned flap
  - Fenestration
  - Vestibular extension
- *Gingival augmentation coronal to recession or root coverage*:
  - Free epithelial autograft
  - Free connective tissue autograft
  - Pedicle autografts:
    - Rotational:
      - Lateral pedicle
      - Double papilla
    - Advanced:
      - Coronally displaced
      - Semilunar
  - Subepithelial connective tissue
  - Subpedicle connective tissue
  - Pouch and tunnel technique
  - Envelope technique
  - Guided tissue regeneration technique

## Epithelial or Free Gingival Graft

In a brief report from Sweden, Bjorn (1963) published the first illustrated success of gingival grafting. Free epithelial grafts are used to create a widened zone of attached gingiva.[5]

### Procedure[5-7]

- *Step I: Inject anesthesia*: Adequate anesthesia is injected on to the recipient as well as donor sites.
- *Step II: Prepare the recipient site*: A firm connective tissue bed is prepared to receive the graft. The recipient site can be prepared by incising at the existing mucogingival junction with a 15 No. blade to the desired depth, blending the incision on both ends with the existing mucogingival line. The incision is extended to approximately twice the desired width of the attached gingiva, which allows for 50% contraction of the graft when healing is complete. Insert 15 No. blade along the cut gingival margin, and separate a flap consisting of epithelium and underlying connective tissue without disturbing the periosteum. The recipient bed should be smooth and essentially free of muscle attachment tissue. At this point, gauze square is packed between the wound and the lip or cheek to limit bleeding and promote hemostasis in the recipient area while the donor tissue is being obtained.
- *Step III: Obtain the graft from the donor site*: Donor site may be gingivectomy tissue, an edentulous ridge, or the palate. The amount of donor palatal tissue needed can be accurately determined by using a foil template. Place the template over the donor site and make a shallow incision around it with a 15 No. blade. All palatal incisions are made in such a fashion so as to create a butt joint margin at the donor site. Insert the blade to the desired thickness at one edge of the graft. Elevate the edge and hold it with tissue forceps. Continue to separate the graft with the blade, lifting it gently, and as separation progresses, visibility increases. A partial-thickness graft consisting of epithelium and a thin layer of underlying connective tissue is used. The ideal thickness of the graft is between 1.0 and 1.5 mm. Thinner graft shrivels and exposes the recipient site while thicker graft jeopardizes the circulation and nutrient diffusion.

- *Step IV: Transfer and immobilize the graft*: Pressure The recipient site is applied to remove the excess clot as a thick clot interferes with the vascularization of the graft. Suture the graft at the lateral borders and to the periosteum to secure it in position. The graft should be immobilized because any movement interferes with healing. Avoid excessive tension, which can distort the graft from the underlying surface.
- *Step V: Protect the donor site*: Once the graft is free, firm pressure should be applied to the donor site with a gauze square. Cover the donor site with a periodontal pack for one week and repeat it if necessary. A modified Hawley retainer is useful to cover the pack on the palate.
- *Step VI: Postoperative instructions*: Instructions to the patient are most important to the graft's success. The patient should be advised not to brush at the recipient site for the week. The patient should not retract the lip or cheek to observe the graft. No postoperative factor will facilitate failure in soft-tissue grafting to the degree that smoking does. Smoking causes constriction of capillaries, diminished blood flow to the area, poor oxygenation of tissue causing sloughing of the graft. Thus, the patient is instructed to quit smoking immediately preoperatively and abstain for the 1st week (preferably for two weeks).
- *Step VII: Suture removal*: Sutures are removed after 7–10 days **(Figs. 53.1A to E)**.

### Drawbacks

Drawbacks of epithelialized palatal graft for the root coverage procedure are as follows:
- Blood supply to the graft is available on only one surface, rather than two, as with the connective tissue graft.
- The color match of the tissues is a problem between the grafted area and the adjacent tissues.
- A palatal wound is more invasive, more prone to hemorrhage, and heal slowly.
- It is a sensitive and time-consuming technique.

### Postoperative Healing

- *Phase I: Plasmatic circulation (0–3 days)*: A thin layer of exudate is present between the graft and the recipient bed. The grafted tissue survives with an avascular "plasmatic circulation" from the recipient bed. The epithelium of the free graft degenerates early in the initial healing phase, and subsequently, it becomes desquamated. The graft area over the avascular root surface receives nutrients from the connective tissue bed that surrounds the recession[8,9] **(Figs. 53.2A to C)**.
- *Phase II: Vascularization (2–11 days)*: Anastomoses establish between the blood vessels of the recipient bed and those in the grafted tissue, which is characterized by capillary proliferation. Thus, the circulation of blood is reestablished in the preexisting blood vessels of the graft. Epithelium from the adjacent tissues proliferates, causing the reepithelialization of the graft **(Fig. 53.2D)**.
- *Phase III: Organic union (11–42 days)*: Tissue maturation phase: The graft's vascular system appears normal. The epithelium gradually matures with the formation of a keratin layer during this stage of healing **(Fig. 53.2E)**.

The two ways of root coverage are primary root coverage and secondary root coverage. Primary root coverage is found initially after grafting, whereas secondary root coverage is through creeping attachment. In 1964, Goldman et al. noted a second mechanism of gaining root coverage by the phenomenon of creeping attachment. This occurs between one month and one year which is the result of coronal migration of newly grafted attached gingiva over the portions of a previously denuded root.

Factors associated with incomplete coverage are as follows:
- Improper classification of marginal tissue recession.
- Improper preparation of the recipient site.
- Inadequate root planing or failure to treat planed root with citric acid.
- *Graft factors*: Inadequate graft size or graft thickness, dehydration of graft, an inadequate adaptation of graft

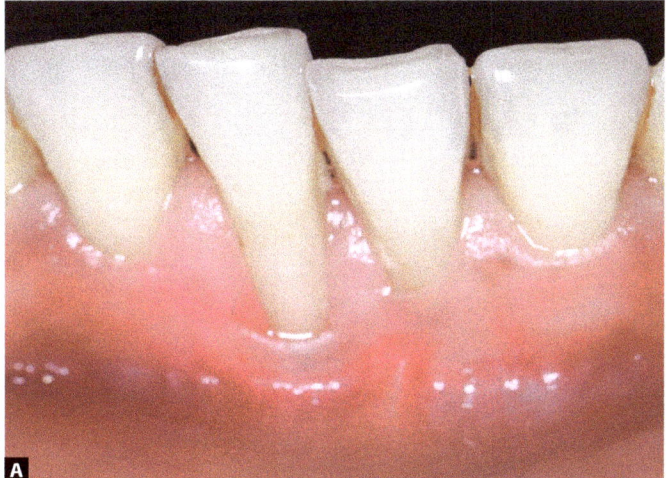
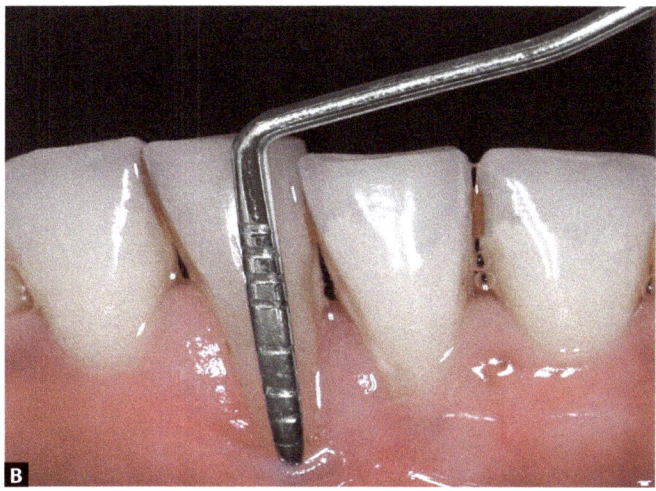

**Figs. 53.1A and B**

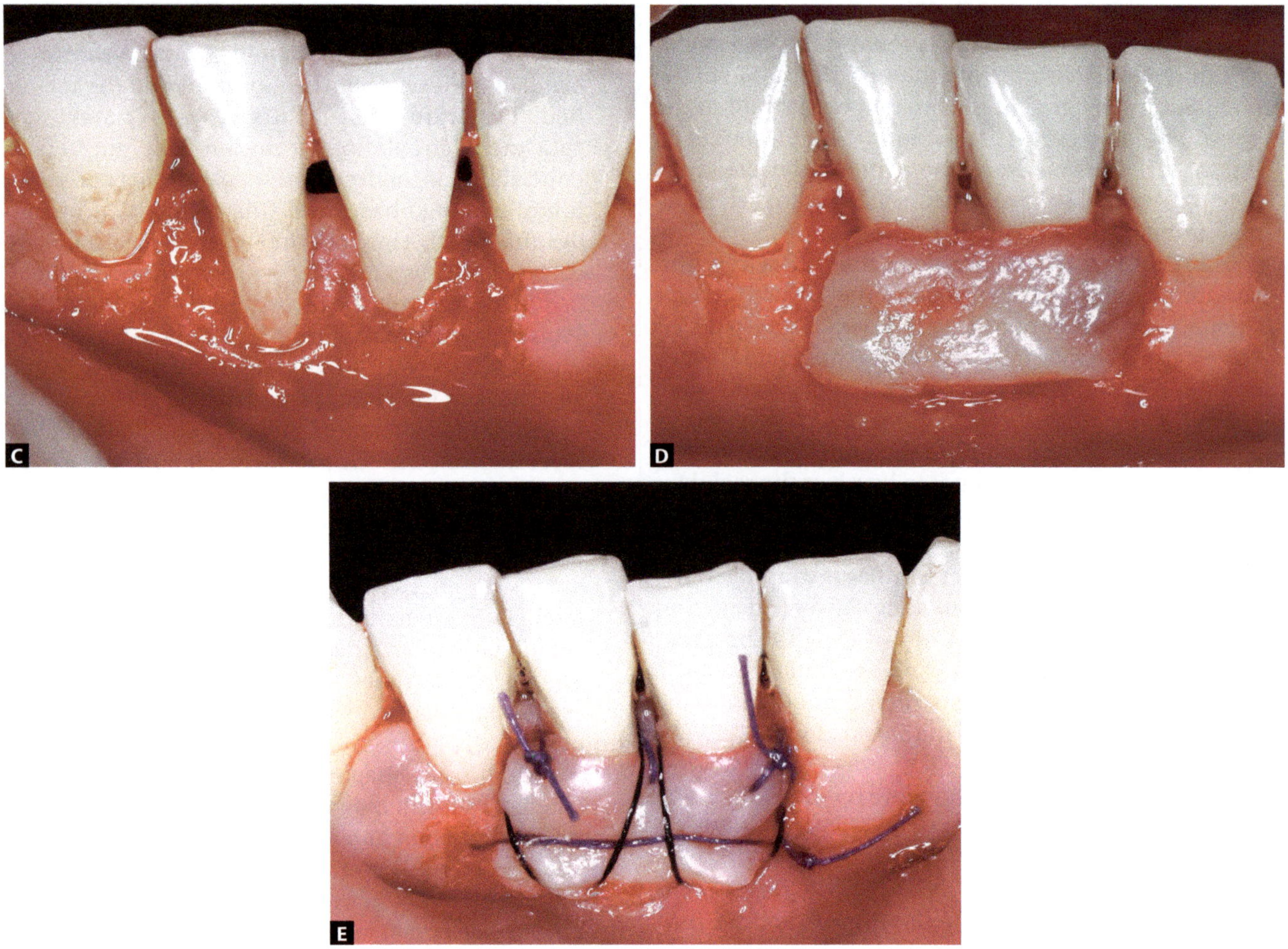

**Section 7:** Treatment: Surgical Therapy

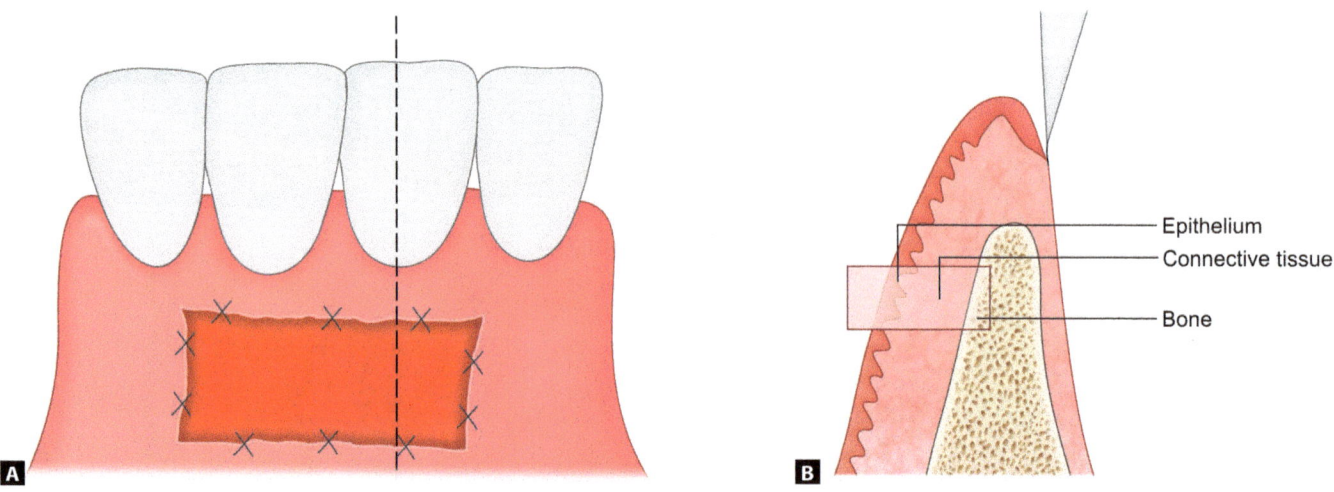

**Figs. 53.1C to E**

**Figs. 53.1A to E:** Clinical picture showing free gingival grafting procedure: (A and B) Preoperative lack of attached gingiva on 41 and 31 (recipient sites); (C) Surgical recipient sites prepared; (D) Free gingival graft placed over recipient site that was procured from palate; (E) Free gingival graft sutured over the recipient sites.

**Figs. 53.1A and B**

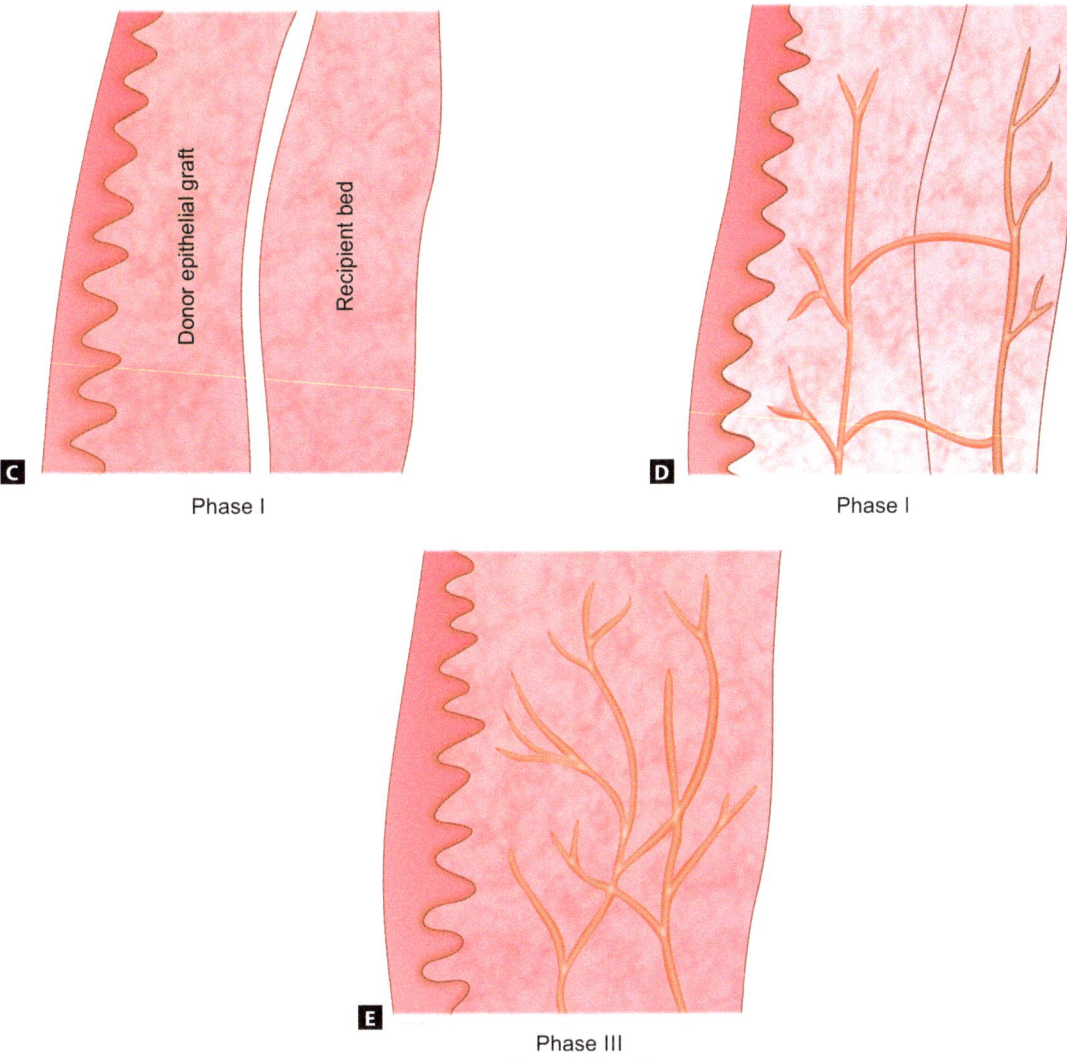

**Figs. 53.2A to E:** Schematic representation showing healing of the free epithelial graft.

to root and remaining periosteal bed, failure to stabilize the graft, excess or prolonged pressure in coadaptation of the graft.
- *Patient factors*: Excessive smoking, alcohol, or noncompliance.

## ROOT COVERAGE GINGIVAL RECESSION

Indications for root coverage procedure are to reduce root sensitivity, improve esthetics, and manage defects resulting from root caries removal or cervical abrasions.

### Etiological Factors
- Anatomical or developmental factors:
  - *Dehiscence*: Abnormal direction of tooth eruption, malposition of teeth, the buccolingual thickness of root more than crestal bone thickness, morphotypes having narrow long teeth and orthodontic tooth movement
  - Fenestration
  - Lack of attached gingiva
  - Abnormal path of tooth eruption
  - Individual tooth shape
  - Tooth eruption compensation
  - Abnormal tooth position in the arch
- *Physiological factors*:
  - Senile atrophy or the aging process
  - Genetic predisposition
  - *Orthodontic movement of teeth*: Controlled and erratic
- *Pathological factors*:
  - Gingivitis or periodontitis
  - *Chronic trauma*: Impaction of foreign bodies against gingiva and factitious injuries, fingernail scratching of the gums, over rigorous and incorrect toothbrushing and occlusal injury
  - Frenal pull
  - Tobacco chewing
  - Acute traumatic injuries
  - *Psychological factors*: Stress and emotions

## Etiopathogenesis

It is based on inflammation and subsequent destruction of the connective tissue of free gingiva. The oral epithelium migrates to the borders of destroyed connective tissue. The thickening of gingival and sulcular basal lamina reduces the quantity of connective tissue between them. Thus, the blood supply is reduced, negatively influencing the repair of the initial lesion. As the lesion progresses, connective tissue disappears and oral epithelium fuse with junctional or sulcular epithelium. In a recession caused by plaque and calculus, an initial ulcer appears in the junctional epithelium, and the destruction of connective tissue occurs from inside out. In toothbrush trauma lesions, destruction occurs from outside in.

## Classifications

- *According to Miller[10] (1985)*: The marginal tissue recession was classified as:
    - *Class I*: Marginal tissue recession not extending to the mucogingival junction. No loss of interdental bone or soft tissue **(Figs. 53.3A and B)**.
    - *Class II*: Marginal tissue recession extends to or beyond the mucogingival junction. No loss of interdental bone or soft tissue **(Figs. 53.3C and D)**.
    - *Class III*: Marginal tissue recession extends to or beyond the mucogingival junction. Loss of interdental bone or soft tissue or malpositioning of the tooth **(Figs. 53.3E and F)**.
    - *Class IV*: Marginal tissue recession extends beyond the mucogingival junction. Loss of interdental bone and soft tissue loss interdentally and/or severe tooth malposition **(Figs. 53.3G and H)**.

- *According to Sullivan and Atkins[11] (1968)*: Gingival recession was classified as follows:
    - Shallow-narrow
    - Shallow-wide
    - Deep-narrow
    - Deep-wide
- *According to Mahajan[12] (2014)*: Gingival recession defects were classified as:
    - Class I Gingival recession defects (GRD) not extending to the mucogingival junction (MGJ)
    - Class II GRD extending to the MGJ/beyond it
    - Class III GRD with bone or soft-tissue loss in the interdental area up to cervical 1/3 of the root surface and/or malpositioning of the teeth
    - Class IV GRD with severe bone or soft-tissue loss in the interdental area greater than cervical $1/3^{rd}$ of the root surface and/or severe malpositioning of the teeth.
    
    Prognosis
    BEST: Class I and Class II with thick gingival profile.
    GOOD: Class I and Class II with thin gingival profile.
    FAIR: Class III with thick gingival profile.
    POOR: Class III and Class IV with thin gingival profile.

### Classification of Soft-tissue Procedures used for Root Coverage

Cohen classified soft-tissue grafting procedures as:
- *Free soft tissue autografts*:
    - Epithelial graft
    - Subepithelial connective tissue graft
- *Contiguous or pedicle soft tissue flap*:
    - *Rotational flap*:
        - Laterally positioned flap

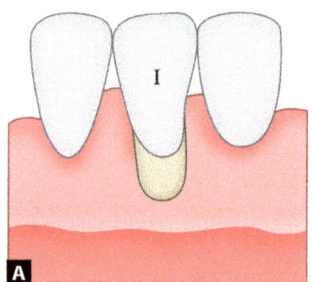 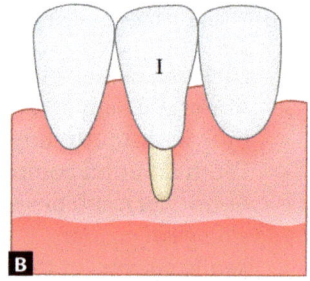 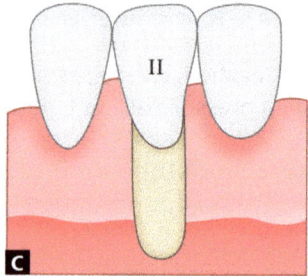 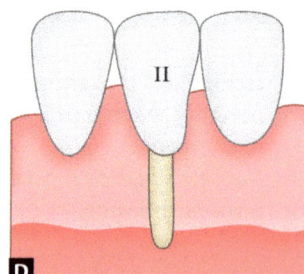
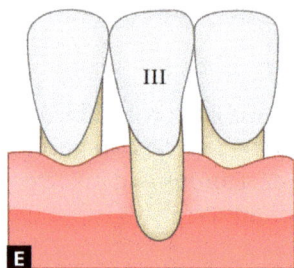 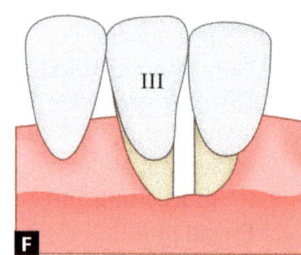 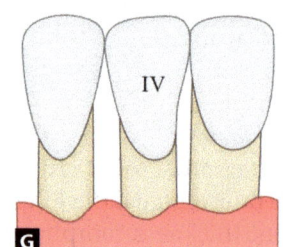 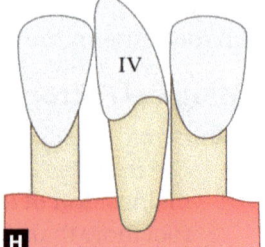

**Figs. 53.3A to H:** Schematic representation showing PD Miller's classification of marginal tissue recession: (A and B) Grade-I; (C and D) Grade-II; (E and F) Grade-III; (G and H) Grade-IV.

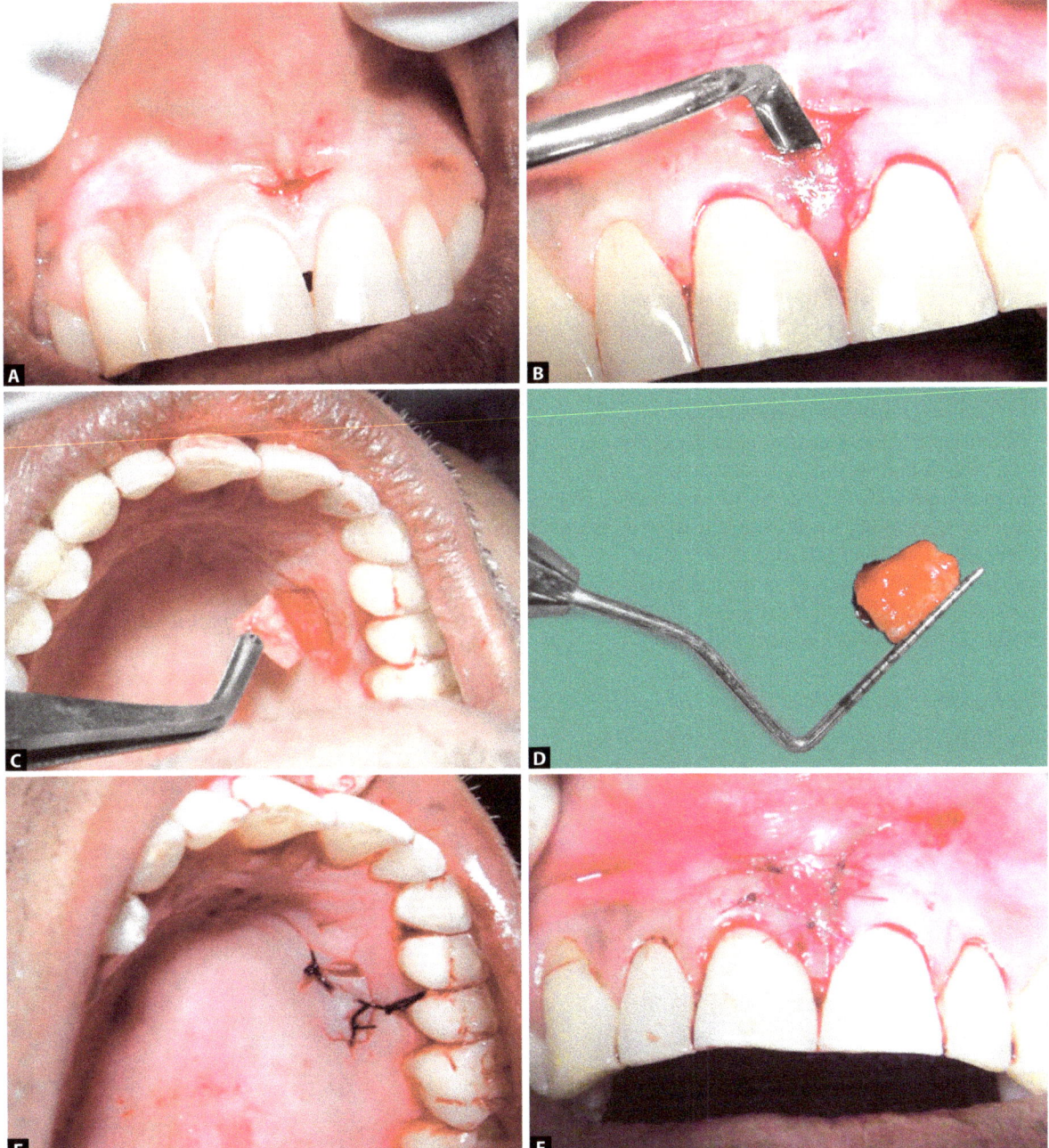

**Figs. 53.4A to F:** Clinical picture showing subepithelial connective tissue graft: (A) Incision is given at the recipient site; (B) Recipient bed is prepared for subepithelial connective tissue graft; (C) Flap is raised and underlying connective tissue to be used as donor tissue; (D) Donor connective tissue; (E) Overlying flap sutured back after taking the donor connective tissue; (F) Donor connective tissue sutured at the recipient site.
(*Courtesy*: Dr Alka Kaushik)

- ♦ Oblique rotated flap
- ♦ Double papillae flap
- *Advanced flap*: Coronally positioned flap.

## Subepithelial Connective Tissue Graft

It was described by Langer and Langer[13] in 1985. This procedure is indicated for larger and multiple defects with good vestibular depth and gingival thickness to allow a split-thickness flap to be elevated. Adjacent to the denuded root surface, the donor connective tissue is sandwiched between the split-flap **(Figs. 53.4A to F)**.

### Procedure

- *Step I: Incisions and flap reflection*: Raise a partial-thickness flap with a horizontal incision 2 mm away from the papilla tip and two vertical incisions 1–2 mm away from the gingival margin of the adjoining teeth. These incisions should extend at least one half to one

tooth wider mesiodistally than the area of gingival recession. Extend the flap to the mucobuccal fold without perforations that could affect the blood supply.
- *Step II: Scaling and planing*: Thoroughly scale and plane the root surface, reducing the root surface's prominence.
- *Step III: Obtaining the graft*: From the palate, obtain connective tissue graft by means of a horizontal incision 5–6 mm from the gingival margin of molars and premolars. The connective tissue is carefully obtained, and all adipose and glandular tissues are removed. The donor site is sutured after the graft is removed.
- *Step IV: Transferring the graft*: Place the connective tissue on the denuded root. Suture it with resorbable sutures to the periosteum. Good stability of the graft must be attained with adequate sutures.
- *Step V: Suturing*: Cover the graft with the outer portion of the partial-thickness flap and suture it interdentally. At least one-half to two-thirds of the connective tissue graft must be covered by the flap for the exposed portion to survive over the denuded root.
- *Step VI: Covering the graft*: Cover the grafted site with dry aluminium foil and periodontal dressing. After 7 days, the dressing and sutures are removed.

### Laterally Positioned Pedicle Flap

It was originally developed by Grupe and Warren[14] in 1956.

### Procedure

Following are the steps for lateral positioned pedicle flap **(Figs. 53.5 and 53.6)**:
- *Step I: Incisions*: Make an incision, resecting the gingival margin around the exposed root. Remove the resected soft tissue and scale and plane the root surface. With the blade held at right angles to the gingiva's surface, a horizontal incision to the depth of the bevel of the blade is made 1–2 mm below the free margin of the gingiva of the donor tooth and extending nearly to the proximal line angle of the next tooth. From that proximal line angle, a vertical incision is made into connective tissue parallel to the exposed root.
- *Step II: Cut-back incision*: It is given at the distal corner of the flap into the alveolar mucosa, pointing in the direction of the recipient site.
- *Step III: Prepare the flap*: A split-thickness flap is then prepared by sharp dissection within the area delineated by these incisions so that a layer of connective tissue is left covering the bone in the donor area when the flap is laterally displaced over the denuded root surface.
- *Step IV: Transfer the flap*: Slide the flap laterally onto the adjacent denuded root, making sure that it lies flat and firm without excess tension on the base. Suture the flap to the adjacent gingiva and alveolar mucosa with interrupted sutures. Sling suture is made around the involved tooth to prevent the flap from slipping apically.

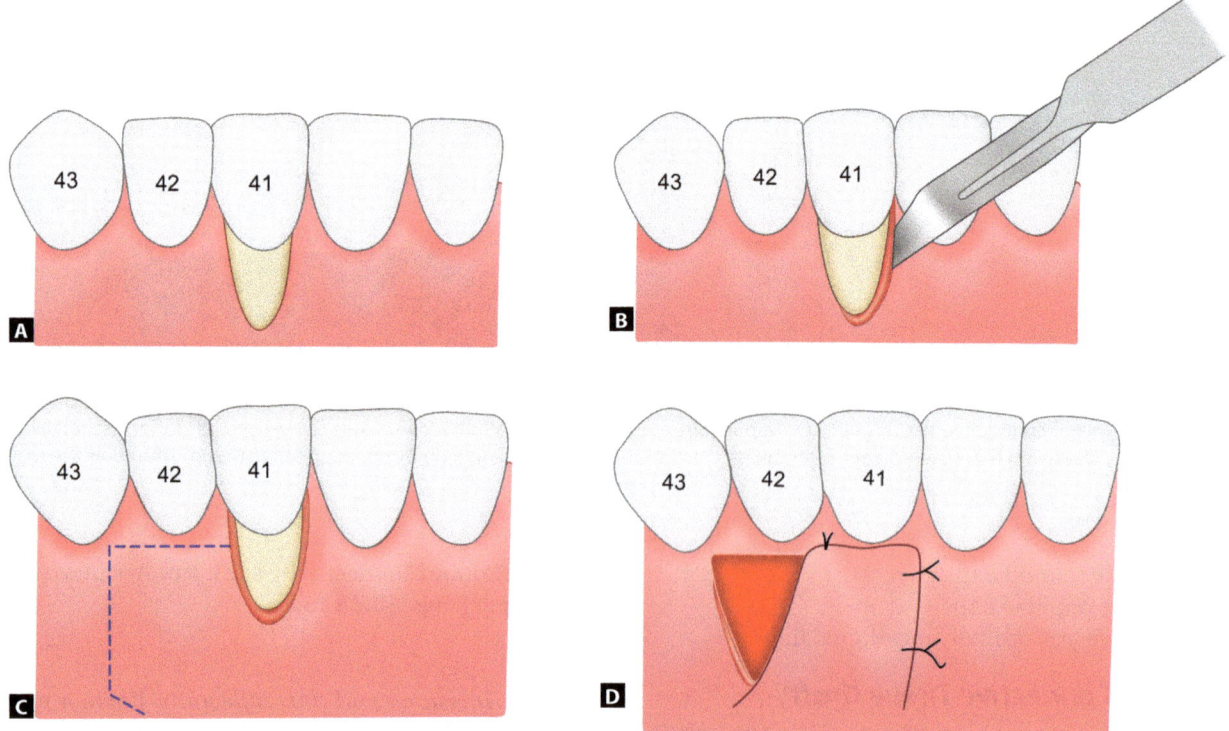

**Figs. 53.5A to D:** Schematic representation showing laterally displaced flap procedure: (A) Grade I recession on 41; 42 and 43 are donor sites with sufficient amount of attached gingiva; (B) Resecting gingival margin around the exposed root of 41; (C) Vertical and horizontal incisions around the donor sites 42 and 43; (D) Flap laterally displaced from 42, 43 to 41 and sutured.

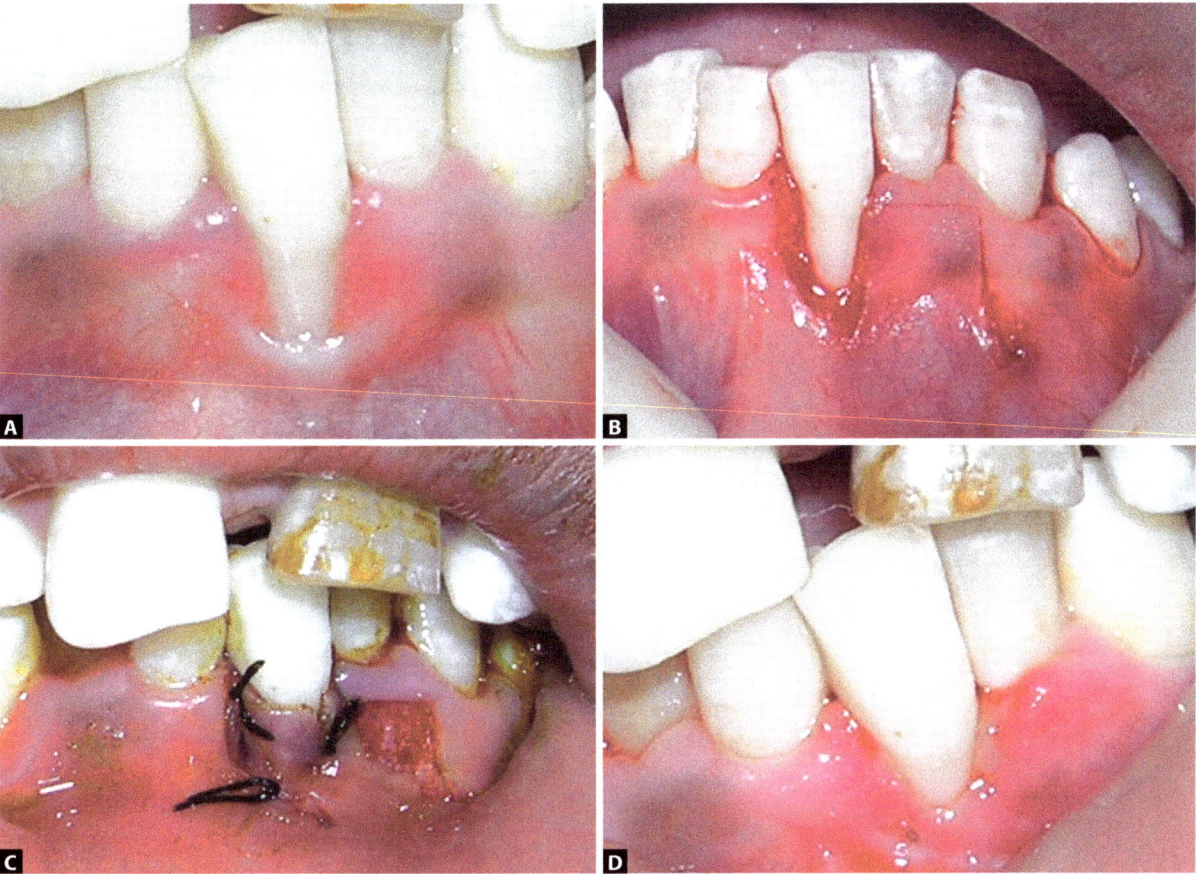

**Figs. 53.6A to D:** Clinical picture showing laterally displaced flap procedure: (A) Preoperative recession site; (B) Vertical and horizontal incisions around the donor site; (C) Flap laterally displaced and sutured; (D) Postoperative site.

- *Step V: Protect the flap and donor site*: Cover the operative field with aluminium foil and periodontal dressing, extending it interdentally and onto the lingual surface to secure it.
- *Step VI: Postoperative instructions*: These are given thereafter.
- *Step VII: Sutures removal*: Sutures are removed after 7–10 days.

*Advantages:*
- Single surgical site
- Esthetic, close color blend
- Good vascularity

*Disadvantages:*
- Dehiscence or fenestration at the donor site
- Possibility of recession at the donor site
- Limited to one or two teeth with a recession

*Contraindications*
- Shallow vestibule
- Lack of keratinized attached gingiva
- Excessive root prominence
- Presence of deep interproximal pockets
- Deep or extensive root abrasion or erosion
- Significant loss of interproximal bone height

### Modifications of Lateral Pedicle Flap

The variants of the lateral pedicle flap are shown in **Figs. 53.7A to E**.
A. Original Grupe design was given in 1956
B. Submarginal incision
C. Cut-back incision was given by Corn in 1964
D. Rotated pedicle flap-without cut back incision was given by Dhalberg in 1969
E. Split-full rotated pedicle flap without cut back incision was given by Goldman in 1982

## Double Papilla Flap Procedures

It is a variant of lateral pedicle flap in which the basic technique is similar except that the donor tissue is mobilized from the two adjacent papillae rather than from a single adjacent tooth papilla.

### Indications
- When the interproximal papillae adjacent to the mucogingival problem are sufficiently wide.
- When the attached gingiva on an approximating tooth is insufficient to allow for a laterally positioned flap.
- When a periodontal pocket is not present.

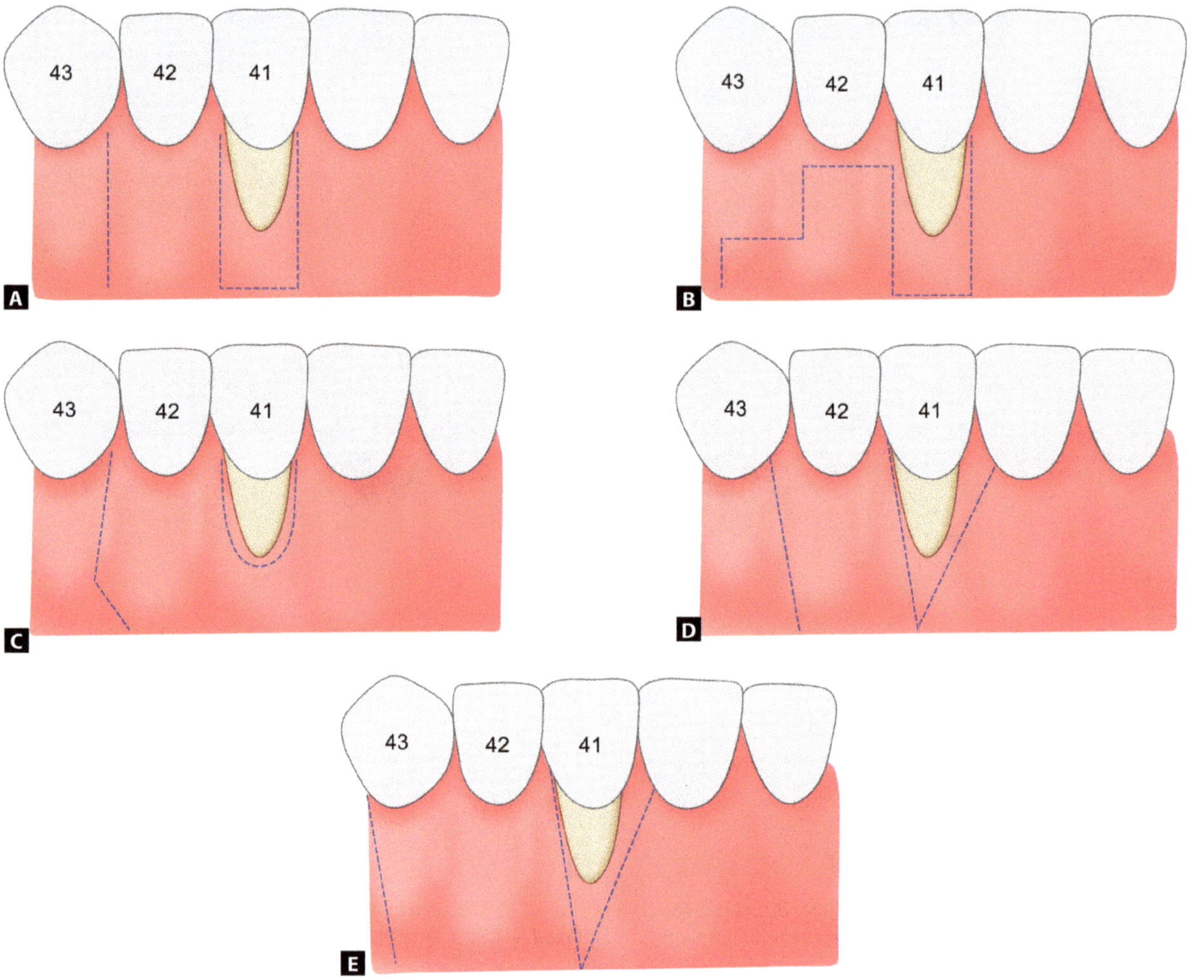

**Section 7:** Treatment: Surgical Therapy

**Figs. 53.7A to E:** Schematic representation showing modifications of lateral pedicle flap.

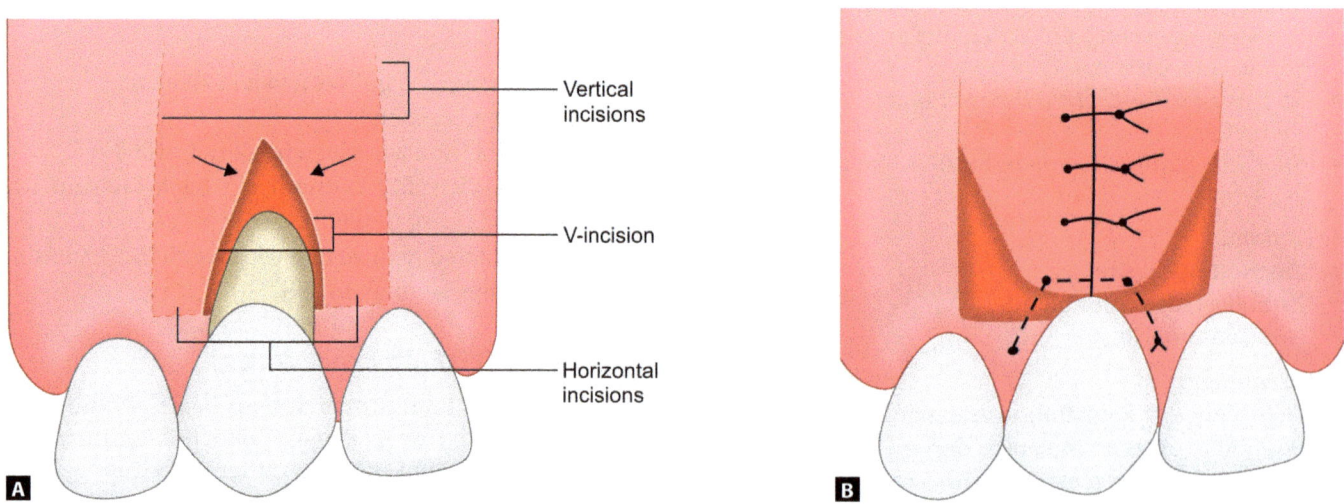

**Figs. 53.8A and B:** Schematic representation showing double papilla flap procedure.

### Procedures

Following are the steps for double Papilla flap procedure[15] **(Figs. 53.8A and B)**.

- *Step I: Incision*: V-shaped incision is made around the recessed gingiva margin to expose connective tissue at its edge. The incision is extended to the depth of, but not including the periosteum. V-section (wedge of gingiva) is then removed, and the root surface is scaled thoroughly.
- *Step II: Lateral releasing or vertical incisions*: These are made at the mesiofacial and distofacial line angles of

the adjacent teeth. Horizontal incisions are made across the top of papillae.
- *Step III: Flap reflection*: The two papillary tissues is grasped with rat-tail tissue pliers and gently lifted as it is separated from its underlying tissue by means of surgical blade No. 15. Care must be taken not to lift the periosteum, puncture, or severe the flap. The two papillary flaps are raised and repositioned to cover the exposed root.
- *Step IV: Suturing*: The flaps are sutured together. The suture needle is passed through the outer surface of the first papilla and on through the second papilla's undersurface. Resorbable 5-0 medium gut sutures are used for suturing.
- *Step V: Postoperative instructions*: These are given thereafter.

*Advantages:*
- The risk of resorption of alveolar bone is minimized because the interdental bone is more resistant to loss than is radicular bone.
- The clinical predictability of the procedure is good.
- Papilla usually supplies a greater width of the attached gingiva than the radicular surface of the tooth.
- Less tension is placed on the donor tissue.

*Disadvantages:*
- Two flaps are sutured over the root surface.
- Manipulation of freed papilla during suture is difficult.

## Coronally Displaced Flap

The purpose of the coronally displaced flap is to create a split-thickness flap in the area apical to the denuded root and position it coronally to cover the root.

### Indication
Cover denuded root surface with adequate width of keratinized gingiva.

### Procedure
- *Step I: Incisions*: Internal bevel incision is given from the gingival margin to the bottom of the pocket on the selected site. At each end of internal bevel incision, vertical incisions are given beyond the mucogingival junction, to delineate the flap.
- *Step II: Flap reflection*: Partial-thickness flap is raised with surgical blade No. 11 or 15.
- *Step III: Scaling and planing*: Scaling and planing are done on the root surface with the help of curettes.
- *Step IV: Suturing*: The flap is then sutured to the level coronal to the pre-treatment position to cover the recession. Cover the area with a periodontal pack.

## Semilunar Coronally Displaced Flap

This technique was given by Tarnow.[16] The technique is very simple and predictably provides 2-3 mm of root coverage, which is successful for the maxilla. It is not recommended for mandibular teeth.

### Procedure
The following are the steps for Semilunar coronally displaced flap procedure[15] **(Figs. 53.9A to C)**.
- *Step I—Incision*: A semilunar incision is made following the curvature of the receded gingival margin and ending about 2-3 mm short of the papillae's tip so that the flap derives all of its blood supply from the papillary areas.
- *Step II—Split-thickness dissection*: Perform a split-thickness dissection of the facially located tissue by an intracrevicular incision extending apically to the level of the semilunar incision.
- *Step III*: The tissue collapse coronally, covering the denuded root. It is then held in its new position and

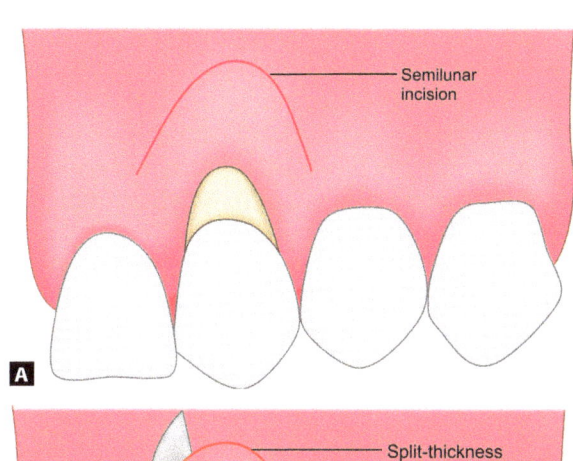

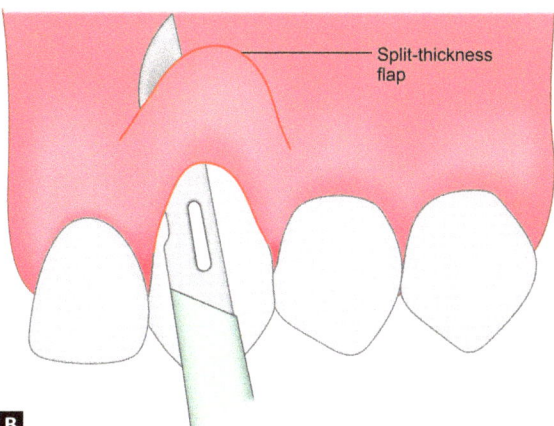

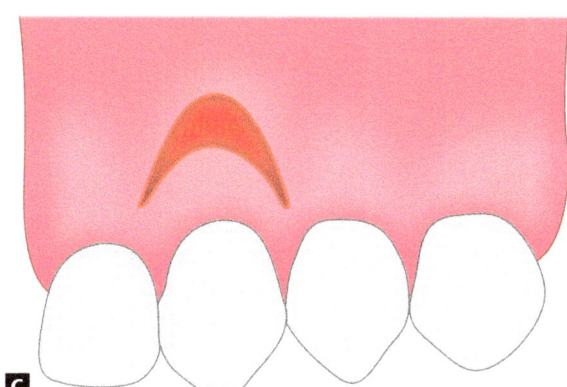

**Figs. 53.9A to C:** Schematic representation showing semilunar coronally displaced flap procedure.

stabilized by light pressure for 5 minutes; there is no need to suture or to pack.

*Advantages:*
- No shortening of the vestibule
- It can treat multiple areas of recession
- Flaps are not under tension and require no sutures

*Disadvantages:*
- Fails if adjacent papillae are not wide enough because flap derives its blood supply from adjacent papillae.
- It cannot be used in mandibular teeth with narrow interdental papillae.

## TECHNIQUES FOR FRENECTOMY

Frena are sickle-shaped folds normally found in the maxillary and mandibular alveolar mucosa in canine, premolar area, and between central incisors.

Morphologic functional classification of labial frenum attachments[17] (Placek Mirko 1974) are as follows:
- Mucosal attachment refers to an attachment of the frenum to the mucogingival junction.
- Gingival attachment refers to an attachment of the frenum within the attached gingiva.
- Papillary attachment refers to an attachment of the frenum within the papilla.
- Papilla penetrating attachment refers to frenal fibers when it crosses the alveolar process and extends up to palatine papilla.

Other variations of normal frenal attachment, according to Kakodhar[18] (2009) are as follows:
- Simple frenum with:
  - A nodule
  - Appendix
  - Nichum
- Bifid labial frenum
- Persistent tectolabial
- Double frenum
- Wider frenum

### Frenectomy

Frenectomy is the complete removal of the frenum, including its attachment to the underlying bone, whereas frenotomy is the incision of the frenum.

### Indications
- *Gingival or papillary frenal attachment*: To eliminate well-developed frenum that penetrates the gingival papilla to its origin on the incisive papilla.
- *High-frenum attachment*: Where oral hygiene is hindered by shallow vestibule caused by high-frenum attachment.
- To facilitate orthodontic treatment, when spacing is there between maxillary central incisors due to thick frenum resisting orthodontic forces.
- *Gingival recession*: Where frenal fibers radiate into marginal gingiva producing gingival retraction and localized gingival recession. Thus, to control the recession of facial gingiva, a frenectomy is combined with vestibuloplasty.
- When lingual frenum interferes with speech.

### Instruments
- Mosquito forceps or hemostat.
- Surgical handle Bard-Parker No. 3 with detachable and replaceable surgical blades No. 15 or 11.

### Procedure
The following are the steps for the frenectomy procedure **(Figs. 53.10A and D)**.
- *Step I—Anesthesia*: Local infiltration is given to anesthetize the selected site.
- *Step II—Extending and gripping*: The lip is extended and, the frenum is gripped with mosquito forceps or hemostat to the depth of the vestibule.
- *Step III—Incisions*: Incisions are made above and below the instrument, the triangular frenum tissue is removed **(Figs. 53.10B and C)**. Underlying fibrous attachment to the bone is exposed **(Fig. 53.10D)**. A horizontal incision is given onto these fibers separating and dissecting from the bone.
- *Step IV—Suturing*: The edges of the wound are undermined slightly and approximated without creating tension and suture, only the incision's mucosal extent.

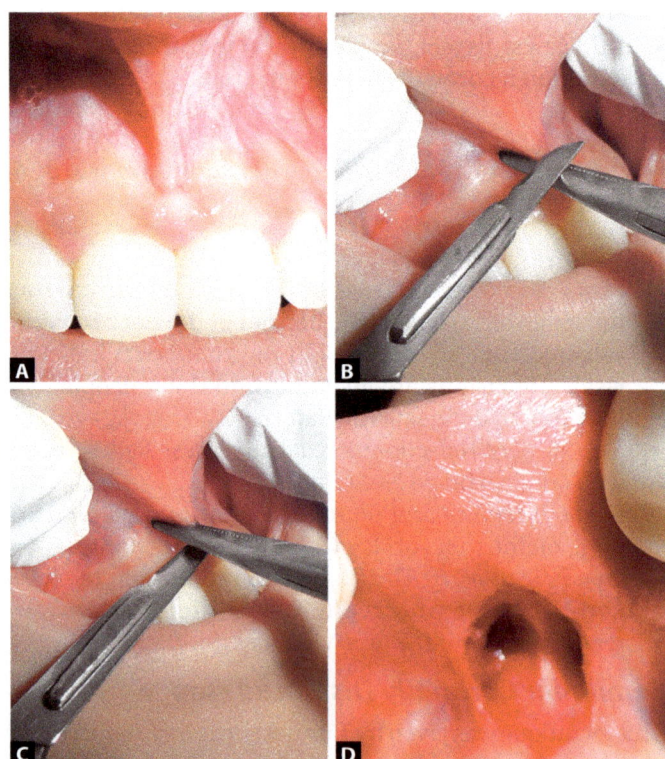

**Figs. 53.10A to D:** Clinical picture showing frenectomy.
(*Courtesy*: Dr Deepak Bala)

The gingival extent is not closed and allowed to heal by secondary intention. Cover the area with dry aluminium foil and then periodontal pack.
- *Step V—Postoperative instructions*: The most important postoperative instruction is to ask the patient not to stretch the lip again and again; thus, avoiding vigorous lip movements after the frenectomy procedure. Rest postoperative instructions are given in "Chapter 46: General Principles of Periodontal Surgery."

### Laser-assisted Frenectomy

The excision of frenum attachments can also be accomplished through a laser. The tendinous frenum attachment is ablated with the laser and often does not require suture reapproximation of the tissue because reepithelialization occurs from the wound margins. Frenectomies completed with the laser often respond well with fewer postoperative complaints of swelling and pain.

## TECHNIQUES FOR VESTIBULAR EXTENSION

The shallow vestibule was one of three original mucogingival problems cited by Friedman in the late 1950s that required the increased apicocoronal dimension of the gingiva. The termination of the orofacial muscles into the soft tissues covering the alveolar process forms the vestibular fornix. Shallow vestibular depth usually interferes with oral hygiene procedures causing ineffective plaque control. Vestibuloplasty is a procedure designed to extend the vestibular fornix. There are three basic procedures for extending the gingiva into the vestibule:
1. Gingival extension using periosteal fenestration.
2. Vestibuloplasty using modified Edlan-Mejchar procedure.
3. Gingival extension with a free epithelial graft.

### Objectives

- To enhance plaque control by allowing space for the effective use of plaque control aids.
- To gain more retention for removable prosthetic appliances by expanding the prosthesis bed.

## Gingival Extension using Periosteal Fenestration

Indications for the vestibular extension with periosteal fenestration include areas where a shallow vestibule puts tension on a broad region of the gingival margin, leading to progressive gingival recession. It is also indicated prior to the construction of partial prosthesis where the prosthesis bed's expansion is needed.

### Procedure

After adequate local anesthesia, an incision is made at or near the mucogingival junction, retaining all of the attached gingiva from the mucogingival junction to the margin of the gingiva. A split-thickness flap is then reflected using a broad surgical blade, with reflection beginning at the mucogingival junction. The muscle fibers and tissue are sharply dissected from the periosteum, freeing the mucosal flap, which is then sutured in the depth of the vestibule. Once the sutures are completed, a strip of the exposed periosteum is removed across the entire surgical area at the level of the original mucogingival junction, leaving a periosteal fenestration exposing bone. A dressing is placed over the surgical site to minimize patient discomfort. Following healing, the vestibular depth is maintained by scar tissue formed in the area of the fenestration.

## Vestibuloplasty using the Edlan–Mejchar Procedure

The Edlan–Mejchar procedure for vestibular deepening results in an increased width of the attached mucosa extending into the fornix. No new attached gingiva develops from this procedure; however, it can provide a widened band of alveolar mucosa extending into the deepened vestibule and fixed to the underlying tissue.[19]

### Indications

Indications for this procedure include the need for expansion of the prosthesis bed and cases of generalized recession over a large arch segment. This procedure is also indicated for the treatment of localized recession or for the elimination of a broad, high frenum.

### Contraindications

The Edlan–Mejchar procedure is contraindicated if a wide band of attached gingiva is needed to cover a recession area.

### Procedures

Two vertical incisions are made from the gingival margin to outline the area of the operative field. This is followed by a horizontal incision 10-12 mm from the alveolar margin into the depth of the vestibule. A mucosal flap is elevated, exposing the periosteum. The periosteum is then separated from the bone beginning at the margin of the alveolar crest, including the muscle fibers. The periosteal flap is then transposed to the lip, and the margins of the flap are sutured to the margin of the incision on the lip. Next, the mucosal flap is sutured at a depth of the vestibule **(Figs. 53.11A to E)**. Caution should be exercised during incisions and flap reflection in the mental foramen area to prevent trauma to the mental nerve or sever the blood vessels in this region. To help adapt the mucosal flap to the denuded bone, a moist gauze square is applied to the flap and held for 3-5 minutes with gentle pressure. This will help to control hemorrhage, reducing the chance of the flap being dislodged by a blood clot. A periodontal dressing is placed and carefully adapted to the vestibular contours.

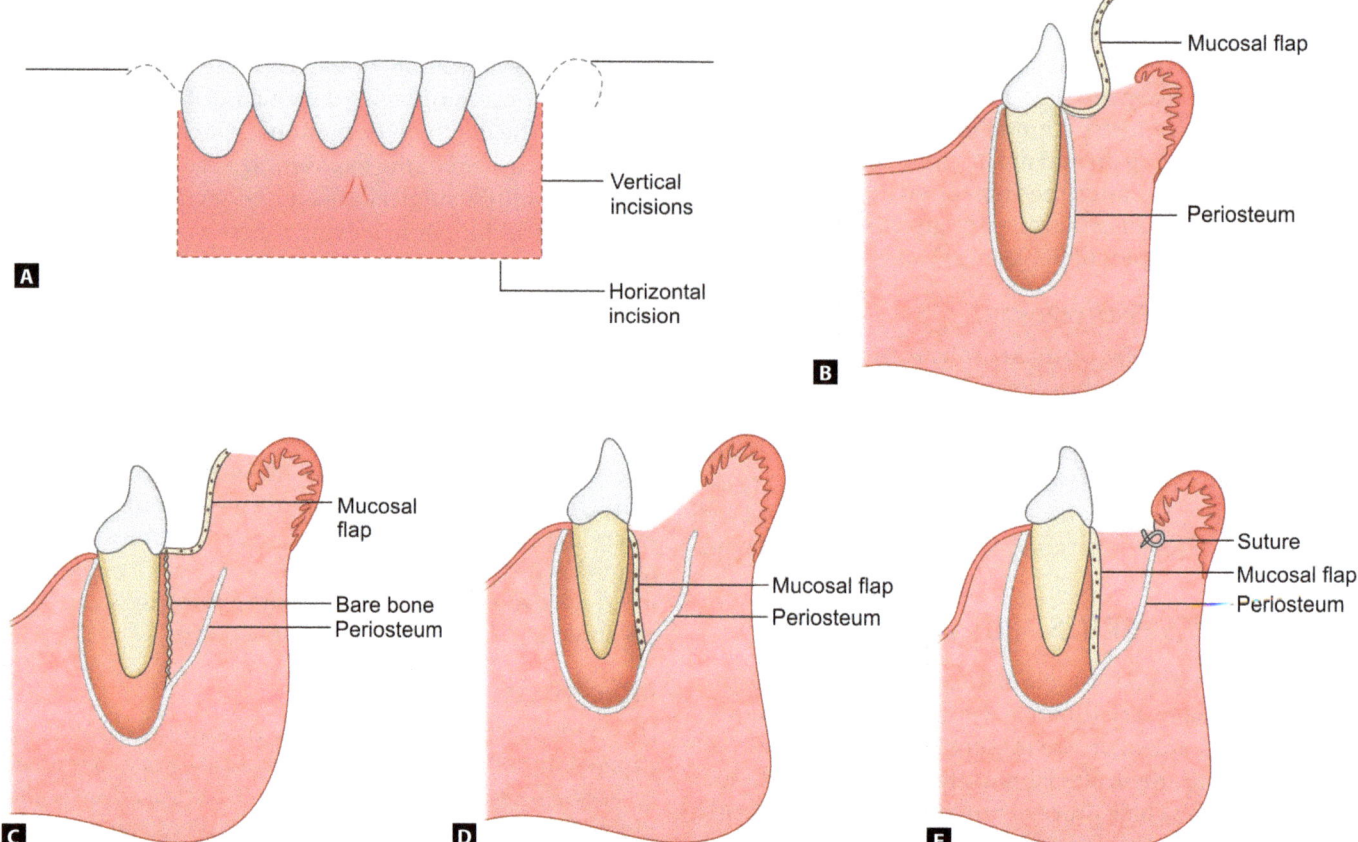

**Figs. 53.11A to E:** Schematic representation showing vestibuloplasty; Edlan–Mejchar operation: (A) Two vertical incisions are joined by horizontal incision; (B) Mucosal flap is elevated, exposing periosteum; (C) Periosteum is separated from bone; (D) Mucosal flap is folded down over the bone; (E) Periosteum is transposed to lip and sutured.
(*Courtesy*: Dr SK Salaria)

## TECHNIQUES FOR PAPILLA RECONSTRUCTION

The loss of a key papilla in an esthetic zone and a black triangle is an indication for papillary reconstruction evaluation. The complete regeneration of lost papillae is unpredictable; therefore, retention of the papilla is of great importance when an aesthetic result is desired from surgical procedures.

### Classification of Papillary Height

According to Nordland and Tarnow[20] (1998) **(Figs. 53.12A to D)**:

- *Normal*: The interdental papilla occupies the entire embrasure space apical to the interdental contact point or area.
- *Class-I*: The tip of the interdental papilla is located between the interdental contact point and the level of the cementoenamel junction (CEJ) on the proximal surface of the tooth.
- *Class-II*: The tip of the interdental papilla is located at or apical to the level of the CEJ on the proximal surface of the tooth but coronal to the level of the CEJ mid-buccally.
- *Class-III*: The tip of the interdental papilla is located at or apical to the level of CEJ mid-buccally.

The causes of loss of interdental papilla are tooth extraction, excessive surgical periodontal treatment, and localized progressive gingival and periodontal lesion.

The effects of loss of interdental papilla are cosmetic deformities, phonetic problems, and lateral food impaction.

### Procedure

The various methods to create interdental papilla are as follows:[21-23]

- *Nonsurgical papilla creation*:
  - If interdental papilla is absent because of diastema, orthodontic closure is the treatment of choice.
  - Orthodontic forced eruption.
  - Repeated scaling, root planing, and curettage procedure.
- *Surgical papilla creation*:
  - Pedicle graft technique utilizing the soft palatal tissues of the interdental area.
  - Semilunar coronally positioned papilla.
  - Envelope type flap with a connective tissue graft.

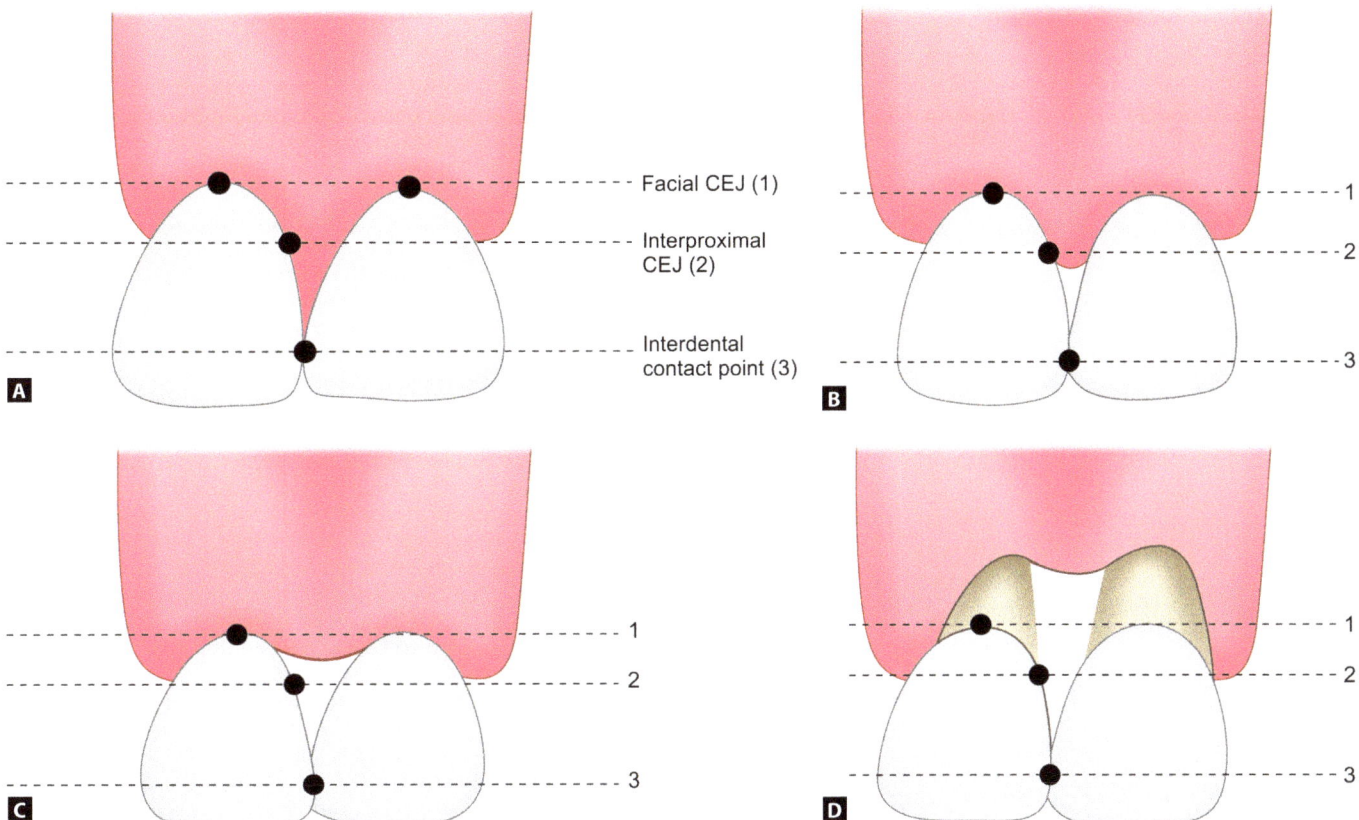

**Figs. 53.12A to D:** Schematic representation showing the classification of papillary height (A) Normal; (B) Class I; (C) Class II; (D) Class III.
(CEJ: cementoenamel junction)

## TECHNIQUES FOR ALVEOLAR RIDGE AUGMENTATION

### Classifications of Ridge Defects

- *According to Seibert[24] (1983)* **(Figs. 53.13A to C)**:
  - *Class I*: Loss of buccolingual width but normal apicocoronal height
  - *Class II*: Loss of apicocoronal height but normal buccolingual width
  - *Class III*: A combination of loss of both height and width of the ridge
- *According to Allen et al., a modification of Seibert classification*:
  - *Type A*: Apicocoronal loss of ridge contour
  - *Type B*: Buccolingual loss of ridge contour
  - *Type C*: Combined loss of ridge contour in both apicocoronal and buccolingual dimensions
- *According to the depth of defect*:
  - *Mild*: Less than 3 mm
  - *Moderate*: 3–6 mm
  - *Severe*: Greater than 6 mm

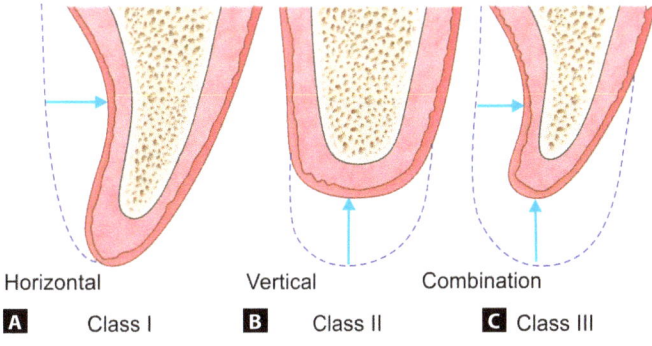

**Figs. 53.13A to C:** Schematic representation showing the classification of ridge defects: (A) Class I: Horizontal; (B) Class II: Vertical; (C) Class III: Combination.

### Procedure

The various approaches for the utilization of soft tissues for ridge augmentation are as follows:
- *Pedicle graft procedure*: Roll flap procedure[25]
- *Free graft procedures*:
  - Pouch graft procedure
  - Interpositional graft procedure **(Figs. 53.14A to D)**
  - Onlay graft procedure

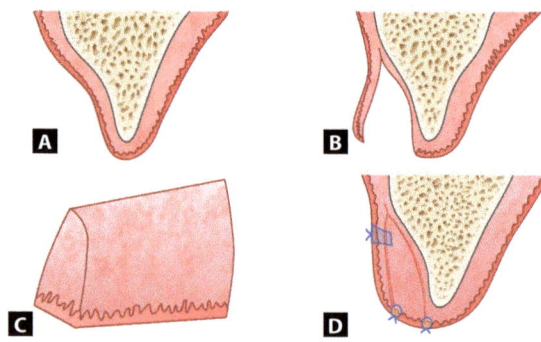

**Figs. 53.14A to D:** Schematic representation showing interpositional graft: (A) Class III combination ridge defect; (B) Split-thickness flap; (C) Free epithelial graft from maxillary tuberosity; (D) Graft sutured in between the split-thickness flap.

### Points to Ponder

- Cut-back incision is given at the distal corner of the laterally displaced flap into the alveolar mucosa, pointing in the direction of the recipient site.
- The free epithelial graft is usually covered by whitish mass, termed as ghost graft, which consists of sloughing epithelial cells after 7–10 days postoperatively. This matter can be rinsed away with a gentle stream of water.
- Pull syndrome: A detaching movement of the marginal gingiva transferred from the lip by the frenum has been termed the pull syndrome (Placek 1974).

## REFERENCES

1. Friedman N. Mucogingival surgery. Texas Dent J. 1957;75:358-62.
2. The American Academy of Periodontology. In: Proceedings of the 1996 World Workshop in Clinical Periodontics. Annals of Periodontology. Chicago: The American Academy of Periodontology; 1996.
3. Miller PD Jr. Periodontal plastic surgery. Curr Opin Periodontol. 1993:136-43.
4. Takei HH, Azzi RR. Periodontal plastic and esthetic surgery. In: Newman MG, Takei HH, Carranza FA (Eds). Carranza's Clinical Periodontology, 9th edition. Philadelphia, PA, USA: WB Saunders; 2003. pp. 851-75.
5. Bjorn H. Free transplantation of gingiva propia. Sven Tandlak Tidskr. 1963;22:684.
6. Hall WB. The free gingival graft. In: Pure Mucogingival Problems: Etiology, Treatment, and Prevention, 1st edition. Chicago, USA: Quintessence Book Publishing; 1984. pp. 127-52.
7. Grant DA, Stern IB, Listgarten MA. Mucogingival surgery. In: Periodontics, 6th edition. St. Louis: CV Mosby; 1988. pp. 883-910.
8. Oliver RG, Loe H, Karring T. Microscopic evaluation of the healing and revascularization of free gingival grafts. J Periodontal Res. 1968;3(2):84-95.
9. Wennstrom JL, Pini Prato GP. Mucogingival therapy: periodontal plastic surgery. In: Lindhe J, Karring T, Lang NP (Eds). Clinical Periodontology and Implant Dentistry, 4th edition. Oxford, UK: Blackwell Munksgaard; 2003. pp. 576-649.
10. Miller PD Jr. A classification of marginal tissue recession. Int J Periodontics Restorative Dent. 1985;5(2):8-13.
11. Sullivan HC, Atkins JH. Free autogenous gingival grafts. 3. Utilization of grafts in the treatment of gingival recession. Periodontics. 1968;6(4):152-60.
12. Mahajan A, Kashyap D, Kumar A, Mahajan P. Reliability study of Mahajan's classification of gingival recession: A pioneer clinical study. J Indian Soc Periodontol. 2014;18: 38-42.
13. Langer B, Langer L. Subepithelial connective tissue graft technique for root coverage. J Periodontol. 1985;56(12): 715-20.
14. Grupe HE, Warren RF. Repair of gingival defects by a sliding flap operation. J Periodontol. 1956;27:92-5.
15. Glover ME. Periodontal plastic and reconstructive surgery. In: Rose LF, Mealey BL, Genco RJ, Cohen DW (Eds). Periodontics: Medicine, Surgery, and Implants, 1st edition. Philadelphia, PA, USA: Elsevier-Mosby; 2004. pp. 405-87.
16. Tarnow DP. Semilunar coronally repositioned flap. J Clin Periodontol. 1986;13(3):182-5.
17. Mirko P, Miroslav S, Lubor M. Significance of the labial frenum attachment in periodontal disease in man. Part I. Classification and epidemiology of the labial frenum attachment. J Periodontol. 1974;45(12):891-4.
18. Kakodkar PV, Patel TN, Patel SV, Patel SH. Clinical assessment of diverse frenum morphology in permanent dentition. Internet J Dent Sci. 2009;7.
19. Edlan A, Mejchar B. Plastic surgery of the vestibulum in periodontal therapy. Int Dent J. 1963;13:593.
20. Nordland WP, Tarnow DP. A classification system for loss of papillary height. J Periodontol. 1998;69(10):1124-6.
21. Azzi R, Etienne D, Carranza F. Surgical reconstruction of the interdental papilla. Int J Periodontics Restorative Dent. 1998;18(5):466-73.
22. Beagle JR. Surgical reconstruction of the interdental papilla: case report. Int J Periodontics Restorative Dent. 1992;12(2):145-51.
23. Han TJ, Takei HH. Progress in gingival papilla reconstruction. Periodontol 2000. 1996;11:65-8.
24. Seibert JS. Reconstruction of deformed, partially edentulous ridges, using full thickness onlay grafts. Part I. Technique and wound healing. Compend Contin Educ Dent. 1983;4(5): 437-53.
25. Abrams L. Augmentation of the deformed residual edentulous ridge for fixed prosthesis. Compend Contin Educ Gen Dent. 1980;1(3):205-13.

### VIVA VOCE

**Q1. What are the effects of loss of interdental papilla?**
**Ans.** The effects of loss of interdental papilla are the following:
- Cosmetic deformities
- Phonetic problems
- Lateral food impaction.

**Q2. What is a creeping attachment?**
**Ans.** In 1964, Goldman et al. noted a second mechanism of gaining root coverage by the phenomenon of creeping attachment. This occurred between 1 month and one year and was the result of coronal migration of newly grafted attached gingiva over the portions of a previously denuded root.

## Chapter 53: Periodontal Plastic Surgery

**Q3.** **Which root coverage grafting procedure is considered the gold standard?**
**Ans.** Connective tissue grafting procedure.

**Q4.** **What is the main disadvantage of epithelial grafting?**
**Ans.** The color difference between the grafted area and the adjacent tissues.

**Q5.** **Which flap technique increases the width of the attached gingiva?**
**Ans.** Apically displaced flap.

**Q6.** **What is the main postoperative instruction given to the patient after the grafting procedure?**
**Ans.** The patient should not retract the lip or cheek to observe the graft.

**Q7.** **Who gave subepithelial connective tissue grafting procedure?**
**Ans.** Langer and Langer in 1985.

**Q8.** **Who originally developed laterally positioned pedicle flap?**
**Ans.** Grupe and Warren in 1956.

**Q9.** **Who gave the semilunar Coronally displaced flap technique?**
**Ans.** Tarnow in 1986.

**Q10.** **What is the basic difference between frenectomy and frenotomy?**
**Ans.** Frenectomy is the complete removal of the frenum, including its attachment to the underlying bone, whereas frenotomy is the incision of the frenum.

# Chapter 54

# Periodontal Microsurgery

*Shalu Bathla, Swantika Chaudhary*

## Chapter Outline

- Historical Perspective
- Principles
- Magnification Systems
- Microsurgical Instruments
- Requirements of the Surgeon
- Role of Microsurgery in Periodontal Procedures

## INTRODUCTION

Microsurgery involves a surgical procedure performed microscopically. It is generally a refinement of the operative technique through which visual acuity is enhanced by using a surgical operating microscope.[1]

It can also be defined as the refinement of the existing basic surgical techniques that are made possible by using the surgical microscope and subsequently improving the visual acuity.[2]

In microsurgery, there is a great reduction in surgical damage to the tissues due to the excellent visualization of the operative field through the microscope; this least traumatic surgical approach being possible because of the magnified surgical field and enhanced dexterity of the surgeons leading to less injury and more meticulous tissue handling.

## HISTORICAL PERSPECTIVE

The concept of microsurgery was introduced in 1922 when Carl Nylén, for the first time, used a binocular microscope for ear surgery. Hence, Nylén is called the Father of microsurgery.[3] From 1921 to 1960, microsurgery was considered as the standard operating procedure in many specialties, including neurology and ophthalmology.[4,5] In dentistry, Apotheker, and Jako were the first to introduce microscope in 1978.[6] In this respect; Carr published an article demonstrating endodontic procedures with the help of surgical microscope in 1992.[7] In the field of oral surgery, Leblanc laid the foundations and used microsuturing nerve repair techniques to treat traumatic injuries to the lower dental nerve. During 1992 this microsuturing nerve repair technique was introduced in the field of periodontics.[8] In 1993, at the Annual Meeting of the American Academy of Periodontology, Shanelec and Tibbetts introduced a course of continuing education in periodontal microsurgery. This leads to the development of centers devoted to teaching "periodontal microsurgery".[9]

## PRINCIPLES

Three important principles of microsurgery are as follows:[10]
1. Improvement in motor skills enhances surgical ability.
2. The use of smaller instruments during microsurgical procedures reduces trauma to periodontal tissues at the surgical site and also decreases the surgical field.
3. Microsurgical principles are useful to enhance the process of passive and primary wound closure. It has good application in the reduction of gaps and dead spaces present at wound edge and facilitation of new tissue formation in order to fill out surgical voids. In such procedures, major emphasis is given on the achievement of passive closure of the wound with proper primary apposition at the wound edges.

## MAGNIFICATION SYSTEMS

There are two types of optical magnification available:
1. *Magnifying loupes*:
    - Simple loupes
    - Compound loupes
    - Prism telescopic loupes
2. Surgical microscope

## Magnifying Loupes

Microsurgical procedures commonly use three types of magnifying loupes. Each type varies significantly in lens construction and design.

### Simple Loupes

These are composed of a pair of solitary, positive, side-by-side meniscus lenses. Each lens has two refracting surfaces. Cost is the sole advantage of the simple loupe. Disadvantages are as follows:
- Spherical and chromatic aberration disturb the image of the object that is being viewed.
- The practical dental application is restricted to a magnification range of 1.5 diameters, where working distances and depths of field are compromised.

### Compound Loupes

Compound loupes use multiple converging lenses, which have intervening air spaces, which help in achieving added refracting power, magnification, working distance, and field depth. The achromatic lens is composed of two joined glass lenses by using clear resin. Compound loupes are commonly mounted in or on eyeglasses (**Fig. 54.1**). Multi-element compound loupes are usually optically not efficient at magnifications of more than 3.0 diameters.

### Prism Telescopic Loupes

These are considered as an optically advanced type of loupes (**Fig. 54.2**). These employ Schmidt or rooftop prisms, which helps in enhancing the path of light through a series of switchback mirror reflections within the lens elements, virtually folding the light in order to shorten the barrel of the loupes.

Advantages of prism telescopic loupes are as follows:
- Good magnification
- Wider field depths
- Enhanced working distances
- Larger view fields compared to other loupe types

The barrels of prism loupes are short enough to be mounted on either eyeglass frames or headbands. However, the enhanced weight of prism telescopic loupes with magnification more than 3× produces more comfortable and stable headband mounting compared to eyeglass frame mounting.

Disadvantages of prism telescopic loupes are as follows:
- Include fixed magnification (lack of magnification variability).
- The potential need for an additional light for magnification levels of 4.0 or greater.
- Since eyes need to converge to view an image, it usually results in eyestrain. Moreover, it can result in vision changes with prolonged use of poorly fitted loupes.

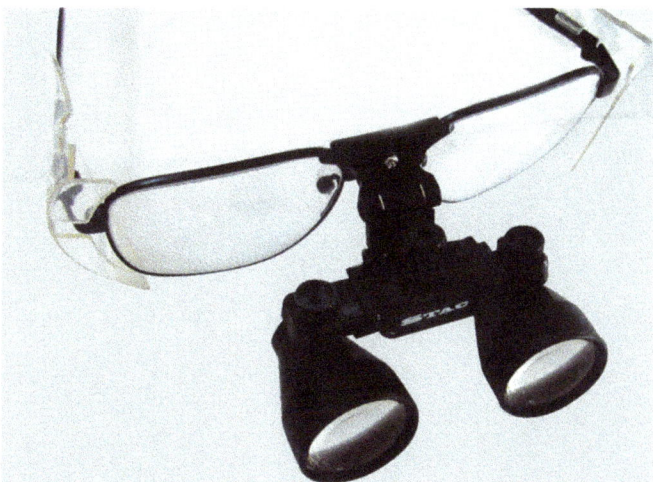

**Fig. 54.1:** Photograph showing Galilean compound loupe (3.5 mm × 420 mm).

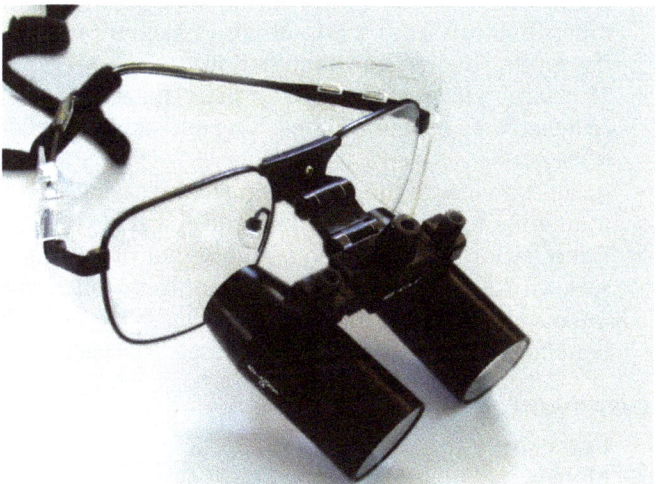

**Fig. 54.2:** Photograph showing prismatic loupe (4.0 mm × 420 mm).

- As the length of the loupe increases to provide more magnification, the lens's weight also increases, which becomes more uncomfortable.

## Surgical Microscope

The surgical microscope or operating microscope is considered as a complicated system of lenses. It allows a binocular view through a magnification of ×4 to ×40 approximately. In a surgical microscope, both beams of light fall parallel onto the observer's retinas. This prevents eye convergence and reduces the excessive demand of eye muscles. It consists of magnification changer, objective lenses, lighting unit, binocular tubes, and eyepieces (**Fig. 54.3**). It is fixable to the floor or mountable on the wall or ceiling as per the operator's convenience.

### Advantages

- It has greater operator eye comfort due to parallel viewing optics provided by the Galilean system.

## Section 7: Treatment: Surgical Therapy

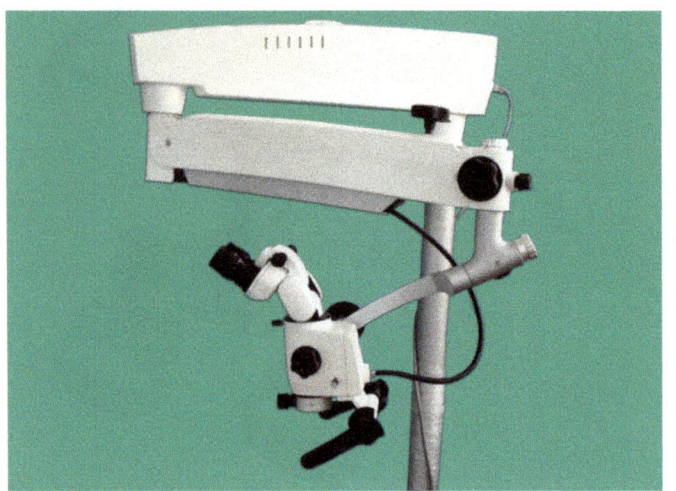

Fig. 54.3: Photograph showing a surgical operating microscope.

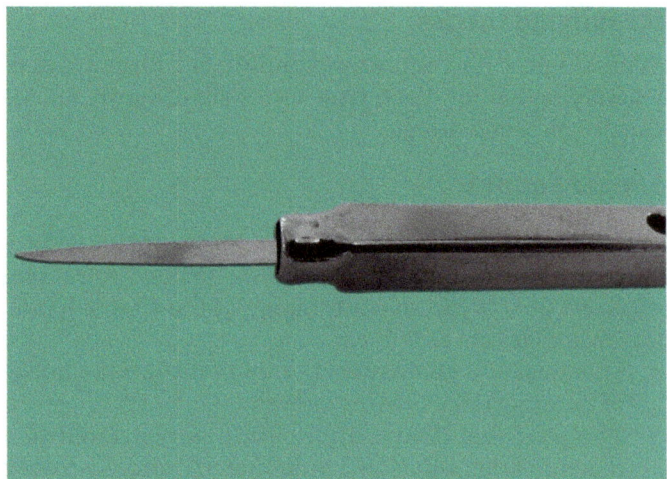

Fig. 54.4: Photograph showing scalpel.

- It offers versatility due to an extended range of variable magnification from 2.5 to 20 and excellent coaxial fiberoptic, shadow-free illumination.
- The same view can be shared with the students or reflected on a monitor for teaching and achieve better teamwork.
- It can even record the surgery due to the availability of numerous accessories for digital still and video images.
- Illumination, magnification, and higher precision in surgical skills are the important advantages of operating microscopes for the clinician. Collectively these three benefits are termed as the "microsurgical triad".[5-8]

### Disadvantages
- Expensive
- More cumbersome to use
- Difficult to master the technique to use

## MICROSURGICAL INSTRUMENTS

### Design of the Micro Instruments

They should be approximately 18 cm long but are much smaller, often by 10-fold. Using these smaller instruments under magnification allows surgeons to refine their movements with the end result of enhanced surgical skills. Their handles have a round cross-sectional diameter to enhance rotary movements using the precision grip. Each instrument weighs to a maximum of 15–20 g to avoid the fatigue of arm and hand muscles. They are made of titanium to reduce weight and prevent magnetization. These instruments have a colored-coating surface, which helps in avoiding the unfavorable metallic glare under the operating microscope.[9,10]

### Scalpel and Blades

Ophthalmic scalpel, blades, and Castroviejo microsurgical scalpel are used. Ophthalmic knives offer the dual advantages of extreme sharpness and minimal size. Because ophthalmic knives are chemically etched rather than ground, their sharper blades produce a more precise wound edge (Fig. 54.4). The other knives used are blade breaker knife, crescent knife, mini crescent knife, spoon knife, lamellar knife, and scleral knife.

### Suture Needles

Atraumatic suture consists of a strand which is firmly connected to the needle through a press-fit swage. The needle is made up of swage, body, and tip. The commonly preferred needles are precision-tipped reverse cutting needles or microtipped spatula needles. Reverse cutting needles are available with a higher degree of firmness compared to round body needles. Hence, reverse cutting needles easily penetrates coarse gingiva. For periodontal microsurgery, the needle body diameter should be flattened for stabilizing the needle in its holder. The use of a 3/8-inch circular needle is sufficient to achieve better results. The lengths which are measured along the needle curvature, from tip to the proximal end of the needle lock, extend from 5 to 13 mm depending on the area applied. Needle length preferred for a papilla suture should range from 11 to 13 mm. A spatula needle is 6.6 mm in length and has a curvature of 140°. The needle track is shallow and provided with a precise purchase point. Suture needles with such characteristics allow accurate apposition, wound closure and immobilization of the connective tissue graft.[9,10]

### Suture Materials

Microsutures 7-0 to 9-0 are used. Polypropylene is a waterproof isotactile thread and remains hydrolytically unchanged in body tissues. It is considered as the optimum suture material for microsurgery.[2,11]

### Suturing

*Principles of micro suturing*:
- The needle angle of entry and exit is slightly less than 90°.

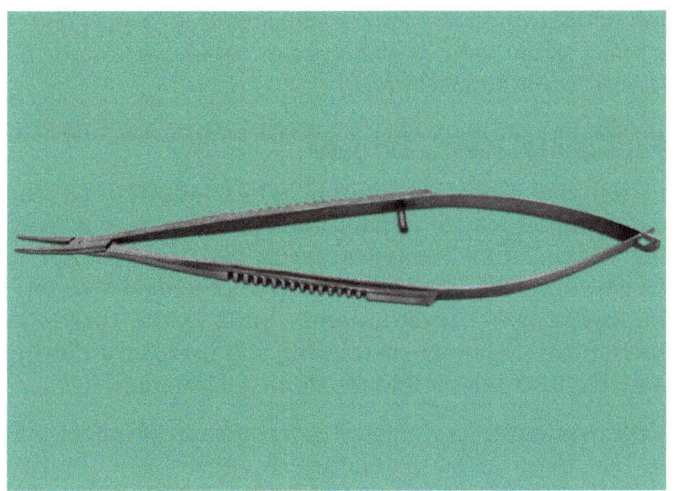

Fig. 54.5: Photograph showing microneedle holder.

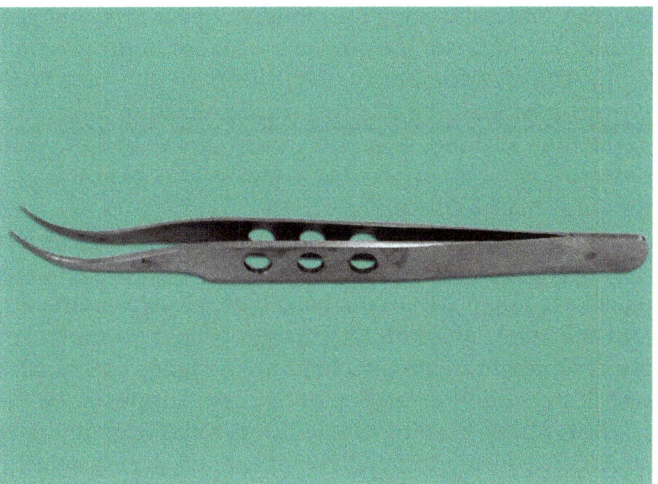

Fig. 54.6: Photograph showing curved jeweler's microforcep.

- Sutures pass across the incision line at oblique/acute angles rather than perpendicularly.
- Suture bite-size should be approximately 1.5 times the tissue thickness.
- Equal bite sizes (symmetry) on both sides of the wound.
- Knot tying using the microscope is done using instrument ties, with a microsurgical needle holder in the operating hand and a microsurgical tissue forceps in the nonoperating hand.

## Microneedle Holder

It is commonly used during the suturing process where it holds the needle, pulls it through the tissues, and utilized for tying knots. The needle is required to be grasped between its middle and lower thirds from its distal tip. It is usually equipped with a precise working lock with a maximum locking force of 50 g only. The exertion of higher locking forces, usually initiate tremors and minimize the feeling for the movement **(Fig. 54.5)**.

## Surgical and Anatomical Forceps

The surgical forceps is designed as a combination instrument with both surgical and anatomical utility. It is designed as an anatomical forceps but converts into a surgical forceps towards the end **(Fig. 54.6)**. This is useful in seizing mucosal flaps and knotting the thread assuredly without changing the instruments. The tips of the forceps are flat-surfaced or finely cross-hatched, which prevents the thread's sliding during knotting. The latter should be designed to grip fine and rough needles. It is designed so that the light is unable to pass through the tips on closing. Locks on the forceps initiate controlled rotation movements on the handles without exerting undue pressure. The tips should be maintained 1–2 mm apart approximately when the forceps is held in hand without any pressure.

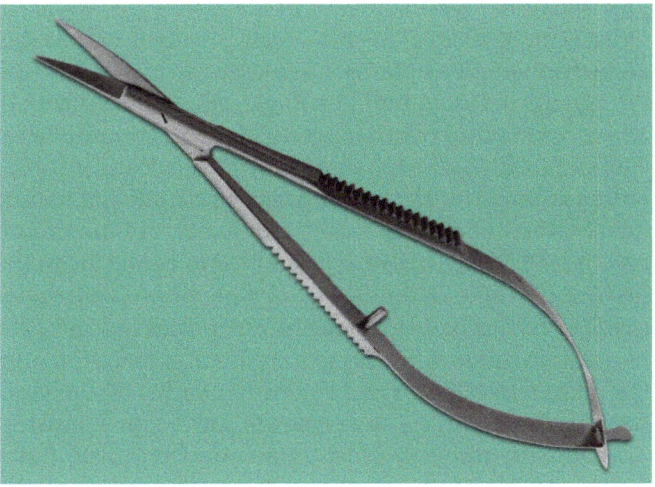

Fig. 54.7: Photograph showing microscissors.

## Microscissors

Laschal microscissors with small beak scissors are regularly used in the dissection of tissues, blood vessels, and nerves. During surgical procedures, the routinely used microscissors are 14 cm and 18 cm long **(Fig. 54.7)**.

## Storage of Instruments

Microinstruments need to store in a sterile container or tray to avoid damage. During sterilization procedures or transportation, precautions must be taken to prevent touching the tips to each other.

## REQUIREMENTS OF THE SURGEON

Microsurgical training is an important aspect of conducting microsurgical procedures. The training focuses on improving the fine-tuning of the hand and arm's motor muscles and enhancing the clinician's cognitive abilities. Ideally 1–2 hours of training per week for approximately 3 months is sufficient for beginners to conduct such procedures. Training involves standardization in the use of the time knotting technique, instrument handling, and dexterity. This helps the surgeon to concentrate entirely on the surgical procedure.[9,10]

The clinician seated position is also an important aspect during surgical procedures. It should be adjusted in a way where the upper part of the body balances symmetrically, and the lower arms and hands get proper support. For microsurgeons, treatment chairs are designed specifically, which permits fine-tuning of the arm supports. In the learning phase, keeping a folded cloth rolls on the patient's shoulders provide sufficient hand support during surgical procedure.[9,10]

## Internal Precision Grip

The pen grip or internal precision grip is the well-known precision grip used in the field of microsurgery because of its excellent stability. The three-digit grip involves grasping an instrument like holding a pen when writing where the thumb and index and middle fingers are used as a tripod. The surgeon should rest her/his hands on an immovable flat surface provided with the support of the ulnar surface of the wrist and forearm. The microsurgical instrument is mainly held by the middle finger with the support of the thumb and index finger, which are positioned in contact with the instrument. The opening and closing of an instrument require very fine hand movements with a minimum number of possible tremors. In this pen or internal precision grip, the relaxation of flexor and extensor muscles of the hand, facilitating accurate movements during procedures. Additionally, proper surgical ergonomics help to minimize back and neck strain.

Moreover, it improves the functional environment to efficiently conduct endodontic microsurgery and avoid esthetic complications. The surgeon should seat in an upright position keeping thighs approximately at a right angle to the knees. The patient and chair position should be adjusted according to the position of operating surgeon and microscope.[9,10]

Microsurgical instrumentation, accurate hand movements with a precision handgrip and correct posture and position are immensely important to prevent back and neck problems in surgeons.

## ROLE OF MICROSURGERY IN PERIODONTAL PROCEDURES

The microsurgery has gained popularity among some periodontists because of less morbidity and superiority to conventional surgery in achieving the end-point appearance. Compared to the conventional approach, microsurgery is associated with cleaner incisions, closer wound apposition, reduced hemorrhage, and reduced trauma at the surgical site.

## Periodontal Plastic Surgery

Periodontal plastic surgery should be conducted, keeping equal importance to esthetic and functional results. With the advanced microsurgical technique, it is possible to achieve optimal esthetic results in microgingival surgery, maintaining other parameters, such as the surgeon's theoretical and practical training, the necessary viewing aids, the instruments and the suture technique.[2,11]

Various microsurgical gingival procedures are as follows:[12-14]
- Tissue grafting procedure to correct the gingival recession.
  - Free epithelial grafting
  - Subepithelial connective tissue grafting
- Papilla reconstruction procedure.
- *Establishing an esthetic smile line*: The achievement of an ideal esthetic smile with harmonious gingival contours requires multiple factors, such as lip position, symmetry, and relative gingival levels of adjacent teeth. Various complex periodontal plastic microsurgeries involve either removal of tissue on some teeth or replacement on others.
- *Restoring the edentulous ridge*: Different techniques are available for ridge augmentation, including guided bone regeneration, block, and particulate grafts, soft tissue grafts, and a combination of these methods.

### Advantages of Microsurgery
- Improved cosmetics
- Rapid healing
- Minimal discomfort
- *Less invasive*: As there is reduced incision size, lessened need for vertical releasing incisions and smaller surgical sites thus, periodontal microsurgery is considered as a less invasive procedure
- Reduces surgical fatigue and development of spinal and occupational pathology of the operator
- Enhanced patient acceptance

### Disadvantages of Microsurgery
- Understanding of optics and surgical techniques required.
- The increased adjustment period and surgical time.
- Limited surgical access.
- High cost.

> **Points to Ponder**
> - Carl Nylén is called as the Father of microsurgery.
> - In periodontal surgery, an ideal magnification is considered as ×4.5 to ×5 for loupe spectacles and ×10 to ×20 for surgical microscopes.

## REFERENCES

1. Shanelec DA. Periodontal microsurgery. J Esthet Restor Dent. 2003;15(7):402-7.
2. Shanelec DA, Tibbetts LS. Recent advances in surgical technology. In: Newman MG, Takei HH, Carranza FA (Eds). Carranza's Clinical Periodontology, 9th edition. Philadelphia, PA, USA: WB Saunders; 2003. pp. 876-81.
3. Dohlman GF. Carl-Olof Nylén and the birth of the otomicroscope and microsurgery. Arch Otolaryngol. 1969;90(6):813-7.
4. Barraquer JI. The history of the microsurgery in ocular surgery. J Microsurg. 1980;1(4):288-99.
5. Serafin D. Microsurgery: past, present, and future. Plast Reconstr Surg. 1980;66(5):781-5.
6. Apotheker H, Jako GJ. A microscope for use in dentistry. J Microsurg. 1981;3(1):7-10.
7. Carr GB. Microscopes in endodontics. J Calif Dent Assoc. 1992;20(11):55-61.
8. Labanc JP, Van Boven RW. Surgical management of inferior alveolar nerve injuries. Oral Maxillofac Surg Clin North Am. 1992;4:425-37.
9. Shanelec DA, Tibbetts LS. The status of periodontal microsurgery: Continuing education course, 79th American Academy of Periodontology Annual Meeting, Chicago, 1993.
10. Shanelec DA. Principles of periodontal plastic microsurgery. In: Rose LF, Genco RJ, Mealey BL, Cohen DW (Eds). Periodontics: Medicine, Surgery, and Implant, 1st edition. St. Louis: Elsevier-Mosby; 2004. pp. 488-501.
11. Hoerenz P. The operating microscope. I. Optical principles, illumination systems, and support systems. J Microsurg. 1980;1(5):364-9.
12. Tibbetts LS, Shanelec D. Periodontal microsurgery. Dent Clin North Am. 1998;42(2):339-59.
13. Belcher JM. A perspective on periodontal microsurgery. Int J Periodontics Restorative Dent. 2001;21(2):191-6.
14. Burkhardt R, Hürzeler MB. Utilization of the surgical microscope for advanced plastic periodontal surgery. Pract Periodontics Aesthet Dent. 2002;12(2):171-80.

## VIVA VOCE

**Q1. What is the microsurgical triad?**
**Ans.** Three elements, i.e., illumination, magnification, and refined surgical skills by instruments, are called the microsurgical triad. Operating microscopes offer these three distinct advantages to the clinician.

**Q2. What are the advantages of loupes over microscopes?**
**Ans.** The advantages of loupes over microscopes are as follows:
- They are less expensive to purchase.
- They are easier to use.
- Loupes tend to be less cumbersome in operating field and less likely to breach a clean operative field.
- They are handy in freelancing practice.

**Q3. Which grip is used for the microsurgical procedure?**
**Ans.** Internal precision grip or pen grip.

**Q4. Which is the optimum suture material for microsurgery?**
**Ans.** Polypropylene.

**Q5. Which is the preferred needle for microsurgery?**
**Ans.** Precision-tipped reverse cutting needle or microtipped spatula needle.

**Q6. Who is called as the Father of microsurgery?**
**Ans.** Nylén.

**Q7. Name various optical magnification are available.**
**Ans.** There are two types of optical magnification—magnifying loupes (simple loupes, compound loupes, prism telescopic loupes) and surgical microscope.

**Q8. What are the disadvantages of a surgical microscope?**
**Ans.** Expensive and cumbersome.

**Q9. Name various knives used in microsurgery.**
**Ans.** Ophthalmic and Castroviejo microsurgical scalpel, blade breaker, crescent, mini crescent, spoon, lamellar and scleral knives are used in microsurgery.

**Q10. What are the advantages of microsurgery compared to conventional approach?**
**Ans.** Microsurgery is associated with cleaner incisions, closer wound apposition, reduced hemorrhage, and reduced trauma at the surgical site.

# Chapter 55

# Periodontal Treatment of Medically Compromised Patients

*Preetinder Singh*

## Chapter Outline

- Cardiovascular Diseases
- Endocrine Disorders
- Renal Diseases
- Liver Diseases
- Pulmonary Diseases
- Immunosuppression and Chemotherapy
- Radiation Therapy
- Prosthetic Joint Replacement
- Pregnancy
- Hemorrhagic Disorders
- Blood Dyscrasias
- Infectious Diseases
- Patients on Bisphosphonate Therapy
- Epileptic Patients

## INTRODUCTION

Often patients seeking dental care have associated medical conditions that change both the course of oral disease and the intended therapy. Hence, for the clinician, the important therapeutic responsibility is identifying the patient's medical problems and the formulation of proper treatment plans. For this detailed medical histories are crucial. If significant findings are unveiled, consultation with or referral of the patient to an appropriate physician may be indicated. This ensures correct patient management and provides medicolegal coverage to the clinician.

Cardiovascular disease (CVD) and diabetes mellitus are the common medical conditions found in elderly and medically compromised patients. The periodontist should identify new cases of these diseases and must be able to provide adequate periodontal care to patients who already received treatment for these problems without endangering their lives.

## CARDIOVASCULAR DISEASES

Cardiovascular disease can be identified by:
- Taking a detailed medical history and a limited physical examination helps to identify physical symptoms and signs associated with CVD.
- Identifying the vital signs, including blood pressure and pulse rate.
- Consultation with a physician, if needed.

### Hypertension

Hypertension is defined as a systolic blood pressure of 140 mm Hg or higher or a diastolic blood pressure of 90 mm Hg or higher.[1,2] However, it is not diagnosed only on a single elevated blood pressure recording. Instead, the average value of three or more blood pressure readings should be taken at three or more appointments. The higher value of either the systolic or diastolic blood pressure determines the patient's classification **(Table 55.1)**.

The periodontal recall system is an ideal method for hypertension detection and monitoring.

Following are the guidelines to do periodontal treatment in hypertensive patient:[3]
- Stress-free, calm, and relaxing environment.
- Short appointments.
- Afternoon appointments: blood pressure generally increases around awakening and peaks at mid-morning.
- A local anesthetic solution containing epinephrine concentration not greater than 1:100,000 should be used.
- Intraligamentary injection is generally contraindicated because hemodynamic changes are similar to intravascular injection.
- An aspirating syringe should be used since epinephrine in the anesthetic solution may get into the blood and may raise blood pressure and precipitate dysrhythmias.
- Epinephrine containing local anesthetic should be used cautiously and only in very small amounts in a

**TABLE 55.1:** Classification of adult blood pressure.

| Classification | Blood pressure (mm Hg) Systolic | Diastolic | Dental treatment modifications |
|---|---|---|---|
| Normal | <130 | <85 | No changes in dental treatment |
| High-normal | 130–139 | 85–89 | No changes in dental treatment |
| **Hypertension:** | | | |
| Stage 1 | 140–159 | 90–99 | Inform patient of findings:<br>❑ Routine medical consultation or referral<br>❑ No changes in dental treatment<br>❑ Minimize stress |
| Stage 2 | 160–179 | 100–109 | Inform patient:<br>❑ Routine medical referral<br>❑ Selective dental care (routine examination, prophylaxis, restorative, nonsurgical endodontics and periodontics); minimize stress |
| Stage 3 | ≥180 | ≥110 | Inform patient<br>❑ Immediate medical consultation or referral<br>❑ Emergency dental care only (to alleviate pain, bleeding, infection)*<br>Minimize stress |

*Risk of providing emergency dental care must outweigh the risk of possible hypertensive complications.

patient taking nonselective beta-blockers, with careful monitoring of vital signs.[4]
- Postural hypotension is common with patients on antihypertensive drugs and can be minimized by slow positional changes in the dental chair.
- Gingival retraction cords containing epinephrine should be avoided.
- General anesthesia should be avoided whenever possible.
- Aspirin may cause sodium and fluid retention and may be contraindicated in severe hypertension or cardiac failure.

## Ischemic Heart Diseases

Ischemic heart disease commonly manifested as angina pectoris and myocardial infarction.
- Following are the guidelines to do periodontal treatment in ischemic heart disease patient:
- The physician should be consulted before elective dental therapy to determine the degree of heart damage or arterial occlusive disease, the stability of the patient's condition, and the potential for infective endocarditis (IE) or graft rejection.
- Dental treatment is generally deferred for at least 6 months following myocardial infarction because the peak mortality rate occurs during this time.
- After the 6-month post-myocardial infarction period, patients are mostly managed with techniques similar to the stable angina patient. Management involves relatively short appointments and a stress reduction protocol where indicated.
- Patients who treat acute anginal attacks with nitroglycerine should be instructed to bring their medication to dental appointments. Nitroglycerine should also be kept in the official emergency medical kit. For particularly stressful procedures, the patient may take a nitroglycerine tablet preoperatively to prevent angina, although this is generally not necessary. The patient's nitroglycerin should be readily accessible on the dental tray in case it is needed during treatment.
- Short appointments.
- *Stress reduction protocol*: Because stress often induces an acute anginal attack, stress reduction is important.
- The maximum allowable dose of epinephrine is 0.04 mg per appointment for a patient with stable angina.
- Intraosseous injection with epinephrine containing local anesthetics should be done cautiously in patients with ischemic heart disease because it results in a transient increase in heart rate and myocardial oxygen demand.
- Prophylactic antibiotics are not usually necessary for cardiac bypass patients unless recommended by the cardiologist.

A patient who has an angina episode in the dental chair should receive the following emergency medical treatment:
- Discontinue the periodontal procedure.
- Administer one tablet (0.3–0.6 mg) of nitroglycerin sublingually.
- Reassure the patient and loosen restrictive garments.
- Administer oxygen with the patient in a reclined position.
- If the signs and symptoms cease within 3 minutes, complete the periodontal procedure if possible, make sure that the patient is comfortable. Terminate the procedure at the earliest convenient time.
- If the anginal signs and symptoms do not resolve with this treatment within 2–3 minutes, administer another dose of nitroglycerin, monitor the patient's vital signs, call his or her physician, and be ready to accompany the patient to the emergency.
- A third nitroglycerin tablet may be given 3 minutes after the second. Chest pain that is not relieved by three tablets of nitroglycerin indicates likely myocardial infarction.
- The patient should be transported to the nearest emergency medical facility immediately.

Pain that persists after three doses of nitroglycerin and lasts more than 15–20 minutes or that is associated with diaphoresis, nausea, vomiting, syncope, or hypotension usually indicate myocardial infarction. It is important to make arrangements for immediate transportation to a hospital, and vital signs should be monitored closely. The patient should continue to receive oxygen and administration of 5–10 mg of morphine sulfate intravenously to manage the pain and anxiety. If the cardiopulmonary arrest occurs while aid is still forthcoming, the dentist and office staff must perform resuscitative measures.

## Congestive Heart Failure

Congestive heart failure (CHF) is a condition in which the heart's pump function is unable to supply sufficient amounts of oxygenated blood to meet the body's needs.[5] Following are the guidelines for periodontal treatment in CHF patients:

- *Semirecumbent or upright position*: The dental chair should be adjusted to a comfortable level for the patient instead of being placed in a supine position. However, it should be adjusted in a comfortable position for the patient, especially semirecumbent or upright.
- Schedule stress free, short appointments. Profound local anesthesia, possibly conscious sedation and use of supplemental oxygen, should be considered.

## Cardiac Pacemakers and Automatic Defibrillators

Patients with cardiac arrhythmias need special attention during periodontal therapy. Cardiac arrhythmias are usually managed with medications. However, some cardiac arrhythmias are treated with implantable pacemakers or automatic defibrillators. Commonly used anti-arrhythmic drugs usually have oral side effects, including gingival overgrowth or xerostomia. Both these have effects on the dentition or periodontium.

Following are the guidelines for periodontal treatment in patients with cardiac pacemakers and automatic defibrillators:

- In patients with refractory arrhythmias, the use of local anesthetics with vasoconstrictors may be contraindicated.
- Periodontal treatment should be completed in a controlled medical setting provided with careful cardiac monitoring.
- The patient's physician's prior opinion allows determination of the underlying cardiac status, the type of pacemaker or automatic defibrillator, and other precautionary measures to be taken. Older pacemakers were unipolar and may be disrupted by dental equipment due to the generation of electromagnetic fields such as ultrasonic and electrocautery units. However, newer units are bipolar and hence usually not affected by dental equipment.
- During periodontal treatment, stabilization of the operating field with bite blocks or other devices helps to avoid unexpected trauma.

## Valvular Heart Disease

The dental patient with valvular heart disease is at increased risks of heart failure, hemodynamically significant arrhythmia, and IE. In these patients, in the view of dentists, the main concern is about the possibility of endocarditis. The term IE is preferred over the previous term bacterial endocarditis because the disease can also be caused by fungi and viruses. α-hemolytic streptococci (e.g., *Streptococcus viridans*) is the most common organism associated with the incidence of IE. Along with it, nonstreptococcal organisms present in the periodontal pocket, including *Eikenella corrodens, Actinobacillus actinomycetemcomitans, Capnocytophaga*, and *Lactobacillus species* increase risk of IE.

Dental procedures involving bleeding may induce transient bacteremia. Hence, the American Heart Association (AHA) recommends antibiotic prophylaxis before performing dental procedures "associated with significant bleeding from hard or soft tissues, periodontal surgery, scaling, and professional teeth cleaning" **(Table 55.2)**.

Following are the preventive measures to reduce the risk of IE:[6,7]

- *Define the susceptible patient*: A careful medical history will disclose the susceptible patients; health questioning should cover the history of all potential categories of risk.
- *Consult the patient's physician*: If any doubt exists, the patient's physician should be consulted.
- *Provide oral hygiene instructions*: Oral hygiene should be practiced with methods that improve gingival health yet minimize bacteremia. In patients with significant gingival inflammation, oral hygiene should initially be limited to gentle procedures (i.e., oral rinses and gentle toothbrushing with a soft brush) to minimize bleeding. As gingival health improves, more aggressive oral hygiene may be initiated.

Oral irrigators are generally not recommended because their use may induce bacteremia. Susceptible patients should be encouraged to maintain the highest level of oral hygiene once soft tissue inflammation is controlled.

Following are the guidelines for periodontal treatment in IE patients:[8,9]

- Consult the patient's physician.
- Recommended prophylactic antibiotic regimens should be practiced with all susceptible patients **(Table 55.2)**.
- All periodontal treatment procedures (including probing) require antibiotic prophylaxis.
- Pretreatment with chlorhexidine mouthrinses is recommended before all procedures, including

## Chapter 55: Periodontal Treatment of Medically Compromised Patients

**TABLE 55.2:** Recommended antibiotic prophylaxis regimens for periodontal procedures in adults at risk for infective endocarditis.

| Regimen | Antibiotic | Dosage |
| --- | --- | --- |
| Standard oral regimen | Amoxicillin | 2.0 g 1 hour before the procedure |
| Alternate regimen for patients allergic to amoxicillin or penicillin | ☐ Clindamycin or<br>☐ Azithromycin or Clarithromycin or<br>☐ Cephalexin or Cefadroxil | 600 mg 1 hour before the procedure<br><br>500 mg 1 hour before the procedure<br>2.0 g 1 hour before the procedure |
| Patients unable to take oral medications | Ampicillin | 2.0 g IM/IV within 30 minutes before the procedure |
| Patients unable to take oral medications and allergic to penicillin | Clindamycin | 600 mg IV within 30 minutes before procedure (must be diluted and injected slowly) |
| | or Cefazolin | 1.0 g IM/IV within 30 minutes before the procedure |

*Note*: Children's dosages are lower.

periodontal probing, to reduce the presence of bacteria on mucosal surfaces.
- When possible, allow at least 7 days between appointments (preferably 10-14 days). If this is not possible, select an alternative antibiotic regimen for appointments within 7 days.
Teeth with severe periodontitis and poor prognosis may require extraction. Teeth with less severe involvement in a motivated patient should be retained, treated, and maintained closely.
- Sutures reabsorbing in a short period like chromic catgut are indicated for patients at risk of IE.
- Regular recall appointments, with an emphasis on oral hygiene reinforcement and periodontal health maintenance, are extremely important in IE patients.

## Cerebrovascular Accident

A cerebrovascular accident (CVA), or stroke, occurs due to ischemic changes (e.g., cerebral thrombosis owing to an embolus) or hemorrhagic phenomena. A stroke results from A sudden interruption of blood flow to the brain deprives the neuronal cells of oxygen and results in the stroke. Hypertension and atherosclerosis are predisposing factors to CVA. They should alert the clinician to evaluate the patient's medical history carefully for the possibility of early cerebrovascular insufficiency and be aware of the disease's symptoms.

Following are the guidelines for periodontal treatment in patients who are seen after a stroke:
- No periodontal therapy (unless for an emergency) should be performed for 6 months because of the high risk of recurrence during this period.
- After 6 months, periodontal therapy may be performed using short appointments with an emphasis on minimizing stress. Profound local anesthesia should be obtained using the minimal effective dose of local anesthetic agents. Concentrations of epinephrine greater than 1:100,000 are contraindicated.
- Light conscious sedation (inhalation, oral or parenteral) may be used for very anxious patients. Supplemental oxygen is indicated to maintain thorough cerebral oxygenation.
- Stroke patients usually need oral anticoagulant therapy. For procedures that entail significant bleeding, such as periodontal surgery or tooth extraction, the anticoagulant regimen often needs adjustment in consultation with the physician.
- Monitor blood pressure carefully. Recurrence rates for CVAs are high, as are rates of associated functional deficits.

## Anticoagulant Therapy

Anticoagulant therapy is commonly administered in patients with prosthetic heart valves, other valvular disorders, or a history of myocardial infarction, CVA, or thromboembolism.

Anticoagulant agents are coumarin derivatives, including dicumarol and warfarin, which are vitamin K inhibitors. These agents lead to depletion of vitamin-K dependent coagulation factors II, VII, IX, and X. Warfarin has a delayed onset of action and a prolonged effect. The effectiveness of warfarin is monitored via the prothrombin time. The commonly administered therapeutic dose of anticoagulant is one that doubles prothrombin time compared to normal clotting time.

For performing dental procedures, the range of 1.5-2.0 times the normal clotting time is considered within the range of safety and less likely to cause bleeding.

Following are the guidelines for periodontal treatment in patients on anticoagulant therapy:
- When procedures are known to be associated with bleeding, it is better to consult the patient's physician for adjusting the dosages that can keep the prothrombin time between 1.5 and 2 times the control. Usually, this adjustment should be initiated 2-3 days prior to the procedure. Moreover, it is necessary to test a prothrombin time in the morning of the dental appointment.
- After dental treatment, the patient should be instructed to continue the anticoagulant as soon as possible (usually the day of the procedure). The prolonged half-life of warfarin makes it suitable for initial wound healing

before the prothrombin time again increases beyond the safe treatment range.
- When local hemostatic measures cannot be effective in the anticoagulated patient, initiate pharmacological manipulation. If the anticoagulated patient can tolerate a wait of several hours or more, vitamin K administration will reverse the effect of warfarin.
- In emergency situations, the patient usually requires a transfusion of fresh-frozen plasma.

## ENDOCRINE DISORDERS

### Diabetes

The diabetic patient requires special precautions before periodontal therapy. Classic signs of diabetes are as follows:
- Polydipsia (excessive thirst)
- Polyuria (excessive urination)
- Polyphagia (excessive hunger, often with unexplained concurrent weight loss).

These clinical features are associated usually with a loss of strength, loss of weight, recurrence of bed-wetting, drowsiness, and malaise. Hence, awareness about these features is necessary among the dental team.

Periodontal therapy has limited success in the presence of undiagnosed or poorly controlled diabetes **(Fig. 55.1)**. If a patient is suspected of having undiagnosed diabetes, the following procedures should be performed:
- Consult the patient's physician.
- *Analyze laboratory tests*: Fasting blood glucose, random glucose, and postprandial blood glucose.
- Rule out acute orofacial infection or severe dental infection, and provide emergency care only until a diagnosis is established.
- Establish the best possible oral health through nonsurgical debridement of plaque and calculus and institute oral hygiene instructions. Limit more advanced care until a diagnosis has been established and good glycemic control obtained.

The glycosylated or glycated hemoglobin assay HbA1c is the primary test used to assess glycemic control in a known diabetic individual. Two different tests available for diabetic detection are the estimation of HbA1 and the HbA1c test. The HbA1c is a more commonly used test.[10] Patients with relatively well-controlled diabetes (HbA1c <8%) usually respond to therapy in a manner similar to nondiabetic individuals. Poorly controlled patients (HbA1c >10%) often have a poor response to treatment, with more postoperative complications and less favorable long-term results.[11]

Following are the guidelines for periodontal treatment in diabetic patients:[12]
- Patients should be instructed to carry their glucometer to the dental office during each appointment.
- Patients should check their blood glucose before any long procedure to get a baseline level.
- Patients with blood glucose levels at or below the lower end of normal before the procedure may become hypoglycemic intraoperatively. It is advisable to have such a patient consume some carbohydrate before starting treatment. For example, if a 2-hour procedure is planned and the pretreatment glucose level is 70 mg/dL (the lower end of normal range), providing 4 oz of juice preoperatively may help prevent hypoglycemia during treatment. If pre-treatment glucose levels are excessively high, the procedure may need to be postponed until better glycemic control is established. After the procedure, the rechecking of blood glucose should be done in order to assess fluctuations over time.
- Any time the patient feels symptoms of hypoglycemic, the glucose should be checked immediately. This may prevent the onset of severe hypoglycemia, a medical emergency.
- Usually, in the diabetic patient, dental appointments should be scheduled in the morning hours. At this time, the patient is well-rested with maximum tolerance for stress. Appointments should be before or after periods of peak insulin activity.
- Patients should follow their usual insulin regimen and take their routine breakfast. The appointment should be scheduled for approximately 1.5 hours following insulin administration and breakfast.
- Certain drugs like aspirin and corticosteroids should be avoided as they can directly affect the diabetic condition.

The most common dental office complication noted in diabetic patients on insulin is experiencing symptomatic low blood glucose or hypoglycemia. Hypoglycemia does not usually occur until blood glucose levels fall below 60 mg/dL. However, in patients with poor glycemic control who have prolonged hyperglycemia (high blood glucose levels), a rapid drop in glucose can precipitate signs and

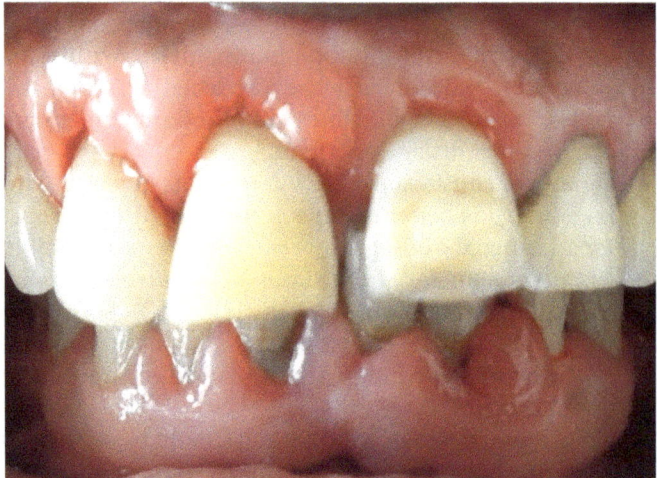

**Fig. 55.1:** Clinical picture showing gingival inflammation in a diabetic patient.

symptoms of hypoglycemia at levels well above 60 mg/dL. Signs and symptoms of hypoglycemia are tremors, sweating, tachycardia, dizziness, seizures, and unconsciousness. Hypoglycemia is more common in patients with better glycemic control. Patients taking insulin are at greatest risk, followed by those on sulfonylurea agents, but metformin and thiazolidinediones generally do not cause hypoglycemia.

Checking the pretreatment glucose with the patient's glucometer, checking again during long procedures, and again at the end of the procedure prevent hypoglycemia.

If hypoglycemia occurs during dental treatment, therapy should be immediately terminated. If a glucometer is available, the blood glucose level should be checked.

Treatment guidelines include the following:
- Provide approximately 15 g of oral carbohydrate to the patient: 4-6 oz of juice or soda; 3 or 4 tsp of sugar; hard candy with 15 g of sugar.
- If the patient is unable to take food or drink by mouth, or if the patient is sedated:
  - Give 25-30 mL of 50% dextrose intravenously, or within 3-5 minutes after injection, the patient should regain consciousness.
  - Give 1 mg of glucagon intravenously (glucagon results in rapid release of stored glucose from the liver). The patient will usually respond to the glucagon.
  - Within 10-15 minutes after the injection, or
  - Give 1 mg of glucagon intramuscularly (if no IV access).
- Management of the unconscious patient usually involves airway maintenance, oxygen administration, and monitoring of vital signs. Patients experiencing periods of unconsciousness should be taken to a hospital for further evaluation and treatment instead of permitting them to leave the office.

## Thyroid Disorders

Periodontal therapy demands minimal alterations in the patient with adequately managed thyroid diseases.[13] Following are the guidelines for periodontal treatment in thyroid disorder patients:
- Patients with thyrotoxicosis and those with inadequate medical management should not receive periodontal therapy until their conditions are stabilized.
- Patients with a history of hyperthyroidism should be carefully evaluated to determine the level of medical management. They should be managed in a way that limits stress and infection. Hyperthyroidism may cause tachycardia and other arrhythmias, increased cardiac output, and myocardial ischemia.
- Avoid epinephrine and other vasopressor amines in thyrotoxicosis, poorly controlled thyroid disorders and hyperthyroidism patients.[14]
- Avoid sedatives and narcotics in hypothyroid patients due to the potential for excessive sedation.

## Adrenal Insufficiency

Acute adrenal insufficiency causes peripheral vascular collapse and cardiac arrest. It is of two types: primary adrenal insufficiency (Addison's disease) and secondary adrenalin sufficiency (most often caused by use of exogenous glucocorticosteroids).

Clinical manifestations are mental confusion, fatigue and weakness, nausea, vomiting, hypertension, syncope, intense abdominal pain, lower back pain, leg pain, loss of consciousness, and coma.

Following are the guidelines for periodontal treatment in adrenal insufficiency patients:
- For patients taking large doses of more than 20 mg cortisol equivalent per day and requiring stressful periodontal procedures, doubling or tripling normal steroid dose 1 hour before the procedure is often recommended.[15]
- For patients on low doses for short periods of time that is less than one month, no supplementation is required.
- In an emergency situation, the increase in steroids' dosage before the procedure may decrease the chances of an acute adrenal crisis.

Following are the guidelines to manage a patient with acute adrenal insufficiency:
- *Conscious patient*:
  - Terminate dental therapy
  - Monitor vital signs
  - Place the patient in the supine position
  - Emergency kit (oxygen)
  - *Administer glucocorticosteroids*: 100 mg Hydrocortisone sodium Succinate IV or IM over 30 seconds.
  - Summon medical assistance.
- *Unconscious patient*:
  - Recognize unconsciousness
  - Place the patient in the supine position
  - Basic life support

## RENAL DISEASES

The most common causes of renal failure are glomerulonephritis, pyelonephritis, cystic kidney disease, renovascular disease, drug nephropathy, obstructive uropathy, and hypertension. Renal failure may result in severe electrolyte imbalances, cardiac arrhythmias, pulmonary congestion, CHF and prolonged bleeding.[16] The patient in chronic renal failure has a progressive disease that ultimately may require kidney transplantation or dialysis. It is preferable to treat the patient before, rather than after, transplant or dialysis.

Following are the guidelines for periodontal treatment in renal disease patients:
- Consult the patient's physician.
- Monitor blood pressure (patients in end-stage renal failure are usually hypertensive).

- *Check laboratory values*: Partial thromboplastin time, prothrombin time, bleeding time, and platelet count; hematocrit; blood urea nitrogen (do not treat if less than 60 mg/dL); and serum creatinine (do not treat if less than 1.5 mg/dL).
- Eliminate areas of oral infection to prevent systemic infection.
  - Good oral hygiene should be established.
  - Periodontal treatment should aim at eliminating inflammation or infection and providing easy maintenance.
  - Questionable teeth should be extracted if medical parameters permit.
  - Frequent recall appointments should be scheduled.
- Drugs that are nephrotoxic or metabolized by the kidney should not be given (e.g., phenacetin, tetracycline, aminoglycoside antibiotics). Acetaminophen may be used for analgesia, and diazepam may be used for sedation. Local anesthetics such as lidocaine are generally safe.

The patients who are receiving hemodialysis require special precautions and treatment planning modifications. These patients have a high incidence of viral hepatitis, anemia, and prolonged hemorrhage. The risk for hemorrhage is related to anticoagulation during dialysis, platelet trauma from dialysis, and the uremia that develops with renal failure. Hemodialysis patients have either an internal arteriovenous fistula or an external arteriovenous shunt. This shunt is often located in the arm and must be protected from trauma. Thus, in addition to guidelines for patients with chronic renal disease, the following recommendation is made for those on hemodialysis:

- Screen for hepatitis B and hepatitis C antigens and antibodies before any treatment.
- Provide antibiotic prophylaxis to prevent endarteritis of the arteriovenous fistula or shunt. Intermittent peritoneal dialysis (IPD) and continuous ambulatory peritoneal dialysis (CAPD) patients do not generally require prophylactic antibiotics).
- Patients receive heparin anticoagulation on the day of hemodialysis. Therefore, provide periodontal treatment on the day *after* dialysis, when the effects of heparinization have subsided. Hemodialysis treatments are generally performed 3 or 4 times a week. (IPD and CAPD patients are not systemically heparinized; therefore, they usually do not have the potential bleeding problems associated with hemodialysis.)
- Be careful to protect the hemodialysis shunt or fistula when the patient is in the dental chair. If the shunt or fistula is placed in the arm, do not cramp the limb; *blood pressure readings should be taken from the other arm*. Do not use the limb for the injection of medication. Patients with leg shunts should avoid sitting with the leg dependent for longer than 1 hour. If appointments last longer, allow the patient to walk about for a few minutes and then resume therapy.
- Refer the patient to the physician if uremic problems develop, such as uremic stomatitis. Refer to the physician if oral infections do not resolve promptly to prevent systemic dissemination.

The renal transplant patient's greatest foe is infection. Transplant patients take immunosuppressive drugs that greatly reduce resistance to infection. Excessive bleeding may occur during or after periodontal treatment due to drug-induced thrombocytopenia, anticoagulation, or both. A periodontal abscess is a potentially life-threatening situation. For this reason, a dental team approach should be used *before* transplantation to determine which teeth can be easily maintained. Many organ transplant centers now include dental examination in their standard pretransplant protocol. Teeth with severe bone and attachment loss, furcation invasion, periodontal abscesses, or extensive surgical requirements should be extracted, leaving an easily maintainable dentition.

In addition to the recommendations for patients with chronic renal failure, the following should be considered for the renal transplant patient:
- Hepatitis B and C screening.
- Determination of the level of immunocompromise derived from antirejection drug therapy.
- Prophylactic antibiotics (using American Heart Association recommendations).

## LIVER DISEASES

Major causes of liver disease include drug toxicity, cirrhosis, viral infections (e.g., hepatitis B and C), and neoplasms.[17] The liver is the site of production for most of the clotting factors. Hence, excessive bleeding can occur during or after periodontal treatment in patients with severe liver disease. Many drugs are metabolized in the liver; thus, liver disease alters normal drug metabolism.

Following guidelines should be used during periodontal therapy:[18]
- Consultation with the physician concerning the current stage of the disease, risk for bleeding, potential drugs to be prescribed during treatment, and required alterations to periodontal therapy.
- Screening for hepatitis B and C.
- Check laboratory values for prothrombin time and partial thromboplastin time.

## PULMONARY DISEASES

The periodontal treatment of a patient with pulmonary disease (asthma, emphysema, bronchitis) may require alteration depending on the nature and the severity of the respiratory problem.[19]

Following guidelines should be used during periodontal therapy:[18,20]
- Identify and refer patients with signs and symptoms of the pulmonary disease to their physicians.
- In patients with known pulmonary disease, consult with their physicians regarding medications (antibiotics, steroids, chemotherapeutic agents) and the degree and severity of the pulmonary disease.
- Avoid elicitation of respiratory depression or distress:
  - Minimize the stress of a periodontal appointment. The patient with emphysema should be treated in the afternoon, several hours after sleep, to allow for airway clearance.
  - Avoid medications that could cause respiratory depression (e.g., narcotics, sedatives, and general anesthetics).
  - Avoid bilateral mandibular block anesthesia, which could cause increased airway obstruction.
  - Position the patient to allow maximal ventilator efficiency, be careful to prevent physical airway obstruction, keep the patient's throat clear, and avoid excess periodontal packing.
- In a patient with a history of asthma, make sure the patient's medication (inhaler) is available.
- Patients with active fungal or bacterial respiratory diseases should not be treated unless the periodontal procedure is an emergency.

## IMMUNOSUPPRESSION AND CHEMOTHERAPY

Immunosuppressed individuals are at greatly increased risk for infection, and even minor periodontal infections can become life-threatening if immunosuppression is severe.

Following guidelines should be used during periodontal therapy:
- The greatest potential for infection occurs during periods of extreme immunosuppression; therefore, treatment should be conservative and palliative. It is always preferable to evaluate the patient before initiation of chemotherapy.
- Teeth having a poor prognosis should be extracted, with thorough debridement of remaining teeth to minimize the microbial load.
- The clinician must emphasize the importance of good oral hygiene. Antimicrobial rinses such as chlorhexidine are recommended, especially for patients with chemotherapy-induced mucositis, to prevent secondary infection.
- If periodontal therapy is needed during chemotherapy, it should be conducted the day *before* chemotherapy is usually given when white cell counts are relatively high. In such cases, coordination with the oncologist is important.
- Dental treatment should be done when white cell counts are above $2,000/mm^3$, with an absolute granulocyte count of $1,000–1,500/mm^3$.[16]

## RADIATION THERAPY

Following are the perioral side effects head and neck radiation therapy:
- *Xerostomia*: The parotid is the most radiosensitive of the salivary glands; saliva may become extremely viscous or nonexistent, depending on the dose delivered to the particular gland. Xerostomia causes a decrease in the normal salivary cleansing mechanisms, buffering capacity of saliva, and pH of oral fluids.
- Oral bacterial populations shift to preponderantly cariogenic forms (e.g., *Streptococcus mutans*, *Actinomyces spp.*, and *Lactobacillus spp.*). Radiation-induced caries may progress very rapidly and affects primarily smooth tooth surfaces.
- *Osteoradionecrosis (ORN)*: ORN is considered as the most severe oral complication. High-dose radiation therapy leads to hypovascularity of irradiated tissues resulting in a reduction in the wound healing capacity. Reduction in vascularity renders the bone less capable of resolving trauma or infection. This leads to severe destruction of bone with resultant ORN. Periodontal disease acts as one of the precipitating factors in ORN.[21,22] Following guidelines should be used during periodontal therapy:
  - *Physician consultation*: The physician should be asked about the amount of radiation to be administered, extent and location of the lesion, nature of any surgical procedures already performed or to be performed, number of radiation ports, exact fields to be irradiated, mode of radiation therapy, and patient's prognosis (i.e., the likelihood of metastasis).
  - *Dental consultation*: Patients scheduled to receive requires dental consultation *at the earliest possible time* to reduce the morbidity of the known perioral side effects.
  - Preirradiation treatment should commence immediately after the physician consultation.
  - Daily topical fluoride application and oral hygiene are the best means of preventing radiation caries in the long-term aspect.
  - Hence, the clinician should address the patient's periodontal disease status before initiating radiation whenever possible.
  - In case of nonrestorable or severely periodontally diseased teeth, it is advisable to extract such teeth, ideally at least two weeks before radiation.
  - Tooth extraction after radiation treatment is associated with a high risk of developing ORN, and hence ideally, surgical flap procedures are discouraged after radiation therapy.

Extractions should be performed in a manner that allows primary closure. Mucoperiosteal flaps should be gently elevated; teeth should be extracted in segments; alveolectomy should be performed, allowing no rough bony spicules to remain; and primary closure should be provided without tension.
- The first decision that should be made relates to possible extractions because radiation can cause side effects that interfere with healing.
  - For head and neck squamous cell carcinomas, the radiation dose is usually 5,000–7,000 cGy (centigrays; 1 cGy = 1 rad) delivered in a fractionated method (150–200 cGy/day over a 6- to the 7-week course).[23]
  - This is considered full-course radiation treatment, and the degree of perioral side effects depends on which tissues are irradiated, i.e., the radiation fields.
  - If this dose is administered to the salivary gland tissues, xerostomia will ensue.

It is unnecessary to extract teeth that can be retained with conservative restorative, endodontic, or periodontal therapy. However, prudence dictates the extraction of questionable teeth because periodontal treatment after irradiation may be limited to nonsurgical forms of therapy. Flap surgery or extraction of teeth after radiation may lead to ORN. Management of ORN is usually difficult and costly and involves the progressively more aggressive treatment, especially when a bone fails to respond to conservative therapy. Costly hyperbaric oxygen therapy is frequently required for complete resolution. During radiation therapy, patients should receive weekly prophylaxis, oral hygiene instruction, and professionally applied fluoride treatments unless mucositis prevents such treatment. Patients should be instructed to brush daily with 0.4% stannous or 1.0% sodium fluoride gel. Custom gel trays allow optimum fluoride application. All remaining teeth should receive thorough debridement (scaling and root planing). Postirradiation follow-up consists of palliative treatment given as indicated. Viscous lidocaine may be prescribed for painful mucositis, and salivary substitutes may be given for xerostomia. A long-term, 3-month recall interval is ideal.

## PROSTHETIC JOINT REPLACEMENT

Antibiotic prophylaxis before dental treatment is not indicated for most patients with prosthetic joint replacements. However, prophylaxis is indicated for almost all patients within the first two years after joint replacement and for so-called "high-risk" patients including those with previous prosthetic joint infections **(Table 55.3)**, immunosuppression, rheumatoid arthritis, systemic lupus erythematosus, type 1 diabetes, and hemophilia.[24]

Before initiating periodontal treatment, it is advisable to consult with the patient's orthopedic surgeon, who may help to assess the risk for joint infection relative to current dental status and type of periodontal treatment planned. Because individuals with significant periodontal disease are considered "high risk," antibiotic prophylaxis before treatment is common in the periodontal practice.

**TABLE 55.3:** Prophylactic antibiotic regimens for prevention of prosthetic joint infections.

| Antibiotic regimens | Patient characteristics |
| --- | --- |
| 2 g cephalexin, cephradine, or amoxicillin orally 1 hour before dental procedure | Patients not allergic to penicillins |
| 600 mg clindamycin orally 1 hour before dental procedure | Patients allergic to penicillins |
| 1 g cefazolin or 2 g ampicillin IM or IV 1 hour before dental procedure | Patients not allergic to penicillins and unable to take oral medications |
| 600 mg clindamycin IV 1 hour before dental procedure | Patients allergic to penicillins and unable to take oral medications |

## PREGNANCY

The aim of periodontal therapy for the pregnant patient is to reduce the potential exaggerated inflammatory response associated with the pregnancy-associated hormonal alterations. Meticulous plaque control, scaling, root planing, and polishing should be the only nonemergency periodontal procedures performed.

The second trimester is considered the safest time to conduct treatment. Long, stressful appointments and periodontal surgical procedures should be postponed up to the postpartum period.

Following precautions should be taken during the treatment of a pregnant patient:[16,25]
- Short appointments served in series to avoid unnecessary fatigue in patients.
- In a pregnant patient, the chair should be gently lowered and straighten because of genuine awkwardness due to new shape and weight gain.
- Place the patient on the left side or elevate the right hip 5–6 inches by placing a pillow or blanket roll underneath. The supine position allows the weight of developing a fetus to bear down directly on vena cava, aorta, and major vessels. The reduction in return cardiac blood supply usually leads to supine hypotensive syndrome with decreased placental perfusion.
- Advice non-alcoholic mouthwash and neutral sodium fluoride rinse.
- Instruct on avoiding brush right after vomiting to prevent erosion because nausea and vomiting are common in the first trimester.
- Recommend use of less strong-flavored dentifrice because of the chances of adverse reaction to strong smells and flavor in the pregnant patient.

- Recommend a small toothbrush; take care of the instrument and radiographic film placement to avoid gagging.
- Ideally, no medications should be prescribed because of the toxic or teratogenic effects of therapy on the fetus.
- The use of dental radiographs during pregnancy should be kept to a minimum. When required during pregnancy, the patient is covered with a lead apron, thyroid collar, and a second apron for the back to prevent secondary radiation from reaching the abdomen.
- The prescribed drugs should be taken just after breastfeeding by nursing mother and then avoid breastfeeding for 4 hours or more. This helps to markedly decrease drug concentration in breast milk.
- *Plaque control*: In the pregnant patient, primary objectives are establishing a healthy oral environment and optimal oral hygiene levels. This can be achieved by recommending a preventive periodontal program. It consists of nutritional counseling and rigorous plaque control measures in the dental office and at home. Scaling, polishing, and root planing are recommended whenever necessary throughout the pregnancy.
- Generally, pregnancy tumors will regress somewhat postpartum, but surgical excision is often required for complete resolution. The tumor is surgically removed in pregnancy only if it is being traumatized by opposing teeth or restoration, causing bleeding.

## HEMORRHAGIC DISORDERS

Patients with a history of bleeding problems either due to disease or drug should be managed appropriately in order to reduce the risks of hemorrhage. Identification of these patients via health history, clinical examination, and clinical laboratory tests is paramount.

Health questioning should cover:
- History of bleeding after previous surgery or trauma
- Past and present drug history
- History of bleeding problems among relatives
- Illnesses associated with potential bleeding problems.

Clinical examinations should detect the existence of jaundice, ecchymosis, spider telangiectasia, hemarthrosis, petechiae, hemorrhagic vesicles, spontaneous gingival bleeding, or gingival hyperplasia.

Laboratory tests include bleeding time (BT), prothrombin time (PT), tourniquet test, complete blood cell count, partial thromboplastin time (PTT), and coagulation time (CT).

Bleeding disorders classified as:
- Coagulation disorders
- Thrombocytopenic purpuras
- Nonthrombocytopenic purpuras

## Patients with Coagulation Disorders

The common inherited coagulation disorders (**Table 55.4**) are as follows:[16,26]
- Hemophilia A results in a deficiency of coagulation factor VIII.
    - Mild hemophiliacs with 6–30% factor VIII rarely bleed spontaneously but may still have hemorrhage after severe trauma or during surgical procedures.
    - Moderate hemophiliacs with 1–5% factor VIII have less frequent spontaneous hemorrhage but still, bleed with minimal trauma.
    - Severe hemophiliacs with less than 1% of normal factor VIII levels may have severe bleeding on the slightest provocation.

Precautions:
- The dentist should seek physician consultation before initiating periodontal treatment. This helps to determine the risk for bleeding and treatment modifications required.
- In order to avoid surgical hemorrhage, levels of factor VIII should be at least 30%. In patients with mild or moderate hemophilia administration of parenteral 1-deamino-8-D-arginine vasopressin (DDAVP) helps to raise factor VIII levels 2 to 3-fold.

**TABLE 55.4:** Inherited coagulation disorders.

| Type | Prolonged | Normal | Treatment |
| --- | --- | --- | --- |
| Hemophilia A | Partial thromboplastin time (PTT) | Prothrombin time (PT) Bleeding time | ❑ DDAVP<br>❑ Factor VIII concentrate or cryoprecipitate<br>❑ Fresh frozen plasma<br>❑ Fresh whole blood<br>❑ Epsilon-aminocaproic acid (EACA)<br>❑ Tranexamic acid |
| Hemophilia B | Partial thromboplastin time | Prothrombin time Bleeding time | ❑ Purified prothrombin complex concentrates<br>❑ Factor IX concentrates<br>❑ Fresh frozen plasma |
| von Willebrand's disease | Bleeding time<br>Partial thromboplastin time<br>Variable Factor VIII deficiency | Prothrombin time Platelet count | ❑ DDAVP (desmopressin)<br>❑ Factor VIII concentrate or cryoprecipitate |

(DDAVP: 1-deamino- 8-D-arginine vasopressin)

- Most moderate and severe hemophiliacs require the infusion of factor VIII concentrate before surgical procedures.
- Hemophilia B/Christmas disease results in the deficiency of factor IX.
  Precautions:
  - Surgical therapy requires a factor IX level of 30–50%
  - Purified prothrombin complex concentrates, or factor IX concentrates is administered.
- Von Willebrand's disease is due to a deficiency of the von Willebrand factor, which is responsible for the adhesion of platelets to the injured vessel wall and initiates primary hemostasis. Von Willebrand factor also carries the coagulant portion of factor VIII in the plasma. Bleeding during dental treatment is considered as the first sign of the underlying disease.
  Precautions:
  - Milder forms respond well to the administration of DDAVP before undertaking periodontal surgery.
  - Severe forms need administration of preoperative factor VIII concentrate or cryoprecipitate infusion.

## Patients with Liver Diseases

Periodontal treatment should be altered as follows:
- Consult physician.
- *Laboratory test*: Prothrombin time, bleeding time, platelet count, and partial thromboplastin time.
- Nonsurgical and conservative periodontal therapy.
- *For periodontal surgery, the patient may require hospitalization*: International normalized ratio (INR) (prothrombin time) should generally be <2.0. For simple surgical procedures, INR < 2.5 is generally safe. Platelet count should be >80,000/mm$^3$.

Perhaps the most common cause of abnormal coagulation is drug therapy. Patients with prosthetic heart valves or histories of myocardial infarction, stroke, or thromboembolism are usually candidates of regular anticoagulant therapy with the use of coumarin derivatives such as dicumarol and warfarin. These drugs are vitamin K antagonists that decrease the production of vitamin K-dependent coagulation factors II, VII, IX, and X. The effectiveness of anticoagulation therapy is monitored via the prothrombin time. The recommended level of anticoagulation for most patients is INR of 2.0–3.0, with prosthetic heart valve patients generally in the range of 2.5–3.5.

## Patients on Anticoagulant Therapy

Periodontal treatment should be altered as follows:
- Consult the patient's physician to determine the nature of the underlying medical problem and the degree of required anticoagulation.
- Determines the acceptable INR:
  - INR <3.0 is required for infiltration anesthesia, scaling, and root planing.
  - INR <2.0 is required for block anesthesia, minor periodontal surgery, and simple extractions.
  - INR <1.5 is required for complex surgery or multiple extractions.
  - The physician should be consulted about discontinuing or reducing anticoagulant dosage until the desired INR is achieved. Frequently, the anticoagulant is discontinued for 2–3 days before periodontal treatment (the clearance half-life of warfarin is 36–42 hours), and the INR is checked on the day of therapy. If the INR is within the acceptable target range, the procedure is done, and the anticoagulant is resumed immediately after treatment.
- Careful technique and complete wound closure are paramount. For all procedures, the application of pressure can minimize hemorrhage. The use of oxidized cellulose, microfibrillar collagen, topical thrombin, and tranexamic acid should be considered for persistent bleeding.
- *Avoid aspirin*: Aspirin binds irreversibly to platelets and thus, interferes with normal platelet aggregation resulting in prolonged bleeding. Since it binds irreversibly to platelets, its effects last for 4–7 days. It does not alter bleeding time if taken in a smaller dose, but higher doses may increase bleeding time and predispose the patient to postoperative bleeding. Thus, aspirin should not be prescribed for patients receiving anticoagulation therapy or have illnesses related to bleeding tendencies.

## Thrombocytopenic Purpuras

Thrombocytopenia occurs when the platelet count is less than 100,000/mm$^3$. Thrombocytopenia induced bleeding may occur in idiopathic thrombocytopenic purpuras, radiation therapy, myelosuppressive drug therapy (e.g., chemotherapy), leukemia, or infections.

Following are the alteration in periodontal therapy for patients with thrombocytopenia:
- A physician referral is indicated for a definitive diagnosis and to determine any alterations in planned therapy.
- Conservative treatment should be done wherever possible. Aggressive therapy should be avoided. Patients should be instructed on regular oral hygiene instructions and frequent maintenance visits.
- Nonsurgical therapy, i.e., scaling and root planing, is usually safe in such cases, except where platelet counts are <60,000/mm$^3$.
- *Surgical therapy*: Surgical procedures are usually contraindicated when the platelet count is <80,000/mm$^3$. Platelet transfusion may be required before surgery. Surgical technique should be as atraumatic as possible along with the application of appropriate local hemostatic measures.

## Nonthrombocytopenic Purpuras

Nonthrombocytopenic purpuras occur as a result of either vascular wall fragility or thrombasthenia (impaired platelet aggregation). The former may result due to hypersensitivity reactions, scurvy, infections, phenacetin, and aspirin. Thrombasthenia occurs in uremia, Glanzmann's disease, aspirin ingestion, and von Willebrand's disease. Both kinds of nonthrombocytopenic purpuras may result in immediate bleeding after the gingival injury.

Following are the alterations in periodontal therapy for patients with nonthrombocytopenic purpuras:
- A physician referral is indicated for a definitive diagnosis and to determine any alterations in planned therapy.
- *Direct local pressure*: Treatment consists primarily of direct pressure applied for at least 15 minutes to control the bleeding.
- Surgical therapy should be avoided unless the qualitative and quantitative platelet problems are resolved.

## BLOOD DYSCRASIAS

Numerous disorders of red and white blood cells may affect the course of periodontal therapy. Alterations in wound healing, bleeding, tissue appearance, and susceptibility to infection may occur. Clinicians should be aware of the clinical signs and symptoms of blood dyscrasias, the availability of screening laboratory tests, and the need for a physician referral.

### Leukemia

Altered periodontal treatment for patients with leukemia is based on such patients' enhanced susceptibility to infections, bleeding tendency, and the effects of chemotherapy.[16]

The treatment plan for leukemic patients is as follows:
- Refer the patient for medical evaluation and treatment. Close cooperation with the physician is required.
- Before chemotherapy, a complete periodontal treatment plan should be developed with a physician.
  - Monitor hematologic laboratory values daily: bleeding time, coagulation time, prothrombin time, and platelet count.
  - Administer antibiotic coverage before any periodontal treatment because the infection is a major concern.
  - Extract all hopeless, non-maintainable, or potentially infectious teeth at least ten days before the initiation of chemotherapy, if systemic condition allows.
  - Periodontal debridement (scaling and root planing) should be performed, and thorough oral hygiene instructions are given if the patient's condition allows. Twice-daily rinsing with 0.12% chlorhexidine gluconate is recommended after oral hygiene procedures. Recognize the potential for bleeding due to thrombocytopenia. Use pressure and topical hemostatic agents as indicated.
- During the acute phases of leukemia, patients should receive only emergency periodontal care. Any source of potential infection must be eliminated to prevent systemic dissemination. Antibiotic therapy is frequently the treatment of choice, combined with nonsurgical or surgical debridement, as indicated.
- Oral ulcerations or mucositis are treated palliatively with agents such as viscous lidocaine. Systemic antibiotics may be indicated to prevent secondary infection.
- Oral candidiasis is common in the leukemic patient and can be treated with nystatin suspensions (100,000 U/mL 4 times daily) or clotrimazole vaginal suppositories (10 mg 4–5 times daily).
- For patients with chronic leukemia and those in remission, scaling, and root planing can be performed without complication, but periodontal surgery should be avoided. Platelet count and a bleeding time should be measured on the day of the procedure.

If either is low, postpone the appointment and refer the patient to a physician.

### Agranulocytosis

Patients with agranulocytosis (cyclic neutropenia and granulocytopenia) have an increased susceptibility to infection. The total white blood cell count is reduced, and granular leukocytes (neutrophils, eosinophils, and/or basophils) are reduced or disappear. These disorders are often marked by early, severe periodontal destruction. In such cases, periodontal treatment should be carried out in the periods of disease remission. Whenever possible, try to opt for conservative treatment with a significant focus on reducing the potential sources of systemic infection. Severely affected teeth should be extracted only after physician consultation. The patient must be instructed on oral hygiene instructions, including the use of chlorhexidine mouthrinses twice daily. Scaling and root planing should be conducted carefully under antibiotic protection.

## INFECTIOUS DISEASES

Because many infectious diseases are occult in nature, and because medical histories are often inaccurate or incomplete, all periodontal patients should be treated as though they have an infectious disease. Protection of patients, clinicians, and office staff requires the use of universal (standard) precautions for each and every patient, maximizing the prevention of infection and cross-contamination. Hepatitis, human immunodeficiency virus (HIV), acquired immunodeficiency syndrome (AIDS), and tuberculosis in relation to the precautions required in periodontal therapy are discussed in this chapter.

## Section 7: Treatment: Surgical Therapy

**TABLE 55.5:** Various types of hepatitis.

| Hepatitis viruses | Source | Primary modes of transmission | Incubation period (in days) | Vaccine available |
|---|---|---|---|---|
| A | Feces | Fecal-oral | 15–50 | Yes |
| B | Blood and body fluids | Percutaneous or per mucosal, sexual | 15–160 | Yes |
| C | Blood and body fluids | Percutaneous or per mucosal | 15–150 | No |
| D | Blood and body fluids | Percutaneous or per mucosal | 15–150 | Yes |
| E | Feces | Fecal-oral | 15–60 | No |
| G | Blood | Percutaneous | Unknown | No |

## Hepatitis

To date, six distinct viruses causing viral hepatitis have been identified: Hepatitis A, B, C, D, E, and G viruses.[27] These forms of viral hepatitis differ in their virology, epidemiology, and prophylaxis **(Table 55.5)**. Because most hepatitis infections are undiagnosed, the clinician must be aware of high-risk groups such as renal dialysis patients, healthcare workers, immunosuppressed patients, and patients who have received multiple blood transfusions, homosexuals, and drugs users, and institutionalized patients.

Guidelines for treating hepatitis patients are as follows:[18]
- If the disease, regardless of type, is active, do not provide periodontal therapy unless the situation is an emergency. In an emergency case, follow the protocol for HBsAg – positive patients (HBV surface antigen).
- For patients with a history of hepatitis, consult the physician to determine the type of hepatitis, course, length of the disease, mode of transmission, and any chronic liver disease or viral carrier state.
- For recovered hepatitis A or E patients, perform routine periodontal care.
- For recovered hepatitis B and D patients, consult with the physician and order HBsAg and anti-HBs (antibody to HBV surface antigen) laboratory tests:
  - If HBsAg and anti-HBs tests are negative, but the hepatitis B virus is suspected, order another HBs determination.
  - Patients who are HBsAg positive are probably infective (chronic carriers); the degree of infectivity is measured via an HBsAg determination.
  - Patients who are anti-HBs positive may be treated routinely (they have antibodies to the HBs antigen).
  - Patients who are HBsAg negative may be treated routinely.
- For hepatitis C patients, consult with the physician to determine the patient's risk for transmissibility and the current status of chronic liver disease.
- If a patient with active hepatitis, positive HBsAg (HBV carrier) status or positive HCV carrier status requires emergency treatment, use the following precautions:
  - Consult the patient's physician regarding status.
  - If bleeding is likely during or after treatment, measure prothrombin time and bleeding time. Hepatitis may alter coagulation; alter treatment accordingly.
  - All personnel in clinical contact with the patient should use full barrier techniques, including masks, gloves, glasses or eye shields, and disposable gowns.
  - Use as many disposable covers as possible, covering light handles, drawer handles, and bracket trays. Headrest covers should also be used.
  - All disposable items (gauze, floss, saliva ejectors, masks, gowns, gloves, etc.) should be placed in one lined wastebasket. After treatment, these items and all disposable covers should be bagged, labeled, and disposed of, following proper guidelines for biohazardous waste.
  - Aseptic technique should be followed at all times. Minimize aerosol production by not using ultrasonic instrumentation, air syringe, or high-speed handpieces; remember that saliva contains a distillate of the virus. Rinsing with chlorhexidine gluconate for 30 seconds prior is highly recommended.
  - When the procedure is completed, all equipment should be scrubbed and sterilized. If an item cannot be sterilized or disposed of, it should not be used.

If a percutaneous or per mucosal injury occurs during an HBV carrier's dental treatment, the current Centers for Disease Control and Prevention guidelines recommend administration of hepatitis B immunoglobulin. The HBV vaccine should also be administered if the injured individual has not previously received it. Unfortunately, postexposure prophylaxis with immunoglobulin or antiviral agents is generally ineffective if a percutaneous injury occurs during the treatment of a hepatitis C carrier.

## HIV and AIDS

Guidelines for treating HIV and AIDS patient are as follows:
- Individuals with known HIV infection may not admit their status in medical history. Therefore, every patient receiving dental treatment should be managed as a potentially infected person, using universal precautions for all therapy.
- Extensive periodontal treatment plans should be taken into account considering their relationship to the patient's systemic health, prognosis, and survival time. The progression of HIV varies considerably among individuals. Hence, an ideal treatment plan usually selected in light of the state of the patient's overall health.

For many HIV-infected patients, few contraindications are commonly encountered in routine dental treatment. Moreover, the periodontal treatment plan is influenced by the patient's overall systemic health and coincident oral infections or diseases. Hence, for the clinicians, it is a must to recognize the previously undiagnosed disease, including oral disorders associated with HIV infection. This knowledge also helps to modify treatment protocols appropriately.[16,28]

## Tuberculosis

Guidelines for treating tuberculosis patients are as follows:
- Any patient who gives a history of poor medical follow-up (e.g., lack of yearly chest radiographs) or shows signs or symptoms indicative of tuberculosis should be referred for evaluation.
- The patient with tuberculosis should receive emergency care only.
- If the patient has completed chemotherapy, his or her physician should be consulted regarding infectivity and the results of sputum cultures for *Mycobacterium tuberculosis*.
- When medical clearance has been given, and the sputum culture results are negative, these patients may be treated normally.[18]

## PATIENTS ON BISPHOSPHONATE THERAPY

Bisphosphonate medications are primarily used to treat cancer (IV administration) and osteoporosis (oral administration). They act by inhibiting osteoclastic activity, which leads to less bone resorption, less bone remodeling, and less bone turnover. The use of bisphosphonates in cancer treatment is aimed at preventing the often-lethal imbalance of osteoclastic activity. In the treatment of osteoporosis, the goal is simply to harness osteoclastic activity to minimize or prevent bone loss. The major difference in the use of bisphosphonates for cancer versus osteoporosis is the potency and administration route. The potency is influenced by the chemical properties and pharmacokinetics of these agents with bone.

Clinically, bisphosphonate-related osteonecrosis of the jaw (BRONJ) presents as exposed alveolar bone occurring spontaneously or after a dental procedure. Individuals treated with high potency, nitrogen-containing bisphosphonates, especially those administered via IV for cancer treatment (e.g., zoledronate), appear to be at greater risk for BRONJ than individuals taking oral bisphosphonates for prevention and treatment of osteoporosis. The risk for individuals treated with oral bisphosphonates for a period of less than three years appears to be minimal or zero. Regular use of oral bisphosphonates for a period greater than 3 years suggests a risk profile that increases with time and length of use.[29]

As with many multifactorial diseases and conditions, the factors in addition to bisphosphonate therapy likely contribute to the individual risk of BRONJ.
- Potential risk factors thought to contribute to the development of BRONJ include systemic corticosteroid therapy, smoking, alcohol, poor oral hygiene, chemotherapy, radiotherapy, diabetes, and hematologic diseases.
- Reported factors or conditions leading to BRONJ include extractions, root canal treatment, periodontal infections, periodontal surgery, and dental implant surgery.

Both periodontal disease and treatment (especially surgery) pose a risk for patients treated with bisphosphonates. The bacterial-induced inflammatory process of periodontitis that causes bone resorption can lead to bone necrosis. Likewise, periodontal treatment, especially surgery, may cause bone necrosis in the presence of bisphosphonates. Caution is warranted for any patient who has been or will be treated with bisphosphonates.[29] Healthcare providers need to evaluate patients carefully, communicate with medical health care providers, inform patients, and consider treatment options and risks carefully:[30]
- A careful intraoral examination is prudent for all patients treated with bisphosphonate therapy (IV or oral) to determine whether bone exposures exist and to assess any local conditions that might predispose them to the development of BRONJ.
- A thorough medical history should be reviewed, evaluated, and recorded with details about any bisphosphonate treatment, including medication type, dose, route of administration, and duration.
- Comorbidities, such as previous and current medications, treatments, and existing disease or pathology, should be considered.
- Radiographs should be carefully evaluated for signs of bisphosphonate toxicity.
- Finally, Marx has suggested that a laboratory blood test for the serum C-terminal telopeptide fragment of type I collagen (CTX) can be used as a means of assessing an individual's risk of developing BRONJ (Table 55.6). He reported that lower CTX values are associated with greater risk. The CTX laboratory test is a measure of the specific C-terminal fragment of type I collagen cleaved by osteoclasts and serves as a good indicator of bone resorption activity. However, its use as a measure of

**TABLE 55.6:** C-terminal telopeptide laboratory risk assessment for bisphosphonate therapy.

| C-terminal telopeptide value | Risk for BRONJ |
| --- | --- |
| 300–600 pg/mL (normal) | None |
| 150–299 pg/mL | None or minimal |
| 101–149 pg/mL | Moderate |
| ≤100 pg/mL | High |

(BRONJ: bisphosphonate-related osteonecrosis of the jaw)

risk for BRONJ is controversial and not confirmed by prospective studies.

Optimal periodontal/oral health should be achieved and maintained for all patients. For individuals treated with IV bisphosphonates, invasive treatment, such as extractions, periodontal surgery, implant surgery, and bone augmentation procedures, should be avoided. Caution and careful consideration of risks must be considered before any treatment for individuals with a history of taking oral bisphosphonates for periods longer than 3 years.

## EPILEPTIC PATIENTS

Following are the guidelines for periodontal treatment in epileptic patients:[31]

- An early hour's appointment should be given to the patient.
- Treatment sessions should be kept short and simple.
- Avoid extreme noise and bright lights.

Following are the guidelines if a seizure occurs while the patient is in the dental chair:[32]

- Stop the treatment and clear all instruments away from the patient. Preventing injury is the primary, most important goal of assistance.
- Place the dental chair in a supported, supine position as near to the floor as possible.
- Place the patient on his or her side (to decrease the chance of aspiration of secretions or dental materials in the patient's mouth).
- Any tight clothing the patient is wearing should be loosened.
- Do not restrain the patient.
- If the seizure lasts longer than 1 minute or for repeated seizures, administer a 10-mg dose of diazepam intramuscularly (IM) or intravenously (IV), or 5 mg of midazolam, IM, or IV.
- Be aware of the possibility of a compromised airway or uncontrollable seizure.

Once the seizure is over, do not undertake further dental treatment that day and do not allow the patient to leave the office if his or her level of awareness is not fully restored. Depending on the post-ictal state, discharge the patient to home with a responsible person. If required, contact his or her family physician or emergency room for further assessment.

### Points to Ponder

- ❏ The second trimester is considered the safest time to conduct treatment in a pregnant patient.
- ❏ Place the pregnant patient on the left side or elevate the right hip 5–6 inches. Avoid placing the pregnant patient in a supine position.
- ❏ Phenacetin, tetracycline, aminoglycoside antibiotics, which are metabolized by the kidney, are avoided in renal disease patients.
- ❏ After the epileptic attack, the patient is placed on his or her side to decrease the chances of aspiration of secretions or dental materials in the mouth.

## REFERENCES

1. Glick M. New guidelines for prevention, detection, evaluation, and treatment of high blood pressure. J Am Dent Assoc. 1998;129 (11):1588-94.
2. Muzyka BC, Glick M. The hypertensive dental patient. J Am Dent Assoc. 1997;128:1109-20.
3. Mask AG. Medical management of the patient with cardiovascular disease. Periodontol 2000. 2000;23:136-41.
4. Yagiela JA. Adverse drug interactions in dental practice: Interactions associated with vasoconstrictors. J Am Dent Assoc. 1999;130(5):701-9.
5. Findler M, Garfunkel AA, Galili D. Review of very high-risk patients in the dental setting. Compendium Contin Educ Dent. 1994;15(1):58.
6. Dajani AS, Taubert KA, Wilson W, Bolger AF, Bayer A, Ferrieri P, et al. Prevention of bacterial endocarditis. Recommendations by the American Heart Association. JAMA. 1997;277(22):1794-801.
7. Dajani AS, Taubert KA, Wilson W, Bolger AF, Bayer A, Ferrieri P, et al. Prevention of bacterial endocarditis. Recommendations by the American Heart Association. J Am Dent Assoc. 1997;128(8):1142-51.
8. Durack DT. Prevention of infective endocarditis. N Engl J Med. 1995;332(1):38–44.
9. Lockhart PB, Schmidtke MA. Antibiotic considerations in medically compromised patients. Dent Clin North Am. 1994;38(3):381-402.
10. Mealey BL. Impact of advances in diabetes care on dental treatment of the diabetic patient. Compendium Contin Educ Dent. 1998;19(1):41-4.
11. Tervonen T, Karjalainen K. Periodontal disease related to diabetic status. A pilot study of the response to periodontal therapy in type 1 diabetes. J Clin Periodontol. 1997;24: 505-10.
12. Rees TD. Periodontal management of the patient with diabetes mellitus. Periodontol 2000. 2000;23:63-72.
13. Sherman RG, Lasseter DH. Pharmacologic management of patients with diseases of the endocrine system. Dent Clin North Am. 1996;40(3):727-52.
14. Yagiela JA. Adverse drug interactions in dental practice: Interactions associated with vasoconstrictors. J Am Dent Assoc. 1999;130:701.
15. Shapiro R, Carroll PB, Tzakis A, Cemaj S, Lopatin WB, Nakazato P. et al. Adrenal reserve in renal transplant recipients with cyclosporine/azathioprine/ prednisone immunosuppression. Transplantation. 1990; 49(5):1011.
16. Mealey BL. Periodontal implications: Medically compromised patients. Ann Periodontol. 1996;1(1): 256-321.
17. Ziccardi VB, Abubaker. AO, Sotereanos GC, Patterson GT. Maxillofacial considerations in orthotopic liver transplantation. Oral Surg Oral Med Oral Pathol. 1991;71(1):21-6.
18. Mealey BL, Klokkevold PR, Otomo-Corgel J. Periodontal Treatment of Medically Compromised Patients. In: Newman MG, Takei HH, Carranza FA (Eds). Carranza's Clinical Periodontology 9th edition. Philadelphia, PA, USA: WB Saunders; 2003. pp.527-50.
19. Scannapieco FA: Respiratory diseases. In: Rose LF, Genco RJ, Mealey BL, Cohen DW (Eds). Periodontal Medicine. 1st edition. Toronto, Canada: BC Decker Publishers, 2000.
20. Scannapieco FA, Bush RB, Paju S. Associations between periodontal disease and risk for nosocomial bacterial pneumonia and chronic obstructive pulmonary disease. A systematic review. Ann Periodontol. 2003;8(1): 5469.
21. Carl W. Local radiation and systemic chemotherapy. Preventing and managing the oral complications. J Am Dent Assoc. 1993;124(3):119-23.

22. Galler C, Epstein JB, Guze KA, Buckles D, Stevenson-Moore P. et al. The development of osteoradionecrosis from sites of periodontal disease activity: report of 3 cases. J Periodontol. 1992;63(4):310-6.
23. Mealey BL, Semba SE, Hallmon WW: The head and neck radiotherapy patient: Part 2. Management of oral complications. Compendium Contin Educ Dent. 1994;15(4):442.
24. American Dental Association, American Academy of Orthopaedic Surgeons: Advisory Statement: Antibiotic prophylaxis for dental patients with total joint replacements. J Am Dent Assoc. 1997;128:1004.
25. Tarsitano BE, Rollings RE. The pregnant patient: Evaluation and management. Gen Dent. 1993;41(3):226-34.
26. Patton LL, Ship JA. Treatment of patients with bleeding disorders. Dent Clin North Am. 1994; 38:465.
27. Gillchrist JA. Hepatitis viruses A, B, C, D, E, and G: Implications for dental personnel. J Am Dent Assoc. 1999;130(4):509-20.
28. Ryder MI. Periodontal management of HIV-infected patients. Periodontol 2000. 2000;23:85-93.
29. Markiewicz MR, Margarone JE, Campbell JH, Aguirre A. Bisphosphonate-associated osteonecrosis of the jaws: A review of current knowledge. J Am Dent Assoc. 2005;136:1669-74.
30. Migliorati CA, Casiglia J, Epstein J, Jacobsen PL, Siegel MA, Woo S-K. Managing the care of patients with bisphosphonate-associated osteonecrosis. J Am Dent Assoc. 2005;136:1658-68.
31. Fiske J, Boyle C. Epilepsy and Oral Care. Dental Update. 2002;29:180-7.
32. Sanders BJ, Weddell JA, Dodge NN. Managing patients Who have seizure disorders: dental and medical issues. JADA. 1995;126(12):1641-7.

## VIVA VOCE

**Q1.** After how much time period of myocardial infarction, dental treatment can be undertaken?
**Ans.** 6 months.

**Q2.** What should be the concentration of Adrenaline in LA while treating hypertensive patients?
**Ans.** Adrenaline concentration should not be greater than 1:100,000.

**Q3.** Which microorganisms are commonly found in periodontal pockets and are implicated as causing IE?
**Ans.**
- *Actinobacillus actinomycetemcomitans*
- *Eikenella corrodens*
- *Capnocytophaga*
- *Lactobacillus species*

**Q4.** What is the preferable time gap between appointments for periodontal treatment in patients with IE?
**Ans.** 10–14 days or at least seven days.

**Q5.** Why 1-deamino- 8-D-arginine vasopressin (DDAVP) is considered the drug of choice in hemophilic patients?
**Ans.** DDAVP has the advantage of avoiding the risk of viral disease transmission from factor VIII infusion.

**Q6.** Why should aspirin be avoided in diabetic patients?
**Ans.** Aspirin decreases glucose levels in diabetic patients and may also enhance the activity of the sulfonylurea hypoglycaemic agents.

**Q7.** In which position the dental chair should be adjusted in CHF patient?
**Ans.** Semirecumbent or upright position.

**Q8.** Name the classic signs of diabetes mellitus.
**Ans.** Polydipsia; Polyuria; Polyphagia.

**Q9.** Why is an epileptic patient placed on his or her side during a seizure?
**Ans.** So as to decrease the chance of aspiration of secretions or dental materials in the patient's mouth.

**Q10.** How do bisphosphonates act?
**Ans.** They act by inhibiting osteoclastic activity, which leads to less bone resorption, less bone remodeling, and less bone turnover.

# Section 8

# Implantology

- Implant Basics
- Implant Surgical Procedures
- Advanced Implant Surgical Procedures
- Peri-implantitis and other Implant-related Complications

# Chapter 56: Implant Basics

*Farhan Durrani, Shalu Bathla*

## Chapter Outline

- Terminologies
- Indications
- Contraindications
- Classifications
- Biomaterials
- Soft Tissue-implant Interface
- Implant—Bone Interface
- Evaluation of Osseointegrated Implants
- Diagnosis and Treatment Planning
- Osseous Considerations

## INTRODUCTION

Implants are now routinely considered as an option in the treatment of partial or complete edentulism. Implant procedures are very technique sensitive and therefore should be undertaken by adequately trained periodontists/surgeons/prosthodontists. The main objective of using dental implants for replacement of missing tooth is the preservation of alveolar bone. The dental implant is positioned into the bone to provide an adequate anchor for the prosthetic device. It also serves as good preventive maintenance procedure for alveolar bone. One basic principle in implant dentistry is that implants are used as replacement for the natural roots. It is therefore, important to understand the similarities and differences between implants and teeth to create strategies that will achieve predictably superior results. Implants and tooth roots have some important similarities and dissimilarities.

## TERMINOLOGIES

Following are the terminologies related to implants (**Fig. 56.1**):[1]

*Body*: The body is that portion of the implant designed to be surgically placed into the bone.

*Cover screw*: In two-stage implant, the first-stage cover screw is positioned on the top of the implant. This avoids

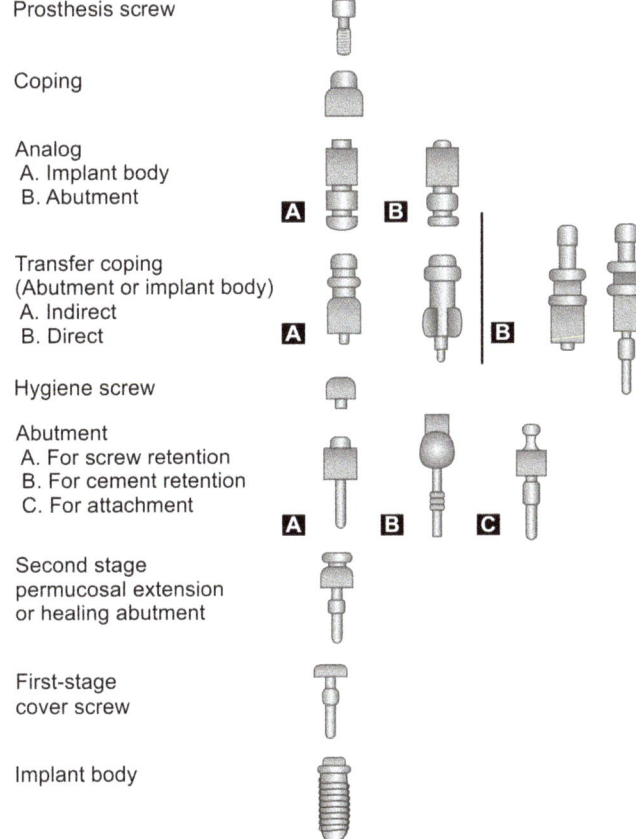

**Fig. 56.1:** Schematic representation showing terminologies related to implant.

the invasion of bone and soft tissue into the abutment connection area during healing process.

*Healing abutment/permucosal extension*: In two-stage implant, a second surgical procedure is conducted to expose implant and provide attachment to a transepithelial portion. This transepithelial portion is called permucosal extension. These are designed to heal or shape tissues after the uncovery procedures. Its purpose is to create an emergence profile in the gingival tissue for the future implant crown.

*Abutment*: The abutment is the implant's part that help to support and/or retain the prosthesis or implant superstructure in position.

According to the method of retention of the prosthesis or superstructure on to the abutment, implant abutments are divided into three main categories:
1. An abutment for screw, uses a screw to retain the prosthesis or superstructure.
2. An abutment for cement, uses dental cement to retain the prosthesis or superstructure.
3. An abutment for attachment, uses an attachment device to retain a removable prosthesis.

Each of the three types of abutments is further classified into straight or angled abutment, which describes the axial relationship between the implant body and the abutment. An abutment for screw type uses a hygiene cover screw positioned over the abutment between prosthetic appointments. This avoids entry of debris and calculus into the internally threaded portion of the abutment.

*Superstructure*: A superstructure is defined as a metal framework that fits the implant abutment (or abutments) and provides retention for the prosthesis.

*Transfer coping/Impression coping/Impression post*: It helps to position an analog in an impression.

*Analog*: An implant analog is helpful in the fabrication of the master cast to replicate the retentive portion of the implant body or abutment.

*Coping*: A coping is a thin covering, specifically designed to fit the implant abutment. It serves as the connection between the abutment and the prosthesis or superstructure. A screw retained prosthesis or superstructure is secured to the implant body or abutment with a coping screw.

## INDICATIONS

- *Edentulous patient*: One of the first indications for dental implant treatment is to treat complete edentulism.
- Partially edentulous patient.
- *Single tooth loss*: Implant maintains bone volume after tooth extraction.
- *Anchorage for the maxillofacial prosthesis*: Patients with maxillofacial deformities uses implant for the maxillofacial prosthesis.
- For rehabilitation of congenital and developmental defects like cleft palate, ectodermal dysplasia, etc.
- For orthodontic anchorage.

## CONTRAINDICATIONS

Following are the extraoral and intraoral contraindications for implant therapy:
- Immunologically compromised patients: Systemic diseases such as developing cancer and AIDS.
- Cardiac diseases: Implant surgery should be carefully considered in patients with heart valve replacements and should not be performed on patients having suffered from recent infarcts, i.e., within the latest 6 months period.
- Deficient hemostasis and blood dyscrasias.
- Anticoagulant medications.
- *Certain psychiatric disorders*: Patients with psychological disorders have difficulties in cooperating and maintaining sufficient oral hygiene.
- Uncontrolled acute infections, as in the respiratory tract, may negatively influence the surgical procedure or may affect the treatment result and are thus, a contraindication for surgical treatment.
- *Recent history of orofacial irradiation*: Irradiation of the jaw may be another potential risk factor for implant treatment, specifically if the jaw has been exposed to irradiation over the level of 50 Gy.
- Heavy smoking and alcohol abuse.
- Various intraoral contraindications are xerostomia, macroglossia and unfavorable intermaxillary occlusal relationship.

## CLASSIFICATIONS

Implants can be classified as follows:[2]
- *According to the shape and position in the jaws*:
  - *Subperiosteal implant*: Custom fabricated framework of metal that is supraalveolar (on top of the bone) but beneath the oral tissues.
  - *Transosteal implant*: These are non-osseointegrated staple implant which are used in mandibular anterior sextant.
  - *Endosseous implant*: Implant is placed directly into the socket which is prepared by using a series of specially prepared drills.
- *According to their body shapes (macrodesign)*[3,4] **(Figs. 56.2A to C)**.
  - *Threaded implants*: These implants are threaded into bone recipient site like a screw with a handpiece or wrench after drilling a hole slightly smaller in diameter than the implant. The threaded implants are more widely used because they usually provide superior initial stability in bone and vertical positioning of the implant during placement can

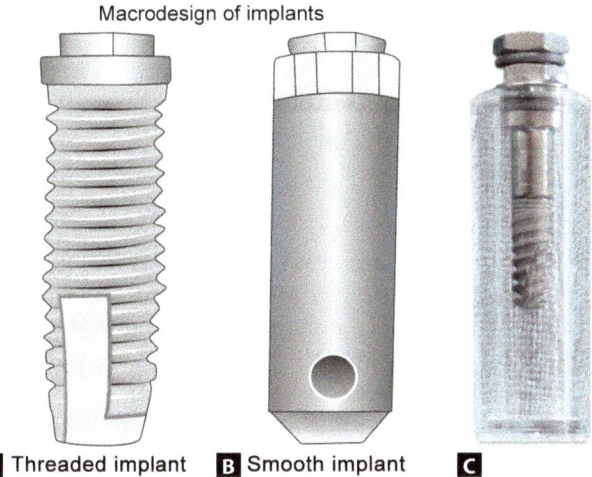

**Figs. 56.2A to C:** Schematic representation and clinical picture showing macrodesign of implants.

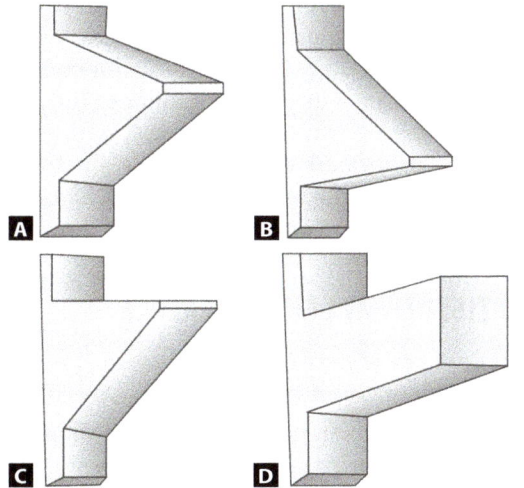

**Figs. 56.3A to D:** Schematic representation showing the four basic thread shapes for implant design: (A) V-thread; (B) Buttress thread; (C) Reverse buttress thread; (D) Square thread.

be more precisely controlled. Tapered threaded implants are useful in placing implants into anterior extraction sockets immediately. There are four basic implant thread shapes namely: V-thread, Buttress thread; Reverse buttress thread and Square thread **(Figs. 56.3A to D)**. Thread Pitch is the distance measured between adjacent threads. Pitch has the most significant effect on changing the surface are on a threaded implant. Smaller the pitch, the more threads. So in D4 bone, decrease the pitch to increase the functional surface area. Thread depth is the distance between major and minor diameter of the thread. Greater the depth – greater the surface area. Tapered implant, has similar minor diameter, but the outer diameter decreases in relationship to the taper, so that thread depth decreases toward the apical region. As a result, tapered implant design has overall less surface area. In D1 Bone, the shallower the thread depth, the easier is to thread the implant in dense bone and less likely bone tapping is required before implant insertion.

- *Threadless/smooth implants*: The cylinder shaped, threadless implants are tapped into a recipient hole that is similar to the diameter of the implant body.
- *According to surface characteristics (microdesign).*[3,4]
  - Additive surface treatment:
    - Titanium plasma spraying (TPS)
    - Hydroxyapatite (HA) coated surface
  - Substractive surface treatment:
    - Blasting with titanium oxide/aluminum oxide
    - Acid-etched surface
  - Modified surface treatment:
    - Laser induced roughened surfaces
    - Ion implantation
    - Oxidized surface treatment

*Titanium plasma spray*: The TPS surface has been reported to increase the surface area of the bone— implant interface and acts similarly to a three-dimensional surface, which may stimulate adhesion osteogenesis. TPS—porous or rough titanium surfaces have been fabricated by plasma spraying a powder form of molten droplets at high temperatures. Molten particles of titanium powder of 0.05–0.1 mm diameter is projected at high velocity of 600 m/sec at 150,000°C onto metal or alloy substrate. The plasma-sprayed layer after solidification provide a thickness of 0.04–0.05 mm.

*Hydroxyapatite coatings*: Hydroxyapatite coatings are available with same roughness and increased functional surface area as TPS.

*Blasted surface*: The surface is blasted with titanium dioxide ($TiO_2$) particles or aluminum oxide ($Al_2O_3$) particles. Blasting technique is used to enhance implant surface topography with micro- to macroscopic hills, valleys and indentations.

*Acid-etched surfaces*: Acid-etching is performed by bathing titanium base in hydrochloric acid (HCl), sulfuric acid ($H_2SO_4$), hydrogen fluoride (HF) and nitric acid ($HNO_3$) in different combinations. The roughness before etching, the acid mixture, the bath temperature and the etching time all affect the acid-etching process. *Sandblasted and acid-etched surfaces*: Implants are blasted with 250–500 µm corundum grit followed by acid-etching in a hot solution of HCl and $H_2SO_4$.

Sandblasting produces macroroughness onto which acid-etching superimposes microroughness.

*Laser*: Laser ablation is a technique that can be used to produce a surface with predetermined reproducible characteristics. Implants are modified to produce a controlled, micron-sized surface, with topographical features on the flanks of the threads. Excimer laser is used to create roughness over the implant surface.

# BIOMATERIALS

Many biologically compatible materials can be used for the manufacturing of implants. The various implant systems are summarized in **Table 56.1**. There are three basic types of biomaterials for dental implants:[5-7]

1. *Metals and alloys*:
   - *Commercially pure titanium (cpTi)*: Titanium is a reactive metal. Under physiological conditions, in presence of air, water or any other electrolyte a spontaneous formation of an oxide occurs and get maintained on the surface of the metal without apparent break-down or corrosion. This mechanism is typically exhibited by titanium and other elements with valency IV, including silicon and zirconium. Commercially pure titanium (cpTi) based on the incorporation of small amounts of oxygen, nitrogen, hydrogen, iron and carbon during purification procedures is available in four different grades- Grade I-IV, each grade has different physical and mechanical properties. Grade IV is having the most (0.4%) and grade 1 the least (0.18%) oxygen content.
   - *Titanium-Aluminum-Vanadium (Ti-6Al-4V)*: It consists of 90% Ti, 6% Al, 4% V. This is also called as Grade V Titanium which is the strongest and thus preferred in posterior maxillary region. The aluminum is responsible for increasing in the strength and reduction of the weight of the alloy. The vanadium acts as an aluminum scavenger and hence possibly avoid the formation of corrosion promoting Ti-Al compounds.[8] Titanium oxidizes (passivates) on contact with room air and normal tissue fluids, which is favorable for dental implant devices.
   - *Cobalt-Chromium-Molybdenum (Co-Cr-Mo) based alloys*: These are used to make custom designs such as subperiosteal frames. Chromium provides corrosion resistance through the oxide surface. Molybdenum provides strength and bulk corrosion resistance.
   - *Iron-Chromium-Nickel (Fe-Cr-Ni) based alloys*: The surgical stainless steel alloy has high strength and ductility. This alloy should be avoided in patients allergic or hypersensitive to nickel.
   - Other metals and alloys are:
     - Gold
     - Niobium
     - Tantalum
2. *Polymers*: These are cross-linked polymers including polymethyl-methacrylate, silicone rubber and polyethylene. These polymers lack adhesion property to living tissues and they sometime show adverse immunological reactions.
3. *Ceramics and Carbons*: These are inorganic, nonmetallic materials manufactured by compacting and sintering at elevated temperatures. This group mainly consists of $Al_2O_3$ (alumina and sapphire) ceramics, carbon and carbon-silicon compounds. HA is considered as a solid material with surface coating properties and hence used widely. Zirconia ($ZrO_2$) is a ceramic material used in implantology because of its biocompatibility, esthetics (because its color is similar to the teeth) and mechanical properties, which are better than alumina. Implants produced with $ZrO_2$ are biocompatible, bioinert, radiopaque and they present a high resistance to corrosion, flexion and fracture.

# SOFT TISSUE-IMPLANT INTERFACE

*Clinical features of peri-implant mucosa*: The clinically healthy gingiva and peri-implant mucosa has a pink color and a firm consistency.

*Radiographic features of peri-implant mucosa*: The alveolar bone crest is usually located about 1 mm apical to a line connecting the cemento-enamel junction of neighboring teeth. The marginal termination of the bone crest is usually close to the junction between the abutment and fixture part of the implant system.

*Histological features of peri-implant mucosa*: The mucosal tissues around intraosseous implants form a tightly

**TABLE 56.1:** Various implant systems.

| System | Design | Surface | Number of surgery stages |
|---|---|---|---|
| Nobel biocare (Brånemark) | Screw and tapered screw | Pure Ti machined and Ti-unite | Two |
| Nobel biocare (Steri-Oss) | Screw, cylinder and tapered screw | Acid-etched, Ti and HA plasma sprayed | Two and one |
| ITI Straumann | Screw, cylinder and basket | Ti plasma-sprayed and SLA | One |
| Paragon/Core-vent | Screw, cylinder and hollow basket | Acid-etched Ti + HA plasma sprayed | Two |
| Friadent | Tapered cylinder and screw | Acid-etched Ti | Two |
| Astra | Screw | Pure Ti blasted | Two |
| 3i | Screw and cylinder | Ossadotite and Ti + HA plasma sprayed | Two and one |

| TABLE 56.2: Comparison of tooth and implant support structures. | | |
|---|---|---|
| | **Tooth (Fig. 56.4)** | **Implant (Fig. 56.5)** |
| Connection | Cementum, bone and periodontal ligament | Osseointegration, bone functional ankylosis |
| Connective tissue | 13 groups: Perpendicular to tooth surfaces | Only 2 groups: Parallel and circular fibers<br>No attachment to the implant surface and bone |
| Biologic width | JE: 0.97–1.14 mm<br>CT: 0.77–1.07 mm<br>BW: 2.04–2.91 mm | JE: 1.88 mm<br>CT: 1.05 mm<br>BW: 3.08 mm |
| Vascularity | Greater; supraperiosteal and periodontal ligament | Less; supraperiosteal |
| Probing depth | 3 mm in health (**Fig. 56.9A**) | 2.5–5.0 mm (depending on soft tissue depth) (**Fig. 56.9B**) |
| Bleeding on probing | More reliable | Less reliable |

(JE: junctional epithelium; CT: connective tissue; BW: biologic width)

adherent band. This band is primarily composed of a dense collagenous lamina propria covered by stratified squamous keratinizing epithelium. The junctional and barrier epithelia are about 2 mm long and the zones of supra-alveolar connective tissues are between 1 mm and 1.5 mm high. Both epithelia are via hemidesmosomes attached to the implant surface. The main attachment fibers (the principal fibers) invest in the root cementum of the tooth, but at the implant site the corresponding collagen fibers are nonattached and run parallel to the implant surface, owing to the lack of cementum. The sulcus around an implant is lined with sulcular epithelium that is continuous apically with the junctional epithelium (**Table 56.2**).[9,10]

## IMPLANT—BONE INTERFACE

One of the two below mentioned mechanisms acts to maintain the relationship between endosseous implants and bone.

- *Fibro-osseous integration*: In this integration soft tissues such as fibers and/or cells get interposed between the two surfaces of implant and bone (**Fig. 56.6**).
- *Osseointegration* (**Fig. 56.7**): Originally, it was defined as direct bone deposition on the implant surfaces, a fact also called "functional ankylosis". Osseointegration is considered as a direct structural and functional connection between ordered living bone and the surface of a load-bearing implant. Brånemark defined osseointegration phenomenon as the "direct contact between the living bone and a functionally loaded implant surface without interposed soft tissue at the light microscope level".[11] The above definition was not clinically applicable, thus a new definition based on implant stability was suggested by Zarb and Albrektsson,

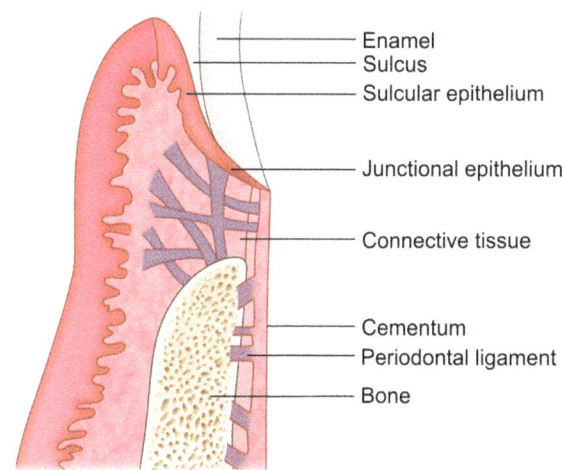

Fig. 56.4: Schematic representation showing attachment apparatus of tooth.

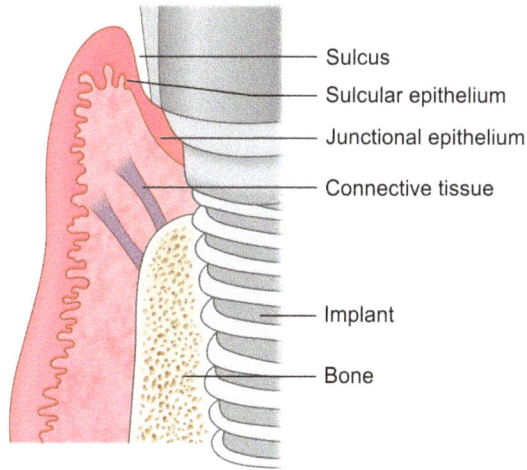

Fig. 56.5: Schematic representation showing attachment apparatus for implant peri-implant mucosa. (No periodontal ligament fibers and cementum).

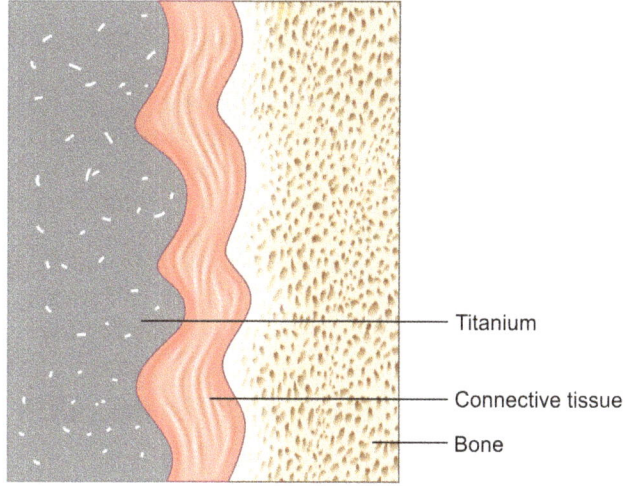

Fig. 56.6: Schematic representation showing fibro-osseous integration.

## Section 8: Implantology

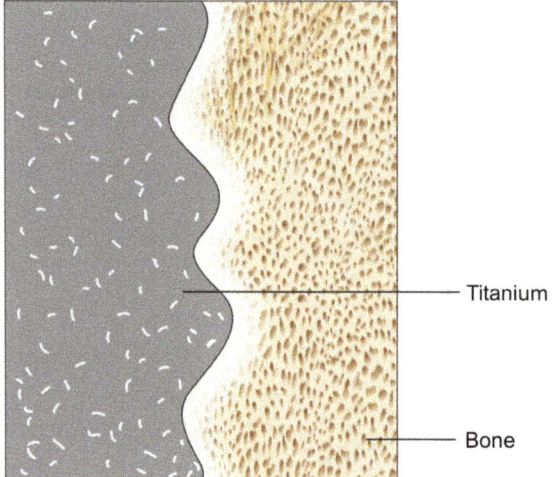

**Fig. 56.7:** Schematic representation showing osseointegration.

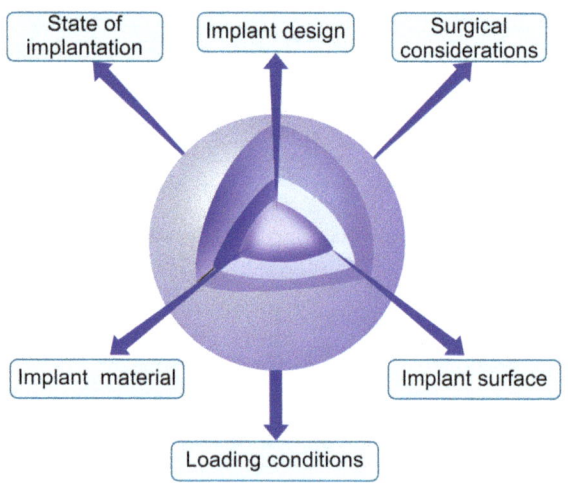

**Fig. 56.8:** Schematic representation showing key factors for osseointegration.

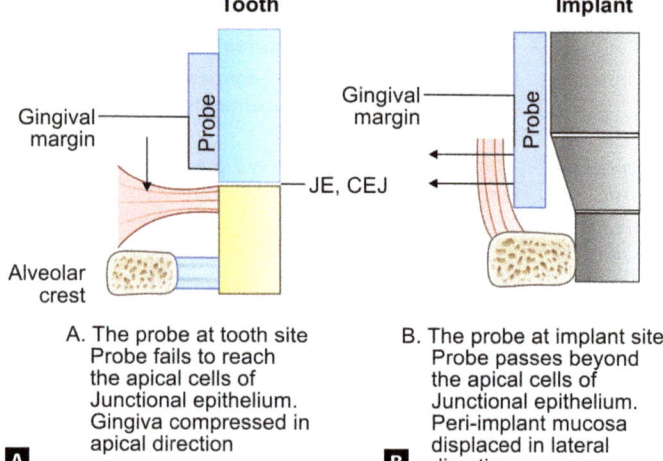

**Figs. 56.9A and B:** Schematic representation showing probe in position at (A) tooth site; (B) implant site (No periodontal ligament fibers and cementum).

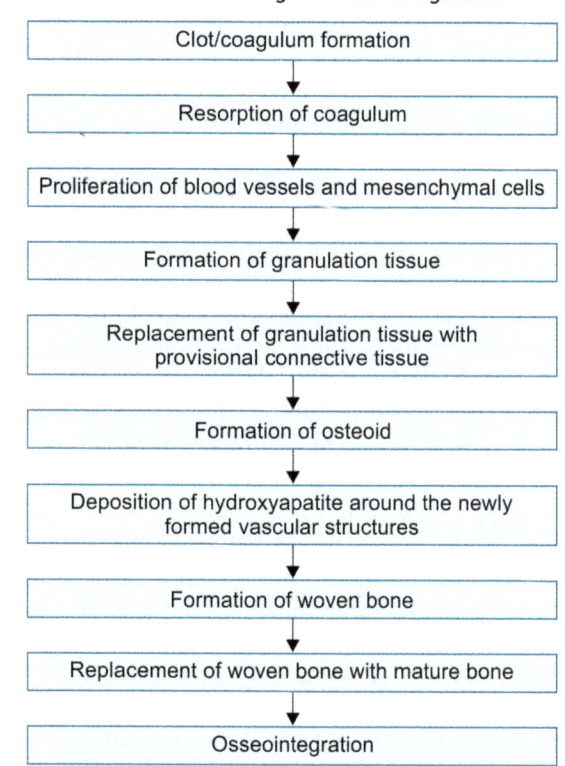

**Flowchart 56.1:** Stages of osseointegration.

"a process whereby clinically asymptomatic rigid fixation of alloplastic materials is achieved and maintained in bone during functional loading".[12]

Key factors leading to successful osseointegration are (**Fig. 56.8**):[15]

Thus, biologically determined program of osseointegration can be subdivided into three stages:
1. Incorporation by woven bone formation.
2. Adaptation of bone mass to load (lamellar and parallel—fibered bone deposition); and
3. Adaptation of bone structure to load (bone remodeling).

Healing of bone around implant[13,14]/stages of osseointegration is well explained in **Flowchart 56.1**.

### EVALUATION OF OSSEOINTEGRATED IMPLANTS

#### Periotest

The periotest method was developed by Schulte and coworkers at the University of Tubingen. The periotest is basically an electronic device. It is designed to conduct quantitative measurements of the damping characteristics of the periodontium. This helps to establish a value for implant mobility. This device measures the braking time following a reproducible impact applied to a tooth crown or implant abutment. The handpiece of the Periotest contains a rod inside and it is held in a low friction bearing that is accelerated until it reaches a nominal speed. The rod flies at a constant speed of 2 m/sec and this speed is maintained by compensation for friction and gravitation until contact with the surface of the implant is made. Automatically the rod

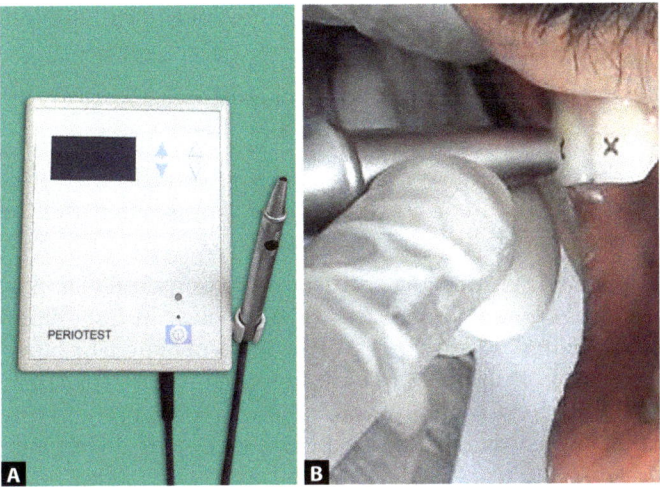

**Figs. 56.10A and B:** (A) Photograph showing periotest mobilometer; (B) Clinical picture showing testing tooth mobility with periotest.
(*Courtesy*: Dr S Chakrapani)

gets drawn back to its starting point and again reaccelerated, achieving 16 defined and reproducible impacts, 4 times/sec. The tapping head of the rod contains a miniature accelerometer, which records the impacts deacceleration during the contact time (braking effect). The greater the stability, the higher the damping effect is noted and faster the deacceleration achieved. The braking time between the implant and the tapping head of the rod is the signal used for analysis by the system.[16] The braking time ranges between 0.3 ms to 2.3 ms which corresponds to periotest values –8 to 50 **(Figs. 56.10A and B)**.

## Resonance Frequency Analysis

Resonance frequency analysis (RFA) is a method purely based on a steady-state, swept frequency technique. RFA has been developed by Meredith and his coworkers. The method uses a small transducer, which is screwed onto an implant or abutment. A steady-state signal is used to excite the transducer and its response is measured. The resonance frequency value of an implant indicates the function of its stiffness in the surrounding bone and the level of the marginal bone. The stiffness of the implant itself, the implant-tissue interface and the surrounding bone affect the overall stiffness of an implant placed in the recipient bone.[17]

## DIAGNOSIS AND TREATMENT PLANNING

Information acquired by medical history, dental history, clinical examination, laboratory tests, diagnostic casts, diagnostic wax-up and diagnostic imaging plays an important role in developing patients treatment plan.

*Medical history*: A thorough medical history is fundamental in preparation for dental implant treatment. Medical history identifies the factors that potentially poses a risk to the patient during the course of periodontal reconstructive and implant surgery. Such factors are history of myocardial infarction, compromised immune system and pro- longed use of steroids, uncontrolled endocrine disorders, alcohol and excessive smoking.

*Dental history*: The timing of and reason for the previous dental extractions will predict the adequacy of bone which is necessary for implant placement.

Dental history is necessary to determine the patient's compliance as maintenance is crucial for long-term implant success. It is also important to know how the extraction socket was treated at the time of extraction.

*Oral examination*: The examination should include a detailed dental and soft tissue evaluation to rule out infection, pathology and deformities. In oral examination following information should be considered:
- Periodontal status and prognosis
- Tooth mobility
- Amount of interocclusal space
- Position of teeth
- Root configuration and crown-to-root ratio
- Space availability
- Ridge morphology width
- Esthetics

*Diagnostic cast*: The study of articulated casts help in diagnosing arch form and arch relationship and implant sites in relation to the remaining teeth. A diagnostic wax up of the final restoration helps in finalizing the treatment plan and in determining the position and number of implants necessary to achieve the desired restoration. The ideal surgical guide is fabricated from a full diagnostic wax-up that is completed on properly mounted diagnostic cast. The cast assists in implant site selection and angulation requirement during surgical phase. Surgical templates are also designed from the diagnostic casts.[18]

*Surgical template*: When adapting the template for surgical use, holes are created in the template to accommodate the various drills used in preparing the implant osteotomy. Thus, surgical template ensures proper implant angulations and positioning relative to adjacent teeth or implants. It should fit passively after surgical flap reflection. Thus, it dictates the implant body placement.

*Diagnostic imaging (presurgical imaging)*:[19] The potential sites for implant placement and the number, length and width of implants to be placed to accommodate the prosthetic design are made with the aid of radiographs. Thus, radiographs are used:
- To determine bone quality and quantity
- To determine implant position and orientation
- To identify the disease
- To verify the absence of pathology
- To identify vital structures such as the floor of the nasal cavity, maxillary sinus, mandibular canal and mental foramen.

Following are the types of imaging modalities—

***Two-dimensional imaging modalities are:***
- Periapical radiography
- Panoramic radiography
- Occlusal radiography
- Cephalometric radiography

***Three-dimensional imaging modalities are:***
- Computed tomography (CT)
- Magnetic resonance imaging (MRI)
- Interactive computed tomography (ICT)

Computed tomography produces images consisting of individual units known as voxels. The density of the image is measured in Hounsfield units (HU), which is named after its inventor Sir Godfrey Hounsfield. Water has a Hounsfield value of 0 and is the standard for comparison. The density of the CT image in HU can be related to the density of the bone. The HU used in CT scan improves the diagnosis of bone quality by providing radiologic densitometric readings of bone.

CT scan, such as Dentascan can provide an accurate three-dimensional representation of maxilla and mandible. Dentascans produces an axial scans parallel to the occlusal plane at 1 mm intervals through maxilla or man- dible. The software program is used to produce segmental oblique cross-sections every 2 mm or 3 mm around the en- tire curvature of alveolar ridge. Each of the cross-sections is sequentially numbered and matched to tick marks on the axial views. Thus, Dentascan helps in planning the position, angulations and size of implant **(Figs. 56.11A to C)**.

## OSSEOUS CONSIDERATIONS

Lekholm and Zarb classified bone quality into four categories based on its radiographic appearance and the resistance at drilling[20] **(Fig. 56.12)**.

*Type 1 bone*: Almost the entire bone is composed of homogeneous compact bone. This type of bone has poor blood supply compared to the rest of the types of bone. The blood supply is usually necessary for the bone to harden or calcify the bone next to the implant. Hence, such type of bone takes approximately 5 months to integrate with an implant.

*Type 2 bone*: Here a thick layer of compact bone surrounds a core of dense trabecular bone. It takes approximately 4 months to integrate with an implant.

*Type 3 bone*: In this bone, a thin layer of cortical bone surrounds a core of dense trabecular bone. In such type of bone, 6 months duration is suggested before loading an implant.

*Type 4 bone*: It is a thin layer of cortical bone surrounding a core of low density trabecular bone of poor strength. Such type of bone takes the longest duration, almost 8 months, to integrate with the implant after its placement.

These differences in bone quality correspond with different areas of anatomy in the upper and lower jaw. In

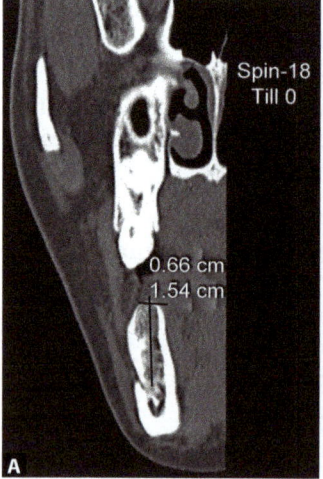 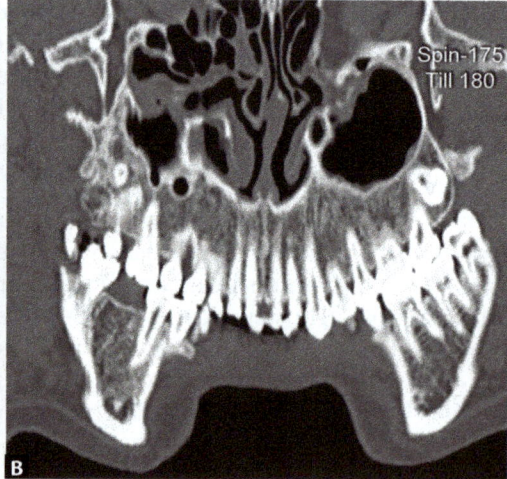 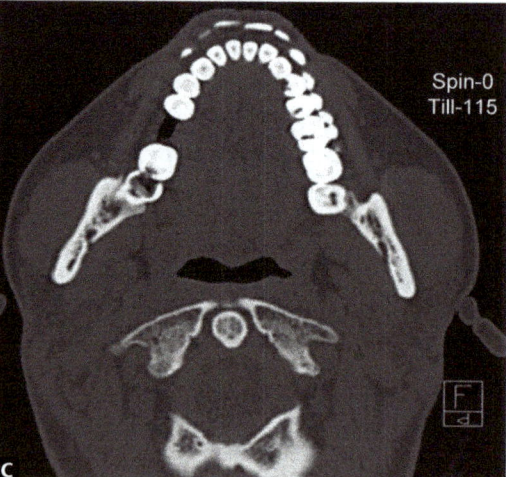

**Figs. 56.11A to C:** Schematic representation showing dentascan. (A) Axial view; (B) Panoramic view; (B) Cross-sectional view.
(*Courtesy:* Dr Rachna Jain)

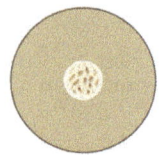 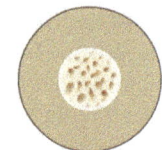 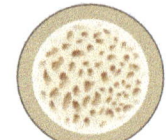 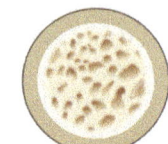

**Type I**
Most of the bone consist of homogeneous cortical bone

**Type II**
Thick compact bone surrounds highly trabecular core

**Type III**
Thin cortical bone surrounds highly trabecular core

**Type IV**
Thin cortical bone surrounds loose spongy core

**Fig. 56.12:** Schematic representation showing bone quality (Lekholm and Zarb classification 1985).

normal scenario, mandibles are more densely corticated compared to maxillas. Both jaws show a tendency towards reduction in their cortical thickness and enhancement in their trabecular porosity as they move posteriorly.

- *Misch and Judy classified available bone into four divisions (A to D)*: Abundant, barely sufficient, compromised and deficient.[21]

*Division A*: Abundant bone requires no augmentation and have
- 5 mm or more width
- 12 mm or more height
- 7 mm or more length

*Division B*: Barely abundant bone which has
- 2.5–5 mm or more width
- 12 mm or more height
- 6 mm or more length
- Less than 20° in angulation

*Division C*: Compromised bone which has
- 0–2.5 mm or more width
- Less than 12 mm height
- More than 30° angulation

*Division D*: Deficient bone—this is the bone with severe atrophy, and it represents as basal bone loss, flat maxilla and pencil-thin mandible.

- *Misch classified cancellous bone density into five grades*:[22]
  - D1: Greater than 1,250 HU
  - D2: 850–1,250 HU
  - D3: 350–850 HU
  - D4: 150–350 HU
  - D5: Less than 150 HU

### Points to Ponder

- Osseocoalescence is defined as the chemical integration of implants in bone tissue. Surface reactive materials like bioactive glasses and calcium phosphate undergo reactions that lead to chemical bonding between bone and implant.[23]
- Biointegration is bonding of living bone to the surface of an implant which is independent of any mechanical interlocking mechanism. Tricalcium phosphate and hydroxyapatite coatings produce bioactive surface that promote bone growth and induce direct bond between the implant and the hard tissues.[24]

## REFERENCES

1. Misch CE. Generic root form component terminology. In: Contemporary Implant Dentistry, 3rd edition. St. Louis, USA: CV Mosby; 2008. pp. 26-37.
2. Iacono VJ. Dental implants. In: Genco RJ, Goldman HM, Cohen DW (Eds). Contemporary Periodontics. St. Louis, USA: CV Mosby; 1990. pp. 653-70.
3. Piattelli A, Misch CE, Pontes AEF, Iezzi G, Scarano A, Degidi M. Dental implant surfaces: A review. In: Misch CE (Ed). Contemporary Implant Dentistry, 3rd edition. St. Louis, USA: CV Mosby; 2008. pp. 599-620.
4. Bernard GW, Carranza FA, Jovanovic SA. Biologic aspects of dental implants. In: Newman MG, Takei HH, Carranza FA (Eds). Clinical Periodontology, 9th edition. Philadelphia, USA: WB Saunders; 2003. pp. 882-8.
5. Donley TG, Gillette WB. Titanium endosseous implant-soft tissue interface: a literature review. J Periodontol. 1991;62(2):153-60.
6. Lemons JE. Dental implant and biomaterials. J Am Dent Assoc. 1990;121(6):716-9.
7. Parr GR, Gardner LK, Toth RW. Titanium: the mystery metal of implant dentistry. Dental materials aspects. J Prosthet Dent. 1985;54(3):410-4.
8. Ellingsen JE, Thomsen P, Lyngstadaas SP. Advances in dental implant materials and tissue regeneration. Periodontol 2000. 2006;41:136-56.
9. Lindhe J, Berglundh T. The transmucosal attachment. In: Lindhe J, Karring T, Lang NP (Eds). Clinical Periodontology and Implant Dentistry, 4th edition. Oxford, UK: Blackwell Munksgaard; 2003. pp. 829-37.
10. Rose LF, Minsk L. Dental implants in the periodontally compromised dentition. In: Rose LF, Mealey BL, Genco RJ, Cohen DW (Eds). Periodontics, Medicine, Surgery and Implants. St. Louis, USA: Elsevier Mosby; 2004. pp. 610-75.
11. Brånemark PI. Introduction to osseointegration. In: Branemark PI, Zarb G, Albrektsson T (Eds). Tissue integrated prostheses. Berlin, New York: Quintessence; 1985. pp. 11-76.
12. Zarb G, Albrektsson T. Osseointegration: a requiem for the periodontal ligament? Guest editorial. Int J Periodontics Restorative Dent. 1991;11:88-91.
13. Salvi GE, Bosshardt DD, Lang NP, Abrahamsson I, Berglundh T, Lindhe J, et al. Temporal sequence of hard and soft tissue healing around titanium dental implants. Periodontol 2000. 2015;68(1):135-52.
14. Schenk RK, Buser D. Osseointegration: a reality. Periodontol 2000. 1998;17:22-35.
15. Albrektsson T, Brånemark PI, Hansson HA, Lindström J. Osseointegrated titanium implants. Requirements for ensuring a long-lasting, direct bone-to-implant anchorage in man. Acta Orthop Scand. 1981;52(2):155-70.
16. Olive J, Aparicio C. Periotest method as a measure of osseointegrated oral implant stability. Int J Oral Maxillofac Implants. 1990;5(4):390-400.
17. Meredith N, Alleyne D, Cawley P. Quantitative determination of the stability of the implant-tissue interface using resonance frequency analysis. Clin Oral Implants Res. 1996;7(3):261-7.
18. Sarment DP, Misch CE. Diagnostic casts and surgical templates. In: Misch CE (Ed). Contemporary Implant Dentistry, 3rd edition. St. Louis, USA: CV Mosby; 2008. pp. 276-92.
19. Resnik RR, Kircos LT, Misch CE. Diagnostic imaging and techniques. In: Misch CE (Ed). Contemporary Implant Dentistry, 3rd edition. St. Louis, USA: CV Mosby; 2008. pp. 38-67.
20. Lekholm U, Zarb GA. Patient selection and preparation. In: Branemark PI, Zarb GA, Albrektsson T (Eds). Tissue-Integrated Prostheses—Osseointegration in Clinical Dentistry. Chicago, USA: Quintessence Publishing; 1985.
21. Misch CE, Judy KW. Classification of partially edentulous arches for implant dentistry. Int J Oral Implantol. 1987;4(2):7-13.
22. Misch CE. Bone density: A key determinant for clinical success. In: Contemporary Implant Dentistry, 2nd edition. St Louis, USA: CV Mosby; 1999. pp. 109-18.
23. Daculsi G, Legeros RZ, Deudon C. Scanning and transmission electron microscopy, and electron probe analysis of the interface between implants and host bone. Osseo-coalescence versus osseo-integration. Scanning Microsc. 1990;4(2):309-14.
24. Meffert RM, Langer B, Fritz ME. Dental implants: a review. J Periodontol. 1992;63(11):859-70.

## VIVA VOCE

**Q1.** Who coined the term osseointegration?
**Ans.** Brånemark.

**Q2.** What does primary stability principally represents?
**Ans.** The primary stability principally represents the mechanical stability with the surrounding bone which an implant achieves immediately after insertion.

**Q3.** Why threaded implants are more widely used?
**Ans.** Threaded implants provide superior initial stability in bone due to increased surface area and thus, vertical positioning of the implant during placement can be more precisely controlled.

**Q4.** Which type of implants are placed immediately in extraction sockets?
**Ans.** Tapered threaded implants.

**Q5.** How much time is required to integrate implant in Type 2 bone?
**Ans.** Approximately 4 months.

**Q6.** What is the purpose of healing abutment/ permucosal extension?
**Ans.** Its purpose is to create an emergence profile in the gingival tissue for the future implant crown.

**Q7.** Posterior maxilla has usually which kind of bone density?
**Ans.** D4

**Q8.** What is implant thread pitch and thread depth?
**Ans.** Implant thread pitch is the distance measured between adjacent implant threads.
Implant thread depth is the distance between major and minor diameter of the implant thread.

**Q9.** Which bone type is ideal for implant placement?
**Ans.** Type 2 bone which takes approximately 4 months to integrate with an implant.

**Q10.** What is Osstell?
**Ans.** It is resonance frequency analysis (RFA) based instrument. The resonance frequency value of an implant indicates the function of its stiffness in the surrounding bone and the level of the marginal bone.

# Chapter 57: Implant Surgical Procedures

*Anuj Gandhi, Shalu Bathla*

## Chapter Outline

- Armamentarium
- Surgical Protocol
- Two-stage Implant Surgery
- One-stage Implant Surgery
- Immediate Implant Placement
- Platform Switching

## INTRODUCTION

A well-performed surgical protocol, based on preoperative examinations and treatment planning, constitutes the prerequisite for a successful future implant treatment result. The placement of the implant within tooth position, both in mesiodistal and buccolingual dimensions, is of prime importance.

## ARMAMENTARIUM

Armamentarium has been classified into following groups:
- Dental implant surgical kit (**Fig. 57.1**).
- Physiodispenser (implant motor).
- Rotary handpiece.

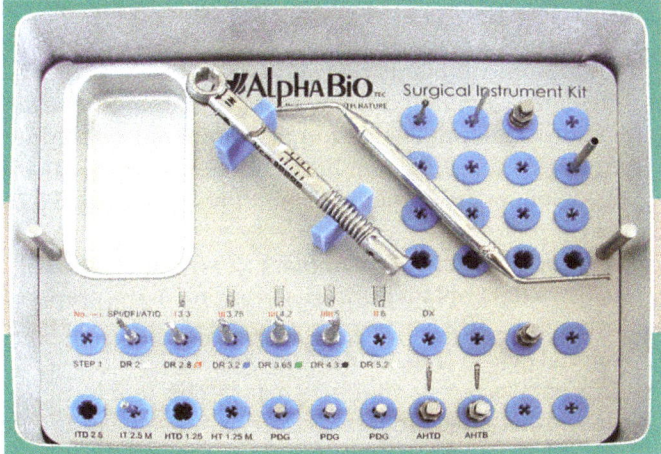

**Fig. 57.1:** Photograph showing dental implant surgical kit.
(*Courtesy:* Dr Anish Manocha)

### Dental Implant Surgical Kit

- *Drills*: All implant surgical kits contain a set of surgical drills which are sequentially used for preparation of osteotomies for different diameter implants of a particular system. These drills can be of the following types:
  - *Small round carbide bur*: It is used to mark the implant site and to make an entry through the hard cortical bone at the ridge crest (**Fig. 57.2A**).
  - *Large round carbide bur*: It is used to remove bony irregularities and to flatten the sharp and irregular ridge crest before osteotomy preparation for the implant.
  - *Lance drill*: After making the osteotomy site with a small round carbide bur and before using the pilot drill, this drill can be used. It is also known as cortical breaker, as it punches through the hard cortex and makes it easy for drilling with pilot drill (**Fig. 57.2B**).
  - *Pilot drill*: This is the first drill which is used to make an entry to the complete depth (**Fig. 57.2C**).
  - *Width increasing or widening drills*: This is a set of the drills sequentially increasing in diameter, used after the pilot drill to widen the osteotomy to the same depth. All the drills (pilot and widening drills) have definite markings along the length of the drills, representing the lengths of different implants available in a particular system. These markings guide the surgeon during drilling, to drill up to a particular depth marking (**Fig. 57.3**).
  - *Countersink drill*: These are crestal bone drills used at a high speed (1,500–2,000 rpm) before implant insertion limited to the crestal part of the bone to

**Section 8:** Implantology

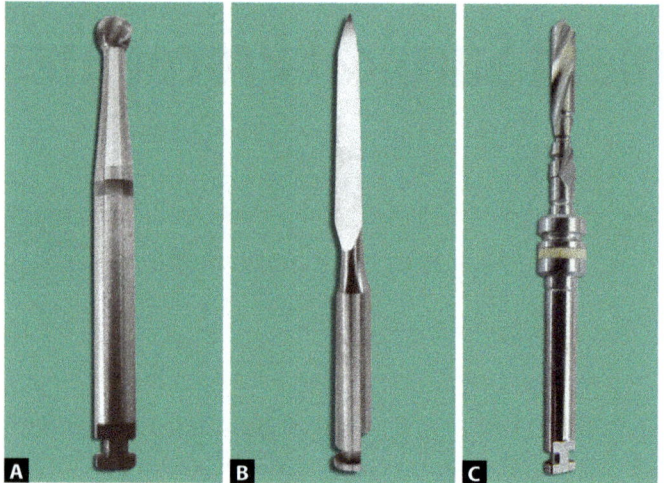

**Figs. 57.2A to C:** Photographs showing (A) Small round bur; (B) Lance drill; (C) Pilot drill.

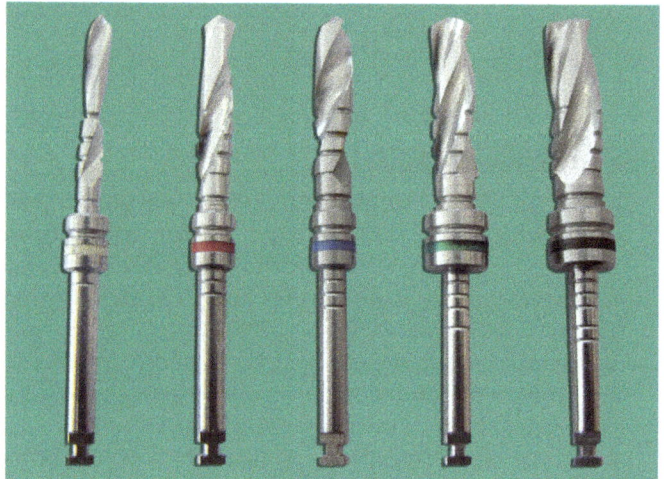

**Fig. 57.3:** Photograph showing various drills used during osteotomy of implant recipient site.

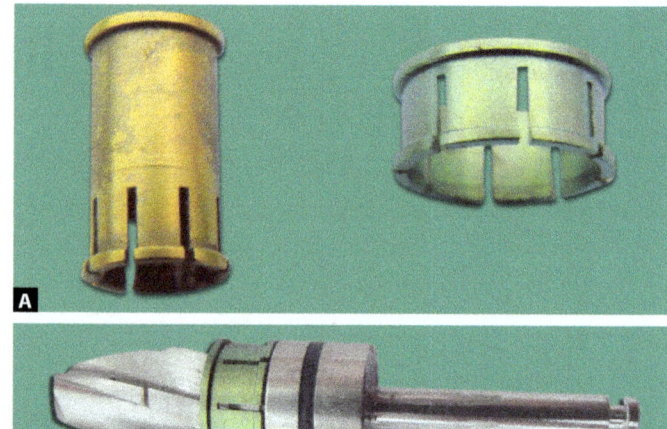

**Figs. 57.4A and B:** Photograph showing drill stoppers.

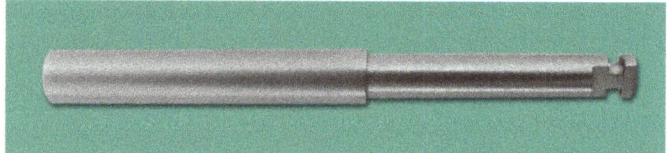

**Fig. 57.5:** Photograph showing drill extender.

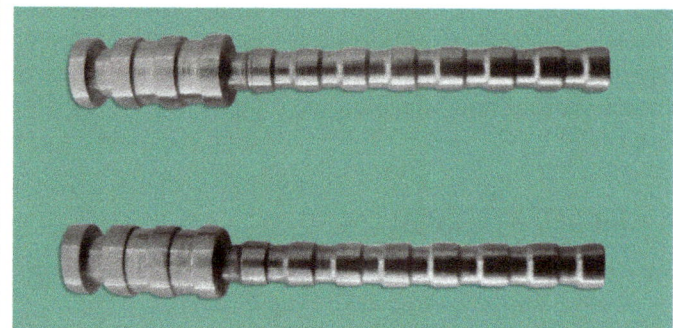

**Fig. 57.6:** Photograph showing parallel guide.

submerge or countersink the wider platform of the implant into the high density cortical part of the ridge crest.
- *Bone tap or thread former*: These are drills which make threads in the bone along the prepared osteotomy walls at very slow speed (20–40 rpm) before implant insertion. These are used when an implant with noncutting or non-self-tapping threads is inserted in a high-density bone to reduce the chances of pressure necrosis of the bone.
- *Drill stoppers*: These stoppers can be fitted to drills with different diameters to prevent overdrilling, especially in the area of vital structures, such as the mandibular canal and the sinus floor **(Figs. 57.4A and B)**.
- *Drill extender*: It can be fitted to any drill to extend its length for easy drilling access in narrow spaces between adjacent teeth **(Fig. 57.5)**.
- *Parallel guide or depth guide*: These guides are used to measure accurately the depth in radiographs taken after pilot drilling and to visualize parallelism during drilling for multiple implants **(Fig. 57.6)**.
- *Implant depth probe*: It has definite markings along its length for depth evaluation of a prepared osteotomy. Any perforation that may have checked by gently moving its tip along the prepared osteotomy walls **(Figs. 57.7A to C)**.
- *Implant insertion tool or implant driver*: This tool is used to drive the implant during its insertion in the prepared osteotomy. This can be rotary handpiece driven or hand ratchet driven **(Fig. 57.8)**.
- *Hex screwdriver or abutment driver*: This tool is used to drive the connection screw, cover screw, gingival former, etc. It can also be used to seat the abutment directly on to the implant. It can be hand driven or rotary handpiece driven **(Fig. 57.9)**.

## Chapter 57: Implant Surgical Procedures

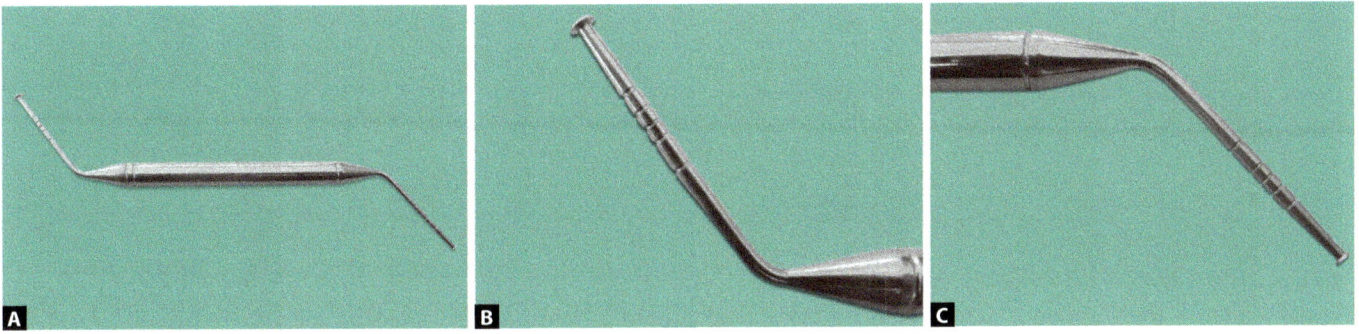

Figs. 57.7A to C: Photographs showing implant depth probe.

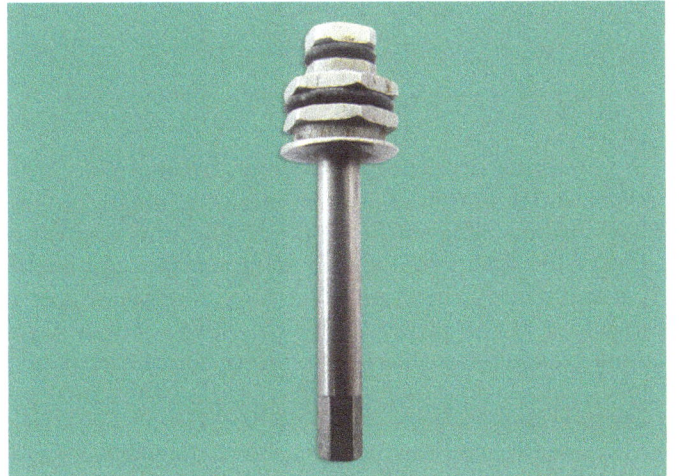

Fig. 57.8: Photograph showing implant driver.

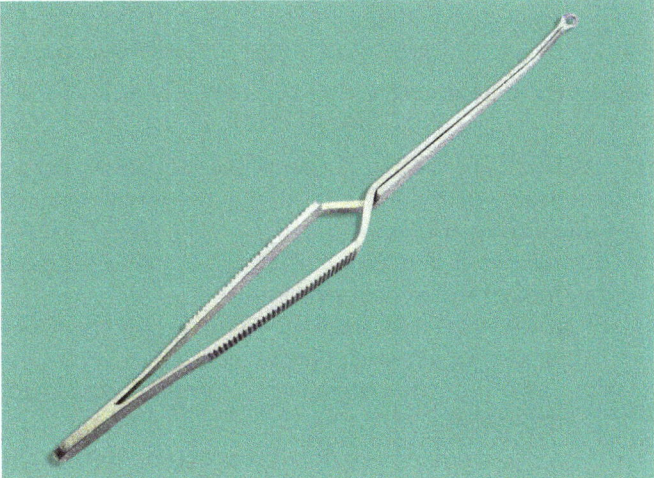

Fig. 57.10: Photograph showing abutment forcep.

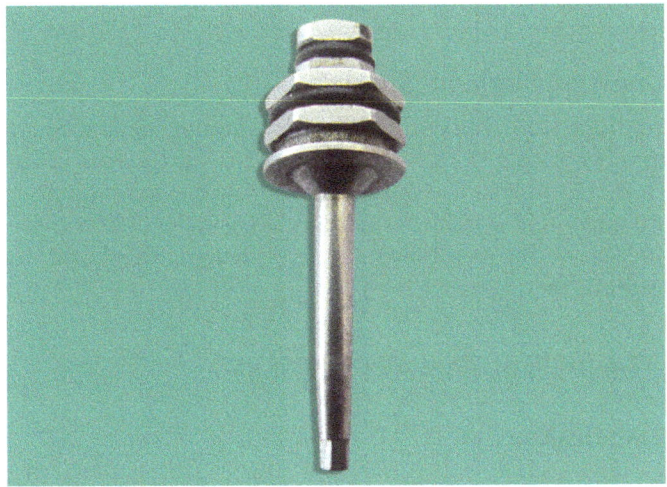

Fig. 57.9: Photograph showing hex screwdriver or abutment driver.

- *Abutment forcep (Hebel-Melton forcep)*: It secures prosthetic parts virtually at any angle. It has self-tensioning handle that keeps parts secure for pick up and transfer **(Fig. 57.10)**.

- *Ratchet*: They are used to insert the implants with the help of implant driver connected to it. It can be of two types:
  1. *Ratchet wrench*: A single ratchet without any torque measurement **(Fig. 57.11A)**.
  2. *Torque ratchet*: It allows the clinician to accurately apply the recommended preload torque. The torque level can be adjusted accordingly to check the primary stability of the inserted implant and tighten the connection screw before final prosthetic loading of the implant **(Fig. 57.11B)**.

## Physiodispenser (Implant Motor)

Physiodispenser is the surgical motor used in the implant surgery. It has following special features:

- *Torque control*: The implant motor usually has torque control from 0 Ncm to 50 Ncm, so that the handpiece does not stop rotating during drilling in hard bone and during implant insertion with handpiece at slow speed.
- *Speed control*: It ranges from 20 rpm (speed required for implant insertion) to 2,500 rpm (speed required for drilling in hard bone).

## Section 8: Implantology

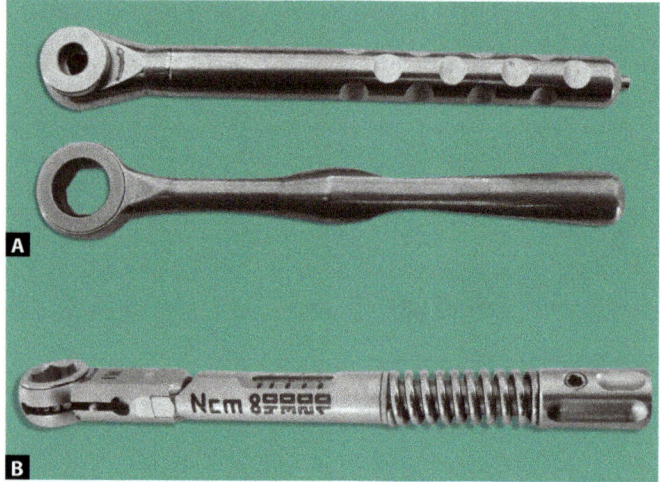

**Figs. 57.11A and B:** Photograph showing (A) Normal ratchet wrench; and (B) Torque ratchet.

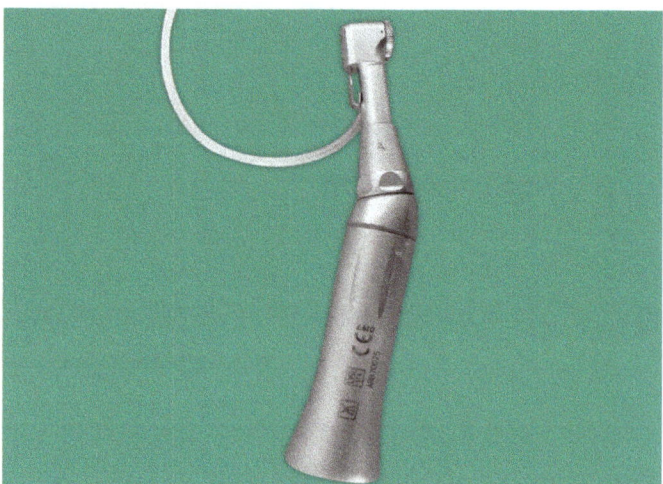

**Fig. 57.12:** Photograph showing contra-angle handpiece.

- *Saline irrigation control*: Controlled saline flow during osteotomy preparation to reduce the overheating of bone during drilling.
- *Handpiece*: It should offer the option of a range of handpieces to be connected to it:
  - At least a 1:1 handpiece for osteoplasty, bone harvesting, sinus window preparation, etc.
  - A 20:1 reduction handpiece for implant osteotomy preparation.
- *Programs*: It usually has different programs that can be set for a particular implant procedure.
- *Forward and reverse functions*: This feature helps in taking the drill or implant out, if it stops in the bone. It is very useful for removing the cover screw and gingival former from the implant.
- *Foot control*: The motor has a foot control with speed, forward and reverse functions.
- *Autoclavable implant motor cord*: This helps in maintaining surgical asepsis.

### Rotary Handpieces

- A 1:1 straight or contra-angle handpiece can be used for osteoplasty, autogenous bone harvesting, sinus window preparation **(Fig. 57.12)**. A 20:1 speed reduction handpiece is a standard one, which is used to prepare osteotomy, bone tapping and implant insertion.
- Newer generation fiber optic handpieces provide better visibility during implant insertion procedure.

## SURGICAL PROTOCOL

Endosseous implant systems can be categorized as either the traditional two stages (submerged) or one-stage (nonsubmerged).

### Two-stage Implant Surgery

The implant is placed and then covered with soft tissue and allowed to be osseointegrated for the defined period. The top of the implant is completely submerged under gingiva and thus also called as submerged implant system. In the second-stage surgical procedure, the implant is exposed to oral environment by using a healing abutment. This approach is recommended when there is extensive bone loss at the implant site or when vertical bone augmentation is necessary or when bone quality is poor.[1-3]

> **Clinical Tip**
> - Relieving incision should be kept vertical and parallel overlying on sound bone. It may be flared at apical extent that too should be on sound bone.[5]
> - Avoid placing oblique relieving incision over prominent root surfaces.
> - Avoid adjacent papilla reflection, to preserve the esthetics which is difficult to reconstruct if lost.

### One-stage Implant Surgery

In this system, the coronal portion stays exposed through gingiva during the healing period. The advantages of the one-stage surgical approach are that the mucogingival management around the implant is easier, patient comfort increases because fewer surgeries are involved and the esthetic management is easier.[4]

## TWO-STAGE IMPLANT SURGERY

### Flap Design

- *Incisions*: Crestal incision is used in the wider alveolar crest while in high and narrow crest, buccal approach (paracrestal incision) is used **(Fig. 57.13)**. In the crestal design flap, the incision is taken along the crest of the ridge to bisect the existing zone of keratinized mucosa. ncision must be extended within gingival crevices of adjacent teeth.[5]
- Flap reflection: In this procedure, a full-thickness flap is required to elevate buccally and lingually to the level of

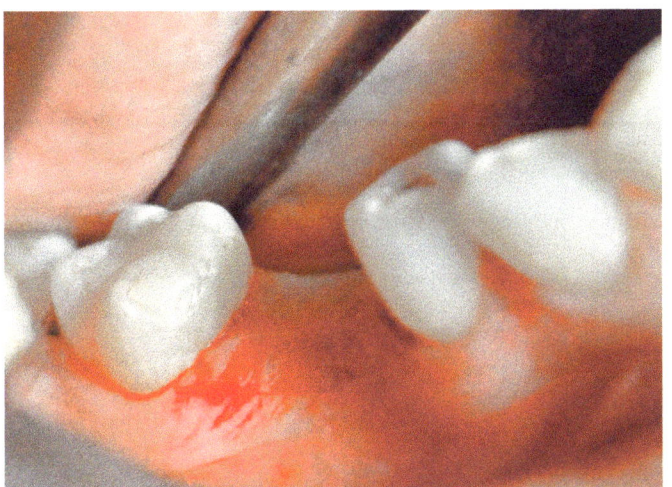

**Fig. 57.13:** Clinical picture showing paracrestal incision.

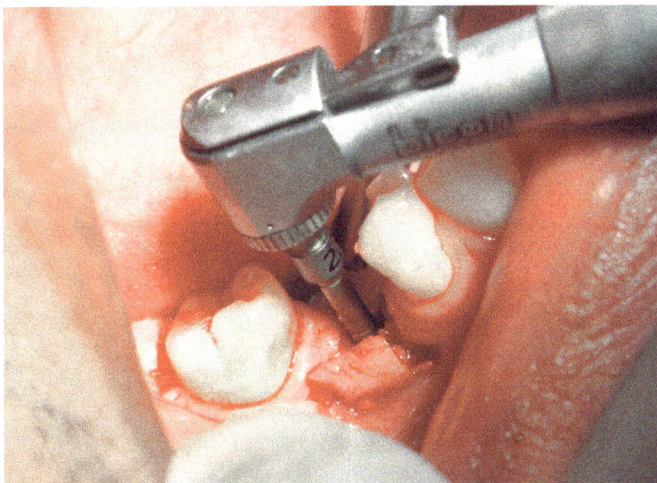

**Fig. 57.14:** Clinical picture showing initial osteotomy preparation with the pilot drill of 2 mm diameter.
(*Courtesy*: Dr Rachna Jain)

the mucogingival junction. This approach exposes the alveolar ridge of the implant sites. Raised flaps either sutured to the buccal mucosa or the opposing teeth in order to keep the surgical site open during the surgery.

## Preparation of Osteotomy Site

Here after reflection of the flap, a surgical guide or stent is positioned intraorally and a small round bur or spiral drill is used to mark the implant site. Then the stent is removed and the site is examined for their appropriate faciolingual location. Osteotomy site is prepared with intermittent drilling and under profuse saline irrigation because osteocytes damage occur above 47°C. A small spiral drill of 2 mm diameter is used to establish depth and align the axis of the implant recipient site **(Fig. 57.14)**. Internal or external irrigation continually washes away bone chips and keeps the drill bits clear of debris. In order to increase the size of the recipient site, a wider diameter pilot drill is used. A final size drill is used to finish the preparation of the recipient site. A countersink drill is used to widen the entrance of the recipient site. A tap is used to create screw threads. Final evaluation of a prepared osteotomy can be done by implant depth probe which has definite markings along its length **(Fig. 57.15)**. Any perforation can be checked by gently moving its tip along the prepared osteotomy walls.

## Implant Placement

Following are the parameters that are correctly addressed to achieve optimal esthetic results and biological health:[6]
- *Vertical positioning*: As a general recommendation, inserted implant should whenever possible be placed so that they engage two cortical layers, i.e. one at the marginal and another at the apical level of the implant.
- *Buccolingual positioning*: It is usually not a critical issue for implant-supported overdentures, but is extremely

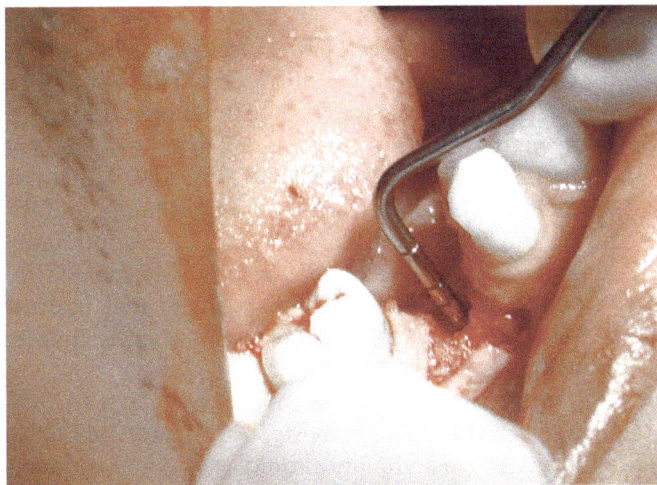

**Fig. 57.15:** Clinical picture showing implant depth probe into prepared osteotomy site.
(*Courtesy*: Dr Rachna Jain)

important for the placement of implants for crown and bridge restorations in areas demanding high esthetic results. The maxillary anterior implant must be positioned far buccally to provide proper esthetics, but not compromising over the thin buccal plate. This bone is responsible for supporting the overlying gingiva, which in turn, affects the esthetics of the restoration by providing soft tissue framing.
- The general principle is to place the implants within tooth position, which means that normally the long axis of the implant should be directed through the crown. The direction of the long axis of mandibular implants will mainly be towards the limbus part of the incisors or the palatal cusps of the teeth in the maxilla. For maxillary implants, the corresponding inclination should be directed towards the incisive edges of incisors or the

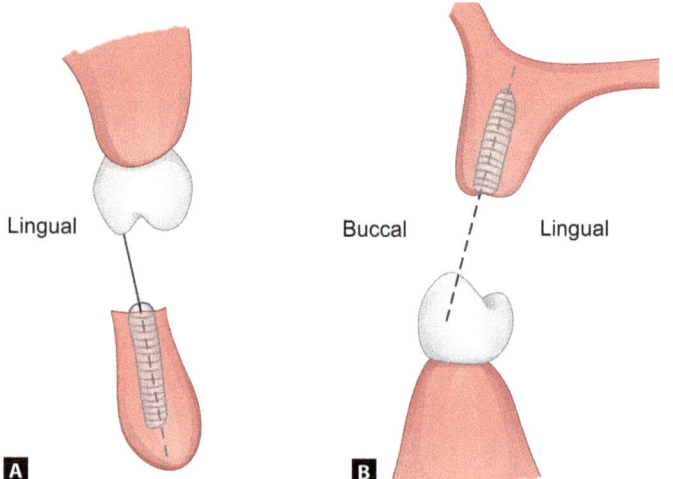
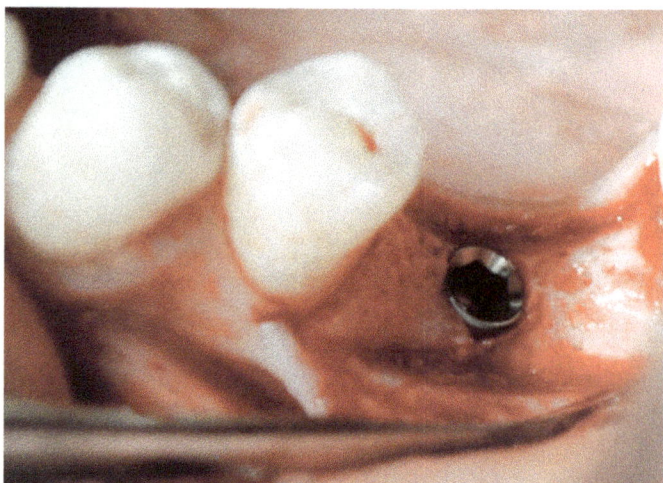

**Figs. 57.16A and B:** Schematic representation showing implant positioning: For placement of (A) Mandibular and (B) Maxillary implants.

**Fig. 57.17:** Clinical picture showing implant seated with its platform at the level of ridge crest.

buccal cusps of the premolars or molars of the mandible **(Figs. 57.16A and B)**.

- *Mesiodistal positioning*: For the mesiodistal dimension, the rule is that the implant site closest to the last tooth is placed parallel to the long axis of the root of that tooth. In the mandible, it is recommended that the most distal implants should be placed in a slightly mesial direction to facilitate the connection of the abutments and the fabricated fixed bridge construction. Correspondingly, when working in the premolar regions of the maxilla, the last implant could be directed slightly distally in order to follow the mesial wall of the maxillary sinus, thereby allowing a longer implant to be placed.

Depending on the specific condition of each site, the surgeon selects the most suitable type of implant. Whenever possible, the longest implant should as a rule be inserted, as shorter implants have a tendency to show less favorable survival rates than longer ones. Consequently, it is the bone quality and not the implant length that is of importance for the outcome of the implant treatment.

The implant is screwed into the recipient site **(Fig. 57.17)** and the cover screw is placed.

## Closure of the Flap

Once the implant is screwed in and the cover screw is placed, the flap is closed with inverted mattress and interrupted sutures over the implant. The inverted mattress sutures approximate the bleeding edges of the flap and the interrupted sutures help to seal the edges.

## Postoperative Care

Written postoperative instructions should be clearly explained and given to the patient. In order to prevent infection, postoperative antibiotics (Amoxicillin 500 mg TID) should start immediately before the surgery and continue it for 7–10 days.

Patient should apply icepacks extraorally intermittently for the first 24 hours. The surgical site should be kept as clean as possible. Chlorhexidine gluconate mouthrinses should be used twice daily. Analgesics are dispensed before surgery and continued after surgery. For the first few days, patients should have a liquid or semisolid diet and then gradually return to normal diet. Patients should completely avoid tobacco and alcohol use for 1–2 weeks postoperatively.

## Healing Period

The general and original principle has been that the softer the bone, the longer the healing time. For mandibular implant, the standard length of healing is 3–4 months for bone of good quality and for the maxilla, the corresponding time is 5–6 months, as the bone is normally more cancellous.

> **Clinical Tip**
> Principles of implant positioning
> - Vertical positioning of the implant in bone.
> - Buccolingual positioning of the implant in bone.
> - Mesiodistal placement of the implant in bone.
> - Trajectory or angle of the implant.

## Second-stage Surgery

It is done to expose the submerged implant ensuring proper abutment seating. Gingiva covering the head of the implant can be punched out or a full-thickness flap can be raised to expose the implant. The cover screw is then removed, the head of the implant is thoroughly cleaned of any soft- or hard-tissue overgrowth and the healing abutment or standard abutment is placed on the fixture. A very simple technique consisting of "+" and "X" incision is sufficient and when adequate attached gingiva is present. This technique would first involve a small crestal incision that will later give place to a cross type [+] incision **(Figs. 57.18A and B)**.

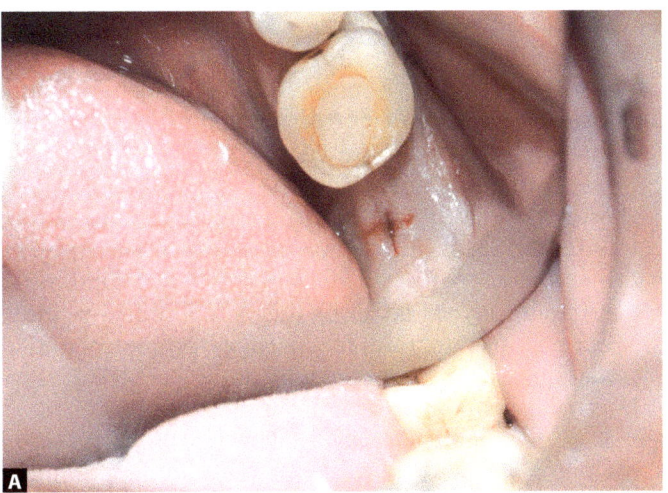 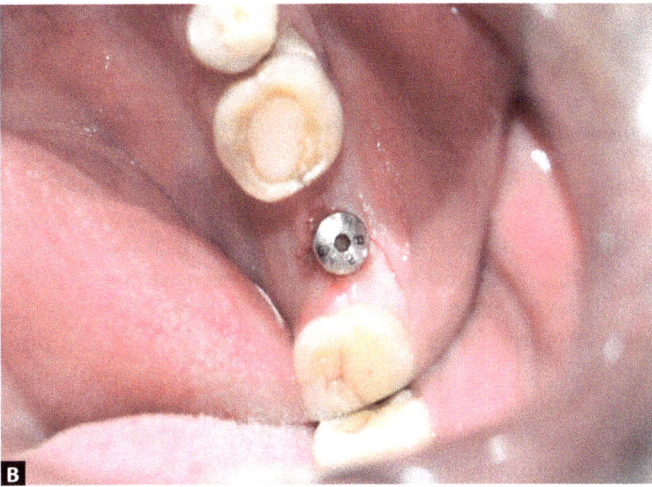

**Figs. 57.18A and B:** Clinical picture showing "+" incisional technique.

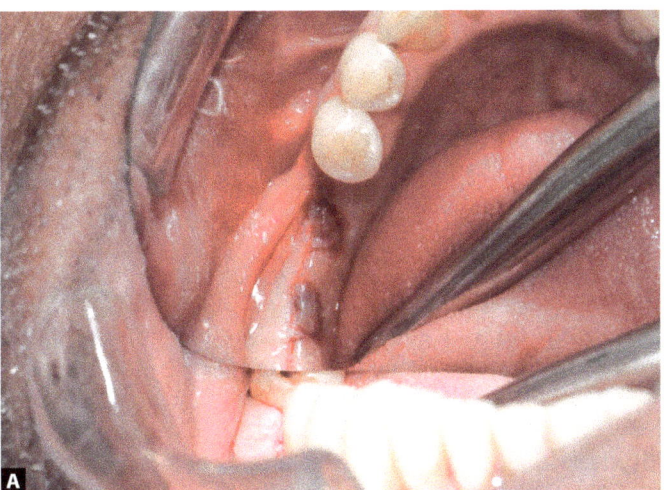 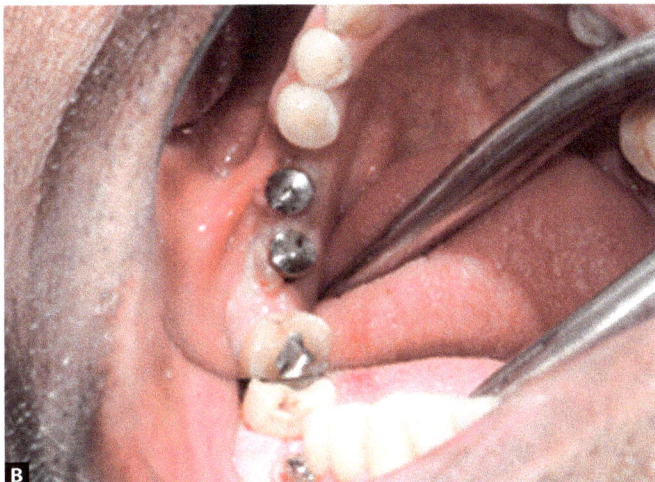

**Figs. 57.19A and B:** Clinical picture showing pouch roll technique.

The flap design for second-stage surgery such as split finger, pouch roll technique **(Figs. 57.19A and B)** appears to have several advantages, such as minimal surgical trauma; flap nutrition preservation; formation of papilla like tissue. Thus, second stage surgery should be given to promote and preserve the soft tissue profile around the implants **(Fig. 57.20)** and not just as a process of uncovering the coverscrew.

## ONE-STAGE IMPLANT SURGERY

Surgical protocol for one-stage implant system is similar to two-stage implant system with the following exceptions:[7]
- The flap design is always a crestal incision bisecting the existing keratinized tissue. Vertical incisions may be needed in one or both ends.
- The only difference in the placement of the implant is that the implant or the healing abutment extension of the implant is placed in such way that the head of the

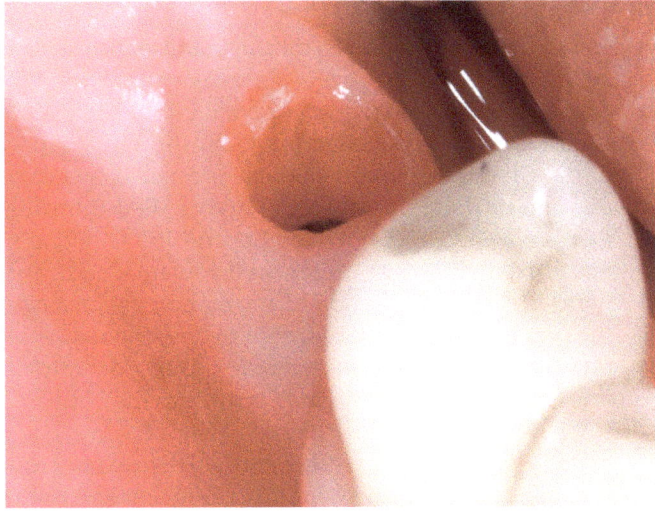

**Fig. 57.20:** Clinical picture showing emergence profile of the gingival tissue after the removal of healing abutment.

implant protrudes about 2–3 mm from the bone crest in one-stage implant system.

## IMMEDIATE IMPLANT PLACEMENT

Following tooth removal, a variable amount of ridge collapse takes place because of bone resorption. This bone resorption either buccolingual or apicocoronal reduces bone available for implant placement. To correct these defects, complex regenerative procedures requiring additional treatment time are required. To avoid these problems, a technique involving simultaneous tooth extraction and immediate implant placement has been introduced.[8-10]

The decision regarding immediate implant placement is determined by three factors:
1. Absence of acute noncontained infection.
2. Achievement of initial stability of the implant.
3. Sufficient quantity and quality of bone present.

### Advantages

Following are the advantages for immediate placement of implant:[11]
- Reduction of surgical procedure.
- Reduction in treatment time.
- Maintenance of ideal soft-tissue contour.
- Preservation of alveolar bone.
- Better implant placement.
- Improvement in the patient's psychological outlook for implant therapy.

### Disadvantages

- Possibility of infection.
- Thin tissue biotype may compromise optimal outcome.
- Procedure is technique sensitive.
- Potential lack of keratinized mucosa for flap adaptation.

### Procedure (Figs. 57.21A to E)

- *Step 1:* Local anesthesia is administrated at the selected surgical site.
- *Step 2—Incision and flap reflection*: Blade No. 15 or 12 is used to create a sulcular incision along the buccal aspect of the planned implant site and a vertical releasing incision to share the adjacent papillae. Full-thickness flap is elevated and extended beyond the anticipated apical extension of the preplanned implant length. This permits careful evaluation of any pathology present at the periapical region of the tooth to be extracted.
- *Step 3—Atraumatic tooth extraction*: Questioned tooth is extracted involving minimal trauma to the bone and surrounding soft tissues. The extraction is accomplished using a periotome directing along the proximal and buccal surfaces of the tooth root. Care is taken not to fracture the thin buccal plate in case of type I thin gingival phenotype.
- *Step 4—Socket debridement*: Socket is then thoroughly degranulated with curettes and diamond rotatory instrumentation to remove all remnants of periodontal ligament and granulation tissue. Depth gauge of various diameters is inserted to ascertain the socket architecture before the initiation of the osteotomy. Initiation of the osteotomy should be performed in a standard fashion with the initial penetration point for the anterior maxillary teeth approximately 2 mm coronal to the extraction apex and along the palatal wall. The initial bur penetration point for maxillary premolars and all mandibular single rooted teeth is directed towards the exact apex of the extraction socket.
- *Step 5—Implant placement*: Following implant insertion, an appropriate healing cap is selected depending on the desire for a submerged, nonsubmerged healing approach.
- *Step 6—Graft placement*: If gap between the wall of extraction socket and surface of implant is more than 2 mm, then osseous grafting membrane is done. To increase soft-tissue volume, a connective tissue graft is placed before flap closure, if required.
- *Step 7: Suturing*: Suture material of 5-0 is used to tie interrupted sutures.

## PLATFORM SWITCHING

Platform switching refers to the use of a smaller diameter abutment on a larger diameter implant collar so as to decrease circumferential bone loss.

The concept of platform switching was discovered accidentally in 1991. Initially, 3i Implant Innovations produced implants of larger diameter before introducing the corresponding abutments of the same measure. After a long period of 14 years, evaluation of cases using abutments of lesser diameter showed better preservation of hard and soft tissues compared to those where matched abutments were used. In 2005, Gardner introduced the term "platform switching" in a case study.[12] In 2006, Lazzara and Porter provided a clinical rationale for this implant design and introduced this concept in the literature.[13]

### Rationale

The mechanisms by which platform switching reduce crestal bone loss are:[14,15]
- *Shifting the inflammatory cell infiltrate inward and away from the adjacent crestal bone:* Microgap at the implant abutment junction provides bacteria with an open channel to penetrate into the implant system and also allows for micro-movement of the abutment within the implant. This micro-movement further creates movements and stresses on the abutment screw, which cause a loosening and micropumping effect that expels additional bacterial by products and toxins at implant soft-tissue interface and eventually at the osseous crest.

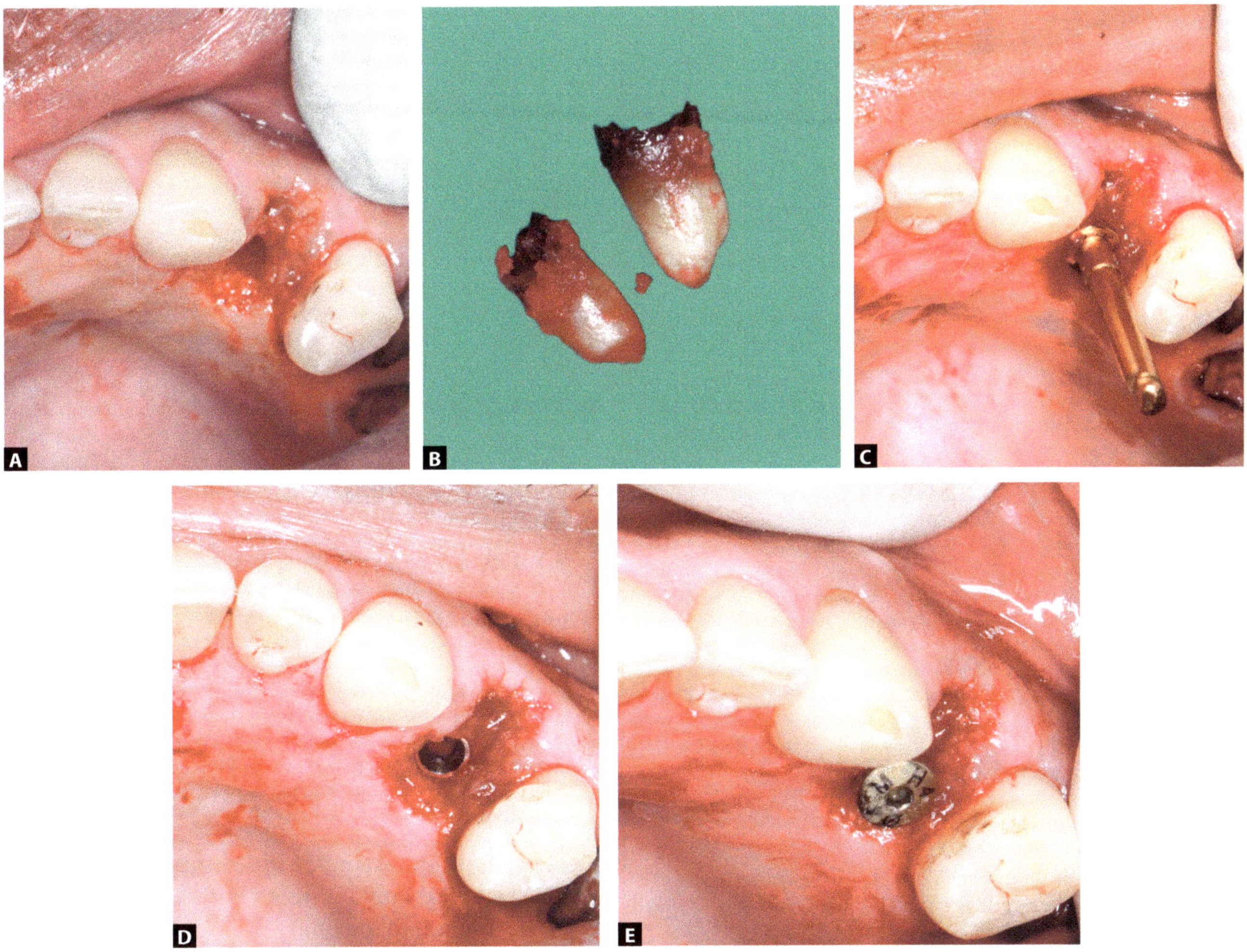

**Figs. 57.21A to E:** Clinical picture showing: (A) Atraumatic extraction; (B) Extracted root stumps; (C) Socket with parallel pin; (D) Immediate implant placed; (E) Healing abutment placed.

- On account of the concentration of toxins, the body defenses come into play increasing the inflammatory response at the crest, causing soft-tissue detachment and crestal bone loss. Lazzara and Porter first theorized that platform switching displaces implant abutment junction horizontally inwards from the perimeter of the implant platform and adjacent bone, thus increasing the distance between the inflammatory response arena at the microgap and the crestal bone, thereby minimizing the effect of inflammation on the crestal bone remodeling.
- *Maintenance of biological width and increased distance of implant abutment junction from the crestal bone level:* The angle or step created between the abutment and implant permits horizontal establishment of the biological width. This results in less vertical bone resorption to compensate for the biological seal **(Figs. 57.22A and B)**.
- *Decreased stress levels in the peri-implant bone:* The stress concentration gets shifted away from the bone-implant interface and it directs the forces of occlusal loading along the axis of the implant.

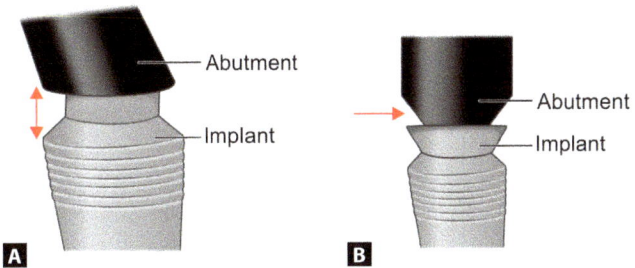

**Figs. 57.22A and B:** Schematic representation showing maintenance of biological width by platform switching: It helps in maintaining (A) Vertical and (B) Horizontal components of biological width.

Platform switching can be achieved by:
- Using abutment with a smaller diameter compared to the implant neck or body width **(Fig. 57.23)**.
- Using an implant design with an increasing neck diameter with respect to the implant body width **(Fig. 57.24)**.
- Using inherently platform-switched implant and conical emergence abutment **(Fig. 57.25)**.

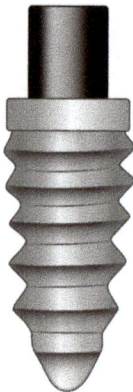

**Fig. 57.23:** Schematic representation showing platform switched implant abutment diameter less than implant platform diameter.

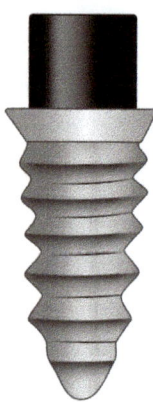

**Fig. 57.24:** Schematic representation showing expanded implant platform with equal implant and abutment diameter.

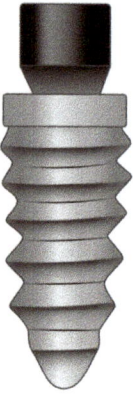

**Fig. 57.25:** Schematic representation showing platform-switched implant using conical emergence abutments.

- Using implants with a reverse conical neck **(Fig. 57.26)**, referred to as bone platform switching which involves an inward bone ring in the coronal part of the implant that is in continuity with the alveolar bone crest.

## Advantages

- Platform switching improves esthetics in anterior zone as it preserves the crestal bone leading to improved esthetics.

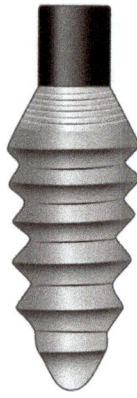

**Fig. 57.26:** Schematic representation showing implant with a reverse conical neck.

- Platform switching facilitates formation of a peri-implant soft-tissue cuff which seals the crestal bone from the oral environment and bacterial invasion.
- Where anatomic structures, such as sinus or nerve, limit the residual bone height, the platform switching approach minimizes bone resorption and increases the biomechanical support available to the implant.
- Improves bone support for short implants.
- Reduces the shear forces exerted on the cortical bone.

## Limitations

- There is undersizing of the components during all phases of the implant treatment, i.e., from placement of the implant to the final restoration.
- It increases the stress in abutment or the abutment screw.
- Sufficient prosthetic space is needed to develop a proper emergence profile.
- It has a positive effect on bone preservation in the 1st year, but after 5 years, the marginal bone change is insignificant.

### Points to Ponder

- ❑ The drilling of the osteotomy site should be performed with a pumping action, in which the drill is moved up and down along the same axis, allowing for bone chips to be expelled and bone tissue and drill to be cooled.
- ❑ At immediate implant placement site, if peri-implant osseous defects resulting in a gap measurable from the wall of extraction socket to the surface of the implant is more than 2 mm, augmentation with bone grafts and membrane is required.
- ❑ Tapered implant is the implant of choice in fresh extraction sites as these implants mimic the shape of natural tooth root.

## REFERENCES

1. Branemark PI, Adell R, Breine U, Hansson BO, Lindstrom J, Ohlsson, A. Intra-osseous anchorage of dental prostheses. I.

Experimental studies. Scand J Plast Reconstr Surg. 1969;3(2):81-100.
2. Arvidson K. A subsequent two-stage dental implant system and its clinical application. Periodontol 2000. 1998;17:96-105.
3. Steenberghe DV, Navert I. The first two stage dental implant system and it's clinical application. Periodontol 2000. 1998;17:89- 95.
4. Han TJ, Park KB. Surgical aspects of dental implants. In: Newman MG, Takei HH, Carranza FA (Eds). Carranza's Clinical Periodontology, 9th edition. Philadelphia, PA, USA: WB Saunders;2003. pp. 897-904.
5. Flap designs for implant surgery. In Palmer RM, Smith BJ, Howe LC, Palmer PJ (Eds). Implants in clinical dentistry. Martin Duntiz. 2002;97-104.
6. Lekholm U. The surgical site. In: Lindhe J, Karring T, Lang NP (Eds). Clinical Periodontology and Implant Dentistry, 4th edition. Oxford, UK: Blackwell Munksgaard; 2003. pp. 852-65.
7. Buser D, Belser UC and Lang NP. The original one stage dental implant system and its clinical application. Periodontol 2000. 1998;17:106-8.
8. Ostman PO. Immediate/early loading of dental implants. Clinical documentation and presentation of a treatment concept. Periodontol 2000. 2008: 47: 90–112.
9. Wilson TG Jr, Schenk R, Buser D et al. Implants placed in immediate extraction sites: a report of histologic and histometric analysis of human biopsies. Int J Oral Maxillofac implants. 1998;13(3):333-41.
10. Becker W, Goldstein M. Immediate implant placement: treatment planning and surgical steps for successful outcome. Periodontol 2000. 2008;47:79-89.
11. Beagle JR. The immediate placement of Endosseous Dental implants in fresh extraction sites. Dent Clin North Am. 2006;50(3):375-89.
12. Gardner DM. Platform switching as a means to achieving implant esthetics. N Y State Dent J.2005;71:34-7.
13. Lazzara RJ, Porter SS. Platform switching: A new concept in implant dentistry for controlling postrestorative crestal bone levels. Int J Periodontics Restorative Dent. 2006;26(1): 9-17.
14. Yang TC, Maeda Y. The biomechanical effect of platform switching on external- and internal-connection implants. Int J Oral Maxillofac Implants. 2013;28(1):143-7.
15. Maeda Y, Miura J, Taki I, Sogo M. Biomechanical analysis on platform switching: Is there any biomechanical rationale? Clin Oral Implants Res. 2007;18:581-4.
16. Wilson TG Jr, Schenk R, Buser D, et al. Implants placed in immediate extraction sites: a report of histologic and histometric analyses of human biopsies. Int J Oral Maxillofac Implants. 1998; 13(3): 333-41.

## VIVA VOCE

**Q1. Which implants are preferred in anterior sockets immediately after extraction?**
Ans. Conical implants are preferred in anterior sockets immediately after extraction.

**Q2. How do we prevent pressure necrosis of the cortical bone?**
Ans. By using bone tap or thread former or countersink drill.

**Q3. What is the use of countersink drill?**
Ans. These are crestal bone drills used at a high speed 1,500–2,000 rpm before implant insertion limited to the crestal part of the bone to submerge or countersink the wider platform of the implant into the high-density cortical part of the ridge crest.

**Q4. What is jumping distance?**
Ans. During immediate implant placement small peri-implant osseous defects result in gap between the wall of the extraction socket and surface of implant. This defect type is called as horizontal defect dimension or jumping distance.[16]

**Q5. What are angled abutments?**
Ans. Due to constrain in bone availability and clinical error, implants may be placed in unfavorable angulation or inclination. To correct this inclination in desired position of screw access holes in superstructure, angulated abutments may be used. For this purpose these days various abutments with various angles (up to 30°) are available which place the superstructure in line with rest of the dentition.

**Q6. Which incision is given during two stage implant surgery?**
Ans. Crestal incision is used in the wider alveolar crest while in high and narrow crest, buccal approach (paracrestal incision) is used.

**Q7. What is the ideal drilling speed and torque used during the implant osteotomy preparation?**
Ans. Ideal drilling speed below 2000 rpm and ideal torque 50 Ncm.

**Q8. What is the minimum distance between implants?**
Ans. The minimum distance between implants is 3 mm.

**Q9. What is the minimum distance between implant and other vital structures?**
Ans.

| Vital structures | Minimum distance (mm) |
| --- | --- |
| Maxillary sinus | 5 |
| Mental nerve | 2 |
| Inferior alveolar nerve | 2 |
| Adjacent tooth | 1.5 |

**Q10. What is the minimum distance between implant and tooth?**
Ans. The minimum distance between implant and tooth is 1.5 mm.

# Advanced Implant Surgical Procedures

*Ramesh Fry, Krishna K Gupta*

## Chapter Outline

- Guided Bone Regeneration
- Socket Preservation
- Ridge Augmentation
- Socket Shield
- Sinus Elevation and Sinus Bone Grafting
- Nerve Repositioning

## INTRODUCTION

Periodontal bone loss, tooth extraction and long-term use of removable appliances lead to advanced alveolar bone loss. This results in disturbance in the placement of implants in an optimal prosthetic position. However, persistent innovations in surgical techniques introduce new advanced implant procedures and bone augmentation procedures to overcome anatomic deficiencies for the optimal placement of dental implants.

## GUIDED BONE REGENERATION

Guided bone regeneration (GBR) was originally developed by Hurley et al.[1] in 1959 and Boyne[2] in 1964. They introduced the use of a microporous cellulose acetate filter for covering bone defects, and were thus able to achieve bone regeneration. Because the objective of GBR is to regenerate a single tissue, namely bone, it is theoretically easier to accomplish than guided tissue regeneration (GTR), which strives to regenerate multiple tissues in a complex relationship.[3]

### Barrier Membranes

Barrier membranes are synthesized from bioinert materials that mainly protect the blood clot and avoid soft tissue cells (epithelium and connective tissue) migration into the bone defect, permitting establishment of osteogenic cells.[4] The ideal properties of a barrier membrane are: (1) biocompatibility, (2) space maintenance, (3) cell occlusiveness, (4) good handling properties and (5) resorbability.

### Generations of Membranes

- *1st Generation (nonresorbable barrier membranes)*: Here a space is maintained under a barrier membrane with bone graft material or tenting screws. This facilitates the regeneration of bone. Stiffer membranes are able to promote significant amount of new bone and maintain sufficient space without the use of supportive devices. Ridge augmentation can be enhanced with a titanium reinforced membrane in conjunction with implant placement in localized bone defects. The disadvantage of a nonresorbable barrier membrane is that subsequent surgical procedure is required to remove it.
- *2nd Generation (resorbable barrier membranes)*: The primary advantage of a resorbable membrane is the elimination of a surgical re-entry for a membrane removal. In case of subsequent implant placement procedure (or exposure surgery), this may not be a significant advantage.
  The disadvantage associated with resorbable membrane is that it sometimes degrades before bone formation is completed and the degradation process is associated with varying degrees of inflammation. Another disadvantage is that resorbable membranes lack in stiffness which results in the collapse of membrane into the large defect area.[5]
- *3rd Generation membrane (with active ingredient)*: These membranes are incorporated with some active ingredients (antimicrobial agents/growth factors) to facilitate predictable bone regeneration.
  - Barrier membranes with antimicrobial activity have drugs incorporated into the membrane which is

released gradually as the membrane is resorbed, thus offering extended window of antimicrobial activity. The drugs used are 25% doxycycline, 2% metronidazole.
- Barrier membranes with bioactive $Ca(PO_4)_3$ contain
- nanocrystalline hydroxyapatite (HA) particles that facilitate bone regeneration.
- Barrier membranes with growth factors (PDGF, FGF,
- IGF, etc.) release have shown to be of great potential for enhance GBR.

- *Recent developments*: Use of 3D printed GTR (e-spinned) membranes harnesses the use of nanotechnology to deliver growth factors at a predetermined rate optimal for periodontal regeneration.

Functionally graded multilayered technique has provided a new concept for GTR membrane design with graded component and graded structures. This technique allows for creation of a single membrane that has two different functional surfaces.

## Bone Graft Materials

Bone graft materials have been used to facilitate bone formation within a given space by occupying that space and allowing the subsequent bone growth (and graft replacement) to take place.
- Osteogenesis occurs when living osteoblasts are part of the bone graft. Given an adequate blood supply and cellular viability, these transplanted osteoblasts form new centers of ossification within the graft like autogenous bone grafts.
- Osteoinduction involves new bone formation via stimulation of osteoprogenitors from the defect (or from the vasculature) to differentiate into osteoblasts and begin forming new bone.
- Osteoconduction is the formation of bone by osteoblasts from the margins of the defect on the bone graft material. Materials that are osteoconductive serve as a scaffold for bone growth. They do not inhibit bone formation, nor do they induce bone formation.

## Autogenous Bone Harvesting

Intraoral sources of autogenous bone include edentulous spaces, maxillary tuberosity, mandibular ramus, mandibular symphysis and extraction sites.[6]

Basic principles that should be followed to harvest autogenous bone graft are:
- Critical radiographic evaluation prior to surgery identifies individuals with the branches of inferior alveolar nerve (IAN) extending anteriorly beyond the mental foramen.
- Use extreme care in making incisions laterally towards the mental nerve, and dissect the area with blunt instruments to locate the foramen.
- Do not elevate and reflect muscle attachments beyond the inferior border of the mandible.

- Avoid overheating of bone and do not exceed temperature beyond 47°C which cause bone necrosis.
- Limit bone cuts to an area at least 5 mm away from the tooth apices, the inferior border of the mandible and the mental foramen. Do not extend cuts or harvest bone deeper than 6 mm, and do not include both labial and lingual cortical plates.
- Suturing should be done in layers (muscle and overlying mucosa separately) to prevent postoperative wound separation.

## SOCKET PRESERVATION

After tooth extraction, the alveolar ridge commonly decreases in volume with associated morphologic changes including soft tissue collapse into the extraction socket. If the resultant loss of bone volume and gingival contour is significant enough, the placement of an implant becomes extremely challenging. Such a case may require bone augmentation techniques followed by implant placement. However, this problem can efficiently be managed by site preservation through socket grafting. This will help to optimize bony fill within the extraction socket, thereby maintaining vertical bone height and helping to stabilize the marginal soft tissues at the site.[7]

This generally results in a healed site, which lends itself well to implant placement with a high degree of predictability as well as improved soft tissue contour. The key to successful socket preservation is minimal hard and soft tissue trauma around the tooth being extracted. The use of a periotome and luxator is instrumental in achieving atraumatic tooth extraction.

## Procedure

Following are the steps for socket preservation procedure **(Figs. 58.1A and B)**:
- *Step 1*: Sulcular incision is given around the tooth to be extracted. No flap or minimal flap is reflected to allow for instrumentation by periotome and luxator.
- *Step 2*: After the tooth/root has been extracted, the socket wall is thoroughly debrided with a surgical spoon curette.

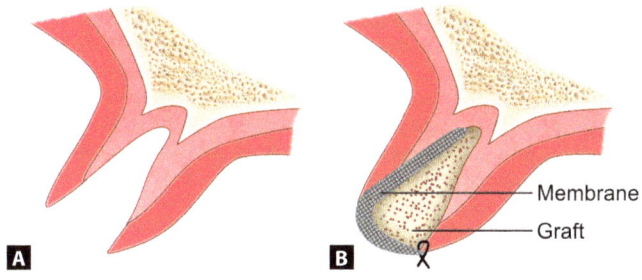

**Figs. 58.1A and B:** Schematic representation showing (A) Atraumatic tooth extraction socket; (B) Membrane placed over the graft and sutured.

Remnants of periodontal ligament fibers may result in fibrous healing and poor graft consolidation.
- *Step 3*: Cortical perforation using a small round bur is done to inducing some bleeding into the socket for good wound healing.
- *Step 4*: A suitable graft material is incrementally packed into the extraction socket to the level of surrounding alveolar bone.
- *Step 5*: Graft containment is done utilizing a resorbable barrier membrane. The edges of the membrane are tucked under the buccal/labial and palatal/lingual flaps and the flap sutures placed over the top of the membrane thereby holding the barrier stable. This is particularly important if there is no primary closure through a coronally advanced flap or the addition of a connective tissue graft.

## RIDGE AUGMENTATION

### Flap Management for Ridge Augmentation

Soft tissue management is a critical aspect of bone augmentation procedures. Incisions, reflection and manipulation should be designed to optimize blood supply and wound closure.

Following are the principles associated with flap management for ridge augmentation:
- *Step 1*: Incisions should be remote relative to the placement of barrier membranes (e.g., vertical releasing incisions should be given at least one tooth away from the site to be grafted).
- *Step 2*: The use of vertical incisions should be minimized wherever possible.
- *Step 3*: Full mucoperiosteal flap elevation at least 5 mm beyond the edge of the bone defect is desirable.
- *Step 4*: Wound closure should incorporate a combination of mattress sutures to approximate connective tissues and interrupted sutures to adapt wound edges.

### Bone Expansion

Ridge bone expansion is the procedure which is used to increase the horizontal dimension of the alveolar bone. **(Figs. 58.2A to D)** In 1992, Simion and colleagues reported the use of a split crest technique in patients receiving immediate implant placement in alveolar ridges that had significantly reduced width.[8]

### Procedure

- *Step 1*: After giving local anesthesia, elevate full-thickness buccal and lingual mucoperiosteal flap to expose the alveolar ridge.
- *Step 2*: Curette the cortical bone to remove all connective tissue and periosteum.
- *Step 3*: Before implant placement, split alveolar ridge longitudinally into two parts, with the help of a small chisel creating a greenstick fracture.

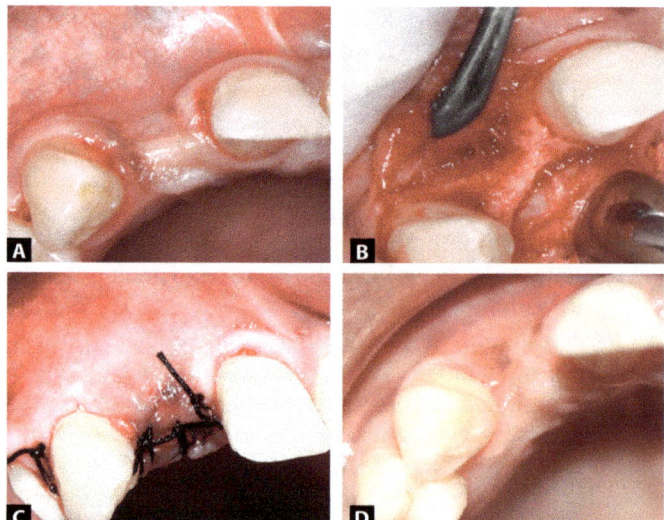

**Figs. 58.2A to D:** Clinical picture showing (A) Preoperative Inadequate horizontal dimensions of bone; (B) Thin ridge; (C) Bone expanded and sutured; (D) Postoperative adequate horizontal bone.

- *Step 4*: To spread the two cortical plates, tap the bone with the chisel and mallet, which is then used as a lever. For preparation of proper implant site and getting primary stabilization of the implants, extend the surgical fracture to a depth of 5-7 mm leaving at least 3-4 mm of intact bone apical to the fracture.
- *Step 5*: Care should be taken to avoid sharp and complete vertical or horizontal fractures of the buccal, palatal, or lingual bone plates.
- *Step 6*: Cover the implants with a contoured non-resorbable barrier membrane extending 3-4 mm over the bone margin of the defects.
- *Step 7*: Remove the membrane at the abutment-connection, in stage two surgery after 6 months of healing.

### Distraction Osteogenesis

The process of generating new bone by stretching is referred to as distraction osteogenesis. It was introduced by Gavriil Ilizarov.[9] In distraction osteogenesis, no second surgical site is needed to harvest bone and the newly created bone has native bone at the crest, which can withstand forces better than fully regenerated bone. This surgical technique has been developed to increase vertical bone height in the deficient jaw site and is in contrast to the more conventional method of bone grafting with or without membranes.[10]

Basic principles developed by Ilizarov have the following three distinct phases:[11]
1. *Latency phase*: Lasts for approximately 7 days of initial postsurgical healing.
2. *Distraction phase*: Consists of gradual incremental separation of two bone pieces at a rate of approximately 1 mm/day.

3. *Consolidation phase*: During which new bone forms in the regenerated zone between the separated bone pieces.

## Procedure

- *Step 1*: Local or general anesthesia.
- *Step 2*: Incision: Mid crestal or vestibular mucosal incision.
- *Step 3*: Full thickness flap is elevated on the buccal aspect only.
- *Step 4*: Horizontal and vertical osteotomies are prepared with either fissure bur or saw.
- *Step 5*: Place and fix the distractor and complete osteotomies.

  *Various distractors are:*
  - *Intraosseous distractors*: ACE surgical distractor; Leibinger endosseous alveolar distraction system (LEAD).
  - *Extraosseous distractors*: KLS Martin distractor.
  - *Veriplant distraction device*: Combination of oral implant and distractor device.
- *Step 6*: Device function is tested to make sure that there are no interferences.
- *Step 7*: Suturing is done with resorbable sutures.
- *Step 8*: Allow 1 week latency healing period.
- *Step 9*: Distraction period: With complete soft tissue closure distraction should be initiated at the rate of up to 1 mm/day.
- *Step 10*: Consolidation phase: Distractor removal and implant placement can be performed during consolidation phase. As a minimum time line for consolidation, long bone literatures have suggested 5 days per 1 mm of distraction.[12]

### Clinical Tips
- Do not reflect lingual flap.
- Take care not to damage lingual periosteum.
- To prevent device interferences, vertical osteotomies should converge slightly to the coronal and to the lingual aspect.

## Growth Factors for Bone Augmentation

### Bone Morphogenetic Proteins

Another adjunct to regenerative therapy is osteogenic stimulating substrates to enhance bone formation. Bone morphogenetic proteins (BMPs) are one of the group which acts as osteogenic stimulating substrates. It belongs to the transforming growth factor β (TGF-β) superfamily. Of this family, recombinant human bone morphogenetic protein (rhBMP-2) has shown significant signs of bone enhancing potential.

### Platelet-rich Plasma

Platelet-rich plasma (PRP) is an autologous source of platelet derived growth factors and TGF. It is derived by sequestering and concentrating platelets by centrifugation. The PRP contains a high mixture of platelets and a concentration of growth factors. This PRP mixture is added to the autologous bone graft and has shown to increase the quality of and reduce the time needed for bone regeneration.

## SOCKET SHIELD

Socket shield technique was introduced by Hurzeler[13] et al., in 2010. In this procedure, a partial buccal root fragment is retained around an immediately placed implant with the aim of avoiding tissue alterations after tooth extraction.

Rationale behind socket shield technique is to prevent the postextraction bone resorption and to support the buccal/facial soft and hard tissues, as most of the bone resorption occurs during the first year postextraction and 2/3rd of bone loss occurs within the first 3 months postextraction.

There are certain indications and contraindications for socket shield immediate implant placement.

### Indications

- Vertical fracture of teeth without pulpal pathologies
- Non restorable asymptomatic tooth with healthy and stable buccal root
- Tooth with healthy gingival tissue
- Adequate amount of bone volume apical to the extraction socket to support implant

### Contraindications

- Absent buccal lamina which develops for instance after vertical root fractures or periodontitis
- Signs of active infection, such as purulent discharge, tenderness related to tooth planned for extraction
- Large osseous defect in the extraction socket
- Mobile tooth with inadequate height or width of bone apical to extraction socket
- Poor quality of bone
- Inadequate marginal soft tissue around the socket

### Steps

Following are the steps for socket shield immediate implantation in the anterior region/aesthetic zone[14] **(Fig. 58.3A to C)**:

1. *Root sectioning*: Tooth root is sectioned along its long axis mesiodistally as far apical as possible with hydrated high speed handpiece and long tapered fissure diamond bur into two halves. The root is split vertically into 1/3rd facial and 2/3rd palatal halves.
2. *Atraumatic root extraction*: Start the extraction of palatal half of the root with thin scalpel blade giving incision within the sulcus around the root, to dissect the connective tissue attachment fibers present above the bone. Later on, atraumatic extraction is to be done with

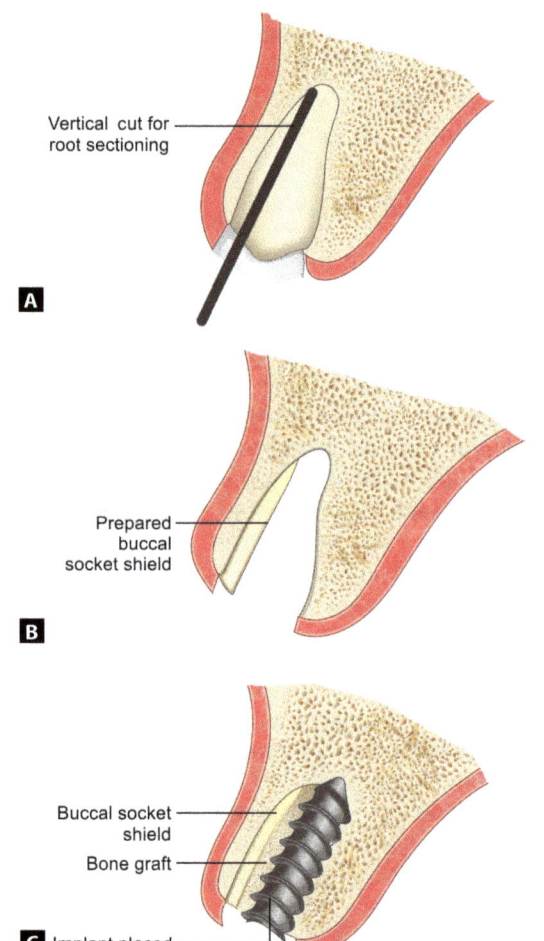

**Figs. 58.3A to C:** (A) Schematic representation showing vertical cut for root sectioning; (B) Schematic representation showing prepared buccal socket shield; (C) Schematic representation showing buccal socket shield, Bone graft and Implant placed.

periotomes, luxators and forceps preserving the facial root section undamaged and attached facial bone and soft tissue to the tooth socket to the greatest possible extent before immediate implantation. Thus, smaller facial root fragment is retained and larger palatal root fragment is removed.

3. *Socket shield preparation*: Buccal socket shield's height is aligned with bone. The rest palatal extraction socket is inspected for any defect under magnification and illumination. Tooth socket's palatal wall and apex should be curetted well to remove any residual infection and granulation tissue. Socket is irrigated with antibiotic (inj Clindamycin 600 mg) followed by 0.12% Chlorhexidine.
4. *Drilling protocol*: In maxillary anterior region, drilling should be done in palatal wall and not in the socket. Round bur is used to prepare the purchase point in the palatal wall. Alternatively, side cutting drill, i.e., Lindemann drill is used.

   Initially, the drill exit at the incisial edge and subsequentially drill is straightened to get palatal access hole and drill exit at the cingulum. It should be done 4 to 5 mm beyond the socket. All the osteotomy drill should be used in the same direction and depth. Final drill should not contact the socket shield. Jumping distance is kept purposefully to ensure bone grafting in the area.
5. *Implant placement*: Root dimensions should be measured to select the implant of appropriate diameter and length. Tapered implants are preferred due to its excellent initial fixation. They require minimal drilling and achieve primary stability even in low density bone. Chances of socket shield perforation is lesser with tapered implants. Cervico-incisally implant should be 3 to 4 mm apical to free gingival margin of adjacent teeth. Implant shoulder should be placed 1 to 2 mm apical to the labial CEJ of adjacent teeth. If recession is there on adjoining teeth, using CEJ as a guide will provide a poor aesthetic result. Specifically the coronal position of maxillary canines and central incisor is located 3 to 4 mm apical to the midpoint of the facial free gingival margin. In maxillary lateral incisor, the normal apical distance from free gingival margin is 2 to 3 mm.
6. *Bone grafting*: Grafting is done in jumping distance present between the implant and socket shield. Autograft, allograft, xenograft or synthetic bone graft can be used as graft. Graft acts as a scaffold to maintain hard and soft tissue volume and also maintains blood clot. Slow-resorbing bone graft is preferred to fill the gap between the socket shield and implant to predictably preserve bone volume till new bone is not formed.
7. *Temporization*: Pre-existing positions of the gingival margin and papillae can be maintained by provisional crown supporting the gingival architecture. Insertion torque of 30 to 40 Ncm should be achieved while placing abutment and provisional crown. The provisional prosthesis should be out of occlusion.
8. *Postoperative instructions and care*: Following postoperative instructions should be provided to the patient in both verbal and written form.

## SINUS ELEVATION AND SINUS BONE GRAFTING

### Maxillary Arthroplasty

The maxillary sinus lift grafting procedure that was originally designed and described by Hilt Tatum,[15] Bob James and Phil Boyne[16] is not the same procedure that is performed today. The maxillary sinus contains a 15-mL volume airspace that resembles a slopped paperweight, with its largest and only flat side composing the medial wall (which also forms the lateral wall of the nasal cavity). The bony walls of the sinus are usually thin, except its anterior wall and the alveolar ridge in the dentate individual. In the edentulous person, the alveolar bone is atrophied and may be only 1–2 mm thick, making it unsuitable as an implant site. Hence, the main objective of sinus lift surgery is the restoration of a sufficient amount of alveolar bone for successful placement of implants. The maxillary sinus is lined with pseudostratified columnar epithelium, which is also called the Schneiderian membrane. The thickness of the maxillary sinus correlates with the degree of pneumatization. Pneumatization helps to minimize or completely eliminate the amount of vertical bone available for endosteal implant placement.[17,18]

Grafting materials that are currently being used for antral floor augmentation include autogenous bone grafts, bone allografts and alloplasts, such as tricalcium phosphate and resorbable and nonresorbable HA. Autogenous bone has high osteogenic, osteoinductive and osteoconductive properties, and has long been considered as the gold standard grafting material.[19, 20]

### Indication

Sinus lift procedure is indicated in maxilla, where insufficient bone height is present.

### Contraindications

- Previous sinus surgery, such as the Caldwell-Luc operation, which often leaves scar tissues is an absolute contraindication.
- Maxillary sinus diseases, such as chronic polypous sinusitis is considered as contraindication for sinus lifting.
- Presence of Underwood's septa/severe sinus floor convolutions forms a relative contraindication for sinus lifting.

### Preoperative Evaluation

Radiological examination including panoramic and sinus radiograph and computed tomography scans are conducted to determine the availability of maxillary alveolar bone height, the location of sinus floor convolutions (septi) and the surgical entry site **(Figs. 58.4A to C)**.

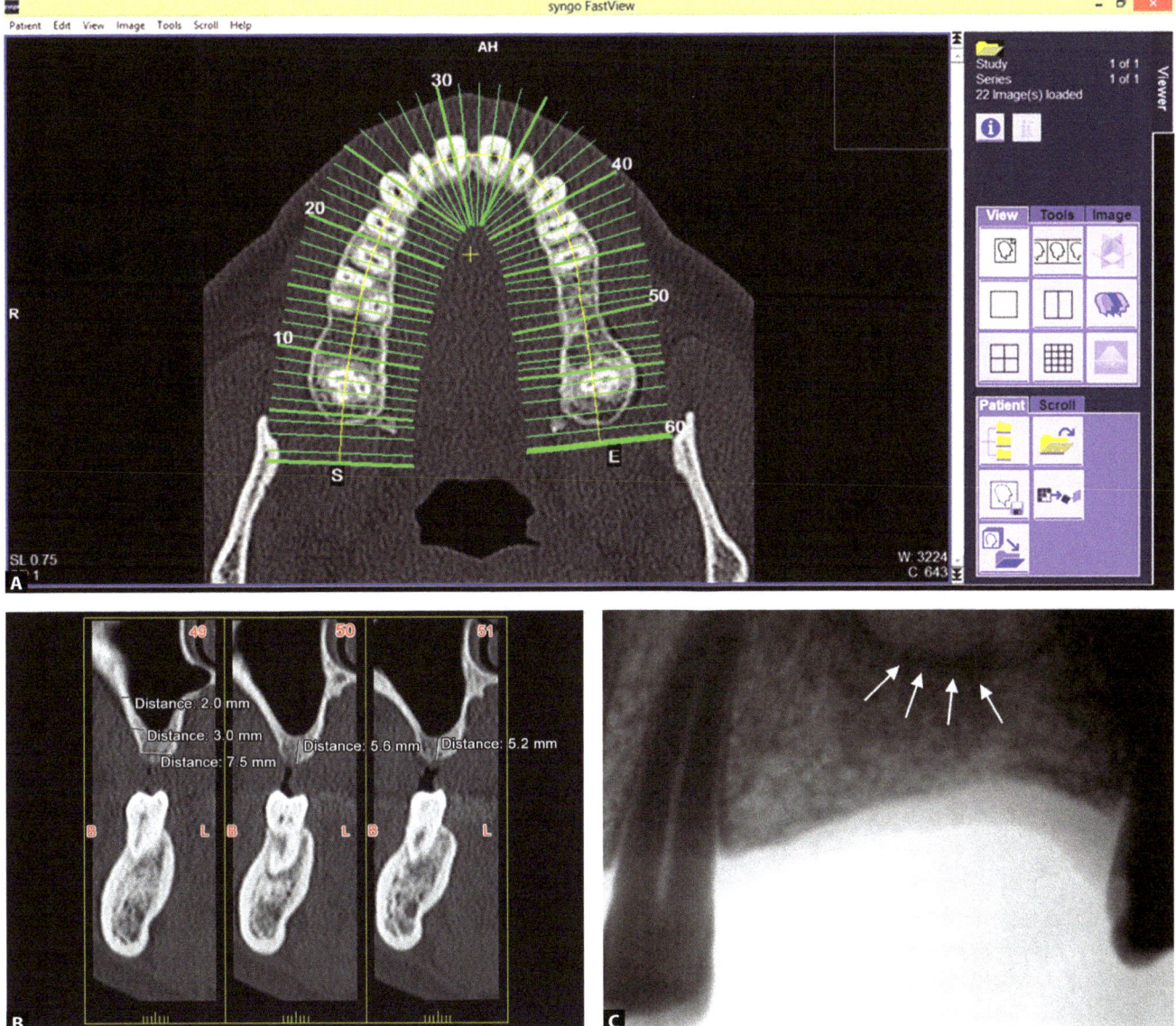

**Figs. 58.4A to C:** (A) Dentascan showing missing teeth (17, 26 and 27); (B) Dentascan showing available bone in the region of 26 and 27; (C) Preoperative radiograph showing membrane.

### Procedure

There are two main approaches for maxillary sinus floor elevation: direct and indirect approach. Direct—lateral window technique and indirect—osteotome sinus floor elevation, bone added sinus floor elevation, minimally invasive transalveolar sinus approach, and antral membrane balloon elevation.[19]

Surgical direct technique involved in the sinus lift procedure is as follows **(Figs. 58.5A to H)**:

- *Step 1*: The surgery can be performed with local anesthesia, i.e., posterosuperior alveolar and greater palatine nerve blocks combined with infiltration.
- *Step 2*: A horizontal incision is made on the crest or palatal aspect of the edentulous ridge and incision is carried forward beyond the anterior border of the sinus. A vertical releasing incision is made in the canine fossa in order to reflect the flap and expose the bone. Such incision will also ensure adequate soft tissue closure over the bone. Reflection of the mucoperiosteal flap superiorly to the level of the molar buttress helps to expose the lateral wall of the maxilla.
- *Step 3*: After the lateral maxillary wall has been completely exposed, a no. 8 round diamond bur should be used at a low speed (100 rpm) to make an oval or semicircular osteotomy in the lateral wall of the maxillary sinus **(Fig. 58.6)**. An oval osteotomy is recommended instead of a rectangular or trapezoidal osteotomy to minimize sharp edges on the bony window, which can cause tears in the underlying Schneiderian membrane.
- *Step 4*: To ensure that the bone has been penetrated all the way around the oval osteotomy, it should be tapped gently and any movement is noted.
- *Step 5*: Thus bone can be either pushed into serve as the root of the graft or removed. This helps to form a window for better visualization and access.
- *Step 6*: At this stage, the underlying Schneiderian membrane gets exposed. Meticulous care should be taken to reflect the Schneiderian membrane superiorly without perforating it **(Fig. 58.7)**. The Schneiderian membrane should be carefully elevated from the floor interiorly, anteriorly and posteriorly through the osteotomy sites. This creates an empty chamber superior to the residual alveolar bone **(Figs. 58.8A and B)**.

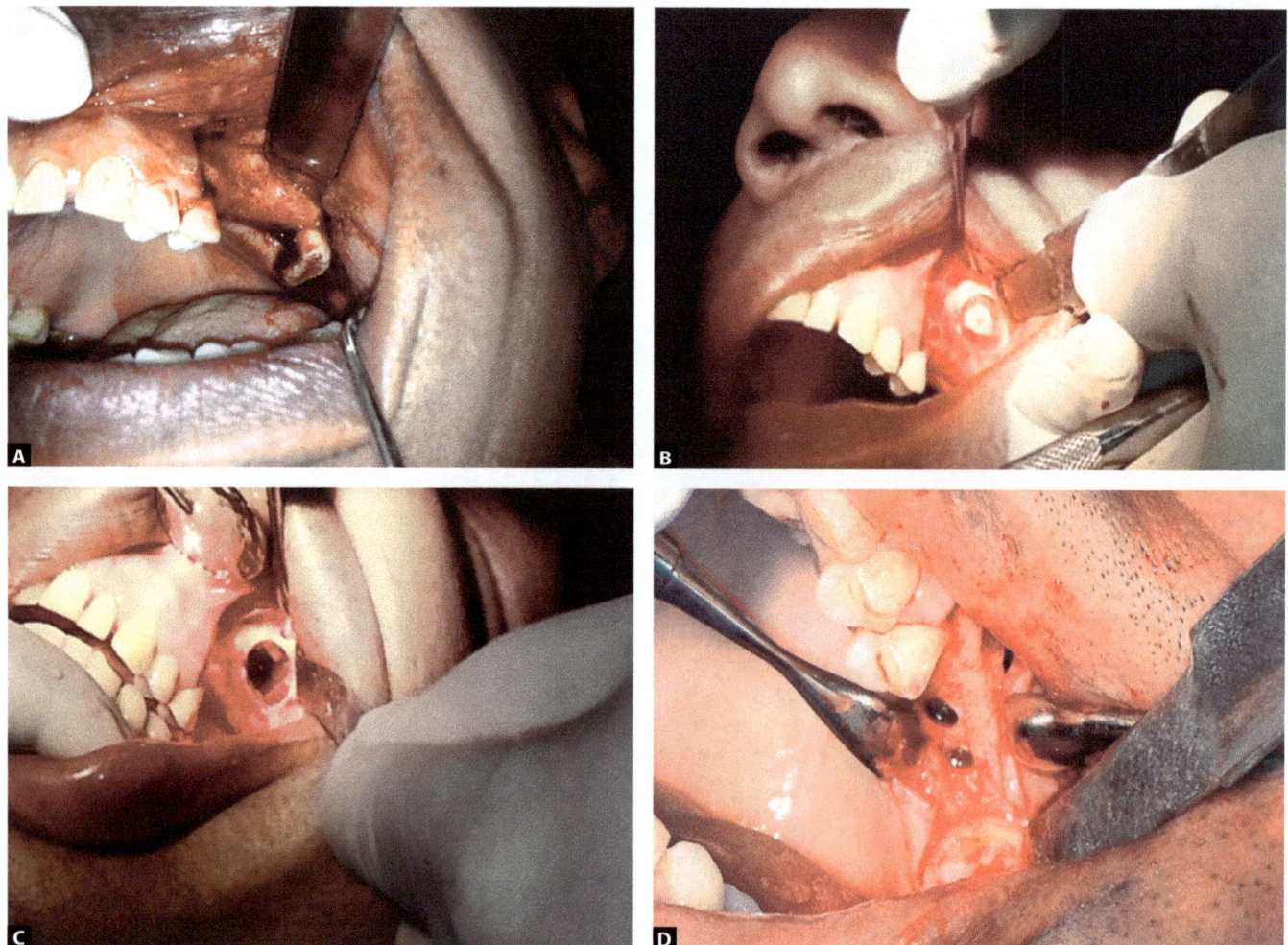

**Figs. 58.5A to D:**

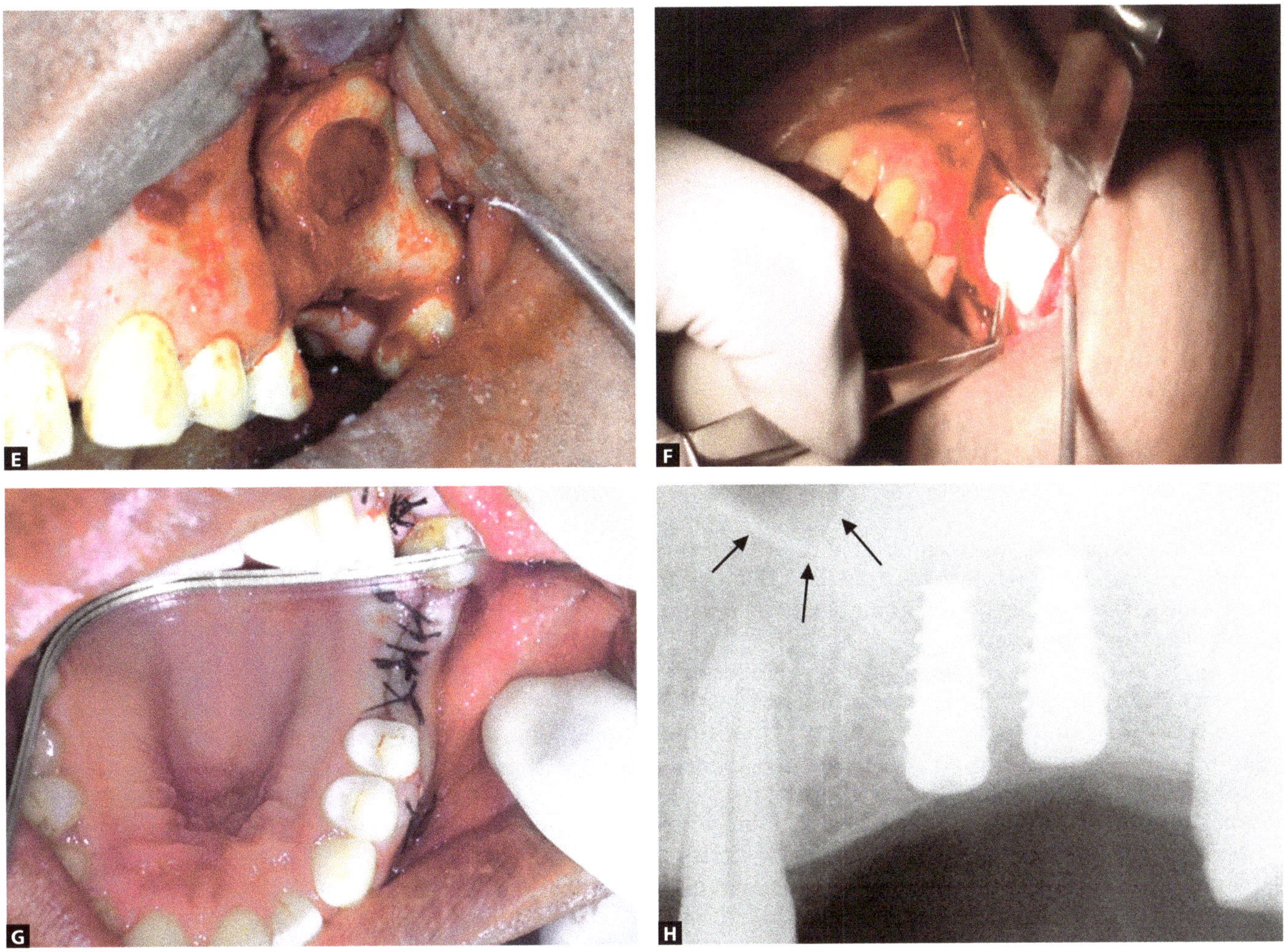

**Figs. 58.5E to H:**

**Figs. 58.5A to H:** Direct sinus lift and implant placement in 26 and 27 region: (A) Clinical picture showing incision given and flap reflected; (B) Clinical picture showing creation of a lateral window; (C) Clinical picture showing moving sinus membrane with inspiration; (D) Clinical picture showing implant placed (4.2 mm × 10 mm) in 26 and 27 region; (E) Clinical picture showing packing the area with bone graft; (F) Clinical picture showing placement of collagen membrane; (G) Clinical picture showing suturing; (H) Postoperative radiograph.

(*Courtesy*: Dr Krishna K Gupta)

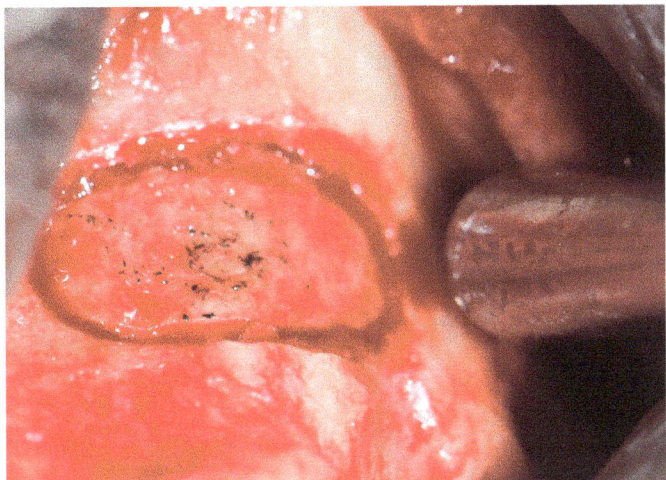

**Fig. 58.6:** Clinical picture showing oval window osteotomy in the lateral wall of maxillary sinus.

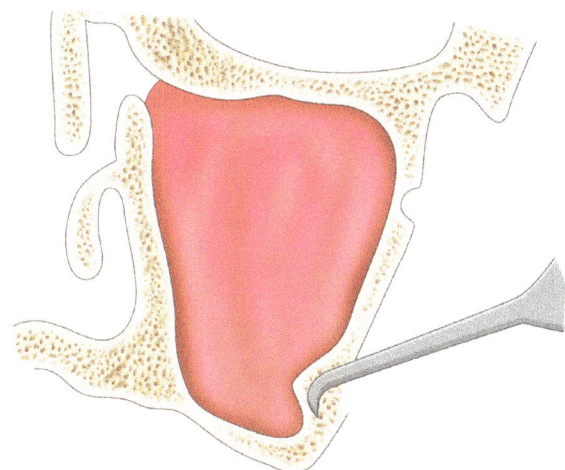

**Fig. 58.7:** Schematic representation showing scrapping sinus membrane off the bone.

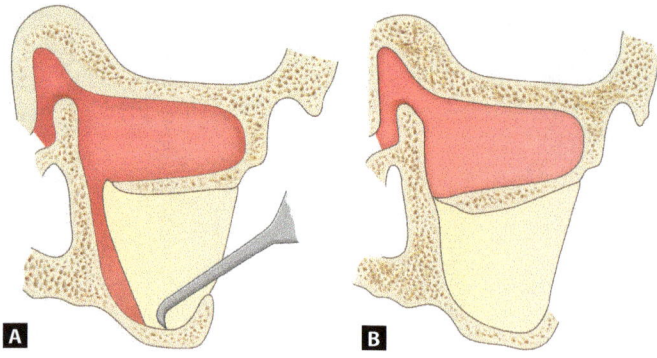

**Figs. 58.8A and B:** Schematic representation showing sinus lift procedure: (A) Sinus curette scratches the floor of the antrum to the medial wall; and (B) The distance from the crest of the ridge to the elevated sinus is increased.

The newly created space i.e., inferior maxillary antrum is then augmented with various types of bone graft materials. These materials may be autografts, allografts, alloplasts or a combination.

- *Step 7: Postoperative instructions*: The postoperative instructions are similar to those for most of the periodontal implant surgery. A chlorhexidine mouthrinse should be used twice a day for 2 weeks to reduce the chances of infection. Blowing the nose, sucking liquid through a straw (which creates negative pressure) and smoking cigarettes should be avoided for at least 2 weeks after surgery. Smoking can also compromise healing. Coughing or sneezing should be performed with an open mouth to relieve pressure. Antibiotic therapy, such as augmentin 500 mg BID for 7–10 days, is continued postoperatively. Before the prosthetic phase begins, 4–6 months should be allowed for the bone graft and implants to integrate. During this period, the patient can wear a conventional prosthesis that has been modified with a soft relining material.

## Complications

The first and most common complication of sinus lift procedure is the perforation of the Schneiderian membrane. Loss of graft or loss of implants into the sinus due to sinus mucosa perforation is another complication noted with this procedure. Sinus graft is a technique sensitive procedure, which requires surgical and prosthodontic skills.

## NERVE REPOSITIONING

To avoid injury to the inferior alveolar nerve (IAN), some authors have advocated the use of local anesthesia as infiltration agents only, rather than as nerve blocks, to leave the patient with some sensation. The damage to the IAN can be lessened by using computer-based navigational systems for drilling in the posterior mandible. Nerve avoidance tactics including slanting the implants in the posterior mandible to incline it downward and laterally from the crestal cortical bone helps to engage the buccal cortical plate at a lower level. These are called as transverse alveolar implants. In the partially edentulous mandibular arch with severely resorbed ridges, a mandibular nerve repositioning is an option. This procedure requires extensive manipulation of the mandibular nerve and often results in extended periods of paresthesia and dysesthesia of the lower lip. In most cases, the patient returns to normal sensation in about 6 months. Patients should be carefully selected for these procedures and clearly informed in writing of all possible side effects.

Two related procedures are:
1. Inferior alveolar nerve lateralization
2. Distalization of mental neurovascular bundle

## Alveolar Nerve Lateralization

### Procedure

Following are the steps for alveolar nerve lateralization:[21,22]

- *Step 1: Anesthesia*: Intravenous sedation or general anesthesia is required for alveolar nerve lateralization. Infiltration and block local anesthesia are also used for the purpose of both vasoconstriction and postoperative pain management.
- *Step 2: Incision*: Soft tissue incision is made slightly buccal to the crest of the residual alveolar ridge. This incision is extended up to the mesial portion of the cuspid tooth. At this point, a vertical releasing incision is made. Anterior vertical releasing incision is carried to the mesial portion of the cuspid tooth to minimize the trauma to the anterior component of the mental neurovascular bundle.
- *Step 3*: At the inferior border of the mandible a full thickness flap is reflected. The inferior alveolar canal usually lies 2 mm below the level of mental foramen in its distal path through the body of the mandible.
- *Step 4*: Anterior border of the osteotomy is created 3–4 mm distal to the mental foramen and extending positively 4–6 mm distal to the most distal implant position.
- *Step 5*: With the help of bur in straight handpiece, trabecular bone is removed with the help of bone chisel. This approach helps to gain entry to the cortical bony layer of inferior alveolar canal. With the help of nerve hook retractor the IAN gets free from its position in canal **(Fig. 58.9)**. Then, elastic type retractor is passed around the nerve bundle and is used to lateralize and retract the neurovascular bundle.
- *Step 6*: Osseous receptor site is prepared using appropriate burs for the placement of implant. The

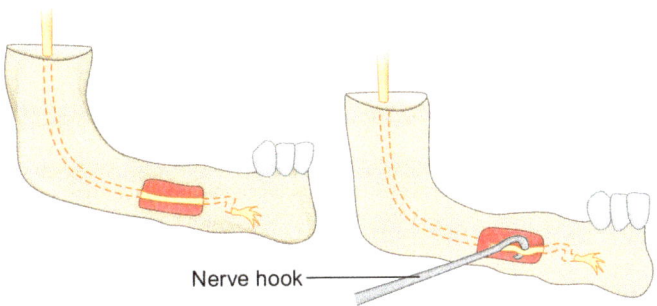

**Fig. 58.9:** Schematic representation showing inferior alveolar lateralization.

apical end of the preparation should be placed inferior to osteotomy site to ensure stabilization and immobilization of implant in bone.
- **Step 7:** After the implant is placed, nerve is repositioned over the lateral aspect of implant.

## Distalization of the Mental Neurovascular Bundle
- **Step 1:** Incision, flap design and reflection are similar to the procedure for lateralization of nerve.
- **Step 2:** The osteotomy is made at the distal wall of the mental foramen for distalization of mental neurovascular bundle. After detecting location of the IAN, the remaining osseous structure between the mental foramen and the osteotomy site is removed by creating a thin groove. As these bony cuts are created, the mental neurovascular bundle is retracted distally, away from the area of the cut using the nerve hook instrument.

### Points to Ponder
- A condition referred to as "witch's chin" occurs when the facial muscles and overlying skin of the chin fall, causing a disfiguring sag of facial tissues after autogenous bone harvesting surgery from the mandibular symphysis.
- In maxillary sinus lift grafting, the configuration of maxillary antrum is changed by rotating the osteotomized window medially and superiorly. The sinus membrane is elevated, creating an empty chamber superior to the residual alveolar bone. The newly created space, i.e., inferior maxillary antrum is then augmented with various types of bone graft materials.

## REFERENCES
1. Hurley LA, Stinchfield FE, Bassett AL, Lyon WH. The role of soft tissues in osteogenesis. An experimental study of canine spine fusions. J Bone Joint Surg Am. 1959;41-A:1243-54.
2. Boyne PJ. Regeneration of alveolar bone beneath cellulose acetate filter implants. J Dent Res. 1964;43:827.
3. Hämmerle CH, Karring T. Guided bone regeneration at oral implant sites. Periodontol 2000. 1998;17:151-75.
4. Klokkevold PR, Jovanovic SA. Advanced implant surgery and bone grafting techniques. In: Newman MG, Takei HH, Carranza FA (Eds). Carranza's Clinical Periodontology, 9th edition. Philadelphia: WB Saunders; 2003. pp.905-21.
5. Misch CE, Suzuki JB. Tooth extraction, socket grafting and barrier membrane bone regeneration. In: Misch CE (Ed). Contemporary Implant Dentistry, 3rd edition. St. Louis: CV Mosby; 2008. pp. 870-904.
6. Becker W, Becker BE, Polizzi G. Autogenous bone grafting of bone defects adjacent to implants placed into immediate extraction sockets in patients: a prospective study. Int J Oral Maxillofac Implants. 1994;9(4):389-96.
7. Chandna S, Kaur K, Kaur N, Manocha A. Socket augmentation. J Int Clin Dent Res Organ. 2015;7(3):73-80.
8. Simion M, Baldoni M, Zaffe D. Jawbone enlargement using immediate implant placement associated with a split-crest technique and guided tissue regeneration. Int J Periodontics Restorative Dent. 1992;12(6):462-73.
9. Ilizarov GA. The tension-stress effect on the genesis and growth of tissues: Part 2. The influence of the rate and frequency of distraction. Clin Orthop Relat Res. 1989;239:263-85.
10. Vega LG, Bilbao A. Alveolar distraction osteogenesis for dental implant preparation: an update. Oral Maxillofac Surg Clin North Am. 2010;22(3):369-85.
11. McAllister BS, Gaffaney TE. Distraction osteogenesis for vertical bone augmentation prior to oral implant reconstruction. Periodontol 2000. 2003;33:54-66.
12. Paley D. Problems, obstacles, and complications of limb lengthening by the Ilizarov technique. Clin Orthop Relat Res. 1990;250:81-104.
13. Hurzeler MB, Zuhr O, Schupbach P, Rebele SF, Emmanouilidis N, Fickl S. The socket-shield technique: a proof of principle report. J Clin Periodontol. 2010;37: 855-62.
14. Bathla S, Fry R, Goyal K, Goyal S, Talnia S. Socket shield technique for immediate implant placement. Int J Periodontol Implantol 2018; 8(3):87-90.
15. Tatum H Jr. Maxillary and sinus implant reconstructions. Dent Clin North Am. 1986;30(2):207-29.
16. Boyne PJ, James RA. Grafting of the maxillary sinus floor with autogenous marrow and bone. J Oral Surg. 1980;38(8):613-6.
17. Misch CE, Resnik RR, Dietsch FM. Maxillary sinus anatomy, pathology and graft surgery. In: Misch CE (Ed). Contemporary Implant Dentistry, 3rd edition. St. Louis: CV Mosby; 2008. pp. 905-74.
18. ten Bruggenkate CM, van den Bergh JP. Maxillary sinus floor elevation: a valuable pre-prosthetic procedure. Periodontol 2000. 1998;17:176-82.
19. Bathla SC, Fry RR, Majumdar K. Maxillary sinus augmentation. J Indian Soc Periodontol 2018; 22:468-73.
20. Tiwana PS, Kushner GM, Haug RH. Maxillary sinus augmentation. Dent Clin North Am. 2006;50(3): 409-24.
21. Babbush CA, Hahn JA, Krauser JT, Rosenlicht JL. Inferior alveolar nerve lateralization and mental neurovascular distalization. In: Dental Implants—The Art and Science, 2nd Edition. Philadelphia, PA, USA: WB Saunders; 2010.
22. Worthington P. Injury to the inferior alveolar nerve during implant placement: a formula for protection of the patient and clinician. Int J Oral Maxillofac Implants. 2004;19(5):731-4.

## Section 8: Implantology

### VIVA VOCE

**Q1. What are the contraindications for ridge split/ridge expansion?**
**Ans.** Ridge width less than 2 mm and alveolar bone height less than 10 mm.

**Q2. What are the instructions given after sinus lift procedure?**
**Ans.** Blowing the nose, sucking liquid through a straw (which creates negative pressure) and smoking cigarettes should be avoided for at least 2 weeks after surgery. Coughing or sneezing should be performed with an open mouth to relieve pressure. Antibiotic therapy, such as Augmentin 500 mg bid for 7 to 10 days, is continued postoperatively. Before the prosthetic phase begins, 4 to 6 months should be allowed for the bone graft and implants to integrate.

**Q3. What are the contraindications for sinus lift procedure?**
**Ans.** Previous sinus surgery, such as the Caldwell-Luc operation, maxillary sinus diseases such as chronic polypous sinusitis and presence of underwood's septa/severe sinus floor convolutions.

**Q4. What is distraction osteogenesis?**
**Ans.** The process of generating new bone by stretching is called as distraction osteogenesis. This surgical technique increases vertical bone height in the deficient jaw site.

**Q5. What is the most common complication of sinus lift procedure?**
**Ans.** Perforation of the Schneiderian membrane.

**Q6. Who originally developed Guided bone regeneration (GBR)?**
**Ans.** Hurley et al. in 1959 and Boyne in 1964

**Q7. What is the thickness of sinus membrane?**
**Ans.** Thickness of the membrane normally varies from 0.13 to 0.5 mm (average 0.8 mm thick).

**Q8. What is the various approaches for maxillary sinus floor elevation?**
**Ans.** There are two main approaches for maxillary sinus floor elevation: Direct and Indirect approach.

**Q9. How to avoid sinus membrane perforation?**
**Ans.** Sinus membrane perforation can be avoided by use of piezosurgery, special non-cutting drills and hydraulic pressure technique.

**Q10. What are the indications of socket shield technique?**
**Ans.**
1. Vertical fracture of teeth without pulpal pathologies.
2. Nonrestorable asymptomatic tooth with healthy and stable buccal root.
3. Tooth with healthy gingival tissue.
4. Adequate amount of bone volume apical to the extraction socket to support implant.

# Peri-implantitis and Other Implant Related Complications

Anil Melath, Veenu M Hans

## Chapter Outline

- Definitions of Peri-implantitis
- Etiology of Peri-implantitis
- Classifications of Peri-implantitis
- Diagnosis of Peri-implantitis
- Management of Peri-implantitis
- Supportive and Maintenance Therapy of Peri-implantitis
- Other Implant Related Complications
- Implant Failure

## DEFINITIONS OF PERI-IMPLANTITIS

Pathological changes of the tissues around the implant are placed in a general category of peri-implant diseases. The term peri-implantitis was introduced in 1987 by Andrea Mombelli to define a destructive inflammatory process which affected the soft and hard tissues around the osseointegrated implants, further resulting in formation of peri-implant pocket and loss of supporting bone. It is a site specific infection yielding many features common with chronic periodontitis.[1]

Albrektsson defined peri-implant mucositis as inflammatory changes, confined to the soft tissue surrounding an implant. It is analogous to gingivitis. Progressive peri-implant bone loss in conjunction with a soft tissue inflammatory lesion is termed peri-implantitis. It is analogous to periodontitis.[2]

Tonetti defined peri-implantitis as an inflammatory bacterial driven destruction of the implant supporting apparatus.[3]

### Peri-implant Mucositis

Peri-implant mucositis is used for describing reversible inflammatory reactions occurring along the mucosa adjacent to an implant.[4] Likewise gingivitis, the etiology for peri-implant mucositis is also a bacterial plaque. The bacterial plaque stimulates an inflammatory cascade in peri-implant mucosa which is almost similar to that in gingiva around tooth.

The clinical features of peri-implant mucositis overlap with gingivitis. The symptoms of inflammation like swelling and redness are also present in peri-implant mucosa. The differences in morphology of peri-implant mucosa and gingiva around tooth and lack of light transmission through metal usually hide the visible signs of inflammation. Assessment of peri-implant mucositis involves assessment of bleeding on probing (BOP) and suppuration. Presence of BOP is suggestive of inflammation in peri-implant sulcus. Suppuration and slight increase in probing pocket depth may also be present in peri-implant mucositis.

## ETIOLOGY OF PERI-IMPLANTITIS

The tissue breakdown associated with peri-implantitis is multifactorial in origin **(Table 59.1)**. However, bacterial infection and biomechanical overload contribute to major tissue damage.[7]

- *Bacterial infection*: The plaque is formed similarly around the implants as it forms around the teeth. When the plaque accumulates around an implant, the inflammatory cells get infiltrate in the subepithelial connective tissue. With the apical extension of the plaque, the appearance of tissue destruction is noted around implants both clinically as well as radiographically. The subgingival flora around diseased implants is usually not the same as that around healthy implants. The microbiology of the implants is similar to that of the bacteria already residing in oral cavity. This suggests that the teeth which are remaining act as reservoirs for bacterial overgrowth in peri-implant tissues. A previous study comparing the microbiota around the successful and failing implants suggest that the latter exhibited significantly elevated proportion of the microorganisms, which were traditionally associated

| TABLE 59.1: Potential risk factors for peri-implantitis.[5,6] |
|---|
| **Local factors** |
| ♦ Thin gingival biotypes |
| ♦ Nonkeratinized tissue |
| ♦ Periodontally involved teeth |
| ♦ Poor bone quality |
| ♦ Surgical trauma |
| ♦ Immediate implants placed into extraction sockets |
| ♦ Improper angulation of the implants |
| ♦ Augmented bone |
| **Restoration related factors** |
| ♦ Over engineered restorations with too many implants |
| ♦ Too closely placed implants making cleaning difficult |
| ♦ Fixed bridges with widespread flanges |
| ♦ Limited embrasure area between implants |
| ♦ Restorations with extensive cantilevers increasing plaque retention |
| **Patient related factors** |
| ♦ Smokers |
| ♦ Poor oral hygiene and compliance |
| ♦ History of parafunction habits (bruxism) |
| **Systemic factors** |
| ♦ Diabetes mellitus |
| ♦ Systemic medications that can affect bone turnover |

with periodontal diseases. Peri-implantitis sites were specifically harbored by gram-negative anaerobic rods, spirochetes and fusiform bacteria in higher proportions in comparison to the healthy sites, which predominantly were composed of coccoid forms.

- *Biomechanical factors*: Biomechanical forces also play an important role in success, survival or failure of dental implants. Excessive presence of biomechanical factors can result in increased stress and microfractures in coronal bone to implant contact. Persistent excessive biomechanical forces lead to lack of osseointegration around the implant neck. This cause is particularly important in case of insufficient bone, poor bone quality, parafunctional activities and misfit of prosthesis. In contrast to bacteria related peri-implantitis, bone loss caused by mechanical overload is not associated with a primary inflammatory response of the surrounding mucosal tissues. As the bone loss progresses, a combination of bacteria-related and loading-related bone loss is seen when the bone loss creates deep pocket that collect plaque, resulting in a secondary microbial related inflammatory reaction leading to bone loss.
- *Other cofactors are*:[8]
    - The relationship between the roughness of implant surface and bacterial colonization play significant role in peri-implantitis. A proportional relationship is found between surface roughness and the rate of bacterial colonization in association with both supragingival and subgingival plaque.
    - Smoking is considered to be an established risk factor for chronic periodontitis and hence associated with enhanced risk of implant loss.
    - Compromised host response
    - Traumatic surgical technique

## CLASSIFICATIONS OF PERI-IMPLANTITIS

Spiekermann has given the following classification of the peri-implant bone loss:[9]
- *Class 1*: Slight horizontal bone loss with minimal peri-implant defect.
- *Class 2*: Moderate horizontal bone loss with isolated vertical defect.
- *Class 3*: Moderate to advanced horizontal bone loss with broad circular bony defect.
- *Class 4*: Advanced horizontal bone loss with broad circumferential vertical defects as well as loss of oral and/or vestibular bony wall.

## DIAGNOSIS OF PERI-IMPLANTITIS

Clinically, the well advanced peri-implantitis lesion is easily identifiable. But, the early lesions are not only the greatest challenge to the clinician but they are also of significant value so as to prevent further bone resorption and subsequently the loss of implant. The diagnosis of peri-implantitis rests on the same parameters as that for diagnosing periodontal diseases. The parameters normally used in the diagnosis of peri-implantitis are the clinical signs, such as suppuration, mobility, BOP, peri-implant probing and peri-implant radiography.[10,11]

- *Clinical assessment*: Peri-implantitis lesions are usually asymptomatic and identified during routine recall appointments. Peri-implant mucosa exhibit swelling and redness due to associated peri-implant infections. Clinical assessment must include the evaluation of the amount of plaque around an implant. Suppuration is usually associated with inflammation of the peri-implant tissues, indicating suppuration as a sign of peri-implantitis. Presence of mobile implant suggests the lack of osseointegration. However, it is one of the final stages of deintegration and hence of no use in the diagnosis of early implant disease.
- *Peri-implant probing*: A blunt and straight plastic periodontal probe (**Fig. 59.1**) is used for probing the peri-implant sulcus which allows the assessment of peri-implant probing depth, soft tissue margin distance and a reference point on the implant for measurement of hyperplasia or recession along with bleeding and suppuration. In long-term monitoring of peri-implant mucosal tissues, probing around oral implants is ideally a reliable and sensitive parameter. A probing depth of more than 4 mm is indicative of peri-implant disease. Bleeding during probing suggest inflammation in the pocket or sulcus with presence of ongoing inflammatory process.

## Chapter 59: Peri-implantitis and Other Implant Related Complications

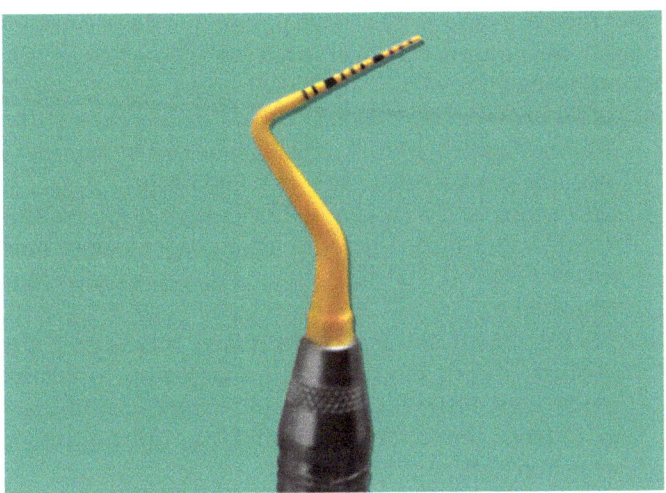

**Fig. 59.1:** Photograph showing plastic probe.

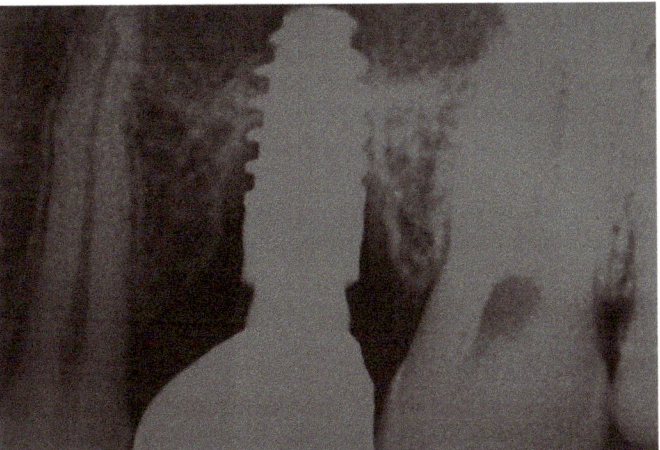

**Fig. 59.2:** Radiographic image showing bone loss around the implant.

- *Peri-implant radiography*: In standardized radiographs, the distance from implant shoulder or apical termination of the cylindrical part till the alveolar bone crest is considered a reliable parameter indicating peri-implantitis. Conventional radiography usually fails to detect minor changes in bone morphology until they reach a significant size **(Fig. 59.2)**. Radiographic evidence of bone to implant contact is not indicative of osseointegration. Digital subtraction radiography has significant sensitivity and hence has a successful use in detection of peri-implantitis.

## MANAGEMENT OF PERI-IMPLANTITIS

The early diagnosis and management of peri-implant pathology is important to prevent further bone loss and subsequent loss of implant. For the therapy of peri-implantitis, Mombelli has suggested five considerations:
1. The disturbance and/or removal of the bacterial biofilm in the peri-implant pocket.
2. Decontamination and conditioning of implant surface.
3. Correction via reduction or elimination of sites that cannot be adequately maintained by oral hygiene measures.
4. Establishment of an effective plaque control regime.
5. Re-osseointegration

The treatment of peri-implantitis is divided into an initial therapeutic phase and surgical phase.[12-14]

### Initial Therapeutic Phase

- *Occlusal therapy*: Analysis of prosthesis and occlusal evaluation is an important aspect of peri-implant diagnosis, as excessive forces also contribute to peri-implant bone loss. Change in the design of the prosthesis and improvement in implant number and position helps to arrest progression of the peri-implant tissue breakdown.
- *Anti-infective therapy*: Nonsurgical anti-infective therapy for peri-implantitis and peri-implant mucositis involves removing plaque deposits using a plastic instrument and polishing all accessible surfaces with pumice. Additionally peri-implant pockets can be irrigated with the help of 0.12% chlorhexidine or local antimicrobials. The initial therapy phase is usually sufficient for re-establishing peri-implant health or occasionally has to be followed by surgical phase.
- *Systemic antibiotics*: Systemic antibiotics can be administered as a supportive therapy for treatment of peri-implant disease. Frequently used antibiotics for this purpose are metronidazole, doxycycline or a combination of metronidazole and amoxicillin.
- *Implant surface preparation*: Peri-implantitis commonly present with contamination of the implant surface with bacteria and bacterial by products. This contamination hampers the wound healing process and inhibits the bone regeneration and re-osseointegration in that area. Therefore, for desirable outcome of bone regeneration implant surface preparation has to be done. This is usually achieved by using an air powder abrasive which is a mixture of sodium bicarbonate and sterile water. This abrasive does not change surface topography of implant and do not produce any adverse effect on cell adhesion. Implant surface preparation can also be done with the application of tetracycline hydrochloride, citric acid for 30–60 seconds and more recently, use of $CO_2$, diode erbium-doped: yttrium aluminum garnet (Er:YAG) lasers has been advocated for implant surface decontamination and preparation.

### Surgical Phase

- *Peri-implant resective therapy*: This is suitable for peri-implant lesion with horizontal or vertical bone loss

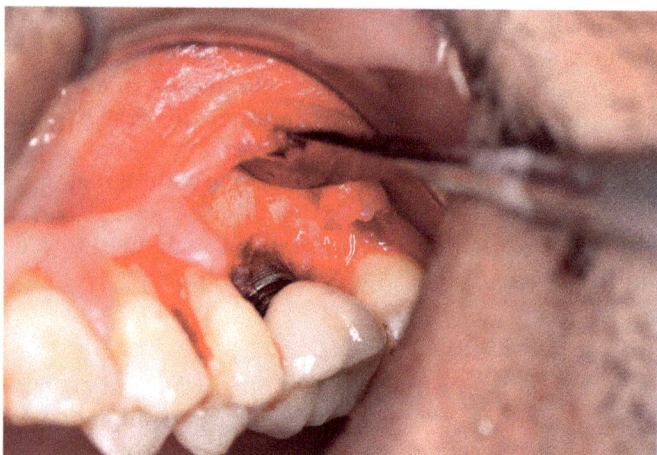

**Fig. 59.3:** Clinical picture showing granulation tissue and peri-implant bone loss after flap elevation.

(<3 mm). In order to access the surgical area, a full thickness flap is raised and degranulation of the defect and resective therapy is done.

- *Implantoplasty*: Implant surfaces presenting with threads, roughened topography, or hydroxyapatite surfaces are treated by using high-speed finishing burs and produce a smooth, polished and continuous titanium surface. It is performed with profuse irrigation before osseous resective therapy.[15]
- *Osseous resective therapy*: Bone around implant is recontoured and flap is apically repositioned and sutured.
- *Peri-implant regenerative therapy*: Use of guided bone regeneration is recommended in cases where moderate to deep vertical defects are seen in peri-implant bone. The surgical therapy includes removal of granulation tissue after elevation of flap **(Fig. 59.3)**, implant surface preparation and use of bone graft and barrier membrane on the defect. The membrane is extended 3–4 mm beyond the defect and flap is closed over it.
- *Re-osseointegration*: The treatment goal of peri-implant regenerative therapy is de novo bone formation at the portion of implant that has lost its osseointegration in the inflammatory process. This increase in height of the bone leads to marginal shift of mucosa thereby, enhancing the soft tissue esthetics.

## SUPPORTIVE AND MAINTENANCE THERAPY OF PERI-IMPLANTITIS

The *cumulative interceptive supportive therapy (CIST)* is a protocol based approach for monitoring the healthy implants and interception of peri-implant diseases. The protocol considers various parameters including BOP, probing depth and radiographic evidence of bone loss. With increase in severity of each parameter, more complex treatment is introduced, with each subsequent treatment incorporating that of the previous protocol.[16]

- *CIST protocol A (mechanical debridement)*: If the probing depth is <4 mm, oral hygiene can be improved by using soft scalers, rubber cup and paste.
- *CIST protocol A + B (antiseptic therapy)*: If the probing depth is 4–5 mm, antiseptic therapy (chlorhexidine rinse or topical chlorhexidine gel daily) is used along with step A.
- *CIST protocol A + B + C (antibiotic therapy)*: If the probing depth is greater than or equal to 6 mm, tetracycline fibers for 10 days and systemic antibiotics for 10 days (amoxicillin + metronidazole) are used along with step A+B.
- *CIST protocol A + B + C + D (regeneration and resective)*: If the CIST protocol A + B + C is used and still considerable amount on bone loss and probing pocket depth are present, surgical therapy is used along with step A + B + C. Regenerative approach (barrier membrane, nonsubmerged) or resective approach (osteoplasty + apically positioned flap) is opted depending on esthetic considerations and morphological characteristics of the lesion.

The main aim of CIST approach is the earliest prevention of peri-implant tissue destruction.

## Maintenance Procedures Performed by the Patient

Plaque control should be started immediately after the implant is exposed to the intraoral environment and monitored over time. Implant superstructures are often bulky and overcontoured, which makes traditional home care procedures more difficult. Patients may find smaller diameter toothbrush heads to be beneficial in areas of difficult access. When single tooth implant is present, it can generally be cleaned just like tooth with a toothbrush and dental floss but when restorations are attached to multiple implants in a splinted fashion, or when hybrid-type prosthesis are present, oral hygiene can become much more difficult for the patient.[17,18]

- Toothbrush should be round ended with soft filaments to prevent damage to peri-implant tissue.
- Dentifrice or other cleaning agents should not be used as it causes abrasion of the titanium or other implant material. Titanium implants are corroded by acidic fluoride preparations.
- Yarn or gauge strips with floss threader are used to clean crossbar of subperiosteal implant and proximal surface of endosseous implants abutment.
- Irrigators can also be used as adjunctive aids.
- Gauze strips can be easily used to clean under posterior cantilever areas using a shoeshine technique.

## Maintenance Procedures Performed by the Therapist

Patient recall should be at 3-month intervals for the 1st year and then on a semi-annual basis. Some patients may require more frequent follow-up care. Recall visits should include: (1) an evaluation of oral hygiene compliance, (2) occlusal harmony, (3) implant and prosthesis stability, (4) overall soft and hard peri-implant tissue health and (5) radiographic follow up. The recommended instrumentation for implant debridement includes plastic, nylon, or special alloy instruments that will not alter the implant surface **(Fig. 59.4)**. Sonic or ultrasonic scalers that use a plastic cap over the metal tip have been shown to be safe and effective. Titanium tipped curettes has been developed for removal of calculus on implant surface.[17,18]

Instruments used for assessment and calculus removal from implant should be made of a material that is softer than the implant material; plastic instrument is most commonly used; some plastic instrument can be sterilized by autoclave for several cycles; following manufacturer's instructions for sterilization and reuse.

## OTHER IMPLANT RELATED COMPLICATIONS

Surgical implant complications are divided into two categories: soft tissue and hard tissue complications:[19-22]

### Soft-tissue Complications

#### Hemorrhage

Types of hemorrhagic patches develop as a result of injury: petechiae (<2 mm in diameter); purpura (2-10 mm); ecchymosis (>10 mm). These patches are nonelevated, rounded, or irregular and initially are red-blue or purplish in color.

Hematoma (contusion) is a collection of blood, which gets clotted in an organ, space, or tissue. It is a result of a break in a blood vessel wall. The excessive fluid may form an elevated, hard lump. If a hematoma develops, ice can reduce the amount of swelling, and it may be advantageous to elevate a bruised site to facilitate blood leaving the area.

Healing of the above conditions follows a predictable pattern of color alterations that is related to hemoglobin breakdown. Initially, lesions are reddish, reflecting the presence of blood. After 1-2 days, the sites appear black and blue (purple). By day 6, the color changes to green, and this reflects the presence of biliverdin. At day 8-9, the site is yellowish-brownish denoting that bilirubin is present. Discoloration usually goes in 2-3 weeks.

The incidence of hemorrhagic patches can be reduced with careful soft-tissue management. Vertical releasing incisions usually sever blood vessels and lead to increase in bleeding. Hence if possible it is better to avoid such type of incisions. During the procedure of flap elevation, care should be taken to rest elevators on bone and not on soft tissue, and suctioning ought to be done on bone as opposed to soft tissue. In addition, after flap replacement, it is advantageous to apply pressure to the tissue for several minutes to minimize blood clot thickness and to ensure that bleeding has stopped. These actions will reduce ecchymosis and hematoma formation.

#### Nerve Injury

During process of osteotomy development, intrusion into the inferior alveolar or mental canal may lead to transection, tearing or laceration of nerves. Insertion of implant may also result in bone compression on the nerve. Additionally, within the soft tissue, the lingual or mental nerve possibly gets injured by compression, stretching, scalpel, or needle penetration.

Whenever there is concern that nerve damage occurred during osteotomy development and the implant was inserted, radiographs should be taken to ascertain the implant's position. If it is intruded into a nerve canal, the authors suggest that the implant should be slightly withdrawn a couple of turns or removed altogether. The next day, if a patient relates symptoms of altered perception, it needs to be determined whether they are due to the presence of the implant or sequelae of soft-tissue manipulation or edema. Whenever it is believed that the implant is the problem, it should be removed. If the twist drill or the implant did not encroach upon the canal, it is possible that bone was compressed, thereby placing pressure on the nerve. The implant should be slightly withdrawn several turns. In the event of uncertainty with regard to implant penetration into a nerve canal, a computed tomography (CT) scan may be needed to provide additional information.

An altered sensation may result due to an inflammatory reaction, especially when an implant is not within a nerve canal. Prescription of steroid therapy or anti-inflammatory medication (ibuprofen, 800 mg, 3 times a day) for 3 weeks is useful in such cases.

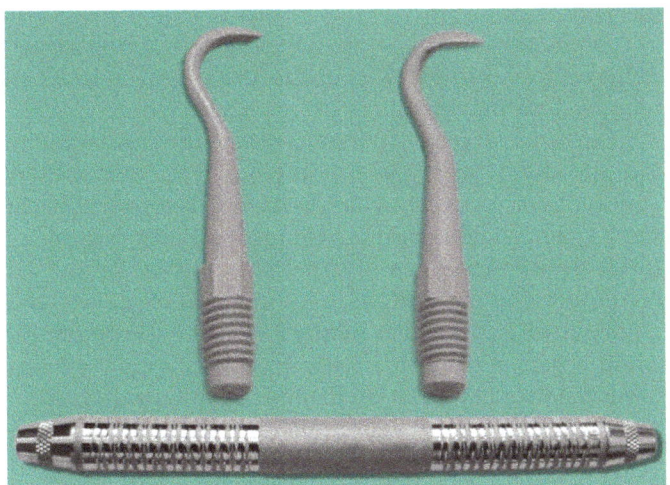

**Fig. 59.4:** Photograph showing Implacare implant instrument.

Determining the location of the inferior alveolar nerve and mental foramen before osteotomy helps to prevent nerve injuries to a great extent. This requires complete evaluation of periapical and panoramic films and a CT scan if needed. Use of the appropriate magnification correction factor is must and placement of drill guards on burs helps to avoid unintentional overpenetration of the drill. As safety margin of 2 mm between the entire implant body and any nerve canal should be maintained.

### Infection

Infection at the implant site may present with edema, exudate and pain. They are caused by bacterial contamination during surgery either directly via accidental contacts with the implants or indirectly from gloves or instruments.

Infection can be reduced by following the surgical principles of asepsis: working under clean and sterile area; disinfection of the perioral skin with povidone-iodine solutions; disinfection of the oral mucosa with 0.2% chlorhexidine; cleansing surgical gloves in sterile saline to remove dust or contaminants.

### Edema

It is the accumulation of excess plasma fluid in the interstitial spaces which may negatively affect healing and create discomfort to the patient.

Edema can be prevented or reduced by following steps: Atraumatic surgical techniques; application of icepacks and administration of corticosteroids.

## Hard-tissue Complications

### Periapical Implant Pathosis and Endodontic

#### Considerations

Incorrect positioning of an implant can lead to striking an adjacent tooth or impingement on the tooth's blood supply or overheating of the bone during the osteotomy. This makes an adjacent tooth nonvital in nature. In such cases, the damaged tooth will usually need endodontic therapy, an apicoectomy, or an extraction. Additionally, a periapical lesion which is a result of devitalization may encroach upon the implant and contaminate it resulting in loss of the implant. Other explanations for the initiation of periapical pathosis around an implant are microbial contamination at the time of placement, bone necrosis due to overheating of bone during osteotomy development and residual foreign bodies in the bone.

To avoid devitalizing an adjacent tooth during osteotomy development, the angulation of adjacent teeth and dilacerations of roots should be assessed radiographically before placement of an implant. A 1.5–2 mm of bone must exist between an implant and the adjacent tooth to prevent such complication.

To reduce the potential of developing retrograde peri-implantitis, it is advisable to avoid immediate placement of an implant into an infected site or when there is a radiographic indication of pathosis. Conversely, thorough debridement and irrigation may be sufficient to provide a proper environment, because it seems that retrograde implantitis only occurs 1% of the time. Implant packages should be opened immediately before placement and should not touch anything other than the bone to avoid transferring contaminants. Osteotomies ought to be flushed and suctioned prior to implant insertion to remove debris. In addition, teeth adjacent to an implant site that need endodontic treatment should be treated prior to implant placement.

### Mandibular Jaw Fracture

There are several factors that predispose a patient to mandibular jaw fracture associated with implant placement: osteoporosis (reduction of bone mass), stress at the implant location and trauma.

When a fracture occurs, the degree of displacement is the critical determinant in selecting the appropriate treatment. If the fracture manifests minimal mobility or displacement, the implant should be maintained.

However, if there is a large amount of displacement, the surgeon needs to decide whether a closed or open fracture reduction is needed with or without retention of an implant along the fracture line.

### Inadvertent Penetration into Maxillary Sinus or Nasal Fossa

The most common problem associated with sinus elevation is perforation of the Schneiderian membrane. Such perforations can be occluded with a bioabsorbable barrier before placing graft material.

Sometimes a tear in the membrane is present along the periphery of the osteotomy and reengaging the membrane seems difficult. Such situation needs to be tackled by extending the osteotomy outline several millimeters past the original window and reestablishing contact with the membrane.

Sometimes during implant insertion, an implant may inadvertently get displaced into the sinus cavity. This requires its removal from cavity.

The removal procedure involves creation of a window into the sinus to retrieve the implant. Administration of antibiotics is necessary if an infection develops within the sinus (pain, redness and tenderness) without fluctuance. If the fluctuance develops, incision and drainage are recommended in addition to administration of systemic antibiotics. It is prudent to culture the infection to determine whether the appropriate antimicrobial therapy is being used. A persistent infection dictates that the graft material may be removed and the sinus flushed out. Presence of fever, facial pain (that increases on leaning forward) and yellow to green purulent discharge from the nose, which may drain posteriorly causing a cough and malaise usually indicate sinusitis. Related symptoms include popping of the ears and muffled hearing. There may be swelling of the periorbital tissues and referred pain to the maxillary teeth. Sinus infections can have serious consequences. Uncommonly, they can progress to unilateral or bilateral pansinusitis or to cavernous sinus involvement.

## IMPLANT FAILURE

From a therapeutic point of view, the distinction between ailing implants, failing implants, failed implants and biologic complications are critical. Ailing implant has been defined as a clinically stable implant showing soft- tissue inflammatory signs, pocketing or mild bone loss. Peri-implant mucositis refers to inflammatory changes involving the soft tissue surrounding an implant. Hence, an implant presenting with peri-implant mucositis is considered as an ailing implant. In few cases, the ailing implant may show early bone loss along with pocketing of soft tissue. An implant that is progressively losing its bone anchorage, but is still clinically stable can be defined as failing. However, a "failing" implant might be saved when recognized and treated properly. The major difference between an ailing and a failing implant is the outcome of the therapy. In other words, the term "ailing" implies a somewhat more favorable prognosis than "failing".

Clinically, lack of osseointegration is generally characterized by implant mobility. Hence, a mobile implant is considered as a failed implant.

The dental implant failure is usually classified into seven categories:[23,24]
1. According to the etiology
2. According to timing of the failure
3. According to the origin of infection
4. According to condition of failure
5. According to responsible personnel
6. According to failure mode
7. According to the tissues involved

## Category I: According to the Etiology

It is concerned with the etiologic reasons of implant failures, which include failure because of host factors, surgical placement, implant selection and restorative problems.

### Host Factors
- *Medical status*: Osteoporosis and other bone disease, uncontrolled diabetes.
- *Habits*: Smoking, parafunctional habits.
- *Oral status*: Poor home care, irradiation therapy.

### Surgical Placement
- Off-axis placement (severe angulation).
- Lack of initial stabilization.
- Impaired healing and infection because of improper flap design or others.
- Overheating the bone and exerting too much pressure.
- Minimal space between implants.
- Placement of implant in immature bone-grafted sites.
- Placement of implant in an infected socket or a pathologic lesion.
- Contamination of the implant body before insertion.

### Implant Selection
- Improper implant in improper bone type.
- Length of the implant (too short-, crown-to-root ratio unfavorable).
- Improper width of the implant.
- Incorrect number of implants.
- Improper implant design.

### Restorative Problems
- Excessive cantilever.
- Improper fit of the abutment.
- Improper occlusal scheme.

## Category II: According to Timing of Failure

- *Before stage II*: It usually occurs as a result of implant malplacement (e.g., placement of the implant in an infected socket, pathological lesion, or immature bone previously augmented or placement of a contaminated implant in the osteotomy), infection or soft-tissue complications, lack of biocompatibility, excessive surgical trauma and/or lack of primary stabilization of the implant.
- *At stage II*: It can fail at the second stage of surgery, during healing or head placement, at abutment connection and before prosthetic placement.
- *After restoration*: This particular timing of failure is the most common. It starts after an integrated implant is loaded. The most common cause is occlusal trauma.

## Category III: According to Origin of Infection

- *Peri-implantitis (infective process, bacterial origin)*: Peri-implantitis was defined by Meffert as the progressive loss of peri-implant bone as well as soft-tissue inflammatory changes. Tonetti and Schmid divided the host's reaction to bacterial invasion into two groups: (1) peri-implant mucositis, which implies that the inflammatory changes are localized only to the surrounding soft tissue; and (2) peri-implantitis, in which the reaction affects the deeper soft tissue and surrounding bone.
- Retrograde peri-implantitis.

## Category IV: According to Condition of Failure (Clinical and Radiographic Status)

Meffert proposed a classification of failure including ailing, failing and failed implants.

## Category V: According to Responsible Personnel

The success and integrity of the dental implant rely on cooperation among dental team that consists of the general dentist, surgeon, prosthodontist, periodontist, laboratory technician and the patient.

## Category VI: According to Failure Mode

- Lack of osseointegration
- Unacceptable esthetics
- Functional problems
- Psychological problems

## Category VII: According to the Tissues Involved

- Soft-tissue problems (lack of keratinized tissues, inflammation)
- Bone loss (radiographic changes, etc.)
- Both soft tissue and bone loss

### Points to Ponder

- Peri-implant mucositis is analogous to gingivitis.
- Peri-implantitis is analogous to periodontitis.

## REFERENCES

1. Mombelli A, Van Oosten MA, Schurch E, Land NP. The microbiota associated with successful or failing osseointegrated titanium implants. Oral Microbiol Immunol. 1987;2(4):145-51.
2. Albrektsson T, Isidor F. Consensus report of session IV. In: Lang NP, Karring T (Eds). Proceedings of the 1st European Workshop on Periodontology. Chicago, USA: Quintessence Publishing; 1994. pp. 365-9.
3. Tonetti M. Peri-implantitis: biological considerations. J Parodontol Implantol Orale. 1996;15:284-96.
4. Berglundh T, Lindhe J, Lang NP, Mayfield L. Mucositis and Peri-implantitis. In: Lindhe J, Karring T, Lang NP (Eds). Clinical Periodontology and Implant Dentistry, 4th edition. Oxford, UK: Blackwell Munksgaard; 2003. pp. 1014-23.
5. Rocchietta I, Nisand D. A review assessing the quality of reporting of risk factor research in implant dentistry using smoking, diabetes and periodontitis and implant loss as an outcome: critical aspects in design and outcome assessment. J Clin Periodontol. 2012;39(Suppl 12):114-21.
6. Peri-implant mucositis and peri-implantitis: a current understanding of their diagnoses and clinical implications. J Periodontol. 2013;84(4):436-43.
7. Jovanovic SA. The management of peri-implant breakdown around functioning osseointegrated dental implants. J Periodontol. 1993;64:1176.
8. Jovanovic SA. Diagnosis and Treatment of Peri-implant complications. In: Newman MG, Takei HH, Carranza FA (Eds). Clinical Periodontology, 9th edition. Philadelphia, USA: WB Saunders; 2003. pp. 931-42.
9. Spiekermann DH, Donath K, Hassell T, Jovanovic S, Ritcher J. Color Atlas of Dental Medicine: Implantology, 1st edition. New York, USA: Thieme Medical Publishers; 1995. pp. 321-2.
10. Mombelli A, Lang NP. The diagnosis and treatment of peri-implantitis. Periodontol 2000. 1998;17:63-76.
11. Klinge B, Hultin M, Berglundh T. Peri-implantitis. Dent Clin North Am. 2005;49(3):661-76.
12. Jovanovic SA. The management of peri-implant breakdown around functioning osseointegrated dental implants. J Periodontol. 1993;64(11 Suppl):1176-83.
13. Smeets R, Henningsen A, Jung O, Heiland M, Hammächer C, Stein JM. Definition, etiology, prevention and treatment of peri- implantitis—a review. Head Face Med. 2014;10:34.
14. Roos-Jansåker AM, Renvert S, Egelberg J. Treatment of peri-implant infections: a literature review. J Clin Periodontol. 2003;30(6):467-85.
15. Zablotsky MH, Diedrich DL, Meffert RM. The ability of various chemotherapeutic agents to detoxify the endotoxin infected HA-coated implant surface. Int J Oral Implantai. 1991;8:45-50.
16. Mombelli A. Etiology, diagnosis and treatment considerations in peri-implantitis. Curr Opin Periodontol. 1997;4:127-36.
17. Al-Sabbagh M. Implant in the esthetic zone. Dent Clin North Am. 2006;50(3):391-407.
18. Lang NP, Lindhe J. Maintenance of the implant patient. In: Lindhe J, Karring T, Lang NP (Eds). Clinical Periodontology and Implant Dentistry, 4th edition. Oxford, UK: Blackwell Munksgaard; 2003. pp.1024-30.
19. Misch K, Wang HL. Implant Surgery Complications: Etiology and Treatment. Implant Dent. 2008;17:159-168.
20. Greenstein G, Cavallaro J, Romanos G and Dennis Tarnow D. Clinical Recommendations for Avoiding and Managing Surgical Complications Associated With Implant Dentistry: A Review. J Periodontol. 2008;79:1317-1329.
21. Esposito M, Hirsch JM, Lekholm U, Thomsen P. Differential Diagnosis and Treatment Strategies for Biologic Complications and Failing Oral Implants: A Review of the Literature. Int J Oral Maxillofac Implants. 1999;14:473-90.
22. Sakka S, Coulthard P. Implant failure: Etiology and complications. Med Oral Patol Oral Cir Bucal. 2011; 16:e42-4.
23. Askary ASE, Meffert RM, Griggin T. Why do dental implants fail? Part I. Implant dentistry. 1999;8:173-83.
24. Askary ASE, Meffert RM, Griggin T. Why do dental implants fail? Part II. Implant dentistry. 1999;8:265-75.

### VIVA VOCE

**Q1.** What is the basic difference between ailing and failing implant?
**Ans.** Ailing implant has been defined as a clinically stable implant showing soft-tissue inflammatory signs, pocketing or mild bone loss. Failing implant is an implant that is progressively loosing its bone anchorage, but is still clinically stable.

**Q2.** Name implant detoxification agents.
**Ans.** Abrasive sodium carbonate air-powder, citric acid and tetracycline HCl.

## Chapter 59: Peri-implantitis and Other Implant Related Complications

**Q3. Name index used to assess marginal mucosal conditions around oral implants.**
**Ans.** Modified and adapted gingival index, i.e., modified gingival index (mGI) was given by Mombelli et al.,

| Score | Description |
|---|---|
| 0 | No bleeding when a periodontal probe is passed along the mucosal margin adjacent to the implant |
| 1 | Isolated bleeding spots visible |
| 2 | Blood forms a confluent red line on mucosal margin |
| 3 | Heavy/profuse bleeding. |

**Q4. What are the main etiological factors for peri-implantitis?**
**Ans.** Bacterial infection and biomechanical overload.

**Q5. Which instruments are used for calculus removal from implants?**
**Ans.** Plastic tipped scalers (implacare implant instrument) or titanium tipped curettes.

**Q6. What is cumulative interceptive supportive therapy (CIST)?**
**Ans.** CIST is a protocol based approach for monitoring the healthy implants and interception of peri-implant diseases. The protocol considers various parameters including bleeding on probing, probing depth and radiographic evidence of bone loss.

**Q7. What is peri-implant mucositis?**
**Ans.** Albrektsson defined peri-implant mucositis as inflammatory changes, confined to the soft tissue surrounding an implant.

**Q8. What is peri-implantitis?**
**Ans.** Progressive peri-implant bone loss in conjunction with a soft tissue inflammatory lesion is termed peri-implantitis.

**Q9. Which parameters are normally used in the diagnosis of peri-implantitis ?**
**Ans.** Suppuration, mobility, BOP, peri-implant probing and peri-implant radiography.

**Q10. With which instrument peri-implant probing is done?**
**Ans.** Blunt and straight plastic periodontal probe.

# Section 9: Interdisciplinary Approach

- Periodontics-Prosthodontics
- Periodontics-Endodontics
- Periodontics-Restorative Dentistry
- Periodontics-Orthodontics
- Periodontics-Pediatric Dentistry
- Periodontics-Oral surgery
- Periodontics-Psychiatry

# Chapter 60: Periodontics-Prosthodontics

*Shalu Bathla*

## Chapter Outline

- Sequence of Treatment
- Application of Periodontics in Prosthodontics
- Periodontal Considerations in Complete Denture and RPD
- Periodontal Considerations in FPD
- Periodontal Maintenance in the Prosthetic Patient

## INTRODUCTION

The association between periodontal health and the restoration of teeth runs parallel to each other. For long-term survival of restorations, the periodontium should be healthy in order to maintain the teeth in the normal position. Similarly, for maintaining healthy periodontium, restorations must be managed adequately in several areas to maintain their harmony with surrounding periodontal tissues.

## SEQUENCE OF TREATMENT

In patients with mutilated dentitions and extensive periodontal disease, the sequence of treatment can be modified as follows: first of all hopeless teeth are extracted which is followed by construction of a temporary partial denture and then, periodontal therapy is performed. Approximately 2 months after periodontal treatment, when gingival health is restored and the location of the gingival sulcus is established, the preparations are modified to relocate the margins in proper relation to the healthy gingival sulcus, and final restorations are constructed.[1]

## APPLICATION OF PERIODONTICS IN PROSTHODONTICS

### Preprosthetic Periodontal Care

Periodontal tissues should be in a state of health prior to preparation of a tooth for any restoration. Inflammation alters the contour, shape, volume and consistency of the marginal gingiva and the interdental papilla, so that when inflammation is present, it is impossible to accurately prepare the tooth because of lack of reference points for the correct placement of the cervical margin of the preparation, and ease of bleeding of the pocket wall. The gingiva should therefore be treated first and after healing has been completed, the preparation should be done. It is the periodontal health that determines when the tooth preparation can be started. Once gingival inflammation and periodontal pockets have been eliminated, the gingival margin will change position and shape. The possibilities of gingival recession after placement of restoration are minimized if the procedure is started with healthy periodontal tissues.

Periodontal disease must be eliminated prior to prosthetic treatment because of the following reasons:[2]

- With completion of periodontal treatment, margins of restorations covered by inflamed gingiva get shrinks. Hence, in order to locate and determine the gingival margin of restoration properly, establishment of the position of the healthy and stable gingival margin is must before tooth preparation.
- The position of teeth get frequently changed in periodontal disease. After treatment, resolution of inflammation and regeneration of periodontal ligament fibers lead to teeth movement, usually back to their original position.
- Inflammation of the periodontium hinders the capacity of abutment teeth to achieve the functional demands.
- With the restoration of periodontal health, partial prosthesis constructed on casts made from impressions of diseased gingiva and edentulous mucosa fails to fit

properly. With the adequate control of inflammation, the contour of gingiva and adjacent mucosa is altered. Shrinkage creates spaces beneath the pontics of fixed bridges and the saddle areas of removable prosthesis again resulting in plaque accumulation.
- Tooth mobility and pain interfere with mastication and function of restored teeth.

Gingival massage is advised to the patient for better healing after extraction. Thus, preprosthetic periodontal treatment and care should create healthy gingivo-mucosal environment and osseous topography necessary for the proper function of single tooth restorations, fixed partial denture (FPD) and removable partial denture (RPD).

## Preprosthetic Periodontal Surgery

The procedure, which aims to treat the periodontal condition and preparing the mouth for the ensuing esthetic, restorative and prosthetic therapy, is called as preprosthetic periodontal surgery. This includes:
- Crown-lengthening surgery
- Correction of deformed ridges
- Ridge augmentation

### Crown-lengthening Surgery

The surgical procedure to expose adequate clinical crown to prevent the placement of the crown margin into the area of the biologic width is called as crown-lengthening surgery.[2]

Biologic width is defined as the dimension of healthy gingival tissue, which is attached to the tooth coronal to the crest of the alveolar tissue. Average length of connective tissue attachment[3] is 1.07 mm and of junctional epithelium is 0.97 mm which makes total biologic width of 2.04 mm (**Fig. 60.1**). The term biologic width was replaced by supracrestal attached tissues in 2017 classification. Significance of supracrestal attached tissues: If the restorative margin is placed into biologic width area then there will be gingival inflammation, pocket formation and loss of crestal bone to re-establish the biologic width.

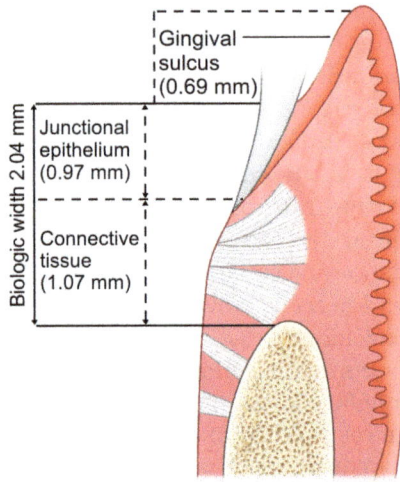

**Fig. 60.1:** Schematic representation showing biologic width.

*Indications for crown-lengthening surgery*
- Subgingival caries or fracture.
- Inadequate clinical crown length for retention.
- Unequal or unesthetic gingival height.

*Surgical methods for crown-lengthening*
Following are the surgical methods for crown lengthening:[4]
- *Gingivectomy*: The external-bevel gingivectomy is suitable procedure when more than adequate attached gingiva is available without any bone involvement. It is one of the method useful in removing excessive pocket depth and/or of exposing additional coronal tooth structure.
- *Apically positioned flap surgery*: A different surgical procedure is needed when there is lack of a sufficient zone of attached gingiva with or without the need for correction of osseous abnormalities which demands reduction of excessive pocket depth and exposure of additional coronal tooth structure. The external-bevel gingivectomy is one of the methods that help to remove all or most of the attached gingiva without leaving anything back except alveolar mucosa. Cases demanding the correction of osseous pathology need internal beveling of the flap in order to expose the supporting alveolar bone.

Both gingivectomy and apically positioned flap surgery without osseous reduction comes with restrictive uses, especially cases requiring compulsory bone removal to provide adequate distance from the osseous crest to the anticipated restoration margin, allowing for biologic width.
- *Apically positioned flap surgery with osseous reduction*: This is the commonly used technique for crown-lengthening surgery. It consists of following steps:
    - *Incisions*: Initial incision is usually reverse or internal bevel incision. It may be intrasulcular in cases of narrow, or scalloped gingival width. Vertical releasing incisions are helpful as it permits better access and apical positioning of the flap. For maintaining proper contour of the gingiva and underlying bone, a neighboring tooth on each side of the tooth needs to be lengthened during the surgical procedure.
    - *Flap reflection*: Full-thickness flap raised with mucoperiosteal elevator.
    - *Osseous recontouring*: Initial osseous recontouring is done with carbide, diamond round burs, and end-cutting burs circumferentially around the tooth. It is completed with the help of chisels and curettes in order to achieve the desired reduction with proper maintenance of a scalloped, parabolic bony contour which may follow the desired contour of the overlying gingiva.
    - Apically positioned flap with ostectomy removes the tooth-supporting bone to lengthen the clinical crown. There should be at least 3 mm distance be-

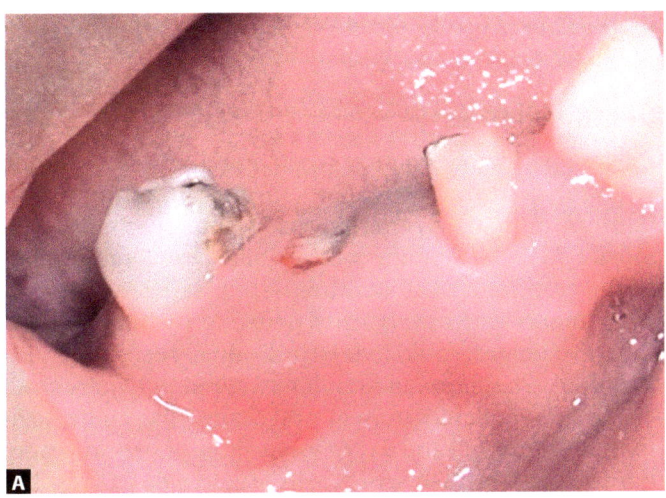
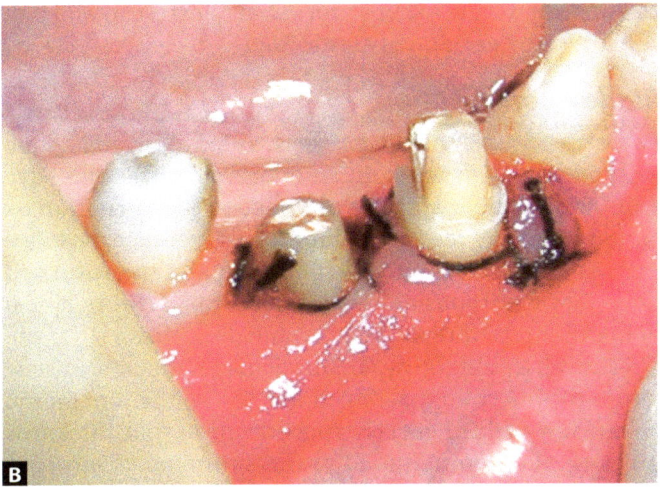

**Figs. 60.2A and B:** Clinical picture showing crown-lengthening procedure.

tween the apical extension of restoration and crest of the alveolar bone[5] **(Figs. 60.2A and B)**. This space permits sufficient room for the supracrestal collagen fibers which form part of the periodontal support mechanism, and provide a gingival crevice of 2–3 mm. The margin of the crown is finally positioned at its correct level, approximately halfway down the gingival crevice. Inability in keeping sufficient space between the crown margin and the alveolar crest height suggests the positioning of finished restoration in the periodontal tissues which can lead to increase in inflammation and pocket formation **(Fig. 60.3)**.

- *Provisional restoration:* The provisional restoration is cemented on to the tooth.
- *Suturing:* The buccal and palatal/lingual flaps are placed at the alveolar bone crest and sutured. A vertical mattress suture is used to close the flaps if crown-lengthening involved a single tooth. If crown-lengthening involved multiple teeth, a continuous sling suture may be used instead. A periodontal dressing is often used to protect the surgical site and to assist in positioning the flap apically.
- *Forced tooth eruption:* Orthodontic tooth movement is suitable for eruption of teeth in adults. With use of moderate eruptive forces, the entire attachment apparatus can move in unison with the tooth. The tooth must be extruded a distance equal to or slightly longer than the portion of sound tooth structure that will be exposed in the subsequent surgical treatment. Once the tooth reaches at the intended position and sufficiently stabilized, a full-thickness flap bone recontouring is conducted to expose sound root structure. The bone and soft-tissue levels at adjacent teeth should remain unchanged for esthetic reasons.[6]

## Correction of Deformed Ridges

*Knife-edged ridge:* Alveolar bone resorption after extractions frequently produces a thin, knife-edged edentulous

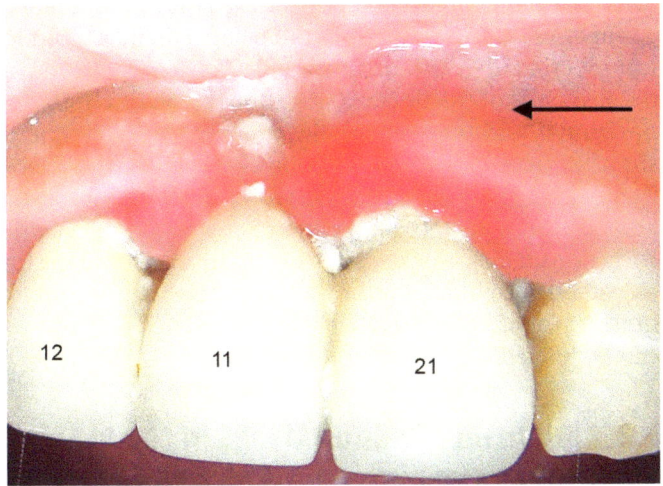

**Fig. 60.3:** Clinical picture showing violation of biologic width: Inflammatory changes on gingiva of crown 11, 21.

ridge with inadequate attached gingiva, especially in the mandibular arch. If there is inadequate attached gingiva on which to place a denture, a tissue substitution procedure can be used to remove the alveolar mucosa on the buccal (or lingual) side of the ridge and substitute in its place an equal zone of masticatory mucosa by employing a free graft from the palate.

*Elimination of ridge undercuts:* To gain a path of insertion for the buccal flange of a prosthesis, a surgical flap and osseous resection procedures have been used to eliminate the bony projection that produce the undercut areas.

*Vestibular extension procedures:* A shallow buccal or lingual vestibule frequently limits the placement of an adequate flange of a removable prosthesis. The masticatory mucosa of the palate functions as a special mucosa to withstand the forces of mastication. It can be used in vestibular extension surgery. The major problem in using the palate as donor site, is the limitation in the amount of donor tissue that can be obtained during a single procedure.[7] Rest is explained in "Chapter 53: Periodontal Plastic Surgery".

### Ridge Augmentation

These procedures correct the excessive loss of alveolar bone that sometimes occurs in the anterior region. This excessive bone loss complicates the prosthetic reconstruction as large space may result in either a long pontic or a space between the apical end of the pontic and the resorbed ridge. These osseous defects may occur in a coronoapical or buccolingual directions or in both directions.

The roll technique by Abrams manages moderate tissue loss in the buccolingual direction.[8] The epithelium on the palatal side of the defect is removed. After a split-thickness incision, the flap denuded of the epithelial covering is rolled beneath the buccal-split flap. The rolled portion of the palatal-split flap augments the ridge in a buccal direction. If the ridge defect is more extensive subepithelial connective donor tissue from the palate can be placed in tunnel created at the recipient site. Vertical incisions at the two ends of the defect and a tunnel made in both the horizontal and the vertical directions create a recipient site that provides excellent blood supply to the donor tissue. This tissue is positioned with gut sutures from the palatal side. The vertical augmentation achieved by this surgery provides an excellent soft-tissue environment for an esthetic-fixed restoration. In larger defects, bone grafts in the form of a monocortical block using fixation screws can be placed.

## PERIODONTAL CONSIDERATIONS IN COMPLETE DENTURES AND RPD

### Impression Materials

In general, completely set hydrocolloid (both reversible and irreversible), polysulfide and silicone impression materials have not been shown to cause any detrimental tissue reactions. The main concern with reversible hydrocolloid is the possibility of burning soft tissue if the material has not been conditioned at the proper temperature. The catalyst of the silicone materials has been known to be chemically irritating. Care should be exerted not to inadvertently leave any impression material, especially the rubber base type, in the gingival crevice. Such residual impression material may lead to a foreign body reaction with severe periodontal implications.[9]

### Design of the Prosthesis

The components of removable partial denture must be designed and fabricated in such a way that the gingiva is not impinged by the prosthesis. Major connector in maxillary and mandibular are kept at 6 mm and 3 mm respectively from the gingival margin. Removable partial dentures covering gingival tissue favor the accumulation of plaque.

### Denture Plastics

Polymethylmethacrylate is the material most commonly used for denture bases. The chronic inflammation, or denture stomatitis, experienced by some patients in the mucosa beneath dentures was attributed to allergic reaction to the components of denture base plastic. Some of the constituents (polymer, benzoyl peroxide, hydroquinone, or the dye pigment) could indeed individually cause chemical irritation. Therefore, incompletely cured polymers could cause some inflammation to oral tissue.[9] Partial dentures that are worn night and day promote more plaque formation compared to those worn only during day time. The removable partial dentures promote quantitative changes in dental plaque and enhance qualitative changes favoring the development of spirilla and spirochetes.

### Partial Denture Framework Alloys

Some patients have been observed to develop mucosal contact stomatitis, general dermatitis or combinations of the two. Reactions have varied from severe to minor. The predominant culprits in these alloys have been nickel, although cobalt and chromium have also been responsible on occasions.[9]

## PERIODONTAL CONSIDERATIONS IN FPD

The ideal goal for prosthodontic work should be to make conditions adjacent to fixed single crowns and bridges as favorable as around natural teeth and not to initiate pathologic processes that may endanger the longevity of abutment teeth.

Certain factors to be considered are:
- Tooth preparation in relation to the gingival margin
- Gingival management for making impressions
- Restoration contours
- Occlusal surface
- Pontic design
- Cementation
- Impression materials

### Tooth Preparation in Relation to the Gingival Margin

Overhanging margins act as ideal locations for plaque accumulation and bring change in the ecologic balance of the gingival sulcus area to one that favors the growth of disease-associated organisms. Thus, such margins contribute significantly to development of periodontal disease. The location of the gingival margin of restoration is directly related to the periodontal health status. Subgingivally located margins contribute to the formation of large amounts of plaque; development of more severe gingivitis and formation of deeper pockets. During subgingival tooth preparation, avoid injury to the gingival tissues, especially where gingiva is thin and delicate. In case of minimal attached gingiva, injuries usually result in recession.[10] Among all the supporting structures, the epithelial attachment is the most susceptible to injury and procedural trauma may lead to its apical migration with development of periodontitis or recession. In crown preparation, basic general principles should be followed:

- Sufficient tooth structure should be removed so that there is a definite cervical area to accommodate a restoration that will reconstruct the anatomy of the tooth in harmony with dental and periodontal environment.
- Subgingival finish lines should be terminated at least 0.5 mm short of epithelial attachment.
- Rotary instruments can severely injure or obliterate the gingiva. This usually results in formation of esthetically poor soft-tissue contours and produces problems in maintaining periodontal health.
- Establishment of the type of subgingival finish line is usually associated with the gingival trauma. Hence, establishment of a shoulder finish line subgingivally can be done by keeping the entire rotary instrument diameter within the peripheral tooth contours.
- The formation of chamfers and beveled shoulders requires that part of rotary instrument diameter be located outside peripheral tooth contours, with greater potential for gingival trauma.[11]

## Gingival Management for Making Impressions

For subgingival preparation margin extending to the appropriate depth in the sulcus, gingival tissue must be protected from abrasion. Gingival retraction cord of appropriate size is useful for the required tissue displacement. During retraction process, electrosurgery is helpful for the removal of any overlying tissue. A fine wire-tip electrode is held parallel to the tooth and against the margin in the sulcus and moved through the overhanging tissue, opening-up the margin and the retraction cord to visual access.[1]

## Restoration Contours

Overcontoured crowns and restorations tend to accumulate plaque and prevent self-cleansing mechanisms of adjacent cheek, lips and tongue. Inadequate or improperly located proximal contacts and failure to reproduce the normal protective anatomy of the occlusal marginal ridges and developmental grooves lead to food impaction. The facial and lingual contours of restorations are also important in the preservation of gingival health. In patients in whom periodontal disease causes the gingival margin to be in a much more apical position than it was during health, the facial and lingual contours become even more significant.

In this particular case, the bulge on the facial contour of the crown, which normally would be subgingival, appears supragingivally. In Class III and IV furcation defect, it is important that the restoration be contoured in such a way as to facilitate access for oral hygiene. In these cases, it is important to emphasize the midfacial groove of the crown so that this groove is confluent with the furcation.[1]

## Occlusal Surface

Occlusal surfaces should be designed to direct masticatory forces along the long axis of the teeth. The anatomy of the occlusal surface should provide well-formed marginal ridges and occlusal sluiceways to prevent interproximal food impaction. Restorations that fail to conform to the occlusal patterns of the mouth result in occlusal disharmonies, which are responsible for injury to the supporting periodontal tissues.[1,12]

## Pontic Design

From a periodontal point of view, pontics in fixed bridges represents a hygienic problem. Therefore, in designing pontic the following requirements should be met:

- All surfaces should be smooth, polished and convex. Soldered points must be polished.
- Pontics should be constructed to permit adequate oral hygiene measures. Principally there should be no contact between the undersurface and the soft tissue, the embrasure should be wide, and the shape of the pontic should be convex in buccolingual as well as mesiodistal direction. There are four pontic designs: (1) sanitary, (2) ridge-lap, (3) modified ridge-lap and (4) ovate pontic designs. The key differences between the four pontic designs relate to the esthetics and access for hygiene procedures. The shape of the undersurface of pontic determines the ease with which plaque and food debris can be removed. The sanitary and ovate pontics have convex undersurfaces that are easy for cleaning. Ridge-lap and modified ridge-lap designs have concave surfaces and hence more difficult to access with dental floss. The ovate pontic serves important periodontal function by maintaining the interdental papilla next to abutment teeth after extraction.[13] Becker et al., reported that the modified ridge-lap in the posterior region and ridge-lap facing design in the anterior region give minimal tissue contact, acceptable cosmetic value, proper check support and accessibility for adequate oral hygiene.[14] This design will allow for a mechanical cleansing of the undersurface and interproximal surfaces of the pontic with an interdental brush.
- Embrasure spaces should be large enough to provide some self-cleansing and allow woodstick to clean through.
- The occlusal table should be of the same width as that of the abutment teeth, and food shedding surfaces of the pontic in harmony with those of the abutments.

## Cementation

During cementation, restoration must be seated as close to the tooth preparation as possible. After cementation, all excess cement should be removed from the sulcus because retained cement particles can lead to gingival inflammation.[1]

## Impression Materials

Inflammatory gingival responses related to the use of alloys containing nickel in dental restorations have been reported. Use of glass ceramics and porcelain veneers have better advantages over other types of restorative material, especially in the maintenance of gingival health. Their fine marginal fit lead to formation of a thin cement line that reduces gingival irritation. It is found that tissues respond more to the differences in surface roughness of the material compared to the composition of the material. Furthermore, nonporous surface of porcelain significantly avoids adherence of bacteria to it.

## PERIODONTAL MAINTENANCE IN THE PROSTHETIC PATIENT

Patient should be instructed to evaluate the effectiveness of his home care periodically. Plaque-disclosing agents are commonly used for this purpose. However, staining of the oral mucosa, restoration margins, fingernails or the wash basins are often undesirable side effects of this procedure and are motivational deterrents. The patient should be given written instructions for the care, cleansing and maintenance of the prosthesis.

## Fixed Partial Prosthesis

- *Toothbrushing*: Microbial debridement of the apical third or neck of the crown has been emphasized in the natural or intracoronally restored dentition because that area represents the major site of microbial activity that is detrimental to the tooth and its periodontium. Charters toothbrushing technique is helpful in cleaning the gingival surface of the pontic from the facial aspect. The filaments can be directed under the pontic to clean the gingival surface. For removal of plaque from proximal crown margins, the use of an interdental cleanser is necessary to reach the middle third of mesial and distal tooth surface. The specific aids indicated or proximal tooth cleaning depend on the size of the gingival embrasures between crowns and on the manual dexterity of the patient. Dental floss is used to remove plaque and loose debris between the abutment and pontic. With dentifrice, dental floss is used with moderate pressure on the undersurface/gingival surface of pontic to remove bacterial plaque. Floss threaders are used to position yarn or gauze bandage strip around an abutment and under fixed prosthesis. Super floss is used for cleaning the under surface of fixed prosthesis **(Fig. 60.4)**. Knitting yarn may also be used for the same. Interdental brushes, single-end tuft brushes, are also used for cleaning interproximal areas. For cleaning crown margins adjacent to extremely large embrasures or sanitary pontics, unitufted brushes are preferred over bottle-brush cleansers.[15]
- A nonabrasive dentifrice is indicated to prevent the possibility of abrasion when pontic or crown facings are made of acrylic. Fluoride containing dentifrice is important for the protection of remaining tooth surfaces, particularly exposed cementum. Acidulated fluoride preparations are contraindicated for porcelain and composite restorations.
- *Oral irrigators*: In dentition with excessive fixed restorations that often provide less than ideal interproximal access for oral hygiene aids, daily oral irrigation with a pulsating stream of water is useful for removing food lodged between crowns and underneath pontics. However, water irrigators are not capable of removing any appreciable amounts of stainable plaque from tooth surfaces and, therefore, should not be recommended for prevention of caries, gingivitis, or periodontitis.[15]

## Removable Partial Prosthesis and Complete Dentures

- Separate denture brush should be used for cleaning removable prosthesis **(Fig. 60.5)**. These are especially designed brush having one group of tufts in a large round arrangement that permits access to the thinner, curved impression surface of the denture. The second group of tufts is arranged to form a rectangular brush for convenient adaptation to the polished and occlusal denture surfaces. These brushes have round end filaments. Edentulous gingiva under removable denture is cleaned by soft manual/power-assisted toothbrush and digital massage.[16]
- Power-assisted brush can also be used but not in between the intricate clasps of removable prosthesis.
- Short brushing strokes further minimize the risk of catching a clasp with the brush. All debris and dentifrice residues on the prosthesis must be brushed-off thoroughly under running water before placing the appliance. This prevents irritation of the oral mucosa. A commercial denture cleaning solution can be used to supplement, but not substitute for mechanical debridement. Cetyl dimethiocone copolymer inhibits the formation of plaque and stain on the surface of acrylic dentures.

# Chapter 60: Periodontics-Prosthodontics

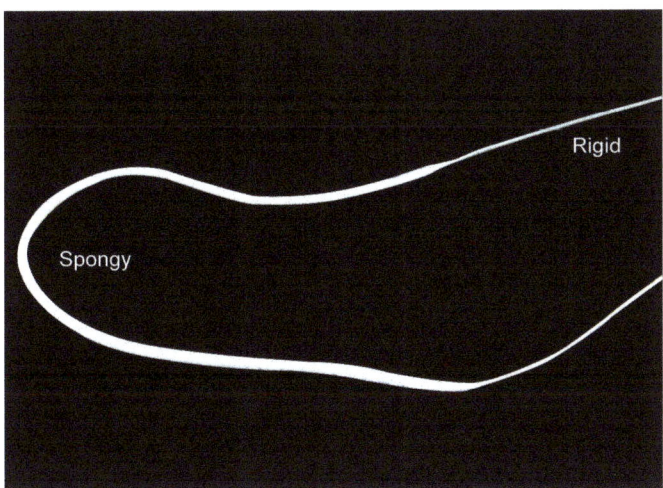

**Fig. 60.4:** Photograph showing super floss.

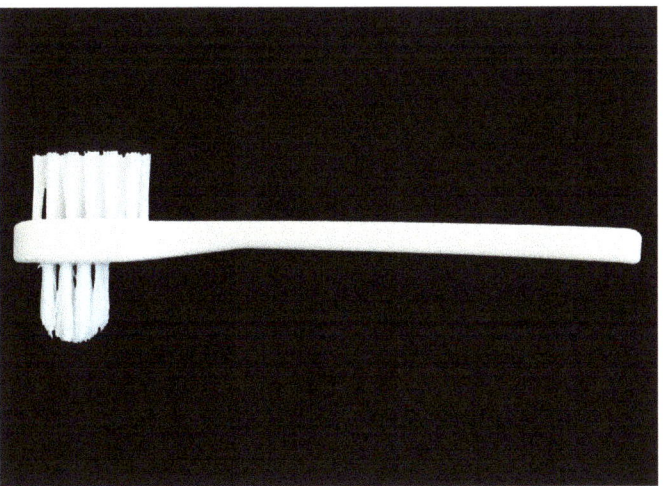

**Fig. 60.5:** Photograph showing denture brush.

- Especially designed narrow, tapered cylindrical brush about 2 inches long that can be adapted to the inner surface of clasps are recommended. Grasp of a partial prosthesis should not be too tight, otherwise it may bend or fracture the clasp or bar. Partial filling of the sink with water or lining of the sink with a face towel is necessary to prevent accidents that cause breakage of prosthesis.

## Recall Schedule

The individual schedule for each patient is determined on the basis of relevant information gathered during the active treatment phase, such as complexity of prosthetic reconstructions, caries activity, formation rate of plaque and calculus, level of manual skills and motivation, and periodontal and general state of health.[17]

### Points to Ponder

- Crown-lengthening surgery is the surgical procedure which exposes adequate clinical crown to prevent the placement of the crown margin into the area of the biologic width.
- Biologic width is defined as the dimension of healthy gingival tissue, which is attached to the tooth coronal to the crest of the alveolar bone.

## REFERENCES

1. McGuire MK. Periodontal-restorative interrelationship. In: Newman MG, Takei HH, Carranza FA (Eds). Carranza's Clinical Periodontology, 8th edition. Philadelphia, PA, USA: WB Saunders; 1996. pp. 723-42.
2. Takei HH, Azzi RR, Han TJ. Preparation of the periodontium for restorative dentistry. In: Newman MG, Takei HH, Carranza FA (Eds). Carranza's Clinical Periodontology, 9th edition. Philadelphia, PA, USA: WB Saunders; 2003. pp. 943-8.
3. Gargiulo A, Wentz F, Orban B. Dimensions and relations of the dentogingival junction in humans. J Periodontol. 1961;32:261-7.
4. Becker W, Ochsenbein C, Becker BE. Crown lengthening: the periodontal-restorative connection. Compend Contin Educ Dent. 1998;19(3):239-40.
5. Brägger U, Lauchenauer D, Lang NP. Surgical lengthening of the clinical crown. J Clin Periodontol. 1992;19(1):58-63.
6. Ingber JS, Rose LF, Coslet JG. The "biologic width"--a concept in periodontics and restorative dentistry. Alpha Omegan. 1977;70(3):62-5.
7. Seibert JS. Surgical preparation for fixed and removable prostheses. In: Genco RJ, Goldman HM, Cohen DW (Eds). Contemporary Periodontics, 1st edition. St. Louis, United States: CV Mosby; 1990. pp. 637-52.
8. Abrams L. Augmentation of the deformed residual edentulous ridge for fixed prostheses. Compend Contin Educ Gen Dent. 1980;1(3):205-13.
9. Caputo AA. Biological implications of dental materials. Dent Clin North Am. 1980;24:331-42.
10. Padbury A, Eber R, Wang HL. Interactions between the gingival and the margin of restorations. J Clin Periodontol. 2003;30(5):379-85.
11. Hall WB. Periodontal preparation of the mouth for restoration. Dent Clin North Am. 1980;24:195-214.
12. Spear FM, Cooney JP. Periodontal restorative interrelationship. In: Newman MG, Takei HH, Carranza FA (Eds). Carranza's Clinical Periodontology, 9th edition. Philadelphia, PA, USA: WB Saunders; 2003. pp. 949-65.
13. Spear FM. Maintenance of the interdental papilla following anterior tooth removal. Pract Periodontics Aesthet Dent. 1999;11(1):21-8.
14. Becker CM, Kaldahl WB. Current theories of crown contour, margin placement, and pontic design. J Prosthet Dent. 2005;93:107-15.
15. Schmid MO. The maintenance phase of dental therapy. Dent Clin North Am. 1980;24:379-93.
16. Wilkins EM. Care of dental prostheses. In: Clinical Practice of the Dental Hygienist, 8th edition. Philadelphia, PA, USA: Lippincott Williams & Wilkins; 1999. pp. 394-410.
17. Thayer HH, Kratochvil FJ. Periodontal considerations with removable partial dentures. Dent Clin North Am. 1980;24:357-68.

## VIVA VOCE

**Q1. What is the dimension of biologic width?**
**Ans.** Connective tissue attachment of 1.07 mm and 0.97 mm of junctional epithelium makes total biologic width of 2.04 mm.

**Q2. What should be the distance between the apical extension of restoration and crest of the alveolar bone?**
**Ans.** At least 3 mm.

**Q3. What are the Thumb rules for placing intracrevicular margins?**
**Ans.**
- If the gingival sulcus is 1.5 mm or less, place the restoration margin 0.5 mm below the gingival tissue crest.
- If the gingival sulcus is between 1.5- 2 mm, place the margin one half the depth of the sulcus below the gingival tissue crest.
- If the gingival sulcus is greater than 2 mm, do crown lengthening procedure (gingivectomy) to create a 1.5-mm sulcus. Then place the restoration margin 0.5 mm below the gingival tissue crest.

**Q4. Name various preprosthetic periodontal surgeries.**
**Ans.** Crown-lengthening surgery; correction of deformed ridges and ridge augmentation.

**Q5. Name various methods for crown lengthening.**
**Ans.** Gingivectomy; apically positioned flap surgery; apically positioned flap surgery with osseous reduction and forced tooth eruption.

**Q6. What are the various pontic designs?**
**Ans.** Sanitary, ridge-lap, modified ridge-lap and ovate pontic designs.

**Q7. Which toothbrushing technique is helpful in cleaning the gingival surface of the pontic from the facial aspect?**
**Ans.** Charters toothbrushing technique.

**Q8. Which interdental aid is used for cleaning the under surface of fixed prosthesis?**
**Ans.** Super floss.

**Q9. What are the indications for crown-lengthening surgery?**
**Ans.** Subgingival caries or fracture; inadequate clinical crown length for retention; unequal or unesthetic gingival height.

**Q10. Which brush is used for cleaning removable prosthesis?**
**Ans.** Special denture brush.

# Chapter 61: Periodontics-Endodontics

*Vineeta N Srivastava, Shalu Bathla*

## Chapter Outline

- Pathways of Communication
- Etiopathogenesis
- Classifications
- Diagnosis
- Treatment and Prognosis

## INTRODUCTION

The term "endo-perio" is an integral part in the dental vocabulary, since 1964, when Simring and Goldberg described the relationship between the periodontal and the endodontic diseases for the first time.[1] Pulp and the periodontium has been derived from a common mesodermal source of the developing tooth bud. Thus, the relationship between the pulpal and the periodontal disease starts to exist right from the embryological development. Ectomesenchymal cells proliferate to form the dental follicle and papilla, acting as precursors of the periodontium and the pulp respectively. These embryonic developments are responsible for the origin of anatomical connections, some of which remains patent throughout their life.

## PATHWAYS OF COMMUNICATION

A very strong relationship is known to exist between the periodontal and the pulpal tissues. Many studies strongly favor the disease transmission between these two by exhibiting significant microbiological similarities between the advanced periodontitis and infected root canals. Microbial findings along with the similarities in the composition of cellular infiltrates favor the presence of communication between the periodontal tissues and the pulp.

The pathways that favor the entry of bacteria and their toxic byproducts into the tissues are usually divided into two categories as anatomical and nonphysiological pathways.[2]

### Anatomical Pathways

These include vascular pathways, such as the apical foramen, accessory canals and tubular pathways (Fig. 61.1).

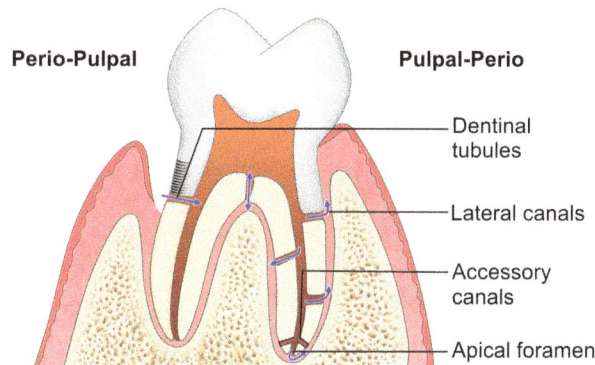

**Fig. 61.1:** Schematic representation showing pathways between pulp and periodontium.

### Apical Foramen

The apical foramen is the main and direct communication route between the pulp and periodontium. Periodontal disease usually exhibits a cumulative damaging effect on the pulp tissue. However, total disintegration of the pulp takes place only when bacterial plaque affects the main apical foramen, including the vascular supply. Irritants arising from a diseased pulp can easily pass through the apical foramen and result in periapical pathosis. This leads to periodontal tissue destruction and resorption of the root and neighboring alveolar bone.

### Accessory Canals

Apart from the apical foramen "accessory canals" are also the route of communication between pulpal and periodontal tissues. These are basically the ramifications of a multitude of branches connecting the main root canal system with the periodontal ligament. With the development of root, ectomesenchymal channels get incorporated, either during the dentin formation which exists around the blood vessels or when there is break in the continuation of the Hertwig's epithelial root sheath, to form lateral or accessory canals. The root's apical part and the molar furcation areas[3] constitute majority of the accessory canals. Bender et al. reported that the presence of more number of accessory canals in the molars leads to frequent periodontal-endodontic problems in the molars compared to the anterior teeth. The percentage of lateral canals in the furcation area is 50–60% in any multirooted teeth, but in 1st molars it is approximately 46%. Gutmann (1978) found 25.5% accessory canals in the furcation areas.[4] Accessory canals, which are patent, cause spread of microorganisms, their toxic byproducts and other irritants, from the pulp to the periodontal ligament and vice versa. This leads to development of inflammatory process in the periodontal and pulpal tissues.

### Tubular Pathways

Presence of the patent dentinal tubules, especially when the cementum layer is denuded, favors the spread of microorganisms between the pulp and periodontal tissues. It is usually associated with various developmental defects, including incomplete union of cementum and enamel at cementoenamel junction (CEJ), disease processes or surgical procedures which involve root surfaces, like scaling and root planing. In areas of denuded cementum, these exposed dentinal tubules act as communicating pathways between pulp and periodontal ligament.

### Nonphysiological Pathways

The nonphysiological pathways are the iatrogenic root canal perforations, traumatic vertical root fractures, and pathways created due to resorption. The restored teeth with intracanal posts and the root canals filled with lateral condensation technique are more prone for root fractures.

## ETIOPATHOGENESIS

## Effect of Periodontal Lesions on the Pulp

### Microbial Agents

In addition to other etiological factors, microbial agents act as the main culprit during the evolution of the perio-endo lesions. After the development of periodontal disease, the bacterial plaque formation upon the denuded root surfaces leads to the induction of pathologic changes in the pulp through accessory or lateral canals. Periodontal lesions have the potential to induce atrophic and degenerative changes on the pulp, which includes dystrophic mineralization, reduced number of pulp cells, reparative dentin formation, fibrosis, inflammation and ultimately resorption.

### Atrophic Changes

Pulpal tissue, which has been periodontally affected exhibits, cells of smaller size and more collagen depositions compared to normal cells. Impairment in nutrition results in gradual degeneration of the pulp cells. The cell death takes place so slowly which can many times diminish the morphologic evidence. Disrupted flow of blood through the lateral canals leading to localized areas of coagulation necrosis in the pulp is the significant cause of these atrophic changes. These areas with poor blood supply eventually get separated from the rest of the healthy pulp tissue by collagen and dystrophic mineralization. With advancement in the periodontal disease, deposition of cementum can lead to obliteration of lateral canals before occurrence of pulpal irritation. Hence, pulpal atrophy and canal narrowing is not found in all periodontally involved teeth. The mobility of these periodontally involved teeth may also lead to pressure atrophy.

### Inflammatory Changes

The causative agents of periodontal diseases are usually present in the gingival sulcus which are persistently challenged by host-defense mechanism. This microbiologic challenge leads to elicitation of an immunologic or inflammatory response, which leads to the formation of granulomatous tissue in the periodontium. With the extension of periodontal disease from the gingival sulcus towards the apex, microorganisms and inflammatory products usually infect the periodontal ligament tissues and the adjacent alveolar bone.

Evidences are lacking in explaining strong correlation between pulpal involvement and progressive periodontal disease. The localized apical granuloma is considered as the most common periodontal lesion produced by the pulp disease. It is developed due to diffusion of bacterial toxic byproducts through the root apex leading to vascular granulation tissue formation. This may result in resorption of the alveolar bone and sometimes of the root itself.

### Resorption

Resorption of root's side is commonly noted adjacent to the granulation tissue overlying the roots. With the development of the deep periodontal lesions, resorption may also occur within the root canals, at the apical foramen and often opposite lateral canals. This resorptive process usually extends into the dentin peripherally towards the pulp, and the activating factors are produced from the periodontal lesion. Hence, this phenomenon is termed as peripheral inflammatory root resorption (PIRR) reflecting its etiology.[5]

## Effect of Periodontal Therapy on the Pulp

### Nonsurgical Periodontal Therapy

*Scaling and root planing*: It involves removal of the bacterial plaque and calculus. Improperly conducted root planing procedure sometimes removes cementum and dentin superficially leading to exposure of dentinal tubules to the oral environment. This favors the microbial colonization of the dentin and subsequently invasion of bacteria into the dentinal tubules leading to the development of inflammatory lesions in the pulp. Initially, patient complaints of sharp pain which is of rapid onset that disappears at the removal of stimulus.[6]

### Surgical Periodontal Therapy

*Acid etching*: During periodontal regenerative therapy, citric acid is commonly used for root conditioning which helps to get rid of anaerobic bacteria and bacterial endotoxins. Root conditioning exposes the collagen bundles, which serve as a matrix for the new connective tissue attachment to the cementum. However, during root conditioning procedure with citric acid there is removal of smear layer, which is an important pulp protector. Application of citric acid may have a detrimental effect on the dental pulp.

## Effect of Endodontic Lesions on the Periodontium

Intrapulpal infection usually promotes downgrowth of the epithelium along a denuded dentinal surface. It has been seen that in experimentally induced periodontal defects around the infected teeth there were 20% more downgrowth of the epithelium compared to the noninfected teeth. Infected teeth exhibited 10% lesser connective tissue coverage than the noninfected ones. Hence, it is recommended that the pulpal tissue infections should be managed prior to proceeding for the periodontal regenerative procedures.

## Effect of Endodontic Therapy on the Periodontium

### Intracoronal Bleaching

Intracoronal bleaching done with 30–35% hydrogen peroxide ($H_2O_2$) has high potential to cause root resorption. Chemical diffuses through dentinal tubules and causes inflammation and necrosis of cementum and periodontal tissues.

### Root Perforation

Iatrogenic root perforation is produced during root canal treatment by rotary instruments or during post-preparation. At perforation site, inflammatory reaction occurs in periodontal tissues leading to formation of endo-perio lesions.

## CLASSIFICATIONS

Periodontal-endodontic lesions have been classified into accordingly:
- Classification according to Weine (1982), based on etiology of the disease **(Flowchart 61.1)**.[7]
- Classification according to Simon, Glick and Frank (1972), which is the most accepted classification, has been explained in **Flowchart 61.2**.[8]
- Classification according to Torabinejad and Trope (1996), based on the periodontal pocket origin **(Flowchart 61.3)**.[9]
- Classification according to World Workshop for Classification of Periodontal Diseases (1999) **(Flowchart 61.4)**.[10]

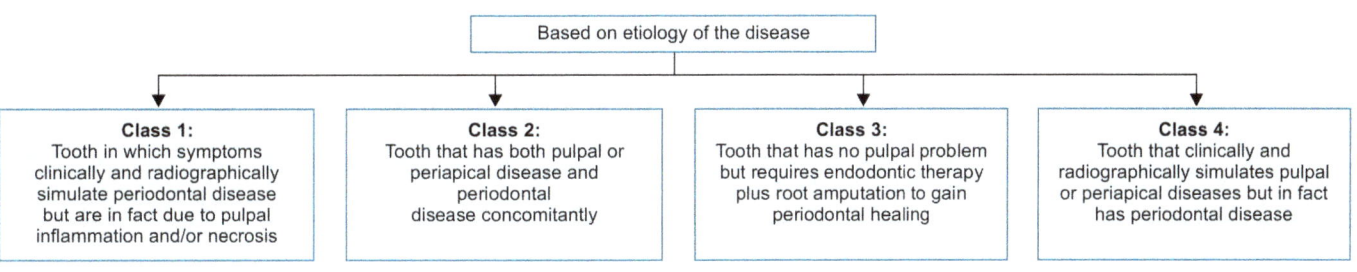

**Flowchart 61.1:** Weine's classification based on etiology of the disease.

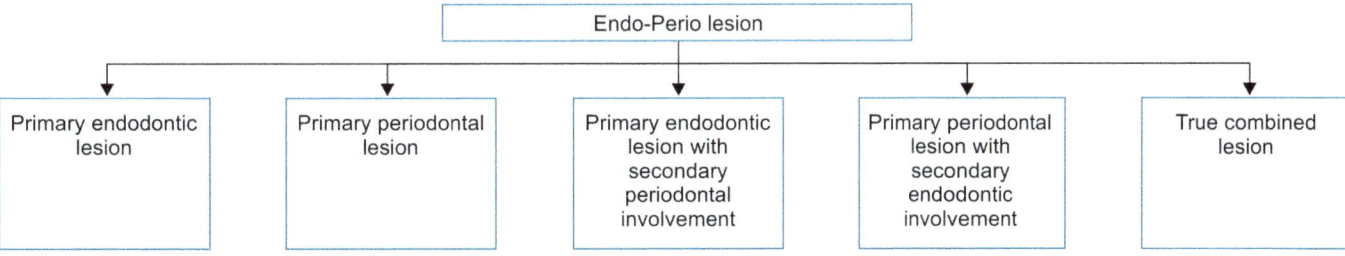

**Flowchart 61.2:** Simon's classification.

## Section 9: Interdisciplinary Approach

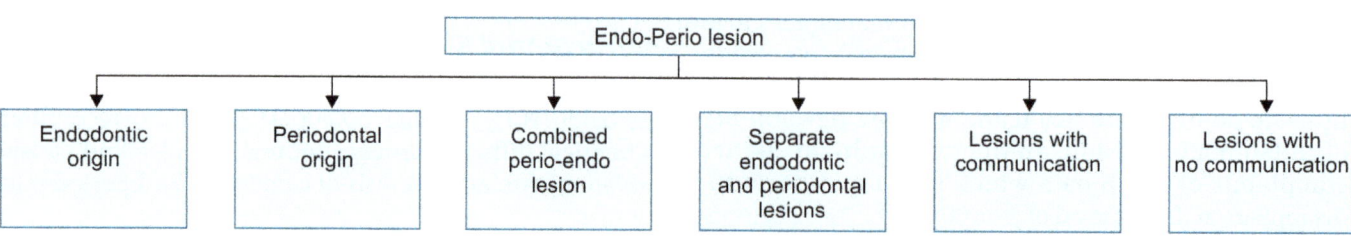

Flowchart 61.3: Torabinejad's classification.

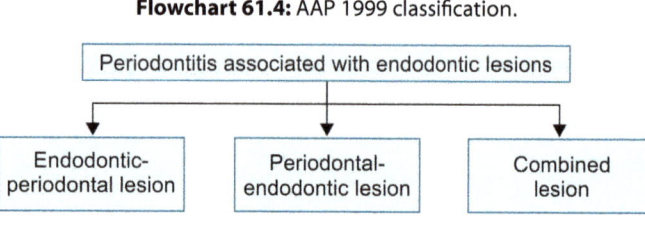

Flowchart 61.4: AAP 1999 classification.

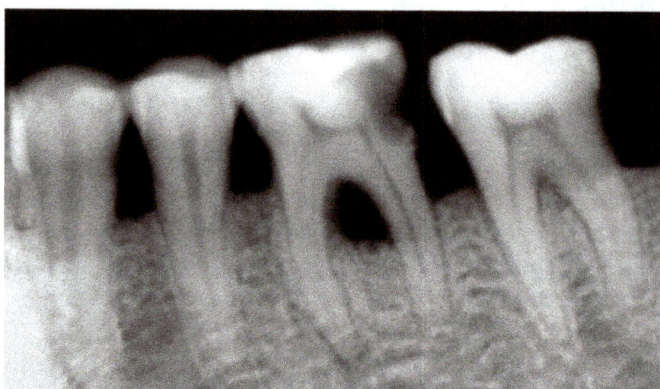

Fig. 61.3: Radiograph showing primary endodontic lesion.

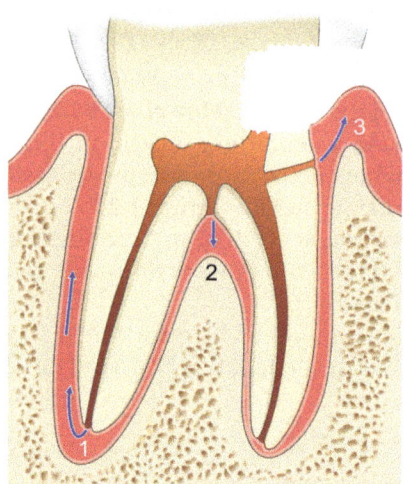

**Fig. 61.2:** Schematic representation showing primary endodontic lesion. Endodontic origin-pulpal infection spreads through: (1) Apical foramen to periodontal ligament; (2) Accessory canals to furcation; and (3) Accessory canals to gingiva.

### Primary Endodontic Lesion

An acute exacerbation of a chronic apical lesion on a tooth in the presence of necrotic pulp usually drains coronally into the gingival sulcus through the periodontal ligament **(Figs. 61.2 and 61.3)**. Root canal therapy proved to be effective in healing primary endodontic lesions. When managed at an early stage, the sinus tract extending into the gingival sulcus or furcation area disappears. With adequate removal of the necrotic pulp, the root canals are well-sealed.[11]

### Primary Periodontal Lesion

These lesions are associated with frequent accumulation of local factors, such as plaque and calculus, and also the presence of deep periodontal pockets. Periodontal pathogens are mainly responsible for the development of such lesions **(Fig. 61.4)**. During this process, chronic

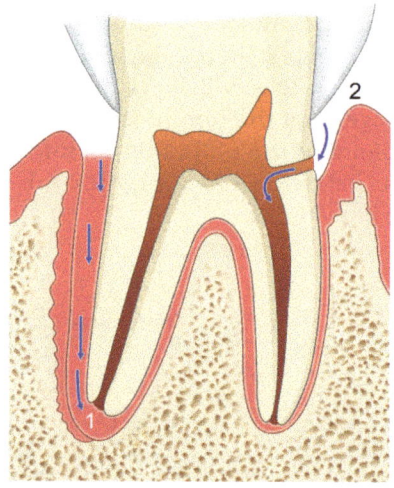

**Fig. 61.4:** Schematic representation showing primary periodontal lesion. Perio-origin-periodontal infection spread through: (1) Apical foramen; (2) Lateral canal to pulp.

periodontitis progression takes place along the root surface, apically. Mostly in such lesions, clinical pulp tests suggest normal pulp reaction.[11]

### Combined Diseases

*Primary endodontic lesion with secondary periodontal involvement*: Untreated primary endodontic lesion usually gets affected secondarily with periodontal breakdown. Long-standing periapical lesion draining through the periodontal ligament can become secondarily complicated leading to retrograde periodontitis **(Fig. 61.5)**.[1,11]

## Chapter 61: Periodontics-Endodontics

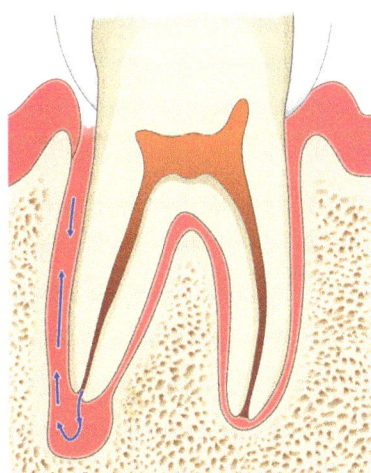

**Fig. 61.5:** Schematic representation showing retrograde periodontitis.

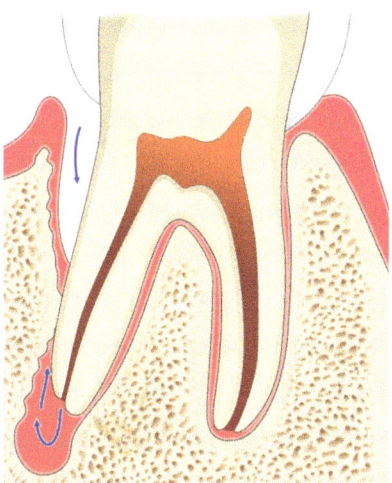

**Fig. 61.6:** Schematic representation showing true combined lesion. Independent endo and perio lesions coexist and eventually fuse with each other.

Accumulation of plaque at the gingival margin of the sinus tract results in the development of plaque-induced periodontitis at that site. Presence of plaque and calculus demands different mode of the treatment of the involved teeth compared to those teeth involved with only endodontic disease. This also affects disease prognosis. Such lesions demand both endodontic therapy and periodontal therapy. Primary endodontic lesion with secondary periodontal involvement can develop during restoration of the crown where pins and posts are misplaced or during the root canal treatment where there is root perforation. Symptoms are acute in origin and can be associated with periodontal abscess formation leading to swelling, pain, pus, periodontal pocket formation and tooth mobility. Chronic response is usually devoid of pain, and presents with sudden appearance of a pocket with exudation of pus or bleeding on probing. Presence of root fractures suggests the primary endodontic lesions with secondary periodontal involvement.

*Primary periodontal disease with secondary endodontic involvement:* Bacterial and inflammatory products of periodontitis can access the pulp via apical foramen, lateral canals, accessory canals, dentinal tubules and this reverse effect is called as retrograde pulpitis. The apical progression of a periodontal pocket may continue until the involvement of apical tissues. Due to entry of infection through the apical foramen or lateral canals, the pulp usually becomes necrotic. Root resection of the involved root can be done in such cases, as all roots usually do not suffer from similar loss of supporting tissue. Single-rooted teeth usually exhibited poor prognosis. Molar teeth are associated with the better prognosis.

With the presence of intact blood supply circulating through the apex, the pulp shows good survival prospects. When the apical foramen is involved, pulpal changes due to periodontal disease occur more commonly. In such cases, the probable source of root canal infection is the bacteria originating from these periodontal pockets.

It has been reported that the treatment of periodontal disease may lead to secondary endodontic involvement. Scaling and root planing or surgical flap procedures are usually associated with opening of dentinal tubules and lateral canals to the oral environment. In such cases, it is common for a blood vessel within a lateral canal to be served by a curette and for the microorganisms to be pushed into the area during periodontal treatment, which favors pulpal infection, inflammation and later on pulpal necrosis.[12]

### True Combined Lesion

Pure combination of endodontic-periodontal diseases is rare as compared to other endodontic-periodontal problems. Such lesions occur due to coronal progression of endodontic lesion, which joins with infected periodontal pocket progressing apically **(Fig. 61.6)**. Such types of lesions are invariably associated with large degree of attachment loss and with guarded prognosis as in single-rooted teeth. Root resection is usually done in molar teeth. The radiographic appearance of combined lesion may mimic to a vertically fractured tooth. In presence of sinus tract, flap should be raised to know the exact etiology of the lesion.[11,12]

## DIAGNOSIS

Determination of the primary lesion, whether pulpal or periodontal, is the important step in diagnosis to avoid selecting wrong treatment or unnecessary overtreatment.[13] Following diagnostic measures are undertaken to establish the correct diagnosis:[14,15]

- *Vitality tests:* The first step would be to examine for vitality by pulp testing and with heat and cold. A nonvital tooth may indicate primary pulpal involvement, although at times, it can indicate secondary pulpal disease. Endodontic treatment (root canal therapy) is required in this situation. A vital tooth indicates primary periodontal involvement, and does not require endodontic therapy. Clinician should be cautious about the possibility of false-positive results also.

- *Radiographic evaluation:* Radiograph may exhibit loss of bone at the alveolar crest, an apical radiolucency, or a continuous bone loss involving both sites. Apical radiolucency indicates primary pulpal disease. Bone loss confined to coronal one-third of the tooth is associated with primary periodontal disease. Finding the cause is more difficult when bone loss is present at both sites. If the tooth has a radiographic furcation involvement that cannot be detected clinically, there is likelihood of pulpal involvement. Gutta-percha points used as probes in sinus tracts can be a valuable aid in tracing the origin of a draining lesion.
- *Pain and abscess formation:* Clinical signs and symptoms will help to differentiate between endodontic and periodontal lesions.
    - Pulpal pain is usually sharp. Periodontal abscess may produce a dull, more even pain, which is accompanied by a feeling of fullness in the area.
    - Pulpal lesion may be difficult to localize when the symptoms start. The periodontal lesion is usually easy to localize.
    - Pulpal lesion is usually drained by a fistula through the alveolar mucosa or gingiva, it rarely fistulates through the sulcus. The periodontal abscess usually drains through the lumen of the pocket.
- *Probing:* In the absence of periodontal disease, the presence of a deep solitary pocket usually suggests lesion to be of endodontic origin or a vertical root fracture. In such cases, periodontal probing adds light to differentiate between periodontal and endodontic lesions. Additionally, it helps in tracking a sinus originating from an inflammatory periapical lesion that extends cervically through the periodontal ligament space. Periodontal lesions are characterized by presence of numerous subgingival calculus deposits and osseous defects throughout the mouth. In a periodontally involved mouth, if pocket does not extend to the apical one-third of the root, it suggests that the lesion is a primary periodontal in nature.
- *Mobility:* In the acute stage of an endodontic infection, mobility involves a single tooth. If lesion is occlusal or periodontal in origin, then generalized mobility may be present in many teeth.
- *Palpation and percussion:* In an individual tooth with a periodontal problem, palpation and percussion tests are usually negative but in case of periapical abscess, these tests are usually positive. Tenderness and pain on percussion and palpation is usually present in tooth with endodontic lesion.

## TREATMENT AND PROGNOSIS

Treatment of primarily periodontal and endodontic lesions involves simple steps of procedures with favorable prognosis. In case of combined forms of the lesions predicting prognosis seems to be more difficult. However, endodontic therapy is more predictable and yields positive effect on periodontal healing, if completed before conducting periodontal procedures. It is usually found that in perio-endo lesions, the endodontic treatment is more predictable than periodontal therapy. For better long-term results, the complete treatment of both aspects, i.e. endodontic and periodontal of lesions are essential.[14,15]

- *Primary endodontic lesion*:
    - Treatment: Root canal treatment.
    - Prognosis: Good.
- *Primary periodontal lesion*:
    - Treatment: Periodontal treatment.
    - Prognosis: Depends upon periodontal treatment and response of the patient.
- *Primary endodontic-secondary periodontal lesion*:
    - Treatment: Root canal treatment first followed by periodontal treatment after 2–3 months.
    - Prognosis: Depends upon endodontic and periodontal treatment and response of the patient.
- *Primary periodontal-secondary endodontic lesion*:
    - Treatment: Endodontic and periodontal treatment [Guided tissue regeneration (GTR)].
    - Prognosis: Depends upon severity of the periodontal disease and periodontal tissue response to treatment.
- *True combined lesion*:
    - Treatment: Endodontic and periodontal treatment including surgical procedures like amputation, hemisection or bicuspidization.
    - Prognosis: More guarded prognosis.

### Points to Ponder

- Periodontal probing, pulp vitality test and radiographs are the cornerstones for diagnosis and classifying endo-perio lesions.
- When fistula with gutta-percha point is traced to radiograph apex, then endodontic etiology can be considered.
- When fistula with gutta percha point is traced to midroot, then periodontal etiology/pulpal necrosis in lateral canal can be considered.
- A long, narrow pocket in a single tooth in a mouth generally free from periodontal disease is usually associated with primary pulpal disease.
- A pocket that does not extend to the apical one third of the root in a periodontally diseased mouth indicates primary periodontal origin.

## REFERENCES

1. Simring M, Goldberg M. The pulpal pocket approach: retrograde periodontitis. J Periodontol. 1964;35:22-48.

2. Zehnder M, Gold SI, Hasselgren G. Pathologic interactions in pulpal and periodontal tissues. J Clin Periodontol. 2002;29(8):663-71.
3. DeDeus QD. Frequency, location, and direction of the lateral, secondary, and accessory canals. J Endod. 1975;1(11):361-6.
4. Gutmann JL. Prevalence, location, and patency of accessory canals in the furcation region of permanent molars. J Periodontol. 1978;49(1):21-6.
5. Gold SI, Hasselgren G. Peripheral inflammatory root resorption. A review of literature with case reports. J Clin Periodontol. 1992;19(8):523-34.
6. Bergenholtz G, Lindhe J. Effect of experimentally induced marginal periodontitis and periodontal scaling on the dental pulp. J Clin Periodontol. 1978;5(1):59-73.
7. Weine FS. Endodontic-periodontal problem in endodontic therapy. In: Endodontic Therapy, 3rd edition. St. Louis: Mosby; 1982. pp. 503.
8. Simon JH, Glick DH, Frank AL. The relationship of endodontic-periodontic lesions. J Periodontol. 1972;43(4):202-8.
9. Torabinejad M, Trope M. Endodontic and periodontal interrelationships. In: Walton RE, Torabinejad M (Eds). Principles and Practice of Endodontics. Philadelphia, PA, USA: WB Saunders; 1996.
10. Armitage GC. Development of a classification system for periodontal diseases and conditions. Ann Periodontol. 1999;4(1):1-6.
11. Ammons WF Jr, Harrington GW. The periodontic-endodontic continuum. In: Newman MG, Takei HH, Carranza FA (Eds). Carranza's Clinical Periodontology, 9th edition. Philadelphia, PA, USA: WB Saunders; 2003. pp. 840-50.
12. Rossman LE. Endodontic-periodontic consideration. In: Rose LF, Mealey BL, Genco RJ, Cohen DW (Eds). Periodontics: Medicine, Surgery, and Implants, 1st edition. St. Louis: Mosby; 2004. pp. 772-89.
13. Harrington GW, Steiner DR, Ammons WF. The periodontal-endodontic controversy. Periodontol 2000. 2002;30:123-30.
14. Bergenholtz G, Hasselgren G. Endodontics and periodontics. In: Lindhe J, Karring T, Lang NP (Eds). Clinical Periodontology and Implant Dentistry, 4th edition. Copenhagen, Denmark: Blackwell Munksgaard; 2003. pp. 318-51.
15. Rotstein I, Simon JH. Diagnosis, prognosis and decision-making in the treatment of combined periodontal-endodontic lesions. Periodontol 2000. 2004;34:165-203.

## VIVA VOCE

**Q1.** What are various anatomical pathways of communication between pulpal and periodontal tissue?
**Ans.** Apical foramen, accessory canals/lateral canals, dentinal tubules and palatogingival grooves.

**Q2.** What are various nonanatomical/nonphysiological pathways of communication between pulpal and periodontal tissue?
**Ans.** Root canal perforations and traumatic vertical root fractures.

**Q3.** What is retrograde periodontitis?
**Ans.** Retrograde periodontitis is long-standing periapical lesion which drains through the periodontal ligament.

**Q4.** What is retrograde pulpitis?
**Ans.** Bacterial and inflammatory products of periodontitis can access the pulp via apical foramen, lateral canals, accessory canals, and dentinal tubules and this reverse effect is called as retrograde pulpitis.

**Q5.** What is the basic difference in the pocket configuration of primary periodontal lesion and primary endodontic lesion?
**Ans.**
- Pocket with broad configuration is suggestive of primarily periodontal lesion.
- Pocket with narrow configuration/tube like pocket is suggestive of primarily endodontic lesion.

**Q6.** Which is the main and direct communication route between the pulp and periodontium?
**Ans.** Apical foramen.

**Q7.** What is true combined lesion?
**Ans.** Lesion which occurs due to coronal progression of endodontic lesion, which joins with infected periodontal pocket progressing apically.

**Q8.** How primary endodontic lesion is treated?
**Ans.** By root canal treatment.

**Q9.** How primary endodontic with secondary periodontal lesion is treated?
**Ans.** Root canal treatment first followed by periodontal treatment after 2–3 months.

**Q10.** What are the cornerstones for diagnosis and classifying endo-perio lesions?
**Ans.** Periodontal probing, pulp vitality test and radiographs.

# Chapter 62: Periodontics-Restorative Dentistry

*Shalu Bathla*

## Chapter Outline

- Inter-Relationship
- Periodontal Considerations
- Maintenance

## INTRODUCTION

Properly constructed restorations are of therapeutic value. Restorations, when improperly constructed, can become risk factor for the periodontal disease. The outer surface of a restoration is of significance from periodontal viewpoint. Proper contact, contour, occlusion, marginal adaptation and surface finish are as important to periodontics as they are to restorative dentistry. Also, periodontal health is critical for both the preservation of the natural dentition and the success of any restorative procedure. Thus, periodontium and the restoration of teeth are intimate and inseparable.

## INTER-RELATIONSHIP

The application of periodontics in restorative dentistry includes:
- Prerestorative periodontal care.
- Periodontal surgery for the placement of restoration.

### Prerestorative Periodontal Care

Active periodontal disease must be treated and controlled prior to any restorative procedure because margins of restorations covered by inflamed gingiva shrink after periodontal treatment. Thus, to locate and determine the gingival margins of restorations properly, the position of the healthy and stable gingival margin must be established prior to tooth preparation.[1,2]

### Periodontal Surgery for the Placement of Restoration

#### Free Gingival Graft and Full Crown Restoration

When the attached gingiva is totally absent and the soft-tissue crown interface has been compromised by recession or inflammation, surgical augmentation to provide a collar of attached gingiva is beneficial. Periodontal plastic surgery (free gingival graft) should be carried out at least 2 months before placement of dental restorations. This allows time for mature tissue to form in the gingival margin so that restorative procedures do not cause the return of clinical inflammation.[3]

#### Crown Lengthening Procedures

These procedures are usually done in cases of subgingival caries, fracture and when there is inadequate clinical crown length for retention. When severe caries approaches or extends below the alveolar crest, a full-thickness flap extending to adjacent teeth and osseous reduction to gain sound tooth structure are required. The apically positioned flap with ostectomy is an excellent means of preserving and often gaining attached gingiva. At least 3 mm should be the least distance between the apical extension of restoration and crest of the alveolar bone, otherwise law of biologic width is compromised.[4] Rest is explained in "Chapter 60: Periodontics-Prosthodontics".

Application of restorative dentistry in periodontics includes:
- Excavation of dental caries and restoration.
- Restorative correction of open gingival embrasures.
- Management of gingival embrasure form with periodontal recession.
- Restoration of root-resected teeth.
- Splinting.

### Excavation of Dental Caries and Restoration

Caries destroy tooth structure, creating open contacts, poor embrasure form and plunger cusps all of which encourage food impaction, plaque retention and periodontal disease.

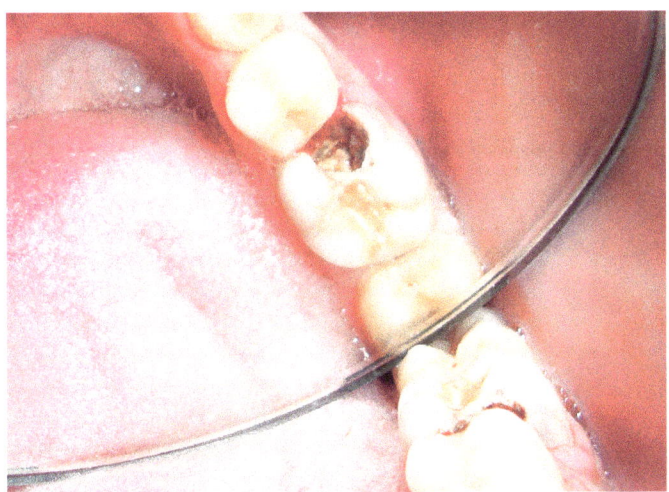

**Fig. 62.1:** Clinical picture showing carious lesion acting as plaque retentive area.

Thus, the removal of dental caries and the restoration of sound tooth structure are necessary components of early treatment (phase I) of a patient with periodontal disease. Restoration of dental caries should be conservative with normal interproximal contacts and proper embrasure space preventing plaque accumulation and creating environment conducive to periodontal health **(Fig. 62.1)**.

## Restorative Correction of Open Gingival Embrasures

There are two causes of open gingival embrasures, either the papilla is inadequate in height due to bone loss, or the interproximal contact is located too high coronally. If the open gingival embrasures is due to high contact and the roots are parallel with the normal papilla, then the problem is probably related to tooth shape, specifically, an excessively tapered form. Restorative dentistry can correct this problem by moving the contact point to the tip of the papilla. Thus, the margins of direct bonded restoration is carried subgingivally 1.0–1.5 mm, and the emergence profile of the restoration is designed to move the contact point towards the papilla while blending the contour into the tooth below the tissue.

## Management of Gingival Embrasure Form with Periodontal Recession

In esthetic areas, it is necessary to carry the interproximal contacts apically towards the papilla to eliminate the presence of large open embrasures. With multiple unit restorations, it is possible to bake porcelain papillae directly on the restoration using tissue-colored ceramics.

## Restoration of Root-resected Teeth

The removal of a root alters the direction of occlusal forces on the remaining resected tooth. Occlusion of that tooth is evaluated and adjusted and then the crown is placed. But before giving permanent restoration the quality of the endodontic filling, residual ledges should be examined radiographically and clinically. A cast post and core may be indicated to create an adequate foundation for the final restoration. Because the remaining roots are often very thin mesiodistally, it is difficult to cement prefabricated posts and have adequate bulk to place a foundation core on the mesial and distal of the post. That is why the one-piece cast post and core restoration is placed. Heavy convexities should be avoided for restoring these teeth for hygiene access. Facially and lingually, the contours should be essentially a straight line from the margin coronally, whereas interproximally, the contour emerges from the margin as a straight line or is slightly convex as it slopes up to the contact point. The gingival embrasure form created in the restoration must be fluted into these areas so that the surfaces can be accessed with an interdental brush.[4-6]

## Splinting

Splinting stabilizes mobile teeth during periodontal surgery and also during the healing period following surgery. Various restorative materials can be used for intra- and extracoronal splintings such as amalgam, acrylic or composite (rest is explained in "Chapter 44: Splinting").

## PERIODONTAL CONSIDERATIONS

These considerations include:
- Margins of restorations.
- Gingival management for making impressions.
- Contour of restoration.
- Occlusal surface.
- Surface finish of restorative materials.
- Restoration of hemisected and resected tooth.
- Restorative procedures.
- Materials.
- Restorative design features for periodontally treated teeth.

## Margins of Restorations

In restoring a tooth with any plastic filling material, accurately contoured and placed matrix bands stabilized by triangular wood or plastic wedge are essential to avoid overhanging margins. In cross section, the base of the triangle will be in contact with the interdental papillae, apical to gingival margin of the proximal cavity. The two sides of triangle coincide with the corresponding two sides (mesial and distal) of the gingival embrasure. The apex of wedge should coincide with the gingival start of the contact area. Thus, wedge defines the gingival extent of the contact area thereby, assuring the health of proximal periodontal tissues. Overhanging margins contribute to periodontal disease by providing ideal locations for plaque

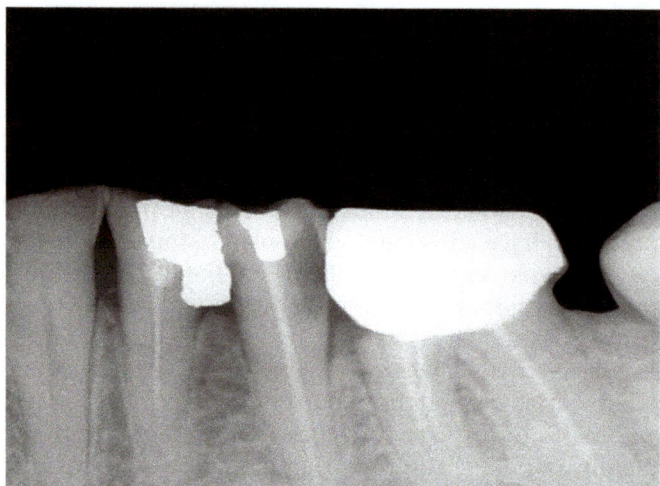

**Fig. 62.2:** Radiograph showing overhanging restoration leading to interproximal bone loss.

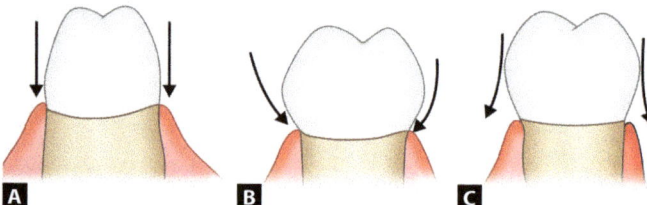

**Figs. 62.3A to C:** Schematic representation showing crown morphology: (A) Undercontoured; (B) Overcontoured; (C) Normal morphology.

accumulation and changing the ecological balance of the gingival sulcus area to one that favors the growth of disease-associated organisms **(Fig. 62.2)**. Overhanging can be removed with the help of files, enamel shavers or EVA prophylaxis system. When overhang cannot be removed, restoration should be replaced.[7] The location of the gingival margin of restoration is directly related to the periodontal health status. Subgingivally located margins are associated with large amounts of plaque, more severe gingivitis and deeper pockets.

## Gingival Management for Making Impressions

For subgingival preparation margin extending to the appropriate depth in the sulcus, gingival tissue must be protected from abrasion. Tissue management is achieved with gingival retraction cords of the appropriate size to achieve the required displacement. Electrosurgery can also be used to remove any overlying tissue in the retraction process. A fine wire tip electrode is held parallel to the tooth and against the margin in the sulcus and moved through the overhanging tissue, opening up the margin and the retraction cord to visual access.

## Contour of Restoration

Over contoured crowns and restorations tend to accumulate plaque and prevent self-cleansing mechanism of adjacent cheek, lips and tongue. The facial and lingual contours of restorations are also important in the preservation of gingival health. In patients in whom periodontal disease causes the gingival margin to be in a much more apical position than it was during health, the facial[7] and lingual contours become even more significant **(Figs. 62.3A to C)**. In this particular case, the bulge on the facial contour of the crown, which normally would be subgingival, appear supragingival. In Class III and IV furcation defects, it is important that the restoration be contoured in such a way so as to facilitate access for oral hygiene. In these cases, it is important to emphasize the midfacial groove of the crown so that this groove is confluent with the furcation.

## Occlusal Surface

Failure to reproduce the normal protective anatomy of the occlusal marginal ridges and developmental grooves lead to food impaction. Occlusal surfaces should be designed to direct masticatory forces along the long axis of the teeth. The anatomy of the occlusal surface should provide well-formed marginal ridges and occlusal sluiceways to prevent interproximal food impaction. Thus, restorations that do not conform to the occlusal patterns of the mouth cause occlusal disharmonies that may be injurious to the supporting periodontal tissues.

## Surface Finish

The surface of restoration should be smooth so as to limit plaque accumulation. Rough restorative surface in subgingival region results in plaque accumulation and thus, results in gingival inflammation. Therefore, all restorative materials placed in gingival environment must have the highest possible polish.

## Restoration of Hemisected and Resected Tooth

### Mandibular Molar

If both parts of hemisected tooth are to be retained, it is essential that an adequate embrasure space must be created between the two halves of the tooth, as it is too narrow. Hemisected teeth are prepared for restorative procedures, adequate tooth material is removed in the areas between the roots, so that a wide embrasure space is constructed, which will allow passage of an oral hygiene device. When a mandibular molar is hemisected and one portion is extracted, the remaining portion serves as abutments for a three unit bridge.

### Maxillary Molars

When a mesiobuccal or distobuccal root has been resected, it is necessary to hollow out the crown contours in the area coronal to the area where root was resected so that adequate access is available for oral hygiene procedures. When palatal root has been resected, the crown is made thinner buccopalatally, with a groove running in the midpalatal surface resembling a mandibular molar.

## Restorative Procedures

Injudicious tooth separation injures the supporting tissues of the periodontium. The use of rubber dam clamps, copper bands, matrix bands and disks may lacerate the gingiva resulting in gingival inflammation. Excessive vigorous condensing of gold foil restorations may also be the source of injury to the periodontium.[2]

## Materials

Inflammatory gingival responses related to the use of alloys containing nickel in dental restorations have been reported. Glass ceramics and porcelain veneers offer a clear advantage over other types of restorative material in the maintenance of gingival health. Their fine marginal fit results in a thin cement line, which lessens gingival irritation. More importantly, tissues respond more to the differences in surface roughness of the material rather than the composition of the material. Moreover, nonporous surface of porcelain does not allow bacteria to adhere significantly.

## Restorative Design Features for Periodontally Treated Teeth

Restoration of badly broken down, periodontally involved teeth or periodontally treated teeth pose a challenge to clinician. Gingival margins of tooth preparation should be placed supragingivally. If the restoration is to replace all occluding surface, the width of occlusal table should be reduced to minimize the amount of forces to be received by the periodontally involved teeth.

## MAINTENANCE

### Restored Teeth

A nonabrasive dentifrice is indicated to prevent the possibility of abrasion of acrylic. Fluoride containing dentifrice is important for the protection of remaining tooth surfaces, particularly exposed cementum. Acidulated fluoride preparations are contraindicated for porcelain and composite restorations.[8]

### Root-resected Restored Teeth

The interproximal areas of root-amputated and hemisected teeth often present with surface concavities on the root trunk, and these areas cannot be adequately cleaned with floss, thus the gingival embrasure form created in the restoration must be fluted into these areas so that the surfaces can be accessed with an interdental brush.

> **Points to Ponder**
> - Overcontoured crowns and restorations accumulate plaque and prevent self-cleansing mechanism of adjacent cheek, lips and tongue.
> - Overhanging can be removed with the help of files, enamel shavers or EVA prophylaxis system.

## REFERENCES

1. Spear FM, Cooney JP. Periodontal restorative interrelationship. In: Newman MG, Takei HH, Carranza FA (Eds). Carranza's Clinical Periodontology, 9th edition. Philadelphia, PA, USA: WB Saunders; 2003. pp. 949-65.
2. McGuire MK. Periodontal restorative interrelationship. In: Newman MG, Takei HH, Carranza FA (Eds). Carranza's Clinical Periodontology, 8th edition. Philadelphia, PA, USA: WB Saunders; 1996. pp. 723-42.
3. Casullo DP. Periodontal considerations in restorative dentistry. In: Genco RJ, Goldman HM, Cohen DW (Eds). Contemporary Periodontics, 1st edition. St. Louis: CV Mosby; 1990. pp. 619-35.
4. Takei HH, Azzi RR, Han TJ. Preparation of the periodontium for restorative dentistry. In: Newman MG, Takei HH, Carranza FA (Eds). Carranza's Clinical Periodontology, 9th edition. Philadelphia, PA, USA: WB Saunders; 2003. pp. 943-48.
5. Ramfjord SP, Ash MM. Periodontal considerations in restorative and other aspects of dentistry. In: Periodontology and Periodontics: Modern Theory and Practice, 1st edition. New Delhi, India: AITBS Publisher and Distributor; 1996. pp. 339-51.
6. Eley BM, Manson JD. Restorative and prosthetic procedures. In: Outlines of Periodontics, 5th edition. Edinburgh, Scotland: Wright Publishing; 2004. pp. 262-74.
7. Grant DA, Stern IB, Listgarten MA. Restorative and prosthetic dentistry. In: Periodontics, 6th edition. Missouri, USA: CV Mosby; 1988. pp. 1045-55.
8. Wilkins EM. Care of dental prostheses. In: Clinical Practice of the Dental Hygienist, 11th edition. Philadelphia, PA, USA: Lippincott Williams & Wilkins; 2012. pp. 394-410.

## VIVA VOCE

**Q1. Why active periodontal disease are treated and controlled prior to any restorative procedure?**
**Ans.** Because margins of restorations covered by inflamed gingiva shrinks after periodontal treatment. Thus, to locate and determine the gingival margins of restorations properly, the position of the healthy and stable gingival margin must be established prior to tooth preparation.

**Q2. How overhanging margins contribute to periodontal disease?**
**Ans.** Overhanging margins provide ideal niche for plaque accumulation and also change the ecological balance of the gingival sulcus area to one that favors the growth of disease associated organisms.

**Section 9:** Interdisciplinary Approach

**Q3. Why dental caries removal and restoration is done in phase I only?**
**Ans.** Carious lesion acts as plaque retentive area.

**Q4. Why periodontal plastic surgery (free gingival graft) should be carried out atleast 2 months before placement of restorations?**
**Ans.** Two months time allows mature tissue to form in the gingival margin so that restorative procedures do not cause the return of clinical inflammation.

**Q5. Which dentifrices are contraindicated for porcelain and composite restorations?**
**Ans.** Acidulated fluoride preparations.

**Q6. How the surface of restoration have effect on plaque accumulation?**
**Ans.** Rough restorative surface in subgingival region results in plaque accumulation and thus, results in gingival inflammation.

**Q7. How overhanging margins are avoided in restoring a tooth with any plastic filling material?**
**Ans.** By placing accurately contoured matrix bands stabilized by triangular wood or plastic wedge.

**Q8. Name various restorative materials used for intra- and extracoronal splintings.**
**Ans.** Amalgam, acrylic or composite.

**Q9. What are the application of periodontics in restorative dentistry?**
**Ans.** Prerestorative periodontal care; periodontal surgery for the placement of restoration.

**Q10. What are the causes of open gingival embrasures?**
**Ans.** Inadequate papilla height due to bone loss; coronally placed interproximal contact.

# Chapter 63: Periodontics-Orthodontics

*Geetanjali Gandhi, Shalu Bathla*

## Chapter Outline

- Indications
- Contraindications
- Benefits of Orthodontic Treatment
- Response to Tooth Movements
- Application of Orthodontics in Periodontics
- Application of Periodontics in Orthodontics
- Effects of Orthodontic Tooth Movement
- Systematics of Combined Treatment
- Maintenance

## INTRODUCTION

Periodontal therapy has entered a new era because of the innovations in adult tooth movement. Severe crowding that strangles the embrasure spaces and tilted and tipped molars, can be resolved by orthodontic treatment. In addition, very difficult surgical situations can be minimized or even eliminated by this multidisciplinary approach of combining periodontal and orthodontic therapy. Hence, orthodontic treatment acts as an adjunctive to periodontal therapy.

Periodontal factors, such as the width and height of alveolar bone; length and shape of the root and the structure of gingiva, are commonly involved in the consideration of orthodontic biomechanics and treatment planning. Orthodontics is a nonsurgical approach to enhance hard- and soft-tissue volume and height before the placement of an implant. Forced eruption can be used not only as a means of atraumatically extracting hopeless teeth, but of "carrying" the surrounding bone and soft tissue into a more coronal position. Periodontal maintenance visits are scheduled in orthodontic visits. Routinely, the mechanical aids, such as powered toothbrushes and interdental brushes are advised during such visits.

## INDICATIONS

Orthodontic treatment for individuals with periodontal disease may be indicated in the following situations:[1]

- *Basic malocclusion*: Crowded, malposed teeth may result in poor gingival form. Deep overbites are accompanied by trauma to maxillary palatal gingiva, and mandibular labial gingiva.
- *Migration*: Tooth migration can contribute to further periodontal breakdown by producing alteration in occlusion. Tooth migration can be caused by habits, such as tongue thrusting, trauma, aggressive periodontitis and gingival hyperplasia.
- *Bony defects*: They sometimes are treated better by combined periodontal-orthodontic measures than by periodontal treatment alone.
- *Preparation for reconstruction*: Fixed splinting requires parallel abutments, pontics require sufficient width and open embrasure. Thus, tilted and protruded teeth are uprighted. When neighboring teeth have drifted into edentulous spaces, orthodontic procedures are useful to create the ideal amount of space for implants and subsequent restorations.
- *Esthetic improvement*: Migration, which is evident in periodontal disease, may be the cause of embarrassment and may compel the patient to seek orthodontic treatment.

## CONTRAINDICATIONS

- No adequate inflammatory control before or lack of maintenance of periodontal health during tooth movement. A far worse situation may be created if inadequate anchorage due to extensive bone loss is there. Thus, the presence of active periodontal disease or existing extensive periodontal destruction is contraindicated for adult tooth movement.

- No adequate occlusal control (occlusal traumatism, parafunctional habits) in periodontally susceptible individuals.
- Short root or idiopathic root resorption.

## BENEFITS OF ORTHODONTIC TREATMENT

Orthodontic therapy offers various advantages in an adult periodontal patient as mentioned below:[2]

- *Reducing plaque retention*: Aligning of crowded or malposed maxillary or mandibular anterior teeth in adult patients offer better access for cleaning all teeth surfaces.
- *Improving osseous form*: In periodontal patients, vertical orthodontic tooth repositioning helps to overcome osseous defects. The tooth movement usually reduces the need for resective osseous surgery.
- *Improving gingival form*: Before restorative dentistry, orthodontic treatment is helpful for maintaining esthetic relationship of the level of maxillary gingival margins. Orthodontically achieved alignment of the gingival margin helps to prevent gingival recontouring, which may demand bone removal and exposure of the roots of the teeth.
- *Facilitating prosthetic replacements*: Orthodontics has a significant beneficial effect in the patient suffering from a fracture occurring at maxillary anterior tooth, which demands forced eruption for the adequate restoration of the root. In such cases, eruption permits the crown preparation in order to achieve sufficient resistance form and retention for final restoration.
- *Improving esthetics*: Orthodontic treatment is useful in the correction of open gingival embrasures to regain lost papilla. When open gingival embrasures are present in maxillary anterior region, they look unesthetic. A combination including orthodontic root movement, tooth reshaping, and/or restoration helps in correction of such unesthetic areas.
- *Orthodontic treatment*: It is helpful in correction of neighboring tooth position preceding to placement of implant or replacement of tooth. It is beneficial in patient whose teeth has been missing since several years and has drifting and tipping of the adjacent dentition.

## RESPONSE TO TOOTH MOVEMENTS

### Extrusion

Extrusion is the bodily movement of the tooth out of the socket. As far as periodontium is considered, it is least hazardous kind of tooth movement. Extrusion followed by clinical crown equilibration is associated with reduction in infrabony defects and pockets **(Figs. 63.1A and B)**. Extrusive tooth movement in areas of one-wall and two-wall bony pockets results in a coronal (favorable) positioning of

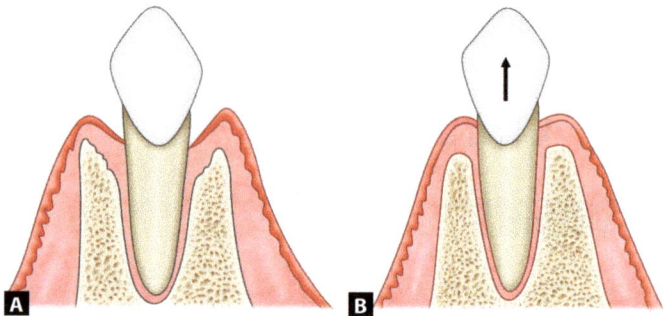

**Figs. 63.1A and B:** Schematic representation showing extrusion reducing infrabony defect and pocket.

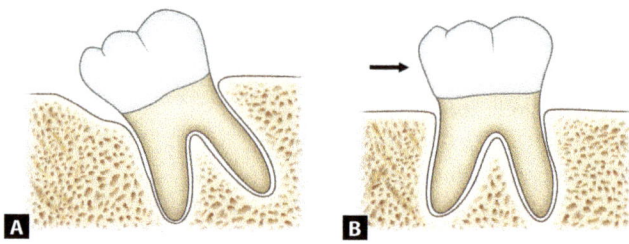

**Figs. 63.2A and B:** Schematic representation showing uprighting.

the intact connective tissue attachment and shallowing of the bony defect. These changes in attachment and bone levels are important issues in uprighting-tipped molars[3] **(Figs. 63.2A and B)**. The use of light, well-controlled forces enables fractured teeth and hemiseptal defects to be treated more easily.

### Intrusion

Intrusion is the bodily movement of a tooth into the socket and bone. It is thought that intrusion can lead to root resorption, deepening of infrabony pockets and bone defects. Thus, benefits of intrusion for improvement of the periodontal condition around teeth are controversial.

### Tipping

Severe epithelial attachment destruction and the loss of crestal bone are induced at the alveolar crest due to the heavy forces. Heavy forces induced at the alveolar crest lead to controlled tipping which may induce high forces in the periodontal ligament due to shifts of fulcrum in more apical position with higher amount of bone loss. Occasionally, cases have been reported where a gingival lesion gets transformed into a periodontal lesion due to injudicious use of tipping movement. Therefore, in tipping movement a lighter force should be used and the area kept plaque-free in order to avoid the formation of angular bony defects.

### Bodily Movement

Movement of a tooth bodily into a periodontal defect has been noted to carry the bone alongside the tooth leading to an improved defect. Recently conducted studies reported that this is an illusion as it leads to only an improved attachment of the connective tissue and actually causes worsening of the bony defect. Thus, this is contraindicated at least until new evidence favors.

## APPLICATION OF ORTHODONTICS IN PERIODONTICS

### Orthodontic Treatment of Osseous Defects

Following are the orthodontic treatments of various osseous defects:[4-6]

- *Hemiseptal defects*: These include one-wall or two-wall osseous defects commonly located around mesially tipped teeth or those which have been supraerupted. With the appropriate orthodontic treatment these defects can be reduced. In case of tipped tooth, uprighting and eruption of the tooth levels the bony defect.[7] In case of supraerupted tooth, intrusion and leveling of the adjacent cementoenamel junctions (CEJs) is useful for leveling the osseous defect **(Figs. 63.3A and B)**.
- *Furcation defects*: Class III furcation defect can be eliminated by hemisecting the crown and tooth root. However, the procedure requires endodontic, periodontal and restorative treatments. Hemisected roots when separated orthodontically permit favorable restoration and splinting. Hemisection, endodontic therapy and periodontal surgery should be performed earlier before starting orthodontic treatment. Bands or brackets and coil springs are placed on the root fragments to be separated. About 7 mm or 8 mm of space is created between the roots of the hemisected molar. This process improves the furcation defects and permits patients to clean the concerned area with more efficiency.[8]
- *Root proximity*: Maintenance of periodontal health and accessibility for restoration of adjacent teeth is usually compromised when roots of posterior teeth come in close proximity.[9] By orthodontic therapy, these roots can be moved apart and bone will be formed between the adjacent roots. Thus, open embrasure beneath the tooth contact provides additional bone support and enhances the patient's access to the interproximal region for hygiene. Brackets must be placed obliquely to facilitate orthodontic movement to separate the roots. Usually, 2–3 mm of root separation leads to adequate bone and embrasure space to achieve periodontal health.
- *Fractured teeth or forced eruption*: If the fracture extends beneath the level of the gingival margin and terminates at the level of the alveolar bone, then erupt the fractured root out of the bone and move the fracture margin coronally so that it can be properly restored. When extension of tooth fracture is at the bone level, it must be erupted at 4 mm. The first 2.5 mm moves the fracture margin far away from the bone in order to avoid a biological width problem. The other 1.5 mm provides a proper amount of ferrule for adequate resistance form of the crown preparation. The orthodontic mechanics necessary to erupt the tooth can vary from elastic traction to orthodontic banding and bracketing. If a large portion of the tooth is still present, then orthodontic bracketing is necessary. If the entire crown has fractured, leaving only the root, then elastic traction from a bonded bar may be possible.
- *Hopeless teeth maintained for orthodontic anchorage*: Hopeless teeth usually prove helpful for orthodontic anchorage when the periodontal inflammation is controlled. Flaps are reflected for debridement of the roots to control inflammation around the hopeless teeth during the orthodontic process. After orthodontic treatment the hopeless tooth may be improved so that it is retained.[10]

### Orthodontic Treatment of Gingival Discrepancies

#### Uneven Gingival Margins

The relationship of the gingival margin of the six maxillary anterior teeth is crucial in maintaining the esthetic appearance of the crowns.[11]

The factors that contribute to the ideal gingival form are as follows:[2]

- The gingival margin should be at the same level as the two central incisors.
- The gingival margin of the central incisors must be located more apically compared to the lateral incisors and maintained at the same level as the canines.
- The contour of the labial gingival margin should be similar to the CEJs of the teeth.
- A papilla should exist between each tooth. Also the height of the papillary tip should be at halfway between the incisal edge and the labial gingival height of contour over the center of each anterior tooth. Hence, the gingival papilla usually occupies almost half of the interproximal contact, and the other half of the contact is made by the adjacent teeth. The relationship between the shortest central incisor and the adjacent lateral incisors should be evaluated. In the case of longer shortest central compared to the lateral incisors, the longer central

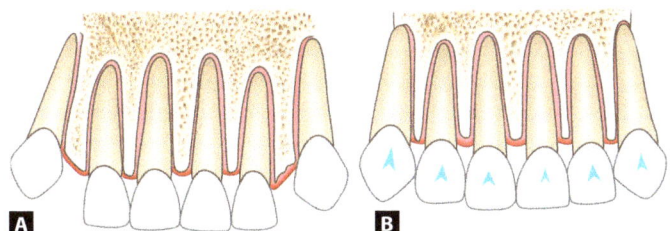

**Figs. 63.3A and B:** Schematic representation showing intrusion: (A) Angular bone topography between canines and incisors before intrusion; (B) Leveling of bone after intrusion.

incisor is extruded and then incisal edge is equilibrated. This helps to reposition the gingival margin coronally and reduces the discrepancy of gingival margin.

### Significant Attrition and Overeruption

If the patient had a protrusive bruxing habit that had caused severe attrition and overeruption of the maxillary anterior teeth, resulting in the loss of over half of the crown length of the incisors, intrusion movement is applied on the four incisors which level the gingival margin apically. Then the incisal edges are restored and final crowns are placed.

### Open Gingival Embrasures

Advanced periodontal disease with loss or cratering of interdental alveolar crest usually leads to loss of the papilla. Thus in such cases, "resurrecting" the gingival papillae is not helpful. However, the esthetics of the situation can be improved by tooth movement. During the movement of these teeth together orthodontically, the gingival tissue present in between the teeth squeezes into the shape of an interdental papilla. The overdivergence of adjacent roots results in missing papilla. This is common in orthodontic cases where mistakes were made in initial bracket placement. Thus, it is mandatory for the operator to immediately verify the mesiodistal root tip with periapical radiographs when such discrepancy is noted. The "missing papilla" can be avoided by simple repositioning of the orthodontic brackets or by judicious wire bending countering the exaggerated root divergence.[12]

## Correction of Pathologic Migration

Three basic appliances that are used for intra-arch tipping movements are: (1) Hawley appliance, (2) Crozat appliance and (3) Spring retainer, thus correcting pathologic tooth migration.[1]

## Implant Placement

Orthodontic extrusion of a single tooth that needs to be extracted is considered as an ideal method for improving the marginal bone levels before proceeding for the surgical placement of single implant **(Figs. 63.4A to D)**. During orthodontic extrusion, both the bone and the soft-supporting tissues will move vertically with the teeth. Hence, orthodontic extrusion of a "hopeless" incisor is also a useful method for esthetic improvement of the marginal gingival levels associated with the implant placement. Through controlled movement of hopeless teeth, the orthodontist can establish an environment that will ultimately house a functional and esthetic restoration. This facilitates immediate implant placement after tooth extraction because an increased volume of peri-implant bone and soft tissue are available.[13]

## APPLICATION OF PERIODONTICS IN ORTHODONTICS

### Preorthodontic Osseous Surgery

The type of defect (i.e., hemiseptal defect, osseous crater, furcation lesion and three wall intrabony defect) determines the extent of the periodontal osseous surgery.

### Osseous Craters

It is an interproximal, two wall defect that usually fails to improve with orthodontic treatment. During orthodontic treatment, shallow craters (i.e., 4-5 mm pocket) can be maintained nonsurgically. But the deep craters are first corrected surgically by reshaping the defect and by pocket depth reduction. This increases the ability to maintain these interproximal areas during orthodontic treatment. Thus, by eliminating the crater before orthodontics, the patient could maintain the area during and after orthodontic treatment.

### Three-wall Intrabony Defects

Regenerative periodontal therapy including bone grafts and barrier membranes has been successful in regenerating the lost periodontium and filling three-wall defects. Orthodontic treatment may be initiated 3–6 months after periodontal surgery if the results remain stable.

### Fiberotomy

Fiberotomy should be done after orthodontic correction of rotated teeth, especially maxillary and mandibular anterior teeth. The procedure should be done before debonding.[14] It reduces the occurrence of rotational relapse. The principal fibers of the periodontal ligament and the supra-alveolar fibers are soft-tissue periodontal entities that influence the stability. The periodontal ligament fibers and transseptal

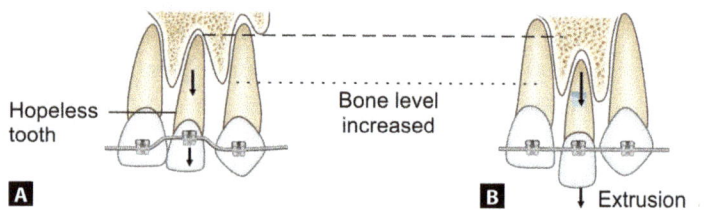 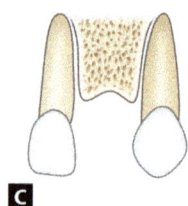 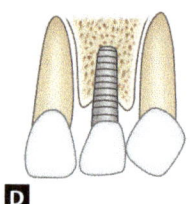

**Figs. 63.4A to D:** Schematic representation showing implant placement: (A) Extrusion of a hopeless tooth; (B) The tooth is stabilized for 4 months prior to extraction; (C) Extraction is done; (D) Implant is placed on a favorable bed.

groups usually remodel efficiently and histologically within 2–3 months after orthodontic rotation of teeth. However, the supra-alveolar fibers are apparently more stable, with a slow turnover. The gingival soft tissues are mainly made up of nonelastic collagenous fibers. Hence, the exact mechanism by which the gingival soft tissues may apply a force responsible for moving the teeth is still not known. Both practically and clinically it is noted that the supracrestal gingival tissues may contribute to rotational relapse as demonstrated by the effect of the circumferential supracrestal fiberotomy (CSF) technique. The technique consists of insertion of a scalpel into the gingival sulcus and severing the epithelial attachment surrounding the involved teeth. Additionally, the blade may transect the transseptal fibers by interdentally entering the periodontal ligament space.[8,15,16]

## Frenectomy

The contribution of the maxillary labial frenum to the etiology of a persisting midline diastema, and to re-opening of diastemas after orthodontic closure, is controversial (Procedure is explained in "Chapter 53: Periodontal Plastic Surgery").

## Preorthodontic Grafting

The periodontal tissues should have a stable relationship around the cervical area of the tooth which is in the process of tooth movement. An adequate amount of attached gingiva should be available for achieving the gingival health and to permit orthodontic forces without producing bone loss and gingival recession. During orthodontics the thin and delicate tissue is more susceptible to exhibit recession compared to normal thick tissue. In such cases, free gingival grafting is done before beginning orthodontic movement.

## Periodontally Accelerated Osteogenic Orthodontics

Wilcko et al., introduced periodontally accelerated osteogenic orthodontics (PAOO) as a clinical procedure that combines selective particulate bone grafting, alveolar corticotomy and the application of orthodontic forces.[17] Theoretically PAOO is based on the bone healing pattern which is also called as the regional acceleratory phenomenon (RAP). It leads to an enhancement in alveolar bone width, reduction in time of treatment, improvement in post-treatment stability and reduction in amount of apical root resorption.[18]

### Principle

In PAOO, during decortications of bone, there is a phase called as osteopenia, where its mineral content gets temporarily reduced. The tissue of the alveolar bone releases rich calcium deposits and new bone begins to mineralize in about 20–55 days. When the alveolar bone is in the transient state, orthodontic force provided with the help of braces helps to move teeth quickly. This is because the bone at this stage is soft and there is lesser resistance to the force of the braces.[18,19]

### Indications

Following are the indications for this technique:
- To resolve crowding and shorten orthodontic treatment time.
- To accelerate canine retraction after premolar extraction.
- To enhance postorthodontic stability.
- To facilitate eruption of impacted teeth.
- To facilitate slow orthodontic expansion.
- For molar intrusion and open bite correction.

### Contraindications

- Patients with active periodontal disease or gingival recession.
- Periodontal accelerated osteogenic orthodontics is not an alternative procedure for surgically assisted palatal expansion in the management of severe posterior crossbite.

### Surgical Technique

Following are the steps for PAOO:[19-21]
- *Step I (Raising of flap)*: Full-thickness flap is raised which gives significant access to the alveolar bone where corticotomies need to be performed.
- *Step II (Decortication)*: With completion of flap elevation, under local anesthesia decortications of bone adjacent to the malpositioned teeth is carried out by using round burs at low speed. Vertical cuts are deepened in the cortical bone of about 1.5–2.0 mm and are joined using the horizontal cuts. It is performed at clinical sites without entering the cancellous bone and by limiting risk of damage to underlying structures including the maxillary sinus and the mandibular canal.
- *Step III (Particulate bone grafting)*: Grafting is performed in all areas which have undergone corticotomies. The most common materials used for grafting are autogenous bone, decalcified freeze-dried bone allograft, or a combination of these.
- *Step IV (Closure)*: The flap should be closed using nonresorbable interrupted sutures without creating excessive tension.
- *Step V (Orthodontic force application)*: The placement of orthodontic brackets and activation of the arch wires are required to be carried out a week before the surgical aspect of PAOO is performed. Initiation of orthodontic force should not be delayed for more than 2 weeks after surgery.

## EFFECTS OF ORTHODONTIC TOOTH MOVEMENT

- *Loss of periodontal attachment and bone relative to orthodontic therapy*: With the absence of periodontal disease and practice of excellent oral hygiene, proper orthodontic treatment leads to no significant long-term effects on periodontal attachment and bone levels. However, in patients mostly adults having active periodontitis with presence of plaque-infected deep pockets as evidenced by bleeding on probing, orthodontic tooth movement may hasten the disease process, even in the presence of good oral hygiene. Because of the reduced volume of the periodontal ligament space in advanced periodontitis, orthodontic forces should be lighter than those used with periodontally healthy teeth. Orthodontic band placement leads to increase in salivary bacterial counts, especially *Lactobacillus*, *Prevotella intermedia* and *Porphyromonas gingivalis*.

- *Gingival recession relative to orthodontic therapy*: An adequate amount of attached gingiva is compulsory which permits appliances both functional and orthopedic to deliver orthodontic forces without resulting in gingival recession. Orthodontic tooth movement per se does not cause gingival recession. In areas of thin labial tissue, however, labial orthodontic tooth movement can result in bone dehiscence, creating an environment in which plaque and/or toothbrush trauma may cause sudden recession.
- *Gingival hyperplasia relative to orthodontic therapy*: In the presence of excellent oral hygiene (provided that the appliances are properly placed, without excessive adhesive flash), no significant hyperplasia should develop as a result of orthodontic tooth movement in adolescents or adults. However, fixed orthodontic appliances in the presence of consistently poor oral hygiene can lead to moderate-to-severe hyperplasia **(Figs. 63.5A and B)**, especially in the lower incisor region **(Fig. 63.5C)**. Severe cases of gingival hyperplasia may lead to attachment loss. Proper band fit or bonding of etching material is necessary so that the patient is able to continue adequate oral hygiene procedures.
- Kokich proposed the possibility of three unesthetic situations developing during orthodontic treatment[12,13] Gingival margin discrepancies, (2) the missing papilla and (3) gummy smile.

## SYSTEMATICS OF COMBINED TREATMENT

Following is the systematic approach of combined periodontal and orthodontic treatment:[22]

### Phase I: Preorthodontic Phase

- *Reduction of marginal inflammation*: Plaque control, scaling and root planing.
- *Soft-tissue augmentation*: Free epithelial graft, connective tissue graft.
- *Hard-tissue augmentation*: Regenerative osseous surgery.

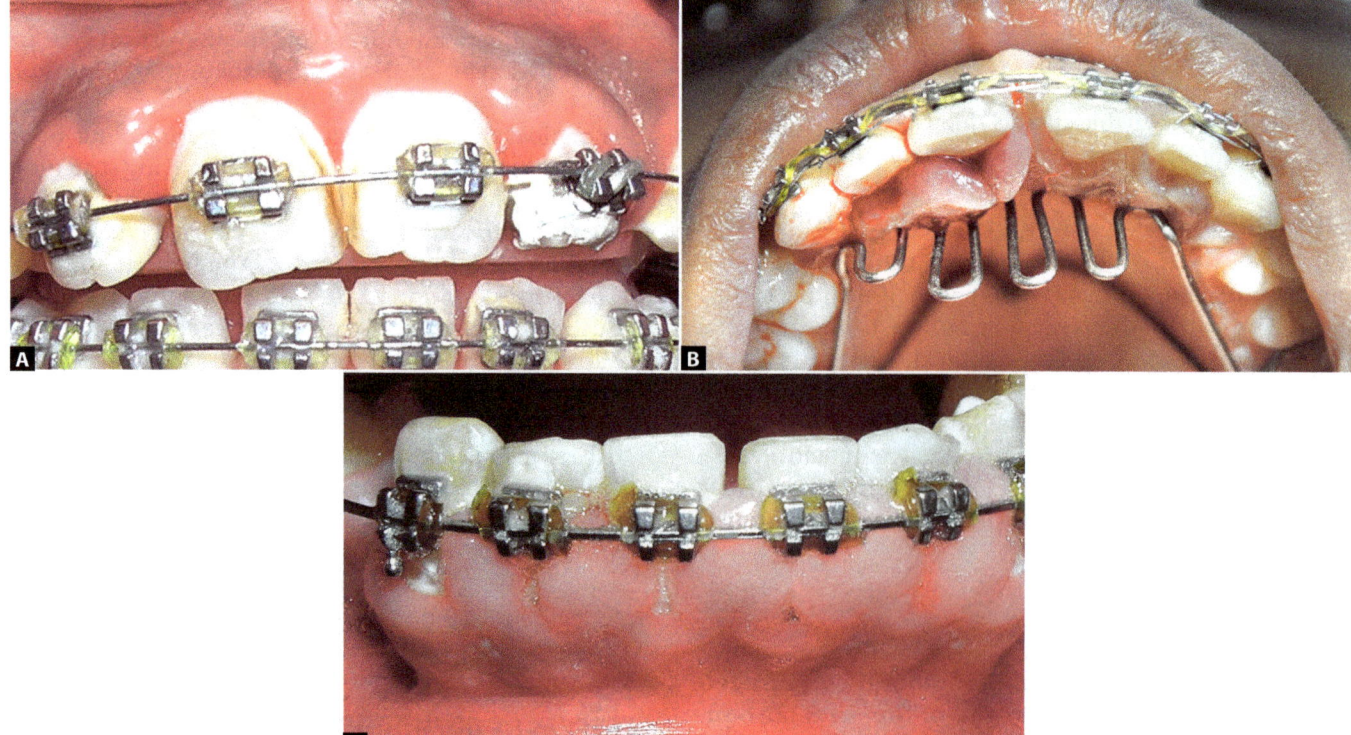

**Figs. 63.5A to C:** Clinical picture showing gingival hyperplasia at the: (A) Facial maxillary gingiva; (B) Palatal maxillary gingiva; (C) Facial mandibular gingiva during fixed orthodontic treatment.

- *Improvement of oral hygiene status*: Caries removal and restorations.
- *Elimination of functional disorders*: Therapeutic position of mandible.

## Phase II: Orthodontic Phase

This phase is determined by following two key factors:
1. *Findings-oriented biomechanics*: Thorough planning of biomechanics reduces the risk of root resorptions, gingival recession and bone dehiscence.
2. Continuous monitoring of periodontal health.

## Phase III: Postorthodontic Phase

This phase should last at least 6 months to complete mineralization of osteoid tissues. This phase includes the following:
- Periodontal reevaluation.
- Definitive restorative therapy.
- Recall schedule.

## MAINTENANCE

### Plaque Control

The presence of fixed orthodontic appliances makes plaque control measures difficult. The orthodontic patient should be reinforced at each visit with the oral hygiene techniques. Soft special bilevel orthodontic brush with rounded-end filaments is generally recommended **(Fig. 63.6)**. These brushes are designed with spaced rows of soft nylon filaments with a middle row that is shorter and can be applied directly over the fixed appliance. It is used with a short horizontal stroke. Sometimes, power-assisted toothbrushes are recommended.[23] Tufted dental floss or yarn used in the floss threader removes plaque more efficiently from the proximal tooth surfaces than regular dental floss. Most orthodontic patients can benefit from the regular use of an irrigator for removal of loose bacterial plaque and food debris and prevention of gingival inflammation.

Removable appliances are cleaned after each meal and before retiring. Brush and rinse teeth and gingival tissue under the appliance each time the appliance is removed. The orthodontic appliance should be properly designed in a way for providing stable anchorage without leading to tissue irritation. Additionally it should be esthetically acceptable. In order to prevent orthodontic appliances-induced accumulation of plaque on the teeth, appliances and mechanics should be kept simple. Outside the bracket bases, it is better to avoid hooks, elastomeric rings and excess bonding resin.

All brackets must use steel ligatures because elastomeric rings are proved to be more plaque attractive as compared to steel ties.

Bonds are preferred over bands, as bonded molars show less plaque accumulation, gingivitis[24] and loss of attachment interproximally. Every attempt should be made to achieve and maintain healthy oral tissues. Also the patient must be motivated to perform thorough daily plaque removal.

### Points to Ponder

- After 4–6 weeks of regenerative osseous therapy, orthodontic treatment can be initiated.
- PAOO is contraindicated in patients with active periodontal disease or gingival recession.
- Fiberotomy reduces the occurrence of rotational relapse.
- In thin gingival biotype, free gingival grafting is done before the beginning of orthodontic movement.

## REFERENCES

1. Carranza FM, Murphy NC. Orthodontics considerations in periodontal therapy. In: Carranza FA, Takei HH, Newman MG (Eds). Carranza's Clinical Periodontology, 8th edition. St. Louis: WB Saunders; 1996. pp. 559-64.
2. Kokich VG. The role of orthodontics as an adjunct to periodontal therapy. In: Newman MG, Takei HH, Carranza FA (Eds). Carranza's Clinical Periodontology, 9th edition. St. Louis: WB Saunders; 2003. pp. 704-18.
3. Vanarsdall RL. Tooth movement as an adjunct to periodontal therapy. In: Genco RJ, Goldman HM, Cohen DW. Contemporary Periodontics, 1st edition. St. Louis: CV Mosby; 1990. pp. 505-19.
4. Brown IS. The effect of orthodontic therapy on certain types of periodontal defects. I. Clinical findings. J Periodontol. 1973;44(12):742-56.
5. Nevins M, Wise RJ. Use of orthodontic therapy to alter infrabony pockets. 2. Int J Periodontics Restorative Dent. 1990;10(3):198-207.
6. Polson A, Caton J, Polson AP, Nyman S, Novak J, Reed B. Periodontal response after tooth movement into intrabony defects. J Periodontol. 1984;55(4):197-202.
7. Ingber JS. Forced eruption: I. A method of treating isolated one and two wall infrabony osseous defects—rationale and case report. J Periodontol. 1974;45(4):199-206.
8. Grant DA, Stern IB, Listgarten MA. Orthodontic measures in periodontal therapy. In: Periodontics, 6th edition. St. Louis: CV Mosby; 1988. pp. 1017-44.

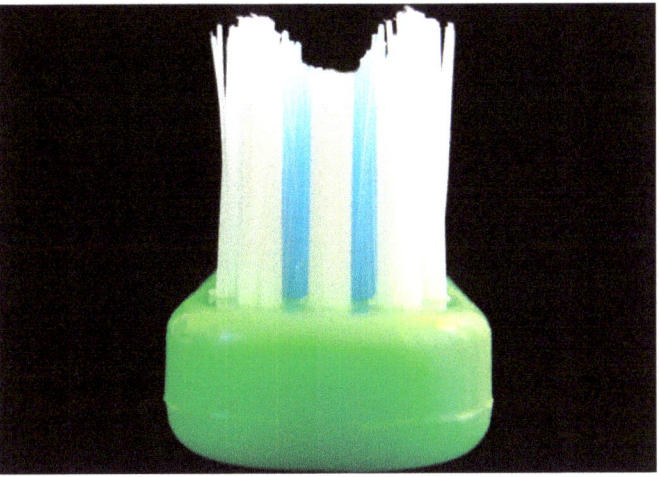

**Fig. 63.6:** Photograph showing orthodontic bilevel toothbrush.

9. Gould MS, Picton DC. The relation between irregularities of the teeth and periodontal disease. Br Dent J. 1966;121:21.
10. Melsen B, Agerbaek N. Orthodontics as an adjunct to rehabilitation. Periodontol 2000. 1994;4:148-59.
11. Keim RG. Aesthetics in clinical orthodontic-periodontic interactions. Periodontol 2000. 2001;27:59-71.
12. Kokich VG. Esthetics and vertical tooth position: orthodontic possibilities. Compend Contin Educ Dent. 1997;18(12):1225-31.
13. Kokich VG, Kokich VO. Orthodontic therapy for the periodontal-restorative patient. In: Rose LF, Mealey BL, Genco RJ, Cohen DW (Eds). Periodontics: Medicine, Surgery, and Implants, 1st edition. St. Louis: Elsevier-Mosby; 2004. pp. 718-44.
14. Edwards JG. A surgical procedure to eliminate rotational relapse. Am J Orthod. 1970;57(1):35-46.
15. Proffit WR. The biologic basis of orthodontic therapy. In: Contemporary Orthodontics, 4th edition. Missouri: Mosby Elsevier; 2007. pp. 331-58.
16. Zachrisson BU. Orthodontics and periodontics. In: Lindhe J, Karring T, Lang NP (Eds). Clinical Periodontology and Implant Dentistry, 4th edition. Copenhagen, Denmark: Blackwell Munksgaard; 2003. pp. 744-80.
17. Wilcko WM, Wilcko MT, Bouquot JE, Ferguson DJ. Accelerated orthodontics with alveolar reshaping. J Ortho Practice. 2000;10:63-70.
18. Wilcko WM, Wilcko MT, Bouquot JE, Ferguson OJ. Rapid orthodontics with alveolar reshaping: two case reports of decrowding. Int J Periodontics Restorative Dent. 2001;21(1):9-19.
19. Wilcko WM, Ferguson OJ, Bouquot JE, Wilcko MT. Rapid orthodontic decrowding with alveolar augmentation: case report. World J Orthod. 2003;4:197-205.
20. Wilcko MT, Wilcko WM, Marquez MG, Ferguson DJ. The contributions of periodontics to orthodontic therapy. In: Dibart S (Ed). Practical Advanced Periodontal Surgery, 1st edition. Ames, IA, USA: Wiley Blackwell; 2007. pp. 23-50.
21. Wilcko MT, Wilko WM, Bissada NF. An evidence-based analysis of periodontally accelerated orthodontic and osteogenic techniques: a synthesis of scientific perspective. Semin Orthod. 2008;14:305-16.
22. Diedrich P, Fritz U, Kinzinger G. Interrelationship between periodontics and adult orthodontics. Perio. 2004;1(3):143-9.
23. Wilkins EM. Care of dental prostheses. In: Clinical Practice of the Dental Hygienist, 8th edition. Philadelphia, PA, USA: Lippincott Williams & Wilkins; 1999. pp. 395-409.
24. Jacobson L. Mouthbreathing and gingivitis. J Periodontal Res. 1973;8(5):269-77.

## VIVA VOCE

**Q1. What is the association of mouth breathing and orthodontic treatment?**
**Ans.** A significant problem in orthodontic patients is added periodontal insult of mouth breathing. The drying effect on the exposed tissue in susceptible patients is associated with enlarged, erythematous labial gingiva, particularly in the maxillary and mandibular anterior region. Although the plaque index is not significantly higher in mouth breathers, an increase in the gingival index has been reported. This increased inflammation should be reduced to minimum before fixed appliances are placed, and is usually accomplished by scaling and root planing.

**Q2. What are the various periodontal factors which affect orthodontic biomechanics and treatment planning?**
**Ans.** Width and height of alveolar bone, length and shape of the root and width of attached gingiva.

**Q3. Which fibers are transected during circumferential supracrestal fiberotomy?**
**Ans.** Supracrestal and transseptal fibers.

**Q4. What are the causes of open gingival embrasures?**
**Ans.**
- Inadequate papilla height due to alveolar bone loss.
- Coronally high interproximal contact due to divergence of root or tapered tooth shape.

**Q5. What are the advantages of PAOO technique?**
**Ans.** Reduction in time for ortho treatment and improvement in post-treatment stability.

**Q6. Which brush is generally recommended to patients with orthodontic brackets?**
**Ans.** Soft special bi-level filaments orthodontic brush or powered brush.

**Q7. Who introduced periodontally accelerated osteogenic orthodontics (PAOO)?**
**Ans.** Wilcko et al.

**Q8. How much root separation is required for adequate bone and embrasure space to achieve periodontal health?**
**Ans.** Approximately 2–3 mm.

**Q9. Why bonds are preferred over bands?**
**Ans.** Bonded molars show less plaque accumulation, gingivitis and loss of attachment interproximally.

**Q10. Which appliances are used for intra-arch tipping movements for correcting pathologic tooth migration?**
**Ans.** Hawley appliance; Crozat appliance and Spring retainer.

# Chapter 64: Periodontics-Pediatric Dentistry

*Nikhil Srivastava, Shalu Bathla*

## Chapter Outline

- Periodontium of Deciduous Dentition
- Gingivitis and Gingival Enlargement
- Periodontitis
- Periodontitis as a Manifestation of Systemic Diseases
- Anatomical Periodontal Problems
- Childhood Diseases Affecting Gingiva
- Maintenance

## INTRODUCTION

The normal periodontium presents with its unique features, which need to be studied carefully for assessment of the oral health of children. Healthy periodontium exhibits lack of inflammatory signs including redness, swelling, exudates and bleeding upon gentle probing along with maintenance of a functional periodontal attachment over a period of time.

## PERIODONTIUM OF DECIDUOUS DENTITION

Following are the differences between the periodontium of deciduous and permanent dentition **(Table 64.1)**:[1-6]

The free gingival margin is thicker and rounder around primary teeth because of prominent cervical bulge and constricted cementoenamel junction. The gingival sulcus depth in permanent dentition is comparatively lesser than that seen in the primary dentition.

The morphology of interdental gingiva is determined by the anatomy and cervical contours of the primary teeth. Most children have well-spaced dentitions with absence of contact points hence there is no chance of interdental col formation. In primary teeth, the presence of widespread interdental spacing results in so-called interdental saddle areas. Lack of interdental contacts leads to fusion of papilla from both sides and formation of interdental saddle areas. These areas are covered with well-keratinized epithelium which is less vulnerable to bacterial infection. Hence, the children might exhibit lower prevalence of periodontal disease compared to adults.

The interdental cleft and retrocuspid papilla are the two unique anatomic features seen in the gingiva of children. The interdental clefts are seen lying apical to the interdental areas while the retrocuspid papilla is present behind the mandibular canine below the marginal gingiva. The retrocuspid papilla decreases with age and should not be confused with any intraoral swelling.

Attached gingiva is wider than permanent dentition.[7] The incidence of stippling in children is said to be around 35%.[8]

The alveolar bone is immature, more elastic and pliable in children. It is less calcified, has fewer trabeculae and larger bone marrow spaces.[10-12]

### Clinical Tip

In young children, stippling is extremely fine, and the greater vascularization gives the attached gingiva a reddish color, making it difficult to distinguish it from the alveolar mucosa. So, jiggle method is used to delineate the mucogingival junction (MGJ).[9]

## GINGIVITIS AND GINGIVAL ENLARGEMENT

### Eruption Gingivitis

Gingivitis associated with tooth eruption is frequent and has given rise to the term "eruption gingivitis". However, tooth eruption per se does not cause gingivitis. The inflammation results from plaque accumulation around erupting teeth. The initiation of gingivitis appears to be related to plaque accumulation rather than to tissue remodeling associated with eruption. Plaque retention around deciduous teeth facilitates plaque formation around juxtaposed permanent teeth. The inflammatory changes accentuate the normal prominence of the gingival margin and may create the

**TABLE 64.1:** Differences between the periodontium of deciduous and permanent dentition.

| Parameters | Deciduous dentition | Permanent dentition |
|---|---|---|
| *Gingiva* | | |
| Color | Pale pink | Coral pink |
| Surface texture | Stippling usually absent | Stippling usually present |
| Consistency | Less fibrous | More fibrous and firm |
| Interdental papilla | Broad faciolingually and narrow mesiodistally | Narrow faciolingually and broad mesiodistally |
| Width of attached gingiva | Less | More |
| Epithelium | Thinner | Thicker |
| Keratinization | Less | More |
| Connective tissues | More vascular | Less vascular |
| *Periodontal ligament* | | |
| Width | More wide | Less wide |
| Direction of periodontal fibers | Principal fibers are parallel to long axis of teeth | They are arranged in different directions |
| Vascularity of periodontal ligament | More | Less |
| *Cementum* | | |
| Thickness | Thinner and less dense | Thicker and more dense |
| *Alveolar bone* | | |
| Lamina dura | Prominent | Less prominent |
| Trabeculae | Fewer but thicker | More but thinner |
| Marrow spaces | Larger | Smaller |
| Crest of interdental septa | Flat | Angulated |
| Radiographic distance between cementoenamel junction and alveolar crest | Approximately 0–2 mm | Approximately 0–4 mm |

impression of a marked gingival enlargement **(Fig. 64.1)**. Partially exfoliated, loose deciduous teeth often cause gingivitis. The eroded margin of partially resorbed teeth favors plaque accumulation which causes gingival changes varying from slight discoloration and edema to abscess formation with suppuration. Management is by good oral hygiene maintenance. Aggressive therapy should not be done unless situation demands (e.g., gingival abscess).

## Factitious Gingivitis

Children may develop localized, nonspecific, acute marginal lesions as a result of faulty toothbrushing, impaction of foreign objects, pricking the gingiva with fingernail or fingernail biting. A traumatic ulcerative gingival lesion in children is often caused by excessive or incorrect toothbrushing and is infected by mixed normal flora of the oral cavity. Clinically the lesions are often localized to area and the gingiva exhibits ulcers that are covered with thin, yellowish or grayish exudate. The patient also complains of pain in the affected area. In such cases, it is important to identify the mechanism of injury which helps to instruct the patient to avoid the injurious behavior. In some cases, the habit or behavior may be associated with certain emotional or psychological problems. In such conditions, referral for psychiatric evaluation and treatment is helpful to improve outcomes.

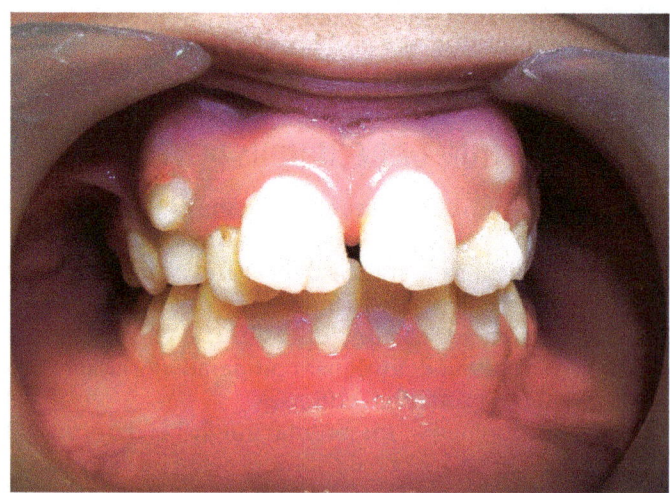

**Fig. 64.1:** Clinical picture showing eruption gingivitis.

## Acute Inflammatory Enlargement

### Gingival Abscess

A gingival abscess is a localized, painful, rapidly expanding lesion with a sudden onset in nature. Gingival abscess is commonly restricted to the marginal gingiva or interdental papilla. It occurs when a foreign substance, including toothbrush bristles, a piece of apple core, or a lobster shell fragment, food grains and popcorn hull gets forcefully embedded into the gingiva. This facilitates the transmission of bacteria into the tissues. In early stages, the lesions appear as a red swelling with a smooth and shiny surface. Such abscesses respond well to debridement.

## Chronic Inflammatory Enlargement

Poor oral hygiene leading to formation of dental plaque over-extended period of time leads to chronic inflammatory enlargement of gingiva. Along with this anatomic abnormalities, irritation by improper restorative and orthodontic appliances can act as other predisposing factors. It may represent from slight ballooning of the interdental papilla and/or the marginal gingiva to the bulge covering most of the crown. The enlargement is usually painless and progresses slowly. It may be localized or generalized. It may occur as a discrete sessile or pedunculated mass on the interproximal or marginal or attached gingiva.

## Conditioned Gingival Enlargement

### Puberty Gingivitis

Enlargement of the gingiva is sometimes seen in both male and female adolescents and appears in areas of plaque accumulation. It is characterized by prominent bulbous interproximal papillae and spontaneous bleeding from the gingiva. It is the degree of enlargement and the tendency to develop massive recurrence in the presence of relatively scanty plaque deposits that distinguish pubertal gingival enlargement from uncomplicated chronic inflammatory gingival enlargement **(Fig. 64.2)**. Management includes scaling, home care and oral hygiene instructions. Usually after puberty, there is spontaneous reduction of enlargement but does not disappear until plaque and calculus are removed.

### Vitamin C Deficiency

It is essentially a conditioned response to bacterial plaque. Acute vitamin C deficiency as such does not cause gingival inflammation itself, but it does cause collagen degeneration, hemorrhage and edema of the gingival connective tissue. These changes modify the response of the gingiva to plaque to the extent that the normal defensive delimiting reaction is inhibited, and the extent of the inflammation is exaggerated. The child with scorbutic gingivitis complains of severe pain and spontaneous hemorrhage. It appears as bluish red, soft, and friable with smooth, shiny surface. There may be surface necrosis with pseudomembrane formation.

### Plasma Cell Gingivitis

It is also called as atypical gingivitis and plasma cell gingivostomatitis. A localized lesion, referred to as plasma cell granuloma, is located in the oral aspect of the attached gingiva and therefore differs from plaque-induced gingivitis. It is considered that plasma cell gingivitis is allergic in origin and might be related to components of chewing gum, dentifrices, or various diet components. There is mild marginal gingival enlargement that extends to the attached gingiva. The gingiva appears red, friable and sometimes granular which bleeds easily. Lesions start to resolve on cessation of exposure to the allergen.

### Nonspecific Conditioned Enlargement (Pyogenic Granuloma)

Pyogenic granuloma is a tumor-like enlargement of gingiva which develops as an exaggerated conditioned response to minor trauma. The exact nature of the systemic conditioning factor has not been known yet. The lesion varies from a discrete spherical, tumor-like mass with a pedunculated attachment to a flattened, keloid-like enlargement with a broad base **(Fig. 64.3)**. It is reddish or bluish, sometimes lobulated, and may be sessile or pedunculated with surface ulceration and purulent exudation. It may develop rapidly and the size varies considerably. Bleeding from the ulcerated lesion is common, but typically it is not painful. Teeth may become separated due to interdental growth of the lesion. Due to its red color, which may sometimes turn

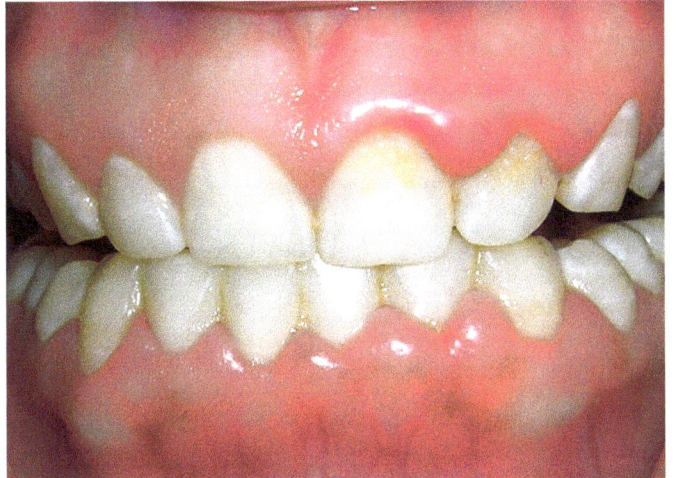

**Fig. 64.2:** Clinical picture showing puberty gingivitis.

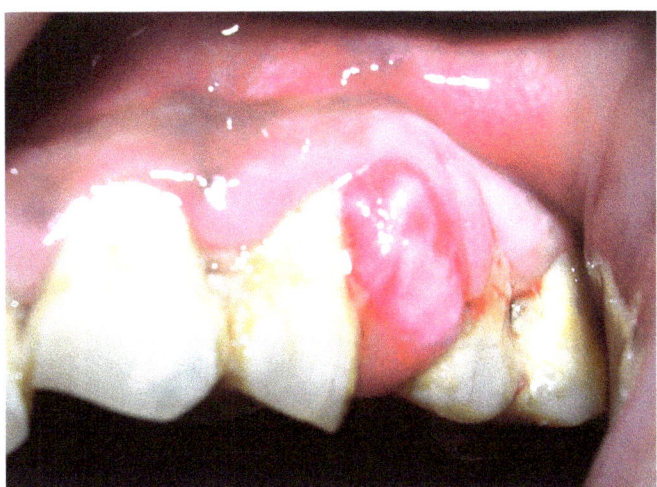

**Fig. 64.3:** Clinical picture showing pyogenic granuloma.

to a cyanotic hue, pyogenic granuloma may be mistaken for giant cell granuloma. Treatment consists of surgical excision of the lesion and the elimination of irritating local factors.

## Drugs-induced Gingival Enlargement

It arises most commonly as a result of ingestion of various medications, such as phenytoin, cyclosporine, nifedipine and amphetamines. Phenytoin is an anticonvulsant drug. Cyclosporine is used to control host rejection of transplanted organs and to treat autoimmune diseases. Nifedipine is a calcium-channel blockers that is sometimes used in children to control hypertension.[13,14] Amphetamines are a class of drugs that were used previously as antiobesity medications but now are used to treat certain subtypes of attention-deficit hyperactivity disorder (ADHD). These conditions affect 5–10% of school-aged children. ADHD with hyperactivity and impulsivity is seen 10 times more frequently in boys than in girls and not only is manifested in childhood but also persists throughout adolescence and sometimes into adulthood.[15] Clinical features are similar for all drugs. Lesions appear within first 2 months of drug therapy as painless enlargement of interdental papillae and marginal gingiva, which becomes lobulated and progress to cover the crowns **(Fig. 64.4)**. They form pseudopockets with a probing depth more than 4 mm. It has a predilection for anterior region. It has increased propensity in children and adolescents. It does not occur in edentulous areas. The gingival enlargement may cause difficulties with esthetics, mastication, tooth eruption, speech. If possible, before the patient initiating drug therapy, an oral hygiene regimen should be established to prevent or to minimize the occurrence of medication-induced gingival enlargements. Treatment includes replacement with alternate drug if possible, in consultation with the physician. The condition regresses or disappears after cessation of drug therapy. Oral prophylaxis and home care are needed. Daily use of chlorhexidine may be beneficial. In some cases, gingivectomy is needed. A 3–4-month recall visit for dental prophylaxis and reinforcement of oral hygiene instructions should be undertaken.

## Idiopathic Gingival Fibromatosis

Idiopathic gingival fibromatosis is also known as gingivostomatitis, hereditary gingival hyperplasia, congenital familial fibromatosis and elephantiasis. It is idiopathic with no known cause and believed to be originated as hereditary form. Sometimes, it occurs as an isolated disease entity or may present as a part of a syndrome. It is associated with tuberous sclerosis, which is characterized by a triad of epilepsy, mental retardation and cutaneous angiofibromas. Fibromatosis involves gingival margin, interdental papillae and attached gingiva of the facial and lingual surfaces of the mandible and maxilla. Clinical manifestations involve large masses of firm, dense, resilient, insensitive fibrous tissue covering the alveolar ridges and extending over the teeth **(Fig. 64.5)**. Color is usually normal or turns erythematous in case of inflammation. If the enlargement is present before tooth eruption, dense fibrous tissue may then interfere with or prevent the eruption. Bulbous enlargement of the gingiva leads to distortion of the jaws and patient complains of functional and esthetic problems. Treatment involves surgical removal by series of gingivectomies. If the volume of the overgrowth is extensive, repositioned flap surgery is done.[16,17]

## Necrotizing Ulcerative Gingivitis

This condition is known by many other terms like ulcerative gingivitis, acute necrotizing gingivitis, Vincent's infection, fusospirochetal disease or trench mouth. Necrotizing ulcerative gingivitis (NUG) is easy to diagnose due to involvement of the interproximal papillae and formation of a pseudomembranous necrotic covering of the marginal tissue. Two microorganisms, *Borrelia vincentii* and fusiform

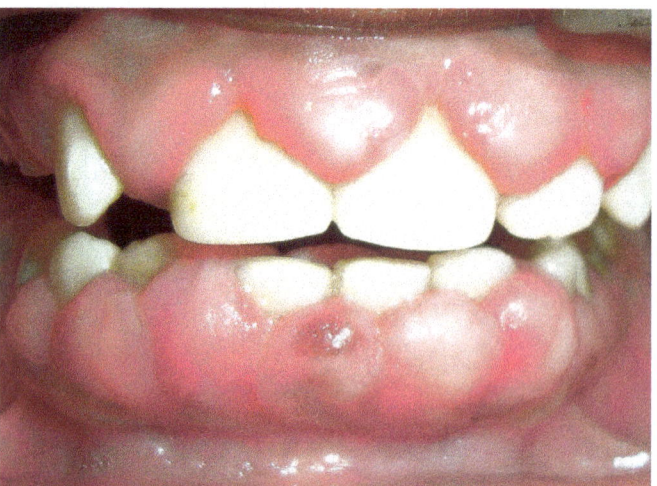

**Fig. 64.4:** Clinical picture showing phenytoin-induced gingival enlargement.

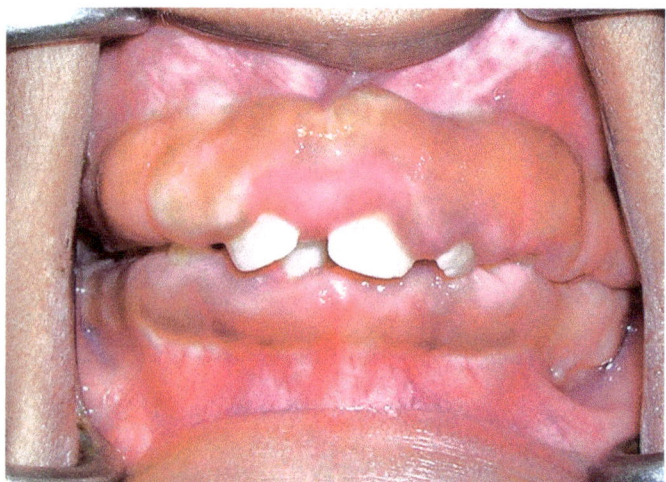

**Fig. 64.5:** Clinical picture showing idiopathic gingival fibromatosis.

bacilli, referred to as spirochete organisms are generally believed to be responsible for the disease. The predisposing factors include malnutrition, stress and lack of sleep. The clinical manifestations of the disease include inflamed, painful, bleeding gingival tissue, poor appetite, fever as high as 40°C (104°F), general malaise, fetid odor and lymphadenopathy. The disease is episodic in progression, each episode lasting 3–12 days. It is characterized by necrotic ulceration of the gingival margins. Involvement is usually restricted to a single tooth, a group of or entire dentition. In the early stages, the papillary gingiva becomes swollen and the tips of the papilla become ulcerated. Patient complains of gingival soreness which is sometimes severe and feeding becomes difficult. There may be spontaneous bleeding of gingiva, metallic taste, excessive salivation and halitosis. Necrotic ulceration of the papillae spreads laterally along the gingival margins. The ulcers are painful to touch and are covered by a yellowish-gray slough or pseudomembrane.

Management includes local debridement (ultrasonic scaling), subgingival curettage and use of mild oxygenating solutions. Antibiotic therapy includes penicillins/erythromycin and metronidazole. Nonsteroidal anti-inflammatory drugs (NSAIDs) may be used for pain relief. Response to antibiotics is usually seen within 24–48 hours and the acute symptoms subside and ulcers heal in 10–14 days. The gingival margins become thickened by fibrous repair and the papillae retain the concave shape of the healed ulcer. This saucer-shaped deformity is characteristic of NUG, thus an episode of previous infection can be diagnosed later. Patients suffering from unexplained recurrences of NUG should undergo medical examination and blood screening.

## Acute Herpetic Gingivostomatitis

It is the most common viral disease that affects the gingiva. The herpes simplex virus type 1 (HSV-1) is the etiological agent for herpetic gingivostomatitis. Though it affects infants and children younger than 6 years of age, it can also be seen in adolescents and adults. It affects male and female patients equally. Clinically, it is presented as a diffuse, erythematous, shiny involvement of the gingiva and the adjacent oral mucosa, with varying degrees of edema and gingival bleeding. The presence of discrete, spherical gray vesicles on the gingiva, labial and buccal mucosa, soft palate, pharynx, sublingual mucosa and tongue is the characteristic feature of this disorder. Approximately after 24 hours the vesicles rupture to form painful, small ulcers with a red, elevated, halo-like margin and a depressed, yellowish- or grayish-white central portion **(Fig. 64.6)**. These are present either in widely separated areas or occur in clusters where confluence occurs. Occasionally, primary herpetic gingivitis develops without overt vesiculation. Clinical picture constitutes diffuse, erythematous, shiny discoloration and edematous enlargement of the gingiva

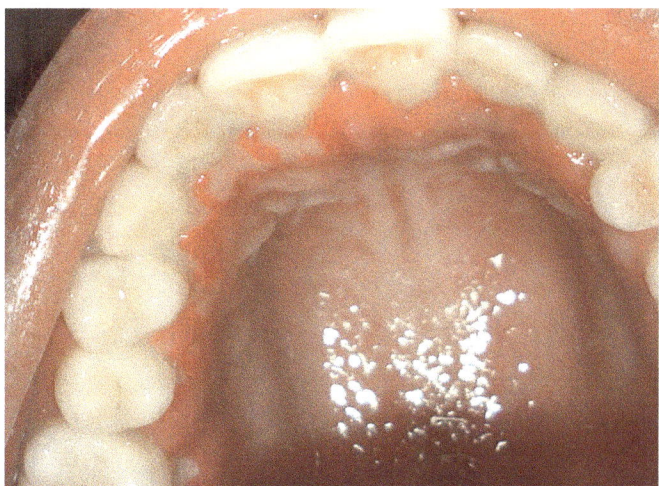

**Fig. 64.6:** Clinical picture showing acute herpetic gingivostomatitis (AHGS).
(*Courtesy*: Dr Gayathri Rao)

with a tendency towards bleeding. Generalized "soreness" of the oral cavity usually interferes with eating and drinking. In case of infants the disease is presented as irritability and refusal to take food. Cervical adenitis, fever as high as 101–105°F (38.3–40.6°C), and generalized malaise are other but common systemic signs and symptoms.[18]

### Management of Acute Herpetic Gingivostomatitis

The disease is self-limiting. It runs a 7–10-day course and heals without scars. Bland food and liquid supplements are recommended. If the patient is experiencing pain of longer duration, aspirin or a nonsteroidal anti-inflammatory agent can be given systemically. Plaque, food debris and superficial calculus are removed to reduce gingival inflammation, which complicates the acute herpetic involvement. Mucosal ointments (orabase) can be applied to lesions with cotton swabs for temporary relief. Especially before meals, topical local anesthetic, such as lidocaine hydrochloride viscous solution can be applied to the affected areas.[18]

Symptomatic treatment consists of bed rest, antipyretics and analgesics to control fever and relieve pain. Topical application of dyclonine HCl (0.5%), lidocaine viscous or a mixture of equal parts of diphenhydramine (benadryl) elixir and kaopectate is done. Encourage lots of oral fluid intake as dehydration may be a problem in young patient. Occasionally intravenous fluids may be necessary. Isolate the patient from siblings and peers to prevent spread of infection. Antibiotics are contraindicated unless there is superinfection. Steroids are also contraindicated as they mask inflammatory signs.

## Pericoronitis

Pericoronitis is a gingival inflammation in relation to the crown of an incompletely erupted tooth. Ideally the

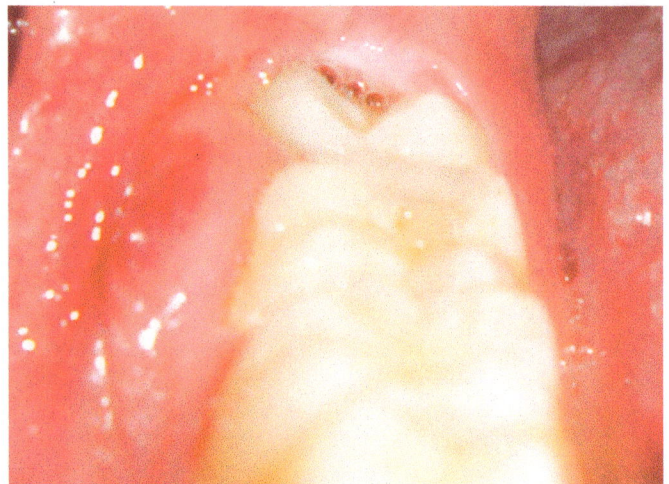

**Fig. 64.7:** Clinical picture showing pericoronitis.

accumulation of food debris and bacterial growth occurs in the space between the crown of the tooth and the overlying gingival flap **(Fig. 64.7)**. Acute pericoronitis is diagnosed with varying degrees of inflammatory involvement of the pericoronal flap and adjacent structures along with presence of systemic complications. The presence of inflammatory fluid and cellular exudate enhances the bulk of the flap, which hinders with complete closure of the jaws, and gets traumatized by contact with the opposing jaw, aggravating the inflammatory involvement.

The patient usually complains of inability to open the jaws more than a few millimeters. This is because of severe tenderness and extreme pain of pericoronitis. It is usually treated by debridement and antibiotic therapy. In some cases surgical removal of pericoronal flap (operculectomy) may be necessary.[18]

# PERIODONTITIS

## Chronic Periodontitis

It mainly affects about one-half of the adult population. However, it can be noted in children and adolescents. Chronic periodontitis commonly involves both primary and permanent dentitions and disease progression is slow in nature. Affected children present with loss of periodontal attachment and bone. The disease originates from development of bacterial plaque and *Porphyromonas gingivalis* is the most commonly associated organism. Host exhibits neutrophil defense mechanism as a part of immune response. Host inflammatory response contributes to the disease process. Localized periodontitis involves less than 30% sites in the mouth and generalized cases exhibit more than 30% involvement.

## Aggressive Periodontitis

This form of periodontitis can affect at different age groups and persists in older adults too. Hence, the initial term of early-onset periodontitis is removed. Localized juvenile periodontitis or localized early-onset periodontitis is now replaced with the term "localized aggressive periodontitis (LAP)". Likewise, generalized early-onset periodontitis is replaced by the new term as "generalized aggressive periodontitis".

### Localized Aggressive Periodontitis

It is a new term for localized juvenile periodontitis. Localized aggressive periodontitis can occur in healthy children and adolescents in the absence of clinical features of systemic disease. The disease is manifested as the rapid and severe loss of alveolar bone around more than one permanent tooth, mainly involving the 1st molars and incisors. Clinically, LAP is presented with little or no tissue inflammation and very little supragingival dental plaque or calculus. In LAP progression of bone loss is 3–4 times faster compared to chronic periodontitis. The radiograph shows localized arc-shaped bone loss around permanent incisors and first permanent molars.

Localized aggressive periodontitis is not thought to be a single disease entity. The causative microbial agents thought to be responsible for LAP are *Aggregatibacter actinomycetemcomitans* or *A. actinomycetemcomitans* in combination with *P. gingivalis, Prevotella intermedia* and *Fusobacterium nucleatum*. A variety of neutrophil defects are seen in patient with LAP.

### Generalized Aggressive Periodontitis

Clinically, generalized aggressive periodontitis is characterized by generalized interproximal attachment loss affecting at least three permanent teeth other than 1st molars and incisors. In generalized aggressive periodontitis there is pronounced episodic nature of the destruction of attachment and alveolar bone. Affected teeth harbor nonmotile, facultative, anaerobic, gram-negative rods.

# PERIODONTITIS AS A MANIFESTATION OF SYSTEMIC DISEASES

In children occurrence of periodontitis as a manifestation of systemic disease is a rare entity. However, it develops between the time of eruption of the primary teeth up to the age of 4 years or 5 years.

## Leukocyte Adhesion Deficiency

Prepubertal generalized aggressive periodontitis is one of the oral manifestations of leukocyte adhesion deficiency (LAD). It occurs as autosomal recessive traits and exists in two forms as LAD I and LAD II. The disease is characterized by defect in leukocyte surface glycoprotein and result in poor leukocyte adherence. Systemic manifestations are present in the form of frequent respiratory, skin, ear and soft-tissue bacterial infections. Severe gingivitis and periodontitis results in periodontal destruction and leads to tooth loss. The rapid attachment and bone loss after eruption lead to early exfoliation of deciduous dentition. In most of the cases disease does not respond to local therapy and bone marrow transplantation remains the only option.

## Down Syndrome

In Down syndrome patients, the prevalence of periodontal diseases is 60–100%. Clinical manifestations of periodontitis can occur in primary dentition with peculiar involvment of mandibular incisors. Down syndrome, a generic form of mental retardation resulting from the presence of three copies of chromosome 21, is accompanied by an increased susceptibility to periodontitis. Various minor immune deficits, particularly in neutrophil function, have been identified in patients with Down syndrome and may be responsible for the increased susceptibility to periodontitis. Severe recession in the mandibular anterior region associated with high frenum attachment is also common in Down syndrome.

## Neutropenia

Neutropenia occurs due to reduced circulating polymorphonuclear cells. Cyclic neutropenia is the severe form of neutropenia. Chronic benign neutropenia of childhood, chronic idiopathic neutropenia and familial benign neutropenia are other types.

Clinical manifestation of neutropenia-associated periodontitis includes severe gingivitis with ulcerations, alveolar bone loss, early loss of deciduous teeth and severe periodontal disease in permanent dentition. There may be a history of other soft-tissue infections. White blood cell differential count leads to diagnosis of this entity.

## Acute Leukemia

In acute myeloblastic leukemia (AML), infiltration with leukemic cells leads to gingival enlargement. The common presenting symptom is presence of hyperplastic, edematous and bluish red gingiva. Petechiae or mucosal ulcerations are the clinical manifestations in any form of leukemia associated with thrombocytes and coagulation abnormalities. Gingival ulceration is common. Complete blood picture is helpful for the initial diagnosis of disease.

## Langerhans Cell Histiocytosis

Abnormal proliferation and dissemination of histiocyte cells of Langerhan's system lead to development of a group of disorders with variable symptoms termed as Langerhan's cell histiocytosis. Generally 10% of them show oral involvement. Bone lesions produce floating teeth. Gingival swelling is seen. The disease is confirmed with biopsy and histopathological examination.

## Acquired Immune Deficiency Syndrome

In children, human immunodeficiency virus (HIV) infection is also associated with necrotizing ulcerative periodontitis. The severity of periodontitis is shown to be associated with a reduction in CD4 lymphocyte levels. In HIV-infected children, a typical gingival inflammation around the marginal gingiva and linear gingival erythema are common presenting features. Along with this, spontaneous gingival bleeding and deep aching pain are also noted. This may progress to cancrum oris or noma in undernourished and debilitated individuals. The prevalence of periodontal disease in children who are not under antiviral therapy is estimated to be around 55%. Orofacial lesions associated with pediatric AIDS include candidiasis, herpes simplex infection, parotid enlargement and recurrent aphthous stomatitis, childhood, chronic idiopathic neutropenia and familial benign neutropenia.

Periodontal involvement is presented in the form of severe gingivitis with ulcerations, alveolar bone loss, early loss of deciduous teeth and severe periodontal disease in permanent dentition. There may be a history of other soft-tissue infections. Diagnosis is confirmed by estimating white blood cell differential count.

## Insulin-dependent Diabetes Mellitus (Type I)

Type I diabetes mellitus is presented with the fasting blood sugar level more than 120 mg/dL. This type of diabetes is associated with increased incidence of gingivitis, increased risk and earlier onset of periodontitis (10–15% teenagers) and alveolar bone resorption. The disease incidence enhances after puberty and with growing age. It is associated with reduced function of neutrophils along with the presence of xerostomia and recurrent gingival abscesses. Reduced salivary flow leads to increase caries risk. Altered oral microflora with increased *Candida albicans*, hemolytic streptococci, and staphylococci is seen. Plaque and calculus levels are comparable to normal controls. There is increased susceptibility to infections and reduced wound healing. Both premature and delayed eruption of permanent teeth are observed. Dental management includes advising the patient to take normal diet before dental appointment to prevent hypoglycemia. If dental procedure is anticipated to be stressful, consult the physician for adjustment in insulin dosage. Prophylactic antibiotic is given before the procedure. If hypoglycemia is encountered during dental treatment, glucose should be given.

## Papillon and Lefèvre Syndrome

In 1924, Papillon and Lefèvre discovered this syndrome. It is a rare autosomal-recessive disorder characterized by mutation in cathepsin C gene located on chromosome 11 (11q14–q21). The disease is characterized by rapid generalized destruction of alveolar bone, palmar-plantar hyperkeratosis, intracranial calcification and retardation of somatic development. It affects both the deciduous and permanent dentitions.[19]

## Chediak–Higashi Syndrome

It is an autosomal-recessive mode of inheritance disease localized to chromosome 1q43. There is a fusion of azurophil and specific granules into giant granules called megabodies in neutrophils. It is characterized by decreased chemotaxis, decreased degranulation, decreased microbial activity of neutrophils. Oral manifestations are severe periodontitis and oral ulceration.

## ANATOMICAL PERIODONTAL PROBLEMS

### Localized Gingival Recession

Gingival recession is often observed in children. There are many causes of gingival recession some of them are toothbrush trauma, tooth prominence, orthodontic tooth movement, oral habits, alveolar bony dehiscence.

In labial version, gingival recession occurs on teeth. It is also noted on those that are tilted or rotated so that the roots project labially **(Fig. 64.8)**. Anterior open bite increases the prevalence of gingival recession. The recession may occur in a transitional phase in tooth eruption process and correct itself with the proper alignment of teeth. Sometimes it is necessary to realign the teeth orthodontically.[20-22]

Intraoral and perioral piercings may cause injury to the gingival tissues, such as inflammation and recession. Constant pressure being applied to a specific area repeatedly may result in severe localized attachment loss. Tongue piercing was a significant factor in the development of lingual recession in the mandibular anterior teeth. Effective educational strategies and cessation programs are needed to target adolescent dental patients who choose to have tongue or lip piercings.[22]

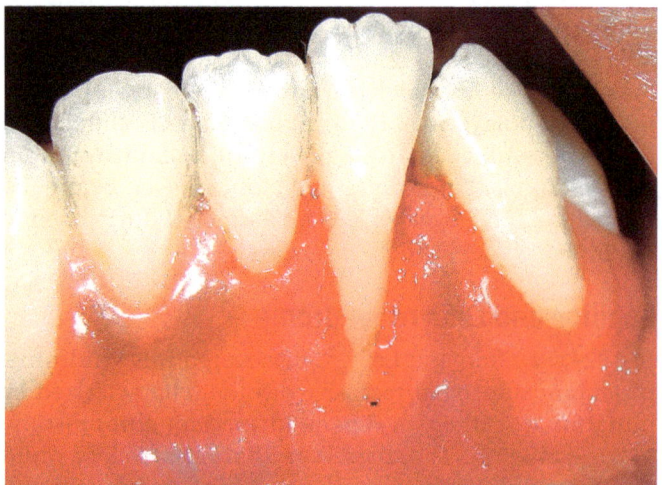

**Fig. 64.8:** Clinical picture showing localized gingival recession.

### Abnormal Frenum Attachment

Abnormal frenum jeopardizes gingival health as it interferes with proper placement of a toothbrush and open gingival crevice by muscle pull. Frenum is judged abnormal when the frenum is unusually broad or there is no apparent attached gingiva in the midline or interdental papilla moves by stretching the frenum.[21,22]

## CHILDHOOD DISEASES AFFECTING GINGIVA

The various common childhood diseases, which present specific alterations in gingival tissues, are as follows:
- *Chickenpox*: Small blisters-like lesions on the gingiva appear which are not particularly painful. These lesions are slightly raised vesicles with the surrounding erythema, which rupture soon after formation and then form small eroded ulcers with red margins
- *Measles*: Palatal petechiae along with the generalized inflammation and focal ulceration of the gingiva are the oral manifestations seen in children suffering from measles.
- *Scarlet fever*: Palatal gingiva appears congested and often fiery red.
- *Diphtheria*: Diphtheritic membrane sometime appears on the gingiva. This membrane is a false membrane which is grayish, thick, fibrinous gelatinous appearing exudate containing dead cells, leukocytes and bacteria. It tends to be adherent and leaves a bleeding surface if stripped away.

## MAINTENANCE

Maintenance of gingival and periodontal health in children can be divided into following phases:[22-25]
- *Infants (Birth to 1 year of age)*.
  - Cleaning of gum pads: Parents should clean gum pads daily before eruption of first primary tooth. A wet clean cloth is wrapped around the index finger and gum pads are massaged.
  - Introduce soft bristled toothbrush.
  - Do not use dentifrices especially containing fluoride.
- *Toddlers (1–3 years of age)*.
  - Introduce soft bristled toothbrush.
  - Use dentifrices around 2 years of age using pea-sized amount.
  - Parents or caregivers should brush children's teeth.
- *Preschool (3–6 years of age)*.
  - Use dentifrices around 2 years of age using pea-sized amount.
  - Dental flossing is recommended in interproximal
  - areas having tooth-to-tooth contact.
  - Children should be assisted by parents or caregivers in toothbrushing.
- *Toothbrush*: The dimension of the handle of an adult is 6 inches and for child it is one-third smaller than adult

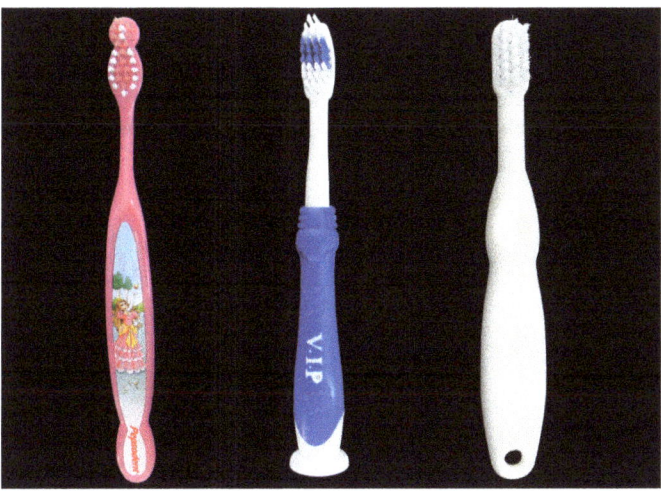

**Fig. 64.9:** Photograph showing small toothbrushes for children.

size **(Fig. 64.9)**. Nylon bristles are of 0.1 mm (0.005 inch) diameter and 8.7 mm (0.344 inch) length.
- Powered toothbrushes are recommended for children with physical or mental disabilities and children with fixed orthodontic appliances.
- *Dentifrice*: Pea-sized amount of dentifrice should be used. Fluoridated dentifrice is recommended as per age and caries status of children. Low-fluoride dentifrice (e.g., 400–500 ppm fluoride) is also available in market for children. Nowadays, dentifrice containing natural protective enzymes like lactoferrin, lactoperoxidase and lysozyme are also available.[26]
- *Toothbrushing method*: Fones or scrub method is usually recommended in school children or young children because of simplicity. Dr Fones advocated this circular method. The method involves closing the teeth and lightly pressing bristles of toothbrush against posterior teeth and gingiva.[27] Brush head should be revolved in a fast circular motion with a large diameter circles. Continue circular motion. Hold maxillary and mandibular teeth apart and continue same circular motion on maxillary lingual surfaces and then on mandibular lingual surfaces.

Diagnosis at early stages ensures the better treatment outcomes. Hence, it is important that children should receive a periodontal examination as part of their routine dental visits.

### Points to Ponder

- Retrocuspid papilla is a circumscribed nodule of the gingival tissue which lies lingual to the mandibular canine in young children. It disappears with age.
- Herpetic gingivostomatitis is the viral infection that affects the gingiva of infants and children younger than 6 years of age.
- Parents should clean gum pads daily before eruption of first primary tooth.
- The dimension of the handle of an adult is 6 inches and for child it is 1/3rd smaller than adult size.

## REFERENCES

1. Itoiz ME, Carranza FA. The gingiva. In: Newman MG, Takei HH, Carranza FA (Eds). Carranza's Clinical Periodontology, 9th edition. Philadelphia, PA, USA: WB Saunders; 2003. pp. 16-35.
2. Bernard GW, Carranza FA. The tooth supporting structures. In: Newman MG, Takei HH, Carranza FA (Eds). Carranza's Clinical Periodontology, 9th edition. Philadelphia, PA, USA: WB Saunders; 2003. pp. 36-57.
3. Bhaskar SN. Maxilla and mandible (alveolar process). In: Orban's Oral Histology and Embryology, 11th edition. St. Louis: CV Mosby; 1991. pp. 239-59.
4. Carranza FA. Gingival disease in childhood. In: Newman MG, Takei HH, Carranza FA (Eds). Carranza's Clinical Periodontology. 9th edition. Philadelphia, PA, USA: WB Saunders; 2003. pp. 308-13.
5. Lindhe J, Karring T, Araujo M. Anatomy of the periodontium. In: Lindhe J, Karring T, Lang NP (Eds). Clinical Periodontology and Implant Dentistry, 4th edition. Oxford, UK: Blackwell Munksgaard; 2003. pp. 3-49.
6. Grant DA, Stern IB, Listgarten MA. Gingiva and dentogingival junction. In: Periodontics, 6th edition. St. Louis: CV Mosby; 1988. pp. 25-55.
7. Bimstein E, Eidelman E. Longitudinal changes in the width of attached gingiva in children. Pediatr Dent. 1988;10;22-4.
8. Soni NN, Silberkweit M, Hayes RL. Histological characteristics of stippling in children. J Periodontol. 1963;34:427-31.
9. Maynard JG Jr, Ochsenbein C. Mucogingival problems, prevalence and therapy in children. J Periodontol. 1975;46(9):543-52.
10. Modéer T, Wondimu B. Periodontal diseases in children and adolescents. Dent Clin North Am. 2000;44(3):633-58.
11. Kinane DF. Periodontal disease in children and adolescents. Periodontol 2000. 2001;26:7-15.
12. Cameron AC, Widmer RP, Australasian Academy of Paediatric Dentistry (AAPD). Handbook of Pediatric Dentistry, 4th edition. St. Louis: Mosby-Elsevier; 1999. pp. 65-72.
13. Doufexi A, Mina M, Ioannidou E. Gingival overgrowth in children: epidemiology, pathogenesis, and complications. A literature review. J Periodontol. 2005;76(1):3-10.
14. Carranza FA, Hogan EL. Gingival enlargement. In: Newman MG, Takei HH, Carranza FA (Eds). Carranza's Clinical Periodontology, 9th edition. Philadelphia, PA, USA: WB Saunders; 2003. pp. 279-96.
15. Hasan AA, Ciancio S. Relationship between amphetamine ingestion and gingival enlargement. Pediatr Dent. 2004;26(5):396-400.
16. Kamolmatyakul S, Kietthubthew S, Anusaksathien O. Long-term management of an idiopathic gingival fibromatosis patient with the primary dentition. Pediatr Dent. 2001;23(6):508-13.
17. Tay YK, Bellus G, Weston W. What syndrome is this? Gingival fibromatosis-hypertrichosis syndrome. Pediatr Dermatol. 2001;18(6):534-36.
18. Carranza FA, Klokkevold PR. Acute gingival infections. In: Newman MG, Takei HH, Carranza FA (Eds). Carranza's Clinical Periodontology, 9th edition. Philadelphia, PA, USA: WB Saunders; 2003. pp. 297-307.
19. Hart TC, Shapira L. Papillon-Lefèvre syndrome. Periodontol 2000. 1994;6:88-100.
20. Zappler SE. Periodontal disease in children. J Am Dent Assoc. 1948;37(3):333-45.
21. Bradley RE. Periodontal lesions in children: their recognition and treatment. Dent Clin North Am. 1961;671-85.
22. Maynard JG Jr, Wilson RD. Diagnosis and management of mucogingival problems in children. Dent Clin North Am. 1980;24(4):683-703.

## Section 9: Interdisciplinary Approach

23. Clerehugh V, Tugnait A. Diagnosis and management of periodontal diseases in children and adolescents. Periodontol 2000. 2001;26:146-68.
24. Studen-Pavlovich D, Ranalli DN. Periodontal and soft tissue prevention strategies for the adolescent dental patient. Dent Clin North Am. 2006;50(1):51-67.
25. del Aguila MA, Anderson M, Porterfield D, Robertson PB. Patterns of oral care in a Washington State dental service population. J Am Dent Assoc. 2002;133(3):343-51.
26. Damle SG. Maintenance of oral hygiene in infants and children. In: Textbook of Pediatric Dentistry, 3rd edition. New Delhi, India: Arya (Medical) Publishing House; 2010. pp. 232-42.
27. Fones AC. Mouth hygiene, 4th edition. Philadelphia, PA, USA: Lea & Febiger; 1934.

### VIVA VOCE

**Q1.** What are the two unique anatomic features seen in the gingiva of children?
**Ans.** Interdental cleft and retrocuspid papilla.

**Q2.** Why in children there is lower prevalence of periodontal diseases as compared to adults?
**Ans.** Children have well-spaced dentitions with absence of contact points hence there is no chance of interdental col formation. In primary teeth, the presence of widespread interdental spacing lead to fusion of papilla from both sides and formation of interdental saddle areas. These areas are covered with well-keratinized epithelium which is less vulnerable for bacterial infection.

**Q3.** Name the various common childhood diseases which affect gingival tissues.
**Ans.** Chickenpox, measles, scarlet fever, diphtheria.

**Q4.** Which tooth brushing method is usually recommended in school children/young children?
**Ans.** Fones or scrub method.

**Q5.** What is the basic difference between the periodontal ligament of deciduous and permanent dentition?
**Ans.** The width of periodontal ligament in deciduous dentition is wider than permanent.

**Q6.** What is the basic difference between the cementum of deciduous and permanent dentition?
**Ans.** Cementum of permanent dentition is thicker and denser than deciduous.

**Q7.** What is Chediak–Higashi Syndrome?
**Ans.** It is an autosomal-recessive mode of inheritance disease localized to chromosome 1q43. There is a fusion of azurophil and specific granules into giant granules called megabodies in neutrophils.

**Q8.** What is Papillon and Lefèvre syndrome?
**Ans.** It is a rare autosomal-recessive disorder characterized by mutation in cathepsin C gene located on chromosome-11 (11q14–q21).

**Q9.** What are the clinical manifestations in any form of leukemia?
**Ans.** Petechiae or mucosal ulcerations.

**Q10.** How gum pads of infants are cleaned?
**Ans.** Parents wrap wet clean cloth around the index finger and gum pads should be massaged daily.

# Chapter 65

# Periodontics-Oral Surgery

*Ramesh Fry, Shalu Bathla*

## Chapter Outline

- Inter-Relationship
- Periodontal Considerations
- Maintenance

## INTRODUCTION

Oral surgery has major contributions in the diagnosis and treatment of oral conditions affecting the jaw and mouth structures which demand surgical intervention. This specialty deals with the surgical removal of teeth and treatment of diseases, deformities and defects of the jaws and associated structures. Because of the close proximity, maxillofacial surgeons have to work in the area which is also under the domain of other surgical specialties, like neurosurgery, otorhinolaryngology, ophthalmology and orthopedics. Apart from this, oral surgeons have to work in an area where other specialties of dentistry have to work afterwards for the complete rehabilitation of the patient, such as prosthodontics, orthodontics, endodontics and periodontics. Though relationship of oral surgery with medical specialties, prosthodontics and orthodontics is much talked about in literature, we do not find much literature on relationship of periodontics and oral surgery.

## INTER-RELATIONSHIP

While doing surgical procedures in the maxillofacial region surgeon is likely to injure the tooth supporting structures, like the gingiva, periodontium and alveolar bone, leading to plaque retention, gingivitis, pocket formation and alveolar bone loss. Thus, perio-oral surgery relationship becomes very important for a successful clinical practice. We can divide perio-oral surgery relationship into two main headings:
1. Inadvertent injury to periodontium during oral surgical procedures.
2. Spread of infection during oral surgical procedures.

### Inadvertent Injury to Periodontium during Oral Surgical Procedures

The most common oral surgical procedures which can cause inadvertent injury to periodontium include:
- Removal of an impacted tooth.
- Fixation of maxillomandibular fixation (MMF) apparatus on the teeth.

#### Removal of an Impacted Tooth

Removal of an impacted tooth is considered as bread and butter procedure for maxillofacial surgeons. Much has been discussed in literature about prevention of major postoperative complications, such as fracture of the jaw, pain, swelling, infection, trismus, etc. The greatest periodontal hazard in oral surgery is development of distal pocket on 2nd molars following extraction of impacted 3rd molars.

The most common complication reported is the iatrogenic damage to the gingiva of the mandibular aspect of 2nd molar. During impaction surgery, the peripheral gingival soft tissues may get damaged on flap elevation, during bone removal or tooth sectioning with rotary instruments. Patient usually complains of pain with loss of the thin band of keratinized gingiva of the 2nd molar. This problem gets worsened due to surgically induced bone defect associated with impaction removal. In case of unerupted tooth, the distal part of the 2nd molar is usually adjacent to the anterior border of the ascending ramus with total lack of clinically evident distobuccal collar of keratinized gingiva. Only a thin band of keratinized gingiva (often <1 mm in width) can be found on the buccal aspect of the tooth. Flap reflection and removal of the impacted mandibular 3rd molar in such patient may lead to destruction of little attached gingiva which was available before surgery. Disruption of the gingival attachment of the 2nd molar and destruction of the fragile attached gingival collar results in an immediate loss in vestibular depth. This is due to the pull of the buccinator muscle insertions on the flap. This usually avoids cervical reattachment of the gingiva to the 2nd molar and disturbs the healing of the remaining nonkeratinized gingiva. This is responsible for plaque retention, inflammation and pocket formation demanding secondary periodontal therapy.[1-3]

### *Fixation of Maxillomandibular Fixation Apparatus on the Teeth*

The main objective of MMF is provision of indirect stabilization of fractures of the maxilla, mandible or both. With the technique of using arch bars, generally 16–22 interdental wires are passed. The patient has to keep his mouth closed from 4 weeks to 6 weeks. Passing of wires and presence of arch bar in the neck of the tooth causes injury to the periodontium. Prolonged MMF also leads to poor oral hygiene status which further aggravates the condition. Though ivy eyelet wiring is a good alternative but still some wires have to be passed through the neck of the teeth leading to injury of periodontium and also there is difficulty in maintaining oral hygiene. It has some limitations like we cannot use this method in severely displaced and impacted fractures as elastic traction cannot be given.

Another alternative can be the use of transalveolar screws. The technique of intraoral transalveolar bone screw fixation begins with local anesthetic administration, followed by the use of a curved mosquito hemostat to perforate the mucosa to the level of the periosteum, then elevation with a periosteal elevator. A 2.1 mm drill bit is used to perforate the bone before the insertion of 2.7 mm self-tapping screws. Screws 18–20 mm long are used in the maxilla while 20 mm long screws are chosen for the mandible. It has many advantages including increased patient compliance, improved oral hygiene, decreased rate of infection and no penetration of wires through gingiva.

### Spread of Infection during Oral Surgical Procedures

As incidence of periodontal diseases are very high in a developing country, like India, a patient requiring maxillofacial surgical procedure may also be suffering from some periodontal disease. Thus, chances of spread of infection from infected periodontium to surgical site are high. As a rule thorough oral prophylaxis should be done prior to any oral surgical procedure. When multiple extractions are to be done, first maxillary teeth should be extracted so that specks of calculus do not fall into fresh mandibular extraction sockets. Whenever cyst or tumor removal warrants extraction of the involved tooth, prior oral prophylaxis should be done so that debris from extracted tooth should not contaminate the surgical area.

Pericoronitis is one of the most common conditions where patient is referred to either oral surgeon or periodontist. Operculectomy should only be done in soft tissue impactions where there is no hindrance in eruption of tooth either from adjacent bone or tooth, otherwise removal of impacted tooth should be sought.[2]

## PERIODONTAL CONSIDERATIONS

### Atraumatic Extraction of Infected Teeth

Teeth should be extracted in an atraumatic manner to conserve alveolar bone. If bone is to be removed to avoid fracturing a tooth or the alveolus, it is best to remove the tooth through a lingual or palatal approach to conserve the remaining buccal plate of bone. The extreme challenge to conserve the soft and hard tissues of the ridge arises when tooth to be extracted has fractured or decayed to the level of gingival margins or crestal bone. The design of soft tissue flaps and plans for osseous resection must be thought carefully to prevent the formation of a deformity in the healed residual ridge. Surgical elevators and forceps must be used with extreme caution in such conditions.[4]

### Postextraction Management of Socket Area

Extraction sockets should be inspected carefully for any sign of infection after the teeth or remaining roots have been removed. Granulomatous tissue should be curette to remove it from its attachment to the walls or the base of the sockets and the area should be irrigated thoroughly to ensure removal of all debris and loose bony spicules. Earlier, clinicians used to apply pressure at the crest of the socket to compress the rim of the alveolar bone. But this practice should be avoided as it results in the collapse of the remaining buccal plate of bone and also hastens the formation of a deformity within the ridge.

## MAINTENANCE

### Preparation of the Mouth Prior to General Inhalational Anesthesia

Plaque control and professional instrumentation aid in reducing the oral bacteria count. Because the mouth is an entrance to the respiratory chamber, the possibility always exists that debris and fluids may be inhaled from the mouth during the administration of an anesthetic or when the patient coughs.

### Patient with Intermaxillary Fixation

All possible attempts should be made to keep patient's mouth clean for good comfort and sanitation. Attempt should also be made for keeping mouth plaque-free in order to prevent disease development. The patient wearing fixation appliances involving only the mandible when suffering from temporomandibular joint injury, finds it difficult to apply a toothbrush to the lingual surface of teeth. Almost all factors including appliances, the condition of the lips, tongue and other oral tissue and the cooperation of the patient affect the extent of oral care. The patient should receive an encouragement for toothbrushing as soon as possible after the surgical procedure. However, before that a plan for care is outlined for a caregiver for providing adequate oral care. The limited access for personal oral care procedures and the effect of the liquid diet required for most cases define the need for special dental hygiene care for the patient with intermaxillary fixation. After removal of appliances, almost all patients experience a degree of muscular trismus that hinders toothbrushing and mastication. When the patient can open mouth normally then plaque control procedures are initiated and complete scaling and root planing can be performed.[5]

### Points to Ponder

- Teeth should be extracted in an atraumatic manner to conserve alveolar bone.
- Clinician should avoid applying pressure at the crest of the socket to compress the rim of the alveolar bone as it results in the collapse of the remaining buccal plate of bone and also hastens the formation of a deformity within the ridge.

## REFERENCES

1. Motamedi MH. A technique to manage gingival complications of third molar surgery. Oral Surg Oral Med Oral Pathol Oral Radiol Endod. 2000;90(2):140-3.
2. Ramfjord SP, Ash MM. Periodontal considerations in restorative and other aspects of dentistry. In: Periodontology and Periodontics: Modern Theory and Practice, 1st edition. New Delhi, India: AITBS Publisher and Distributor; 1996. pp. 339-51.
3. Richardson DT, Dodson TB. Risk of periodontal defects after third molar surgery: An exercise in evidence-based clinical decision-making. Oral Surg Oral Med Oral Pathol Oral Radiol Endod. 2005;100(2):133-7.
4. Seibert JS. Treatment of moderate localized alveolar ridge defects. Preventive and reconstructive concepts in therapy. Dent Clin North Am. 1993;37(2):265-80.
5. Wilkins EM. The oral and maxillofacial surgery patient. In: Clinical Practice of the Dental Hygienist, 2nd edition. Philadelphia, PA, USA: Lippincott Williams & Wilkins; 1999. pp. 707-20.

### VIVA VOCE

**Q1.** Why mouth preparation is done prior to general inhalational anesthesia?
**Ans.** Plaque control and professional instrumentation aid in reducing the oral bacteria count. As mouth is an entrance to the respiratory chamber, the possibility always exists that debris and fluids may be inhaled from the mouth during the administration of an anesthetic.
**Q2.** Which oral surgical procedures can cause inadvertent injury to periodontium?
**Ans.** Removal of an impacted tooth and fixation of maxillo-mandibular fixation apparatus.
**Q3.** What is the greatest periodontal hazard related to extraction of impacted third molar?
**Ans.** Development of distal pocket on second molar.
**Q4.** In which kind of impactions, operculectomy is indicated?
**Ans.** In soft tissue impactions where there is no hindrance in eruption of tooth either from adjacent bone or tooth.
**Q5.** What is the main disadvantage related to prolonged maxillomandibular fixation (MMF)?
**Ans.** Prolonged MMF leads to poor oral hygiene status.
**Q6.** Which are possible structures that can be injured during the surgical procedures in the maxillofacial region?
**Ans.** Gingiva, periodontium and alveolar bone.
**Q7.** What is the length of the screws that are used for MMF?
**Ans.** 18–20 mm long screws are used in the maxilla; while 20 mm long screws are chosen for the mandible.
**Q8.** Which teeth should be extracted first, in case of multiple extractions?
**Ans.** First maxillary then mandibular.
**Q9.** What is the main indication of operculectomy?
**Ans.** Soft tissue impactions.
**Q10.** Why oral prophylaxis is done before extraction of the involved tooth?
**Ans.** So that debris from extracted tooth should not contaminate the surgical area.

# Periodontics-Psychiatry

*Jagdish C Bathla, Manish Bathla, Shalu Bathla*

## Chapter Outline

- Parafunctional Habits
- Psychosomatic Disorders
- Necrotizing Ulcerative Gingivitis and Stress
- Periodontal Aspects of Psychiatric Patients
- Implications of Psychiatric Medications
- Doctor–Patient Relationship

## INTRODUCTION

Biological and behavioral risk factors have been demonstrated as the significant etiological agents in chronic periodontitis. Other factors contributing to chronic periodontitis are smoking, oral hygiene, systemic conditions and age. However, these factors in a whole fail to explain a significant proportion of the variation in disease severity.[1] Psychosocial factors play an important role in addition to the other factors, thus explaining the remaining variance in disease causation. Freud's *Oral Stage of Psychoanalytic Theory* places great importance on the relationship of the oral cavity to the psyche. It is also hypothesized that the psychological and social factors are involved in diseases of the oral cavity.

## PARAFUNCTIONAL HABITS

Parafunctional habits, defined as any oral nonfunctional activity or behavior involving the masticatory system, are neither uncommon nor are they always harmful.[2] These habits represent perversion of occlusion that is potentially injurious to the periodontal tissues, masticatory muscles and temporomandibular joint. They are referred to as "parafunction" which designates tooth contacts in other than chewing and swallowing.

### Classifications of Parafunctional Habits

- *According to the cause, these are classified in three ways*:
    - Tooth to tooth function, e.g., bruxism.
    - Tooth to soft tissue, e.g., digit-sucking.
    - Tooth to foreign object, e.g., chewing of pens and pencils.
- *According to Sorrin and Cheek, the habits are classified into*:
    - Neurosis:
        - Lip biting
        - Fingernail biting
        - Tongue thrusting
        - Pencil or pen biting
    - Occupational habits:
        - Holding of nails in the mouth by cobblers, upholsterers and carpenter
        - Pressure of a reed during the playing of musical instruments
    - Miscellaneous habits:
        - Mouth breathing
        - Thumb sucking
        - Pipe or cigarette smoking
        - Incorrect methods of toothbrushing

### Bruxism, Clenching, and Tapping

Bruxism is a stereotyped oral motor disorder, characterized by teeth grinding and clenching during sleep as well as during wakefulness.[3] The bruxing movement are rhythmic or sustained-tonic contractions of the masseter and other jaw muscles, usually occurs without patient's awareness.[4]

Bruxism consists of aggressive, repetitive or continuous grinding or gritting of the teeth during the day or night or both, i.e., constant or intermittent occlusal contact of the teeth, aside from mastication, swallowing or speech. It often occurs without any neurological disorders or defects and can be viewed as a phenomenon present in healthy individuals. Some individuals are predisposed to bruxism, which seems to have no functional significance.

Clenching is a continuous or intermittent closure of the jaws under pressure.

Tapping or doodling is repetitive tooth contact made on isolated prominent tooth surfaces or dental restorations when mandible is in eccentric occlusion.

According to the International Classification of Sleep Disorders, the diagnostic criteria for sleep-related bruxism are as follows:[5]

- Presence of regular or frequent tooth grinding sounds occurring during sleep.
- Presence of one or more of the following clinical signs:
  - Abnormal tooth wear consistent with above reports of tooth grinding during sleep.
  - Transient morning jaw muscle pain or fatigue; and/or temporal headache; and/or jaw locking on awakening consistent with above reports of tooth grinding during sleep.

### Etiology of Bruxism

- Occlusal disharmonies or prematurities represent struggling movements of the mandible in an attempt to wear away or push aside the offensive tooth surfaces. This is accompanied by abnormal muscle activity and both disappear when occlusal disharmonies are corrected.[6]
- Emotional tension, anxiety and deep-seated aggression could cause or aggravate bruxism, clenching and tapping. The profile of the bruxistic patient to be anxious, aggressive, hyperactive, with intrinsic hostility, and unable to vent frustration outwardly.[7,8] Psychiatrists explain this neurosis as the oral outlet for subconscious aggression.
- *The psychological explanation for bruxism*: All persons have drive that are associated with life goals. When these drives are blocked the resultant frustration produces rage. Rage must have an outlet, i.e., an enraged child does not hesitate to bite. When the child learns that such biting behavior is socially unacceptable, the biting is repressed. When the rage cannot be suppressed, new outlets for its dissipation must be found. Substitute satisfaction (sublimation) may be employed. When the substitution is inadequate, one may still resort to biting to gain satisfaction. This satisfaction may be gained surreptitiously and symbolically on an unconscious level by bruxing or clenching or tapping.
- *Current hypotheses*: The current hypotheses proposed on the etiology of sleep bruxism mentioned the functions of the central and autonomic nervous systems in the genesis of oromandibular activity during sleep. It supports the sleep-related mechanisms under the influence of brain chemicals. Maintenance of airway patency during sleep probably helps to enhance motor activity underlying the genesis of sleep bruxism and rhythmic masticatory muscle activity, the motor manifestation of sleep bruxism preceding tooth grinding during sleep.[9]
- *The role of neurochemicals*: The linking of tooth grinding to a chemical substance in the brain was first reported in a case report of Parkinsonism. Here, a patient of Parkinson disease was treated for tooth grinding with L-3,4-dihydroxyphenylalanine (L-DOPA), a catecholamine precursor.[10]

### Symptoms of Bruxism[11,12]

- Jaw pain and limitation of movement
- Neck pain
- Back pain
- Frequent headaches
- Affects parotid salivary flow (also known as parotid-masseter syndrome)
- Sensitive and sore teeth
- Tooth mobility
- Muscle pain

### Signs of Bruxism[13]

- Morning jaw stiffness
- Tooth or teeth sensitivity
- Hypertrophied masseter and temporalis muscles
- Abfractions
- Fractures
- Flattening of the condyle
- Enlargement of the posterior mandibular ramus angle
- Appearance of intrusion of the posterior dentition
- Indentations or scalloping of the lateral tongue borders
- Ridging of the buccal mucosa
- Exostosis present in the mandible and maxilla

### Consequences of Bruxism on Periodontium

- Excessive tooth wear characterized by polished facets on tooth surfaces with exaggerated facets in normal functional areas.
- Flat inclined planes.
- Widening of occlusal surfaces.
- Reduction in vertical dimension.
- Eccentric occlusion and mandibular deviation.
- The periodontium often responds favorably to the increased function by thickening of the periodontal ligament and increased density of the alveolar bone.
- Aggravates existing periodontal diseases.
- Tooth mobility.
- Muscle fatigue.
- Causes temporomandibular joint disorders secondary to hypertonicity of masticatory muscles.
- Radiographic changes of the mandibular condyles and articular fossas.

### Treatment of Bruxism

Treatment for these habits include:
- Bite appliances (anterior and posterior bite plane)
- Selective grinding
- Orthodontic therapy
- Restorative therapy
- Use of psychotherapy or psychotropic drugs

## Lips, Cheek, and Tongue Biting

The inadvertent habit of biting or chewing of lips, cheek, or tongue can affect periodontal health. Chewing the mucosa on the interior lip or cheek usually results in a keratinized bite line in the affected area. In a Class II Division I malocclusion, the degree of overjet frequently carries the incisal edges of maxillary incisor past the vermilion border of the lower lip. This establishes a wedging force from the labial and circumoral musculature against the lingual aspects of maxillary anteriors. Migration, mobility and degeneration of the labial attachment apparatus can occur.

## Thumb or Hand Sucking

Thumb or hand sucking can be a problem in periodontics only if it continues into the post-childhood years as seen in some congenital diseases or mental retardation. Thumb or hand sucking has profound effect in childhood and contributed to arch displacement and malocclusion. The periodontal result will be the same as those seen in lip, tongue or cheek biting.

## Tongue Thrusting

It entails persistent forceful wedging of tongue, against the teeth particularly in the anterior region. Instead of placing the tongue against the palate with the tip behind the maxillary teeth during swallowing, the tongue is thrust forward against the mandibular anterior teeth, which tilt and also spread laterally. It is usually associated with an abnormal swallowing habit (reverse swallow). It may develop in infancy as a result of bottle feeding or nasopharyngeal diseases.

### Consequences

- It causes excessive lateral pressure, which may be traumatic to the periodontium.
- Spreading and tilting of anterior teeth with open bite anteriorly, posteriorly or in premolar area **(Fig. 66.1)**.

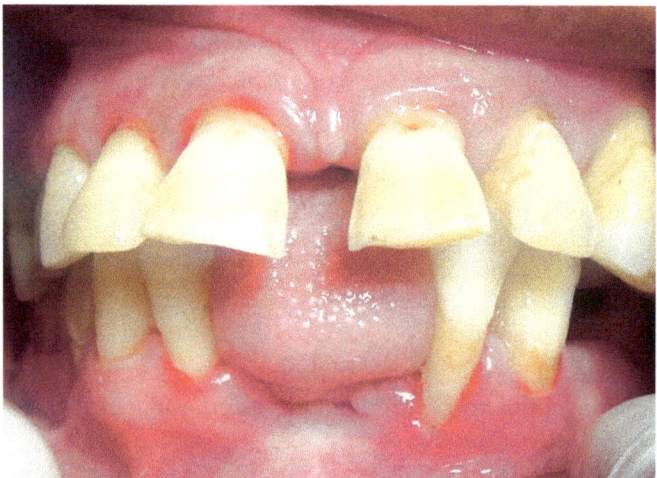

**Fig. 66.1:** Clinical picture showing tongue thrusting which leads to pathologic tooth migration.

- Altered inclination of maxillary anterior teeth results in the change in direction of functional forces, which aggravates the labial drift and undesirable labiolingual rotational forces.
- The antagonism between the forces that direct the tooth labially, and inward pressure from the lip, may lead to tooth mobility.
- Altered inclination of the teeth also interferes with food excursion and favors the accumulation of food debris at gingival margin.
- Loss of proximal contact leads to food impaction.
- Pathological tooth migration.

### Treatment of Tongue Thrusting

It can be performed with appliance therapy, myofunctional and speech therapy, or a combination. Restorative therapy alone will not resolve the damage caused by tongue thrusting. The treatment of the overt anterior thrust must include comprehensive attention to the circumoral as well as the glossal musculature.

## Mouth Breathing

Gingivitis is often seen associated with mouth breathing. The gingival changes include erythema, edema, enlargement and a diffuse surface shininess in the exposed areas. Maxillary anterior region is the most common site of involvement. Its harmful effect is generally attributed to irritation from surface dehydration.

## Factitial Habits

A self-inflicted injury of the periodontal tissues can occur with repeated voluntary trauma to a localized area. This injury can be caused by pacifiers, fingernails, pens, pencils, eyeglass stems and many other provocative objects. Factitial habits, as they are called, can cause a local mechanical injury that invites bacterial contamination and results in inflammatory disease. These habits could proceed from localized recession to bone loss if left unattended. The psychological profile of an individual with a factitial habit should be considered in the treatment plan.

## Cigarette Smoking

Smoking potentially acts by affecting tissue moisture or temperature that has been related to the etiology for necrotizing ulcerative gingivitis (NUG) and other oral diseases as well. Smoking is also inversely related to many psychosocial variables associated with mental health. Hence, an adequate patient management demands better understanding of the cytotoxic effects of tobacco use and the nature of nicotine dependence.

## Dental Problems Associated with Musical Wind Instruments

Wind instruments create forces on the teeth that may injure the periodontium and cause loosening and pathological migration of teeth.

# PSYCHOSOMATIC DISORDERS

Psychosomatic disorders are diseases which involve both mind and body, i.e., there are some physical diseases which are known to be precipitated, aggravated or worsen by mental factors.

Psychosomatic dentistry is defined as the relationship of the mental well-being to the health and integrity of the oral tissues.

In the oral cavity, psychosomatic disorder may be induced by two ways:[14]
- The direct effect of the autonomic nervous system on the physiological tissue balance **(Flowchart 66.1)**.
- The development of habits which are injurious to the periodontium.

## Psychosomatic Factors

- Stress
- Oral hygiene negligence
- Bruxism
- Oral habits
- Smoking and other harmful habits
- Changes in dietary intake
- Lowered host resistance
- Gingival circulation

**Flowchart 66.1:** The role of psychosocial stressors in initiating periodontal diseases.

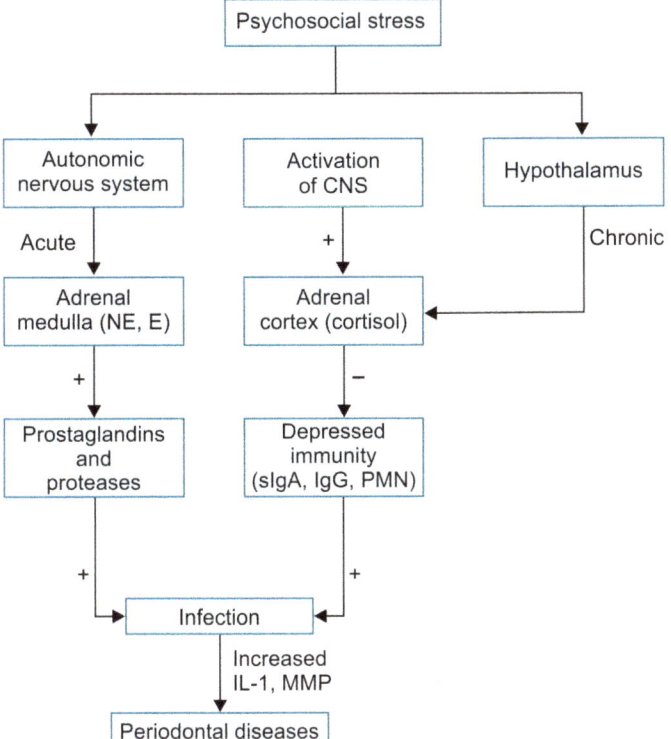

(CNS: central nervous system; NE: norepinephrine; E: epinephrine; IgG: immunoglobulin G; PMN: polymorphonuclear leukocyte; IL-1: interleukin-1; MMP: matrix metalloproteinase)

- Alteration in salivary flow and components
- Others.

## Stress

Selye coined the term "Stress". He defined stress as a total transaction from demand to resolution in response to an environmental encounter that requires appraisal, coping and adaptation by the individual. Coping is the mechanism by which an individual responds to stress (emotionally and physically).

According to Selye, the initial hypothalamic-pituitary-adrenal axis (HPA) response to stress was beneficial. However, if the stressor (mental or physical) persists for prolonged period, it can induce detrimental effects on the body. The body usually responds by reducing the ability to a perceived threat or challenge. This phenomenon was described by Selye as the general adaptation syndrome (GAS).[15,16] GAS is a set of nonspecific physiologic reactions to stress. Response to prolonged stress is a part of the individual's adaptive mechanism which may lead to clinical signs and symptoms called the GAS.

The pioneers who suggested that psychological stress might play a role as an etiological agent of periodontal disease were Dean and Dean (1945) and Schluger (1949). According to these researchers, stress, distress and coping behaviors are considered as crucial factors for development of periodontal disease. Psychosocial factors in association with behavioral changes, such as oral hygiene, smoking, dietary intake, bruxism and drug use, can modify the periodontal status.[17]

Stress and psychosomatic influences are considered to be separate but parallel factors in the causation of disease. The pituitary and adrenal hormones together play a role in regulating the response to stress, involving a feedback mechanism.

Psychosocial stress makes the individual more vulnerable to periodontal diseases, influences the host defenses and hence exerting an immunosuppressive effect. Some of the well-known psychosocial stressors that cause the "vicious cycle" of severe forms of advanced periodontal inflammation and disease are: The consequences of behavioral change, extending from neglect of oral hygiene to dietary inadequacies, poor sleep patterns, use of tobacco products and other substance of abuse.[17]

The less common form of periodontal disease, such as aggressive periodontitis and periodontal disease associated with diabetes, are likely associated with a myriad of intra- and interpersonal stressors. These stressors act as significant risk factors for exacerbation of the underlying periodontal disease condition[18] **(Flowchart 66.2)**.

## Oral Hygiene

A practice of good oral hygiene is partially dependent on the mental health status of the patient. The personal hygiene usually gets neglected in the psychologically disturbed or

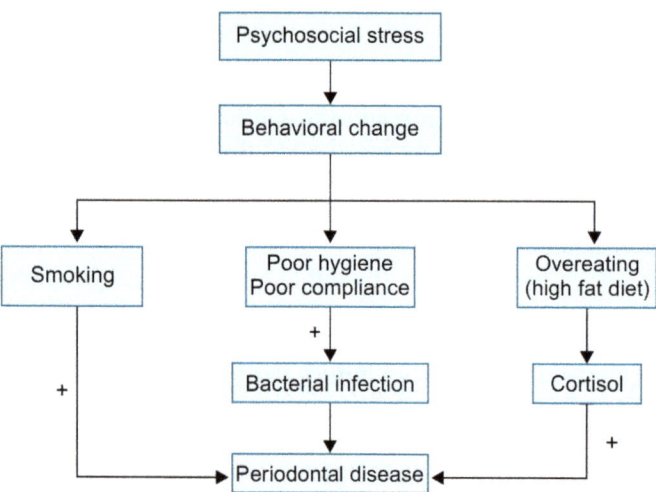

**Flowchart 66.2:** Behavior change as a result of psychosocial stress and its effect on periodontal disease.

distracted patient. Sometimes patients may intentionally ignore oral hygiene because of the result of obsessive thoughts or may be a loss of energy to complete the task. Periodontal disease in such patients might be the result of poor oral hygiene caused by the psychological disturbance.

Oral hygiene may be neglected during depression, anxiety and rebellion against authority or may be a result of passive aggression. However, study data reports little direct effect of depression on plaque accumulation.

Dependent individuals may exhibit chronic neglect as if they were expecting such care to be the responsibility of others. The dentist's instructions concerning oral hygiene may be ignored as a form of "parental defiance".

### Bruxism

Bruxism is explained earlier in section "Bruxism, Clenching, and Tapping" in this chapter.

### Oral Habits

Neurotic needs usually affect oral expression. In neurotics, the mouth may be a way to get satisfaction, to express dependency or hostility, and to inflict or receive pain sensations. In cases of thumb sucking, tongue thrusting, infantile swallowing, and biting of tongue, lip, cheek, or finger nail involving mouth activities like sucking, biting, sensing or feeling may become habitual. These types of actions and activities are also occurring in bruxing, clenching, tooth doodling and smoking. Such habits probably results in tooth migration, occlusal traumatism and occlusal wear.[19]

Coffee drinking is another habit that may act extrinsically (through thermal or chemical properties) and intrinsically (through caffeine content). It is more frequent among smokers and has also been shown to be greater among patients with NUG than among those with healthy gingiva.

### Smoking and Other Harmful Habits

Smoking and other harmful habits are explained in "Chapter 16: Smoking and Periodontium".

### Changes in Dietary Intake

Choice of food is determined by the psychological state of mind. The physical consistency of diet, the consumption of excessive quantities of refined carbohydrates and softer diets that require less vigorous mastication predisposing to plaque accumulation at the proximal risk sites. These factors may have a direct or indirect influence on the periodontium.

### Lowered Host Resistance

Stress and its biochemical mediators can modify the immune response to microbial challenge. This results in decreased defense against periodontal disease. As a result of stress there is release of hormones, such as adrenaline and noradrenaline. These hormones induce a decrease in blood flow. It is also suggested that these hormones possibly reduce those blood elements which are necessary for maintaining resistance to disease-related microbes.[19]

### Gingival Circulation

The emotions may alter the tonus of smooth muscle of blood vessels by the autonomic nervous system, e.g., the prolonged contraction possibly changes the supply of oxygen and nutrients to the tissues.[20] Both smoking and stress play a crucial role in decreasing gingival blood flow. This can enhance the possibility of necrosis of tissues with subsequent reduction in resistance to plaque.[21]

### Alteration in Salivary Flow and Components

Phrases like "spitting mad", "frothing at the mouth" and "drooling in anticipation" shows that salivation has psychiatric implications. Psychological factors are known to influence the rate of secretion and composition of saliva. Saliva has been implicated in plaque formation, calculus deposition, antibacterial and proteolytic activities, all of which have significant impact on periodontal disease. A transient reduction of salivary flow and changes in the salivary enzyme count as a result of mental activity, stress, muscular efforts or emotional disturbances makes the individual more susceptible to oral diseases and disorders. Level of pH has also been observed to go up as salivation increases. These relationships between salivary physiology and psychological status fail to demonstrate causation of periodontal disease. However, such association exhibits a pathway in which periodontal health is affected by salivary changes.[22]

### Other Factors

Patients may have unrealistic attitudes or protective mechanisms that lead them to deny their dental illness. Some patients seeking cosmetic surgery or dental surgery because of somatic delusions may displace their dissatisfaction on the therapist. The acceptance of treatment and its course and success for some patients depends on the therapist's interaction with the patient and management of their psychological status.

## NECROTIZING ULCERATIVE GINGIVITIS AND STRESS

Necrotizing ulcerative gingivitis is a disease that may have an emotional basis. It often occurs in association with stressful situations **(Fig. 66.2)**. Increased adrenocortical secretion and psychological disturbances are common in patients with NUG. Significant correlation between disease incidence and two personality traits, i.e., dominance and abasement, suggests the presence of a NUG-prone personality. The mechanisms whereby psychological factors create or predispose to gingival damage have not been established, but alterations in digital and gingival capillary responses suggestive of increased autonomic nervous activity have been demonstrated in patients with NUG. It can be concluded that opportunistic bacteria are the primary etiologic agents of NUG in patients that demonstrate immunosuppression.

Stress, smoking and preexisting gingivitis are common predisposing factors. Stress has been identified as one of the contributing factors for NUG. Hence, the incidence of NUG increases during periods of physiological and emotional stresses.

The negative effect of stress on the periodontium is possibly due to:[23]
- Altered behaviors, such as poor oral hygiene.
- Smoking.
- Impaired immune function, altogether makes an individual more susceptible for such disease.

Habit of smoking is usually common in such patient population. Increased smoking may be stress associated and commonly leads to vasoconstriction and localized ischemia.

Deinzer et al.[24] reported an increase in the levels of proinflammatory cytokine in stressed gingivitis subjects. Additionally, they strongly believed that stress could probably contribute in the development of NUG and other periodontal diseases. Moreover, stress plays a crucial role in modification of the response to periodontal treatment.

## PERIODONTAL ASPECTS OF PSYCHIATRIC PATIENTS

Some evidences support that patients with mental illness are more susceptible to dental neglect and poor oral health. Dental caries (tooth decay) and periodontal disease (gum disease) are the two commonly noted diseases having a significant impact on the oral cavity.[25]

Advanced dental diseases are commonly noted in patients with psychiatric illnesses, especially schizophrenia probably for following reasons:[26]
- Disease-associated impairments in planning and performing oral hygiene procedures.
- Antipsychotic medications induced adverse effects, such as xerostomia or dry mouth.
- Limited access to treatment due to financial constraints and inadequate number of dentists comfortable in providing care.

### Effect of Depression on Periodontal Health

A web of interactions ensures much adaptive plasticity, so that in most situations, stress induces brain changes that are transient and routinely normalized. At other times, through interactions among genetics, the intensity and duration of stress, along with previous life experiences lead to dysfunction and depression. This results in increased catecholamine secretion which in turn leads to increased proinflammatory cytokine production that enhances the inflammatory reactions in periodontium that may lead to periodontal diseases.[27]

Depression is commonly associated with a lack of interest in oral hygienic procedures, consumption of cariogenic diet, diminishing in salivary flow, rampant dental decay, advanced periodontal disease and oral dysesthesias.[28]

### *Direct Effect of Depression (Stress)*

Affects host resistance factors.

### *Indirect Effects of Depression (Stress)*

- Negligence in performing oral hygiene procedures.
- Increased smoking and use of alcohol.
- Altered food intake.
- Clenching, grinding of the teeth.
- Failure to seek dental care.

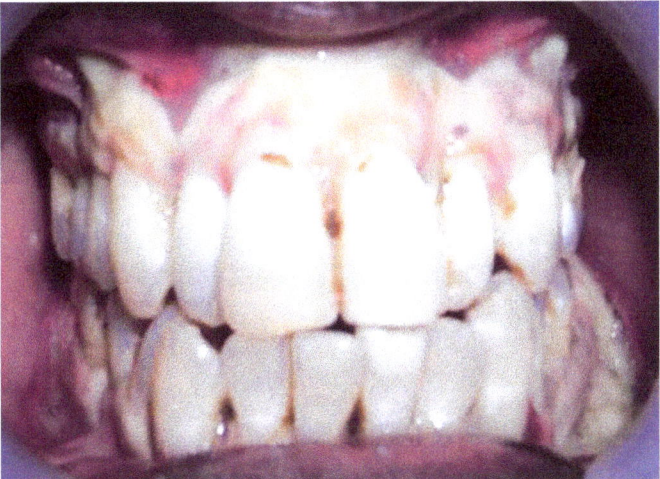

**Fig. 66.2:** Clinical picture showing necrotizing ulcerative gingivitis (NUG).

(*Courtesy*: Dr Ambika Gupta)

## Effect of Anxiety on Periodontal Health

Oral health problems associated with anxiety disorders includes:
- Dry mouth
- Lichen planus
- Canker sores.

People with anxiety disorders may disregard their oral health, hence makes the person more susceptible for periodontal disease and bruxism. Being anxious of a needle can also complicate periodontal procedure.

## Effect of Mental Retardation and Down's Syndrome on Periodontal Health

Prevalence of dental disease in people with Down's syndrome and mental retardation is same as that in general population; these people are more prone to develop more severe form of periodontal disease. Aggressive and generalized periodontitis, along with the subsequent destruction of the supporting tissues and loss of teeth at an early age is usually seen in individuals with Down's syndrome and comorbid mental retardation.

Khocht et al.[29] in their study compared 55 dentate patients suffering from Down's syndrome; 74 with mental disability non-Down's and 88 control subjects. Both groups with Down's syndrome and mental disability non-Down's exhibited significantly more missing teeth, more bleeding on probing, and higher gingival index and plaque index levels compared to the control group. Patients with Down's syndrome showed more attachment loss compared to the other two groups.

Following factors triggers bruxism in individuals with Down's syndrome:
- A state of chronic anxiety.
- Temporomandibular joint dysfunction due to laxity of the supporting ligaments.
- Dental malocclusion.
- Underdeveloped nervous control.

Poor motor development in Down's syndrome frequently leads to dental trauma. Fracture or luxation of the anterior teeth is common and associated with loss of tooth vitality.

## IMPLICATIONS OF PSYCHIATRIC MEDICATIONS

Oral side-effects of psychiatric medications:[25]
- Gingival enlargement or hyperplasia
- Xerostomia
- Altered taste sensation
- Halitosis
- Sialorrhoea
- Dental Caries
- Bruxism
- Parkinsonism and abnormal facial movements (Tics/Orofacial dyskinesia).

Many of the psychiatric medications produce side effects known as medication induced movement disorder. Most common among these are parkinsonism, tardive dyskinesia, and other abnormal facial movements (such as tics and orofacial dyskinesia). These are the side-effects of psychiatric medication for example haloperidol, chlorpromazine, trifluperazine and risperidone.

There is increased prevalence of gingivitis and dental diseases, diurnal and nocturnal sialorrhea and drooling, xerostomia, orofacial pain, the burning mouth syndrome and bruxism.

## Gingival Enlargement or Hyperplasia

Phenytoin-induced gingival overgrowth or enlargement is one of the most serious side-effects noticed with the administration of phenytoin. In the patients on long-term use of phenytoin, enlargement may develop in approximately 50% of the population.[30]

It is mostly marked on the labial surfaces of anterior teeth (**Fig. 66.3**). It usually does not affect edentulous areas. Initial period of 6 months after the administration of treatment with phenytoin plays significant role in the development of gingival enlargement. However, it can be preventable in cooperative patients with regular dental prophylaxis and frequent recalls for reinforcement of plaque control methods.

Initiation of good oral care before the beginning of phenytoin therapy helps to avoid gingival enlargement. However, dental plaque elimination after the appearance of lesion only change the size of enlargement.[26] A preventive dental program involving frequent dental prophylaxis and oral hygiene reinforcement was thought to be effective in reducing enlargement.[31]

Other anticonvulsant drugs causing gingival enlargement are:[32] Carbamazepine, sodium valproate, primidone, vigabatrin. Other non-anticonvulsant drugs causing gingival

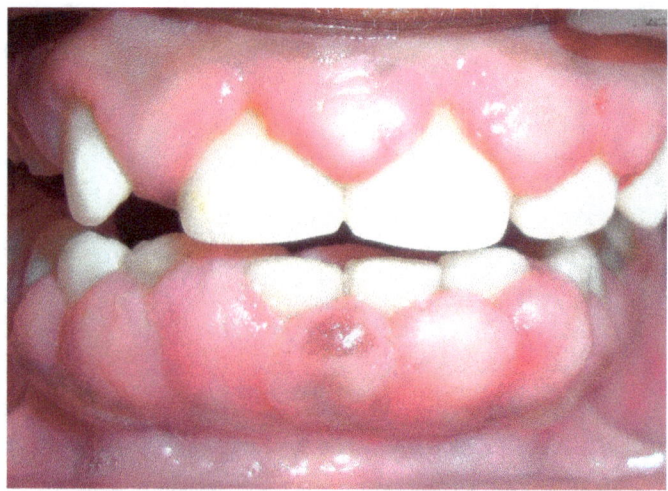

**Fig. 66.3:** Clinical picture showing phenytoin-induced gingival overgrowth or enlargement.

enlargement are: Calcium-channel blockers (nifedipine, amlodipine).

## Xerostomia

Xerostomia is the most common side-effects noted with medications used to treat the psychiatric disorder. It is reported to enhance the incidence of dental diseases. Dryness of mouth being a common adverse effect of tricyclic antidepressants (TCAs) as well as selective-serotonin-reuptake inhibitors (SSRIs); TCAs and SSRIs are the two group of antidepressants most commonly being used.[24]

Xerostomia leads to a change in the oral flora, reduced self-cleaning of the tissues, a loss of buffer capacity, an increased risk of plaque accumulation, gingivitis, periodontitis, caries, candidiasis and sialadenitis.[33] Most of the time hyposalivation is a reversible drug-induced side-effect.

### Medications Producing Xerostomia[25,34]

- *Psychotropic medication*:
  - Tricyclic antidepressants
  - Other antidepressants (e.g., SSRIs)
  - Lithium carbonate
  - Butyrophenones
  - Phenothiazines
  - Sedatives (including benzodiazepines)
- *Nonpsychotropic medication*:
  - Antihistamines
  - Antihypertensives
  - Anticholinergics
  - Diuretics.

## Altered Taste Sensation

Following are the psychiatric medications causing altered taste sensation:[35,36]
- *Anticonvulsants*: Carbamazepine, phenytoin.
- *Antidepressants*: Amitriptyline, clomipramine, desipramine, doxepin, imipramine, nortriptyline.
- *Mood stabilizer*: Lithium.
- *Antipsychotics*: Clozapine, trifluoperazine.
- *Others*: Anti-Parkinsonian, CNS stimulants, migraine medications and hypnotics.

## Halitosis

Following are the psychiatric medications causing halitosis:[37]
- *Antianxiety*: Lorazepam, hydroxyzine, chlordiazepoxide, diazepam, alprazolam.
- *Anticonvulsants*: Carbamazepine, lamotrigine.
- *Antidepressants*: Amitriptyline, desipramine, doxepin, imipramine, amoxapine, fluoxetine, bupropion, clomipramine, fluvoxamine.
- *Antipsychotics*: Clozapine, haloperidol, pimozide, trifluoperazine, chlorpromazine.
- *Sedatives*: Flurazepam.

## Sialorrhea

Sialorrhea is the overproduction of saliva. It is unpleasant for the patient as well as for others. It is commonly noted side-effect of clozapine associated with drooling and soreness of the face. The conditions get improved after reduction in the dose. Anticholinergic medications are recommended to treat sialorrhea in cases where clozapine has to be continued.[25]

## Dental Caries

Depressed patients receiving antidepressants are more vulnerable to increased caries activity.

## Bruxism

Drugs causing bruxism are those drugs that stimulate the central dopaminergic activities such as:
- Cocaine
- Hallucinogens
- SSRIs: Antidepressant medications (citalopram, fluoxetine, paroxetine, sertraline)
- Other antidepressants (buspirone and venlafaxine)
- Chronic use of L-DOPA in Parkinson patients
- Chronic use of neuroleptics by psychiatric patients
- Amphetamine abuse.

## Parkinsonism and Abnormal Facial Movements

The pathogenesis of these disturbances in parkinsonism diseases may be multifactorial:
- Some disorders occur due to general motor impairment and hypokinesia (dental and periodontal diseases due to difficulties in maintaining oral hygiene).
- Others may be a manifestation of involuntary movements (facial dyskinesias/dystonia), due to medication (xerostomia), as a part of sensory dysfunction (taste impairment) or in relation to depressive symptoms (burning mouth syndrome, orofacial pain).

# DOCTOR–PATIENT RELATIONSHIP

## Interview

### Rapport

The doctor–patient relationship begins to form when the patient first meets the dentist. The interview gives the dentist an opportunity to establish rapport, to introduce patient education, and to make the patient familiar with the way in which the practice is conducted. During the interview the chief complaint, the medical history and the dental history are obtained. Simultaneously, the patient is observed for the purpose of making a preliminary evaluation of the individual.

## Observation

A good share of observation consists of being attentive to the patient's manner of response; patient's choice of words; voice tone, pitch, tempo; facial expression and movements during the time of interview. These reactions tend to be heightened in the dental office, since a visit to a dental clinic represents a stressful situation to many patients. Do not lecture the patient on the subject of dentistry.

## Questioning

When the patient asks questions concerning dentistry, he/she may be expressing anxiety rather than an interest in dentistry. The more experienced practitioner will sense this anxiety and reassure the patient. Do not deliver long details on dentistry that does not satisfy the patient's need, leaving the patient with a feeling of frustration.

## Psychological Factors

Qualities of sensitivity, perception and insight can be nurtured by devoting adequate time to the interview. Some knowledge of these qualities is as important to the dentist as it is to the physician.

Responses are clues to the unconscious mind. The unconscious is generally well hidden, and the patient is unaware of its influence on his/her behavior, but the observer can detect the behavior and through it interpret the unconscious mind.

The dentist must deal with the patient's psychological structure and the mouth as a center for emotional manifestations.

## Psychiatric Manifestations during Therapy

### Value Judgements

The dentist should treat the patient with friendliness and respect, not with criticism or condemnation. The patient should be treated with tact and courtesy. The dentist must be sincerely concerned with the welfare of the patient and this should take precedence over dentistry as a business. He/she should try to understand the patient as well as the patient's dental illness. The dentist is often not sufficiently well prepared to meet the psychological demands of the patient or guide the development of new attitudes in patients concerning treatment and health. Although the dentist should conduct a practice in a psychologically sensitive manner, he/she should not attempt psychotherapy per se.

> **Clinical Tip**
> Along with dental examination, a careful history taking for identifying an underlying stress or psychological disorder will help to find out the potential source of stress. In such cases, careful interview is the best source to collect information about the root cause of patient's symptoms. Patient should be referred to a psychiatrist for help.

### Referral

If the dentist perceives a rising level of nervousness or anger, he/she would be best advised to try to determine what he/she or the patient may be doing to precipitate this state of events and if possible deal with its basic cause. When the situation appears to be unmanageable, the patient should be referred to another dentist or physician. The dentist feels less angry when there is no compulsion to comply with impossible demands. This can be done by setting limits for the patient's behavior. The dentist should not view the patient as a threat to himself/herself or his/her competence. The patient should be reassured, not threatened.

## Patient Compliance in Health Care

No other area in health care has more psychological overtones than patient compliance with prescription for medication, smoking, drinking and plaque control. Measures to increase patient compliance with home-care instructions are needed. Self-care motivation is a necessary basis for successful preventive dentistry.

> **Points to Ponder**
> - Psychosomatic disorder in the oral cavity may be caused by either the development of habits that injure the periodontium, or the direct effect of the autonomic nervous system.
> - Psychosocial factors can modify the periodontal status through behavioral changes regarding oral hygiene, smoking, dietary intake, bruxism and drug use.
> - Jacobson's progressive muscle relaxation (JPMR), breathing exercises and guided imagery are simple ways of relieving stress and achieving well-being as a whole.[37]

## REFERENCES

1. Monteiro da Silva AM, Oakley DA, Newman HN, Nohl FS, Lloyd HM. Psychosocial factors and adult onset rapidly progressive periodontitis. J Clin Periodontol. 1996;23(8):789-94.
2. Rugh JD, Ohrbach R. Occlusal parafunctions. In: Mohl ND, Zarb GA, Carlsson GE, Rugh JD (Eds). A Textbook of Occlusion. Chicago, IL, USA: Quintessence Publishing; 1988. p. 249.
3. Lobbezoo F, Van Der Zaag J, Naeije M. Bruxism: Its multiple causes and its effects on dental implants—an updated review. J Oral Rehabil. 2006;33(4):293-300.
4. Bader G, Lavigne G. Sleep bruxism: An overview of an oromandibular sleep movement disorder. Review article. Sleep Med Rev. 2000;4(1):27-43.
5. American Academy of Sleep Medicine, European Sleep Research Society, Japanese Society of Sleep Research, Latin American Sleep Society. Sleep-related bruxism. In: The International Classification of Sleep Disorders, Revised: Diagnosis and Coding Manual, 2nd edition. Westchester, IL, USA: American Academy of Sleep Medicine; 2005. pp. 189-92.
6. Ramfjord SP. Bruxism, a clinical and electromyographic study. J Am Dent Assoc. 1961;62:21-44.
7. Laberge L, Tremblay RE, Vitaro F, Montplaisir J. Development of parasomnias from childhood to early adolescence. Pediatrics. 2000;106(1 Pt 1):67-74.

8. Manfredini D, Ciapparelli A, Dell'Osso L, Bosco M. Mood disorders in subjects with bruxing behavior. J Dent. 2005;33(6):485-90.
9. Klasser GD, Rei N, Lavigne GJ. Sleep bruxism etiology: The evolution of a changing paradigm. J Can Dent Assoc. 2015;81:f2.
10. Winocur E, Gavish A, Voikovitch M, Emodi-Perlman A, Eli I. Drugs and bruxism: A critical review. J Orofac Pain. 2003;17(2):99-111.
11. Goulet JP, Lund JP, Montplaisir J, Lavigne G. Daily clenching, nocturnal bruxism, and stress and their association with TMD symptoms. J Orofac Pain. 1993;7:89-120.
12. Christensen LV. Facial pain from experimental tooth clenching. Tandlaegebladet. 1970;74(2):175-82.
13. Takagi I, Sakurai K. Investigation of the factors related to the formation of the buccal mucosa ridging. J Oral Rehabil. 2003;30(6):565-72.
14. Genco RJ, Ho AW, Kopman J, Grossi SG, Dunford RG, Tedesco LA. Models to evaluate the role of stress in periodontal disease. Ann Periodontol. 1998;3(1):288-302.
15. Morgan CT, King RA, Weisz JR, Schloper J. Emotion and stress. In: Introduction to Psychology, 7th edition. New Delhi, India: Tata McGraw Hill Publishing Company Limited; 1993. pp. 307-38.
16. Stanford TW, Rees TD. Acquired immune suppression and other risk factors/indicators for periodontal disease progression. Periodontol 2000. 2003;32:118-35.
17. Preeja C, Ambili R, Nisha KJ, Seba A, Archana V. Unveiling the role of stress in periodontal etiopathogenesis: An evidence-based review. J Investig Clin Dent. 2013;4(2):78-83.
18. LeResche L, Dworkin SF. The role of stress in inflammatory disease, including periodontal disease: Review of concepts and current findings. Periodontol 2000. 2002;30:91-103.
19. Goyal S, Gupta G, Thomas B, Bhat KM, Bhat GS. Stress and periodontal disease: The link and logic!! Ind Psychiatry J. 2013;22(1):4-11.
20. Manhold JH, Doyle JL, Weisinger EH. Effects of social stress on oral and other bodily tissues. II. Results offering substance to a hypothesis for the mechanism of formation of periodontal pathology. J Periodontol. 1971;42(2):109-11.
21. da Silva AM, Newman HN, Oakley DA. Psychosocial factors in inflammatory periodontal diseases. A review. J Clin Periodontol. 1995;22(7):516-26.
22. Gupta OP. Psychosomatic factors in periodontal disease. Dent Clin North Am. 1966:11-9.
23. Kinane DF, Peterson M, Stathopoulou PG. Environmental and other modifying factors of the periodontal diseases. Periodontol 2000. 2006;40:107-19.
24. Deinzer R, Granrath N, Stuhl H, Twork L, Idel H, Waschul B, et al. Acute stress effects on local Il-1beta responses to pathogens in a human in vivo model. Brain Behav Immun. 2004;18(5):458-67.
25. Cormac I, Jenkins P. Understanding the importance of oral health in psychiatric patients. Adv Psychiatr Treat. 1999;5:53-60.
26. Friedlander AH, Marder SR. The psychopathology, medical management and dental implications of schizophrenia. J Am Dent Assoc. 2002;133(5):603-10.
27. Azmi SA, Fatima Z, Bay A, Gupta ND, Sharma V. Depression and periodontal diseases. Del Psychiatr J. 2014;17(1):7-10.
28. Friedlander AH, Friedlander IK, Gallas M, Velasco E. Late-life depression: Its oral health significance. Int Dent J. 2003;53(1):41-50.
29. Khocht A, Janal M, Turner B. Periodontal health in Down syndrome: Contributions of mental disability, personal, and professional dental care. Spec Care Dentist. 2010;30(3):118-23.
30. Steinberg SC, Steinberg AD. Phenytoin-induced gingival overgrowth control in severely retarded children. J Periodontol. 1982;53(7):429-33.
31. Pihlstrom BL, Carlson JF, Smith QT, Bastien SA, Keenan KM. Prevention of phenytoin associated gingival enlargement: A 15-month longitudinal study. J Periodontol. 1980;51(6):311-7.
32. Dongari-Bagtzoglou A; Research, Science and Therapy Committee, American Academy of Periodontology. Drug-associated gingival enlargement. J Periodontol. 2004;75(10):1424-31.
33. Turner LN, Balasubramaniam R, Hersh EV, Stoopler ET. Drug therapy in Alzheimer disease: An update for the oral health care provider. Oral Surg Oral Med Oral Pathol Oral Radiol Endod. 2008;106(4):467-76.
34. Madinier I, Jehl-Pietri C, Monteil RA. Drug-induced xerostomia. Ann Med Interne (Paris). 1997;148(5):398-405.
35. Douglass R, Heckman G. Drug-related taste disturbance: a contributing factor in geriatric syndromes. Can Fam Physician. 2010;56(11):1142-7.
36. Bromley SM. Smell and taste disorders: A primary care approach. Am Fam Physician. 2000;61(2):427-36, 438.
37. Chandna S, Bathla M. Stress and periodontium: A review of concepts. J Oral Health Comm Dent. 2010;4(Spl):17-22.

## VIVA VOCE

**Q1. What is general adaptation syndrome? Who described this phenomenon?**

**Ans.** General adaptation syndrome (GAS) is a set of nonspecific physiologic reactions to stress. Response to prolonged stress is a part of the individual's adaptive mechanism which may lead to clinical signs and symptoms called the GAS. This phenomenon was described by Selye.

**Q2. What are the possible ways by which the stress affects the periodontium?**

**Ans.** The stress affects the periodontium possibly by: (a) Altered behaviours, such as poor oral hygiene; smoking and (b) Impaired immune function. These factors altogether makes an individual more susceptible for periodontal disease.

**Q3. Which psychiatric medications cause halitosis?**

**Ans.** Following are the psychiatric medications that may cause halitosis:
- Antianxiety: hydroxyzine, chlordiazepoxide, diazepam, alprazolam.
- Anticonvulsants: Carbamazapine, lamotrigine.
- Antidepressants: Amitriptyline, desipramine, doxepin, imipramine, amoxapine, fluoxetine, bupropion, clomipramine, fluvoxamine.
- Antipsychotics: Clozapine, haloperidol, pimozide, trifluoperazine, chlorpromazine.
- Sedatives: Flurazepam.

**Section 9:** Interdisciplinary Approach

**Q4. Which muscles and joints are involved in bruxism?**
**Ans.** Muscles involved in bruxism are the muscles of the face and jaw especially masseter. Joint involved is temporomandibular joint.

**Q5. How are parafunctional habits classified according to the cause?**
**Ans.** According to the cause, parafunctional habits are classified in three ways: (a) Tooth to tooth function, e.g., bruxism; (b) Tooth to soft tissue, e.g. digit-sucking; (c) Tooth to foreign object, e.g., chewing of pens and pencils.

**Q6. Which stage of Freud's places great importance on the relationship of the oral cavity to the psyche?**
**Ans.** Freud's oral stage of psychoanalytic theory.

**Q7. Which is the most common condition associated with mouth breathing.**
**Ans.** Gingivitis

**Q8. Define psychosomatic dentistry.**
**Ans.** Psychosomatic dentistry is defined as the relationship of the mental well-being to the health and integrity of the oral tissues.

**Q9. Who coined the term "stress"?**
**Ans.** Selye.

**Q10. Which oral health problems are associated with anxiety disorders?**
**Ans.** Dry mouth; lichen planus; Canker sores.

# Section 10: Recent Advances

- Recent Advancements in Periodontics

# Chapter 67

# Recent Advancements in Periodontics

*Sana Farista, Veenu M Hans*

## Chapter Outline

- Lasers
- Photodynamic Therapy
- Tissue Engineering
- Gene Therapy
- Nanotechnology
- Periodontal Vaccine
- Minimally Invasive Surgery
- Piezosurgery

## LASERS

### Introduction

Light amplification by stimulated emission of radiation (LASER) is the well-known procedure in modern medicine.

*Light*: Laser light is monochromatic, i.e., it is of one specific color and that color may be visible or invisible. It also has other properties of coherency and collimation. *Coherency* suggests the production of light waves all in phase with one another with identical wave shapes; means, all the peaks and valleys are equivalent. *Collimation* means that beam has specific spatial boundaries. This ensures that the beam which is emitted from the laser cavity is of constant shape and size.

*Amplification*: The mirrors at each end of the active medium of a laser device reflect photons back and forth to allow further stimulated emission and increase the power of the photon beam.

*Stimulated emission*: The term "stimulated emission" has its origin in the quantum theory of physics. A quantum, the smallest unit of energy, is absorbed by the electrons of an atom or molecule, leading to a brief excitation. Afterward, a quantum is released and process is termed as "spontaneous emission". According to theory by Albert Einstein, an additional quantum of energy traveling in the field of the excited atom having the same excitation energy level would result in a release of two quanta, a phenomenon called as stimulated emission. These photons are capable to energize more atoms, which further emit additional identical photons, stimulating more surrounding atoms **(Fig. 67.1)**.

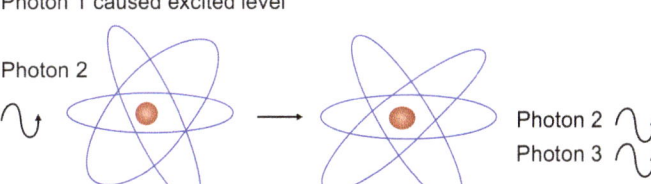

**Fig. 67.1:** Schematic representation showing stimulated emission.

*Radiation*: It refers to the light waves produced by the laser as a specific form of electromagnetic energy. All available dental laser devices have emission wavelengths of approximately 0.5–10.6 μm (500–10,600 nm). They are therefore, within the visible or the invisible infrared nonionizing portion of the electromagnetic spectrum and emit thermal radiation.[1,2]

### Historical Perspective

In 1960, Maiman developed the first laser prototype. Maiman's device is based on the use of crystal medium of ruby that emitted a coherent radiant light from the crystal when stimulated by energy. This gives origin to the ruby laser. Just 1 year thereafter, in 1961, Snitzer published the prototype for the Nd: YAG (Neodymium: yttrium-aluminum-garnet) laser. The first use of laser to dental tissues was reported by Goldman et al. However, the existing relationship of dentistry with the laser is known to originate from an article published in 1985 by Myers and Myers. This article describes the in-vivo removal of dental caries with use of a modified ophthalmic Nd: YAG laser. Four years later, Nd: YAG laser was reported to be used for oral soft-tissue surgery. This discovery successively leads to the current relationship between lasers and clinical periodontics.

## Basic Structure of a Laser Device

An optical cavity of a laser device usually lies at its center. The core of the cavity contains chemical elements, molecules or compounds and is termed as the active medium. Lasers are generically named according to the material of the active medium. The active medium can be a container of crystal, gas, or solid-state semiconductors. There are two gaseous active medium lasers used in dentistry: argon and $CO_2$. The remainder that are available are solid-state semiconductor made with multiple layers of metals, such as gallium, aluminum, indium and arsenic or solid rods of garnet crystal grown with various combinations of yttrium, aluminum, scandium and Ga and then doped with the elements of chromium, neodymium, or erbium. There are two mirrors, one at each end of the optical cavity, placed parallel to each other. The parallelism of the mirrors confirms that the light is collimated. One of the mirrors is selectively transmissive and permits the sufficient energy light to leave the optical cavity. Surrounding this core is an excitation source, either a flash lamp device or an electrical coil, which provides the energy into the active medium. There is some heat generated in the process and the optical cavity must be cooled. A cooling system, focusing lenses and other controls complete the mechanical components[1-3] **(Figs. 67.2 and 67.3)**.

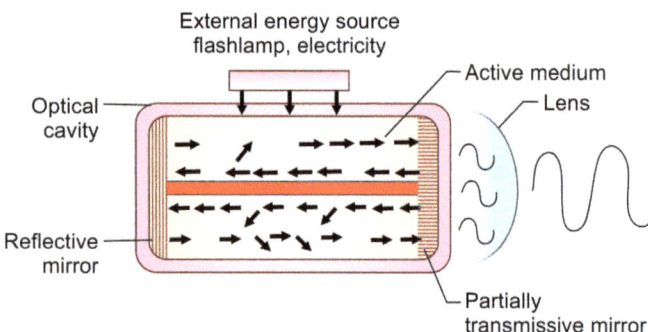

**Fig. 67.2:** Schematic representation showing basic components of laser.

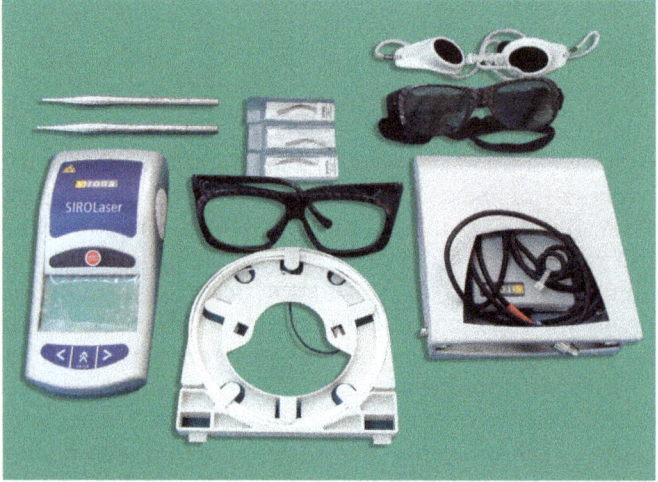

**Fig. 67.3:** Photograph showing laser parts.

## Laser Delivery Systems

### Articulated Arm Delivery Systems

Articulated arm delivery systems consist of a series of rigid hollow tubes with mirrors at each joint (called a knuckle) that reflect the energy down the length of the tube. The disadvantages are that they are bulky, have noncontact systems and there is difficulty in removing discrete lesions within the oral cavity.

### Flexible Hollow Waveguide or Tube

Flexible hollow waveguide or tube comes with an interior mirror finish. The laser energy gets reflected along the tube and exits through a handpiece located at the surgical end with the beam striking the tissue in a noncontact fashion. An accessory tip of sapphire or hollow metal can be connected to the end of the waveguide for contact with the surgical site.

### Glass Fiberoptic Cable

Glass fiberoptic cable is more pliant, lighter and shows lesser resistance to movement as compared to the waveguide. Its diameter is also smaller. The glass component is commonly encased in a resilient sheath. However, it can be fragile and hence unable to bend into a sharp angle. Glass fiber fits snugly into a handpiece and can be used in contact or noncontact mode.

The dental laser device can emit the light energy in two modalities as a function of time:
- Continuous wave where the beam is emitted at one power level only for as long as the operator presses the foot switch.
- Pulsed on and off:
    - *Gated-pulse mode*, where there are periodic alternations of the laser energy, similar to a blinking light.
    - *Free-running pulsed mode*, sometimes called as "true pulsed". This emission is unique where large peak energies of laser light gets emitted for a short time span, usually in microseconds and followed by a relatively long-time in which the laser is off.

The light energy that strikes the tissue for a certain period of time and thus produces a thermal interaction is the main principle of laser emission mode. In case of a pulsed mode type of a laser, the targeted tissue gets some time to cool before the next pulse of laser energy is emitted. While in continuous wave mode, the operator needs to cease the laser emission manually in order to bring thermal relaxation of the tissue. Similarly, when using hard-tissue lasers, a water spray helps to prevent microfracturing of the crystalline structures and reduces the possibility of carbonization.[1-4]

## Classification

LASERS are classified accordingly:
- *Based on state of the medium*:
    - Solid
    - Gas

- Excimer
- Diode
- *Based on output energy*:
  - Low output, soft or therapeutic: A thermic low-energy laser emitted at wavelength which is supposed to stimulate cellular activity, e.g., He-Ne, Ga-As, Ga-Al-As.
  - High output, hard or surgical: A thermic laser emitted at wave length in visible, infrared and ultraviolet (UV) range utilized to cut, coagulate, vaporize and carbonize, e.g., $CO_2$-Ar, Nd:YAG.
- *Based on oscillation mode*:
  - Continuous wave
  - Pulsed wave

## Laser Energy and Tissue Temperature

The principle effect of laser energy is photothermal. This thermal effect of laser energy on tissue depends on the degree of temperature rise and the corresponding reaction of the interstitial and intracellular water. As the laser energy is absorbed, heating occurs.

In the first event, hyperthermia occurs due to rise in the tissue temperature above normal temperature but tissues do not get destroyed. At 60°C temperatures, proteins start to denature without producing any vaporization of the underlying tissue. This phenomenon is important in cases of surgically removed diseased granulomatous tissue. This is because of the control of tissue temperature which helps to maintain the biologically healthy portion as intact. Soft-tissue edges should be "welded" together with maintenance of a uniform heating at 70–80°C. This allows the adherence of the layers because of the stickiness of collagen molecules. When the temperature of target tissue containing water is elevated to a 100°C, vaporization of the water within tissues occurs and the process is termed as "ablation". If the tissue temperature continues to be raised to about 200°C, it is dehydrated and then burned in the presence of air **(Table 67.1)**. Carbon is the end product of the process and absorbs all wavelengths. When laser energy is applied continuously, the surface carbonized layer commonly absorbs the incident beam and becomes a heat sink to prevent normal tissue ablation.

## Laser-tissue Interactions

Laser light can have four different interactions with the target tissue, depending on the optical properties of that tissue **(Fig. 67.4)**.
- *Absorption:* Absorption of the laser energy by the intended tissue. The amount of energy that is absorbed by the tissue depends on the tissue characteristics, such as pigmentation and water content, and also on the laser wavelength and emission mode.
- *Transmission:* Laser energy directly passes through the tissue with no effect on the target tissue, the inverse of absorption. Transmission effect depends upon the wavelength of laser light.

**TABLE 67.1:** Thermal effects of laser energy on tissue.

| Tissue temperature (°C) | Observed effect |
|---|---|
| 37–50° | Hyperthermia |
| 60–70° | Coagulation, protein denaturation |
| 70–80° | Welding |
| 100–150° | Vaporization, ablation |
| >200° | Carbonization |

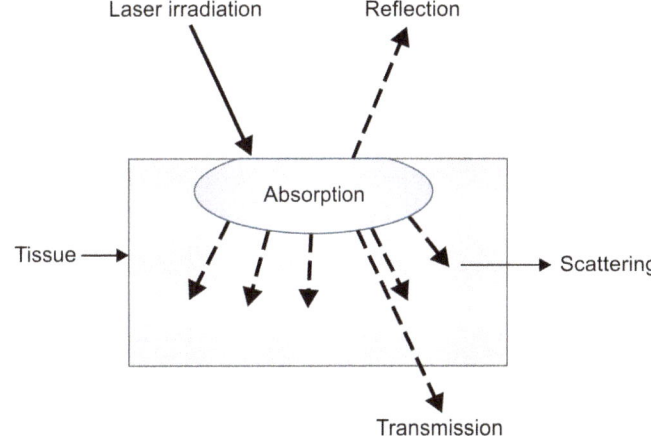

**Fig. 67.4:** Schematic representation showing laser tissue interactions.

- *Reflection:* It is the beam redirecting itself off of the surface, having no effect on the target tissue. This reflection can be dangerous because the energy is directed to an unintentional target, such as the eyes. This forms a major safety concern for laser operation.
- *Scattering:* Scattering of the laser beam, weakens the intended energy, producing no useful biologic effect. It also leads to heat transfer to the tissue adjacent to the operated site resulting in undesirable damage.

## Laser Wavelengths Used in Periodontics

Laser devices that have applications in periodontics are described in **Table 67.2**.

## Laser Uses in Periodontics

### Lasers in Diagnosis

#### Caries Detection

Caries detection with laser works on the principle of differential florescence between healthy tooth and diseased tooth. Such a system has become commercially available (DIAGNOdent). It operates at a wavelength of 655 nm. At this specific wavelength, clean healthy tooth structure exhibits little or no fluorescence, resulting in very low-scale readings on the display. However, carious tooth structure will exhibit fluorescence, proportionate to the degree of caries, resulting in elevated scale readings on the display.[5-8]

#### Calculus Detection

Same laser wavelength of 655 nm can also be used for calculus detection. The commercially available device for

## Section 10: Recent Advances

**TABLE 67.2:** Laser wavelengths used in periodontics.

| Laser | Wavelength | Wave form | Delivery tip | Application |
|---|---|---|---|---|
| Argon | 488–514 nm | Gated or continuous | Flexible fiberoptic system | Soft-tissue incision and ablation |
| Diode | 635–950 nm | Gated or continuous | Flexible fiberoptic system in contact mode for most of the procedures | Soft-tissue incision and ablation, soft-tissue curettage and bacterial elimination |
| Neodymium: yttrium-aluminium garnet | 1.064 µm | Pulsed | Flexible fiberoptic system in contact mode for most procedures | Soft-tissue incision and ablation; subgingival curettage and bacterial elimination |
| Erbium: yttrium-aluminium garnet | 2.94 µm | Free running pulsed | Flexible fiberoptic system or hollow waveguide; contact mode for most procedures | Soft-tissue incision and ablation; subgingival curettage; scaling and root planing; osteoplasty and ostectomy |
| Holmium yttrium-aluminium garnet | 2.1 µm | Pulsed | Flexible fiberoptic system in contact mode for most procedures | Soft-tissue incision and ablation; subgingival curettage and bacterial elimination |
| Carbon dioxide | 10.6 µm | Gated or continuous | Hollow waveguide; beam focused when 1–2 mm from target surface | Soft-tissue incision and ablation; subgingival curettage |

caries detection provides a separate tip for the detection of calculus in the subgingival area. Calculus fluoresces (glows) differently than healthy tissue. The device senses the difference and sends the signal to the numerical display and also presents an audible signal, indicating that calculus has been identified.[5-8]

### Mobility Assessment

Laser has also been applied for the assessment of the mobility of teeth. Laser Doppler vibrometry can be used to assess even small movements in the tooth. This technique is being developed for commercial purposes.

## Lasers in Prevention

### Laser Toothbrush

Laser toothbrush is designed to provide an antibacterial effect in oral cavity using an irradiating laser beam of 630 nm low-output semiconductor laser. It works with a programmed tooth management system that turns on the laser for a recommended treatment period with one-touch mode switch. It does not need toothpaste but directly radiates laser on teeth. This semiconductor medical laser helps to decrease plaque, relieves dentinal sensitivity, toothache and inflammation. It also treats halitosis and can be used in dental bleaching.[5-8]

## Lasers in Nonsurgical Pocket Therapy

### Laser Bacterial Reduction

Laser bacterial reduction is a simple nonsurgical procedure to eliminate or at least reduce the number of viable bacteria in the gingival sulcus. In this procedure, a diode laser is used with a thin fiber-optic fiber. Photonic laser energy is then emitted into the sulcus through this optic fiber reducing the microbes and periodontal pathogens present within.

### Calculus Removal

The most difficult step that ultimately determines the success or failure of the periodontal therapy is the removal of the diseased tissue from the surgical site. If the calcified accretions on the root surface are not removed, the therapy is doomed to fail. Lasers now are being used for this procedure. Not only does the laser remove the calculus on the root surface, it also alters the cementum surface in such a way that it makes it favorable for fibroblast attachment. Diode and Nd: YAG lasers may be used for initial periodontal therapy but both of these wavelengths have a significant interaction with the root surface and may produce craters on it. Erbium: yttrium-aluminum-garnet (Er: YAG) treatment leaves no craters on the root surface. Also, the Er: YAG laser provides selective subgingival calculus removal on a level equivalent to that provided by scaling and root planing. Studies have shown the ability of the Er: YAG laser to remove lipopolysaccharides, smear layer and calculus from root surfaces. The American Academy of Periodontology has stated that the Er: YAG laser demonstrated the best application of laser use directly on hard tissue, leaving the least thermal damage and creating a surface biocompatible for soft-tissue attachment.[5-8]

### Photodynamic Therapy

The use of photo activatable compounds or photosensitizers to cause photodestruction of oral bacteria has been demonstrated, indicating that photodynamic therapy (PDT) could be a useful alternative to mechanical means in eliminating periopathogenic bacteria. In PDT, the dye is applied to the treatment area. The dye is called as a photosensitizer, as this dye after absorbing the light sensitizes the organisms to visible light and induces damage. There is production of free-oxygen radicals due to the application of light, which are cytotoxic. Periowave™ is a photodynamic disinfection system that uses low-intensity lasers (Diode) and wavelength-specific, light-activated compounds to precisely target and kill microorganisms.

### Lasers in Treatment of Hypersensitivity

Low-level laser therapy (LLLT) has reported to induce anti-inflammatory, analgesic and cellular effects in cases of both hyperemia and inflammation of the dental pulp. For the treatment of hypersensitivity, a 780-nm diode laser can

be used at power of 30 mW, or Nd: YAG laser at low power can be used. The laser therapy usually produces following effects on hypersensitive teeth:
- *Primary or immediate effect*: It involves remission of painful symptoms.
- *Secondary or late effect*: It involves intense cellular metabolic activity, proliferation of odontoblasts and production of dentin.

Low-level laser therapy interferes with peripheral nerve signal transmission to the central nervous system, where the signals are interpreted. Sealing of dentinal tubuli, which impede the internal communication of the pulp with external oral fluids, helps to maintain the analgesic state of the dentin. Both process, the coagulation of the hydroxyapatite crystals and formation of reparative dentin following laser stimulation, leads to this sealing.[9,10]

## *Lasers in Surgical Therapies*

Most soft-tissue laser procedures can be categorized into one of three simple processes: (1) incision, (2) excision, or (3) ablation. Whether the dentist is using any of these, the basic process is the same regardless of the wavelength. The difference depends on the ability of the target tissue to absorb the laser energy which depends on its pigmentation, vascularity and water content.

### Advantages of Laser Therapy

Wigdor et al., described the advantages of lasers over conventional surgical procedures as:[11]
1. Dry and bloodless surgery
2. Instant sterilization of the surgical site
3. Reduced bacteremia
4. Reduced mechanical trauma
5. Minimal postoperative swelling and scarring
6. Minimal postoperative pain

Other advantages are being high patient acceptance, less need for suturing and faster healing.

The type and wavelength of laser for a particular procedure depends on the personal preference of the clinician. Some may prefer diode laser for its compact size and portability while other may prefer Nd: YAG for its deeper depth of penetration. Many dentists now prefer the erbium family of lasers for soft tissue due to their high absorption in water and lack of thermal penetration. Following procedures can be carried out with the use of above mentioned lasers:

### Laser-assisted New Attachment Procedure (LANAP)

In this procedure, laser is used to remove the epithelial lining of the sulcus as well as junctional epithelium. With the use of laser, it has been observed that there is retardation of epithelial downgrowth providing more time for connective tissue attachment on the root surface.

### Subgingival Curettage

In this procedure, granulation tissue is removed from within the sulcus and pocket area without raising a flap with the help of a soft-tissue laser.

### Minor Surgeries

- Nonosseous gingival surgeries, like labial frenectomy, **(Figs. 67.5A to D)**, lingual frenectomy to treat ankyloglossia **(Figs. 67.6A to D)**, frenotomy, gingivectomy, gingivoplasty, operculectomy and vestibuloplasty **(Figs. 67.7A to C)** can be performed.
- Biopsy and excision of soft-tissue pathologies.

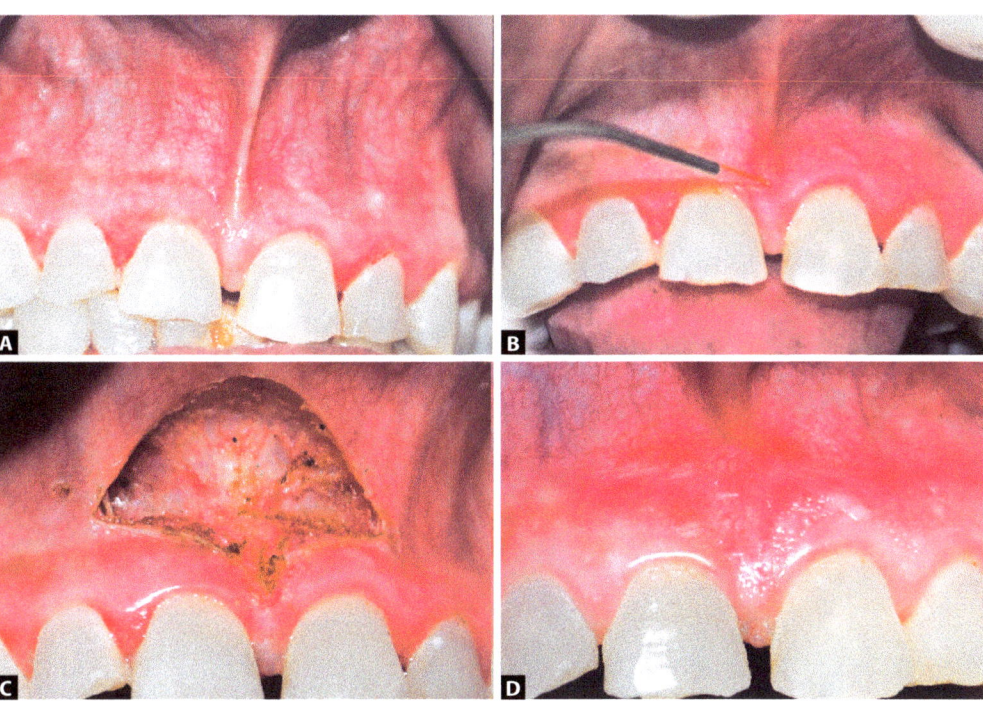

**Figs. 67.5A to D:** Clinical picture showing labial frenectomy with diode LASERS.

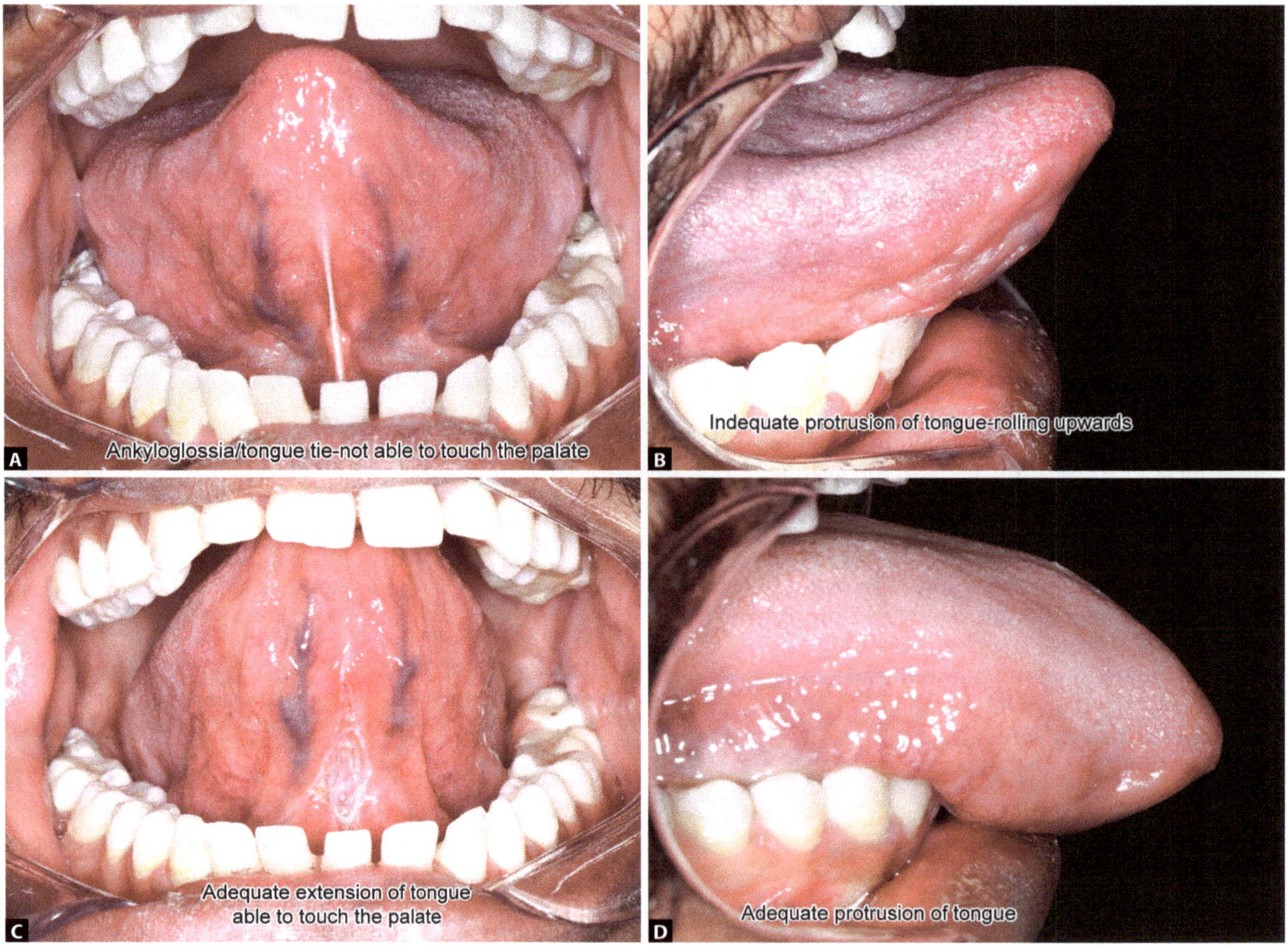

**Figs. 67.6A to D:** Clinical picture showing treatment of ankyloglossia (lingual frenectomy) with diode LASERS.

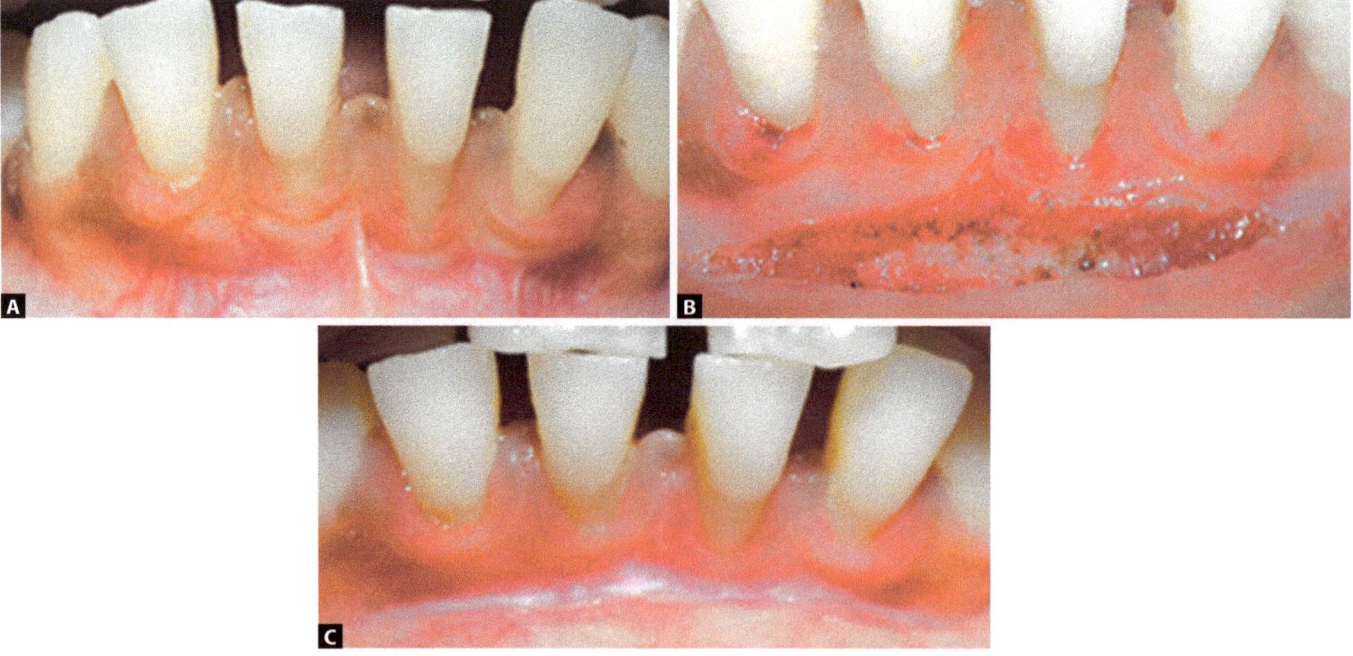

**Figs. 67.7A to C:** Clinical picture showing vestibuloplasty with diode LASERS.

### De-epithelialization

The use of lasers to retard epithelial downgrowth has been investigated. $CO_2$ laser has been used for this purpose. The epithelialization of the $CO_2$ irradiated side is delayed by at least 7 days, allowing for new connective tissue to grow. $CO_2$ laser deepithelialization technique has the ability to obtain new clinical attachment with bone fill in previously diseased sites. The results are even better than that obtained through conventional osseous grafting alone. Also, this technique is less technically demanding and more time efficient than other currently known methods of epithelial retardation.

### Osseous Recontouring

The only wavelengths cleared by the FDA for osseous surgery are the erbium family of lasers. Er:YAG and Er:Cr:YSGG are the only wavelengths that have the ability to ablate osseous tissue safely.

### Removal of Granulation Tissue

Soft-tissue lasers are a good choice for removal of granulation tissue. The soft tissue lasers including argon (488 nm, 514 nm), diode (800–830 nm, 980 nm) and Nd: YAG (1064 nm) get well absorbed by melanin and hemoglobin and other chromophores present in periodontally diseased tissues. The laser energy is transmitted through water and poorly absorbed in hydroxyapatite. Hence, soft-tissue lasers become an excellent choice of use in a periodontally involved sulcus which is usually associated with dark inflamed tissue and pigmented bacteria.

### Periodontal Regeneration Surgery

Lasers are also being used for periodontal regenerative procedures. The most effective method of regenerative periodontal surgical techniques is a double-wavelength technique. This technique uses the Er: YAG to debride the open surgical site, clean and sterilize the root surface and prepare the root surface for the adhesion of fibroblasts.

The $CO_2$ laser would remove the epithelium, which would allow the fibroblasts to adhere and proliferate, creating new attachment. Such a procedure will result in new attachment on previously diseased site.

## Lasers in Esthetic Surgeries

### Depigmentation

Laser peel can be used for depigmentation of gingiva. A $CO_2$ laser can be used at continuous wave in a defocused mode. By using the laser in this manner, it is possible to separate the epithelium from the underlying connective tissue by forming blisters. As melanocytes are found in the basement membrane of the epithelium, they will be permanently eliminated with the tissue that is removed providing a long-term result[12] **(Figs. 67.8A to C)**.

### Crown Lengthening

Crown lengthening or soft-tissue management around short clinical crowns/abutments can be done by LASERS **(Figs. 67.9A to C)**.

## Lasers in Implants

### Second-stage Recovery

The tissue over the implant can be ablated using a $CO_2$ laser. Because the surgical site is so small, the area tends to form a char layer quickly. This char must be removed during surgery. If the char is not removed during surgery, then absorption of the laser energy will cease and scattering of the laser beam will occur, possibly heating up the tissue

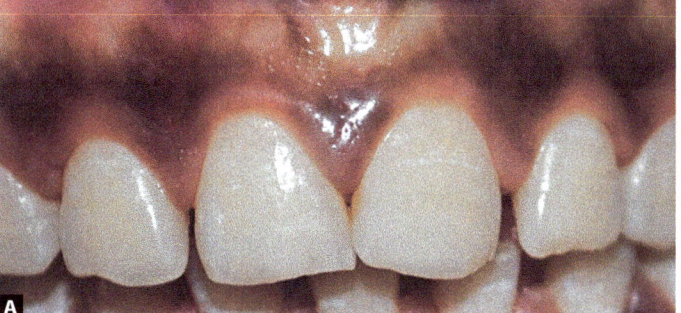
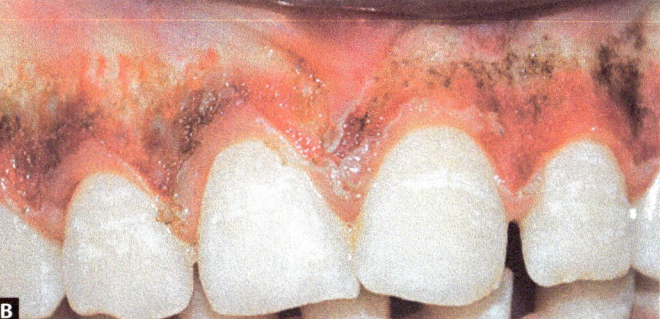
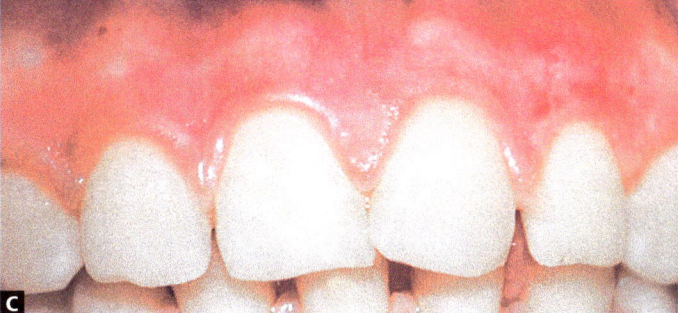

**Figs. 67.8A to C:** Clinical picture showing depigmentation with diode LASERS.

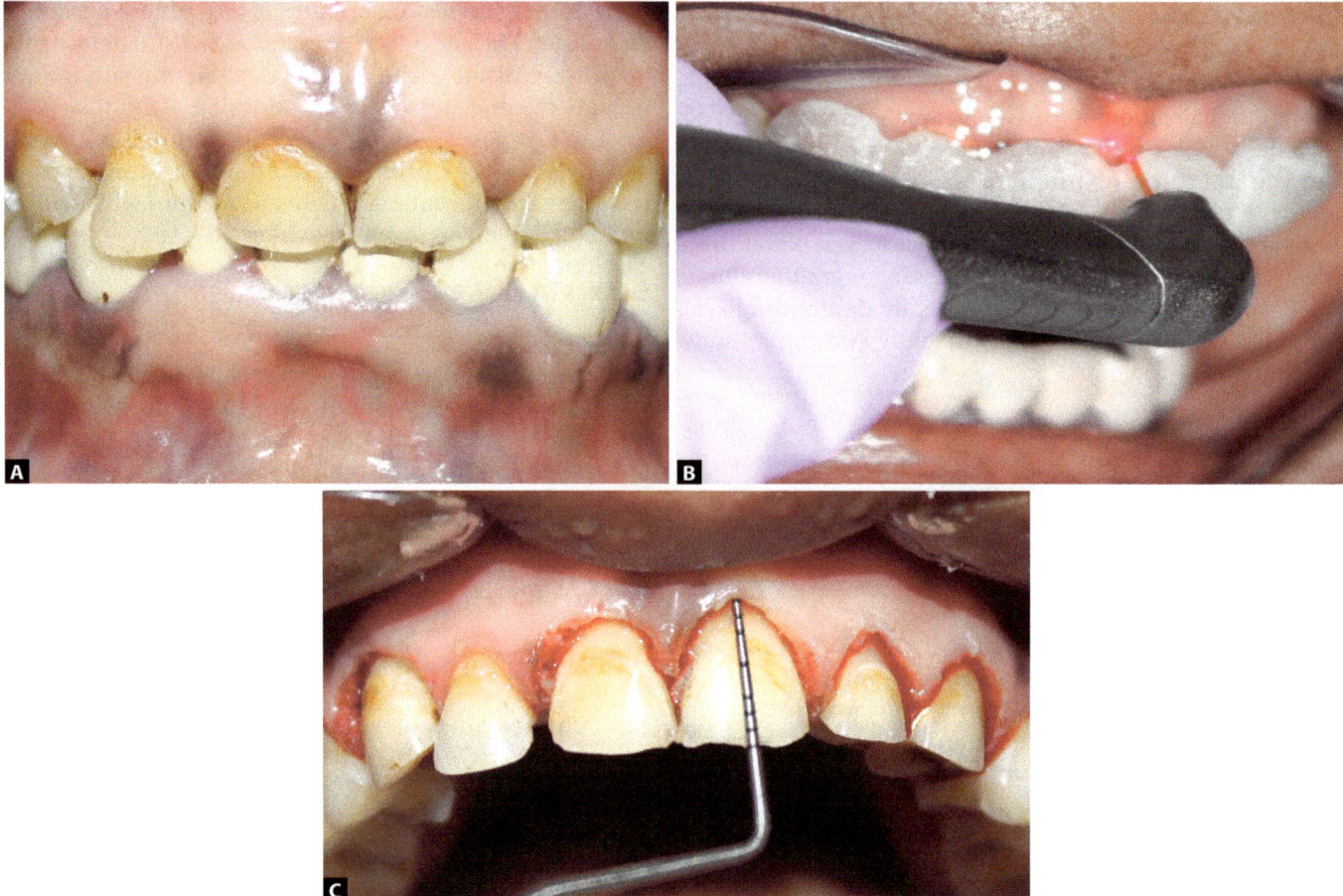

**Figs. 67.9A to C:** (A) Preoperative view of short clinical crowns; (B) Soft tissue and osseous recontouring with LASERS; and (C) Immediate postoperative view of adequate clinical crowns.
(*Courtesy*: Dr Sana Farista)

surrounding the implant and possibly damaging the implant. After the implant is exposed, the cover screw can be removed and a healing abutment is placed. The advantage of using a laser to uncover the implant is that it avoids an incision that would extend through the interproximal papillae located next to the adjacent teeth. By avoiding this incision, a better cosmetic result can be assured.

### Peri-implantitis

Er-YAG laser can be used for managing peri-implantitis, because Er-YAG laser is very well suited for both hard- and soft-tissue treatment. Also, it disinfects implant along with implant surface treatment. The objective in managing peri-implantitis is to achieve a "surgically clean" interface which is indistinguishable from the sterile implant when it was originally placed.[13] The ablative laser is the only instrument which helps to achieve this objective. Lasers kill the microbes during the cleaning of infected area leaving the area free from infection. Even $CO_2$ laser is being researched for this purpose. Pulsed or continuous $CO_2$ laser is effective in removing the granulation and infected tissue. The laser does not lead to overheating of the implant even when its beam hits on the implant within reasonable time and power settings.[14]

### Lasers in Residual Ridge Modification

- Tuberosity reduction
- Torus reduction

## Dental Laser Safety

Laser hazard classification according to American National Standards Institute (ANSI) and Occupational Safety and Health Administration (OSHA) standards has been described in **Table 67.3**.

Following are the various types of Laser hazards:
- *Ocular injury*: Laser has the potential to cause eye injury in case of direct emission from the laser or reflection from the mirror-like surface or convex-curved instruments. The damage usually presents as an injury to sclera, cornea, retina and aqueous humor and may lead to cataract formation.
- *Tissue damage*: Thermal interaction of radiant energy of Lasers with the tissue proteins may damage the skin

**TABLE 67.3:** Laser hazard classification according to American National Standards Institute (ANSI) and Occupational Safety and Health Administration (OSHA) standards.

| Class | Powered | Safety |
|---|---|---|
| I | Low | Safe |
| IIa | Low | Visible lasers; hazardous if viewed directly for >1,000 seconds |
| IIb | Low | Visible lasers; hazardous if viewed for > 0.25 seconds |
| IIIa | Medium | Not hazardous if viewed for less <0.25 seconds without magnifying optics |
| IIIb | Medium (0.5 W maximum) | Hazardous if viewed directly |
| IV | High (> 0.5 W) | Hazardous; can produce ocular, skin and fire hazards |

and other nontarget tissues. Temperature elevation of above normal body temperature (37°C) may induce cell destruction by denaturation of cellular enzymes and structural proteins.

- *Environmental hazards*: Surgical application of lasers may lead to potential inhalation of airborne biohazardous materials. Chemicals, like formaldehyde, methane and benzene, are present in the laser plume and proved to be injurious on inhalation.
- *Combustion hazards*: Flammable solids, liquids and gases used within the clinical setting can easily catch fire on exposure to the laser beam.
- *Electrical hazards*: Currently used dental lasers usually demand very high currents and high voltage. These can result in electrical shock or even explosion hazards.

## Safety Precautions

- *Beam alignment*: Beam should be aligned properly at the treatment area before switching on Laser, to prevent undue injuries to patient as well as practitioner.
- *Laser control*: Foot pedal control of Laser should have a protective hood to prevent an accidental depression by assisting staff.
- *Reflected energy*: Anodized instrument should be used to prevent reflection of Laser light. Also, mirror should be avoided in path of laser beam.
- *Fire protection*: All the flammable substances should be kept away from the operating area to prevent accidental fire hazard.
- *Eye protection*: Safety goggles should be worn by the operating person as well as the assistant. If safety goggles are not available for patient, wet gauge pieces should be kept on closed eyes of the patient for prevention.
- *Plume control*: Laser filtration masks should be worn by the clinician as well as the assistant. The pore size of 0.1 μm has been shown to be effective. A high-volume evacuator or a special laser plume evacuator should be used for the purpose.

## PHOTODYNAMIC THERAPY

### Introduction

The susceptibility of microorganisms to the damaging action of visible light in the presence of a dye has been known since 20th century when microbiologist started using acridine. More recently, PDT has been introduced for its antimicrobial action and also for selective killing of tumor cells. It is also known as photoradiation therapy, phototherapy or photochemotherapy. It uses a photoactive dye, which is photosensitizer in nature and gets activated by exposure to light of a specific wavelength in the presence of oxygen, to form free-radical species that kill targeted microbes.

Photodynamic therapy is now being considered as a possible treatment for periodontal diseases, which are caused by the overgrowth of pathogenic microflora around teeth. It can be a valuable alternative to traditional scaling and root planing as well as antibiotic therapy.[15,16] It offers a new treatment modality that is required since periodontal infection tends to recur after scaling and root planing and also because of widespread drug resistance to antibiotics.

### Historical Perspective

Photodynamic therapy was discovered accidently at the beginning of the 20th century and was then applied in the medical field for the light-induced inactivation of cells, microorganisms or molecules. In 1904, Professor Hermann von Tappeiner introduced the term "photodynamic action" (Photodynamische Wirkung). He is considered as the pioneers of photobiology. It is still unclear why he termed the process as "dynamic". It is thought that this biological phenomenon must be distinguished from the reactions taking place in the photographic process that had been discovered a few years earlier. During the period of 1903-1905, the group of Von Tappeiner for the first time attempted to apply PDT in treatment of tumors and other skin diseases.

US Food and Drug Administration in 1999 approved PDT as a treatment modality to treat the precancerous skin lesions of the face or scalp. Thus, PDT rapidly started to gain popularity in dentistry in the treatment of oral cancer, bacterial and fungal infections and also in the photodynamic diagnosis (PDD) of the malignant transformation of oral lesions.

### Materials Used for Photodynamic Therapy

#### Light Source

A diode laser system is commonly used for PDT since it is easy to handle, portable and cost effective. For treatment of larger areas, noncoherent light sources, such as tungsten filament, quartz halogen, xenon arc, metal halide and phosphor-coated sodium lamps, are used. Nowadays, light-emitting diodes (LEDs) are commonly used because they are small, highly flexible, light in weight and cheaper as compared to the typical light sources.

### Delivery Unit

The light from the source is delivered according to the location and morphology of the lesion. Usually, fiberoptic catheters are used. These fiber tips can be mold into different shapes, permitting diffusion in all directions.

### Photosensitizers

Photosensitizers are usually dyes which get activated in presence of light of specific wavelength to form free radicals which kill the unwanted microbes or tumor cells.

#### Classification of Photosensitizers

- *First-generation photosensitizers*: Phenothiazine dyes, porphyrin-chlorin-phthalocyanine platforms, hematoporphyrin derivatives.
- *Second-generation photosensitizers*: Benzoporphyrin derivative, 5-aminolevulinic acid (ALA), temoporfin [(meta-tetra (hydroxyphenyl)chlorin (mTHPC)], lutetium texaphyrin, talaporfin sodium and tinethyletiopurpurin.

An ideal photosensitizer must exhibit local toxicity only after illumination. The majority of the sensitizers used clinically are phenothiazine dyes or porphyrin-chlorin-phthalocyanine platforms. Untill now Photofrin (dihematoporphyrin ether) is the most extensively studied and clinically used photosensitizer. Foscan (temoporfin) is the most potent second-generation photosensitizer and reported to be 100 times more active compared to Photofrin in animal studies **(Table 67.4)**.

## Applications

Applications of PDT in dentistry are as follows:
- *Photodynamic diagnosis of malignant transformation of oral lesions*: A topical application of ALA is a relatively new approach in the diagnosis of oral lesions.
- *Treatment of premalignant and malignant oral lesions*: Premalignant and malignant lesions in the oral cavity can be successfully managed by topical application of ALA-based PDT. PDT already proved its effectiveness in the treatment of oral lichen planus, oral leukoplakia and squamous cell carcinoma of the lip and tongue. However, PDT of the oral mucosa can lead to superficial necrosis leaving little scarring and no cumulative toxicity. ALA-based PDT seems as an effective approach in treatment for oral leukoplakia; which is because of its good tolerance, low invasiveness, ability to treat multifocal lesions, excellent cosmetic effects and low risk of toxicity after repeated use.
- *Chemotherapy [photodynamic antimicrobial chemotherapy (PACT)] for biofilms*: Dental plaque is a complex aggregation of microorganisms present on the tooth surface in the form of a biofilm. Thus, the organisms are usually located in an extracellular polymeric matrix. A high level of resistance is exhibited by the biofilm- associated bacteria to environmental stresses, to the antibiotics and to the immune defense mechanisms of their host.[17] Moreover, the limited access of topical agents into the plaque and the development of antibiotic resistance have created a situation to search new strategies for adequate plaque control and to treat gingivitis, caries and periodontal disease. In such cases, PACT is proved to be effective against antibiotic-resistant and susceptible bacteria. Repeated photosensitization does not induce the selection of resistant strains.
- *Oropharyngeal candidiasis*: It is a commonly noted opportunistic infection in immunocompromised patients, including the individuals infected with human immunodeficiency virus (HIV). Along with this, Candida associated denture stomatitis is another common disease in people using dentures. *Candida albicans* has great potential to form biofilms on mucosal surfaces and also on the prosthetic devices leading to recurrent infections and failure of antifungal therapy. The increasing resistance of *C. albicans* to antifungal agents increases interest of researchers in photodynamic treatments. Likewise to other yeasts, *C. albicans* is potentially difficult to kill by PACT compared to gram-positive bacteria. Ryan F Donnelly and his colleagues at Queen's University Belfast in the UK demonstrated significant role of mucoadhesive patches containing toluidine blue O as a potential delivery system in oral candidiasis.

## Photodynamic Antimicrobial Chemotherapy

Photodynamic antimicrobial chemotherapy (PACT) is an alternative antibacterial, antiviral and antifungal treatment significantly useful against microbes that are resistant to drug. This is because bacteria would unable to develop resistance to the cytotoxic action of singlet oxygen or free radicals. Hence, the bacteria that are growing in the biofilms are also susceptible to PACT.

### Mechanism of Action

In PDT, a photosensitizer or its metabolic precursor is administered to the patient. Most photosensitizers are

**TABLE 67.4:** Photosensitizers used for photodynamic antimicrobial chemotherapy (PACT).

| Platform | Example |
| --- | --- |
| Phenothiazine dyes | Methylene blue, toluidine blue O |
| Phthalocyanines | Aluminum disulfonated-phthalocyanine cationic, Zn (II)-phthalocyanine chlorines, chlorine 6, Sn (IV) chlorine 6, chlorine 6-2.5, N-methyl-D-glucamine, polylysine and polyethyleneimine conjugates of chlorine 6 |
| Porphyrins | Hematoporphyrin HCl, Photofrin (dihematoporphyrin ether), 5-aminolevulinic acid (ALA) |
| Xanthenes | Erythrosine |
| Monoterpene | Azulene |

activated by light between 630 nm and 700 nm. With light irradiation of a specific wavelength, the photosensitizer undergoes a transition from a low-energy ground state into an excited singlet state. With the subsequent use the photosensitizer gets decay back to its ground state and may emit fluorescence, or may undergo a transition to a higher-energy triplet state. The triplet state can react with endogenous oxygen and produce singlet oxygen and other radical species. These free radicals lead to a rapid and selective destruction of the target microorganisms.[18]

### Photodynamic Antimicrobial Chemotherapy in Periodontitis

Photodynamic antimicrobial chemotherapy can be applied in periodontics by using low-intensity lasers and wavelength-specific, light-activated compounds that particularly target and destroy the microbial pathogens and eliminates the disease symptoms. The photosensitive compounds are usually applied topically in the area of gingival sulcus and then laser is used to activate the compounds to achieve complete disinfection.[19,20]

The bacterial photosensitivity is usually associated with the charge of the sensitizer. In routine practice it is reported that neutral or anionic photosensitizers binds efficiently to and also inactivate gram-positive bacteria. However, they bind to some extent to the outer membrane of gram-negative bacteria and do not inactivate them after illumination. A relatively porous layer of peptidoglycan and lipoteichoic acid outside the cytoplasmic membrane of gram-positive species permits diffusion of the photosensitizer into sensitive sites. The outer membrane of gram-negative bacteria forms a physical and functional barrier between the cell and its environment. The affinity of negatively charged photosensitizers for gram-negative bacteria is increased by linking of the sensitizer to a cationic molecule [e.g., poly-L-lysine-chlorin(e6)], by the use of membrane-active agents (e.g., treatment with Tris- EDTA), or by conjugating the sensitizer with a monoclonal antibody that binds to cell-surface-specific antigens.

### Advantages of Photodynamic Antimicrobial Chemotherapy

- The antimicrobial activity of photosensitizers is commonly mediated by singlet oxygen and hence, PACT is effective in inducing direct effect on extracellular molecules. This facilitates the photodamaging of polysaccharides of an extracellular polymeric matrix. Antibiotics do not exhibit such activity and hence, this activity is considered as a significant advantage of PACT.
- The development of resistance to PACT appears to be unlikely, since, in microbial cells, singlet oxygen and free radicals interact with several cell structures and have different metabolic pathways.
- Photodynamic antimicrobial chemotherapy is equally effective against antibiotic-resistant and antibiotic-susceptible bacteria and repeated photosensitization has not induced the selection of resistant strains.
- The potencies of some key virulence factors (lipopolysaccharide and proteases) have also been shown to be reduced by photosensitization.[21]
- Antioxidant enzymes, such as superoxide dismutase and catalase, protect against some oxygen radicals, but not against singlet oxygen.
- Process is noninvasive and convenient for the patient.
- Photodynamic antimicrobial chemotherapy can be carried out in outpatient or day-care (inpatient) settings.
- Photodynamic antimicrobial chemotherapy can be targeted accurately and selectively in localized diseases.
- Repeated doses are suitable without the need for total-dose limitations.

## TISSUE ENGINEERING

### Introduction

Tissue engineering is a new and advancing field of science which deals with developing newer techniques for the fabrication of new tissues to replace the old damaged tissues. This field works on the principles of cell and developmental biology and the biomaterial science. Initially, the term tissue engineering was used to signify the process of construction in the laboratory of a device containing viable cells and biological mediators in a synthetic or biological matrix which, when implanted in patients facilitates regeneration of a particular tissue. More recently the definition has been broadened to refer to any attempt to regenerate tissues whether in laboratory or patients by adding appropriate biologic mediators and matrices.

### Principles of Tissue Engineering

#### Strategies to Tissue Engineering

Following are the recent strategies employed to engineer tissue:
- *Conductive approach*: It utilizes biomaterials in a passive manner to facilitate the growth or regenerative capacity of existing tissue, e.g., use of barrier membranes in guided tissue regeneration (GTR).
- *Inductive approach*: This approach uses a biodegradable polymer scaffold as a vehicle to deliver growth factors and genes to the host site. The growth factors or genes can be released at a controlled rate based on the breakdown of the polymer which induces regeneration at the site.
- *Cell transplantation approach*: It uses same biodegradable polymer scaffold vehicle for delivery in order to transplant cells and partial tissues to the host site.

The appropriate levels and sequencing of regulatory signals, the presence and numbers of responsive progenitor cells and an appropriate extracellular matrix or cellular carrier constructs are the essential requirements for

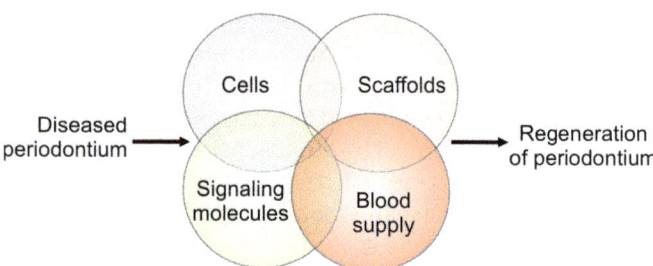

**Fig. 67.10:** Schematic representation showing periodontal tissue engineering.

producing an engineered tissue. Regeneration of the periodontium requires recruitment of progenitor cells. This is because progenitor cells have innate capacity to differentiate into specialized regenerative cells, followed by their proliferation and synthesis of specialized components which requires repair. The tissue engineering strategy employed for regeneration of periodontium needs growing of these cells within a three-dimensional construct and subsequent implantation into the defect.[22,23]

Reconstruction of the lost periodontal tissue commonly needs the combination of cells, scaffolds, signaling molecules, and adequate blood supply. All these factors play significant role in the healing process and associated with the generation of new tissues **(Fig. 67.10)**.

## Scaffolds for Tissue Engineering

Scaffolds act as a delivery vehicle for cell transplantation and as a three-dimensional template for tissue regeneration. It also provides specific clues to regulate bone formation. Naturally derived and synthetic scaffold materials have been used to exploit the regenerative capacities of host tissues or transplanted cells. The specific requirements for scaffold material include biocompatibility, mechanical support, controlled degradation and adequate interstitial fluid flow. Scaffold characteristics, such as porosity, topography and material composition, dictate certain of these features. Matrices that resemble the extracellular matrix of the tissue to be engineered can be used as scaffolds.[24-27]

### *Types of Scaffolds*

#### Nonresorbable Materials

Membranes made from expanded polytetrafluoroethylene (ePTFE) are used to nurture the specific cells. These cells get expanded ex vivo and then delivered to a defect site. Some ceramic materials have also been used as a scaffold. These ceramics have good biocompatibility, are porous and possess osseointegrative capabilities. Hydroxyapatite is a ceramic material with good mechanical properties. Porous hydroxyapatite which lacks interconnectivity of the pores, blocks out the neovascularization of any implant. Nowadays some biodegradable porous ceramic materials have been developed and investigated. One of them is beta-tricalcium phosphate which possesses high biocompatibility and biodegradability. Beta-tricalcium phosphate exhibits good mechanical properties in relation to elasticity and stiffness. Moreover, such material is relatively easy to handle during the surgical placement. Another nonresorbable material with promising outcome is titanium mesh. The absence of bioresorbability of this material proved to be effective in the management of large osseous defects **(Flowchart 67.1)**.

#### Resorbable Materials

The alpha-hydroxy acid polymers that include poly (L-lactic acid), polyglycolic acid and copolymers of poly(lactic-coglycolic acid) which are used for cell seeding. These polymers degrade by nonenzymatic means and fail to elicit a foreign body response which results in massive macrophage infiltration and chronic inflammation. These materials can also be improved chemically to modify its period of degradation depending on clinical need. The disadvantage of these material is difficult attachment or entrapment of cell due to their hydrophobic nature and processing under stringent conditions.

Alginate beads can also serve as a cell carrier for tissue engineering. The basic principal of this technique is the entrapment of individual cells and tissues into an alginate droplet and their transformation into a rigid bead by gelation in a divalent cation-rich solution. In this way, transplanted cells are immune-protected and isolated from host tissue via a nondegradable, selectively permeable barrier.

Due to the significant role of hyaluronate in development and organogenesis, it has considerable potential for tissue engineering. Hyaluronate can be modified with esterification and cross-linking which provides structure and rigidity to gel for cell seeding purpose. Another biopolymer chitosan that structurally resembles naturally occurring glycosaminoglycans can also be used as tissue engineering scaffold. Collagen scaffolds also offer several advantages, such as excellent biocompatibility, safety and easy seeding of cells.

Synthetic hydrogels, such as polyethylene oxide and polyethylene glycol, are useful as a three-dimensional (3D) scaffold for cell delivery. Currently the US FDA has approved polyethylene oxide for several indications in medicine. Along with polyglycolic acid, it is one of the most common synthetic materials used for tissue engineering. Extracellular matrix extracts or derivatives are available as commercial products for cell delivery, including Matrigel™, Epidex™ and Dermagraft™ that allow the incorporation of ex vivo expanded cells. Main disadvantage of using these materials is that they are animal-derived products and/ or allogeneic tissues. Hence, these products can acts as a potential source of pathogens and rarely used as cell delivery devices in the longer term **(Flowchart 67.1)**.

## Cells for Tissue Engineering

Cells harvested for tissue engineering may be heterologous (different species), allogeneic (same species, different

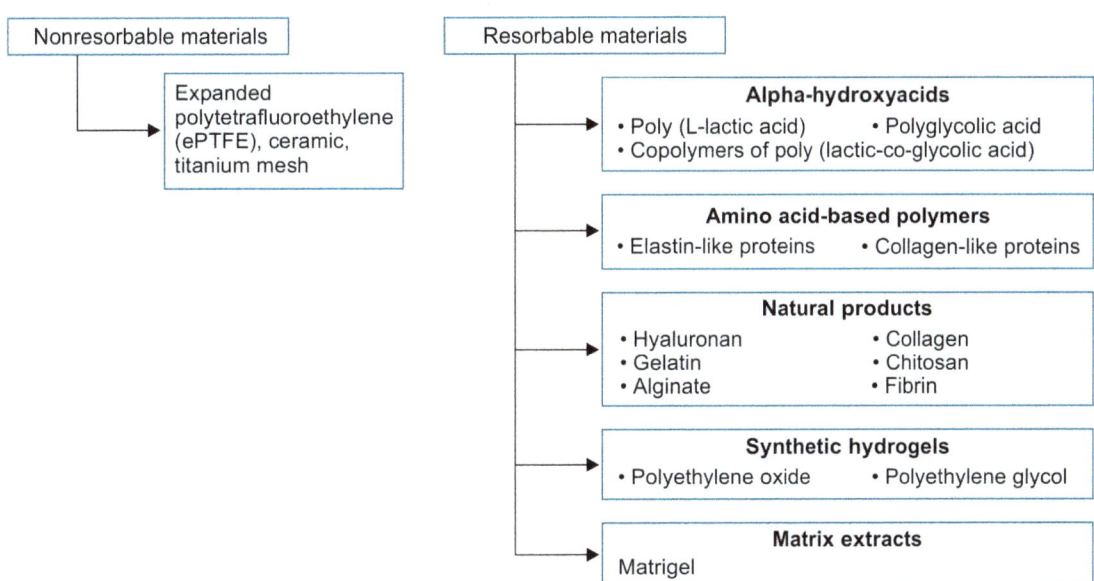

**Flowchart 67.1:** Types of scaffolds.

individual), or autologous (same individual). When cells are used for tissue engineering, a small piece of donor tissue is dissociated into individual cells. These cells are either implanted directly into the host or are expanded in culture, attached to a support matrix and then reimplanted into the host after expansion. Autologous cells are usually selected because they lack an immunologic response and hence useful in preventing the deleterious side effects of immunosuppressive agents.

Stem cell therapy has introduced a new source for harvesting cells for tissue engineering. Stem cells have the ability to self-replicate for indefinite periods. Under right conditions or given right signals stem cells can differentiate into many cell types. Stem cells can be grouped into either embryonic or the adult. Embryogenic stem cells are derived from the blastocyst stage of the embryonic development prior to implantation in uterine wall. These cells are clonogenic that is they are capable of unlimited self-renewal by symmetric division, one daughter cell resembling its mother and other daughter giving rise to multiple types of differentiated cells representing all three germ layers. Incorporating these stem cells in a bioengineered matrix with appropriate mediators can be used for filling periodontal defects.[28]

## Biological Mediators and Signaling Molecules

The bioactive molecules are incorporated into the scaffolding materials; this may facilitate sustained factor release for a period of time, so as to enhance the in-vivo efficacy. The bioactive molecules that are incorporated directly into a bioresorbable scaffold get released by a diffusion controlled mechanism. This mechanism is usually regulated by the size of the pores. The type and rate of degradation of the delivery device and the rate of growth factor diffusion through pores of the scaffolds determines the rate of growth factor release.

Several bioactive molecules play important role in promoting periodontal wound repair in both preclinical and clinical studies. These bioactive molecules include insulin growth factor (IGF-I), platelet-derived growth factor (PDGF), transforming growth factor (TGF), fibroblast growth factor (FGF-2), enamel matrix derivative (EMD)[29] and bone morphogenetic protein (BMP)-2, BMP-4, BMP-7 and BMP-12. These molecules have demonstrated to exhibit positive results in promoting periodontal wound repair and stimulating periodontal regeneration.

## Requirements

Following are the requirements for successful periodontal tissue engineering:

### *Biomechanical Requirements*

#### Space Maintenance

If the space is maintained and the soft-tissue ingrowth is prevented into the provided adjacent tissue space, the bone grows in. This can be used when bioengineered matrices are placed for regeneration. The scaffold should have the ability of easy molding and consistency suitable for easy handling. Additionally, it should be of sufficient rigidity to bear soft-tissue collapse into the defect.[30]

#### Barrier or Exclusionary Function

The engineered tissue must provide sufficient barrier to the ingrowth of unwanted tissues and selectively permit the ingrowth of regenerative tissues. This can be achieved by scaffolding the external surface exclusionary with maintaining the internal scaffold conducive for new tissue ingrowth. Principle aim of tissue engineering for periodontium is the total exclusion of epithelium which helps to form a rapid and successful biological seal.

### *Biological Requirements*

#### Biocompatibility

The bioengineered tissue should be either biodegradable which favors gradual replacement with regenerated tissue and biocompatible with the tissues to be regenerated. Also, the size of the pore and porosity of the scaffold material should allow migration of cells and regeneration of tissues.

#### Incorporation of Cells

It should be possible that the cells with periodontal regenerative phenotype be cultured and subsequently incorporated into a scaffold for immediate incorporation into the periodontal defect. Likely source for these cells can be progenitor cells harvested from the host site, i.e., periodontal ligament, cementum or the bone.[28,31]

#### Incorporation of Instructive Messages

The synthetic matrix must favor adsorption of appropriate growth factors and other instructive molecules which are normally present in regenerating tissues. These materials will later release slowly from the matrix and initiate and propagate regenerative events.

## GENE THERAPY

### Introduction

Periodontitis is a complex disease which affects the human population worldwide. Over the years, many treatment modalities have been suggested to control this disease. Recently, new treatment modalities to regenerate lost periodontium have been developed like GTR with newer materials, like Emdogain and rh-BMP, etc. With advancing knowledge in biological science and better understanding of disease progression, gene therapy contributes significantly in the enhancement of existing therapy and radically recast approaches to the management of periodontal disease. Here, we discuss the gene therapy and its impact on periodontium.

Originally, gene therapy is a technique utilized for correction of defective genes responsible for disease development. The technique uses purified preparations or a fraction of a gene for the treatment of diseases. In gene therapy, the common approach is the identification of a malfunctioning gene and supplementing the patient with functioning copies of that defective gene. The main aim of gene therapy is the introduction of therapeutic material into the target cells, where it becomes active and exerts the intended therapeutic effect.[32]

### Approaches for Gene Therapy

The common approaches used for correcting faulty genes are as follows:
- The most common approach is the insertion of a normal gene into a nonspecific location within the genome to replace a nonfunctional gene.
- Swapping of an abnormal gene for a normal gene through homologous recombination.
- Repairing of the abnormal gene through selective reverse mutation, which returns the gene to its normal functional status.
- The regulation (the degree to which a gene is turned on or off) of a particular gene could be altered.
- *Somatic and germline gene therapy*: Gene therapy can target somatic (body) or germ (egg and sperm) cells. In somatic gene therapy, the recipient's genome is changed, but the change is not passed on to the next generation; whereas with germline gene therapy, the newly introduced gene is passed on to the offspring.[33]

### Gene Transfer Techniques

Gene transfer techniques have been described into following groups:
- *In-vivo gene transfer*: During this technique, the foreign gene is injected into the patient by viral and nonviral methods:
  - Viral
  - Non-viral:
    - Cationic liposomes
    - Microseeding gene therapy
    - Gene-activated matrices
    - Macromolecular conjugate
- *Ex-vivo gene transfer*: The ex-vivo gene transfer involves transduction of a foreign gene into cells of a tissue biopsy, outside the body which results in genetically-modified cells. These cells are then transplanted back into the patient.

### *In-vivo Gene Transfer Technique*

#### Viral Approach

Viral approach is quite efficient method of gene transfer. A virus is used as a vector to introduce therapeutic gene into patient's target cell. Thus, here virus acts as a natural infectious agent for transferring genetic information.

Some of the viruses that can be used as vector are:
- *Retrovirus*: Their genetic material is ribonucleic acid (RNA) through which they can create deoxyribonucleic acid (DNA) that can be integrated into chromosomes.
- Adenoviruses are viruses with double-stranded DNA genomes.
- Herpes simplex viruses are double-stranded virus that can infect a particular cell.

- Adeno-associated viruses are single-stranded DNA viruses that insert genetic material at specific site on chromosome 19.
- Lenti or hybrid viruses combine the traits of two or more viruses.

These vectors are administered either intravenously or injected directly into a specific tissue in the body. The culture cells are exposed to the vector and then reintroduced into the patient.

### Non-viral Approach

*Cationic liposomes*: In this technique, artificial lipid spheres are created with an aqueous core. The liposome, which carries the therapeutic DNA, is capable of passing the DNA through the target cell's membrane.

*Microseeding gene therapy*: This is the simplest method of gene therapy. It involves the direct introduction of therapeutic DNA into target cells using a gene gun. However, this procedure requires large amount of DNA to bring out desired effect and can be used only with certain tissues, hence restricting its use.

*Gene-activated matrices*: It employs polymer matrix sponges to deliver naked DNA to the target cells.

*Macromolecular conjugates*: In this technique, DNA is linked to a molecule that binds to special cell receptors. Once bound, the therapeutic DNA is engulfed by the cell membrane and passed into interior of target cell. This delivery system is less effective than others.[32]

## Applications

Following are the application of gene therapy in periodontics:
- *In prevention of periodontal disease*:[34-37]
  - *Periodontal vaccination*: Research is going on for vaccination techniques to prevent periodontal diseases. Gene transfer research has also started contributing to achieve vaccination against periodontal disease. In this technique, plasmids containing DNA encoding antigens of periodontal pathogens can be injected to the host which results in production of immunoglobulins against the pathogens as a host response thus, preventing periodontal disease, e.g., hemagglutinin is a significant virulence factor of *Porphyromonas gingivalis*. Gene related to it has been identified, coded, cloned and expressed in *Escherichia coli*. This recombinant gene when injected in rats showed increased serum immunoglobulin G (IgG) antibody response against *P. gingivalis* and gave protection against bone loss.
  - *Control of biofilm antibiotic resistance*: It has been observed that biofilm bacteria are 1,000-fold more resistant to antibiotics compared to planktonic counterpart, making them hard to control. Recently, a gene has been identified in *Pseudomonas aeruginosa* which encodes for glycosyl transferase which facilitates synthesis of periplasmic glucans which in turn protects it from effects of antibiotics. With the help of gene therapy, researchers have developed mutant of this gene capable of forming a biofilm but lacking periplasmic glucans, therefore rendering biofilm more susceptible to antibiotic therapy.
  - *Alveolar remodeling*: Periodontal tissues react to stimuli, such as stress and inflammation by active remodeling which facilitates the expression of various molecules. Use of transfer genes which are responsible for various remodeling molecules (Lac Z gene) along with electroporation (electric impulse) for driving gene into cell help to achieve predictable alveolar bone remodeling.
- *To control periodontal disease progression*:[34-37]
  - *Antimicrobial gene therapy*: If a gene which encodes for an antimicrobial peptide is inserted into the host, it can drastically enhance the host-defense mechanisms. It is reported that infection of a host cells in-vivo with a-defensin-2 gene via a retroviral vector favors a potent antimicrobial activity.
  - *Tight adherence gene*: *Aggregatibacter actinomycetemcomitans* is a potent periopathogen which expresses a "tight adherence gene" for its adherence to host tissue and virulence. Researchers have developed a mutant strain of this pathogen lacking this gene. This is might be helpful in controlling periodontal disease progression by limiting colonization and pathogenesis of *A. actinomycetemcomitans*.
- *In treatment of periodontal disease*:
  - *Gene-enhanced tissue engineering*: In general, tissue engineering is helpful in supplementing the regenerative site with therapeutic protein-like growth factor. Growth factor usually undergoes proteolytic breakdown and solubility of delivery vehicle. Gene therapy provides longer exposure of the growth factor for at least 2 weeks to the periodontal wound as compared to tissue engineering. Thus overcomes the shorter lifespan of growth factor associated with tissue engineering. Genetically engineered mesenchymal stem cell, when placed into an osseous defect, induced new bone and blood vessels formation by expressing BMP-2.[38,39] The cells have a capability to engraft, differentiate and display regulatory behaviors.[40] Similarly, platelet-derived growth factor (PDGF) has a potent effect on regeneration of hard and soft tissues and hence, useful for tissue engineering.[41,42]

## Limitations and Difficulties

- *Gene delivery*: Successful gene delivery is difficult to perform and unpredictable, even in single-gene disorders, e.g., the genetic basis of cystic fibrosis is well known, but the presence of mucus in the lungs increases physical complications in delivery of genes to the target lung cells.

- *Durability and integration*: Some of the gene therapy approaches have a long-term durability. This can be achieved in two possible ways. First, is the use of multiple rounds of gene therapy and second is the integration of the therapeutic genes so that they remain active for some time. Integrating therapeutic DNA can induce possible undesirable side effects.
- *Immune response*: Body immunity can identify viral vector as foreign and induce immune attack by stimulating the immune system. This usually reduces the efficacy of gene therapy or induces serious side effects.
- *Safety of the vectors*: Viruses that are used as a vector in gene therapy are associated with various problems to the patient, e.g., immune and inflammatory responses, toxicity, gene control and targeting issues. Moreover, a viral vector can recover its ability to induce disease.
- *Cost factor*: At present, gene therapy is very expensive. This may restrict its use and benefits in only a class of patients and not to wider population.
- *Ethical restrictions*: Applying gene therapy to protect from disabilities or diseases definitely poses an ethical problem. Also, the question of till where and how we can restrict gene therapy is a serious one.

## NANOTECHNOLOGY

### Definitions

Norio Taniguchi of the Tokyo Science University for the first time defined the term "nanotechnology" in a paper published in 1974 as follows: nanotechnology mainly consists of the processing of, separation, consolidation and deformation of materials by one atom or one molecule. Now, the definition of nanotechnology has been expanded to include features as large as 100 nm. In addition to this, the concept of nanotechnology embracing the structures exhibiting quantum mechanical aspects, like quantum dots, has further expanded its definition. Later, the term "nanotechnology" was independently coined and popularized by Eric Drexler.

According to definition provided by National Nanotechnology Initiative, nanotechnology is the research and development of materials, devices and system exhibiting physical, chemical and biological properties that are different from those found on a larger scale.

Molecular nanotechnology (MNT) is the concept of engineering functional mechanical systems at the molecular scale designed and built atom-by-atom.

It would make use of positionally-controlled mechanosynthesis guided by molecular machine systems. It involves combining physical principles demonstrated by chemistry, other nanotechnologies, and the molecular machinery of life with the systems engineering principles found in modern macroscale factories.

### Generations of Nanotechnology Development

Four generations of nanotechnology development has been introduced by Mike Roco of the US National Nanotechnology Initiative **(Fig. 67.11)**. The first era is of passive nanostructures which include materials designed to perform one task. The second phase is of active nanostructures for multitasking, e.g., drug delivery devices and sensors. The third generation was introduced around 2010 and is thought to feature nanosystems with thousands of interacting components. In coming years, the first integrated nanosystems, functioning similar to mammalian cell with hierarchical systems within systems, are expected to be developed.[43,44]

### Properties of Nanomaterials

Following are the properties of nanomaterials:
- Nanomaterials are those materials with components less than 100 nm in at least one dimension.
- They have significant surface effects, size effects and quantum effects exhibiting better performance properties compared to traditional materials.
- They have special chemical, optical, magnetic and electro-optical properties that are different from similar material either individual molecule or at larger scale.
- They have an important property of self-assembly. They autonomously organize themselves into patterns or structures without intervention. This property of self-assembly is typically manipulated and facilitated through correct setting of conditions. Electrostatic attractive interactions between positive and negative charges are the main driving forces for self-assembly.[43,44]

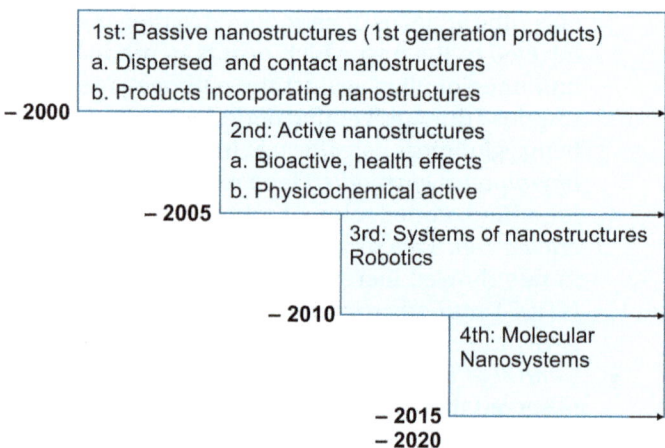

**Fig. 67.11:** Schematic representation showing generations of nanotechnology.

## Nanomaterial Assemblies

- *Multilayer assemblies*: It is the layer-by-layer adsorption of individual atoms to form multilayered structures of various shapes and sizes.
- *Core shell assemblies*: Core shells of particular size, topology and composition are formed by removal of core by either dissolution to produce hollow particles or decomposition to give hollow shells.
- *Nanorods/nanowires/nanofibers*: These are linear structures with a very small diameter formed by linear arrangement of atoms.
- *Nanotubes*: Carbon nanotubes are the most researched nanomaterial. A sheet of carbon atoms can be rolled into a tube forming a carbon nanotube. Properties of carbon nanotube depend on the pattern in which sheet is rolled. The right arrangement of atoms helps to form a carbon nanotube which is 100 times stronger than steel, but 6 times lighter.
- *Nanobuds*: Carbon nanobuds are a newly created material combining two previously discovered allotropes of carbon; carbons nanotubes and fullerene buckyball. A fullerene buckyball is a molecule composed entirely of carbon in the form of a hollow sphere. In Nanobuds fullerene buckyball-like buds are covalently bonded to the outer sidewalls of the underlying carbon nanotube
- *Nanotorus*: A nanotorus is described as carbon nanotube bent into a torus (doughnut shape). Nanotori are predicted to have many unique properties, such as magnetic moments 1,000 times larger than previously expected for certain specific radii.[43,44]

## Applications in Periodontics

Following are the application of nanotechnology in periodontics:[45,46]

- *Treatment of dentin hypersensitivity*: Reconstructive dental nanorobots, using native biological materials, could selectively and precisely occlude-specific tubules within minutes, offering patients a quick and permanent cure.
- *Nanorobotic dentifrices (dentifrobots)*: Nanorobotic dentifrices are suitable to deliver by mouthwash or toothpaste. Guarding with these dentifrobots in all supragingival and subgingival surfaces at least once a day metabolized trapped organic matter into harmless and odorless vapors and help in continuous calculus debridement. Additionally, they are useful in identifying and destroying pathogenic bacteria in plaque and allowing the growth of harmless bacteria. Dentifrobots would also be able to cure halitosis by preventing putrefaction of organic material in oral cavity.
- *Nanofibers*: Nanotechnology is producing nanofibers that have much better properties than conventional fibers. These nanofibers are available with larger surface area per unit mass and allow an easier addition of surface functionalities compared to polymer microfibers. These nanofibers are commonly used in drug delivery systems and tissue engineering scaffolds.
- *Nano biomineralization*: Biomineralization refers to minerals formed biologically, which differ in structure and properties from laboratory formed materials, for example that in bone. Bone formation and structure is also being analyzed at nanolevel to construct a synthetic bone graft substitute with a nanostructured architecture that resembles natural bone. Crystals are manipulated at nanolevels and embedded into collagen fibers to form organic inorganic composite, possessing unique mechanical properties. Body can easily accept such synthetic grafts very well and will guide body cells for mending of bone defects.
- *Tooth repair (biomimicry)*: Nanotechnology can also be applied to synthesize both mineral and cellular components of tooth. Such a technique has been developed by Chen et al., to form dental enamel. They used highly organized microarchitectural units of nanorod-like calcium hydroxyapatite crystals arranged roughly parallel to each other. It is expected that within a span of time we would be able to mimic the periodontal tissues also and would be able to repair them in a natural way with the help of nanotechnology.
- Tissue engineering scaffold.
- Nanotextured implant surface.

## Other Applications

### Inducing Anesthesia

For this, a colloidal solution of millions of dental nanorobots will be instilled on the patient's gingiva. These nanorobots will reach dentin by migrating into gingival sulcus and passing through cementoenamel junction. Through dentin they proceed towards the pulp either by biological guides or through instructions from outside computers. Inside pulp they control nerve impulse traffic inducing anesthesia. These robots will then come out after completion of task through natural pathways. Such a technique will offer more patient comfort, greater selectivity, a faster complete and reversible analgesic effect.

### Tooth Repositioning

Orthodontic nanorobots will be able to manipulate the periodontal tissues which favor painless and fast tooth movements within hours.

### Nanocomposites

It is one of the dental products designs with nanotechnology which is commercially available today. It is composed of non-agglomerated discrete nanoparticles mixed homogenously with resins or coatings to produce nanocomposites. Various advantages of nanocomposites are superior flexible

strength, superior hardness, high esthetic appeal and excellent finish.
- *Nanosolutions*: Nanoparticles homogenously dispersed into various solvents and polymers form nanosolutions. Such solutions provide superior properties than the parent materials. This technique is being applied in bonding agents to provide superior hold of filling materials.
- *Femtolasers*: They are like a pair of nanoscissors producing sharp cuts in the tissue. They act by vaporizing tissue locally while leaving adjacent tissue unharmed. This technique is being applied in plastic and ophthalmic surgery as well as individual chromosome surgery. In near future, we can hope for its use in periodontal plastic surgery.
- *Nanomedical tests*: Chris Backous is developing a Lab-on-chip which is helpful to doctors in getting immediate results for medical tests. It will also be able to analyze genetic information of individual cells. This will provide instant results and would be able to help with the diagnosis. Similar chips could also be designed for diagnosis of periodontal diseases in near future.

## PERIODONTAL VACCINE

### Introduction

The invention and development of periodontal vaccine to prevent periodontal disease is a big advancement in the field of preventive dentistry. It is administered either parenterally, intramuscularly, subcutaneously, intradermally or orally by which the host accepts well and the antibodies reach the destined target areas. The vaccine is tested in canine bearers and other mammals for the immune response and the inflammatory inhibition. Periodontal disease leads to destruction of the tissues and later tooth loss at an early or middle age and bone loss reduces the chances of replacement with a proper prosthesis. Administering the vaccine, in early adolescent age before there is any sign of periodontitis, helps in prolonging the healthy life of the periodontium and risk of any inflammation is reduced.[47,48]

The vaccine development program involves identifying the bacterial peptides and proteins that trigger the immune response, and using these as the basis of vaccines. The vaccines are being trialed in mouse models of periodontal disease and following a positive response, a vaccine will progress to clinical trials.

The increasing prevalence of periodontitis in the populations, especially in the developing countries, demands administering vaccines for periodontitis in large numbers of people. In order to restrict the transmission and/or intraoral dissemination of periodontopathic bacteria, the vaccine should induce immunity at following three levels for better protection:[47,48]
1. Local mucosal secretory immunoglobulin A (IgA)
2. Local draining lymph nodes
3. Circulating specific T and B cell responses

### Active Immunization

Exposure to a foreign antigen induces active immunization. Active immunization involves activation of lymphocytes to produce antibodies against the antigen. The immune system of the host actively responds to the antigen to produce effective antibodies. Previous studies in non-human primate models with ligature-induced experimental periodontitis reported development of active immunization against *P. gingivalis* due to antibody production. Such active immunity can be induced, enhanced, and obtained over time. Whole bacterial cell and purified protein preparations are reported as ideal vaccine candidates and have been evaluated in various animal models producing active immune responses.

Data collected from previous studies suggest that active immunization is helpful in reduction of the rate and severity of bone loss. Additionally, such immunization is noted to temporarily alter the composition of the subgingival microflora. Natural active immunization by therapeutic interventions not only enhances the antibody titer, but also potentially improves treatment outcomes.

Three types of vaccines were employed for the control of periodontal disease:[49]
1. Vaccines prepared from pure cultures of streptococci and other oral organism.
2. Autogenous vaccines were prepared from the dental plaque of patients with destructive periodontal diseases. Plaque samples were removed and sterilized by heat by immersion in formalin solution and reinjected into same patient.
3. Stock vaccines,[50] e.g., Inava Endocorps vaccine, Goldenberg's vaccine, VanCott's vaccine.

Inava Endocarps vaccine was made of mixture of seven microorganisms.[51]

The future vaccine of periodontal disease will likely contain a mixture of adhesins from the most prominent periodontopathogens. Inhibition of the lectin results in loss of ability of the bacteria to adhere to various surfaces. The lectin is a potent immunogen but it is not known if antibodies against the lectin prevent streptococcal adhesion in experimental animals.

### Passive Immunization

Passive immunization involves direct administration of antibodies via lymphocytes or serum from immunized individuals or monoclonal antibodies against specific pathogen. Passive immune response is short-lived and effective only for the time period, the injected antibody persists in the body. However, passive immunization is considered as comparatively safer than active immunization. Passive immunization of humans using *P. gingivalis monoclonal* antibodies temporarily avoids colonization of *P. gingivalis*.[52-55] Along with this, use of probiotic therapy is noted as an alternative approach. For human periodontal vaccine trials, administration of antibodies are associated with regulatory and safety issues. Additionally, shared infectious etiology between periodontitis and other systemic disorders also increases efforts in effective vaccine developments.[56-58]

## MINIMALLY INVASIVE SURGERY

### Introduction

In 1990, a noninstrument-based surgical procedure started to take its origin. Wickham and Fitzpatrick for the first time introduced the techniques of using smaller incisions as "minimally invasive surgery" (MIS). The term "periodontal" describes a smaller more precise surgical technique for periodontal surgery. MIS for periodontal bone grafting was first described by Harrel in 1999.[59] This technique utilizes very small incisions with minimal reflection to achieve pocket depth reduction and, attachment level gain with minimal recession in operated site. In 2007, Cortellini and Tonetti gave a modified surgical approach to minimally invasive surgical technique (MIST) in treating isolated intrabony defects with periodontal regeneration.[60] Later, in 2008 they described a MIST in treatment of multiple adjacent deep intrabony defects. More recently, in 2009, Trombelli et al., has described a single flap approach (SFA) in conjunction with GTR for intraosseous defects characterized by an extension prevalent either on buccal or lingual sides.[61] These techniques have so far shown promising results with GTR procedures and use of materials like Emdogain.

### Rationale of Minimally Invasive Surgical Techniques

- Reduction of surgical trauma
- Increase in flap or wound stabilization
- Improvement of primary closure of wound
- Reduction of surgical chair time
- Minimization of intraoperative and postoperative patient discomfort and morbidity
- Prevention of postoperative gingival recession

### Minimally Invasive Surgery

In 1999, Harrel used a minimally invasive surgical approach for periodontal bone grafting.[59] The MIS is different from traditional approach in the use of much smaller incisions to gain surgical access and debridement of the periodontal defect before placing bone graft and membrane. MIS was found to be effective in terms of mean clinical attachment gain and minimal recession. Later, this technique was used with Emdogain giving similar results.[62] MIS is different from traditional approach in the technique of accessing the periodontal defect, soft-tissue flaps handling procedures, debridement method and wound closure. Hence, MIS needs different technical skills and instruments to handle soft-tissue access, debridement of the periodontal defect and root surfaces as compared to traditional periodontal surgery.

### Indications

- An isolated interproximal defect significantly not extending beyond the interproximal site is the ideal site for bone grafting with MIS technique.
- A periodontal defect that borders on an edentulous area.
- A defect extending from the interproximal area to the buccal and lingual is less ideal site. However, this technique is suitable in such areas.
- The technique is suitable for many isolated defects as long as the incision at one site fails to connect with incision at other site and become a continuous incision.

### Contraindications

- Generalized horizontal bone loss
- Multiple interconnected vertical defects

### Surgical Procedure

- The area intended for surgery is anesthetized with local anesthesia with epinephrine 1: 100,000.
- *Incisions*: Intrasulcular incisions are made on teeth adjacent to defect separately to retain more interproximal papillary tissue and tissue height. A single horizontal incision is placed 2–3 mm from the crest of the papilla to connect two intrasulcular incisions. When the surgery involved an esthetic area, the horizontal incision should be placed in the palatal aspect of the papilla to preserve the shape of the papilla and the graft site is covered by soft tissue. However, for nonesthetic area, horizontal incision is given either on the buccal or lingual side whichever better covers the grafted site with soft tissue.
- *Tissue reflection*: Tissue is elevated using sharp dissection with a smaller sized Orban's knife. Sharp dissection minimizes trauma to flap and preserves blood supply to the tissues. The maintenance of adequate blood supply helps in soft-tissue healing and induces minimal postoperative soft-tissue changes.
- *Visualization*: During MIS, visualization of field requires some form of magnification for which surgical telescopes with magnification of minimum 3.5x are recommended. Visualization of the defect from several angles during MIS makes the use of an operating microscope cumbersome.
- *Defect debridement*: Removal of granulation tissue in MIS is significantly different from traditional surgery. After performing minimal flap reflection, tip of the curette is directed vertically into the defect and the shank is held parallel to long axis of the tooth. Granulation tissue is then removed with the tip of the curette. When the curette is used in usual manner by placing the shank horizontal to long axis of the tooth, the shank will impinge and fold the small gingival flap. This may traumatize the gingiva. Remaining granulation tissue is fragmented with use of

ultrasonic scaler and then removed with degranulator, a mechanical granulation tissue removal instrument. It consists of a sharpened tube useful as curette, a vacuum used to pull the fragmented granulation tissue and a rotating bur for cutting the granulation tissue. Vacuum removes the granulation tissue and keeps the surgical field free of blood providing better visualization. Smoothing of the root surface is achieved in a manner similar to closed root planing. Final root planing and smoothing can be performed with a high speed surgical length finishing bur.

- *Placement of grafting material*: Root conditioning is optional before placing a bone graft. Any combination of grafting material with GTR membrane can be used to regenerate the defect. The graft is positioned into the defect with a modified amalgam gun. The curved tip of the amalgam gun facilitates easier entry into the defect through the MIS opening. A trimmed membrane is laid over the bone graft and margins of the membrane are kept below the buccal and lingual flaps. This stabilizes the graft and keeps it from escaping through incisions. Nonresorbable membranes are usually contraindicated due to the need for second-stage procedure.[63]
- *Wound closure*: To close interproximal site, vertical mattress suture is given. Though any type of suture material is suitable for closing site but 4-0 plain gut suture is commonly used. The suture is placed in the body of the papilla and should be kept away from the tip of the papilla. This suture will help to pull the buccal and lingual tissues together at the base of the flaps. Dressing is not mandatory with MIS techniques.
- *Postoperative instructions and care*: Postoperative instructions are given thereafter. It includes antibiotic coverage and chlorhexidine mouthwash for 1 week.

### Advantages

- Minimally invasive surgery improves probing depths and attachment levels much similar to those obtained with regenerative procedures performed with a traditional surgical approach.
- There is improvement in the rate of healing since smaller incision will heal faster.
- A lesser postoperative pain and discomfort than that with a larger incision.
- Excellent patient acceptance to the procedure.

## PIEZOSURGERY

### Introduction

Piezosurgery is a relatively new technique that utilizes ultrasonic vibration for osteoplasty and osteotomy. The ultrasonic frequency is modulated from 10 cycles/seconds, 30 cycles/seconds and 60 cycles/seconds (Hz) to 29 kHz. The low frequency enables cutting of only mineralized structures, leaving soft tissue. Power can be adjusted from 2.8 W to 16 W, with preset power settings for various types of bone density. The piezosurgery tip vibrates within a range of 60–200 mm, which allows clean cutting with precise incisions.

Dr Tomaso Vercellotti in 1998 invented piezosurgery device for harvesting a bone graft.[64] Jonathon Schofield and Amit Patel reported that the surgical control in mobilizing a block graft is easier by piezosurgery than by conventional methods.[65] The force necessary to produce a cut is much less compared to rotational burs, trephines or reciprocating microsaws. The piezosurgery inserts (tips) vibrate within a width of 60–210 µm with an advanced oscillation controlled module. Therefore an increase in temperature is avoided, which ultimately reduces the risk of bone damage as a result of overheating.

When bur is used for bone cutting there is quite bone wastage resulting in smaller harvested block. However, trephine makes very fine cut with very little bone wastage. But, it allows a circular corticocancellous block harvesting, which is not ideal. The piezosurgery osteotomy makes a narrow cut with little bone wastage. It also allows a block of bone to be cut to match the size of the recipient site.

Thus, piezosurgery offers:

- *Micrometric cutting*: Precise cutting actions with an excellent surgical tactile control.
- *Selective cutting*: Minimizes the risk of adjacent soft-tissue damage.
- *Cavitation effect*: Offers maximum intraoperative visibility.

The unit consists of handpiece, foot switch, ultrasound, control, dynamometric wench and peristaltic pump. Each piezosurgery unit is supplied with two handpieces. It is connected to the main unit, which has holders for the handpiece and irrigation fluids. The liquid is drawn from a bag hanging from the provided rod. The insert tips are tightened to the handpiece with the dynamometric wrench. High-frequency oscillations of 24,000 Hz and 29,500 Hz, modulated with a low frequency between 10 Hz and 60 Hz, enables efficient and controlled use. The unit is controlled solely by means of the keyboard. Each command selected is shown on a display. The sterile tube inserted into the pump contains the liquid. It is used for cooling with a jet of solution that discharges from the insert with an adjustable flow of 0–60 mL/min and removing debris from the bone cutting area.

The Insert Kits-Kit containing the insert tips can be used for various procedures. The insert tips are either steel or gold colored. The steel tips are used to treat roots of teeth or soft tissues, whereas the gold tips are used to treat bone. The golden color of the insert tips is obtained by the titanium nitride coating to improve the surface hardness. Following are the various tips available:

- *Smoothing insert tips*: These tips have diamond surfaces enabling precise and controlled work on the bone structures. Preparation of a sinus window or access to a nerve can be done easily with smoothing insert tips.

- *Sharp insert tips*: These are used in osteoplasty and osteotomy procedures, whenever a fine and well-defined cut in the bone structure concerned is required.
- *Blunt insert tips*: These are used to prepare the soft tissue, e.g., for elevating Schneider's membrane or for lateralizing nerves. These insert tips are also used for root planing.

## Advantages

- *Superior precision*: Piezosurgery requires lesser hand pressure compared with traditional rotary instrumentation. As a result there is enhanced operator sensitivity and control.
- *Safer*: The instrument sections only mineralized structures selectively, leaving adjacent soft tissues. Soft tissues remain intact even in case of accidental contact.
- *Better healing*: Healing is much better with piezosurgery because cutting action is minimally invasive and thus produces less collateral tissue damage.[66-68]
- *Reduced bleeding*: Piezosurgery creates a virtually bloodless surgical site due to its cavitation effect on physiological solutions (blood).
- *Greater visibility*: Due to reduction of bleeding at the site, piezosurgery makes visibility much clearer than other conventional bone cutting instruments.
- *Reduced postoperative necrosis*: Piezosurgery inserts do not become hot remain cool only unlike conventional microsaws and burs, reducing the risk of postoperative necrosis.[69]

## Disadvantages

- *Slow*: Cutting very dense bone with ultrasound can take up to 4 times longer than with a rotary bur.
- *Tip breakage*: The frequency of tip breakage is greater.
- *Expensive*: These are expensive than other mechanical osteotomes.

## Contraindication

Piezosurgery is contraindicated in both patient and operator with pacemakers.

## Applications

Following are the application of piezosurgery in periodontics and implantology:
- Root planing
- Osteoplasty and osteotomy procedures
- Regenerative reconstructive surgery
- Bone harvesting for regenerative surgery (chips or blocks)
- Preparation of implant site
- Expansion of ridge
- Schneiderian's membrane elevation
- Bony window osteotomy during sinus lift procedure
- Extraction for immediate implant positioning

### Points to Ponder

- LANAP is laser assisted new attachment procedure in which laser is used to remove the epithelial lining of the sulcus as well as junctional epithelium. This leads to retardation of epithelial downgrowth providing more time for connective tissue attachment on the root surface.
- Various biologic mediators used in tissue engineering are insulin growth factor (IGF-I), platelet-derived growth factor (PDGF), transforming growth factor (TGF), fibroblast growth factor (FGF-2), enamel matrix derivative (EMD) and bone morphogenetic protein (BMP)-2, BMP-4, BMP- 7 and BMP-12.
- Piezosurgery is contraindicated in both patient and operator with pacemakers.

## REFERENCES

### Lasers

1. Bader HI. Use of lasers in periodontics. Dent Clin North Am. 2000;44(4):779-91.
2. Rossmann JA, Cobb CM. Lasers in periodontal therapy. Periodontol 2000. 1995;9:150-64.
3. Cobb CM, Low SB, Coluzzi DJ. Lasers and the treatment of chronic periodontitis. Dent Clin North Am. 2010;54(1): 35-53.
4. Coleton S. Lasers in surgical periodontics and oral medicine. Dent Clin North Am. 2004;48(4):937-62.
5. Gimbel CB. Hard tissue laser procedures. Dent Clin North Am. 2000;44(4):931-53.
6. Cobb CM. Lasers in periodontics: a review of the literature. J Periodontol. 2006;77(4):545-64.
7. Ishikawa I, Aoki A, Takasaki AA, Mizutani K, Sasaki KM, Izumi Y. Application of lasers in periodontics: true innovation or myth? Periodontol 2000. 2009;50:90-126.
8. Midda M. The use of lasers in periodontology. Curr Opin Dent. 1992;2:104-8.
9. Schwarz F, Arweiler N, Georg T, Reich E. Desensitizing effects of an Er:YAG laser on hypersensitive dentine. J Clin Periodontol. 2002;29(3):211-5.
10. Slot DE, Kranendonk AA, Paraskevas S, Van der Weijden F. The effect of a pulsed Nd:YAG laser in non-surgical periodontal therapy. J Periodontol. 2009;80(7):1041-56.
11. Wigdor HA, Walsh JT Jr, Featherstone JD, Visuri SR, Fried D, Waldvogel JL. Lasers in dentistry. Lasers Surg Med. 1995;16(2):103-33.
12. Sun G. The role of lasers in cosmetic dentistry. Dent Clin North Am. 2000;44(4):831-50.
13. Renvert S, Lindahl C, Roos Jansåker AM, Persson GR. Treatment of peri-implantitis using an Er:YAG laser or an air-abrasive device: a randomized clinical trial. J Clin Periodontol. 2011;38(1):65-73.
14. Deppe H, Horch HH, Neff A. Conventional versus $CO_2$ laser-assisted treatment of peri-implant defects with the concomitant use of pure-phase beta-tricalcium phosphate: a 5-year clinical report. Int J Oral Maxillofac Implants. 2007;22(1):79-86.

### Photodynamic Therapy

15. Andersen R, Loebel N, Hammond D, Wilson M. Treatment of periodontal disease by photodisinfection compared to scaling and root planing. J Clin Dent. 2007;18(2):34-8.

16. Azarpazhooh A, Shah PS, Tenenbaum HC, Goldberg MB. The effect of photodynamic therapy for periodontitis: a systematic review and meta-analysis. J Periodontol. 2010;81(1):4-14.
17. Schneider M, Kirfel G, Berthold M, Frentzen M, Krause F, Braun A. The impact of antimicrobial photodynamic therapy in an artificial biofilm model. Lasers Med Sci. 2012;27(3):615-20.
18. Takasaki AA, Aoki A, Mizutani K, Schwarz F, Sculean A, Wang CY, et al. Application of antimicrobial photodynamic therapy in periodontal and peri-implant diseases. Periodont 2000. 2009;51:109-40.
19. Moslemi N, Heidari M, Bouraima SA. Antimicrobial photodynamic therapy as an adjunctive modality in the treatment of chronic periodontitis. J Lasers Med Sci. 2012;3(4):141-6.
20. Chan Y, Lai CH. Bactericidal effects of different laser wavelengths on periodontopathic germs in photodynamic therapy. Lasers Med Sci. 2003;18(1):51-5.
21. Komerik N, Nakanishi H, MacRobert AJ, Henderson B, Speight P, Wilson M. In vivo killing of *Porphyromonas gingivalis* by toluidine blue-mediated photosensitization in an animal model. Antimicrob Agents Chemother. 2003;47(3):932-40.

## Tissue Engineering

22. Bartold PM, McCulloch CA, Narayanan AS, Pitaru S. Tissue engineering: a new paradigm for periodontal regeneration based on molecular and cell biology. Periodontol 2000. 2000;24:253-69.
23. Bartold PM, Xiao Y, Lyngstaadas SP, Paine ML, Snead ML. Principles and applications of cell delivery systems for periodontal regeneration. Periodontol 2000. 2006;41:123-35.
24. Vats A, Tolley NS, Polak JM, Gough JE. Scaffolds and biomaterials for tissue engineering: a review of clinical applications. Clin Otolaryngol Allied Sci. 2003;283(3):165-72.
25. Yang S, Leong KF, Du Z, Chua CK. The design of scaffolds for use in tissue engineering. Part I. Traditional factors. Tissue Eng. 2001;7(6):679-89.
26. Taba M Jr, Jin Q, Sugai JV, Giannobile WV. Current concepts in periodontal bioengineering. Orthod Craniofac Res. 2005;8(4):292-302.
27. Vogel V, Baneyx G. The tissue engineering puzzle: a molecular perspective. Annu Rev Biomed Eng. 2003;5:441-63.
28. Lynch SE, Genco RJ, Marx RE, Nevins M, Wisner-Lynch LA. Tissue Engineering: Applications in Maxillofacial Surgery and Periodontics, 2nd revised edition. Carol Stream, IL, USA: Quintessence Publishing; 2008.
29. Whitaker MJ, Quirk RA, Howdle SM, Shakesheff KM. Growth factor release from tissue engineering scaffolds. J Pharm Pharmacol. 2001;53(11):1427-37.
30. Butler DL, Goldstein SA, Guilak F. Functional tissue engineering: the role of biomechanics. J Biomech Eng. 2000;122(6):570-5.
31. Hsiong SX, Mooney DJ. Regeneration of vascularized bone. Periodontol 2000. 2006;41:109-22.

## Gene Therapy

32. Mammen B, Ramakrishnan T, Sudhakar U, Vijayalakshmi. Principles of gene therapy. Indian J Dent Res. 2007;18(4):196-200.
33. Meager A, Griffiths E. Human somatic gene therapy. Trends Biotechnol. 1994;12(4):108-13.
34. Baum BJ, O'Connell BC. The impact of gene therapy on dentistry. J Am Dent Assoc. 1995;126(2):179-89.
35. Baum BJ, Kok M, Tran SD, Yamano S. The impact of gene therapy on dentistry: a revisiting after six years. J Am Dent Assoc. 2002;133(1):35-44.
36. Karthikeyan BV, Pradeep AR. Gene therapy in periodontics: a review and future implications. J Contemp Dent Pract. 2006;7(3):83-91.
37. Mahale S, Dani N, Ansari SS, Kale T. Gene therapy and its implications in periodontics. J Indian Soc Periodontol. 2009;13(1):1-5.
38. Jin QM, Anusaksathien O, Webb SA, Rutherford RB, Giannobile WV. Gene therapy of bone morphogenetic protein for periodontal tissue engineering. J Periodontol. 2003;74(2):202-13.
39. Dunn CA, Jin QM, Taba M Jr, Franceschi RT, Brue Rutherford R, Giannobile WV. BMP gene delivery for alveolar bone engineering at dental implant defects. Mol Ther. 2005;11(2):294-9.
40. Wikesjö UM, Sorensen RG, Kinoshita A, Jian Li X, Wozney JM. Periodontal repair in dogs: effect of recombinant human bone morphogenetic protein-12 (rhBMP-12) on regeneration of alveolar bone and periodontal attachment. J Clin Periodontol. 2004;31(8):662-70.
41. Anusaksathien O, Webb SA, Jin QM, Giannobile WV. Platelet-derived growth factor gene delivery stimulates ex vivo gingiva repair. Tissue Eng. 2003;9(4):745-56.
42. Lin Z, Sugai JV, Jin Q, Chandler LA, Giannobile WV. Platelet-derived growth factor-B gene delivery sustains gingival fibroblast signal transduction. J Periodontal Res. 2008;43(4):440-9.

## Nanotechnology

43. Nano A. The A to Z of Nanotechnology and Nanomaterials. The Institute of Nanotechnology, Azom Co Ltd; 2003.
44. Patil M, Mehta DS, Guvva S. Future impact of nanotechnology on medicine and dentistry. J Indian Soc Periodontol. 2008;12(2):34-40.
45. Kong LX, Peng Z, Li SD, Bartold PM. Nanotechnology and its role in the management of periodontal diseases. Periodontol 2000. 2006;40:184-96.
46. Mitra SB, Wu D, Holmes BN. An application of nanotechnology in advanced dental materials. J Am Dent Assoc. 2003;134(10):1382-90.

## Periodontal Vaccine

47. Persson GR. Immune responses and vaccination against periodontal infections. J Clin Periodontol. 2005;32(Suppl 6):39-53.
48. Page RC. Vaccination and periodontitis: myth or reality. J Int Acad Periodontol. 2000;2(2):31-43.
49. Grant DA, Stern IB, Listgarten MA. Microbiology (plaque). In: Periodontics, 6th edition. St. Louis: CV Mosby; 1988. pp. 147-97.
50. McGehee WHO. Stock vaccines in the treatment of pyorrhea alveolaris. Dent Cosmos. 1912;54:997-1002.
51. Casto TD. The treatment of periodontoclasia with a polyvalent vaccine (goldenberg inava endocorps vaccine). Dent Cosmos. 1925;67:689-91.
52. Booth V, Ashley FP, Lehner T. Passive immunization with monoclonal antibodies against Porphyromonas gingivalis in patients with periodontitis. Infect Immun. 1996;64(2):422-7.
53. Abiko Y. Passive immunization against dental caries and periodontal disease: development of recombinant and human monoclonal antibodies. Crit Rev Oral Biol Med. 2000;11(2):140-58.
54. Nakagawa T, Saito A, Hosaka Y, Ishihara K. Gingipains as candidate antigens for *Porphyromonas gingivalis* vaccine. Keio J Med. 2003;52(3):158-62.

55. Lee JY, Yi NN, Kim US, Choi JS, Kim SJ, Choi JI. *Porphyromonas gingivalis* heat shock protein vaccine reduces the alveolar bone loss induced by multiple periodontopathogenic bacteria. J Periodontal Res. 2006;41(1):10-4.
56. Inagaki S, Ishihara K, Takahashi J, Nakagawa T, Yamada S, Okuda K. Antibody response to gingipain R of *Porphyromonas gingivalis* in periodontitis patients. J Dent Res. 2001;80:651.
57. Schenck K, Helgeland K, Tollefsen T. Antibodies against lipopolysaccharide from *Bacteroides gingivalis* before and after periodontal treatment. Scand J Dent Res. 1987;95(2):112-8.
58. Shin EA, Lee JY, Kim TG, Park YK, Langridge WH. Synthesis and assembly of an adjuvanted *Porphyromonas gingivalis* fimbrial antigen fusion protein in plants. Protein Expr Purif. 2006;47(1):99-109.

## Minimally Invasive Surgery

59. Harrel SK. A minimally invasive surgical approach for periodontal regeneration: surgical technique and observations. J Periodontol. 1999;70(12):1547-57.
60. Cortellini P, Tonetti MS. A minimally invasive surgical technique with an enamel matrix derivative in the regenerative treatment of intra-bony defects: a novel approach to limit morbidity. J Clin Periodontol. 2007;34(1):87-93.
61. Trombelli L, Farina R, Franceschetti G, Calura G. Single-flap approach with buccal access in periodontal reconstructive procedures. J Periodontol. 2009;80(2):353-60.
62. Cortellini P, Nieri M, Prato GP, Tonetti MS. Single minimally invasive surgical technique with an enamel matrix derivative to treat multiple adjacent intrabony defects: clinical outcomes and patient morbidity. J Clin Periodontol. 2008;35(7):605-13.
63. Harrel SK, Nunn ME, Belling CM. Long-term results of a minimally invasive surgical approach for bone grafting. J Periodontol. 1999;70(12):1558-63.

## Piezosurgery

64. Vercellotti T. Technological characteristics and clinical indications of piezoelectric bone surgery. Minerva Stomatol. 2004;53(5):207-14.
65. Schofield J, Patel A. Using piezosurgery to harvest a block bone graft from the symphyseal region: a clinical case presentation. Implant Dentistry Today. 2007;1(4):20-4.
66. Aro H, Kallioniemi H, Aho AJ, Kellokumpu-Lehtinen P. Ultrasonic device in bone cutting. A histological and scanning electron microscopical study. Acta Orthop Scand. 1981;52(1):5-10.
67. Vercellotti T, Crovace A, Palermo A, Molfetta A. The piezoelectric osteotomy in orthopedics: clinical and histological evaluations (Pilot Study in Animals). Mediterr J Surg Med. 2001;9:89-96.
68. Vercellotti T, Nevins ML, Kim DM, Nevins M, Wada K, Schenk RK, et al. Osseous response following resective therapy with piezosurgery. Int J Periodontics Restorative Dent. 2005;25(6):543-9.
69. Horton JE, Tarpley TM Jr, Wood LD. The healing of surgical defects in alveolar bone produced with ultrasonic instrumentation, chisel, and rotary bur. Oral Surg Oral Med Oral Pathol. 1975;39(4):536-46.

## VIVA VOCE

**Q1.** What are various LASER tissue interactions?
**Ans.** Laser light have four different interactions with the target tissue namely absorption, transmission, reflection and scattering.

**Q2.** What is the function of scaffolds?
**Ans.** Scaffolds act as a delivery vehicle for cell transplantation and as a three-dimensional template for tissue regeneration.

**Q3.** What is stem cell?
**Ans.** A single cell that can replicate itself and differentiate into many cell types.

**Q4.** Name various stem cells present in pulpal and periodontal tissues.
**Ans.** Dental pulp stem cells, dental follicle stem cells, stem cells from apical papilla, stem cells from exfoliated deciduous teeth, gingival mesenchymal stem cells, epithelial cell rests of Malassez and periodontal ligament stem cells.

**Q5.** What is nanotechnology?
**Ans.** Nanotechnology is the research and development of materials, devices and system exhibiting physical, chemical and biological properties that are different from those found on a larger scale.

**Q6.** What is the principle behind piezosurgery?
**Ans.** Piezosurgery utilizes low ultrasonic frequency which enables cutting of only mineralized structures, leaving soft tissue. It is used mainly in osteoplasty and osteotomy procedures.

**Q7.** Name the esthetic surgeries that can be done using LASER.
**Ans.** Depigmentation; Crown lengthening

**Q8.** Give an example of phenothiazine dyes used for PACT.
**Ans.** Methylene blue, toluidine blue O

**Q9.** Who introduced the generations of nanotechnology development?
**Ans.** Mike Roco

**Q10.** What are the contraindications for MIS?
**Ans.** Generalized horizontal bone loss and multiple interconnected vertical defects.

# Section 11: Maintenance Phase

- Supportive Periodontal Therapy

# Chapter 68

# Supportive Periodontal Therapy

*Kanteshwari I Kumathalli*

## Chapter Outline

- Aims
- Maintenance Interval
- Maintenance Compliance
- Maintenance Program
- Retreatment of Selected Areas
- Maintenance for Implant Patient

## INTRODUCTION

After phase I therapy is completed, patients are placed on a schedule of periodic recall visits for maintenance care to prevent recurrence of the disease. Transfer of the patient from active treatment status to a maintenance program is a definitive step in total patient care that requires time and effort on the part of the dentist, staff and patient. Thus, the maintenance phase has been described as the cornerstone of successful periodontal therapy **(Flowchart 68.1)**.

The continuing, periodic assessment and prophylactic treatment of the periodontal structures permitting early detection and treatment of new and recurring disease has been commonly referred to as periodontal maintenance or recall. The Third World Workshop of the American Academy of Periodontology (1989) has renamed this maintenance treatment phase as "supportive periodontal therapy" (SPT).[1] This term expresses the essential need for therapeutic measures to support the patient's own efforts to control the periodontal infections and to avoid reinfection. SPT is considered more descriptive and, currently, is the accepted term.

## AIMS

Two major aims of SPT are to prevent the occurrence of new disease and recurrence of previous disease. More specifically, the American Academy of Periodontology's position paper on SPT lists its three goals.[1]

They are:
- To prevent or minimize the recurrence and progression of periodontal disease in patients who have been previously treated for gingivitis, periodontitis and peri-implantitis.
- To prevent or reduce the incidence of tooth loss by monitoring the dentition and any prosthetic replacements of the natural teeth.
- To increase the probability of locating and treating, in a timely manner, other diseases or conditions found within the oral cavity.

## MAINTENANCE INTERVAL

Various methods of determining maintenance intervals have been investigated. The 3-month interval is the most

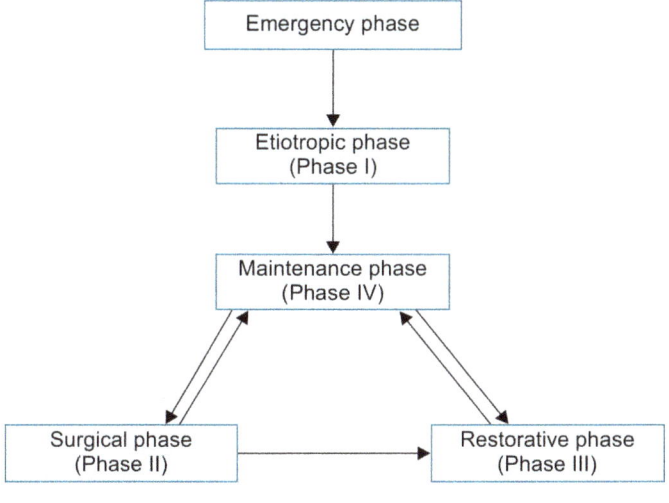

**Flowchart 68.1:** Sequence of periodontal therapy.

## Section 11: Maintenance Phase

| TABLE 68.1: Recall intervals for various classes of recall patients.[2] | | |
|---|---|---|
| **Merin classification** | **Characteristics** | **Recall interval** |
| First year | *First year patient*: Routine therapy and uneventful healing or | 3 months |
| | *First year patient*: Difficult case with complicated prosthesis, furcation involvement, poor crown-to-root ratios, or questionable patient cooperation | 1–2 months |
| Class A | • Excellent results well-maintained for 1 year or more.<br>• Patient displays good oral-hygiene, minimal occlusal, no occlusal problems, no complicated prosthesis, no remaining pockets, and no teeth with <50% of alveolar bone remaining | 6 months to 1 year |
| Class B | Generally good results maintained reasonably well for 1 year or more, but patient displays some of the following:<br>• Inconsistent or poor oral hygiene<br>• Heavy calculus formation<br>• Systemic disease that predisposes to periodontal breakdown<br>• Some remaining pockets<br>• Occlusal problems<br>• Complicated prosthesis<br>• Ongoing orthodontics therapy<br>• Recurrent dental caries<br>• Some teeth with <50% of alveolar bone support<br>• Smoking<br>• Positive family history or genetic test | 3–4 months |
| Class C | Generally, poor results after periodontal therapy and/or several negative factors from the following:<br>• Inconsistent or poor oral hygiene<br>• Heavy calculus formation<br>• Systemic disease that predisposes to periodontal breakdown<br>• Many remaining pockets<br>• Occlusal problems<br>• Complicated prosthesis<br>• Recurrent dental caries<br>• Periodontal surgery indicated but not performed for medical, psychological, or financial reasons<br>• Many teeth with <50% of alveolar bone support<br>• Condition which cannot be improved by periodontal surgery<br>• Smoking<br>• Positive family history or genetic test<br>• More than 20% of pockets bleed on probing | 1–3 months |

frequently used, but can be shortened or lengthened based on an individual patient's clinical parameters and needs **(Table 68.1)**.[2,3] The 3-month rationale is based on the time required for bacterial repopulation of the subgingival environment after mechanical debridement and multiple studies that have shown clinical success with this interval. A regular schedule of periodontal maintenance, thus, appears critical for sustaining health.

## MAINTENANCE COMPLIANCE

Patient compliance with maintenance program is an ongoing problem in dental practices and thus, various strategies for improvement have been investigated. Reasons for noncompliance have been varied and include fear, cost of therapy, type of treatment received, lack of patient motivation and smoking.[4-6]

## MAINTENANCE PROGRAM

The recall hour should be planned to meet the patient's individual needs. The time required for a recall visit for patients with multiple teeth in both arches is approximately 1 hour comprising of three parts **(Fig. 68.1)**.

## First Part (Approx. 10–15 Minutes)

### Examination

Periodontal examination includes an evaluation of the probing depths, bleeding on probing, mobility, the health of the gingival tissues, amount of additional recession, furcation involvement and incidence of suppuration. Determining the percentage of sites with bleeding on probing can be helpful and repeated site-specific bleeding on probing may indicate an individual area of periodontal breakdown. Any desired microbial monitoring can be accomplished at this stage of the appointment. The therapist is continually re-evaluating the success of the periodontal therapy and determining future maintenance procedures with the assessment of these clinical parameters.

### Radiographs

Periodic vertical bitewing radiographs are taken to monitor for any radiographic bone loss or caries; these

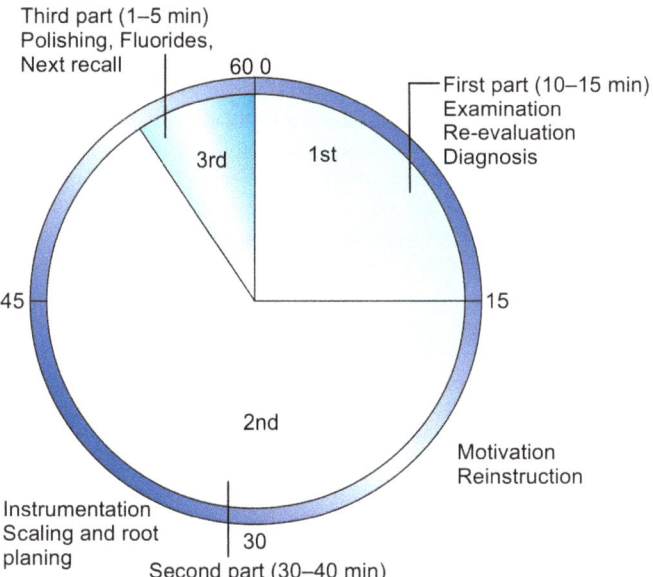

**Fig. 68.1:** Schematic representation showing maintenance program SPT recall hours divided into three parts: (I) The first part is concerned with examination and re-evaluation of the patient's current oral health; (II) The second part includes the necessary motivation, reinstructions and maintenance treatment and (III) The third part involves scheduling the patient for the next recall appointment, additional periodontal treatment (polishing), or restorative dental procedures (fluoride application).

radiographs are compared with previous radiographs. During maintenance therapy, a full-mouth series of radiographs may be beneficial approximately every 5 years to be able to accomplish a complete radiographic evaluation. If general periodontal deterioration is noted from the clinical parameters, then radiographs can be ordered at any appointment. Conversely, if the patient maintains excellent periodontal stability, a full-mouth series of radiographs may not be needed every 5 years.

A plaque assessment using disclosing solution can indicate areas that the patient consistently misses in their daily hygiene regimen and may indicate a needed change in patient hygiene techniques or instrumentation.

## Second Part (Approx. 30–40 Minutes)

Patients frequently need reinforcement of instructions and motivation to continue diligent oral hygiene. An overall increase in gingival inflammation with a generalized increase in the bleeding index may indicate continual poor patient oral hygiene efficiency. A significant increase in the bleeding index with an acceptable plaque index at the maintenance appointment may indicate that the patient had performed adequate oral hygiene for only a few days before the appointment.

Debridement procedures including scaling, root planing and polishing vary depending on the clinical parameters and any presence of deteriorating sites. If significant deposits of subgingival calculus are detected, this may indicate a need for nonsurgical retreatment of selected areas. If multiple sites are found to need additional scaling and root planing, the patient may need to be reappointed for additional treatment because the actual time for debridement during a maintenance visit is limited.

In some instances, a locally delivered antimicrobial agent may be indicated. Topical fluoride treatment for caries prevention is often indicated. Caries and restoration assessments are accomplished at every appointment because exposed root surfaces resulting from periodontal disease can be at risk for root caries.

## Third Part (Approx. 1–5 Minutes)

Scheduling the patient for the next recall must be based on the patient's risk assessment. Polishing the entire dentition to remove all remaining soft deposits and stains provides freshness to the patient and facilitates the diagnosis of early carious lesions. Following polishing, fluorides should be applied in high concentration in order to replace the fluorides which might have been removed by instrumentation from the superficial layers of the teeth. Fluoride or chlorhexidine varnishes may also be applied to prevent root surface caries, especially in areas with gingival recession.

## RETREATMENT OF SELECTED AREAS

During the maintenance visit, areas of periodontal breakdown may be indicated by increasing probing depth, increased attachment loss, increase in bleeding on probing, radiographic bone loss, progressing mobility. The various causes for recurrence of periodontal disease are:[7]

- Inadequate plaque control on the part of the patient or failure to comply with recommended SPT schedules.
- Inadequate or insufficient treatment that has failed to remove all the potential factors favoring plaque accumulation.
- Inadequate restorations placed after the periodontal treatment was completed.
- Failure of the patient to return for periodic checkup.
- Presence of some systemic diseases that may affect host resistance to previously acceptable levels of plaque.

Retreatment is defined as the therapy given after recurrent periodontal destruction has been diagnosed in patients involved in maintenance program. Retreatment may include medications, nonsurgical or surgical procedures.

Treatment schedule varies depending on the following findings:

- If the cause of the generalized breakdown is poor patient plaque control, then surgical therapy should be delayed until nonsurgical therapy is reaccomplished and an adequate plaque control level is maintained by the patient.

- Retreatment of a single failing site will generally include scaling and root planing, with or without local drug delivery. If the area has not responded by the next maintenance appointment, localized surgical therapy may be necessary.
- If health of multiple adjacent sites is not improving, surgical therapy in the area often is indicated. Surgical retreatment is indicated when pockets greater than 5 mm are identified along with bleeding on probing or when probing depths have increased by 3 mm with bleeding on probing over three successive SPT appointments.
- If there is a generalized loss of attachment detected, a thorough analysis for any possible systemic disease should be accomplished. At this retreatment, systemic antibiotics may be considered as an adjunct to the scaling and root planing of the affected areas, with re-evaluation for any possible surgical intervention.
- If increasing mobility is detected, a thorough occlusal evaluation should be done to determine if any occlusal adjustment is necessary.

## MAINTENANCE FOR IMPLANT PATIENT

Maintenance for implant patient is explained in "Chapter 59: Peri-implantitis and other Implant related complications".

### Points to Ponder

- The goals of periodontal and maintenance therapies are identical, i.e., healthy, comfortable, esthetic and functional dentition with stable probing depths.
- The maintenance appointment consists of data collection and the re-evaluation of all clinical parameters.
- Retreatment is needed at times and is considered a part of the maintenance phase of periodontal therapy.

## REFERENCES

1. Supportive periodontal therapy (SPT). J Periodontol. 1998;69(4):502-6.
2. Merin RL. Supportive Periodontal Treatment. In: Newman MG, Takei HH, Carranza FA (Eds). Carranza's Clinical Periodontology, 9th edition. Philadelphia, PA, USA: WB Saunders; 2003. pp. 966-77.
3. Shick R. Maintenance phase of periodontal therapy. J Periodontol. 1981;52(9):576-83.
4. Wilson TG Jr, Glover ME, Schoen J, Baus C, Jacobs T. Compliance with maintenance therapy in a private periodontal practice. J Periodontol. 1984;55(8):468-73.
5. Wilson TG Jr. Compliance. A review of the literature with possible applications to periodontics. J Periodontol. 1987;58(10): 706-14.
6. Wilson TG Jr, Glover ME, Malik AK, Schoen JA, Dorsett D. Tooth loss in maintenance patients in a private periodontal practice. J Periodontol. 1987;58(4):231-5.
7. Wilson TG Jr, Kornman KS. Retreatment: for patients with inflammatory periodontal disease. Periodontol 2000. 1996;12:119-21.

### VIVA VOCE

**Q1. What is the rationale behind SPT?**
**Ans.** There is a sound scientific basis for SPT because systematic observations have shown prevention of recurrence and progression of periodontal disease with due maintenance program.

**Q2. When does the SPT begin?**
**Ans.** After re-evaluation of Phase I Therapy.

**Q3. What are the signs and symptoms of recurrence of periodontitis?**
**Ans.** Areas of periodontal breakdown may be indicated by progressive increase in attachment loss, bleeding on probing, probing depths, radiographic bone loss and tooth mobility.

**Q4. What procedures constitute maintenance program?**
**Ans.** It includes therapy with medicaments, nonsurgical debridement, topical fluoride applications on exposed roots and reassessment of restorations.

**Q5. What was the previous name of "supportive periodontal therapy"?**
**Ans.** Maintenance treatment phase.

**Q6. What are the goals of SPT?**
**Ans.** a. To prevent or minimize the recurrence and progression of periodontal disease
b. To prevent or reduce the incidence of tooth loss
c. To increase the probability of locating and treating diseases or conditions

**Q7. What all is done in first part of recall hour?**
**Ans.** Examination and re-evaluation of the patient's current oral health.

**Q8. What all is done in second part of recall hour?**
**Ans.** Motivation, reinstructions and maintenance treatment.

**Q9. What all is done in third part of recall hour?**
**Ans.** Scheduling the patient for the next recall appointment, additional periodontal treatment (polishing), or restorative dental procedures (fluoride application).

**Q10. What is the rationale behind the 3-month interval?**
**Ans.** The 3-month rationale is based on the time required for bacterial repopulation of the subgingival environment after mechanical debridement and multiple studies that have shown clinical success with this interval.

# Section 12

# Miscellaneous

❖ Miscellaneous

# Chapter 69

# Miscellaneous

Shalu Bathla

## Chapter Outline

- Sterilization
- Discoveries in Periodontics
- Prefix "Perio" Used in Periodontics

## STERILIZATION

### Basic Personal Protective Barrier Equipment

Basic personal protective barrier equipment (PPE) include facemask, protective eyewear, gloves and clinical gown **(Fig. 69.1)**. Facemask should be positioned first when preparing for clinical care procedure, then the protective eyewear and after that hands are washed or scrubbed prior to gloving **(Table 69.1)**.

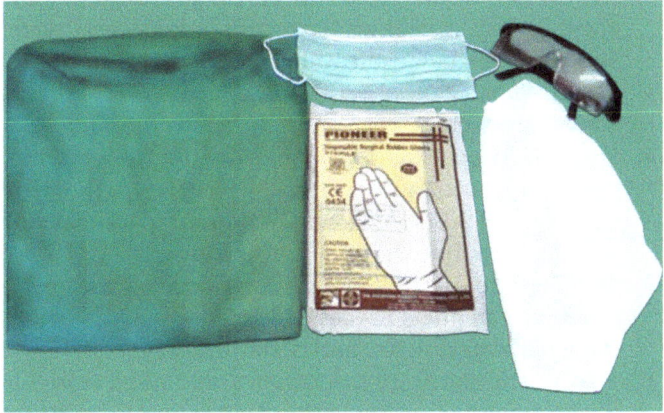

**Fig. 69.1:** Photograph showing personal protective barrier equipment (PPE).

**TABLE 69.1:** Personal protective barrier equipment (PPE): application and removal sequences.

| PPE application sequence | PPE removal sequence |
|---|---|
| I. Eyewear | I. Gloves |
| II. Facemask | II. Facemask |
| III. Gloves | III. Eyewear |

### *Facemask*

Do's and do not's while wearing facemask.

**Do's**

- Adjust the mask and position the eyewear before scrub or handwash.
- Should fit snugly with no gaps.
- Change mask each hour or more frequently when it becomes wet.
- Use fresh mask for each patient.
- Grasp side elastic or tie strings to remove.

**Do Not's**

- Do not wear mask only over mouth (but also on nose).
- Never place the mask under chin.
- Never handle the outside of a contaminated mask with gloved or bare hands.
- Mask should not be worn longer than 1 hour.
- Should not leave the treatment area with the mask hanging around the neck.

### *Handwashing*

There are three methods of handwashing: (1) short scrub, (2) short standard handwash and (3) surgical scrub. Jewelry should be removed before commencing handwash. Finger nails should be cleaned with brushes.

A scrubbing should be done with chlorhexidine soap or povidone-iodine soap at least 3–5 minutes. Chlorhexidine is a broad spectrum rapidly active agent with persistent activity. However, povidone-iodine has a relatively short duration of action. The ideal handwashing technique consists of thorough washing of hands up to the elbows, with removal of the soap in the direction from hand to elbow.

A steady and methodical method of massage along with proper drying is essential for adequate handwash.

### Gloves

Various types of gloves are:
- *Examination or procedure gloves*: Available as:
  - Sterile or nonsterile latex
  - Vinyl latex-free synthetic
- *Over gloves*: These are thin vinyl or copolymer gloves placed over examination gloves to prevent cross contamination, e.g., to retrieve additional supplies from a drawer, use a pen to make treatment notation or press button during X-ray taking.
- *Utility gloves*: These are heavy gloves worn during handling of any chemicals or infectious waste; cleaning of contaminated surfaces instruments or materials and environmental surface. Gloves made of nitrile rubber have an increased resistance to instrument punctures and can be autoclaved.
- *Dermal under gloves*: These gloves are worn to reduce irritation from latex or nonlatex.

#### Procedure of Wearing Gloves

Following steps are followed while wearing gloves (**Figs. 69.2A to G**):
- Right hand grasps inside cuff surface of left glove.
- Left glove is pulled into place.
- Gloved fingers of left hand are inserted into cuff (outer surface) of right glove.
- Right glove is pulled into place.
- Cuff of left glove is unfolded.

#### Procedure of Removal of Gloves

Following steps are followed while removing the gloves (**Figs. 69.3A and B**):
- Use left fingers to pinch right glove near edge to fold back.
- Fold edge back without contact with clean inside surface.
- Use right fingers to contact outside of left glove at the wrist to invert and remove.
- Bunch glove into the palm.
- With ungloved left hand, grasp inner noncontaminated portion of the right glove to peel it off, enclosing other glove as it is inverted.

### Decontamination of Dental Instruments

Dental instruments laying out for use during the day should be adequately cleaned and sterilized at the end of the day, whether or not they are actually used. This is because simple placing of the instruments in a dental office favors bacterial collection and other contaminants. It can facilitate transmission of infection among the patient if they are used without proper cleaning and treatment. Hence, dental instruments must be adequately cleaned, sterilized and stored in order to prepare them for future use (**Flowchart 69.1**).

- Cleaning is a process which removes contamination but does not necessarily destroy microorganisms. However, it is an important prerequisite of decontaminating equipment before proceeding for sterilization or disinfection.
- Sterilization results in complete destruction or removal of all viable microorganisms including spores and viruses. In practice, it is difficult to accomplish complete sterilization. The process is applicable to solid objects including instruments and equipment, but not on skin.
- Disinfection reduces the number of viable microorganisms but will not necessarily inactivate viruses and bacterial spores. It may be classified into:
  - *High level*: Cidal to spores, bacteria and viruses.
  - *Medium level*: Cidal to bacteria and viruses.
  - *Low level*: Cidal to only bacteria and viruses of low resistance.

This process is suitable to delicate instruments that can get damaged by sterilization.

The efficiency of decontamination depends on the:
- Nature of microorganisms
- Load of microorganisms
- Duration of exposure to the agent
- Temperature

### Steps to Sterilize Dental Instruments

- *Step I*: To start for sterilization of the dental instruments, first clean them manually or through mechanical means, such as thermal washer disinfector or an ultrasonic bath. For this they should be immersed in lukewarm water and scrubbed below the water surface and then rinsed.
- *Step II*: After cleaning dental instruments as mentioned above, dry them with a disposable cloth.
- *Step III*: Afterwards pack the dried instruments into medical grade sterilization wraps or sterilization cassettes. All the items should be properly packed before loading them into the heat sterilization unit.
- *Step IV*: The instruments can be sterilized with heat, steam, or chemical process. In a dental setting, heat is the most common method of sterilization.
- *Step V*: The sterilized instruments should be stored in their intact packaging. According to the Centers for Disease Control and Prevention, the packaging should stay sealed and undamaged to maintain the sterile nature of the instrument. In case if the dentists find packaging as wet, torn or damaged in some way, the instrument should be sterilized again through the same process.

Dental assistants are the responsible person for preparing treatment rooms both before and after each patient. They should clean and disinfect surfaces along with

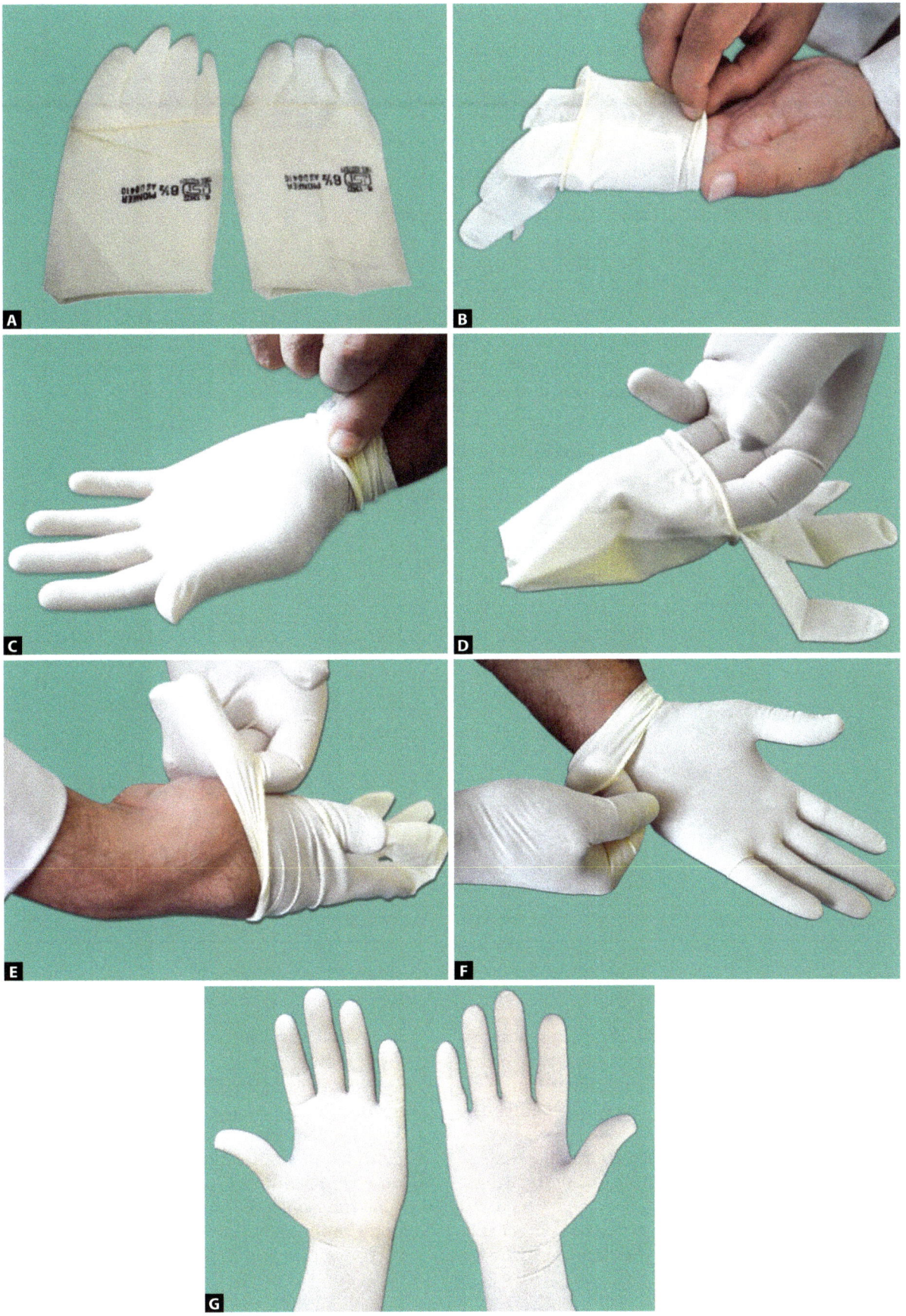

**Figs. 69.2A to G:** Photograph showing wearing of gloves.

### Section 12: Miscellaneous

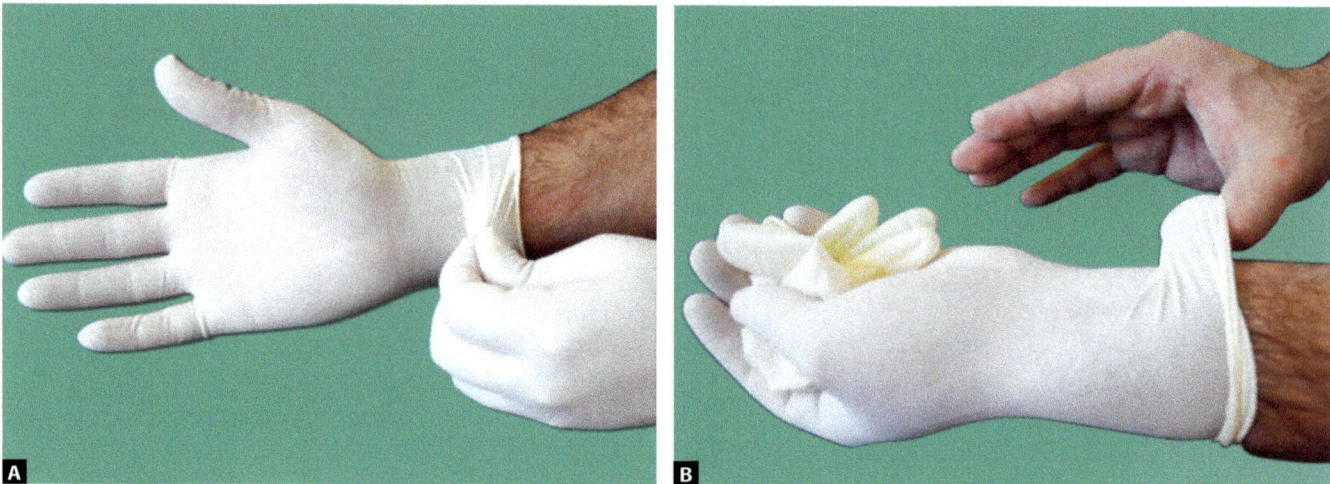

**Figs. 69.3A and B:** Photograph showing removing of gloves.

**Flowchart 69.1:** Decontamination steps.

```
                        Cleaning
                    /            \
            Sterilization      Disinfection
           /     |     \       /    |     \
    Steam    Dry    Chemical  High  Intermediate  Low
    under   heat             level   level        level
    pressure                 disinf. disinf.      disinf.
                    \
                    Use/storage
```

proper cleaning, disinfection and sterilization of instrument. Always select the appropriate product for the task in order to avoid damage to instruments and equipment. This also helps to avoid danger for both health care workers and their patients.

Patient care items are usually categorized as disposable, critical, semicritical and noncritical objects/items **(Flowchart 69.2 and Table 69.2):**

- *Critical objects*: These items penetrate or contact soft tissue, bone and bloodstream. They are sterilized or disposed, e.g., periodontal scalers, forceps, scalpels and surgical burs.
- *Semicritical objects*: These items usually come into contact with mucous membranes and nonintact skin. They are sterilized or high level disinfected, e.g., handpieces, mouth mirrors, reusable impression trays, ultrasonic handpiece and radiographic bite block.
- *Noncritical objects*: These objects do not touch mucous membrane. They are disinfected, e.g., light handles, safety eyewear and X-ray machine parts.

**Flowchart 69.2:** Sterilization of disposable, critical, semicritical and noncritical items.

```
                        Patient care items
         ┌──────────────┬──────────────┬──────────────┐
   Disposable      Noncritical     Semicritical      Critical
     items           items             items           items
       │               │                │               │
     Dispose         Clean            Clean           Clean
                       │                │               │
                   Dry and         High level      Sterilization
                    store          disinfection         │
                                  sterilization     Dry and
                                       │             store
                                   Dry and
                                    store
```

| TABLE 69.2: Sterilization methods and their applications. | |
|---|---|
| **Objects** | **Methods of sterilization** |
| Disposable syringes | Gamma radiations and ethylene oxide |
| Nondisposable syringes | Autoclave, hot air oven and infrared radiation |
| Glasswares | Autoclave and hot air oven |
| Metal instruments (scalers, curettes) | Autoclave, hot air oven and infrared radiation |
| Operation theater, inoculation hood and cubical entrance | Ultraviolet radiation |

## DISCOVERIES IN PERIODONTICS

Various discoveries in periodontics are described in **Table 69.3**.

| TABLE 69.3: Discoveries in periodontics. | | |
|---|---|---|
| **Year** | **Name** | **Discovery/invention** |
| 1535 | Paracelsus | Introduced the term "tartar" and developed "Doctrine of Calculus" |
| 1815 | Levi Spear Parmly | Invented dental floss |
| 1823 | Alphonse Toirac | Gave the term "pyorrhea alveolaris" |
| 1844 | Gunnel | First reported pericoronitis |
| 1846 | William Sharpey | Described Sharpey's fibers |
| 1868 | Paul Langerhan | Described Langerhan cell |
| 1875 | Friedrich Sigmund | Described Merkel cells |
| 1877 | Wilkerson | First hydraulic dental chair |
| 1882 | Metchnikoff | Discovered the mechanism of phagocytosis |
| 1884 | Robiecsek | Gingivectomy with straight incision |
| 1885 | Malassez | First described epithelial rests of Malassez cell |
| 1897 | Vincentini | Described corncob structure of plaque |
| 1898 | GV Black | First used the term plaque in dental context |

## Section 12: Miscellaneous

| Year | Name | Discovery/invention |
|---|---|---|
| 1899 | Talbot | Initially proposed bass method of toothbrushing |
| 1904 | Hartzell | Coined the term "pyogenic granuloma or granuloma pyogenicum" |
| 1914 | Grace Rogers Splading and Gillette Hayden | Founded the American Academy of Periodontology |
| 1918 | Leonard Widman | Described original Widman flap procedure |
| 1918 | Zentler | Described gingivectomy with scalloped incision |
| 1923 | Hegedus | First used bone grafts for reconstruction of bone defects produced by periodontal disease |
| 1923 | Abraham Wesley Ward | Introduced periodontal dressing wonder pack |
| 1923 | Gottlieb | Introduced the term "diffuse atrophy" of alveolar bone |
| 1928 | Gottlieb | Introduced the term "deep cementopathia" |
| 1931 | Kirkland | Described modified flap operation |
| 1932 | Prinz | Coined the term "chronic desquamative gingivitis" |
| 1932 | Paul R Stillman | Described Stillman toothbrushing technique |
| 1934 | Alfred Fones | Described circular toothbrushing technique known as Fones method |
| 1935 | William J Charters | Described Charters toothbrushing method |
| 1936 | Charles HM Williams | Introduced William's probe |
| 1938 | Dupont | Created nylon toothbrush bristle |
| 1938 | Wannenmacher | Introduced the term "periodontitis marginalis progressive" |
| 1940 | Thoma and Goldman | Introduced the term "paradontosis" |
| 1940 | Charles Cassidy Bass | Developed Nylon floss |
| 1942 | Orban and Weinmann | Introduced the term "periodontosis" |
| 1950 | Nathan Friedman | Gave the term "mucogingival surgery" |
| 1951 | Goldman | Introduced the term "Gingivoplasty" |
| 1954 | Nabers | Developed apically repositioned flap |
| 1954 | Muhlemann | Developed macroperiodontometer |
| 1955 | Friedman | Introduced the term "osteoplasty" |
| 1956 | Grupe and Warren | Originally described laterally displaced flap |
| 1956 | Russell | Developed periodontal index |
| 1957 | Ariaudo and Tyrrell | Later modified the apically repositioned flap |
| 1959 | Ramfjord | Introduced periodontal disease index |
| 1959 | Cohen | First described Col |
| 1960 | Green and Vermillion | Developed oral hygiene index |
| 1961 | Garguilo | Found biologic width to be 2.04 mm |
| 1962 | Friedman | Proposed the term "apically repositioned flap" |
| 1962 | Schroder | Described antiplaque property of chlorhexidine |
| 1962 | Gross and Lapiere | Discovered matrix metalloproteinases (MMPs) in the tail of metamorphosing tadpole |
| 1963 | O'Leary and Rudd | Developed microperiodontometer |
| 1963 | Bjorn | Initially described free gingival autograft |
| 1963 | Brannstrom | Gave "Hydrodynamic Theory of Dentin Hypersensitivity" |
| 1964 | Corn | Described cut-back incision |
| 1964 | Silness and Loe | Developed plaque index |
| 1964 | Green and Vermillion | Gave simplified oral hygiene index (OHI-S) |
| 1964 | Simring and Goldberg | First described relationship between periodontal and pulpal disease |
| 1965 | Morris | Introduced internal bevel incision |
| 1965 | Ewen | Introduced bone swaging as autogenous bone grafting |
| 1965 and 1969 | Morris (1965) and Dahlberg (1969) | Described sling suture |
| 1966 | Nabers | Introduced gingival grafts |
| 1966 | Staffileno | Described split thickness flap |
| 1967 | Marshall Urist | Discovered bone morphogenetic protein (BMP) |
| 1967 | Chaput et al. | Introduced the term "juvenile periodontitis" |
| 1968 | Cohen and Ross | First described double-papilla procedure |

| Year | Name | Discovery/invention |
|---|---|---|
| 1968 | Podshadley and Haley | Developed patient hygiene performance (PHP) index |
| 1969 | Robinson | Devised osseous coagulum technique as autogenous bone grafting |
| 1969 | L Hench | Invented bioactive glass |
| 1969 | Stahl | Gave no pack philosophy |
| 1971 | Jones | Coined the term "Corncob structure of plaque" |
| 1971 | Muhlemann and son | Developed sulcus bleeding index (SBI) |
| 1972 | Diem et al. | Described bone blend as autogenous bone grafting technique |
| 1972 | O'Leary, Drake and Naylor | Developed plaque control record index |
| 1972 | Eversol and Robin | Coined the term "peripheral ossifying fibroma" |
| 1974 | Ramfjord and Nissle | Modified Widman flap procedure |
| 1974 | Italian geneticist Ferruccio Ritossa | Discovered heat-shock proteins (HSPs) |
| 1974 | Ingber | Gave the concept of forced orthodontic eruption for treatment of 1-wall and 2-wall osseous defects |
| 1975 | Bernimoulin | Gave two-step procedure for free gingival graft followed by coronally positioned flap |
| 1975 | Ainamo and Bay | Developed gingival bleeding index (GBI) |
| 1976 | Loesche | First defined specific plaque hypothesis |
| 1978 | Bill Costerton | Coined the term "biofilm" |
| 1978 | Dr Paul | Gave Keyes technique or Keyes salt-out technique |
| 1979 | Max Goodson et al. | Developed controlled intrapocket antimicrobial drug deliveries |
| 1979 | Maynard and Wilson | Coined the term "marginal tissue recession" |
| 1979 | Jan Lindhe et al. | First introduced the concept of host modulation therapy |
| 1982 | Nyman et al. | Pioneered guided tissue regeneration (GTR) technique |
| 1985 | Langer and Langer | Described subepithelial connective tissue graft |
| 1985 | Takei | Gave papilla preservation technique |
| 1986 | Gottlow | Coined the term GTR |
| 1986 | Tarnow | Described semilunar coronally positioned flap |
| 1987 | Nelson | Described subpedicle connective tissue graft |
| 1991 | Philip D Marsh | First defined ecological plaque hypothesis |
| 1993 | Miller | Proposed periodontal plastic surgery |
| 1999 | Prosser | Discovered quorum sensing in biofilms |
|  | Gibbon and Nygaard | Discovered interspecies coaggregation of plaque |
|  | Pini Prato | Described GTR for root coverage in recession |
|  | Edel | Originally described free connective tissue autograft |
|  | Klingsberg | Reported the application of sclera as nonbone graft material |
|  | Kwan and Lekovic | Described periosteum as GTR material |
|  | Rateitschak | Described accordion technique of free gingival autografts |
|  | Han and associates | Developed strip technique of free gingival autografts |
|  | Friedman | Described beveled flap |
|  | Edlan and Mejchar | Described vestibular extension technique |
|  | David Sackett | Gave the term "evidence-based dentistry" |
|  | Scandinavian Group | Jens Waerhaug and coworkers |
|  | Michigan Group | Ramfjord and coworkers |
|  | Gothenburg Group | Lindhe and coworkers |

## PREFIX "PERIO" USED IN PERIODONTICS

- *Perio-aid*: It is a toothpick holder, which is one of the most effective aids available for cleaning exposed furcation after periodontal therapy.
- *Perioalert*: Immunoassay to detect serum antibodies to specific bacterial pathogens, monocytes response to lipopolysaccharide (LPS) and peripheral neutrophil function. Site of sample is peripheral blood.
- *Periocare*: It is a zinc oxide non-eugenol periodontal dressing available in the form of paste, gel and setting occurs by chemical reaction. Paste consists of zinc oxide, calcium hydroxide, magnesium oxide and vegetable oils; gel consists of resins, fatty acid, ethyl cellulose, lanolin and calcium hydroxide.

- *Periocheck*: It is rapid chairside test kit developed to detect neutral proteases in gingival crevicular fluid (GCF).
- *Periochip*: It is a small, pale orange chip of baby's thumb nail 4 mm × 5 mm × 350 μm size, weighing 7.4 mg. The prescription chip contains 2.5 mg of chlorhexidine gluconate, biodegradable hydrolyzed gelatin matrix, cross-linked with glutaraldehyde and also containing glycerin and water.
- *Periocline*: It is subgingival delivery system of 2% minocycline hydrochloride in syringeable gel suspension formulation.
- *Periodex*: It contains 0.12% chlorhexidine gluconate.
- *Periodontometer*: It is an instrument used for detecting tooth mobility.
- *Periogard*: Rapid chairside test kit for aspartate aminotransferase (AST). GCF collected is placed in tromethamine hydrochloride buffer, which is allowed to react with mixture of L-aspartic and α-ketoglutaric acids for 10 minutes. If AST is present the aspartate and α-glutarate are catalyzed to oxaloacetate and glutamate.
- *Periogard*: It contains 0.12% chlorhexidine gluconate.
- *Perioglass*: Bioactive glass alloplast consisting of sodium and calcium salts, phosphates, silicon dioxide of irregular particles of 90–170 μm.
- *Periograft*: It is a nonporous hydroxyapatite alloplast.
- *Periopac*: It is premixed zinc oxide non-eugenol dressings. It contains calcium phosphate, zinc oxide, acrylate, organic solvents, flavoring and coloring agents, when this material is exposed to air or moisture, it sets by the loss of organic solvents.
- *Periopaper*: It is blotter on which GCF is collected.
- *Periopik*: Tip used for subgingival irrigation. It is a rigid metal cannula inserted into the pocket to release irrigant for subgingival irrigation performed by an oral health professional before scaling, simultaneously with scaling or directly after scaling.
- *Perioplaner or periopolisher*: They are powered devices for removal of plaque and calculus with reciprocating motion.
- *Perio-probe*: This is an electronic probe with a tip diameter of 0.5 mm and uses standardized probing force of 0.3–0.4 N.
- *Perioscan*: It is chairside diagnostic kit using BANA benzoyl-DL arginine-naphthylamide (BANA) reaction to identify *Tannerella forsythia*, *Porphyromonas gingivalis*, *Treponema denticola* and *Capnocytophaga* species.
- *Perioscopy*: It consists of 0.99 mm-diameter reusable fiberoptic endoscope over which is fitted a disposable sterile sheath. The new fiberoptic endoscope instrument fits into specially designed periodontal explorers with 24–46 power magnification and fiberoptic illumination; this device allows clear visualization into deep subgingival pockets and in furcation areas.
- *PerioStar 2000 and PerioStar 3000*: They are automatic sharpening instruments.
- *Periostat*: It is subantimicrobial dose of doxycycline hyclate capsule of 20 mg prescribed for patients with chronic periodontitis twice daily.
- *Periotemp*: It is probe, which detects pocket temperature differences of 0.1°C from a referenced subgingival temperature. It consists of copper-nickel thermocouple connected to a digital thermometer attached to metal probe.
- *Periotest*: It is device for determining tooth mobility by measuring the reaction of the periodontium to a defined percussion force which is applied to the tooth and delivered by a tapping instrument. Periotest scale ranges from –8 to 50:
    - - 8 to 9: Clinically firm teeth.
    - 10 to 19: First distinguishable sign of movement.
    - 20 to 29: Crown deviates within 1 mm of its normal position.
    - 30 to 50: Mobility is readily observed.
- *PERIO-TOR*: These are the instrument tips for scaling and root planing causing minimal removal of tooth structures.
- *Periotriever*: It is the highly magnetized instrument designed for retrieval of broken instrument tips from the periodontal pocket.
- *Periotron*: It is the electronic machine used for measuring the amount of fluid or GCF collected on filter paper.
- *Perio 2000 system*: Diamond probe is a recently developed instrument, which combines the features of a periodontal probe with the silver sulfide sensor for detection of volatile sulfur compounds.
- *Periowave™*: It is a photodynamic disinfection system developed by Ondine Biopharma Corporation that utilizes low-intensity lasers and wavelength-specific, light-activated compounds to specifically target and destroy microbial pathogens and reduce the symptoms of disease. The photosensitive compounds are topically applied in the gingival sulcus and the laser is used to activate the compounds and complete the disinfection.
- *Periodontology*: The science that deals with the structures and behavior of the periodontium in health and disease is called periodontology.
- *Periodontics*: The branch of dentistry concerned with prevention and treatment of periodontal diseases is called periodontics.

## VIVA VOCE

**Q1. What are basic personal protective barrier equipment (PPE)?**
**Ans.** PPEs include facemask, protective eyewear, gloves and clinical gown.

**Q2. What is the sequence of wearing PPEs?**
**Ans.** Clinical gown, then facemask, then the protective eyewear and after that hands are washed or scrubbed prior to gloving.

**Q3. Name three methods of handwashing.**
**Ans.** Short scrub, short standard handwash and surgical scrub.

**Q4. What are over gloves?**
**Ans.** These are thin vinyl or copolymer gloves placed over examination gloves to prevent cross contamination.

**Q5. What are critical objects?**
**Ans.** These objects penetrate or contact soft tissue, bone and bloodstream. Examples are scalpels and surgical burs.

**Q6. What are semicritical objects?**
**Ans.** These items usually come into contact with mucous membranes and nonintact skin. They are sterilized or high level disinfected.

**Q7. Give examples of semicritical objects.**
**Ans.** Handpieces, mouth mirrors, reusable impression trays, ultrasonic handpiece and radiographic bite block.

**Q8. What are noncritical objects?**
**Ans.** Objects which does not touch mucous membrane. They are disinfected. e.g., light handles, safety eyewear and X-ray machine parts.

**Q9. What is Perioglass?**
**Ans.** Bioactive glass alloplast consisting of sodium and calcium salts, phosphates, silicon dioxide of irregular particles of 90–170 μm.

**Q10 What is Periotemp?**
**Ans.** It is probe, which detects pocket temperature differences of 0.1°C from a referenced subgingival temperature. It consists of copper-nickel thermocouple connected to a digital thermometer attached to metal probe.

# University Questions

## Chapter 1: Gingiva
1. Describe the histologic picture of gingival epithelium. *(MUHS, Nashik Paper IV, December 2014).*
2. Discuss the microscopic structure of gingiva. *(RGUHS Paper II, October 2010).*
3. Write short essay on microcirculation of gingiva. *(RGUHS Paper I, May 2010).*
4. Discuss importance of gingival biotypes in periodontics. *(Pt BD Sharma University of Health Sciences, Rohtak Paper I, April 2014).*
5. Write short note on:
   a. Hemidesmosomes. *(Pt BD Sharma University of Health Sciences, Rohtak Paper I, April 2014).*
   b. Importance of attached gingiva. *(Paper I, 2012).*
6. Write short essay on adequacy of width of attached gingiva. *(RGUHS Paper II, May 2010).*
7. Describe in detail junctional epithelium. *(MJPRU, Bareilly Paper I, 2010; MJPRU, Bareilly Paper I, 2009; RGUHS Paper I, RS November 2012; RGUHS Paper I, April 2008; MMDU Paper I, 2019).*
8. Write short essay on factors affecting gingival pigmentation. *(RGUHS Paper I, April 2008).*
9. Discuss the importance of adequate width of attached gingiva. *(RGUHS Paper III, April 2005).*
10. Write short essay on:
    a. Dentogingival unit. *(RGUHS Paper II, March 2004).*
    b. Attached gingiva—Significance in periodontal health. *(RGUHS Paper II, March 2000).*

## Chapter 2: Periodontal Ligament
1. Write short notes on:
   a. Nerve supply of periodontal ligament. *(Pt. BD Sharma University of Health Sciences, Rohtak Paper I, April 2014).*
   b. Sharpey's fibers. *(MJPRU, Bareilly Paper I, 2012).*
   c. Blood supply to the periodontium. *(RGUHS Paper I, April 2008).*
2. Discuss in detail the functions of periodontal ligament. *(RGUHS Paper I, RS May 2013).*
3. Discuss structure and function of periodontal ligament. *(Pt. BD Sharma University of Health Sciences, Rohtak Paper I, 2012).*

## Chapter 3: Cementum
1. Write short note on biochemistry of cementum. *(Pt. BD Sharma University of Health Sciences, Rohtak Paper I, 2012).*
2. Discuss cementum in health and disease. *(RGUHS Paper IV, October 2009).*
3. Give brief account of:
   a. Hyaline layer of Hopewell Smith. *(Ramachandra Medical Deemed University Paper I, June 2004).*
   b. Cementoenamel junction (CEJ) and its clinical importance. *(BFUHS, Faridkot University Paper I, 2015; Ramachandra Medical Deemed University, Paper I, June 2004).*
4. Discuss "dental cementum: the dynamic tissue covering the root". *(Bombay University Paper I, November 2002).*

## Chapter 4: Alveolar Bone
1. Describe the structure of alveolar bone. *(MJPRU, Bareilly Supplementary Paper IV, 2013; RGUHS Paper II, November 2012; RGUHS Paper I, 1999).*
2. Write short essay on:
   a. Bone remodeling. *(RGUHS Paper I, RS November 2011).*
   b. Periosteum and endosteum. *(RGUHS Paper II, September 2005).*
   c. Lamina dura *(RGUHS Paper II, March 2004 and 2000).*

## Chapter 5: Aging and Periodontium
1. Write short essay on age changes in periodontium. *(Rajasthan University, Paper I 2015; MJPRU, Bareilly Paper I, 2009; RGUHS Paper II, March 2000; MMDU Paper I, 2018).*

## Chapter 6: Classification of Periodontal Diseases
1. Give the current classification of periodontal diseases and discuss the controversies in the classification of the same. *(MUHS, Nashik Paper II, December 2014).*

## Chapter 7: Epidemiology
1. Write long essay on definition and classify indices. Discuss various indices used in evaluation of periodontal diseases. *(RGUHS Paper II, May 2010).*
2. Write note on indices to measure plaque. *(Pt. BD Sharma University of Health Sciences, Rohtak Paper II, April 2013).*
3. Write short essay on periodontal indices. *(RGUHS Paper II, November 2012; RGUHS Paper II, March 2004).*
4. Write short note on:
   a. Community periodontal index for treatment needs (CPITN). *(RGUHS Paper I, April 2008).*
   b. Russell's periodontal index (PI). *(RGUHS Paper II, September 2005).*

## Chapter 8: Periodontal Microbiology
1. Write short essay on:
   a. Microbial complexes. *(JSS University, Mysuru, Paper II 2015; RGUHS Paper II, October 2010; RGUHS Paper II, May 2010).*
   b. Role of viruses in periodontal disease. *(Vinayaka Missions University, Salem Paper II, April 2015; Sumandeep Vidyapeeth Deeemed University Paper II, April 2015; MJPRU, Bareilly Paper I, 2012).*
   c. Gingipain. *(RGUHS Paper II, RS May 2009).*
   d. *Actinobacillus actinomycetemcomitans. (RGUHS Paper III, March 2000).*
2. Evaluate the role of the following microorganism in the etiopathogenesis of periodontal disease:
   a. *Actinobacillus actinomycetemcomitans.*
   b. *Porphyromonas gingivalis.*
   c. Spirochetes. *(MMU Paper II, 2010).*
3. Write briefly on *Porphyromonas gingivalis. (RGUHS Paper II, November 2012; MMU Paper II, 2009).*
4. Discuss the role of red complex bacteria in the etiopathogenesis of periodontal dieases. *(MMDU Paper I, 2020).*

## Chapter 9: Dental Plaque
1. Write composition and mechanism of plaque formation. *(Rajasthan University, 2015).*
2. Write short essay on:
   a. Plaque hypothesis *(MJPRU, Bareilly Paper III, 2013; RGUHS Paper II, November 2012).*
   b. Environmental plaque hypothesis. *(MJPRU, Bareilly Paper II, 2011).*
3. Write specific and nonspecific hypothesis and their current concepts. *(RGUHS Paper II, RS 2, May 2009; RGUHS Paper II, April 2008).*

## Chapter 10: Dental Calculus
1. Write a short essay on:
   a. Mode of attachment of calculus *(RGUHS Paper II, RS November 2012).*
   b. Theories of calculus formation. *(RGUHS Paper IV, October 2009; RGUHS Paper II, April 2008).*
2. Discuss pathogenic potential of calculus in periodontal disease. *(Pt. BD Sharma University of Health Sciences, Rohtak Paper I, 2012).*
3. Write a long essay on:
   a. Restorations as iatrogenic factors in the etiology of periodontitis. *(MMU Paper II, April 2015; RGUHS Paper II, November 2012).*
   b. Role of iatrogenic factors in periodontal diseases. *(Pt. BD Sharma University of Health Sciences, Rohtak Paper II, April 2013; RGUHS Paper II, May 2010).*

## Chapter 11: Immunity and Inflammation
1. Write short essay on:
   a. Role of neutrophils in periodontal diseases. *(MJPRU, Bareilly Paper II, 2011).*
   b. Cells of the immune system. *(MJPRU, Bareilly Paper I, 2010; MMDU Paper I, 2019).*
   c. Role of leukocytes in defense. *(MMDU Paper I, 2020).*

## Chapter 12: Pathogenesis and Host Response
1. Discuss the host response in periodontal disease. *[MJPRU, Bareilly Paper III, 2013; Paper II(S) 2013; Paper IV 2009].*
2. Describe virulence factors of *P. ginigivalis* [MMDU Paper I, 2020].

## Chapter 13: Genetic Basis of Periodontal Diseases
1. Write short essay on interleukin-I polymorphism and periodontal disease. *(Vinayaka Missions University, Salem Paper II, April 2015).*
2. Discuss nutrigenomics and its role in periodontal diseases. *(MMU Mullana, Paper 2015; BFUHS, Faridkot University, Paper IV, 2015).*

## Chapter 14: Systemic Factors and Periodontium
1. Discuss influence of systemic diseases on periodontium. *(MUHS, Nashik Paper II, December 2014).*
2. Elaborate on the various nutritional deficiencies and their role in the initiation and progression of periodontal diseases. *(RGUHS Paper I, RS November 2012).*
3. Describe the role of nutrition in periodontal disease. *(MMU Paper IV, 2011).*
4. Write short essay on:
   a. Free radicals and antioxidants. *(Pt. BD Sharma University of Health Sciences, Rohtak Paper I, April 2014; RGUHS Paper III, RS November 2011; MMU Paper I, 2011).*
   b. Hormonal influences on gingival tissues. *(Pt. BD Sharma University of Health Sciences, Rohtak Paper I, April 2013; RGUHS Paper II, October 2010).*
   c. Vitamin C and the periodontium. *(MJPRU, Bareilly Paper I, 2013; MJPRU, Bareilly Paper III, 2011; Pt. BD Sharma University of Health Sciences, Rohtak Paper I, 2012; RGUHS Paper I, May 2013; RGUHS Paper I, April 2008; MMDU Paper I, 2020).*
   d. Oral mucosa and vitamin A. *(RGUHS Paper I, RS May 2009).*
   e. Diabetes and the periodontium. *(RGUHS Paper II, April 2008).*
   f. Idiopathic thrombocytopenic purpura (ITP). *(RGUHS Paper I, 2001).*

## Chapter 15: Periodontal Medicine
1. Write short essay on:
   a. Diabetes and the periodontium. *(RGUHS Paper II, April 2008).*
   b. Periodontal disease and preterm low birth weight. (PLBW) *(MJPRU, Bareilly Paper III, 2013).*
2. Discuss on diabetes and periodontal disease: a two-way relationship. *(Pt. BD Sharma University of Health Sciences, Rohtak Paper II, 2012).*
3. Discuss about periodontal medicine: impact of periodontal infection on systemic health. *(BFUHS, Faridkot University, Paper II, 2015; MJPRU, Bareilly Paper III, 2013; Pt. BD Sharma University of Health Sciences, Rohtak Paper IV, 2012; MMDU Paper II, 2019).*
4. Discuss about periodontitis and atherosclerosis. *(RGUHS Paper II, RS November 2012).*

## Chapter 16: Smoking and Periodontium

1. Write short essay on:
   a. Smoking and periodontal disease. *(Vinayaka Missions University, Salem Paper II, April 2015).*
   b. Effect of smoking on periodontal disease. *(BFUHS, Faridkot University, Paper II, 2015).*

## Chapter 17: Defense Mechanisms of Gingiva

1. Write short note on gingival crevicular fluid (GCF). *(Rajasthan University, Paper I, 2015).*
2. Describe composition and functions of saliva. *(MMDU Paper I, 2020).*

## Chapter 18: Gingival Inflammation

1. Discuss pathogenesis of gingival bleeding. *(MMU Paper II, 2011).*
2. Write short essay on factors affecting gingival pigmentation. *(RGUHS Paper I, April 2008).*

## Chapter 19: Gingival Enlargement

1. Discuss in detail the etiopathogenesis of gingival enlargements. *(RGUHS Paper II, RS November 2012).*
2. Classify gingival enlargement. Write in detail about drug-induced gingival enlargement. *(RGUHS Paper II, RS November 2011).*
3. Discuss the etiopathogenesis, histopathology, clinical features and management of drug-induced gingival enlargement. *(Bombay University Paper II, November 2002).*
4. Discuss the different conditioned gingival enlargements. *(RGUHS Paper IV, March 2004).*

## Chapter 20: Acute Gingival Conditions

1. Discuss about acute necrotizing ulcerative gingivitis (ANUG) in the light of present literature. *(BFUHS, Faridkot University, Paper III, 2015).*
2. Write short essay on:
   a. Management of acute gingival lesions. *(MJPRU, Bareilly Supplementary Paper III, 2013).*
   b. Pericoronitis. *(MJPRU, Bareilly Paper I, 2013).*
   c. Acute gingival infections. *(MJPRU, Bareilly Paper III, 2009).*
   d. Treatment of herpetic gingivostomatitis. *(RGUHS Paper IV, March 2004).*

## Chapter 21: Soft and Hard Tissue Lesions

1. Discuss clinical features, histopathology and management of chronic desquamative gingivitis. *(Paper I, 1998).*
2. Write note on desquamative lesions of gingiva. *(Paper III, 2015).*
3. Define tumors. Classify them. Write in detail any tumor of the oral cavity. *(NTR University Paper I, 2003).*

## Chapter 22: Periodontal Pocket

1. What is infrabony pocket? Describe the pathogenesis of pocket. *(RGUHS Paper II, RS November 2011).*
2. Write short essay on:
   a. Periodontal pockets. *(RGUHS Paper III, October 2009).*
   b. Pathogenesis of periodontal pocket. *(RGUHS Paper III, March 2004).*

## Chapter 23: Periodontal Abscess

1. Write short essay on periodontal abscess. *(RGUHS Paper II, April 2008).*

## Chapter 24: Bone Defects

1. Mechanism of bone destruction in periodontal diseases. *(MMU paper III April 2015; RGUHS Paper II, RS May 2009; RGUHS Paper III, March 2000).*
2. Write short essay on patterns of bone destruction. *(RGUHS Paper II, RS November 2012; RGUHS Paper IV, October 2009).*

## Chapter 25: Periodontitis

1. Write clinical features of aggressive periodontitis. *(MUHS, Nashik Paper II, December 2014).*
2. Describe the role of chemotherapeutic agents in treatment of aggressive periodontitis. *(MUHS, Nashik Paper III, December 2014).*
3. Write short essay on alteration of neutrophil function in localized aggressive periodontitis. *(RGUHS Paper II, RS November 2012).*
4. Discuss the role of genetics in the etiopathogenesis of aggressive periodontitis. *(RGUHS Paper II, October 2010).*
5. Discuss in detail localized aggressive periodontitis. *(RGUHS Paper III, RS May 2009).*
6. Briefly describe risk factors for chronic periodontitis. *(Pre-Paper II, MMU 2015).*

## Chapter 26: AIDS and Periodontium

1. Write short note on:
   a. AIDS and periodontium. *(BFUHS, Faridkot University, Paper II, 2015).*
   b. AIDS in periodontics: the role of HIV in periodontium. *(RGUHS Paper III, October 2009).*

## Chapter 27: Trauma from Occlusion

1. Describe in detail periodontal response to external forces. *(JSS University Mysuru, Paper III, April 2015).*
2. Write short essay on:
   a. Trauma from occlusion *(Vinayaka Missions University, Salem Paper II, April 2015; RGUHS Paper III, March 2000).*
   b. Pathologic migration. *(MUHS, Nashik Paper II, December 2014; RGUHS Paper II, RS November 2012).*
3. Classify Trauma from occlusion and explain its role in periodontal disease. *(MMDU Paper I, 2019).*

## Chapter 28: Sex Hormones and Periodontium

1. Discuss in detail the periodontal therapy in the female patient. *(RGUHS Paper III, RS November 2012).*
2. Write short essay on hormonal influences on gingival tissues. *(RGUHS Paper II, October 2010).*

3. Discuss the influence of female sex hormones over the periodontium. *(BFUHS, Faridkot University, Paper II, 2015; RGUHS Paper III, April 2005; MMDU Paper I, 2020).*

## Chapter 29: Clinical Diagnosis

1. Discuss the difference between pocket and clinical attachment loss. *(RGUHS Paper III, September 2005).*

## Chapter 30: Radiographic Diagnostic Aids

1. Write short note on subtraction radiography. *(Pt. BD Sharma University of Health Sciences, Rohtak Paper III, 2012).*

## Chapter 31: Microbiological Diagnostic Aids

1. Discuss the role of GCF as a biochemical marker for periodontal disease. *(MMU Paper I, 2009).*
2. Write short note on:
   a. DNA probe. *(MJPRU, Bareilly Paper I, 2012; RGUHS Paper III, April 2008).*
   b. Polymerase chain reaction (PCR). *(MMU Paper II, 2011).*

## Chapter 32: Clinical Risk Assessment

1. Discuss the risk factors of periodontal disease. *(MJPRU, Bareilly Paper II, 2011; RGUHS Paper II, September 2005).*

## Chapter 33: Prognosis

1. Explain the factors which influences prognosis and treatment plan in periodontal diseases. *(JSS University Mysuru, Paper III, April 2015; RGUHS Paper III, May 2010).*
2. Write short essay on:
   a. Individual tooth prognosis. *(MUHS, Nashik Paper II, December 2014).*
   b. Prognosis. *(RGUHS Paper III, October 2009).*

## Chapter 34: Treatment Plan

1. Write essay on periodontal treatment planning in the current scenario of multifactorial etiology of periodontal disease. *(Paper IV, 2015)*

## Chapter 35: Halitosis

1. Write short essay/note on:
   a. Halitosis. *(Pt. BD Sharma University of Health Sciences, Rohtak Paper III, April 2013; RGUHS Paper III, March 2000).*
   b. Recent concepts in etiology and diagnosis of halitosis. *(MMU Paper II, 2010).*
   c. Management of halitosis. *(RGUHS Paper III, RS November 2011; RGUHS Paper III, October 2009).*

## Chapter 36: Dentin Hypersensitivity

1. Write short essay on dentinal hypersensitivity. *(BFUHS, Faridkot University, Paper III, 2015; MJPRU, Bareilly Paper II, (S) 2013; RGUHS Paper I, October 2010; RGUHS Paper I, 2001).*
2. Write short note on management of dentinal hypersensitivity. *(Pt. BD Sharma University of Health Sciences, Rohtak Paper III, April 2013; MJPRU, Bareilly Paper III, 2013).*
3. Define hypersensitivity. Describe in detail the etiology of hypersensitivity and mode of action of desensitizing agents. *(JSS University Mysuru, Paper III, April 2015).*

## Chapter 37: Mechanical Plaque Control

1. Describe the development and evolution of the toothbrush. Discuss the role of toothbrush in preventive periodontics. *(Bombay University Paper IV, November 2002).*
2. Write short essay on:
   a. Powered toothbrushes. *(RGUHS Paper III, RS November 2012).*
   b. Motivation in periodontal practice. *(RGUHS Paper IV, April/May 2007).*
3. Discuss the various disclosing agents used. *(MJPRU, Bareilly Paper I, 2012; MJPRU, Bareilly Paper III, 2011; RGUHS Paper IV, March 2004).*
4. Write short note on:
   a. Oral irrigation devices. *(Pt. BD Sharma University of Health Sciences, Rohtak Paper III, 2012).*
   b. Hawthorne effect. *(MMU 2014).*

## Chapter 38: Chemotherapeutic Agents

1. Write a long essay in detail about the use of systemic antibiotics in the management of periodontal disease. *(RGUHS Paper III, October 2010; RGUHS Paper I, October 2009; MJPRU, Bareilly Paper I, 2009; RGUHS Paper IV, March 2004).*
2. Write short essay on:
   a. Antiplaque agents. *(MJPRU, Bareilly Paper I, 2013; RGUHS Paper I, October 2009).*
   b. Periochip. *(RGUHS Paper III, November 2012).*
   c. Metronidazole. *(Vinayaka Missions University, Salem Paper III, April 2015; RGUHS Paper I, RS May 2009).*
   d. Chemical plaque control. *(MUHS, Nashik Paper IV, December 2014; RGUHS Paper III, May 2010).*
   e. Tetracycline. *(Sumandeep Vidyapeeth Deemed University Paper I April 2015).*
3. Describe the local drug delivery system in periodontitis. *(Vinayaka Missions University, Salem Paper III, April 2015; MJPRU, Bareilly Supplementary Paper IV 2013; MJPRU, Bareilly Paper III, 2009).*
4. Discuss the role of drugs in periodontitis. *(MJPRU, Bareilly Paper III, 2012; MJPRU, Bareilly Paper I, 2010).*
5. Discuss the role of chlorhexidine in periodontal therapy. *(MJPRU, Bareilly Paper I, 2011).*

## Chapter 39: Host Modulation

1. Write short note on pharmacological agents affecting bone resorption. *(Pt. BD Sharma University of Health Sciences, Rohtak Paper I, 2012).*
2. Write short essay on:
   a. Host modulation therapy in periodontal therapy. *(RGUHS Paper III, May 2010).*
   b. Nonsteroidal anti-inflammatory drugs (NSAIDs). *(RGUHS Paper I, RS November 2012; MMU Paper I, 2011).*
   c. Chemically-modified tetracyclines. *(RGUHS Paper I, March 2004; MMDU Paper II, 2020).*
3. Discuss host modulation in periodontics. *(RGUHS Paper IV, May 2010).*
4. Discuss about the role of host modulating agents. *(MMU Paper I 2009; MMDU Paper III, 2019).*

# University Questions

## Chapter 40: Periodontal Instruments

1. Discuss the various instruments and devices used in the treatment of periodontal diseases. Enumerate its various advantages and disadvantages. *(NTR Health University, Paper III, June 2003; MMDU Paper III, 2019).*

## Chapter 41: General Principles of Instrumentation

1. Explain general principles of periodontal instrumentation. *(Pre- Paper II, MMU 2015).*

## Chapter 42: Manual Scaling and Root Planing

1. Discuss the pros and cons of hand scaling and ultrasonic scaling. *(Paper III, RGUHS).*

## Chapter 43: Sonic and Ultrasonic Scaling

1. Write short essay on:
   a. Ultrasonic scalers. *(MUHS, Nashik Paper IV, December 2014).*
   b. Aerosols in dental practice. *(RGUHS Paper I, November 2012).*
   c. Role of ultrasonic in periodontal therapy. *(RGUHS Paper III, RS November 2012; RGUHS Paper III, April 2008).*
   d. Sonics and ultrasonics in periodontics. *(Bombay University Paper IV, November 2002).*

## Chapter 44: Splinting

1. Write short essay on:
   a. Role of splints in periodontal therapy. *(RGUHS Paper III, RS November 2012; MMU Paper III, 2009).*
   b. Splints in periodontal therapy. *(MJPRU, Bareilly Paper III, 2012; RGUHS Paper III, 2008).*

## Chapter 45: Surgical Anatomy

1. Discuss the general considerations of surgical anatomy in relation to periodontics. *(JSS University, Mysuru Paper III, April 2015; RGUHS Paper I).*
2. Describe muscles of mastication. *(JSS University, Mysuru Paper I, April 2015; NTR Health University Paper I, June 2003).*
3. Write short note on anatomy of mandible. *(Pt. BD Sharma University of Health Sciences, Rohtak Paper I, April 2013).*
4. Write short essay on:
   a. Maxillary sinus. *(RGUHS Paper I, May 2013; RGUHS Paper I, RS November 2011).*
   b. Mandibular division of the trigeminal nerve. *(JSS University, Mysuru Paper I, April 2015; RGUHS Paper I, May 2010).*
5. Describe fascial spaces of periodontal interest. *(Sumandeep Vidyapeeth Deemed University Paper III, April 2015; MMU Paper I, 2011).*

## Chapter 46: General Principles of Periodontal Surgery

1. Discuss preoperative considerations in periodontal surgery. *(MMU Paper III, 2010).*
2. Write short essay on:
   a. Complications following flap surgery. *(RGUHS Paper III, May 2010).*
   b. Hemostasis. *(RGUHS Paper I, October 2010).*
   c. Agents used to control bleeding during surgery. *(RGUHS Paper I, October 2009).*

## Chapter 47: Gingival Curettage

1. Define curettage. Mention its indications. *(Paper III, October 1997).*

## Chapter 48: Gingivectomy

1. Write short essay on gingivectomy techniques. *(RGUHS Paper III, October 2009).*

## Chapter 49: Periodontal Flap

1. Discuss in detail the various surgical techniques for pocket elimination. *(MJPRU, Bareilly Paper III, 2013).*
2. Write short essay on palatal flap. Discuss its relevance and principles during periodontal surgeries. *(MJPRU, Bareilly Supplementary Paper III, 2013).*
3. Discuss different periodontal flap techniques from inception to the present status. *(MJPRU, Bareilly Paper IV, 2011).*

## Chapter 50: Resective Osseous Surgery

1. Write short essay on resective osseous surgery. *(Vinayaka Missions University, Salem Paper III, April 2015).*
2. Describe in detail healing after resective osseous surgery. *(MUHS, Nashik Paper III, December 2014).*

## Chapter 51: Regenerative Osseous Surgery

1. Write short essay on:
   a. Materials used in guided tissue regeneration. *(GTR) (RGUHS, Paper III, 2008).*
   b. Bioresorbable membranes. *(MJPRU, Bareilly Supplementary Paper III 2013).*
   c. Platelet rich plasma. *(MJPRU, Bareilly Supplementary Paper III, 2013; RGUHS, Paper III, October 2010; MJPRU, Bareilly Paper III, 2009).*
   d. Platelet rich fibrin *(RGUHS, Paper III November 2012)*
   e. Bone morphogenetic proteins (BMPs). *(Pt. BD Sharma University of Health Sciences, Rohtak Paper III, 2012; MMU, Paper III, 2011).*
   f. Root biomodification. *(RGUHS, Paper III, November 2012; RGUHS, Paper III May 2010; RGUHS, Paper III, September 2005).*
   g. Techniques in harvesting autogenous bone grafts. *(RGUHS, Paper III October 2010).*
   h. Current status of alloplasts in periodontal regeneration. *(RGUHS, Paper III May 2010).*
   i. Bone grafts. *(NTR, Health University Paper IV, June 2003).*
2. Discuss on the recent advances in periodontal regeneration therapy. *(MMU, Paper IV, 2011).*
3. Write short note on bone augmentation. *(Pt. BD Sharma University of Health Sciences, Rohtak, Paper III, 2012).*
4. Describe in detail about classifications of various bone grafting materials. *(RGUHS, Paper III, October 2009).*
5. Discuss reconstructive periodontal surgery. *(RGUHS, Paper III 1999).*
6. Discuss osseous grafts and their healing. *(BFUHS, Faridkot University, Paper III, 2015).*

## Chapter 52: Furcation

1. Write short essay on:
   a. Classification of furcation involvement. *(MJPRU, Bareilly Paper III, 2013).*
   b. Treatment of furcation involvement. *(RGUHS, Paper III, October 2010; RGUHS Paper III, 2008).*
2. Give the classification of furcation involvement and its management. *(MJPRU, Bareilly Paper III, 2009).*

## Chapter 53: Periodontal Plastic Surgery

1. Write short essay on:
   a. Healing of free clinical autografts. *(MJPRU, Bareilly Supplementary Paper III, 2013).*
   b. Reconstruction of interdental papilla. *(MMU paper III, April 2015; RGUHS Paper III, November 2012).*
   c. Define and classify gingival recession. *(RGUHS Paper IV, October 2009).*
   d. Vestibular extension procedure and its indications. *(RGUHS Paper III, October 2009).*
   e. Periodontal plastic and esthetic surgical procedures. *(RGUHS Paper IV, April 2008).*
2. Write short note on free gingival grafts. *(Pt. BD Sharma University of Health Sciences, Rohtak Paper III, 2012; RGUHS Paper III, September 2005).*
3. Describe in detail the various procedure used in the management of gingival recession. Add a note on the recent advances in surgical periodontal therapy. *(RGUHS Paper IV, RS November 2012).*

## Chapter 54: Periodontal Microsurgery

1. Describe periodontal microsurgery. *(RGUHS Paper IV, November 2012; Ramachandra Medical Deemed University Paper III, June 2004).*

## Chapter 55: Periodontal Treatment of Medically Compromised Patients

1. Write short essay on:
   a. Infective endocarditis: prophylaxis. *(RGUHS Paper I, May 2013).*
   b. Laboratory investigations for diabetes. *(RGUHS Paper I, RS May 2013).*
2. Discuss management of immunocompromised patients. *(Pt. BD Sharma University of Health Sciences, Rohtak Paper III, 2012).*

## Chapter 56: Implant Basics

1. Write a long essay defining osseointegration. Also write in detail about the mechanism of osseointegration of dental implants. *(RGUHS, Paper III, October 2010).*
2. Explain the biological aspects of dental implants. *(MMU Paper III, 2009).*
3. Give brief account of osseointegration. *(Ramachandra Medical Deemed University, Paper III, June 2004).*
4. Write a short essay on osseous consideration for implant placement. *(MJPRU, Bareilly Paper III, 2011).*
5. Discuss the biological aspects of dental implants. *(MJPRU, Bareilly Paper III, 2011).*

## Chapter 57: Implant Surgical Procedures

1. Write short essay on:
   a. Platform switching. *(MMU Paper III, April 2015).*
   b. Implant failure: causes and remedy. *(MJPRU, Bareilly Paper III, 2009).*

## Chapter 58: Advanced Implant Surgical Procedures

1. Describe the role of guided bone regeneration in periodontal and implant therapy. *(RGUHS Paper IV, November 2012).*
2. Write short essay on ridge augmentation for implant placement. *(RGUHS Paper III, October 2010).*

## Chapter 59: Peri-implantitis and Other Implant Related Complications

1. Define peri-implantitis and discuss it. *(MMU paper II, April 2015; RGUHS Paper IV, March 2004).*
2. Discuss peri-implant diseases and its management. *(RGUHS Paper III, May 2010; RGUHS Paper III, September 2005; MMDU Paper II, 2020).*
3. Write a short note on diagnosis of peri-implant defects. *(Pt. BD Sharma University of Health Sciences, Rohtak Paper III, April 2013).*
4. Write a short essay on maintenance schedule for the implant patient. *(RGUHS Paper III, April 2008).*

## Chapter 60: Periodontics-Prosthodontics

1. Write short essay on crown-lengthening. *(RGUHS Paper III, RS November 2011; MJPRU, Bareilly Supplementary Paper III, 2013; Ramachandra Medical Deemed University Paper III June 2004).*
2. Write an essay on perioprosthetic considerations. *(Bombay University Paper IV, November 2002).*

## Chapter 61: Periodontics-Endodontics

1. Write short note on periodontic-endodontic continuum. *(Pt. BD Sharma, University of Health Sciences, Rohtak Paper III, April 2013).*

## Chapter 62: Periodontics-Restorative Dentistry

1. Explain Periodontal - Restorative interrelationship. *(Paper IV; Pre- Paper II, MMU 2015).*
2. Discuss the role of faulty dentistry as a causative factor for periodontal diseases. *(MGR paper II, October 2002).*

## Chapter 63: Periodontics-Orthodontics

1. Write short note on role of orthodontics appliances in periodontal diseases. *(Paper I, 2015).*

## Chapter 64: Periodontics-Pediatric Dentistry

1. Discuss periodontal diseases in children. *(Paper II, April 1998).*

## Chapter 65: Periodontics-Oral surgery

1. Discuss Perio-oral surgery relationship. *(Pre- Paper II, MMU 2015).*

2. Discuss the role of faulty dentistry as a causative factor for periodontal diseases. *(MGR paper II, October 2002).*

## Chapter 66: Periodontics-Psychiatry

1. Discuss the role of stress in the etiopathogenesis of periodontal diseases. *(Paper II, Bombay university Nov 2002).*
2. Discuss the psychosomatic influences in periodontitis. *(Paper II, MGR university November 2002).*

## Chapter 67: Recent Advancements in Periodontics

1. Describe the type of lasers and their role in clinical periodontitis. *(MJPRU, Bareilly Supplementary Paper III, 2013).*
2. Discuss in detail LASER in periodontics. *(RGUHS Paper IV, RS November 2011).*
3. Write short essay on photodynamic therapy. *(RGUHS Paper III, November 2012; MJPRU, Bareilly Paper III, 2012).*
4. Discuss approaches for periodontal tissues engineering. *(RGUHS Paper III, RS November 2011).*
5. Discuss the recent advances in periodontal surgery. *(MMDU Paper IV, 2018).*

## Chapter 68: Supportive Periodontal Therapy

1. Write long essay on supportive periodontal therapy. *(RGUHS Paper IV, October 2010; MMU Paper III, 2009).*
2. Describe the role of maintenance phase in periodontitis. *(MJPRU, Bareilly Paper III, 2013; RGUHS Paper IV).*
3. Write short essay on maintenance schedule for the implant patient. *(RGUHS Paper III, April 2008).*

## Chapter 69: Miscellaneous

1. Write essay on sterilization and disinfection. *(Vinayaka Mission university Salem Paper I, 2015).*

www.ingramcontent.com/pod-product-compliance
Ingram Content Group UK Ltd.
Pitfield, Milton Keynes, MK11 3LW, UK
UKHW050813220425
457743UK00008B/55